This book is due for return on or before the last date shown below

- 5 SEP 2013		

INTERVENTIONAL NEPHROLOGY

INTERVENTIONAL NEPHROLOGY

Arif Asif, MD, FASN, FNKF
Professor of Medicine
Chief, Division of Nephrology and Hypertension
Albany Medical College
Albany, New York

Anil K. Agarwal, MD, FACP, FASN, FNKF
Professor of Medicine
Director, Interventional Nephrology
Wexner Medical Center
The Ohio State University
Columbus, Ohio

Alexander S. Yevzlin, MD
Associate Professor of Medicine (CHS)
Director, Interventional Nephrology
and Vascular Access Program
University of Wisconsin, Madison
Madison, Wisconsin

Steven Wu, MD, FASN
Director, Interventional Nephrology
Medical Director, Vascular Access Program
Associate Director, Vascular
Interventional Radiology (HD Access)
Massachusetts General Hospital
Instructor in Medicine
Harvard Medical School
Boston, Massachusetts

Gerald A. Beathard, MD, PhD, FACP, FCAP, FASN
Vice-President
Lifeline Vascular Access
Clinical Professor
University of Texas Medical Branch
Galveston, Texas

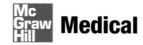

New York   Chicago   San Francisco   Lisbon   London   Madrid   Mexico City
Milan   New Delhi   San Juan   Seoul   Singapore   Sydney   Toronto

Interventional Nephrology

1 2 3 4 5 6 7 8 9 0   CTP/CTP   17 16 15 14 13 12

ISBN 978-0-07-176932-7
MHID 0-07-176932-3

This book was set in Berling by Thomson Digital.
The editors were Christine Diedrich and Brian Kearns.
The production supervisor was Catherine Saggese.
Project management was provided by Charu Bansal, Thomson Digital.
The designer was Alan Barnett; the cover designer was Thomas De Pierro.
China Translation & Printing Services, Ltd. was printer and binder.

This book is printed on acid-free paper.

Library of Congress Cataloging-in-Publication Data

Interventional nephrology / Arif Asif ... [et al.].
   p. ; cm.
 Includes bibliographical references.
 ISBN 978-0-07-176932-7 (hardcover : alk. paper)
 ISBN 0-07-176932-3 (hardcover : alk. paper)
 I. Asif, Arif.
 [DNLM: 1. Kidney—surgery. 2. Catheters, Indwelling. 3. Endovascular
Procedures—methods. 4. Kidney Diseases—surgery. WJ 368]
 617.4'61—dc23
                                                           2012008863

DEDICATIONS

To my parents, Fatima, Harris, Salman as well as my teachers, students and friends, who continue to be my guiding stars.

— *Arif Asif*

To the ever inspiring memory of my parents, Mr. Harish Chandra and Mrs. Kailashwati Agarwal, and to my family for their love, support, and patience.

—*Anil K. Agarwal*

Dedicated to my parents, Tony and Lora Yevzlin, whose support, love, and friendship are the foundation of my career.

—*Alexander S. Yevzlin*

To my parents, wife and children who are most precious to me and keep my dreams alive!

—*Steven Wu*

Dedicated to all of the wonderful patients who have taught me over the years.

—*Gerald A. Beathard*

CONTENTS

SECTION I

SECTION II

SECTION III

CONTRIBUTORS

▶ **Kenneth Abreo, MD**
Professor of Medicine, Chief, Nephrology Section
LSU Health Sciences Center
Shreveport, Louisiana

*History of Interventional Nephrology from
    a Global Perspective*
*Adverse Reactions to Radiocontrast
    Agents in Vascular Access Centers*
Peritoneal Dialysis Catheter Insertion

▶ **Zulqarnain Abro, MD**
Assistant Professor of Medicine
LSU Health Sciences Center
Shreveport, Louisiana

*Adverse Reactions to Radiocontrast Agents in
    Vascular Access Centers*

▶ **Anil K. Agarwal, MD, FACP, FASN, FNKF**
Professor of Medicine
Director, Interventional Nephrology
Wexner Medical Center
The Ohio State University
Columbus, Ohio

*Accreditation and Certification in
    Interventional Nephrology*
*Vascular Access for Hemodialysis: Types,
    Characteristics, and Epidemiology*
Accessory Veins: Recognition and Management
Central Vein Stenosis
Establishing a Vascular Access Center
*Research Opportunities in Interventional Nephrology:
    Why, What, and How!*

▶ **Stephen R. Ash, MD, FACP**
Director of Dialysis
Associate Professor of Clinical Medicine
Indiana University Health Arnett and Director
    of R & D for Ash Access Technology, Inc. and
    HemoCleanse, Inc.
Lafayette, Indiana

*Tunneled Catheter Designs and the Placement
    Conundrum*

▶ **Arif Asif, MD, FASN, FNKF**
Professor of Medicine
Chief, Division of Nephrology and Hypertension
Albany Medical College
Albany, New York

Vascular Mapping
Stent Placement in Hemodialysis Access
Cardiac Rhythm Devices in Renal Patients
Complications of Peritoneal Dialysis Catheter Procedures
Antibiotic Prophylaxis for Dialysis Access Interventions
Secondary Arteriovenous Fistula
Etiology and Management of Cephalic Arch Stenosis

▶ **Rupak K. Banerjee, PhD, PE,
    ASME Fellow**
Professor of Mechanical Engineering
School of Dynamic Systems
University of Cincinnati
Cincinnati, Ohio

Flow Dynamics, Maturity, and Access Failure

▶ **Carlo Basile, MD**
Division of Nephrology
Miulli General Hospital
Acquaviva delle Fonti
Italy

Heart Failure and Left Ventricular Hypertrophy

▶ **Gerald A. Beathard, MD, PhD,
    FACP, FCAP, FASN**
Vice-President
Lifeline Vascular Access
Clinical Professor
University of Texas Medical Branch
Galveston, Texas

History of Interventional Nephrology in the United States
Basic Anatomy for Dialysis Vascular Access
Physical Examination of the Hemodialysis Access
Early and Late Fistula Failure
Arteriovenous Graft Stenosis and Thrombosis
Venous Angioplasty
Pseudoaneurysm and Aneurysm Formation
Cardiac Rhythm Devices in Renal Patients
Sedation and Analgesia for Endovascular Procedures
*Fluoroscopy Basics: Theory, Equipment, and Use in
    Vascular Access Intervention*
Fluoroscopy Clinical: Radiation Exposure and Safety
Complications of Endovascular Dialysis Access Procedures
Antibiotic Prophylaxis for Dialysis Access Interventions

▶ **Bryan Becker, MD, MMM**
AVP Health Affairs
University of Illinois
Chicago, Illinois

*The American Society of Diagnostic and Interventional
Nephrology and Collaboration with other Professional
Societies and Organizations*

▶ **Anatole Besarab, MD**
Director of Clinical Research
Professor of Medicine
Division of Nephrology
Henry Ford Health System
Professor of Medicine, Wayne State School of Medicine
Detroit, Michigan

Vascular Access Monitoring and Surveillance

▶ **Pierre Bourquelot, MD**
Department of Angioaccess Surgery
   Clinique Jouvenet
Paris, France

*Hemodialysis Access-Induced Distal Ischemia (HAIDI):
   Surgical Management*

▶ **Mary Buffington, MD, JD**
Assistant Professor
Department of Medicine
Nephrology Section
Louisiana State University Health Sciences Center
Shreveport, Louisiana

Peritoneal Dialysis Catheter Insertion

▶ **Micah R. Chan, MD, MPH**
Assistant Professor
Department of Medicine
Division of Nephrology
University of Wisconsin School of Medicine
   and Public Health
Madison, Wisconsin

Vascular Access in Special Populations
*The Role of Pharmacologic Agents in
   Preserving Vascular Access*

▶ **Eric S. Chemla, MD**
St George's Healthcare NHS Trust
London, United Kingdom

*Surgical Options for Arteriovenous Access in
   Patients with Exhausted Veins*

▶ **Diego Covarrubias, MD**
Vascular Interventional Radiology
Department of Radiology
Massachusetts General Hospital
Harvard Medical School
Boston, Massachusetts

Peripheral Arterial Disease

▶ **Rajiv K. Dhamija, MD**
Interventional Nephrology
Clinical Associate Professor of Medicine
Western University of Health Sciences
Pomona, California

*Antibiotic Prophylaxis for
   Dialysis Access Interventions*

▶ **Ramanath Dukkipati, MD**
Assistant Professor of Medicine
Medical Director, Interventional Nephrology
David Geffen School of Medicine at UCLA
Harbor-UCLA Medical Center
Los Angeles, California

Etiology and Management of Cephalic Arch Stenosis

▶ **Amy Dwyer, MD**
Associate Professor of Medicine
Director, Interventional Nephrology
University of Louisville
Louisville, Kentucky

*Developing an Academic Curriculum for
   Interventional Nephrology Training*
Surface Coatings for Tunneled Catheters

▶ **Stan Frinak, MSEE**
Division of Nephrology
Henry Ford Health System
Detroit, Michigan

Vascular Access Monitoring and Surveillance

▶ **Dirk Hentschel, MD**
Brigham and Women's Hospital
Harvard Medical School
Boston, Massachusetts

*Research Opportunities in Interventional Nephrology:
   Why, What, and How!*

▶ **Peter Ivanovich, MD**
Professor
Division of Nephrology/Hypertension
Department of Medicine
Northwestern University Feinberg
   School of Medicine
Chicago, Illinois

*Origins of Hemodialysis Access:
   The Scribner Experience*

▶ **Jennifer Joe, MD**
Division of Nephrology
Department of Medicine
Massachusetts General Hospital
Harvard Medical School
Boston, Massachusetts

Hand Ischemia

▶ **Kaveh Kian, MD, MRCP**
Denver Nephrology
Denver, Colorado

*Etiology and Management of
 Cephalic Arch Stenosis*

▶ **Michael J. Kallok, PhD,
 FACC, FAHA**
Chief Executive Officer
Phraxis, Inc.
St. Paul, Minnesota

Device Innovation

▶ **Jariatul Karim, MD**
Assistant Professor of Medicine
Wayne State University
Division of Nephrology
Henry Ford Health System
Detroit, Michigan

*Vascular Access Monitoring and
 Surveillance*

▶ **Klaus Konner, MD**
Retired Nephrologist
Member of Interdisciplinary Vascular Access Center
University Hospital
Cologne (Köln) Germany

Sites and Types of Arteriovenous Fistulae

▶ **Timmy Lee, MD, MSPH**
Associate Professor of Medicine
Department of Internal Medicine
Division of Nephrology and Hypertension
University of Cincinnati
Cincinnati, Ohio

Neointimal Hyperplasia
*Pharmacological Approaches to
 Vascular Access Dysfunction*

▶ **Edgar V. Lerma, MD, FACP, FASN,
 FAHA, FASH, FNLA, FNKF**
Clinical Associate Professor of Medicine
Section of Nephrology
Department of Medicine
University of Illinois at Chicago College of Medicine
Associates in Nephrology, S.C.
Chicago, Illinois

Renal Ultrasonography

▶ **Carlo Lomonte, MD**
Division of Nephrology
Miulli General Hospital
Acquaviva delle Fonti
Italy

Heart Failure and Left Ventricular Hypertrophy

▶ **Marko Malovrh, MD, PhD**
Professor
Department of Nephrology
University Medical Centre Ljubljana
Ljubljana, Slovenia

*Emerging Role of Vascular Ultrasound in
 Arteriovenous Dialysis Access*

▶ **Rick Mishler, MD**
Interventional Nephrologist
Arizona Kidney Disease and
 Hypertension Centers Surgery Center
Phoenix, Arizona

Sites and Types of Arteriovenous Fistulae
Creation of Arteriovenous Fistulae by Nephrologists

▶ **Shahriar Moossavi, MD, PhD**
Associate Professor of Nephrology
Wake Forest University
School of Medicine
Winston-Salem, North Carolina

*Exit-Site, Tunnel Infection, and
 Catheter-Related Bacteremia*

▶ **Vandana Dua Niyyar, MD, FASN**
Assistant Professor of Medicine
Division of Nephrology
Department of Internal Medicine,
Emory University
Atlanta, Georgia

Catheter Lock Solutions

▶ **Jeffrey Packer, DO, FACOI, FASN**
Co-Site Director/Medical Director
AKDHC, LLC, Interventional Nephrology Program
Phoenix, Arizona

Accreditation and Certification in Interventional Nephrology
Sites and Types of Arteriovenous Fistulae
Creation of Arteriovenous Fistulae by Nephrologists

▶ **Timothy A. Pflederer, MD**
University of Illinois College of Medicine at Peoria
Peoria, Illinois
Renal Care Associates, SC
Peoria, Illinois

Quality Assurance and Outcomes Monitoring

▶ **Karthik Ramani, MD**
Assistant Professor of Clinical
Medicine, Division of Nephrology
University of Cincinnati
Cincinnati, Ohio

Pharmacological Approaches to Vascular Access Dysfunction

▶ **Jamie Ross, MD**
Professor of Clinical Medicine
UC Davis, School of Medicine
Sacramento, California

Temporary Hemodialysis Catheters

▶ **Prabir Roy-Chaudhury, MD, PhD**
Professor of Medicine
Division of Nephrology
University of Cincinnati
Cincinnati, Ohio

Medical Director
UC Health Vascular Access Center
West Chester, Ohio

Flow Dynamics, Maturity, and Access Failure
Pharmacological Approaches to Vascular Access Dysfunction
Research Opportunities in Interventional Nephrology:
    Why, What, and How!

▶ **Bharat Sachdeva, MD**
Assistant Professor
Department of Medicine
Nephrology Section
Louisiana State University
Shreveport, Louisiana

History of Interventional Nephrology
    from a Global Perspective
Peritoneal Dialysis Catheter Insertion
Peritoneal Dialysis Catheter Removal

▶ **Wissam Saliba, MD**
Division of Nephrology and Hypertension
University of Wisconsin, Madison
Madison, Wisconsin

Origins of Hemodialysis Access: The Scribner Experience

▶ **Loay Salman, MD**
Assistant Professor of Medicine
University of Miami Miller School of Medicine
Miami, Florida

Vascular Mapping
Cardiac Rhythm Devices in Renal Patients
Complications of Peritoneal Dialysis Catheter Procedures
Antibiotic Prophylaxis for Dialysis Access Interventions

▶ **Rajiv Saran, MBBS, MD, MRCP, MS**
Associate Professor of Medicine
Division of Nephrology
Department of Internal Medicine
Associate Director, University of Michigan Kidney
    Epidemiology and Cost Center
Ann Arbor, Michigan

Epidemiology of Vascular Access for
    Hemodialysis: A Global Perspective

▶ **Donald Schon, MD**
Chair
Public Policy American Society Diagnostic
    and Interventional Nephrology
Paradise Valley, Arizona

Establishing a Vascular Access Center
Coding and Reimbursement for Vascular
    Access Procedures: Past, Present, and Future

▶ **Adrian Sequeira, MD**
Assistant Professor of Medicine
LSU HSC
Shreveport, Louisiana

Adverse Reactions to Radiocontrast Agents in
    Vascular Access Centers
Peritoneal Dialysis Catheter Insertion

▶ **Larry Spergel, MD, FACS**
Director, Dialysis Management Medical Group
Clinical Director, A-V Fistula First Breakthrough Initiative
San Francisco, California

Secondary Arteriovenous Fistula

▶ **Aris Urbanes, MD**
Lifeline Vascular Access
Vernon Hills, Illinois

Training in Diagnostic and Interventional Nephrology

▶ **Tushar J. Vachharajani, MD, FASN, FACP**
Chief, Nephrology Section
W. G. (Bill) Hefner Veterans Affairs Medical Center
Salisbury, North Carolina

Epidemiology of Vascular Access for Hemodialysis:
    A Global Perspective
Accessory Veins: Recognition and Management
Catheter Dysfunction—Recirculation, Thrombosis,
    and Fibroepithelial Sheath
Radiocontrast and Carbon Dioxide Angiography:
    Advantages and Disadvantages

▶ **Luigi Vernaglione, MD**
Division of Nephrology
Giannuzzi Hospital
Manduria, Italy

Heart Failure and Left Ventricular Hypertrophy

▶ **Davinder Wadehra, MD**
Assistant Professor of Medicine
Department of Internal Medicine
Division of Nephrology and Hypertension
University of Cincinnati
Cincinnati, Ohio

Neointimal Hyperplasia
Pharmacological Approaches to Vascular
    Access Dysfunction

▶ **Shouwen Wang, MD, PhD**

Arizona Kidney Disease and Hypertension Centers
Surgery Center
Phoenix, Arizona

Creation of Arteriovenous Fistulae by Nephrologists

▶ **Steven Wu, MD, FASN**

Director, Interventional Nephrology
Medical Director, Vascular Access Program
Associate Director, Vascular Interventional Radiology
(HD Access)
Massachusetts General Hospital
Instructor in Medicine
Harvard Medical School
Boston, Massachusetts

Hand Ischemia
Peripheral Arterial Disease
Kidney Biopsy

▶ **Alexander S. Yevzlin, MD**

Associate Professor of Medicine (CHS)
Director, Interventional Nephrology
and Vascular Access Program
University of Wisconsin, Madison
Madison, Wisconsin

Origins of Hemodialysis Access: The Scribner Experience
Academic Societies, Industry Partnerships, and
Conflict of Responsibility
Arterial Intervention in Hemodialysis Access and Chronic
Kidney Disease
Stent Placement in Hemodialysis Access
Vascular Access Science—What Does the Future Hold?

If riding on a train that is progressing down the track at a rapid rate of speed, one might argue, from a philosophic viewpoint, as to whether one is actually moving or sitting still while the train moves. If you convert this analogy to the situation represented by Interventional Nephrology today, the answer is clear—both are moving and moving rather rapidly.

Since the beginnings of dialysis, vascular access has been a problem that has necessitated procedures, surgical and eventually interventional, for salvage and maintenance. With the rapid growth of the dialysis population, the performance of vascular access procedures has grown almost exponentially. Advances in the approach to these types of problems and the technology designed to manage them have also increased. With the advent of the KDOQI practice guidelines in 1997 and the National Vascular Access Improvement Initiative (Fistula First) in January 2003, coupled with technological developments such as ultra-high pressure balloons and newer guidewire, catheter and stent designs, the train has been moving rapidly.

Interventional nephrologists have not been sitting still. Our activity has gone from its humble beginnings within the private practice sector to a full-fledged subspecialty of nephrology. It has moved from a small group discussing dreams of progress to a vibrant active society with all of the attributes that such an endeavor should have.

We cannot allege that the development of interventional nephrology can be compared in any way to a speeding train; it has taken over 20 years to arrive at its current status which can, at best, still be considered only a beginning.

However, it is picking up speed. Nephrology represents the most rapidly advancing specialty currently performing dialysis access interventional procedures. The numbers of academic centers having dedicated programs continues to grow as do our numbers and the membership of our professional society. By analogy, while the train is moving so is the passenger; moving ever forward.

For a group that is dedicated to a specialized area of medicine to be vibrant and progressive, it must generate a relevant body of literature. This should consist of pertinent, well-constructed scientific publications and text from which knowledge can be shared. This is the group's life-blood. This publication, *Interventional Nephrology*, represents what should be viewed as the next important step in the development of *Interventional Nephrology: A Dedicated Textbook*.

Interventional Nephrology represents a collaborative effort by a number of experts in their field. Without their contributions, this effort would not have been possible. The co-editors are grateful and indebted to them for their time and efforts. Without them this project would have not been possible.

Arif Asif, MD, FASN, FNKF
Anil K. Agarwal, MD, FACP, FASN, FNKF
Alexander S. Yevzlin, MD
Steven Wu, MD, FASN
Gerald A. Beathard, MD, PhD, FACP, FCAP, FASN

ACKNOWLEDGMENTS

"We acknowledge our patients, teachers and colleagues
who helped us acquire the knowledge and experience in writing this book."

ABOUT THE EDITORS

ARIF ASIF

Arif Asif is a Professor of Medicine and Chief of Nephrology and Hypertension at Albany Medical College, Albany, New York. He has published over 200 articles in scientific journals, book chapters, abstracts and has received multiple awards for his services to Interventional Nephrology. He has been an invited speaker for numerous national and international scientific conferences. He has been very active in promoting Interventional Nephrology and has co-chaired multiple scientific conferences. He is the past president of the American Society of Diagnostic and Interventional Nephrology. In addition to being on the editorial board of multiple journals Dr. Asif also serves as the editor for the Interventional Nephrology section of Seminars in Dialysis.

ANIL K. AGARWAL

Anil K. Agarwal, MD, FACP, FASN, FNKF is currently a Professor in the nephrology division of the Department of Medicine at The Ohio State University College of Medicine and Public Health in Columbus, Ohio, where he is also the director of interventional nephrology. After receiving his MD at MLB Medical College in Jhansi, India, Dr Agarwal completed training in India as well as at The Ohio State University. Dr Agarwal has researched in chronic kidney disease and its complications, dialysis, and interventional nephrology. Dr Agarwal has published books, chapters, articles, and abstracts, and has lectured extensively nationally and internationally. He has been recognized in Best Doctors in America and Top Doctors. He serves in many key leadership positions at The Ohio State University and in organizations such as the American Society of Diagnostic and Interventional Nephrology, American Society of Nephrology, and National Kidney Foundation.

ALEXANDER S. YEVZLIN

Alexander S. Yevzlin, MD is currently an Associate Professor in the nephrology division of the Department of Medicine of the University of Wisconsin School of Medicine and Public Health, where he is the director of interventional nephrology. After receiving his undergraduate degree magna cum laude from Dartmouth College. Dr. Yevzlin has published or presented over 150 manuscripts, abstracts, and invited lectures focusing on novel techniques and device innovation. He is currently President Elect of the American Society of Diagnositic and Interventional Nephrology.

STEVEN WU, MD, FASN

Dr. Steven Wu is the Director of Interventional Nephrology, Medical Director of Vascular Access Program, and Associate Director of Vascular Interventional Radiology (Vascular Access) at Massachusetts General Hospital, and Instructor in Medicine at Harvard Medical School. He is councilor at American Society of Diagnostic and Interventional Nephrology (ASDIN), co-chair of the 7th and 8th ASDIN annual scientific meetings, and the editor of "ASDIN Core Curriculum for Peritoneal Dialysis Catheter Procedures". Dr. Wu graduated from Wuhan Tongji Medical University in China. He completed his Nephrology fellowship at the Harvard joint program of Brigham and Women's Hospital/Massachusetts General Hospital, followed by a Vascular Interventional Radiology fellowship at Department of Radiology of Massachusetts General Hospital.

GERALD A. BEATHARD

Gerald A. Beathard received his MD and PHD degrees from the University of Texas Medical Branch in Galveston, Texas. He is board certified in Internal Medicine, Nephrology, Pathology and Allergy and Immunology. Dr Beathard has practiced Nephrology for 45 years and has been actively engaged in Interventional Nephrology for 27 years. He currently limits his practice to Interventional Nephrology. He is founder and past president of ASDIN. Currently he is a medical director of Lifeline Vascular Access, engaged in physician training and is a Clinical Professor at the University of Texas Medical Branch.

SECTION I

History of Interventional Nephrology: Birth of a New Specialty

ORIGINS OF HEMODIALYSIS ACCESS: THE SCRIBNER EXPERIENCE

WISSAM SALIBA, ALEXANDER S. YEVZLIN, & PETER IVANOVICH

LEARNING OBJECTIVES

1. Understand the historical origins of hemodialysis access.
2. Describe the early experience of hemodialysis delivery.
3. Understand the key elements of the Scribner shunt.
4. Discuss the evolution of modern vascular access from the Scribner shunt.

THE PRE-SCRIBNER ERA

Thomas Graham, a physician-scientist from Glasgow, Scotland, was the first to use the term "diffusion" to describe the principle of solute transport across a semipermeable membrane in 1854.[1] In October 1924, George Haas[2] (Giessen, Germany) performed the first hemodialysis on humans, which lasted 15 minutes. Haas tried a series of different dialyzers made of materials from vegetable and animal membranes. He finally developed a dialyzer consisting of organic tubes and a dialysate bath placed in a glass cylinder. He was able to obtain blood from the radial artery through a glass cannula and return it to the antecubital vein. He used hirudin as anticoagulant, which caused severe side effects and was later replaced by heparin in 1928.

Subsequently, on 17 March 1943, Willem Kolff performed the first "effective" hemodialysis on a 29-year-old housemaid with uremia, malignant hypertension, and congestive heart failure.[3] He constructed a rotating drum artificial kidney by wrapping 20 m of cellophane tubing around a horizontal drum. The lowest half of the drum was immersed in a large bath with dialysate. The blood was first obtained through venipuncture needles and consisted of either a vein-to-vein or artery-to-vein circuit. Subsequently, Kolff used a glass cannula that was placed in the radial artery through a small incision. He used large amount of heparin as anticoagulant. Glass tubes connected by small flexible rubber components were used in this access setup. Nils Alwall, from Lund, Sweden, enclosed the Kolff drum artificial kidney concept in a stainless steel canister.[4] This enabled him to apply positive pressure to the blood and therefore remove greater quantity of fluid by ultrafiltration. He also tried arteriovenous shunting in rabbits using glass cannulae but was unable to transfer the innovation to meet human vascular access needs. He supervised the delivery of 1500 dialysis treatments from 1946 to 1960.

In the above instances, arterial cannulation was required to sustain adequate blood flow for hemodialysis. Since arterial cannulation is painful and leads to scarring of a vital source of blood supply to an extremity, this method could only be used as mean of access for acute, limited dialytic treatment. Hemodialysis did not evolve into a chronic, life-sustaining therapy until the pioneers of vascular access were able to device a means of repeated, nontraumatic access of a high-flow vascular circuit.

THE ORIGINS OF MODERN VASCULAR ACCESS FOR HEMODIALYSIS

Belding Scribner and colleagues modified the glass arteriovenous shunt originally tried by Alwall by making them from Teflon. Teflon was heated and shaped as needed to fit the arterial size at the site of cannulation. Two Teflon 1/8 inch tubes were used to cannulate the radial artery and an adjacent cephalic vein at the wrist. These Teflon

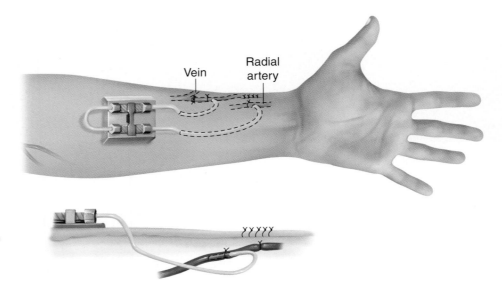

Figure 1-1. Diagram of Scribner shunt. (Modified with permission from Quinton W, Dillard D, Scribner B. Cannulation of blood vessels for prolonged hemodialysis. *ASAIO J.* 1960;6:1.)

tubes were subcutaneously tunneled to minimize the risk of infection and dislodgement.[5] The cannulae emerged from the skin through two tight-fitting puncture wounds, 1 inch apart, a few centimeters away from the site of vessels cannulation. This technique was mainly used for patient with chronic renal failure needing dialysis. In this case, time was available to allow healing of the two tunnels, thus preventing a major bleeding problem, often encountered if this technique was applied for patients with acute renal failure.

The two Teflon tubes external ends were tapered and connected to the dialyzer at the time of dialysis. They allowed a blood flow of 100–200 mL/min. When not in use for dialysis, a special fitting U-shaped device over an arm plate was used to connect the two external ends and shunt blood from the radial artery to the forearm vein (Figure 1-1).

The arm plate consisted of a stainless steel plate of 5 cm × 4.7 cm mounted with two 1/8-inch Teflon tubes that fit snugly into two stainless steel tubes.[6] The function of this arm plate and stainless steel tubing system was mainly to maintain accurate alignment between the two Teflon tubes inside and thus reduce the chance of irregularities and blood clotting. The space between the stainless steel tubing and the Teflon tubing was also filled with sterile silicone grease to decrease the dead space, and therefore blood collection, pooling, and clotting.

The Scribner shunt represents the single most important advance in the history of hemodialysis access: (1) the tunneled Teflon tubing was a strong barrier to infection; (2) the stainless steel connector decreased the risk of thrombosis (no anticoagulation was required to keep the shunt open when not in use for dialysis); (3) the Teflon tubing's unique inner luminal characteristics were a marked improvement over Alwal's glass tubing vis-à-vis blood-foreign material surface interactions and thrombosis.

In addition, with the Scribner shunt, dialysis could be performed anytime, simply by placing a pressure cuff in the arm above the elbow and inflating it above arterial pressure, and then removing the shunt and connecting the cannulae to the dialyzer after greasing their tips with sterile silicone. The blood pressure cuff could then be released allowing blood to run. This was a very simple procedure compared to the methods used before, consisting of repetitive surgeries for cannulations prior to each dialysis therapy.

The Scribner shunt allowed dialysis to be carefully planned to suit the need of each patient. This prevented long hours of dialysis used with conventional cannulation methods, done to delay the next dialysis as much as possible. Such long dialysis can cause a rapid decrease in urea concentration, which may result in cerebral edema and death, especially in severely uremic patients. With Scribner shunt in place, patients could be initiated on dialysis slowly and for a short time, allowing urea concentrations to equalize between the cerebral fluid and the blood few hours after each dialysis session. Most importantly, the Scribner shunt made *maintenance* chronic hemodialysis possible.

Clyde Shields was the first patient who was dialyzed using the Scribner shunt for vascular access on March 9, 1960. He was a 39-year-old machinist with 7-year-history of chronic kidney disease and proteinuria.[7] Starting with once weekly 24 hours hemodialysis treatment, Scribner later decreased the duration of hemodialysis and increased its frequency to twice weekly, and then three times weekly, a schedule that remains ubiquitous at present. Clyde Shields thrived for 11 years on this hemodialysis regimen and died in 1971 after experiencing a massive myocardial infarction. Ten weeks after the first dialysis of Clyde Shields, Scribner published a "Preliminary Report on The Treatment of Chronic Uremia by Means of Intermittent Hemodialysis" and described another case of successful hemodialysis treatment using his method for cannulation.[8] Clairvoyantly, he also discussed medical problems for patients on chronic hemodialysis therapy including malnutrition, hypertension, anemia, and weight loss.

The original Scribner shunt was sustainable for about 2 months, mainly due to the stiffness of the Teflon tubing that continuously irritated the intima of the artery and vein. Later, the replacement of the Teflon bypass tubes by flexible silicon rubber tubing gave the new shunt a lifespan up to years.

In 1962, together with Dr. James Havilland, then President of the King County Medical Society, Scribner established the "Seattle Artificial Kidney Center," the first outpatient dialysis center in the world. It was later renamed the "Northwest Kidney Centers." This created an ethical question on who should be dialyzed, since the demand for hemodialysis far exceeded the capacity of the six machines that were available at the center. This, known as the "Seattle experience," led to the creation of one of the first bioethical committees.

In 1966, Clark and Parsons reviewed the Scribner shunt technique and modified it to decrease risk of complications, including bleeding, clotting, infection, and extrusion of the tubes.[9]

THE LEGACY OF SCRIBNER

Once validated as a possible modality, hemodialysis access was aggressively and creatively pursued by those that followed. The legacy that Scribner left behind, however, transcends vascular access (Table 1-1).

To become independent from the surgeons placing the shunt, Stanley Shaldon (London, UK) established vascular access from percutaneously cannulating the femoral artery and vein using the Seldinger technique in 1961.

He used catheters hand-made from Teflon with a bonded silicon rubber attachment and a plastic nylon adapter.[10] Later, he cannulated vessels in different sites including the subclavian vein.

The multiple potential complications associated with the Scribner shunt, including clotting, local infection, sepsis, dislodgment, and patients' anxiety, led to the creation of the first natural arterio-venous fistula by Drs. Cimino, Brescia, and the surgeon Dr. Appell at Bronx, VA, New York, in 1965. This was a relatively easy procedure consisting of a 3- to 5-mm incision near the wrist and a side-to-side anastomosis between the radial artery and the cephalic vein.[11] This was another major step in the history of hemodialysis access. The new technique gained wide widespread acceptance, and Scribner was the first nephrologist to refer patients from Seattle to New York for creation of an AV fistula.

Over the next few years, several modifications of the Cimino fistula occurred. In 1967, Sperling introduced the technique of end-to-end anastomosis between the radial artery and the cephalic antebrachial vein in the forearm.[12] This was technically challenging mainly due to the difference in diameters between the artery and the vein.

In 1968, Lars Röhl (Heidelberg, Germany) successfully performed radial-artery-side-to-vein-end anastomosis.[13] This technique offered the advantage of being able to use a more lateral antebrachial cephalic vein, which would not have been suitable for a side-to-side anastomosis. This technique has become a standard of practice today.

In 1969, George Thomas (Seattle, USA) attached two silastic cannulae to the walls of the femoral artery and vein using Dacron patches to avoid vessel occlusion by the cannulae and therefore decrease the risk of thrombosis and infection.[14] A Teflon tube then connected the

---

TABLE 1–1

Personal Recollections of Belding Scribner by Peter Ivanovich

Belding H. Scribner, above all, was a compassionate clinician and a dedicated humanitarian. During the 1960s, I was fortunate to be a fellow in his division at the University of Washington and participated in his groundbreaking investigation of the severe metabolic bone disease encountered in the early chronic hemodialysis patients. Dr. Scribner epitomized the unselfish dedication to patient care and the advancement of technology to benefit patients with acute and chronic kidney disease without regard for monetary gain or personal aggrandizement. Professor Robin Eady, one Dr. Scribner's earliest patients, told me when I was drafting my reminiscences: "He was a natural leader who attracted people from all over the world." Dr. Eady received a kidney transplant in 1988 after 25 years as a home hemodialysis patient in Great Britain. Eady's story is illustrative of the countless CKD patients, who live today, thanks to Dr. Scribner.

Dr. Scribner's leadership qualities were also evident in the way in which he managed his Division. Be they clerical personnel, laboratory or dialysis technicians, or nurses, he viewed every person in the Division as a committed member of his team. "Scrib" addressed each with respect and recognized all for their contributions. Some members of his team were so important to the program that they were coauthors in publications. With that high degree of regard for his technical staff, Scrib encouraged me and other medical trainees to learn all aspects of dialysis from them.

The knowledge I gained from him, his training program, and his technical coworkers inspired me to devote my early research at Northwestern to blood–membrane interaction and to facilitate vascular access in hemodialysis patients. It was, however, Scrib's devotion to those renal patients for whom dialysis meant an improved quality of life—even a chance at living—that remains his everlasting inspiration and legacy for those of us fortunate enough to have trained with him.

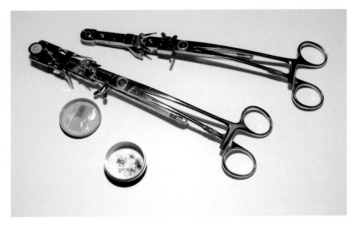

Figure 1-2. Inocuchi device used by neophrologists to create AVFs via anastomotic stapling.

two external tips of the cannulae about 10 cm from the original wound.

In 1970, Gilberto Flores Izquierdo (Mexico City) and James May[15] (Sydney, Australia) used the saphenous vein to connect the brachial artery and an adjacent vein in a U-shape way near the elbow, in patients with minimal peripheral vascular access available.

In1971, Peter Ivanovich, a former trainee of Dr. Scribner ion vascular access placement, traveled to Japan and visited university medical centers in Tokyo, Osaka, Nagoya, Hiroshima, and several other cities where patients were being treated with chronic hemodialysis. As a result of the close cooperation established with the Japanese physicians and surgeons Northwestern University's renal/hypertension division was given a gift of an Inokuchi Vascular Stapling Instrument (Figure 1-2).[16] Dr. Ivanovich, trained in the use of the instrument in the Inokuchi's department's animal surgical research laboratory, demonstrated the use of the instrument by performing anastomoses of animal blood vessels in the United States.[17] The instrument became the primary method for AV fistula placement at the Lakeside VA Medical Center in Chicago, IL. Forearm cephalic veins were carefully assessed to assure unimpeded cephalad flow. A negative Allen test was a critical component of preoperative assessment. Routine laboratory tests, ECG, and chest film were prerequisites of the outpatient procedure. All of the Inokuchi forearm vascular access procedures were performed using local anesthesia exclusively. Acute kidney injury patients requiring dialytic therapy had vascular access surgery performed at bedside in the ICU setting, and the AVFs created were access immediately for acute hemodialysis in many of the patients.

All of these subsequent innovations and developments represent refinements of the technique pioneered by Scribner and colleagues. The seminal innovation that fostered all subsequent techniques was the creation of a means of repeated, nontraumatic access of a high-flow vascular circuit: the Scribner shunt.

CONCLUSION AND FUTURE DIRECTIONS

All of these subsequent innovations and developments represent refinements of the technique pioneered by Scribner and colleagues. The seminal innovation that fostered all subsequent techniques was the creation of a means of repeated, nontraumatic access of a high-flow vascular circuit: the Scribner shunt.

In the era of the Fistula First Breakthrough Initiative, we have witnessed a profound increase in the placement of AVFs in the United States. This increase has been attended by an increase in failure of native AVFs to mature from a historical baseline of 10% reported by Konner[18] to a staggering 40% reported by some US academic centers.[19] Perhaps the future solution of this dilemma rests in the use of the Scribner shunt as a bridge to permanent AVF, thus avoiding catheter use while allowing the veins to hypertrophy prior to creation of a permanent access to allow immediate cannulation. In addition, the outcomes achieved by European Nephrologists, who create arteriovenous access de novo, have led some luminaries in the field to suggest that we return to the visionary practice of Scribner as primary creators of vascular access for hemodialysis,[20] a process that is well underway.[21]

REFERENCES

1. Graham T. The Bakerian lecture: on osmotic force. *Philos Trans R Soc Lond.* 1854;144:177–228.
2. Wizemann V, Benedum J. Nephrology dialysis transplantation 70th anniversary of haemodialysis—the pioneering contribution of Georg Haas (1886–1971). *Nephrol Dial Transplant.* 1994;9(12):1829–1831.
3. Kolff WJ. First clinical experience with the artificial kidney. *Ann Int Med.* 1965;62:608–619.
4. Kjellstrand CM. Dedication to Nils Alwall. *Nephron.* 1985;39(2):71–72.
5. Quinton WE, Dillard DH, Scribner BH. Cannulation of blood vessels for prolonged hemodialysis. *Trans Am Soc Artif Intern Organs.* 1960;6:104–113.
6. Scribner BH, Saner JE, Buri R, Quinton W. The technique of continous hemodialysis. *Trans Am Soc Artif Intern Organs.* 1960;6:88–103.
7. Scribner BH. A personalized history of chronic hemodialysis. *Am J Kidney Dis.* 1990;16:511–519.
8. Scribner BH, Buri R, Caner JEZ, Hegstom R, Burnell JM. The treatment of chronic uremia by means of intermittent hemodialysis: a preliminary report. *Trans Am Soc Artif Intern Organs.* 1960;6:114–122.
9. Clark PB, Parsons FM. Routine use of the Scribner shunt for haemodialysis. *Br Med J.* 1966;1(5497):1200–1202.
10. Shaldon S, Chiandussi L, Higgs B. Haemodialysis by percutaneous catheterization of the femoral artery and vein with regional heparinization. *Lancet.* 1961;II: 857–859.
11. Brescia MJ, Cimino JE, Appel K, Hurwich BJ. Chronic hemodialysis using venipuncture and a surgically created arteriovenous fistula. *N Engl J Med.* 1966;275: 1089–1092.

12. Konner K. History of vascular access for haemodialysis. *Nephrol Dial Transplant*. 2005;20(12):2629–2635.

13. Röhl L, Franz HE, Möhring K, et al. Direct arteriovenous fistula for hemodialysis. *Scand J Urol Nephrol*. 1968;2: 191–195.

14. Thomas GI. A large vessel applique A-V-shunt for hemodialysis. *Trans Am Soc Artif Intern Organs*. 1969;15:288–292.

15. May J, Tiller D, Johnson J, Stewart J, Sheil AGR. Saphenous vein arteriovenous fistula in regular dialysis treatment. *N Engl J Med*. 1969;280:770.

16. Inokuchi, K. A new type of vessel-suturing apparatus. *Arch Surg*. 1958;77:954.

17. Ivanovich, P. Kahan, B. Bergan, J, et al. *Trans Am. Soc. Artif. Intern. Organs*. 1977;23:716–718.

18. Konner K. Vascular access in the hemodialysis patient—personal experience and review of the literature. *Hemodial Int*. 2003;7(2):184–190.

19. Peterson WJ, Barker J, Allon M. Disparities in fistula maturation persist despite preoperative vascular mapping. *Clin J Am Soc Nephrol*. 2008;3(2):437–441.

20. Konner K. Should nephrologists be in charge? *Contrib Nephrol*. 2005;149:121–130.

21. Mishler R, Yevzlin AS. Outcomes of arteriovenous fistulae created by a U.S. interventional nephrologist. *Semin Dial*. 2010;23(2):224–228.

HISTORY OF INTERVENTIONAL NEPHROLOGY IN THE UNITED STATES

GERALD A. BEATHARD

INTRODUCTION

In order to discuss the history of interventional nephrology (IN), one must first define exactly what is meant by the term interventional nephrology. It is actually a little difficult to do so precisely because it is still in the process of being defined. If one considers that a nephrologist is a medical specialist who deals with that branch of medicine related to kidney function and disease, then by analogy, an interventional nephrologist would be a medical specialist who deals with interventional procedures that relate to the kidney and its diseases. According to this definition, it is obvious that an interventional nephrologist would not have to be a nephrologist. However, in reality, most are nephrologist first and then become an interventionalist.

Classically, nephrologists have performed kidney biopsies and inserted temporary dialysis catheters. However, over the past two decades, an increasing number of nephrologists have begun to perform a variety of procedures relating to the establishment and maintenance of both peritoneal and hemodialysis access. These procedures have been so widely practiced that the term interventional nephrology has come to be defined as a medical specialist who deals with the establishment and maintenance of dialysis access, particularly arteriovenous access.

THE BEGINNINGS

IN owes its origins to efforts that began in the private sector in the mid-1980s. This is understandable because with most dialysis patients being cared for by nephrologists in private practice, the increasingly deplorable state of hemodialysis vascular access was most obvious there. I can remember very well one particular day when I stood in front of a young dialysis patient with a dysfunctional access, staring at it and wondering what it was, what it was doing, what was going wrong, and what I could do about it. Unfortunately, I could not offer an answer to any of these questions and, even worse, I had no idea where to turn for the answers. I had returned from a meeting where angiograms of dysfunction dialysis accesses had been shown. I was struck by the appearance of the stenotic lesions that were demonstrated. I decided that this information would be valuable in guiding the surgical treatment that our patients were receiving when they had a problem.

Having a radiology department across the hall from the primary dialysis facility at our clinic, I started doing angiograms on dysfunctional cases by simply injecting radiocontrast through a dialysis needle left in place at the end of the patient's treatment. I saw the same types of lesions that had been demonstrated at the meeting that I had attended. I called one of our consulting vascular surgeons on one of the first cases that I evaluated. The patient had an area of severe stenosis in the basilic vein draining a forearm loop graft. He agreed to see the patient in order to schedule surgery, but I was dismayed when I offered to send the radiographs to his office and he stated that he did not really need them. We did not know at the time that we were taking the first steps in starting a new subspecialty nor was this our goal at that time. We only wanted to understand a major problem that was affecting our patient's ability to dialyze.

REQUIREMENTS FOR A NEW SPECIALTY

In order to start a new specialty or subspecialty several requirements must be met. Among these are need, interest, opportunity, support, academic involvement, and organization. IN is still evolving but it has followed this basic course in its development.

▶ Need

The great nemesis of hemodialysis when it first became a practical reality for the treatment of renal failure in the 1950s and early 1960s was vascular access. The first attempt at a workable long-term vascular access was offered by a nephrologist in the early 1960s, the Scribner shunt.[1,2] This arteriovenous connection was a major advance, but was associated with frequent problems of thrombosis and infection. Nephrologists became very adept at doing shunt thrombectomies and thus became the first interventional nephrologists in the sense in which the term is used today.

The Brescia-Cimino fistula was a major advance in dialysis access. The technique for creating this access and its use in clinical cases was reported in 1966.[3] Both Brescia and Cimino were nephrologists (they were from the renal service; this was actually before nephrology became a formal subspecialty). The first angiogram of a fistula was published in 1968 by Hurwic,[4] a nephrologist who had been a coauthor of the original fistula report with Brescia and Cimino.

In 1972, legislation was passed that established the end stage renal disease (ESRD) program which provided benefit within Medicare for the provision of dialysis treatments. This made the creation of dialysis vascular access a priority for nephrologists with the rapidly increasing numbers of cases requiring dialysis care. At that time, less than 50% of patients were felt to be candidates for a Brescia-Cimino fistula. The bovine arterial heterograft, having been first used as a conduit for arterial bypass surgery, was applied to this problem. It was introduced initially for use in cases in which fistulas could not be established or maintained; however, encouraging early experience led some to advocate its use as the initial means of providing access for hemodialysis.[5] With continued use, reports of long-term complications and failures were increasingly reported,[6] damping the initial enthusiasm with which this material was met.

The expanded polytetrafluoroethylene (PTFE) graft for dialysis vascular access was introduced in 1976,[7] and in large part, IN owes its beginnings to this event (or at least to the problems that grew out of this event). This material had many advantages. It was relatively inexpensive, readily available, and could be placed in a variety of configurations to provide a large cannulation surface area to permit adequate blood flow for efficient dialysis therapy. The PTFE graft however proved to be a double-edged sword.

By the mid-1980s, the predominant type of arteriovenous access used for hemodialysis was the PTFE graft.

As a result of such widespread use, a high incidence of complications was seen. Infection was a significant problem, but recurrent clotting was the major issue. The life expectancy of a PTFE graft was only 50% to 60% at 2 years with 80% of grafts being lost in conjunction with an episode of thrombosis.[8-11] This problem related to the fact that venous stenosis was developing in association with these grafts. The standard approach to dialysis access was to place a PTFE graft without the benefit of vascular studies; it was not until much later that vascular mapping began.[12] It was unusual in most locales to even try to identify candidates for a fistula. If the graft thrombosed, it was declotted with no use of imaging to detect and correct stenotic lesions. If a stenotic lesion became too problematic, a revision was done or the graft was replaced. The dysfunctional dialysis access was a major cause of patient morbidity and even mortality as potential access sites were progressively lost. Neither vascular surgery nor nephrology training programs at the time dealt with dialysis vascular access. Very little was known about this subject by anyone in any specialty. No one was doing anything. The attitude was simply—when it is broken fix it. There was no collaborative effort to do better, no prospective planning, and no progress in an area that was so critical to the welfare of the dialysis patient.

▶ Interest

There was interest, at least the beginnings of interest. A few papers were appearing. Dialysis patients are unique and they have unique problems. Nephrologists have been trained to address and generally aggressively pursue all of the dialysis patient's problems, whether they relate to hematology, endocrinology, nutrition, or any of the other medical issues that beset this special group of patients. The only real exception was vascular access. This was relegated to consultants with no dialysis experience and, in most cases, virtually no nephrology involvement. This situation was not working well and this fact caused nephrologists to become interested and to begin to search for a remedy.

It was into this milieu that IN was born. Angioplasty was relatively new in the 1980s. The first balloon catheter angioplasty of a peripheral artery was done in 1976 by Gruntzig, a cardiologist,[13] who did the first coronary balloon angioplasty in 1977,[14] other vessels soon followed.[15] In the early 1980s, the first reports of the application of this technique to the dysfunctional dialysis access graft appeared.[16-19] However, the technique was not widely applied nor was any large series reported only small anecdotal reports.

▶ Opportunity

Interest is important, but opportunity is critical. Not everyone who is interested actually gets an opportunity to develop that interest. Unfortunately, the opportunities to get involved and at least participate in a solution to the problems of dialysis vascular access were very limited in many locales. However, I was in a unique situation and being in private practice, I was not faced with many of the administrative restrictions which can affect those in academia. I saw a need, had the opportunity, and was able to act on it.

▶ Support

It is very difficult for an individual to stand alone. This is especially true if what he is doing represents a major departure from the accepted norm. The beginning of a new idea or movement often begins with a single individual who sees a need. However, it cannot stay isolated if it is to survive. The idea must attract others. A group of individuals is necessary to develop a body of supportive literature, establish standards of practice, develop practice guidelines, and ultimately develop training programs. A new specialty does not necessarily develop all at once, but by bits. The basics come first, the details and embellishments appear later. This is how change frequently occurs; it takes a group of individuals with a common interest and common goals. Thus, it was with IN.

I was able to get started initially because of local support from associates and the radiologists and surgeons with whom I worked. Shortly after I started doing access angiogram, a new cardiologist arrived at our clinic who was the first in our area to do coronary angioplasty. Because of our interest in the lesions we were seeing, we convinced him to do a few dialysis access cases. We were pleased with the result. It should be noted that at that time no one was doing surveillance and we were doing only the most severe, obvious cases. Very soon this cardiologist became too busy to do our cases so we were back where we started, but with a level of heightened interest because of the results which we had observed.

We were associated with two very talented interventional radiologists, but they were busy and were not convinced that this was a worthwhile activity. I decided that in order to provide the potential patient benefit that I felt existed, I would simply need to do the procedures myself. At that time, credentialing, privileging, and turf issues were not as great as they later became. In fact, one would have to say that local turf conflict was almost nonexistent. I was able to get provisional privileges to do dialysis access angioplasty with a cardiologist proctor without any formal training. Basically, I learned as I went. I worked in the hospital's angiography suite where a wide variety of procedures were performed. I was also fortunate to work with several very knowledgeable radiology technologists who were extremely encouraging and helpful.

In 1989, Schwab et al[20] published a paper on using venous pressure for dialysis access graft surveillance, a technique referred to as dynamic venous pressure monitoring. They used a venous dialysis pressure greater than 150 mm Hg measured early in dialysis at a blood flow of 200 mL/min. In this study, 86% of patients who had an elevated pressure and in whom a venogram was performed were found to have significant venous stenosis. We applied this technique to our patient population and found a similar result. Encouraged by the results that we were obtaining with this type of surveillance and prospective angioplasty, we began to collect data and present our results. Although preliminary data was presented earlier, our first comprehensive paper was published in 1992.[21]

Very shortly after our first reports at meetings and especially after our first publications, we began to have nephrologists from all over the United States and even some outside of the United States contact us to arrange for training. Several of these outstanding physicians have since become leaders in the IN field.

Other physicians have played major defining roles in helping establish the core of activities that come under the heading IN. Stephen Ash developed a technique for the placement of peritoneal dialysis catheters using peritoneoscopy. He started a training course in the late 1980s. Many of the interventional nephrologists that place peritoneal dialysis catheters are products of that training. Charles O'Neill ushered in the practice of diagnostic renal ultrasound by nephrologists by establishing a course at Emory University in the mid-1950s.

In 2000, the American Society of Nephrology (ASN) and the Renal Physicians Association (RPA) published position papers on credentialing in nephrology addressing what they recognized as an emerging area of competency know as interventional nephrology.[22] Specifically, this document stated, "Interventional Nephrology encompasses procedures that are essential to the management of the patient with renal disease, and as such represent an appropriate component of the nephrologist's scope of practice." This support was extremely important in the development of IN.

One would have to acknowledge the fact that if such widespread and enthusiastic support had not been there, IN would never have become a reality. It is misleading to look at an avalanche and point to the first pebble that began to roll down hill; the net effect of an avalanche is related to all of the pebbles, rocks, and even boulders that take up the charge. The development of IN has seemed to be very much analogous to such an avalanche.

▶ Academic Involvement

Academic involvement is essential to the final development of any specialty. This is even more important if the first seeds of development have been sown in a private practice setting. Academic training programs are essential for credibility. They are expected to be the primary source for the body of scientific literature that forms a necessary basis for the new area of emphasis. Formal training programs are also essential to ultimate long-term success. A physician who has trained in an accredited training program is much more easily accepted than one who has been trained through a proctored program in a private practice setting. Academic interest began very early; however, it has moved at a slow pace for two basic reasons. Firstly, being new, there has been a shortage of qualified faculty to develop programs. Secondly, many academic nephrology programs do not have large dialysis patient populations. It requires a large program to support an interventional training facility. Nevertheless, academic involvement has continued to grow and centers of excellence have been established in a number of institutions.

▶ Organization

In order to function as an entity, a new specialty must have organization. A society for this area of special emphasis, The American Society of Diagnostic and Interventional Nephrology (ASDIN), was established on October 12, 2000 at a meeting of the American Society of Nephrology, Toronto, Canada. The Society was incorporated on June 13, 2000. The first annual meeting of the Society was held on February 20, 2001 in New Orleans, LA, in conjunction with the Annual Conference on Dialysis. The first national meeting of ASDIN convened on February 12, 2005 in Scottsdale, AZ.

ASDIN has played an important role in establishing and nurturing excellence in IN. One of the first actions of this Society was to establish a certification program. This, along with training program accreditation and the development of a training curriculum, has been important in the development of IN as a respected subspecialty.

One cannot minimize the role that Inventional Radiology has played in the development of this specialty. Their role was twofold. Firstly, much of the body of scientific knowledge upon which IN rests has been derived from the excellent work of a number of radiologists who have been dedicated to dialysis vascular access. Secondly, they have as a group held nephrologist up to a high standard by assuming the role of a critical observer.[23] One cannot over estimate the importance of either of these roles.

IN is still in its early stages; development and advancement continue to occur as it should in any specialty. In 2004, data were presented on over 14,000 basic dialysis access procedures performed by 29 different nephrologists, showing that these physicians could do this work safely, effectively, and efficiently.[24] This report caused one radiologist who had been critical earlier to conclude that "interventional nephrology was headed in the right direction" and that "a challenge was laid down and the interventional nephrology community rose to it,"[25] During the period from 2001 to 2008, an increase in the incidence of dialysis access angioplasty of 171% was observed. The number of cases performed by nephrologists rose by 1481%. This was in contrast to an increase of 55% of these cases being done by radiologists. Thrombectomies rose by 52% with an increase in nephrology performed cases of 713% and a 2% increase for radiologists.

Recently, nephrology interventionists have started to do more complex arterial work in cases with dysfunctional dialysis access and even treat renal artery lesions in nephrology patients in whom the problem is found to need correction.[26] Additionally, some nephrologists have expanded their procedural repertoire to include the creation of arteriovenous fistulas.[27,28]

Interventional nephrology is emerging as a new area of competency in nephrology. The nephrologist who performs procedures that are critical to the management of patients being maintained on dialysis has becoming a reality. Standardized criteria for certification have been developed, national nephrology organizations have become involved, and a national subspecialty organization has been established. Nephrologists are assuming an ever greater role in the care of their patients who have a dysfunctional dialysis access.

REFERENCES

1. Quinton W, Dillard D, Scribner BH. Cannulation of blood vessels for prolonged hemodialysis. *Trans Am Soc Artif Intern Organs*. 1960;6:104–113.
2. Hegstrom RM, Quinton WE, Dillard DH, Cole JJ, Scribner BH. One year's experience with the use of indwelling teflon cannulas and bypass. *Trans Am Soc Artif Intern Organs*. 1961;7:47–56.
3. Brescia MJ, Cimino JE, Appel K, Hurwich BJ. Chronic hemodialysis using venipuncture and a surgically created arteriovenous fistula. *N Engl J Med*. 1966;275: 1089–1092.
4. Hurwich BJ. Brachial arteriography of the surgically created radial arteriovenous fistula in patients undergoing chronic intermittent hemodialysis by venipuncture technique. *Am J Roentgenol Radium Ther Nucl Med*. 1968;104:394–402.
5. Butt KM, Rao TK, Maki T, Mashimo S, Manis T, Delano BG, Kountz SL, Friedman EA. Bovine heterograft as a preferential hemodialysis access. *Trans Am Soc Artif Intern Organs*. 1974;20A:339–342.
6. Burbridge GE, Biggers JA, Remmers AR, Jr., Lindley JD, Saries HE, Fish JC. Late complications and results of bovine xenografts. *Trans Am Soc Artif Intern Organs*. 1976;22: 377–381.
7. Baker LD, Jr., Johnson JM, Goldfarb D. Expanded polytetrafluoroethylene (PTFE) subcutaneous arteriovenous conduit: an improved vascular access for chronic hemodialysis. *Trans Am Soc Artif Intern Organs*. 1976;22:382–387.
8. Sabanayagam P, Schwartz AB, Soricelli RR, Chinitz JL, Lyons P. Experience with one hundred reinforced expanded PTFE grafts for angioaccess in hemodialysis. *Trans Am Soc Artif Intern Organs*. 1980;26:582–583.
9. Munda R, First MR, Alexander JW, Linnemann CC, Jr., Fidler JP, Kittur D. Polytetrafluoroethylene graft survival in hemodialysis. *JAMA*. 1983;249:219–222.
10. Palder SB, Kirkman RL, Whittemore AD, Hakim RM, Lazarus JM, Tilney NL. Vascular access for hemodialysis. Patency rates and results of revision. *Ann Surg*. 1985;202:235–239.
11. Kherlakian GM, Roedersheimer LR, Arbaugh JJ, Newmark KJ, King LR. Comparison of autogenous fistula versus expanded polytetrafluoroethylene graft fistula for angioaccess in hemodialysis. *Am J Surg*. 1986;152:238–243.

12. Silva MB, Jr., Hobson RW, 2nd, Pappas PJ, Jamil Z, Araki CT, Goldberg MC, Gwertzman G, Padberg FT, Jr. A strategy for increasing use of autogenous hemodialysis access procedures: impact of preoperative noninvasive evaluation. *J Vasc Surg*. 1998;27:302–307; discussion 307–308.

13. Gruntzig A. Die perkutane rekanalisation chronischer arterieller verschlusse mit einen neuen doppelumigen dilatationskatheterr (Dotter-Prinzip). *ROEFO*. 1976;124:80–86.

14. Gruntzig A. Transluminal dilatation of coronary-artery stenosis. *Lancet*. 1978;1:263.

15. Gruntzig A, Kuhlmann U, Vetter W, Lutolf U, Meier B, Siegenthaler W. Treatment of renovascular hypertension with percutaneous transluminal dilatation of a renal-artery stenosis. *Lancet*. 1978;1:801–802.

16. Lawrence PF, Miller FJ, Jr., Mineaud E. Balloon catheter dilatation in patients with failing arteriovenous fistulas. *Surgery*. 1981;89:439–442.

17. Kalman P, Hobbs B, Colapinta R. Percutaneous transluminal dilatation of a stenotic arteriovenous bovine graft. *Dial Transplant*. 1980;9:777.

18. Martin EC, Diamond NG, Casarella WJ. Percutaneous transluminal angioplasty in non-atheroscklerotic disease. *Radiology*. 1980;135:27–33.

19. Gordon DH, Glanz S, Butt KM, Adamsons RJ, Koenig MA. Treatment of stenotic lesions in dialysis access fistulas and shunts by transluminal angioplasty. *Radiology*. 1982;143:53–58.

20. Schwab SJ, Raymond JR, Saeed M, Newman GE, Dennis PA, Bollinger RR. Prevention of hemodialysis fistula thrombosis. Early detection of venous stenoses. *Kidney Int*. 1989;36:707–711.

21. Beathard GA. Percutaneous transvenous angioplasty in the treatment of vascular access stenosis. *Kidney Int*. 1992;42:1390–1397.

22. RPA/ASN Position on Credentialing in Nephrology, Approved as Revised by the Renal Physician's Association and American Society of Nephrology, January 22, 2000.

23. Trerotola SO, Gray R, Brunner M, Altman S. Interventional care of the hemodialysis patient: it's about quality. *J Vasc Interv Radiol*. 2001;12:1253–1255.

24. Beathard GA, Litchfield T. Effectiveness and safety of dialysis vascular access procedures performed by interventional nephrologists. *Kidney Int*. 2004;66:1622–1632.

25. Beathard GA, Trerotola SO, Vesely TM, Schimelman B, Zimmerman R, Himmelfarb J, Work J. What is the current and future status of interventional nephrology? *Semin Dial*. 2005;18:370–379.

26. Yevzlin AS, Schoenkerman AB, Gimelli G, Asif A. Arterial interventions in arteriovenous access and chronic kidney disease: a role for interventional nephrologists. *Semin Dial*. 2009;22:545–556.

27. Mishler R. Autologous arteriovenous fistula creation by nephrologists. *Adv Chronic Kidney Dis*. 2009;16:321–328.

28. Mishler R, Yevzlin AS. Outcomes of arteriovenous fistulae created by a U.S. interventional nephrologist. *Semin Dial*. 2010;23:224–228.

3

HISTORY OF INTERVENTIONAL NEPHROLOGY FROM A GLOBAL PERSPECTIVE

KENNETH ABREO & BHARAT SACHDEVA

LEARNING OBJECTIVES

1. Review history of interventional nephrology.
2. Understand the motivation that led nephrologists to start performing interventional procedures.
3. Study the role of the American Society of Interventional and Diagnostic Nephrology (ASDIN) in promoting the field of interventional nephrology.
4. Recognize the challenges ahead for interventional nephrology.

INTRODUCTION

Pioneering work by nephrologists in the 19th century: invented the dialysis machine, constructed arteriovenous shunts and fistulas, and designed vascular/peritoneal catheters to provide their patients with long-term dialysis. As the number of dialysis patients grew, the construction and care of vascular access was abandoned by nephrologists to surgeons and radiologists. 1980s and 1990s saw a decline in the number of fistulas and with that an increase in vascular complications. Vascular access was not the first priority for the non-nephrologists and this set the stage for the emergence of diagnostic and interventional nephrologists. These self-taught nephrologists trained others, resulting in a critical mass of subspecialists who founded the Society of Diagnostic and Interventional Nephrology. This chapter traces the origin of this exciting field from its pioneers to the society as it exists today. The future of this society depends on academic nephrology fellowship programs fostering training and research in this field.

EARLY YEARS: FROM SHUNTS TO FISTULAS

Willem Johan "Pim" Kolff, a nephrologist from the Netherlands, developed the first clinically useful hemodialyzer in 1943.[1] From 1943 to 1945, following several attempts at dialyzing patients, he succeeded in saving the life of a 67-year-old woman who was in uremic coma [She lived for seven more years].[1] A major limitation of this prototype dialyzer was its inability to remove fluid and patients with acute renal failure would die from acute pulmonary edema. Kolff migrated to the United States in the 1950s and shared his invention with several universities. Dr. Nils Alwall (Figure 3-1) modified the Kolff kidney by enclosing it inside a stainless steel canister allowing the removal of fluids, by applying a negative pressure to the outside canister; thus, making it the first truly practical device for hemodialysis. On September 3, 1946, at the University Hospital in Lund, Dr Alwall dialyzed a comatosed 47-year-old man. The patient regained consiousness after treatment but died of pneumonia within 24 hours. Dr Alwall and Kloff worked independently, but this initial work led to the manufacture of the next generation of Kolff's dialyzer, a stainless steel Kolff-Brigham kidney, which paved the way for the first commercially available dialysis machine in 1956.

The hemodialysis procedure required a cut down to an artery and vein followed by ligation of these vessels at the termination of the treatment. Patients would run out of vascular access sites after a few hemodialysis treatments. Vascular access had become the "Achilles' heel" of the dialysis patient.

In 1949, Alwall and his colleagues adapted an arteriovenous glass shunt used in rabbit experiments to humans for hemodialysis.[2] The glass shunt was abandoned because

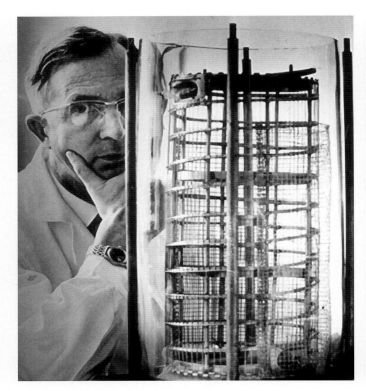

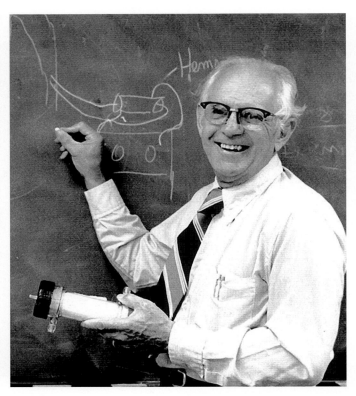

Figure 3-1. Dr. Nils Alwall. Alwall was arguably the inventor of the arteriovenous shunt for dialysis. He reported this first in 1948, where he used such an arteriovenous shunt in rabbits.

Figure 3-2. Dr. Belding Scribner. (Courtesy of University of Washington, School of Medicine.)

of frequent clotting and infection, but the concept of an arteriovenous cannula system for repeated hemodialysis was born. In honor of Alwall's advancements and achievements, *The Nils Alwall Prize* was awarded every year for groundbreaking research in the field of kidney replacement therapy.[3]

In 1960, Belding Scribner, a visionary nephrologist from Seattle, Washington, re-introduced the concept of the "shunt" when he was confronted with the plight of a patient named Joe Sanders who was admitted to the University of Washington Hospital in Seattle for acute renal failure. Scribner wrote:

> When he entered the hospital, he was in coma, and his heart failure was so bad that foam was oozing out of his lungs and mouth. Yet one week [after dialysis began] Joe was up and about, feeling amazingly well as a result of several treatments on the artificial kidney... and yet despite this amazing result all was not right. Mr. Saunders had not passed any urine in a week, a fact that made the original diagnosis suspect. A biopsy of his kidney revealed the tragic answer. The original diagnosis was wrong. Mr. Saunders had a disease which had totally and irreversibly destroyed his kidneys. They would never function again. What to do? We did the only thing we could do. We had an agonizing conversation with

Mrs. Saunders and told her to take her husband back home to Spokane where he would die. Then one morning about 4:00 AM, I woke up and groped for a piece of paper and pencil to jot down the basic idea of the shunted cannulas which would make it possible to treat people like Joe Saunders again and again with the artificial kidney without destroying two blood vessels each time.[4]

Shortly after this episode, Scribner and engineer Wayne Quinton designed a Teflon arteriovenous shunt (Figures 3-2 to 3-4) that was inserted into the radial artery and cephalic vein of the wrist in their first patient, Clyde Sheilds, on March 9, 1960.[5] A testament to the success of the arteriovenous shunt, Shields went on to live for 10 years on intermittent hemodialysis.[5,6] Although Scribner shunts provided long-term access for hemodialysis, they were plagued with episodes of clotting and infection resulting in a short life span. A major breakthrough came in 1966, when a pioneering nephrologist Brescia (Figures 3-5) and his team created the first series of radiocephalic arteriovenous fistulas, called the Brescia-Cimino fistula.[7] Interesting to note that the first ever report of successful use of arteriovenous fistula suggested flows of 250–300 mL/min.[7] This concept of the arteriovenous fistula first introduced by William Hunter in 1757, 250 years ago, could now be used to save the lives of patients with renal failure.[8]

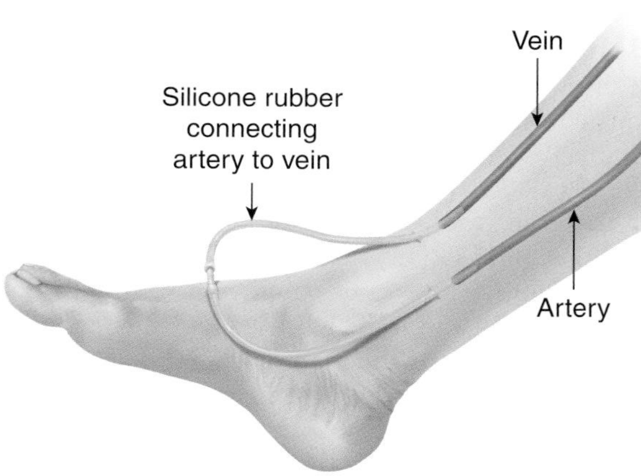

EARLY YEARS: HEMODIALYSIS CATHETERS

Stanley Shaldon designed his own handmade catheters for placement in the artery and vein of patients for immediate dialysis. He was forced to use catheters because he was unable to find surgeons in London to place arteriovenous shunts for his patients with renal failure.[9] Later, he switched to veno-venous catheterization because of excessive bleeding from the artery following removal of the catheter.[10] The Shaldon catheter was the prototype of the temporary hemodialysis catheters that are in common use today. Scribner, Shaldon, and Brescia were the pioneering interventional nephrologists who made seminal contributions to vascular access for hemodialysis patients.

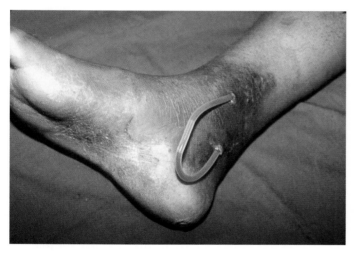

Figure 3-4. Scribner shunt in a hemodialysis patient's leg. (Courtesy Dr. Sundar, Bangalore, India.)

THE DAWN OF PERITONEAL DIALYSIS

The first patient ever treated with peritoneal dialysis was a female with ureteral obstruction due to uterine carcinoma reported by Ganter in 1923.[11] From 1923 through 1950, Ganter, Frank and Seligman, and Odel and Farris used a rubber or steel inlet tube and a rounded glass or steel "sump" drain with multiple side holes for drainage.[12] Grollman[13] at Southwestern medical school in Dallas introduced the concept of placing a flexible catheter into the abdominal cavity through a cannula using an external guide or stylet. Doolan et al[14] adopted the Grollman technique for peritoneal dialysis. He modified the catheter to facilitate easy insertion; his catheter had features that avoided omental obstruction, maximized drainage, and enhanced patient comfort. Subsequently, many other investigators contributed to this method from 1951 to 1973 to improve the design of this initial catheter that had holes at the tip of catheter to optimize flow of peritoneal fluid. This technique improved patient comfort during catheter insertion but afforded little protection from bowel puncture.

Weston and Roberts in 1965[15] described an internal stylet for placement of the semirigid "acute" peritoneal catheter. The blunt shape but sharp point of the stylet tip minimized bowel perforation. A pliable straight rubber tube with side-holes was used by a number of authors beginning in 1962 through 1982. In 1964, Gutch was first to use silicone rubber in a peritoneal dialysis catheter (straight) and placed 1 mm side holes to allow adequate fluid drainage without omental obstruction. Also, in 1964, Palmer reported the successful use of a silicone rubber catheter with a coiled internal portion, a subcutaneous silicone step, and a very long subcutaneous tunnel.

In 1965, Tenckhoff, another visionary nephrologist in Seattle, started a peritoneal dialysis program in Seattle, WA, for end-stage renal disease (ESRD) patients who were not candidates for hemodialysis in Scribner's program. Being a consummate interventionalist, he placed temporary stiff peritoneal catheters in ESRD patients at their homes on weekends.[16] The catheters lasted less than a week, were removed by patients and their families, and had to be frequently re-inserted for continuation of dialysis. In 1968,

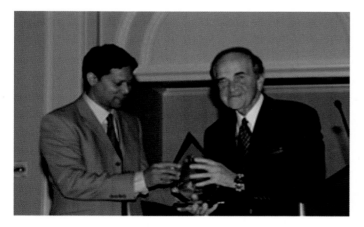

Figure 3-3. Schematic diagram of Scribner-Quinton shunt. (Courtesy Dr. Sundar, Bangalore, India.)

Figure 3-5. Dr. Brescia receiving the ASDIN Lifetime Achievement award from Dr. Asif, President of the ASDIN.

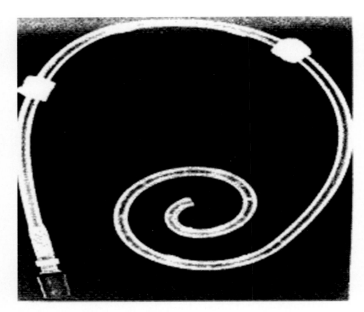

Figure 3-6. The original Tenckhoff-Quinton coiled silicone catheter with cuffs.

Tenckhoff described the advantages of addition of Dacron cuffs to silicone rubber straight and curled catheters. His histologic studies (performed on himself) showed progressive granulation tissue and fibrous tissue ingrowth to these cuffs, without evidence of calcification. The purpose of the deep cuff was to fix the catheter in position, prevent fluid leak around the catheter, and create a barrier to passage of bacteria around the catheter in case of peritonitis. The superficial cuff would prevent bacterial passage from the skin exit site to the subcutaneous tunnel. Tenckhoff also described the proper course of the subcutaneous tunnel, which is in an arc upward from the deep cuff and then downward at the superficial cuff.[17] Tenckhoff and Schechter devised the double-cuff silicone catheter with multiple side holes for long-term use, designed the trochar to introduce the catheter, prepared peritoneal dialysis solutions, and ran a successful home peritoneal dialysis program.[18] Numerous other excellent suggestions for placing and caring for peritoneal catheters are recorded for history in Tenckhoff's excellent Chronic Peritoneal Dialysis Manual.[19] The peritoneal dialysis catheter that bears his name today is not very different from the one he devised in the early 1960s (Figure 3-6).

DECLINE OF FISTULAS AND THE INCREASE OF AV GRAFTS

In the 1970s and 1980s, there was decreased interest in vascular access management by nephrologists as other areas of nephrology seemed scientifically more rewarding.[20] There were a few nephrologists who continued to be involved with the construction and maintenance of arteriovenous fistulas such as Konner in Europe.[21] During this period, the

number of fistulas placed in the United States receded and the access of choice became the graft. Bovine hetro-grafts provided options for patients with advanced vascular disease and were used in the late 1960s in the construction of arteriovenous fistulas for chronic dialysis.[22–26]

Gore-Tex® (W. L. Gore and Associates, Flagstaff, AZ), a synthetic material, was developed and patented in 1976 by Wilbert L. "Bill" Gore and his son Robert W. Gore [Bob]. W. L. Gore & Associates modest beginnings date back to January 1, 1958, when Bill and Genevieve celebrated the New Year and their 23rd wedding anniversary by launching a business in the basement of their home. In 1969, Bob Gore independently discovered expanded polytetrafluoroethylene (ePTFE) and introduced it to the public under the trademark Gore-Tex®. Following the initial experience of Baker et al in 1974,[27] by 1977 use of ePTFE in vascular access graft placement had gained wide popularity despite its obvious limitations.[28,29]

Marketing and reimbursement may have played an initial role in the increased placement of PTFE grafts but with time newly trained surgeons did not have experience in constructing arteriovenous fistulas. In 1999, 49% of patients dialyzed with an arteriovenous graft, 28% with fistulas and 26% with catheters in the United States.[30] In the seven countries that participated in Phase I of the DOPPS study (France, Germany, Italy, Spain, the United Kingdom, Japan, and the United States), substantial differences in the type of vascular access used were seen. Globally, 70–90% of prevalent dialysis patients were using an arteriovenous fistula compared to 24% of patients in the United States (Figure 3-7).[31] Moreover, when surveyed, grafts were the preferred access type for 21% of medical directors and 40% nurse managers.[28] Patients in facilities in which the medical director or nurse manager expressed a preference for grafts were more than twice as likely to have a graft than a fistula (OR = 2.3, $P < 0.01$; reference group = facilities that did not prefer grafts), suggesting that facility preferences influenced the type of access created.[32]

The United States Renal Data System (USRDS) show that the number of patients receiving treatment for ESRD increased sevenfold following the introduction of Medicare coverage for ESRD in 1973. The number of new patients added per year also increased dramatically, approximately fourfold. The gradual acceptance of elderly and diabetic patients led to an increase in the median age of new patients from 46 to 61 years and a 12-fold increase in the incidence of hemodialysis treatment in patients with ESRD due to diabetes.[33] Given the broad acceptance of sicker and older patients, access creation took a backseat.

This ever-increasing dialysis patient population, with predominantly arteriovenous grafts in the 1970–1980s, created a pressing demand for access care. Interventional techniques were underutilized and care of dysfunctional access was primarily surgical. Feldman[34] and others[35,36] reported that access-related morbidity accounted for almost 25% of all hospital stays for ESRD patients and contributed to as

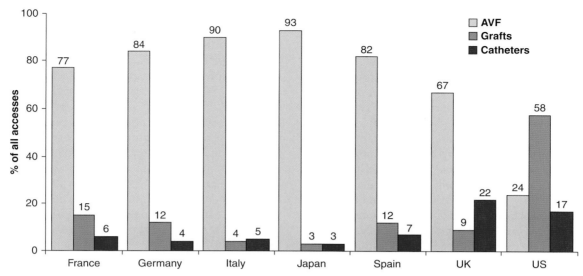

Figure 3-7. Vascular Access Use Among Prevalent HD Patients in the DOPPS: Europe, Japan, and the United States. Catheters include both temporary catheters and PermCaths; Europe (*n* = 2455), Japan (*n* = 2158), the United States (*n* = 3813). The Dopps report: October 2002 Status of DOPPS in 12 Countries; Research on Vascular Access. Available at: http://www.dopps.org/newsletters.aspx. Accessed May 2011.

much as 50% of all hospitalization costs.[34–36] Unfortunately, whereas access dysfunction was of critical and immediate importance to the United States nephrology community, it was not always a priority for surgeons and radiologists, creating both a need and an opportunity for improvement in care.[37]

Since 1982, percutaneous transluminal angioplasty (PTA) with high pressure balloon catheters was the initial approach to restore patency of ePTFE (expanded polytetrafluoroethylene, Gore-Tex) hemodialysis vascular access grafts.[38] PTA was shown to prolong the life of PTFE vascular access grafts and could be easily performed on an outpatient basis, eliminating the need for hospitalization that was usually required for surgical revision. Radiologists began to recognize access problems and applied interventional skills to maintain patency.[39] New advancements in biomedical technology, such as mechanical thrombectomy devices, high-pressure angioplasty balloons, and high performance hemodialysis catheters, stimulated interest in hemodialysis-related percutaneous procedures within the interventional radiology community.[40] As radiologists got busy with the ever-growing field of interventional radiology, dialysis patients were neglected again. The only way dialysis patients would receive timely care was for their nephrologists to provide this facet of their care.

INNOVATIONS IN PERITONEAL DIALYSIS

On the peritoneal dialysis front, Steven Ash made a major contribution by designing and describing the peritoneoscopic technique of Tenckhoff catheter placement in 1981.[41] The ability to view the peritoneal space during catheter insertion made the procedure more reliable and safe. As a founding interventional nephrologist, he set up a peritoneal dialysis insertion course in Indiana that gained popularity and acceptance by nephrologists. This technique had the distinct advantage of viewing the peritoneal cavity for optimal catheter placement. However, it requires investment in a peritoneoscope and special materials for catheter placement. Since interventional nephrologists are familiar with the use of ultrasound and fluoroscopy for vascular access procedures and materials available for tunneled catheter placement are readily available in the interventional suite, a fluoroscopic technique has become popular in recent years.[42,43]

ESTABLISHMENT OF INTERVENTIONAL NEPHROLOGY

Beathard should be credited with laying the foundation of Interventional Nephrology as it is practiced today. In Austin, TX, in the late 1980s, he honed his interventional skills, meticulously collected and published his data in premier nephrology journals,[44,45] generously invited and trained nephrologists in the field, and single handedly wrote a training manual that is now the ASDIN Interventional Nephrology Curriculum.[46] Most importantly, he instilled in his colleagues a sense of confidence, that they were just as capable of doing these procedures as their counterparts in radiology.[47] This came at a time when some of the latter questioned the competence of nephrologists doing access cases.[48] Publications in the literature over the past 10 years have shown the proficiency, effectiveness, and safety of nephrologists performing interventions on dysfunctional accesses.[47,49–58]

In Beathard's words "As second-generation interventional nephrologists brought these techniques to their practices, the field of interventional nephrology was born." Many of the nephrologists trained by Beathard took national leadership roles and they eventually formed the core group that would lay the foundation of American Society of Diagnostic and Interventional Nephrology (ASDIN).

In 1994, O'Neill started an academic program in renal ultrasound at Emory University, Atlanta, GA, and offered courses to practicing nephrologists.[59] He trained nephrology fellows to use ultrasound guidance for renal biopsies by the bedside.[59] Now, ultrasound could be used by nephrologists for the diagnosis of renal diseases and vascular access dysfunction as well as for guidance in placing catheters and performing kidney biopsies. This combination of diagnostic and interventional skills was a prerequisite for the interventional nephrologist and became the major goal of the Society.

THE SOCIETY

Prior to 1990, very few nephrologists other than the pioneers and founders performed access procedures and these were generally outside of academic training programs. These individuals, self-taught and with no formal training or standardization, laid the foundation for endovascular procedures in this field. The National Kidney Foundation played a prominent role by offering a workshop at their 1996 Annual Meeting on renal sonography and hemodialysis catheter placement. The skills of Ash in peritoneal dialysis catheter insertion (1983), Beathard in vascular access (1988), and O'Neill in renal sonography (1994) laid the foundation of skills taught in Interventional Nephrology Training Programs. Because of political issues within academic centers, the establishment and growth of academic interventional nephrology was slow. The first academic training program in Interventional Nephrology was established at Louisiana State University Health Sciences Center (LSUHSC), Shreveport, LA, in the late 1990s by faculty members (Jack Work, M.D., et al) under the tutelage of Beathard. The LSUHSC-Shreveport program is unique in that it offers all Nephrology Fellows the opportunity to train in Interventional Nephrology (all Senior Fellows spend 4 months in the Interventional Suite). There has been a steady growth of academic interventional nephrology programs in the past decade offering Nephrology Fellows opportunities to train in this discipline. Each center had to design its own model using existing and new resources and collaborate with other disciplines such Interventional Radiology or Cardiology.[60]

A milestone in Interventional Nephrology occurred at the American Society of Nephrology Annual Meeting in 1998, when the founders were invited to present a precourse on Interventional Nephrology. This successful course brought together nephrologists with expertise in a wide array of procedures, led to a clarion call to form a society for like-minded nephrologists, and ASDIN was born in 2000 (www.asdin.org). Since the inception of the Society more than 20 centers offer formal training in sonography or dialysis access procedures (http://www.asdin.org/Visitors/Education/training.cfm). The Seminars in Dialysis became the Society's academic journal as it devoted a complete section to the publication of original articles, reviews, editorials, and forthcoming events in interventional nephrology. The first compendium of diagnostic and interventional nephrology was published as an issue of Seminars in Nephrology in 2002.[61] The goal of the Society was to promote the skillful performance of procedures by nephrologists that would lead to substantial improvements in the care of patients. Activities of the Society included the establishment of practice standards, certification of physicians in specific procedures, accreditation of training programs in specific procedures, development of training tools and techniques, sponsoring symposia and training courses, and the dissemination of information through periodic meetings and through print and other media. Renal Physician Association (RPA) and American Society of Nephrology (ASN) published position paper recognizing the need for standardizing the training and credentialing requirements for interventional nephrology.[49] Trainees needed to demonstrate mastery of various aspects of interventional nephrology and demonstrate clinical competence by performing a minimum number of cases as the primary operator.[49] In 2007, Beathard wrote an easy to read, practical guide covering all aspects of vascular interventional nephrology procedures that formed the ASDIN Vascular Access Core Curriculum for Interventional Nephrology.[62] In 2011, Wu edited the ASDIN Peritoneal Dialysis Core Curriculum, a multi-authored collection of techniques for peritoneal dialysis catheter placement and management.[63]

INTERNATIONAL GROWTH

Nephrologists from all parts of the globe have noted the advantages of providing comprehensive access care for their patients. The one-stop-shop concept calls for providing both the access and dialysis to the ESRD patient. Years of fragmented care, often causing delay in providing necessary intervention, fueled once again the growth of Interventional Nephrology in other countries. The International Society of Nephrology (ISN) established an Interventional Nephrology Committee with the vision of promoting and advancing dialysis access care. The first Interventional International Nephrology Symposium was held in Cordoba, Argentina in 2005[64] and the World Congress of Nephrology incorporated Interventional Nephrology sessions in their annual meetings. (http://www.wcn2011.org/monday). The Interventional Nephrology Committee at the ISN also promoted several focused regional courses on renal ultrasound, placement of tunneled dialysis catheter for hemodialysis and placement of peritoneal dialysis catheters.[64] The desire to be trained in Interventional Nephrology can be gauged from a survey where 9/10 practicing nephrologists in Brazil expressed interest in further teaching.[65]

Interest has grown in all parts of the world with national and regional nephrology societies incorporating interventional nephrology training (http://isn-nzc.com/conf_details.jsp [India], http://anzsn2011.com.au/AdditionalMeetings.pdf [Australia/New Zealand], http://www.msn.org.my/main.jsp?1=1&pageid=279567 [Malaysia], http://www.sahf.org.uk/uploads/docs/files/42.pdf [Singapore], http://www.eurolink-tours.co.uk/Nephrology_congress/5th-isn-update-course-in-nephrology-2011-6-792.html [United Arab Emirates]).

THE FUTURE

The future of diagnostic and interventional nephrology will depend largely on the number and quality of its training programs. The Society will grow in proportion to the number of newly trained nephrologists entering the field. Academic nephrology training programs will have to acknowledge that interventional nephrology is here to stay and that investing in it will accrue clinical, academic, and financial rewards. Nephrology fellowship training program directors are aware that their programs will have an edge in recruiting excellent fellowship candidates if they can offer access training. As the demand for training in interventional nephrology increases, they will have to fight "turf battles" to set up interventional nephrology programs in their institutions. This movement is already under way in several academic centers where program directors are setting up interventional suites and recruiting well-trained candidates to run these programs. The establishment of sound and strong academic programs will lead to innovative research that is sorely needed in this field. Multicenter clinical randomized control trials will then become possible in order to answer best practice questions. Expansion of basic research such as the work of Roy-Chaudhury on access stenosis in animal models will add a scholastic dimension to the field and encourage young researchers to investigate the pathology of access dysfunction and failure.[66] Using the interventional cardiology model interventional nephrology could get accredited as an optional third-year program accreted by the Accreditation Council on Graduate Medical Education (ACGME). The core ASDIN curricula for vascular access and peritoneal dialysis will become the ACGME required curriculum for the third-year nephrology fellowship. A broader approach ("kidneycentric") whereby nephrology-related procedures currently delegated to other specialties will be performed by nephrologists is a vision held by a growing number of nephrologists.[67] The future of diagnostic and interventional nephrology looks very bright despite all the inevitable challenges and its success will improve the care of dialysis patients and be rewarding to nephrologists.

REFERENCES

1. Kolff, WJ. *New Ways of Treating Uraemia: The Artificial Kidney, Peritoneal Lavage, Intestinal Lavage*, Vol 112. London: J&A Churchill; 1947:112.
2. Alwall N, Norvitt L, Steins AM. On the artificial kidney. Clinical experiences of the dialytic treatment of uremia. *Acta Med Scand.* 1949;132:587.
3. Available at: http://www.bio-pro.de/magazin/wissenschaft/archiv_2006/index.html?lang=en&artikelid=/artikel/00486/index.html. Accessed July 15, 2011.
4. Peitzman SJ. Chronic dialysis and dialysis doctors in the United States: a nephrologist-historian's perspective. *Semin Dialysis.* 2001;14:200–208.
5. Quinton WE, Dillard DH, Scribner BH. Cannulation of blood vessels for prolonged hemodialysis. *Trans Am Soc Artif Intern Organs.* 1960;6:104–113.
6. Scribner BH, Buri R, Caner JEZ, Hegstom R, Burnell JM. The treatment of chronic uremia by means of intermittent hemodialysis: a preliminary report. *Trans Am Soc Artif Intern Organs.* 1960;6:114–122.
7. Brescia MJ, Cimino JE, Appel K, Hurwich BJ. Chronic hemodialysis using venipuncture and a surgically created arteriovenous fistula. *N Engl J Med.* 1966;275:1089–1092.
8. Beathard GA. History of vascular access. *ASDIN Core Curriculum for Interventional Nephrology*, 13th ed. 2007:1–8.
9. Shaldon S, Chiandussi L, Higgs B. Haemodialysis by percutaneous catheterization of the femoral artery and vein with regional heparinization. *Lancet.* 1961;II:857–859.
10. Shaldon S. Percutaneous vessel catheterization for hemodialysis. *ASAIO J.* 1994;40:7–19.
11. Ganter G. Ueber die Beseitigung giftiger Stoffe aus dem Blute durch Dialyse. *Munch Med Wochschr.* 1923;70:1478.
12. Ash S, Agarwal A. Peritoneal dialysis catheter designs and placement techniques. In *ASDIN Core Curriculum for Peritoneal Dialysis Catheter Procedures*. 1st ed, Chapter 2, 2010.
13. Grollman A, Turner LB, McLEAN JA. Intermittent peritoneal lavage in nephrectomized dogs and its application to the human being. *AMA Arch Intern Med.* March, 1951;87(3):379–390.
14. Doolan PD, Murphy WP, Wiggins RA, Carter NW, Cooper WC, Watten RH, Alpen EL. An evaluation of intermittent peritoneal lavage. *Am J Med.* 1959;26:831–844.
15. Weston R, Roberts M. *Arch Intern Med.* 1965;115(6):659–662.
16. Tenckhoff H, Shilipetar G, Boen ST. One year's experience with home peritoneal dialysis. *Trans Am Soc Artif Intern Organs.* 1965;11:11–17.
17. Tenckhoff H. Catheter implantation. *Dial & Transplant* August/September 1, 1972;18–20.
18. Tenckhoff H, Schechter H. A bacteriologically safe peritoneal access device. *Trans Am Soc Artif Intern Organs.* 1968;14:181–187.
19. Tenckhoff H. *Chronic Peritoneal Dialysis Manual.* Seattle, WA: University of Washington, School of Medicine, 1974.
20. Saad T. Interventional nephrology for hemodialysis vascular access: insight about an evolving branch. *Saudi J Kidney Dis Transplant.* 2004;15:239–250.
21. Konner K, Nonnast-Daniel B, Ritz E. The arterio-venous fistula. *J Am Soc Nephrol.* 2003;14:1669–1680.
22. VanderWerf BA. Bovine graft arteriovenous fistulas for hemodialysis. *Proc Clin Dial Transplant Forum.* 1973;3:12.

23. Johnson JM, Kenoyer MR. Bovine graft arteriovenous fistula for hemodialysis. *Am J Surg*. 1974;128:728.

24. Haimov M, Jacobson JH, II. Experience with the modified bovine arterial heterograft in peripheral vascular reconstruction and vascular access for hemodialysis. *Ann Surg*. 1974;180:291.

25. Zincke H, Hirsche BL, Amamoo DG, et al. The use of bovine carotid grafts for hemodialysis and hyperalimentation. *Surg Gynecol Obstet*. 1974;139:350.

26. Merickel JH, Anderson RC, Knutson R, et al. Bovine carotid artery shunts in vascular access surgery. Complications in the chronic hemodialysis patient. *Arch Surg*. 1974;109:245.

27. Baker LD, Jr., Johnson JM, Goldfarb D. Expanded polytetrafluoroethylene (PTFE) subcutaneous arteriovenous conduit: an improved vascular access for chronic hemodialysis. *Trans Am Soc Artif Intern Organs*. 1976;22:382.

28. Elliott MP, Gazzaniga AB, Thomas JM, Haiduc NJ, Rosen SM. Use of expanded polytetrafluoroethylene grafts for vascular access in hemodialysis: laboratory and clinical evaluation. *Am Surg*. 1977;43(7):455–459.

29. Baker LD Jr, Johnson JM, Goldfarb D. Expanded polytetrafluoroethylene (PTFE) subcutaneous arteriovenous conduit: an improved vascular access for chronic hemodialysis. *Trans Am Soc Artif Intern Organs*. 1976;22:382–387.

30. Goodkin DA, Bragg-Gresham JL, Koenig KG, et al. Association of comorbid conditions and mortality in Europe, Japan, and the United States: The Dialysis Outcomes and Practice Patterns Study (DOPPS). *J Am Soc Nephrol*. 2003;14:3270–3277.

31. The Dopps Report: October 2002 Status of DOPPS in Twelve Countries; Research on Vascular Access. Available at: http://www.dopps.org/newsletters.aspx. Accessed May 2011.

32. Young EW, Dykstra DM, Goodkin DA, Mapes DL, Wolfe RA, Held PJ. Hemodialysis vascular access preferences and outcomes in the Dialysis Outcomes and Practice Patterns Study (DOPPS). *Kidney Int*. 2002;61:2266–2271.

33. Port FK. The end-stage renal disease program: trends over the past 18 years. *Am J Kidney Dis*. 1992;20(1 suppl 1):3–7.

34. Feldman, HI, Held, PJ, Hutchinson, JT, Stoiber, E, Hartigan, MF, Berlin, JA. Hemodialysis vascular access morbidity in the United States. *Kidney Int*. 1993;43:1091–1096.

35. U.S. Renal Data System: X. The cost effectiveness of alternative types of vascular access and the economic cost of ESRD. *Am J Kidney Dis*. 1995;26:S140–S156.

36. Carlston, DM, Duncan, DA, Naessens, JM, Johnson, WJ. Hospitalization in dialysis patients. *Mayo Clin Proc*. 1984;59:769–775.

37. O'Neill WC. The new nephrologist. *Am J Kidney Dis*. 2000;35:978–979.

38. Gordon DH, Glanz S, Butt KMH, Adamsons RJ, Koenig MA. Treatment of stenotic lesions in dialysis access fistulas and shunts by transluminal angioplasty. *Radiology*. 1982;143:53–57.

39. Valji K, Bookstein JJ, Roberts AC, Davis GB. Pharmacomechanical thrombolysis and angioplasty in management of clotted hemodialysis grafts: early and late clinical results. *Radiology*. 1991;178:243–247.

40. Vesely TM. What is the Current and Future status of Interventional Nephrology? *Semin Dialysis*. 2005;18:373–375.

41. Ash SR, Wolf GC and Block R. Placement of the Tenckhoff peritoneal dialysis catheter under peritoneoscopic visualization. *Dialysis Transplant*. 1981;10(5):383–386.

42. Zaman F, Pervez A, Atray N, Aslam A, Murphy S, Zibari G, Abreo K. Fluoroscopy-assisted placement of peritoneal dialysis catheters by nephrologists. *Semin Dialysis*. 2005;18:247–251.

43. Maya I. Ultrasound/fluoroscopy assisted placement of peritoneal dialysis catheters. *Semin Dialysis*. 2007;20:611–615.

44. Beathard GA. Percutaneous transvenous angioplasty in the treatment of vascular access stenosis. *Kidney Int*. 1992;42:1390–1397.

45. Beathard GA. Mechanical versus pharmacomechanical thrombolysis for the treatment of thrombosed dialysis access grafts. *Kidney Int*. 1994;45:1401–1406.

46. Available at: http://www.asdin.org/Visitors/Publications/index.cfm. Accessed April 27, 2009.

47. Beathard GA, Litchfield T. Effectiveness and safety of dialysis access procedures performed by interventional nephrologists. *Kidney Int*. 2004;66(4):970–972.

48. Trerotola SO, Gray R, Brunner M, Altman S. Interventional care of the hemodialysis patient: it's about quality. *J Vasc Interv Radiol*. 2001;12:1253–1255.

49. Renal Physicians Association/American Society of Nephrology position on credentialing in Nephrology. Available at www.renalmd.org/members_online/members/downloads Approved as revised 22 January 2000. Accessed April 25, 2009.

50. Schon D, Mishler R. Salvage of occluded autologous arteriovenous fistulae. *Am J Kidney Dis*. 2000;36:804–810.

51. Beathard GA, Welch BR, Maidment HJ. Mechanical thrombolysis for the treatment of thrombosed hemodialysis access grafts. *Radiology*. 1996;200:711–716.

52. Faiyaz R, Abreo K, Zaman F, Pervez A, Zibari G, Work J. Salvage of poorly developed arteriovenous fistulae with percutaneous ligation of accessory veins. *Am J Kidney Dis*. 2002;39:824–827.

53. Beathard GA, Arnold P, Jackson J, Litchfield T. Aggressive treatment of early fistula failure. Physician Operators Forum of RMS Lifeline. *Kidney Int*. 2003;64:1487–1494.

54. Asif A, Gadalean FN, Merrill D, Cherla G, Cipleu CD, Epstein DL, Roth D. Inflow stenosis in arteriovenous fistulas and grafts: a multicenter, prospective study. *Kidney Int*. 2005;67:1986–1992.

55. Nassar GM. Endovascular management of the "failing to mature" arteriovenous fistula. *Tech Vasc Interv Radiol*. 2008;11(3):175–180.

56. Chan MR, Bedi S, Sanchez RJ, Young HN, Becker YT, Kellerman PS, Yevzlin AS. Stent placement versus angioplasty improves patency of arteriovenous grafts and blood flow of arteriovenous fistulae. *Clin J Am Soc Nephrol*. 2008;3(3):699–705.

57. Maya ID, Allon M. Outcomes of thrombosed arteriovenous grafts: comparison of stents versus angioplasty. *Kidney Int*. 2006;69:9347.

58. O'Neill WC, ed. Interventional nephrology. *Semin Dialysis*, 2003;16:289–346.

59. Nass K, O'Neill WC. Bedside renal biopsy: ultrasound guidance by the nephrologist. *Am J Kidney Dis.* 1999;34:955–959.

60. TJ Vachharajani, S Moossavi, L Salman, S Wu, ID Maya, Alex S. Yevzlin, A Agarwal, KD Abreo, Jack Work, A Asif. Successful models of interventional nephrology at academic medical centers. *Clin J Am Aoc Nephrol.* 2010;5:2130–2136.

61. O'Neill WC. Diagnostic and interventional nephrology. *Semin Nephrol.* 2002;22:181–185.

62. Beathard J. *ASDIN Core Curriculum for Interventional Nephrology. RMS Lifeline Training Manual of Interventional Nephrology.* 13th ed. ASDIN; 2007.

63. Wu S, ed. *ASDIN Core Curriculum for Peritoneal Dialysis Catheter Procedures.* ASDIN; 2011.

64. Herrera-Felix JP, Orias M. Emergence of interventional nephrology at the international level. *Adv Chronic Kidney Dis.* September 2009;16(5):309–315.

65. Nascimento MM, Chula D, Campos R, Nascimento D, Riella MC. Interventional nephrology in Brazil: current and future status. *Semin Dial.* March–April 2006;19(2):172–175.

66. Roy-Chaudhury P, Kelly BS, Miller MA, Reaves A, Armstrong J, Nanayakkara N, Heffelfinger SC. Venous neointimal hyperplasia in polytetrafluoroethylene dialysis grafts. *Kidney Int.* 2001;59:2325–2334.

67. Atray N, Vachhrajani T. Interventional nephrology in federal health care system. *AJKD.* 2003;42:1105.

4

EPIDEMIOLOGY OF VASCULAR ACCESS FOR HEMODIALYSIS: A GLOBAL PERSPECTIVE

TUSHAR J. VACHHARAJANI & RAJIV SARAN

LEARNING OBJECTIVES

1. Understand the global trends and variations in vascular access practices in hemodialysis.
2. Understand the impact of practice variations on vascular access-related morbidity and mortality.
3. Identify clinical approaches to increase the percentage of patients dialyzed with an arteriovenous fistula in order to improve patient outcomes.

INTRODUCTION

An ideal vascular access for hemodialysis should provide safe and effective therapy by enabling the removal and return of blood via the extracorporeal circuit. Such a vascular access should be easy to use, reliable, and pose minimal risk to the individual receiving hemodialysis. However, an ideal and optimally functioning vascular access remains challenging to achieve in practice. The complications and health care costs related to vascular access creation and related complications are major hurdles faced by the end-stage renal disease (ESRD) team.

There are three main types of access for maintenance hemodialysis: native arteriovenous fistula (AVF), synthetic arteriovenous graft (AVG), and tunneled central vein catheter (CVC). Guidelines from several countries recommend AVF as the access of first choice[1-3] (UK Renal Association Guidelines, 2011). In the United Sates, the Centers for Medicare and Medicaid Services and ESRD Networks established the Fistula First Breakthrough Initiative (FFBI) outlining the goals of creating AVF as the primary vascular access for both incident and prevalent hemodialysis patients while simultaneously reducing CVC usage[4]

(www.fistulafirst.org). Despite similar guidelines from multiple global communities, there is a wide variability in the proportion of patients receiving hemodialysis with AVF. Data from several countries provides consistent evidence that AVF use is associated with lower incidence of complications such as infection, hospitalization, and mortality compared with AVG and CVC.[5-11] Thus, it is imperative to understand the practice patterns and strategies employed in different countries to increase the overall AVF rate both in the incident and prevalent hemodialysis population.

GLOBAL TRENDS AND VARIATION IN VASCULAR ACCESS USE

International data and comparative insights into various hemodialysis-related practice patterns are largely available from the Dialysis Outcomes and Practice Patterns Study (DOPPS), an international prospective observational study of hemodialysis patients. The data was collected from multiple, randomly selected hemodialysis facilities in 12 nations from 1996 to 2007 in three different phases.[12] DOPPS Phase 4 is presently ongoing and extension to other countries such as China, Saudi Arabia, and others is currently in progress or being actively planned. DOPPS collects detailed aspects of demographics, comorbid conditions, laboratory values, prescriptions, and dialysis practices at both patient and facility level.[13] The utilization of vascular access for hemodialysis has been shown to vary widely across countries.[8,14] In Europe, hemodialysis patients were threefold more likely to receive AVF per DOPPS data.[14] Several patient-related factors have been associated with AVF use compared to AVG. For example, AVF use is lower in patients who are elderly, female, have peripheral artery disease, coronary artery disease, obesity, diabetes mellitus, and poor functional capacity.[15-19]

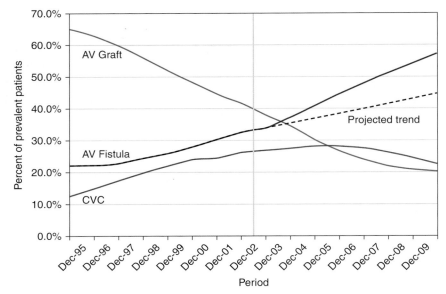

Figure 4-1. U.S. trends in AV fistula, AV graft, and total CVC use, December 1995 through October 2010, with trend in AV fistula use prior to FFBI projected forward. (Adapted from www.fistulafirst.org. Annual report 2010.)

DOPPS data have shown that the vascular access use in the hemodialysis population varies widely across the world when compared to recommended guidelines.[14,18,20]

▶ AVF versus AVG Use

AVF use in the United States among the prevalent hemodialysis population since the inception of FFBI has improved from 32% in July 2003 to 58% in March 2011 (www.fistulafirst.org), but the goal of 66% is yet to be achieved. The current trends for the different types of vascular access in the United States are shown in Figure 4-1.

Notably, however, a high incidence of primary AVF maturation failure has been reported recently in a large multicenter trial involving 877 patients in the United States,[21] which is in contrast to 7.6% failure rate in more than 5000 new fistulas created in Japan.[22]

The distribution of hemodialysis access types varies widely between regions included in DOPPS. Figure 4-2 shows the median percentage of patients dialyzing with an AVF across facilities in Europe and Australia–New Zealand, Japan, and North America.

The change in vascular access use over time is evident when data from different phases of DOPPS are compared. AVF use has declined in Spain, Germany, and Italy ranging from 4% to 13% with a simultaneous increase in AVG placements. The AVG placement in Japan has increased from 3% to 7% with a decline in AVF from 93% to 90%.[23]

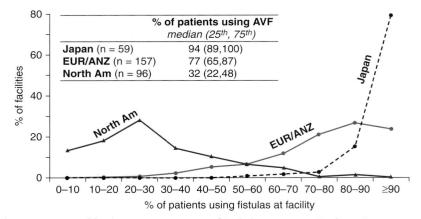

Figure 4-2. Distribution of percentages of facility patients using a fistula by region in Dialysis Outcomes and Practice Patterns Study II (DOPPS II). Percentages of facility fistula use were determined from access use in a prevalent cross-section of hemodialysis (HD) patients within each facility at entry. Analyses were restricted to 312 facilities reporting vascular access use at study entry for a minimum of 13 patients (median, 27 patients, with 20–40 patients in >90% of facilities). Values in inset are median (25th, 75th percentile). Abbreviations: AVF, arteriovenous fistula; North Am, Canada and United States; EUR/ANZ, Belgium, France, Germany, Italy, Spain, Sweden, United Kingdom, Australia, and New Zealand. (Adapted from Pisoni et al.[5])

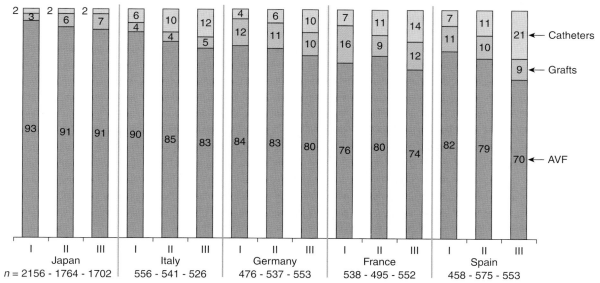

Prevalent patient cross-sections; cuffed catheters comprise 80–95% of catheter use in countries;
A DOPPS I (1996–2000), DOPPS II (2002–2003), DOPPS III (2005–2007)

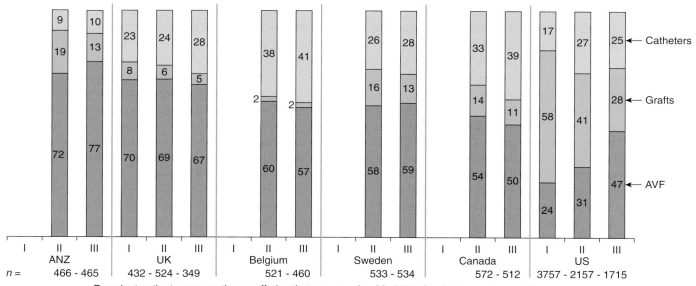

Prevalent patient cross-sections; cuffed catheters comprise 80–95% of catheter use in countries;
B DOPPS I (1996–2000), DOPPS II (2002–2003), DOPPS III (2005–2007)

Figure 4-3. (**A**) Trends in vascular access use (arteriovenous fistula, catheter or graft) at study entry in DOPPS I, II, and III (1996–2007) among prevalent patient cross-sections in Japan, Italy, Germany, France, and Spain. (**B**) Trends in vascular access use (arteriovenous fistula, catheter or graft) at the study entry in DOPPS I, II, and III (1996–2007) among prevalent patient cross-sections in Australia and New Zealand (ANZ) the United Kingdom, Belgium, Sweden, Canada, and the United States. (Adapted and reprinted with permission from Ethier et al.[23])

In the United States, AVG placement has declined over the past 10 years from 58% to 28% (Figure 4-3).

▶ Central Vein Catheters

Despite recognition of the fact that patients using CVC suffer higher morbidity and mortality, CVC use among incident hemodialysis patients in the United States has remained more than 80% (www.usrds.org). The KDOQI guideline recommends <10% CVC in the prevalent hemodialysis population, but the rate remains higher than 20% in several countries including United Kingdom, Belgium, Sweden, Canada, and the United States. In fact, the proportion of hemodialysis patients using CVC increased in Canada, United States, and several European countries (Figure 4-3) and CVC use increased two to three times in Italy, Germany, France, and Spain between DOPPS phase I and III.

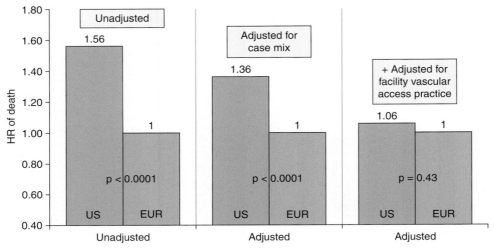

Figure 4-4. Case-mix–adjusted mortality hazard ratio (HR) for hemodialysis (HD) patients in the United States versus Europe (EUR), with and without adjustment for differences in facility vascular access use. The HR of mortality for HD patients in the United States versus EUR (n = 24,398) stratified by study phase is shown after different levels of adjustment: unadjusted; adjusted for patient age, sex, black race, number of years with end-stage renal disease, body weight, 14 summary comorbid conditions, whether treated in a hospital-based unit, facility median treatment time, facility percentage of patients with serum phosphorus level >5.5 mg/dL, and facility percentage of patients with serum calcium level >10 mg/dL; and further adjusted for percentage of facility vascular access use plus the previous 23 adjustments. All models accounted for facility clustering effects. EUR refers to France, Germany, Italy, Spain, and the United Kingdom. (Data from Pisoni RL, Arrington CJ, Albert J, et al. Facility hemodialysis vascular access use and mortality in countries participating in DOPPS: an instrumental variable analysis. *Am J Kidney Dis.* 2009;53:475–491.)

In ESRD patients who remain CVC dependent beyond 180 days, per DOPPS data, 1% had never received a permanent access, 56% had one permanent access, 25% had received two and 10% had received three and about 8% had received four or more permanent access.[23] The demographic characteristics leading to CVC dependence and more than three prior permanent accesses include female, black race, congestive heart failure, hypertension, recurrent gangrene, a psychiatric disorder, longer duration with ESRD, time to first cannulation more than 2 months or in facilities not performing vascular access procedures. The odds of permanent access failure were higher in the United States compared to Japan (adjusted odds ratio = 0.67, p = 0.03). Further, likelihood of CVC dependency of more than 180 days was consistent in patients who were older, obese with higher body mass index, diabetes mellitus, peripheral vascular disease, or recurrent cellulitis.[23]

VASCULAR ACCESS-RELATED MORBIDITY AND MORTALITY

The higher risk of morbidity and mortality in patients using CVC and AVG compared to AVF as a vascular access has been well documented in the literature.[5,9,24–27] The adjusted relative risk of mortality for patients using CVC was 1.45 and 1.14 for patients with AVG compared with patients using AVF.[5] In this context, the higher mortality among dialysis patients in the United States compared to those in Japan and Europe has been recognized[28] and only partly explained by higher comorbidity burden among dialysis patients in the United States.[29] The mortality risk was no

longer significantly different when adjusted for case-mix and facility vascular access use (Figure 4-4),[30] suggesting that it might be possible to eliminate the difference in mortality between Europe and the United States with improvements in facility-level vascular access practices in the United States, ie, by increasing the proportion of AVF and concomitantly reducing CVCs.

The risk of mortality is highest with CVC followed by AVG and least with AVF.[31] The mortality risk improves with conversion of vascular access from CVC to a permanent access.[31,32] Similar to mortality risk, the morbidity with AVF is least compared to AVG and CVC. Infection and hospitalizations (all-cause as well as infection-related) were higher with CVC and AVG compared to AVF.[5] Vascular access-related infection risk was five- to sevenfold higher with CVC compared to AVF.[33]

Along with the higher morbidity associated with CVC as a vascular access, the healthcare costs are also higher. The costs related to vascular access event per patient per year in US dollars were $3194 for patients with AVF, $5960 for patients with AVG, and $7451 for patients with catheters (www.USRDS.org).

▶ Effect of Change in Vascular Access Overtime

Conversion from CVC to AVF/AVG and *vice versa* is a frequent occurrence in clinical practice. Catheters are associated with higher hospitalization from sepsis and all-cause mortality compared to AVF or AVG.[34] The risk of all-cause mortality was lower with conversion from CVC to AVF/AVG compared to AVF/AVG to CVC in a random sample of incident hemodialysis patients from the United States (adjusted mortality HR 0.69 vs 1.81).[32] The effect of conversion from AVF to CVC was associated with a twofold increase in death rate compared to those who had a functioning AVF through a 1-year study period among patients enrolled in the Hemodialysis (HEMO) Study.[11,32] In the same study patients who were switched from CVC to AVF had 1.4-fold reduction in death risk compared to 3.4-fold among patients who continued to use CVC. In a large cohort of nearly 80,000 prevalent hemodialysis patients from the United States, over a short period of 8 months, the risk of death was reduced by 30% among patients who were converted from CVC to a permanent access. The study also found worsening of death risk in patients who were converted to CVC due to failed permanent access.[31]

▶ Factors/Practices Associated with Prolonged CVC Use

Timely referral to a trained and committed vascular access surgeon is critical to the number of patients initiating hemodialysis with a CVC. A wide variation between countries was observed with respect to the median time from referral to vascular access creation. The median time was 5–6 days in Japan, Italy, and Germany and 40–43 days in Canada and the United Kingdom. Starting hemodialysis with a CVC was likely to be higher with longer duration between referral and evaluation by surgeon (adjusted odds ratio = 0.89/5 days longer) as well as between evaluation and access creation (adjusted odds ratio = 0.94/5 days longer).[23]

▶ Timing between AVF Creation and Cannulation for Prolonged CVC Use

The timing of first cannulation was widely different in different countries ranging from <4 weeks in Japan, Italy, Germany, and France to 8–12 weeks in the United States, Canada, and the United Kingdom.[23]

FACTORS ASSISTING WITH OPTIMIZING VASCULAR ACCESS CARE

▶ Facility Preference for Vascular Access

DOPPS analysis of patients in the United States revealed that dialysis facility staff preference for AVF or AVG was the single most factor strongly associated with likelihood of using AVG or AVF.[12] The guidelines from KDOQI and FFBI have slowly changed this attitude and by 2003, only 7% of US DOPPS nurse managers preferred AVG.[35] The ongoing system wide efforts to educate patients and the dialysis community at large is probably the single most important factor responsible for this change in the United States.[36]

▶ Surgical Training and Experience

DOPPS data have also highlighted the critical role of training received by surgeons for successful AVF placement and outcomes.[37] The AVF patency was statistically higher when a surgical trainee had placed at least 25 AVF during their training period (Figure 4-5). Moreover, greater degree of

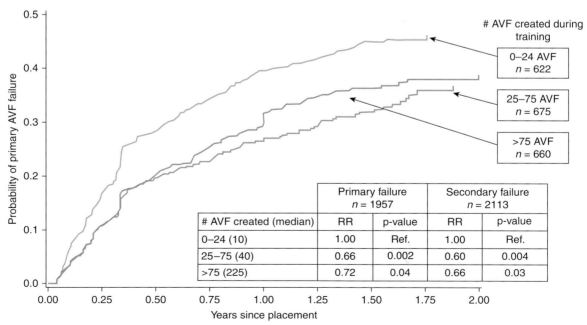

Figure 4-5. Time to primary fistula failure in hemodialysis patients for tertiles of the number of AVF created by the facility's primary surgeon during surgical training. Model accounted for facility clustering effects and was adjusted for age, sex, black (vs. other) race, 14 comorbid conditions, body mass index, time with ESRD, prior catheter use, and country (n = 1957). Primary failure reflects the first intervention to salvage an access; secondary failure represents irreparable failure of an access (results pertaining to secondary fistula failure are also shown in the table insert within the figure). (Adapted and printed with permission, Saran et al.[37])

surgical training in placement of AVF was associated with lower probability of AVG (vs AVF) placement. In DOPPS data, surgical training was widely different in the participating centers from 12 countries. On average, surgeons from the United States reported placing the least number of AVF during their training compared with surgeons from other countries.[37]

DOPPS data further analyzed the success of AVF placement by analyzing following other factors during the training period: emphasis on type of access, specialty of the surgeon (vascular surgeons, general surgeons, or urologist).[37] Interestingly, nephrology trainees at some centers in Italy get extensively trained in creating AVF. On average, a nephrology trainee in Italy performs two surgeries per week during the 5-year training period and masters the AVF surgery in 4–6 months. Besides, the nephrology trainee also learns preoperative clinical assessment that includes ultrasound mapping of blood vessels for suitable AVF site selection.

▶ Vascular Access Maturation and Timing of first Cannulation

A vascular access is considered to be mature often by clinical judgment based on physical examination by experienced dialysis personnel. The rule of 6's as suggested by KDOQI for AVF maturation is often impractical and utilized only in selected clinical scenarios. DOPPS evaluated the timing of first cannulation in an AVF and AVG and the blood flow rate as potential predictors of vascular access failure. First cannulation timing of AVG varied from less than 2 weeks to 4 weeks. 62% of facilities in the United States and 61% of European centers cannulated the AVG between 2 and 4 weeks. 65% of AVG were cannulated in Japan within 3 weeks. The risk of AVG failure was not found to be related to the timing of cannulation.

The timing for cannulating the AVF was widely different across various continents. 74% of Japanese centers, 50% of European centers, and only 2% of US centers cannulated AVF in < 1 month. Almost a third of US centers cannulated AVF after 3 months of placement.[38] The first cannulation timing of AVF was not identified to be a risk factor in vascular access failure despite different practice patterns.

Dialysis pump blood flow rate (BFR) was studied by DOPPS as a predictor for vascular access failure. The median BFR used to dialyze patients in Europe, Japan, and United States was 300, 196.5, and 412 mL/min. A higher BFR seemed to be associated higher AVG failure rate was not found to be statistically significant.[38]

Epidemiological data looking at vascular access maturity and blood flow certainly can guide toward early transition from temporary access to a permanent access without clinically significant deleterious effects on the vascular access.

SUMMARY

There is considerable heterogeneity in dialysis vascular access care across countries. Studying variation in practice patterns provides an insight into various factors that can ultimately affect patient outcome. Larger epidemiological studies have provided the basis for confirming and crafting guidelines that are adopted in improving care of ESRD patients. A significantly lower complication rate associated with AVF use has led to universal acceptance of AVF as the most desirable form of dialysis vascular access. Morbidity and mortality trends among different countries with differences in vascular access care have assisted in setting and optimizing management goals. Well-conducted, large epidemiological studies remain an acceptable and efficient, real-world alternative to "gold standard" randomized-controlled studies. They have the distinct advantage of leveraging much larger sample sizes and variation in practice patterns, ability to study time trends, relating study consequences to changing practices, thereby providing the basis for ongoing comparisons across geographic regions or dialysis facilities and highlighting best practices.

REFERENCES

1. Tordoir J, Canaud B, Haage P, et al. EBPG on vascular access. *Nephrol Dial Transplant*. May 2007;22(suppl 2): ii88–ii117.
2. Clinical practice guidelines for vascular access. *Am J Kidney Dis*. July 2006;48(suppl 1):S248–S273.
3. Clinical practice guidelines for vascular access- UK Renal Association. 2011. Available at: http://www.renal.org/Libraries/Guidelines/Vascular_Access_for_Haemodialysis_-_FINAL_VERSION_-_05_January_2011.sflb.ashx. Accessed January 16, 2012.
4. Fistula First. Available at: http://www.fistulafirst.org/. Accessed January 16, 2012.
5. Pisoni RL, Arrington CJ, Albert JM, et al. Facility hemodialysis vascular access use and mortality in countries participating in DOPPS: an instrumental variable analysis. *Am J Kidney Dis*. March 2009;53(3):475–491.
6. Canaud B, Combe C, Bragg-Gresham JL, Eichleay MA, Pisoni RL, Port FK. [DOPPS estimate of patient life years attributable to modifiable hemodialysis practices in France]. *Nephrol Ther*. July 2008;4(4):256–265.
7. Besarab A. Resolved: Fistulas are preferred to grafts as initial vascular access for dialysis. *Pro. J Am Soc Nephrol*. September 2008;19(9):1629–1631.
8. Pisoni RL, Young EW, Mapes DL, Keen ML, Port FK. Vascular access use and outcomes in the U.S., Europe, and Japan: results from the Dialysis Outcomes and Practice Patterns Study. *Nephrol News Issues*. May 2003;17(6): 38–43, 47.
9. Dhingra RK, Young EW, Hulbert-Shearon TE, Leavey SF, Port FK. Type of vascular access and mortality in U.S. hemodialysis patients. *Kidney Int*. October 2001;60(4):1443–1451.

10. Thomson PC, Stirling CM, Geddes CC, Morris ST, Mactier RA. Vascular access in haemodialysis patients: a modifiable risk factor for bacteraemia and death. *QJM*. July 2007;100(7):415–422.

11. Allon M, Daugirdas J, Depner TA, Greene T, Ornt D, Schwab SJ. Effect of change in vascular access on patient mortality in hemodialysis patients. *Am J Kidney Dis*. March 2006;47(3):469–477.

12. Young EW, Dykstra DM, Goodkin DA, Mapes DL, Wolfe RA, Held PJ. Hemodialysis vascular access preferences and outcomes in the Dialysis Outcomes and Practice Patterns Study (DOPPS). *Kidney Int*. June 2002;61(6):2266–2271.

13. Pisoni RL, Gillespie BW, Dickinson DM, Chen K, Kutner MH, Wolfe RA. The Dialysis Outcomes and Practice Patterns Study (DOPPS): design, data elements, and methodology. *Am J Kidney Dis*. November 2004;44 (5 suppl 2):7–15.

14. Pisoni RL, Young EW, Dykstra DM, et al. Vascular access use in Europe and the United States: results from the DOPPS. *Kidney Int*. January 2002;61(1):305–316.

15. Stehman-Breen CO, Sherrard DJ, Gillen D, Caps M. Determinants of type and timing of initial permanent hemodialysis vascular access. *Kidney Int*. February 2000;57(2):639–645.

16. Marcus RJ, Marcus DA, Sureshkumar KK, Hussain SM, McGill RL. Gender differences in vascular access in hemodialysis patients in the United States: developing strategies for improving access outcome. *Gend Med*. September 2007;4(3):193–204.

17. Wang W, Murphy B, Yilmaz S, Tonelli M, Macrae J, Manns BJ. Comorbidities do not influence primary fistula success in incident hemodialysis patients: a prospective study. *Clin J Am Soc Nephrol*. January 2008;3(1):78–84.

18. Kats M, Hawxby AM, Barker J, Allon M. Impact of obesity on arteriovenous fistula outcomes in dialysis patients. *Kidney Int*. January 2007;71(1):39–43.

19. Kurella M, Covinsky KE, Collins AJ, Chertow GM. Octogenarians and nonagenarians starting dialysis in the United States. *Ann Intern Med*. February 6 2007;146(3): 177–183.

20. Rayner HC, Pisoni RL, Gillespie BW, et al. Creation, cannulation and survival of arteriovenous fistulae: data from the Dialysis Outcomes and Practice Patterns Study. *Kidney Int*. January 2003;63(1):323–330.

21. Dember LM, Beck GJ, Allon M, et al. Effect of clopidogrel on early failure of arteriovenous fistulas for hemodialysis: a randomized controlled trial. *JAMA*. May 14 2008;299(18):2164–2171.

22. Ohira S, Kon T, Imura T. Evaluation of primary failure in native AV-fistulae (early fistula failure). *Hemodial Int*. April 2006;10(2):173–179.

23. Ethier J, Mendelssohn DC, Elder SJ, et al. Vascular access use and outcomes: an international perspective from the Dialysis Outcomes and Practice Patterns Study. *Nephrol Dial Transplant*. October 2008;23(10):3219–3226.

24. Polkinghorne KR, McDonald SP, Atkins RC, Kerr PG. Vascular access and all-cause mortality: a propensity score analysis. *J Am Soc Nephrol*. February 2004;15(2):477–486.

25. Pastan S, Soucie JM, McClellan WM. Vascular access and increased risk of death among hemodialysis patients. *Kidney Int*. August 2002;62(2):620–626.

26. Astor BC, Eustace JA, Powe NR, Klag MJ, Fink NE, Coresh J. Type of vascular access and survival among incident hemodialysis patients: the Choices for Healthy Outcomes in Caring for ESRD (CHOICE) Study. *J Am Soc Nephrol*. May 2005;16(5):1449–1455.

27. Inrig JK, Reed SD, Szczech LA, et al. Relationship between clinical outcomes and vascular access type among hemodialysis patients with Staphylococcus aureus bacteremia. *Clin J Am Soc Nephrol*. May 2006;1(3): 518–524.

28. Held PJ, Brunner F, Odaka M, Garcia JR, Port FK, Gaylin DS. Five-year survival for end-stage renal disease patients in the United States, Europe, and Japan, 1982 to 1987. *Am J Kidney Dis*. May 1990;15(5):451–457.

29. Goodkin DA, Bragg-Gresham JL, Koenig KG, et al. Association of comorbid conditions and mortality in hemodialysis patients in Europe, Japan, and the United States: the Dialysis Outcomes and Practice Patterns Study (DOPPS). *J Am Soc Nephrol*. December 2003;14(12): 3270–3277.

30. Goodkin DA, Pisoni RL, Locatelli F, Port FK, Saran R. Hemodialysis vascular access training and practices are key to improved access outcomes. *Am J Kidney Dis*. December 2010;56(6):1032–1042.

31. Lacson E, Jr., Wang W, Lazarus JM, Hakim RM. Change in vascular access and mortality in maintenance hemodialysis patients. *Am J Kidney Dis*. November 2009;54(5):912–921.

32. Bradbury BD, Chen F, Furniss A, et al. Conversion of vascular access type among incident hemodialysis patients: description and association with mortality. *Am J Kidney Dis*. May 2009;53(5):804–814.

33. Combe C, Pisoni RL, Port FK, et al. Dialysis Outcomes and Practice Patterns Study: data on the use of central venous catheters in chronic hemodialysis. *Nephrologie*. 2001;22(8):379–384.

34. Rayner HC, Pisoni RL, Bommer J, et al. Mortality and hospitalization in haemodialysis patients in five European countries: results from the Dialysis Outcomes and Practice Patterns Study (DOPPS). *Nephrol Dial Transplant*. January 2004;19(1):108–120.

35. Rayner HC, Besarab A, Brown WW, Disney A, Saito A, Pisoni RL. Vascular access results from the Dialysis Outcomes and Practice Patterns Study (DOPPS): performance against Kidney Disease Outcomes Quality Initiative (K/DOQI) Clinical Practice Guidelines. *Am J Kidney Dis*. November 2004;44(5 Suppl 2):22–26.

36. Kulawik D, Sands JJ, Mayo K, et al. Focused vascular access education to reduce the use of chronic tunneled hemodialysis catheters: results of a network quality improvement initiative. *Semin Dial*. November–December 2009;22(6):692–697.

37. Saran R, Elder SJ, Goodkin DA, et al. Enhanced training in vascular access creation predicts arteriovenous fistula placement and patency in hemodialysis patients: results from the Dialysis Outcomes and Practice Patterns Study. *Ann Surg*. May 2008;247(5):885–891.

38. Saran R, Dykstra DM, Pisoni RL, et al. Timing of first cannulation and vascular access failure in haemodialysis: an analysis of practice patterns at dialysis facilities in the DOPPS. *Nephrol Dial Transplant*. September 2004;19(9):2334–2340.

SECTION II

Ethics, Public Policy and Practice Guidelines

5

ACADEMIC SOCIETIES, INDUSTRY PARTNERSHIPS, AND CONFLICT OF RESPONSIBILITY

ALEXANDER S. YEVZLIN

INTRODUCTION

Collaborations between physicians or medical researchers and pharmaceutical, medical device, and biotechnology companies can benefit society by promoting the discovery and development of new technologies that improve individual and public health. Nowhere is this observation truer than in the nascent discipline of interventional nephrology (IN), which, like any procedural specialty, relies heavily on close working relationships with device manufacturers. Financial ties between medicine and industry, however, may create situations that have traditionally been described as conflicts of interest. A conflict of interest (COI) has been traditionally defined as any set of relationships that present the risk of undue influence on professional judgments and thereby may jeopardize the integrity of scientific investigations, the objectivity of medical education, the quality of patient care, and the public's trust in medicine.[1]

In an effort to prevent these types of situations, many academic medical centers, professional societies, medical journals, and other institutions have adopted policies on COI. Indeed, the Institute of Medicine recently appointed the Committee on Conflict of Interest in Medical Research, Education, and Practice to examine conflicts of interest in medicine and to recommend steps to identify, limit, and manage conflicts of interest without negatively affecting constructive collaborations. The committee recommends that medical institutions—including academic medical centers, professional societies, patient advocacy groups, and medical journals—establish conflict of interest policies that require disclosure and management of both individual and institutional financial ties to industry.[2]

The American Society of Diagnostic and Interventional Nephrology (ASDIN) is the main professional society that influences the practice of IN. As such, it has recently implemented a COI policy. The purpose of this chapter is to summarize the policy, to discuss how it may apply to the daily practice of private and academic IN, and to describe its philosophical foundation.

THE ARGUMENT FOR CONFLICT OF INTEREST POLICIES

Although collaborations with industry by individuals and societies can be beneficial, the Institute of Medicine (IOM) recommends that researchers should not conduct research involving human participants if they have a financial interest in the outcome of the research. Likewise, to reduce the risk for bias within the learning environment, academic medical centers and teaching hospitals should prohibit faculty from accepting gifts, making presentations that are controlled by industry, claiming authorship for ghostwritten publications, and entering into consulting arrangements that are not governed by written contracts for expert services to be paid for at fair market value. Medical centers also should restrict visits by industry sales people and limit use of drug samples to patients who lack financial access to medications.

Furthermore, acceptance of meals and gifts and other relationships with industry are also common among physicians who practice outside medical centers. Data suggest that these relationships may influence physicians to prescribe a company's medicines even when evidence indicates another drug would be more beneficial.[3] Therefore, the IOM recommends eliminating these problematic relationships between physicians and industry.[1] Additionally, the IOM suggests that community physicians should also follow the restrictions described previously regarding gifts, meals, etc.[1]

Clinical practice guidelines influence physician practice, quality measures, and insurance coverage decisions. Given this influence, clinical practice guidelines need to be developed with greater transparency and accountability. Societies who publish practice guidelines, such as the ASDIN, should therefore pay close attention to conflicts of interest from the panels that draft the guidelines. In addition, these groups should make public their conflict of interest policies, their funding sources, and any financial relationships panel members have with industry, regardless of whether the funding is going directly into guideline creation or not.[1]

The philosophical justification for this strict policing of COI is as follows: society traditionally has placed great trust in physicians and researchers, granting them the considerable leeway to regulate themselves. However, there is growing concern among lawmakers, government agencies, and the public that extensive breaches of conflict of interest in medicine exist. Responsible and reasonable conflict of interest policies will reduce the risk of bias and the loss of trust between government agencies and physicians, and, more importantly, patients and physicians.

THE ARGUMENT AGAINST CONFLICT OF INTEREST POLICIES

In our era of litigation and mistrust, it is difficult to argue against a position that aims to fortify the rigorous standards of impartiality that most COI policies are striving to uphold. Indeed, the argument against COI policies is an unpopular one in today's academic environment. Intellectual honesty, clarity of thought, and fearless introspection must, however, drive this debate, regardless of popularity.

There is overwhelming evidence that physicians, consciously or subconsciously, tend to prescribe more medications that are produced by industry sponsors of CME activities than those medications that are produced by other companies.[4-10] This potential bias has been articulated for all gifts, independent of value. A recent publication explicitly posed questions to a group of physicians in the language of ethics in order to determine whether physicians make ethical distinctions on the basis of the monetary and educational value of gifts from pharmaceutical companies.[11] Most respondents tended to make distinctions about the ethical appropriateness of gifts on

the basis of the monetary value and type of gift. That is to say, physicians think that the more expensive the gift, the more likely it is to be a breach of an ethical understanding between physician and society.

This makes a great deal of sense. But no matter how nice the industry sponsored dinner may be, this type of gift cannot influence our practice of medicine to the extent that a third party can if it were paying physicians directly to influence their decision making. Indeed, the criminal anti-kickback statute prohibits the knowing and willful offer or payment of anything of value to induce referrals to the federal health care programs.[12,13]

Yet, in procedural disciplines such as IN, this exact scenario plays out daily. We are being asked to objectively assess a patient's need for a procedure, while knowing explicitly that performing that procedure would result in a direct or indirect payment to ourselves. How can pens from a third party be so influential in our clinical decision making process, but our own bank accounts not be?

Thus, the argument against limitations and regulations of industry sponsored CME activities is simply that they are irrelevant compared to the fundamental conflict inherent in our medical payment system.

A NEW PERSPECTIVE ON CONFLICT

The ASDIN is a professional individual membership association many members of which have relationships with other entities, including pharmaceutical and device manufacturers, dialysis facility owners, and other entities. Leaders of the ASDIN must ensure that when they consider any specific issue on behalf of the ASDIN, they do not have a substantial conflict of interest. Therefore, the ASDIN recently put forward a policy on COI that deals with some of the inconsistencies described above.

▶ Definitions

Traditionally, a potential conflict between an individual's *personal* interests and a duty to an independent entity has been seen through the prism of "conflict of interest." The ASDIN recognizes that, because our leaders may be leaders of other organizations as well, potential conflict of "interest" must be understood to extend beyond the *personal* interest of a single individual or his immediate family. To elaborate, "conflict of interest" *per se* can be defined as any *personal* gain that can be obtained by an individual from the decisions made on behalf of another entity that are expected to be made objectively. Examples of this form of conflict may range from honoraria for industry sponsored educational activities to the very reimbursement that specialists obtain from payers each time they decide to perform a procedure.

As distinct from this definition of "conflict of interest," the policy articulated by the ASDIN attempts to apply more broadly to "conflict of responsibility." Conflict of responsibility is the concept that a leader's source of potential conflicts extends beyond the personal. Many ASDIN leaders are also councilors of other organizations to whom they also have distinct responsibilities. Because these sets of responsibilities may often conflict, the ASDIN refers to its conflict policy as a "Conflict of Responsibility Policy."

The ASDIN considers a serious potential conflict of responsibility to exist when an ASDIN leader has a relationship with or engages in any activity that creates a situation such that the professional judgment or actions of an ASDIN leader regarding the ASDIN's mission, purpose, best interest, or core values may be unduly and inappropriately compromised.

In a practical sense, a serious perceived conflict of responsibility was defined as that level of involvement with outside relationships which may cause questions or concerns related to the leader's motives with regard to executing ASDIN business, be they of a personal nature or not (conflict of personal interest is a subset of conflict of responsibility).

▶ General Principles Outlined in the ASDIN Policy

1. Disclosure
   a. The ASDIN will develop and maintain processes that document, review, and track potential conflicts of responsibility for its leaders.
   b. A Conflict of Responsibility Form will be executed by July 1 each year by each member of the Council and Chairs of Standing Committees.
   c. The disclosure statement will name all leadership positions in dialysis organizations, industry, sponsored research, and other medical or professional organizations.
   d. The disclosure will include all financial relationships with these organizations, direct or indirect for the individual or his/her spouse including salaries, royalties, consultancies, speaker's bureaus, honoraria, income-generating relationships with health care facilities, or other funding sources. Holdings in retirement funds or mutual funds will not be reported. The fee for Medical Directorship(s) of Dialysis Facilities is also excluded. Three categories of financial disclosure will be requested:
      i. Less than $10,000/year
      ii. $10,000–$50,000/year
      iii. Greater than $50,000/year
   e. Ownership positions, stock holdings, or partnerships in organizations doing business in renal medicine will be disclosed when such positions exceed $50,000 in value.
   f. Members of the ASDIN leadership will recue themselves from discussion and voting when conflicts of responsibility or the appearance of conflicts of

responsibility are present. In cases where there is uncertainty regarding conflict of responsibility, the burden of proof that there is no conflict rests with the individual leader. Therefore, a conservative and cautious evaluation of one's potential conflicts is recommended.

2. Transparency and Standardization
   a. A uniform policy on potential bias and conflicts of responsibility will be reviewed annually by the ASDIN Industry Relations Committee.
   b. All Potential Conflicts of Responsibility Forms will be made available to all members of the ASDIN upon request.
   c. All potential conflicts of interest will be published on the ASDIN website.

3. Evaluation
   a. The Industry Relations Committee will review the Potential Conflict of Responsibility forms each year, and will make recommendations to the Council concerning any actions needed to maintain the integrity of the ASDIN.
   b. A document outlining the principles this committee will follow will be prepared and reviewed annually by the ASDIN Council.

CONCLUSION

The ethical dilemmas that each procedural specialist encounters on a daily basis can also be viewed through the prism of "Conflict of Responsibility," as articulated above. The Interventional Nephrologist has a *responsibility* to his patients to try to make an impartial decision, to his family to provide an acceptable standard of living, to society to practice medicine free of undue influence, etc. Similarly, IN's close relationship with industry can be regarded from the perspective of conflict of responsibility: in a discipline with very few devices designed specifically for our purpose, creative interventional nephrologists have a *responsibility* to their patients to promote innovation and device development. Recasting the fundamental question as "Conflict of Responsibility" rather than "Conflict of Interest" within the medical profession as a whole may function to generate more light and less heat compared to the traditional view of conflict.

REFERENCES

1. Institute of Medicine (IOM). 2009. Committee on Conflict of Interest in Medical Research, Education, and Practice. Board on Health Sciences Policy. *Conflict of Interest in Medical Research, Education, and Practice.* Washington, DC: National Academy Press.
2. Austad K. Financial conflicts of interest and the ethical obligations of medical school faculty and the profession. Perspectives in biology and medicine. *Autumn.* 2010;53(4): 534–544.

3. Radley DC, Finkelstein SN, Stafford RS. Off-label prescribing among office-based physicians. *Arch Intern Med.* 2006;166:1021–1026.

4. Chren MM, Landefeld CS, Murray TH. Doctors, drug companies, and gifts. *JAMA.* 1989;262:3448–3451.

5. Shaughnessy AF, Slawson DC, Bennett JH. Separating the wheat from the chaff: identifying fallacies in pharmaceutical promotion. *J Gen Intern Med.* 1994;9:563–568.

6. Waud DR. Pharmaceutical promotions: a free lunch? *N Engl J Med.* 1992;327:351–353.

7. Margolis LH. The ethics of accepting gifts from pharmaceutical companies. *Pediatrics.* 1991;88:1233–1237.

8. Goodman B. It's time to just say no to drug reps. *Soc Gen Intern Med Forum.* 1999;22(7):10, 18.

9. Panush RS. Not for sale, not even for rent: just say no: thoughts about the American College of Rheumatology adopting a code of ethics. *J Rheumatol.* 2002;29: 1049–1057.

10. Wazana A. Physicians and the pharmaceutical industry: is a gift ever just a gift? *JAMA.* 2000;283:373–338.

11. Brett AS, Burr W, Moloo J. Are gifts from pharmaceutical companies ethically problematic? A survey of physicians. *Arch Intern Med.* 2003;163:2213–2218.

12. 42 U.S.C. § 1320a-7b(b).

13. Morris L, and Taitsman JK. The agenda for continuing medical education—limiting industry's influence. *N Engl J Med.* 2009;361:2478–2482.

THE AMERICAN SOCIETY OF DIAGNOSTIC AND INTERVENTIONAL NEPHROLOGY AND COLLABORATION WITH OTHER PROFESSIONAL SOCIETIES AND ORGANIZATIONS

BRYAN BECKER

LEARNING OBJECTIVES

1. Understand a framework for looking at academic societies and other specialty organizations.

2. Examine value of collaborative efforts between specialties or other healthcare society organizations.

3. Identify obstacles that alter the potential effectiveness of specialty or other healthcare society organizations in collaboration.

4. Review possible approaches to collaboration that focus on success—"win-win" situations for the collaborating groups.

PROFESSIONAL ORGANIZATIONS IN MEDICINE AND HEALTHCARE

Professional organizations in healthcare may have a variety of designations and home environments (Figure 6-1). They can be specialty-focused groups. The American College of Cardiology and the American College of Surgeons are two such groups. They can be patient-centered. Organizations that fit that category include the American Cancer Society and the National Kidney Foundation (NKF). They can be professional organizations supporting multiple groups of providers. The American Medical Association is an example of one such organization. They can also be academic organizations such as the American Society of Clinical Investigation.

While within each category, professional organizations have some commonality to their missions; in general, the organizations overall have different missions and often will have unique features to their organizational structures. Certainly, all such organizations have different foci at the surface and have a diversity of constituents that may or may not overlap depending on the organizational spheres of interest.

The American Society of Diagnostic and Interventional Nephrology (ASDIN) was founded in 2000 to promote the proper application of new and existing procedures in the practice of nephrology with the goal of improving the care of nephrology patients. The ASDIN is a relatively new organization whose mission is facilitated by close cooperation with other academic and professional societies.

The purpose of this chapter is to describe the complex interplay of surgical, interventional, academic, and patient-centered societies and to articulate a pathway toward a collaborative synergy among the latter.

COLLABORATION

When two or more of these organizations in the medical world choose to collaborate on an issue, they bring tremendous professional weight including the valuable effort of combined membership and a focused agenda from the parties. The expanded network of governmental

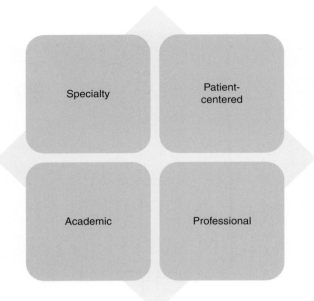

Figure 6-1. General categorization of professional organizations and societies. They included organizations with different missions, different organizational structures, different foci and of course, different people.

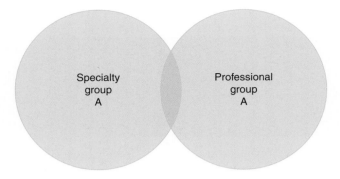

Where collaboration might not work

Figure 6-2. Where collaboration might fail. There may be differing leadership-specific agendas, issues particular to subspecialties that do not cross over into others, complex issues where it is difficult to approach consensus and contradictory goals and objectives.

and regulatory contacts that each organization[1] can leverage expands their influence across differing sectors of the healthcare and legislative arena. Moreover, in some instances, multiple organizations when working together can directly influence legislation or policy. The Centers for Medicare and Medicaid Services (CMS) regularly experience the impact of this effect with the feedback directed toward aspects of healthcare reform.

There are several logical intersections for collaboration between professional organizations. These include policy issues, issues, or topics related to science, innovation, and technology as well as care guidelines and clinical management.

Collaborations are often the result of key leaders playing roles in more than one organization. Collaborations are also the result of common perspectives on an agenda or policy topic or the logical coordination of several organizations that have a vested interest in the topic at hand.

DOOMED TO FAILURE

Where collaborations might not work are in areas in which organizational leadership has moved ahead in a singular direction on a topic (Figure 6-2). Other areas where there might be difficulties in achieving successful collaboration include issues relevant to discrete subspecialty aspects of medicine; complex issues with multiple layers that can differentially affect specialties or even physicians and other providers within the same specialty; lastly, there are topics that might be mutually contradictory for organizations to address.

If professional organizations want to consider collaboration, they must first address a set of challenges to coordinate their efforts. The simplest areas include distance and communication, each overcome with contemporary technologies. Internal alignment is critical and all that much easier for collaboration if positions on issues or policy are already in sync with organizational priorities. If not, then degrees of compromise within organizations much occur for successful efforts across different organizations. Furthermore, organizations have to wrestle with internal priorities and determine if collaboration with other entities is in coordination with internal priorities. Additionally, organizations have to consider whether collaboration will detract from other internal priorities, thus affecting their ability to advance their primary mission.

MODELS FOR ORGANIZATIONAL COLLABORATION

Collaborations can be initiated between professional organizations through initial discussion of pertinent practice issues or topics such as quality items. Organizations usually assess an issue after addressing it, sizing up the ramifications of various positions that might advance an organizational priority locally, regionally, nationally, or even on a global scale. Organizations then look for potential partner groups that might share their perspective or who would be strategic as allies in certain venues such as the legislative arena. The potential partner organizations then determine whether they are in alignment on that particular issue.

COMMUNICATION

The emphasis on communication between organizations cannot be stressed enough. All potential positions that would benefit from collaboration between professional

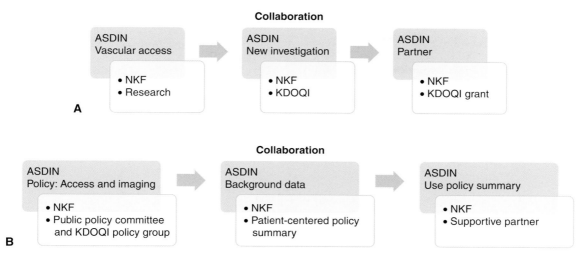

Figure 6-3. (**A** and **B**) Model scenarios using the American Society of Diagnostic and Interventional Nephrology (ASDIN) and the National Kidney Foundation (NKF) as organizations that could collaborate on particular topics.

organizations require large volumes and multiple modalities of communication. Administrative and leadership staff engages across written, telephonic, and electronic communication vehicles. Often face-to-face communication further advances the collaborative effort, especially when timed after an early in-depth communication. The follow-up communication that ensues solidifies and reinforces the decision to collaborate or exposes weaknesses in the potential solidity that give each organization an exit strategy from pursuing further collaborative effort on the particular issue of interest.[2]

A MODEL SCENARIO

A model case illustrates how professional organizational collaboration could occur (Figures 6-3A and B). This case is hypothetical and is constructed as an example. The ASDIN[3] has as its mission: to promote the appropriate application of new and existing procedures in order to improve the care of patients with kidney disease. The NKF has as its mission: enhancing the lives of everyone with, at risk of or affected by kidney disease.[4]

One method of collaboration is to integrate individuals from one organization into a directed effort of the other. NKF has led an effort over the last two decades to review evidence and develop clinical practice guidelines for nephrology care. Vascular access is one area of great importance. NKF can invite a member of ASDIN to participate in a work group and contribute to the creation of the guideline. Similarly, with the guideline product completed, NKF can ask ASDIN to review and comment upon the guideline.

In a different vein, ASDIN, focused on vascular access, could raise ideas related to access in the context of research. NKF could identify an intersecting area of interest with both groups and work together to fund a combined grant

proposal or commission a particular research product that would benefit both entities. Similarly, ASDIN could focus on areas of clinical practice policy and solicit NKF as a potential partner. NKF engaged regularly with its public policy committee and Kidney Disease Outcomes Quality Initiative (KDOQI) policy group could then work with ASDIN on the specific area of policy advancement, focusing on present status, impact assessment, and combined information approaches to entities such as the Congressional Kidney Caucus or CMS to present information and the suggested changes in policy. This type of scenario would have highly positive impact when both ASDIN and NKF would be examining and formulating patient-centered policies for instance. ASDIN could advance those policies into practice with both organizations taking advantage of a broader combined lobbying base to advance those same policies in legislative and regulatory venues.

SUMMARY

Collaboration between professional societies or organizations is moving to a new level of need and skill as healthcare policy and reform takes shape in the United States. Traditional, mission-focused organizations have to develop new ways to partner with similar organizations to leverage their experience, membership expertise, and history to advance healthcare and professional issues in multiple venues. Methods of collaboration are diverse and obstacles can arise at various times. The latter most often are the result of differing organizational missions and leadership direction. The influence and effectiveness of professional society interactions can be significant and may, if properly cultivated, lead to synergistic cooperation in meeting each societies' mission in the future.

REFERENCES

1. Benton CV, Richter F-J, Takai T, ed. *Meso-Organizations and the Creation of Knowledge: Yoshiya Teramotot and His Work on Organization and Industry Collaborations.* Westport, CT: Greenwood Publishing Co.; 2004.

2. Berman S. Collaboration will give pediatric organizations a louder voice. *AAP News.* 2000;17:244.

3. Available at: http://www.asdin.org/. Accessed December 28, 2011.

4. Available at: http://www.kidney.org/. Accessed December 29, 2011.

TRAINING IN DIAGNOSTIC AND INTERVENTIONAL NEPHROLOGY

ARIS URBANES

LEARNING OBJECTIVES

1. Understand the competencies required to ensure the optimal role of the interventional nephrologist in the planning and management of the dialysis patient.
2. Understand the multidisciplinary approach needed to ensure optimal access care for the dialysis patient.
3. Understand the educational and certification requirements for interventional nephrology as outlined by the American Society of Diagnostic and Interventional Nephrology.

Certification in diagnostic and interventional nephrology is available for hemodialysis vascular access, hemodialysis and peritoneal dialysis catheter insertion, and sonographic evaluation of the kidney and urinary bladder. The scope of the discipline, however, is potentially wider and includes native and transplant kidney biopsy, performance and interpretation of vascular access ultrasound, and bone biopsy. There is no separate certification for kidney biopsy but this is a procedural competency that is included in the postgraduate fellowship training program for nephrology. For this discussion, we will limit training to the areas where separate certification in diagnostic and interventional nephrology is available.

▶ Role of the Interventionalist

The strengths of the interventional nephrologist stem from the core foundation of clinical nephrology. Armed with a solid understanding of the physiology and pathology of chronic kidney disease (CKD), the clinical nephrologist makes decisions regarding diagnostic and interventional needs in the context of an appreciation and compassion for the unique needs of the dialysis patient. From this perspective, there is a seamless integration of the patient's needs from CKD, to whatever modality of renal replacement therapy is chosen, and into renal transplantation. The interventionalist advocates for early vein preservation, advises, and collaborates in decisions regarding modality and vascular access, communicates with all interested parties regarding procedural findings, treatment, outcome and prognosis, and counsels patient regarding treatment options. Understanding the role and responsibilities of the interventional nephrologist are essential to optimizing resources and managing health care costs of the dialysis patient.

▶ Qualities of the Interventional Nephrologist

Because interventional nephrology is largely a procedural-based subspecialty, it is imperative that the trainee possess and develop significant dexterity and eye-hand coordination. The tools and skills employed by the interventionalist, from fluoroscopic imaging equipment and radiation safety to endovascular skills and techniques, are unfamiliar to most nephrologists commencing training. Frequent, effective, and clear communication between interventionalist and patient, physician colleagues, team members, and dialysis facility staff is mandatory. Possessing superior grasp of diagnostic and interventional nephrology, he must investigate, appraise, and assimilate evolving scientific evidence and incorporate this into his practice. Medical records must be accurate, complete, and on time and all pertinent findings and recommendations should be appropriately discussed with all vested parties. This is considered part of one's commitment to carrying out professional responsibilities and adherence to highest ethical standards. Finally, there must be an on-going awareness of diagnostic

TABLE 7–1	
Active/Current ASDIN Certifications as of June 2011	
Hemodialysis vascular access procedures	261
PD catheter procedures	22
Renal ultrasound	19
Limited tunneled hemodialysis catheter only	2

TABLE 7–2
Suggested Medical and Nephrologic Historical Data for Inclusion in History
• Current and past vascular accesses, their creation, prior interventions, outcomes, and complications
• Central venous and peripherally inserted central catheters, duration of placement, and complications
• Cardiac history including dysrhythmias, heart failure, ischemic states, certain congenital conditions (eg, patent foramen ovale), and cardiac implantable devices
• Arterial insufficiency
• Arm, facial, neck, or chest swelling
• Difficulties encountered during or problems with dialysis, including missed or abbreviated treatments
• History of hemiparesis, limited range of motion or contractures, mastectomy, and other relevant medical conditions

and interventional discipline within the larger context of health-care delivery to a challenged and challenging population of patients, and appreciate the implications to the manner in which he delivers care.

With this background, the training in interventional nephrology has evolved from a purely apprentice-based paradigm to a more rigidly scholastic program with general educational and specific instructional objectives, a core curriculum with accompanying manual and didactics, graduated independent, proctored and supervised hands-on learning, regular feedback and testing, and critical assessment of interdisciplinary literature relevant to the field. Currently, training in diagnostic and interventional nephrology can be divided into three major categories, with separate certification requirements for each as outlined by the specialty society, the American Society of Diagnostic and Interventional Nephrology (ASDIN).[1] These are:

I. Hemodialysis vascular access procedures

II. Peritoneal dialysis catheter procedures

III. Solid organ renal ultrasound.

The same general categories are recognized as part of the IN core curriculum[2] published as a series of codified skills and competencies (Table 7-1).

HEMODIALYSIS ACCESS PROCEDURES

▶ General Overview and Approach

The trainee will master the basic and relevant variant surface and clinical and surgical anatomy for dialysis vascular access. Eliciting an access history is essential and includes pertinent medical and nephrologic data (Table 7-2).

The indications and contraindications for evaluation and treatment are carefully explored. Access site infection and contraindications based on general medical status and declared drug allergies are considered.

The interventionalist must master the tools at his disposal. It is the judicious, safe, and efficient use of these tools that will permit him to accurately diagnose and appropriately treat various pathological states and complications that may be encountered in the course of the procedure. The appropriate setting in which each of these tools are employed is stressed and the assembly, introduction and application are demonstrated. The trainee must have sufficient working knowledge of the technical properties of each tool to appreciate possible advantages and disadvantages and to enable him to assess innovations and changes in hardware design as they evolve.

Drug reactions, and especially those related to radiocontrast administration, are carefully elicited. The patient's historical experience with sedation and analgesia is crucial because endovascular procedures are commonly performed under conscious sedation in order to control and manage the patient's discomfort. For any given previous dose of medications, effectiveness and duration of sedation and pain control as well as need for rescue or reversal are important parameters in formulating a treatment plan for the patient. Supplemental oxygen needs are noted and examination of the airways is stressed. The importance of this part of the assessment cannot be over-emphasized as it will have direct implications on the patient's ability to handle sedation and analgesia and on the unlikely need for resuscitation.

Management of complications including drug reactions and anaphylaxis; pneumothorax; retained foreign body; venous and arterial vessel rupture; and airway, ventilatory, or hemodynamic compromise are reviewed. Because it is important that the specialty track procedure-related complications, the manner in which these are reported and tracked is reviewed. The two classification methods that are currently in use,[3,4] and their advantages and disadvantages, are discussed.

Included in the general interventional training are sterile and aseptic technique and infection control. Specially, because this population of patients have a perturbed systemic immune response and because the procedures may involve placement of hardware in the vascular bed, the trainee must be cognizant of and apply all current CDC or WHO recommendations as they pertain to his particular practice setting. Knowledge of and adherence to best practice guidelines for blood-borne infection and occupationally related body fluid contamination are also part of the one's responsibility to the patient, coworkers, and the community at large.

The endovascular interventional needs of the dialysis patient will very likely be a recurrent one throughout the life of the access. Because these procedures are performed under guidance of fluoroscopy and digital subtraction angiography, radiation safety is an important aspect of the training curriculum. The various imaging techniques and equipment are similarly discussed. The patient's exposure to radiation, as well as those of the physician's and the staff's must be as low as reasonably allowed to obtain accurate diagnosis and perform the procedure quickly and completely. The recommended dose recording and tracking methods are discussed,[5] as are the clinical manifestations of radiation injury and methods employed to minimize the risk are thoroughly reviewed.[6,7]

Cognizant of the interdisciplinary nature of interventional nephrology, cross-talk among multiple specialties is essential and must be conducted using nomenclature that is as standardized as possible. Current and updated reporting standards[8,9] and quality improvement guidelines[3] are discussed and used in the survey and analysis of literature and in physician medical records whenever appropriate.

Because of the ease with which it is performed[10] and the accuracy and predictability of the findings,[11–14] the physical examination of the vascular access is emphasized. As a preprocedure tool, it allows one to establish a basis upon which any improvements or complications can be judged, and plan a course of action and treatment approach based upon anticipated pathology. A careful and thorough examination of the access can infrequently lead to a decision that intervention is not warranted, thereby saving the patient significant discomfort and unnecessary exposure to medications and radiation. As a postprocedure tool, it confirms that the radiologic improvements are accompanied by clinical resolution of symptoms or/and signs with which the patient presented. As an example, following percutaneous angioplasty of an access suspected of having an outflow obstruction because of hyperpulsatility on examination, this symptom should resolve after successfully dilating the stenotic effluent segment.

Before the procedure is commenced, the trainee will have formulated a treatment plan and approach that includes location of the anticipated culprit lesions, the cannulation site, probable mode of intervention and potential of complications.

▶ Basic Procedures

The procedures that are considered standards of practice for all interventional nephrologists and include:

1. peripheral dialysis vascular access angiography, angioplasty, and thrombolysis;
2. tunneled and nontunneled central venous dialysis catheter placement; and
3. vascular mapping as part of access planning.

ASDIN does not include vascular mapping as part of the certification process for basic hemodialysis vascular access

---

TABLE 7–3
Essential Basic Skills

- Cannulation, including ultrasound-guidance and balloon-entrapment
- Wire selection and passage
- Choice and use of guiding catheters
- Choice and use of dialysis catheters
- Angiography utilizing different imaging modalities and projections
- Thrombolysis utilizing a variety of techniques and tools
- Angioplasty of arterial and peripheral and central venous stenoses
- Hemostasis

---

endovascular work[1] but this remains, nonetheless, an essential procedural skill that has potentially significant impact on fistula creation (Table 7-3).

The reader is referred to the most recently updated ASDIN training and certification guidelines for hemodialysis vascular access procedures for the required number of each procedure to be eligible for certification.[1] At the time of this writing, it is required that the applicant must have performed as the primary operator in a minimum of 25 angiographic procedures, 25 angioplasties, and 25 thrombolysis procedures of both arteriovenous grafts and autogenous fistulae under the supervision of a qualified interventionalist.

The essential skills involved with placement of a tunneled or nontunneled dialysis catheter are the same as those enumerated above, but include the use of ultrasound-guided cannulation of the vein. Use of ultrasound guidance for central venous access results in lower technical failure, a reduction in complications, and faster access[15] and its use considered mandatory by K/DOQI.[16] Other procedures related to dialysis catheter management include catheter exchange over-the-wire and creation of new tunnel or exit site. At the time of this writing, it is required that the applicant must have performed as the primary operator in a minimum of 10 de novo tunneled cuffed long-term dialysis catheter placements under the supervision of a qualified interventionalist.[17]

Vascular mapping involves bimodal study of the arteries and veins that may potentially be used in the creation of a fistula. Doppler duplex ultrasound interrogation of the extremity arteries and of the veins will reveal caliber, depth, calcification, distensibility and compressibility and phasicity of signals. Venography of the extremity and central veins will allow for evaluation of contiguity of vessels, important collateral or side branches, and the presence of central venous obstruction that will flavor one's decision on laterality of the vascular access.

▶ Advanced Procedures

These procedures include accessory vein/side branch obliteration, and endovascular stent placement.

In addition to assessing the hemodynamic relevance of side branches, the trainee will learn basic surgical techniques of percutaneous ligation and cut down and vein isolation. The trainee will also learn the placement of endovascular coils to embolize the target side branch.

Alongside the elective and urgent indications for stent placement, contraindications, stent construction, and choice of stent, the expected outcomes and possible complications are also discussed. The trainee will learn the procedure for stent deployment.

At the time of this writing, it is required that the applicant must have performed as the primary operator in a minimum of five endovascular stent placements and five side-branch obliterations under the supervision of a qualified interventionalist.[1]

PERITONEAL DIALYSIS CATHETER INSERTION

Many of the cognitive skills involved in vascular access work are applicable to PD catheter management. These include medical history and physical examination, management of conscious sedation, radiation safety, and appropriate use of various imaging modalities (Table 7-4).

To complement practice and observational placements, ASDIN requires the placement of six peritoneal catheters under the supervision of a physician who meets the criteria for certification in PD catheter insertion and should be performed within a 1-year period.[17]

RENAL (SOLID-ORGAN) SONOGRAPHY

The procedural skill of ultrasonography is partly applicable from the trainee's experience with vascular access work. Use of the sonographic equipment, transducer and console controls, and image storage hardware and processing software are similar. Positioning of the patient and assuring

TABLE 7–4
Cognitive and Procedural Skills Specific to PD Catheter Placement and Management
• Normal and variant abdominopelvic anatomy • Physiology of peritoneal transport and dialysis • Catheter construction and components, assembly, and proper location • Peritoneoscopic technique, including interpretation of images visualized through the peritoneoscope • Fluoroscopy-guided technique, including images visualized by fluoroscopy or with administration of small amounts of intraperitoneal radiocontrast • Insertion using only surface anatomy • Recognition and correction of problems, malfunction, or complications during placement

TABLE 7–5
Cognitive and Procedural Skills Specific to Renal Sonography Include
• Normal and variant sonographic appearance of the kidney and urinary system • Renal pathology, clinical presentation, and natural history • Preparation of patient to optimize sonographic windows and maneuvers to elicit or delineate different variables • Complete study of the kidneys, the associated collecting systems, and urinary bladder • Evaluation for simple and complex cysts, hydronephrosis, chronic kidney disease, renal allograft, urolithiasis, guidance for percutaneous kidney biopsy, and measurement of urinary bladder volume

reasonable comfort during the examination is, of course, different from that of the examination of the vascular access (Table 7-5).

The reader is referred to the ASDIN[17] for specific criteria for certification in renal sonography. The criteria include a specific amount of training time and number and kinds of cases that have been performed. Also, there is separate certification available for limited sonography of the renal allograft.

CONCLUSION

As diagnostic and interventional nephrology has become mainstream components of nephrology practice, it is the expectation that training in this arena will move progressively to a fellowship-based program, with full accreditation by ACGME and ABMS. Significant and momentous strides in vascular access care have been taken in the past 10 years and it has matured into an essential aspect of the care of the dialysis patient. Training the next generation of nephrologists in the clinical and procedural aspects of vascular access, peritoneal dialysis catheter management and renal sonography will enable the clinician to provide the nonfragmented vision that the patients deserve.

REFERENCES

1. O'Neill WC, Ash SR, Work J, Saad TF. Guidelines for training, certification and accreditation for hemodialysis vascular access and endovascular procedures. *Semin Dial.* 2003;16(2):173–176.
2. Niyyar VD, Work J. Interventional nephrology: core curriculum 2009. *Am J Kidney Dis.* 2009;54(1):169–182.
3. Aruny JE, Lewis CA, Cardella JF, Cole PE, Davis A, Drooz AT, et al. Quality improvement guidelines for percutaneous management of the thrombosed or dysfunctional dialysis access. *J Vasc Interv Radiol.* 2003;14(9):S247–S253.

4. Vesely TM, Beathard G, Ash S, Hoggard J, Schon D. Classification of complications associated with hemodialysis vascular access procedures. *Semin Dial.* 2007;20(4): 359–364.

5. Miller DL, Balter S, Dixon RG, Nikolic B, Bartal G, Cardella JF, et al. Quality improvement guidelines for recording patient radiation dose in the medical record. *J Vasc Interv Radiol.* 2009;20(7S):S200–S207.

6. Koenig TR, Mettler FA, Wagner LK. Skin injuries from fluoroscopically guided procedures: part 2 review of 73 cases and recommendations for minimizing dose delivered to patient. *Am J Radiology.* 2001;177:13–20.

7. Koenig TR, Wolff D, Mettler FA, Wagner LK. Skin injuries from fluoroscopically guided procedures: part 1, characteristics of radiation injury. *Am J Radiology.* 2001;177:177–173.

8. Gray RJ, Sacks D, Martin LG, Trerotola SO. Reporting standards for peructaneous interventions in dialysis access. *J Vasc Interv Radiol.* 2003;14(9):S433–S442.

9. Sidawy AN, Spergel LM, Besarab A, Allon M, Jennings WC, Padberg FT, et al. Recommended standards for reports dealing with arteriovenous hemodialysis access. *J Vasc Surg.* 2002;35(3):603–610.

10. Beathard GA. An algorithm for the physical examination of the early fistula failure. *Semin Dial.* 2005;18(4): 331–335.

11. Asif A, Leon C, Orozco-Vargas LC, Krishnamurthy G, Choi KL, Mercado C, Merrill D, Thomas I, Salman L, Artikov S, Bourgoignie JJ. Accuracy of physical examination in the detection of arteriovenous fistula stenosis. *Clin J Am Soc Nephrol.* 2007;2(6):1191–1194.

12. Leon C, Asif A. Physical examination of arteriovenous fistulae by a renal fellow: does it compare favorably to an experienced interventionalist? *Semin Dial.* 2008;21(6): 557–560.

13. Leon C, Orozco-Vargas LC, Krishnamurthy G, Choi KL, Mercado C, Merrill D, et al. Accuracy of physical examination in the detection of arteriovenous graft stenosis. *Semin Dial.* 2008;21(1):85–88.

14. Campos RP, Chula DC, Perreto S, Riella MC, do Nascimento MM. Accuracy of physical examination and intra-access pressure in the detection of stenosis in hemodialysis arteriovenous fistula. *Semin Dial.* 2008;21(3):269–273.

15. Hind D, Calvert N, McWilliams R, Davidson A, Paisley S, Beverley C, Thomas S. Ultrasoic locating devices for central venous cannulation: a meta-analysis. *Br Med J.* 2003;327(7411):361–368.

16. Clinical Practice Guidelines for Vascular Access. *Am J Kidney Dis.* 2006;48:S176–S247.

17. Ash S. American Society of Diagnostic and Interventional Nephrology: Guidelines for training, certification and accreditation. *Semin Dial.* 2002;15(6):440–444.

DEVELOPING AN ACADEMIC CURRICULUM FOR INTERVENTIONAL NEPHROLOGY TRAINING

AMY DWYER

LEARNING OBJECTIVES

1. Define the ideal qualities of an academic interventional nephrologist.
2. List the major topics of academic interventional nephrology training.
3. Define the ideal training period for academic interventional nephrology.
4. Understand the six core competencies defined by the Accreditation Council for Graduate Medical Affairs.
5. Discuss the education goals of an ideal training program curriculum for academic interventional nephrology.
6. Understand the importance of physician certification by the American Society of Diagnostic and Interventional Nephrology.
7. List the types of physician certification offered by the American Society of Diagnostic and Interventional Nephrology.
8. Discuss the criteria for physician certification by the American Society of Diagnostic and Interventional Nephrology.
9. Understand the importance of Training Program Accreditation by the American Society of Diagnostic and Interventional Nephrology.
10. Discuss the criteria for Training Program Accreditation by the American Society of Diagnostic and Interventional Nephrology.

INTRODUCTION

Nephrologists enjoy an unusually close and extended relationship with their patients, often lasting decades through their evolution of chronic kidney disease to eventual long-term management of end-stage renal disease. Their unique perspective on the importance of dialysis access has expanded an intense interest in the field resulting in the emergence of a new subspecialty: interventional nephrology.

Studies show that nephrologists performing access procedures not only improve convenience for patients but also improve patient outcomes by providing more timely effective, efficient, and safe treatment.[1-3] Beathard reviewed more than 14,000 procedures by interventional nephrologists. The success rate was 96.18% with a very low complication rate of 0.28%[3] (Table 8-1), confirming the proficiency of appropriately trained nephrologists.

The growth of interest has also spurred growth in academic centers nationally. Currently, there are fourteen academic centers in the United States that are dedicated to training fellows in the field of interventional nephrology (Table 8-2). In order to stimulate education, clinical research, and translational and basic science research as part of the interventional nephrology training process, the Interventional Nephrology Advisory Group of the American Society of Nephrology has recently established a training curriculum which could potentially be used by such centers.

The purpose of this chapter is to briefly describe a comprehensive curriculum for academic-based interventional nephrology training programs, outline educational goals, identify core areas of training, and describe certification/accreditation pathways available to trainees.

TABLE 8–1

Summary of Procedures, Beathard et al[4]

Procedure Type[a]	Procedure Number	Successful Procedure	Failed Procedure	Aborted Procedure	Complications	
					Minor	Major
TDC placement	1765	98.24%	1.08%	0.68%	1.36%	0.06%
TDC exchange	2262	98.36%	1.11%	0.53%	1.37%	0.04%
AVF — PTA	1561	96.58%	2.63%	0.83%	4.29%	0.19%
Graft — PTA	3560	98.06%	1.52%	0.42%	1.04%	0.11%
AVF thrombectomy	228	78.10%	16.67%	5.26%	6.07%	0.44%
Graft thrombectomy	4671	93.08%	5.07%	1.84%	5.99%	0.62%
TOTAL	14,067	96.18%	2.94%	1.06%	3.26%	0.28 %

[a]TDC placement = tunneled dialysis catheter placement; TDC exchange = tunneled dialysis catheter exchange; PTA = percutaneous transluminal angioplasty; AVF-PTA = arteriovenous fistula angioplasty; graft-PTA = graft angioplasty; AVF thrombectomy = arteriovenous fistula thrombectomy

IDEAL QUALITIES OF AN INTERVENTIONAL NEPHROLOGIST

Three main attributes are required in a competent interventional nephrologist:[5,6]

1. strong commitment to dialysis access,
2. thorough understanding about the technical aspects of dialysis treatments, and
3. expertise in the procedures required to maintain dialysis access patency.

In addition, it is also important that interventional physicians and vascular access centers have the flexibility to accommodate the challenging dialysis patient schedules and be available for both routine and emergency vascular access procedures at least 5 days per week. Most importantly, it is critical that an interventionalist have the insight to plan ahead for future vascular access sites (ex. secondary fistula).

TRAINING PRINCIPLES

Previous published reports have suggested curriculum guidelines for interventional nephrology.[7–9] However, at the present time, there is no national, standardized curriculum for training in interventional nephrology. The Interventional Nephrology Advisory Group (INAG), convened by the American Society of Nephrology, has been assigned to review this important issue. The following principles of training and education goals are based upon the INAG preliminary academic training program curriculum that has not yet been published.

1. The training should include all major topics of interventional nephrology including:
   - Endovascular procedures
   - Hemodialysis catheter procedures
   - Peritoneal catheter procedures
   - Ultrasound of the kidney and bladder

TABLE 8–2

Academic Interventional Nephrology Training Programs

University	Location	Training Program Director
[a]University of Louisville	Louisville, KY	Amy Dwyer, MD
University of Miami	Miami, FL	Arif Asif, MD
University of Wisconsin	Madison, WI	Alexander Yevzlin, MD
Wake Forest University	Winston-Salem, NC	Tushar Vachharajani, MD
Emory University	Atlanta, GA	Jack Work, MD
[a]University of Alabama	Birmingham, AL	Roman Shingarev, MD
Harvard Medical School	Boston, MA	Steven Wu, MD
Louisiana State University	Shreveport, LA	Kenneth Abreo, MD
Ohio State University	Columbus, OH	Anil Agarwal, MD
[a]University of Arizona	Phoenix, AZ	Rick Mishler, MD
University of Nebraska	Omaha, NE	Marius Florescu, MD
[a]University of California at Davis	Sacramento, CA	Jamie Ross, MD
St. Louis University	St. Louis, MO	Kevin Martin, MD

[a]Denotes Accreditation by the American Society of Diagnostic and Interventional Nephrology.

- Ultrasound vessel mapping
- Radiation
- Research
- Office management.

2. The training period should be 12 months.

3. The curriculum should be based upon six core competencies defined by the Accreditation Council for Graduate Medical Affairs:[10]

   a. Patient care that is compassionate, appropriate, and effective for the treatment of health problems and for the general well being of patients.

   b. Medical knowledge about the application of established and evolving biomedical, clinical, epidemiological and social-behavioral sciences to patient care.

   c. Practice-based learning and improvement that incorporates effective utilization of technology to manage information for patient care and self-improvement.

   d. Interpersonal and communication skills that result in effective information exchange with patients, their families, and other health professionals.

   e. Professionalism as demonstrated by a commitment to ethical principles, diverse patient populations and by consistently considering the needs of patients, families, and colleagues.

   f. Systems-based practice as demonstrated by effectively using systematic a approaches to reduce errors and improve patient care.

EDUCATION GOALS

- The training will establish the foundations for a broad knowledge base in interventional nephrology by providing exposure and opportunities to manage all types of interventional nephrology procedures.
- Each trainee will demonstrate the ability to manage an independent interventional nephrology care center.
- Each trainee will complete a research project in the field of interventional nephrology.
- By the end of the training period, trainees will have completed a sufficient number of procedures to qualify for certification by the American Society of Diagnostic and Interventional Nephrology.

INTERVENTIONAL PROCEDURES

Interventional nephrologists perform procedures on hemodialysis vascular accesses, perform procedures related to peritoneal dialysis catheters, and perform and interpret renal, bladder, and urinary collecting system ultrasound. Some interventional nephrologists also perform ultrasound vessel mapping and venography for preoperative permanent vascular access planning.

▶ Endovascular Procedures

- *Angiogram*: intravenous contrast injection to evaluate blood vessels for areas of stenosis, thrombus, or other problems.
- *Angioplasty*: insertion of a balloon catheter across an area of vascular stenosis, inflation of the balloon in order to open the stenotic area.
- *Thrombectomy*: removal of clotted blood from the vascular circuit.
- *Obliteration of accessory vessels*: occluding side branch vessels that divert blood from the main fistula channel.
   1. Percutaneous ligation: external suture placement
   2. Endovascular coil placement: intravascular insertion of a coil device
- *Stent placement*: insertion of a self-expanding or expandable metal coil across an area of stenosis to open the vessel and maintain patency.

▶ Catheter Procedures

- *Tunneled catheter placement*: insertion of a large lumen hemodialysis catheter with the mid-portion subcutaneous.
- *Tunneled catheter exchange*: replacement of a dysfunctional tunneled catheter using the original exit site, tunnel, and venipuncture site.
- *Tunneled catheter removal*.
- *Nontunneled catheter placement*: insertion of a temporary large bore dialysis catheter (hospital inpatient use only recommended).

▶ Renal and Bladder Ultrasound

- Native kidney ultrasound
- Transplant kidney ultrasound
- Urinary bladder and collecting system ultrasound

▶ Peritoneal Catheter Procedures

- Peritoneal catheter insertion
- Peritoneal catheter exchange
- Peritoneal catheter removal

▶ Vascular Mapping & Venography

- Using imaging to evaluate vessels, including both arteries and veins, in patients with chronic kidney disease to prepare for permanent vascular access placement.

CERTIFICATION

The American Society of Diagnostic and Interventional Nephrology (ASDIN) has taken the lead in developing guidelines to standardize training and certification to maximize patient safety and to improve patient outcomes.[11-13] To date, the ASDIN is the only society to certify both physicians and training programs in interventional nephrology procedures. At the present time, physicians are not required to achieve ASDIN certification to perform procedures; however, since most hospitals require documentation of ability and proof of certification, including board certificates, ASDIN certification may streamline the application to obtain credentials for performing interventional procedures in a hospital setting.

There are three types of ASDIN certification available depending the trainee's desired goals: endovascular procedures, peritoneal catheter procedures, and renal ultrasound. An important requirement for each certification is that the trainee performs a certain number of procedures as "Primary Operator." The definition of "Primary Operator" is very specific. The role of Primary Operator means that a trainee can complete a procedure *independently* from start to finish without any Attending Physician intervention or help. For example, if a trainee cannot successfully cannulate the clotted access but can complete the remainder of a thrombectomy of a vascular access, he/she would not qualify as the Primary Operator.

Since detailed guidelines for training, certification, and accreditation have previously been published by the ASDIN, the following will provide an overview of their criteria.

ASDIN CERTIFICATION TYPES AND CRITERIA

There are three categories of certification by the ASDIN:

1. Vascular access procedures
   a. Endovascular procedures
   b. Tunneled catheter procedures
   c. Advanced procedures
2. Renal ultrasound
3. Peritoneal dialysis catheters

▶ Vascular Access Procedures

There are three categories of certification in vascular procedures: endovascular procedures, dialysis catheter procedures, and advanced procedures.

To obtain ASDIN certification in vascular access procedures, the following three criteria are required:

- The applicant must have active certification by the American Board of Internal Medicine (ABIM) in Nephrology, or board certification in Surgery or Radiology.
- The applicant must have completed a formal training program or be practicing as an interventional nephrologist, interventional radiologist, or surgeon for at least 1 year.
- The applicant must be able to show *continued* practice as an interventional nephrologist, interventional radiologist, or surgeon.

a. ASDIN endovascular procedure certification

Applicants are required to obtain the three broad certification criteria and also have documentation of the additional following number of cases as *primary operator*:

1. Angiogram of both fistula and grafts (25)
2. Angioplasty including both fistula and grafts (25)
3. Thrombolysis/thrombectomy including both fistula and grafts (25)
4. Tunneled dialysis catheter insertion (25)

b. ASDIN catheter procedure certification

Applicants are required to obtain the three broad certification criteria and also have documentation of the additional following criteria as *primary operator*:

Documentation of 25 cases of tunneled dialysis catheter insertion

c. ASDIN advanced procedure certification

Applicants are required to obtain the three broad certification criteria and also have documentation of the additional following number of cases as *primary operator*:

1. Subcutaneous port management (5)
2. Stent placement (5)
3. Obliteration of accessory vessels (5)

▶ ASDIN Certification in Renal Ultrasound

To obtain ASDIN certification in renal ultrasound, the criteria are different for practicing physicians and fellows:

Fellows: 6 weeks of training in an *ASDIN Accredited* Training Program
Practicing Nephrologists: 50 hours minimum of formal training in an *ASDIN Accredited* Training Program

Both fellows and practicing nephrologists must perform 125 ultrasound studies as *primary operator*. A submission of study types performed is also required (Table 8-3).

TABLE 8-3	
Ultrasound Studies Required for Certification by the American Society of Diagnostic and Interventional Nephrology	
Standard Certification	**Transplant Only Certification**
Normal kidney	Normal allograft
Chronic kidney disease	Guidance for biopsy
Renal cysts	Peritoneal fluid collection
Hydronephrosis	Hydronephrosis
Nephrolithiasis	Ureteral stent
Guidance for percutaneous renal biopsy	Measurement of bladder volume
Renal allograft	
Measurement of bladder volume	

TABLE 8–4

Training Programs Accredited by the American Society of Diagnostic and Interventional Nephrology

Program	Location	Training Program Director
American Access Care Physicians	Brooklyn, NY	Greg Miller, MD
Bamberg County Hospital	Bamberg, SC	John Ross, MD
Dialysis Access Center, Inc.	Oakland, CA	Oliver Khakmahd, MD
[a]University of Louisville Kidney Disease Program	Louisville, KY	Amy Dwyer, MD
Nephrology Associates of Mobile	Mobile, AL	Stephen Wilber, MD
Norton Audubon Hospital Vascular Access Center	Louisville, KY	Peter Wayne, III, MD
RMS Lifeline	Vernon Hills, IL	Gerald Beathard, MD, PhD, FASN
Renal Intervention Center	Morton, IL	Timothy Pflederer, MD
[a]University of Alabama at Birmingham	Birmingham, AB	Roman Shingarev, MD
[a]University of Arizona/AKDHC	Phoenix, AZ	Rick Mishler, MD, FACP
[a]University of California, Davis	Sacramento, CA	Jamie Ross, MD

[a]Denotes University-based, Academic Programs.

▶ ## ASDIN Certification in Peritoneal Catheter Procedures

To obtain ASDIN certification in peritoneal catheter procedures, the criteria are as follows:

- Active certification by the American Board of Internal Medicine in Nephrology
- Observation of peritoneal catheter placement
- Performance of peritoneal catheter placement with models/animals
- Placement of PD catheters in six patients with documentation of patient outcomes
- Submission of 10 peritoneal catheter procedures for review

ASDIN ACCREDITED TRAINING PROGRAMS

There are 11 ASDIN Accredited Training Programs in the United States (Table 8-4).

To achieve ASDIN Training Program Accreditation, programs must meet specified requirements related to facilities, institutional support, physician expertise and experience, and personnel directed toward training in diagnostic and interventional nephrology.

There are three categories of ASDIN Training Program Accreditation:

1. Endovascular procedures on hemodialysis vascular access (AV fistulas and grafts, and chronic central venous catheters for dialysis)

2. Peritoneal catheter placement

3. Sonography of kidneys and urinary bladder

COMMON REQUIREMENTS TO BE CONSIDERED FOR ASDIN TRAINING PROGRAM ACCREDITATION

- Evidence of a source of funding sufficient to support the program
- At least one full time, ASDIN certified interventional faculty member
- At least one full time faculty equivalent committed to the program
- Documentation of a formal, written training curriculum that includes
  - didactic instruction
  - proctored training
  - trainee evaluation
- Performance of minimum required number of procedures
- Proper medical record storage
- Maintain an ongoing Quality Assurance program
- A site visit by an ASDIN Member to review program and tour center
- Application fee.

RECERTIFICATION

The ASDIN offers a 5-year recertification for hemodialysis endovascular access procedures and catheter procedures. At this time, recertification for peritoneal catheter procedures and renal ultrasound is not required. The following is an overview of the recertification process.

1. Active ASDIN certification in hemodialysis vascular access procedures *and* provide documentation of current activity doing interventional procedures.

2. Active board certification in Nephrology, Surgery, or Radiology

3. Documentation of at least 7 hours of Continuing Medical Education (CME) involving interventional nephrology within the past 3 years.

4. Documentation of a Continuous Quality Improvement program

5. Documentation that the following minimum procedures have been performed as *primary operator* within the last year:

▶ Hemodialysis Vascular Access Procedures

- Catheter placements (25)
- Endovascular procedures (50)

▶ Catheters Only Recertification

- Catheter placements (25)

SUMMARY AND RECOMMENDATIONS

At the present time, there is no national, standardized interventional nephrology training curriculum or specific individual requirements for physicians to practice interventional nephrology. However, there are guidelines that have been carefully developed by leaders in the field. To ensure optimal training, at this time, the best recommendation would be to pursue training by an ASDIN Certified physician in an ASDIN Accredited program.

REFERENCES

1. Asif A, Merrill D, Briones P, et al. Hemodialysis vascular access: percutaneous interventions by nephrologists. *Semin Dial.* 2004;17(6):528–534.

2. Gadallah M, Pervez A, el-Shahawy MA, et al. Peritoneoscopic versus surgical placement of peritoneal dialysis catheters: a prospective randomized study on outcome. *Am J Kidney Dis.* 1999;33(1):118–122.

3. Nass K, O'Neill WC. Bedside renal biopsy: ultrasound guidance by the nephrologist. *Am J Kidney Dis.* 1999;34(5):955–959.

4. Beathard G, Litchfield T, Physician Operators Forum of RMS Lifeline, Inc. Effectiveness and safety of dialysis vascular access procedures performed by interventional nephrologists. *Kidney Int.* 2004;66:1622–1632.

5. Beathard G. What is the current and future status of interventional nephrology? *Semin Dial.* 2005;18(5):370–371.

6. Beathard G. Interventional nephrology: a part of the solution. *Semin Dial.* 2006;19(2):171.

7. Niyyar VD, Work J. Interventional nephrology: core curriculum 2009. *Am J Kidney Dis.* 2009;54(1):169–182.

8. Maya I, Allon M. Vascular access: core curriculum 2008. *Am J Kidney Dis.* 2008;51(4):702–708.

9. O'Neill WC, Baumgarten DA. Core curriculum in nephrology: imaging. *Am J Kidney Dis.* 2003;42(3):601–604.

10. Graduate Medical Education, ACGME Competencies. Available at: http://www.umm.edu/gme/core_comp.htm. Web September 23, 2010.

11. American Society of Diagnostic and Interventional Nephrology. Guidelines of training, certification and accreditation on placement of permanent tunneled and cuffed peritoneal dialysis catheters. *Semin Dial.* 2002;15(6):440–442.

12. American Society of Diagnostic and Interventional Nephrology. Guidelines for training, certification, and accreditation in renal sonography. *Semin Dial.* 2002;15(6):442–444.

13. American Society of Diagnostic and Interventional Nephrology: education and training. Available at: http://www.asdin.org. Web. September 6, 2010.

9

ACCREDITATION AND CERTIFICATION IN INTERVENTIONAL NEPHROLOGY

JEFFREY PACKER & ANIL K. AGARWAL

LEARNING OBJECTIVES

1. To explain the meaning of accreditation and the process that a training center must follow to obtain this status.

2. To understand the meaning of certification in areas of interventional nephrology and the requirements that must be met to obtain individual certification.

3. To describe the governance process of ASDIN regarding accreditation and certification.

4. To explore future areas of interventional nephrology expertise that may be candidates for accreditation and certification.

INTRODUCTION

Various modalities for renal replacement therapy were developed during the last century. It was quickly realized that vascular access, primarily created and maintained by the surgeons and the radiologists, was central to the performance of hemodialysis. There was a long lag time before formal guidelines for vascular access care were developed in 1997 by the Kidney Disease Outcomes Quality Initiative work group. These opinions and evidence-based guidelines garnered the interest of nephrologists and regulatory agencies, which was further intensified by the Fistula First Initiative that was initiated in 2003. An interest in defragmenting vascular access care paved the way for development of Interventional Nephrology as a distinct subspecialty toward the turn of the century.

Interventional nephrology remains a growing field of endeavor. With increasing numbers of those aspiring to become practitioners in this specialty, a need for more training opportunities has developed. This has, in turn, created a need for standardization of training and a need for the development of minimum standards for that training. Accreditation is defined as "The process by which a (non-) governmental or private body evaluates the quality of a higher education institution as a whole or of a specific educational program in order to formally recognize it as having met certain predetermined minimal criteria or standards. The result of this process is usually the awarding of a status (a yes/no decision), of recognition, and sometimes of a license to operate within a time-limited validity."[1]

The American Society of Diagnostic and Interventional Nephrology (ASDIN) was established in year 2000 with a stated mission to "promote the appropriate application of new and existing procedures in order to improve the care of patients with kidney disease."[4] This organization, therefore has established both an institutional accreditation program and a practitioner certification process for a variety of skills that would fall under its venue. These areas include hemodialysis and vascular access procedures, hemodialysis catheter procedures, peritoneal dialysis catheter procedures, and diagnostic sonography. An overview of institutional accreditation and of individual practitioner certification in each of these areas is presented with discussion of possible future directions. A number of centers have been accredited by ASDIN based on these criteria (Table 9-1)[2].

Apart from the need for accreditation of training centers, certification of individual practitioners of Interventional Nephrology has become necessary to ensure the safety of such procedures. Several curricula for their training have also been developed and published including the "Training Manual for Interventional Nephrology" by the American Society of Diagnostic and Interventional Nephrology (ASDIN).[3] The American Society of Nephrology

TABLE 9–1

Number of ASDIN Accredited Centers from 2003 to August 2010

Year	Applications Received	Accredited Centers
2003	1	1
2004	2	0
2005	3	3
2006	1	0
2007	1	2
2008	1	0
2009	7	3
2010	0	3

Source: ASDIN. Personal Communication August 23, 2010.

is also in the process of developing a comprehensive curriculum for academic training in all types of procedures, core competencies for the trainees in all areas of Interventional Nephrology and evaluation parameters for the

trainees (discussed in detail in Chapter 8). A number of individuals have been certified in the fields of hemodialysis vascular access (HVA), peritoneal dialysis (PD), renal ultrasound or tunneled hemodialysis catheter certification only (Figure 9-1).

TRAINING CENTER ACCREDITATION

In order to promote the development of interventional nephrology skills in patient care, minimal criteria for training programs were established by ASDIN in 2000.[4] These programs can be designed to train nephrology fellows or practicing nephrologists in practice and must have necessary resources and meet specific requirements to provide appropriate training. Attention to the facility, the level of available expertise, and the availability of personnel with the necessary experience all are required for an institution to become accredited. Delivery of safe and effective patient care by qualified operators with appropriate staff and equipment is a necessity. An institution may then pursue an application with appropriate documentation followed

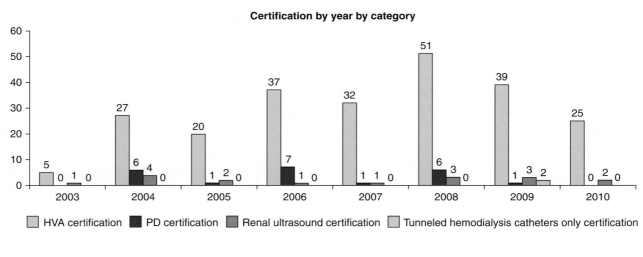

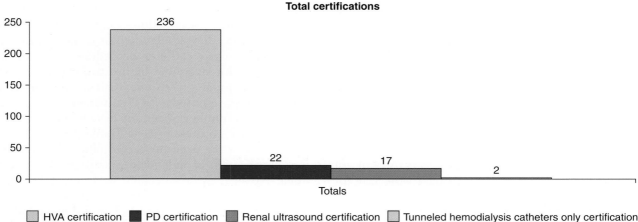

Figure 9-1. Number of Individuals Certified by ASDIN in Various Disciplines of Interventional Nephrology from 2003 to 2010. *Source:* ASDIN. Personal Communication May 25, 2011.

by a site visit before a recommendation for accreditation can be made to the society.

There are several components that are required for accreditation of a training center depending upon the types of procedures performed at the training center. Documentation of adequate funding, adequate faculty, adequate equipment, a sufficient number of procedures performed and ongoing assessment of the trainee and quality assurance all are important criteria for accreditation.

▶ Accreditation for Hemodialysis and Vascular Access Procedures

Funding

The training program must be well-funded to be able to sustain excellence in training and meet the needs of modernization to stay current with the developments in this rapidly evolving field. Currently, the mechanisms of this funding are evolving and may vary from academic or commercial sponsorship to joint venture.

Faculty

Dedicated faculty must be available to train Nephrology fellows or physicians already in practice. The stated goal is the ability to provide ample experience and education to allow the trainee to develop expertise in the field. At least one full-time faculty member must demonstrate sufficient experience to meet the certification requirements of the American Society of Diagnostic and Interventional Nephrology and a given facility must demonstrate at least one full-time equivalent faculty member involved in that area of practice.[5]

Facility

A training program must be associated with an interventional facility that is designed and equipped to deal with the problems associated the hemodialysis access. The space must be adequate to provide patient waiting area, patient dressing area, preoperative/recovery area, and patient procedure area. There should be sufficient space for storage of the needed supplies and equipment. The facility must have appropriate equipment to perform safe and effective procedures. This includes fluoroscopy for imaging of vascular procedures, equipment to create and maintain permanent records of those images, a procedure table that allows fluoroscopy, ultrasound apparatus for vascular imaging and catheter placement, and needed equipment for monitoring of the patient.[5] Supplies for the interventions performed in that facility must be available. An inventory and ordering mechanism must be in place to ensure adequacy of those supplies. Sufficient space must be available for storage of such supplies.[5]

In order to safely and effectively perform those procedures specified in the application, there must be adequate staffing. The staff must be adequately and appropriately trained. At a minimum, an ACLS certified Nurse must be present to monitor the patient during the procedure. In addition, a scrub technician must be available to assist the operator in performing the procedures. A technician must be present to manage the radiology equipment and it is recommended that this person be a Radiology Technician.

Volume of procedures and record maintenance

Adequate training entails the involvement of the trainee in a sufficient number of cases to gain expertise. Therefore, accreditation criteria state that a given facility must be actively performing interventional cases on an ongoing basis with a minimum annual caseload of 300 angiograms, 300 angioplasties, 100 thrombolysis/thrombectomies, and 100 tunneled long-term catheter placements. All procedures must have a report generated that is placed in the patient's permanent medical record with each trainee able to maintain documentation of each procedure performed with outcomes and complications. Several computerized access databases have been developed at individual centers that can facilitate such record keeping.

Quality assurance

An ongoing quality assurance program is a requirement of any interventional facility. A program designed to improve and maintain the delivery of quality care is an important part of a training program. Ongoing assessment of outcomes must be performed with attention to appropriateness of therapy, costs, adverse outcomes and medical necessity. A quality improvement process should also be in place. Practice guidelines should be developed and monitored. This should be based on the collection and assessment of data on an ongoing basis. A reliable system of maintaining this data should exist.

Application for accreditation and site visit

Once all of the requirements noted above have been fulfilled by the center, an application for accreditation should be filed. A site visit will be performed by a representative of the ASDIN Accreditation Subcommittee. This visit will occur not less than 6 months after a program is initiated. The visitor will review the program with attention to the above criteria. The site visit report will then be reviewed by the Subcommittee with a recommendation made to the ASDIN on the basis of the entire application for accreditation.[5]

Ongoing accreditation

Once a program receives accreditation as a training facility in Hemodialysis Vascular Access Procedures, the interval of that approval will last 5 years. At the end of this interval, a facility may submit an application to be reaccredited.

▶ Accreditation for Diagnostic Renal Ultrasound

Renal ultrasonography is an important tool in the diagnosis and management of renal disease.[6] Since the inception of ASDIN, there has been an emphasis on training practitioners to perform and interpret this study. In that regard, accreditation of a facility allows the standardization necessary to ensure adequate exposure to sonography.

Funding

There must be a documented and sustainable funding mechanism for a training facility in renal ultrasonography. This is important for maintenance and modernization of the facility and equipment as well as for provision of adequate staff.

Faculty

To be accredited as an institution that trains in renal ultrasonography, a dedicated faculty is required. At least one full-time faculty member certified by ASDIN must be involved in the training process, with at least 25% of a full-time equivalent dedicated to renal Ultrasonography by that trainer. All faulty members must be identified formally with a curriculum vitae for each trainer submitted with the facility application.[7]

Facility

A training program in renal ultrasonography must provide adequate space for patient waiting area, dressing area, procedure area, preoperative/recovery area, and storage area for equipment and supplies. There should be adequate supplies and staff available for these activities. An accredited training facility will have sufficient scanning equipment that is properly maintained with an adequate ability to store images for review. A minimum of one dedicated scanner should be appropriate for abdominal imaging with probes in the 3 to 6 MHz range (for adults) and include the ability to store images in either a hardcopy or digital format. This storage should be dedicated to that purpose and should be available to the trainee for review. Teaching files or images should be accumulated and maintained. A library including books and other resources is necessary for an approved training facility.

Curriculum, volume of procedures, and record maintenance

Any facility requesting accreditation in renal ultrasonography must have an organized and formalized training program that includes didactic training, proctoring of trainees, and evaluation mechanisms to ensure adequate competence. The didactic program may be written or may consist of formal presentations that cover: the basics of ultrasound physics, an overview of ultrasound instrumentation, the basics of ultrasound interpretation, and the interpretation of renal pathology. Trainees must be adequately supervised and proctored until their proficiency is such that they may make interpretations and demonstrate sufficient skills that they may perform renal ultrasonography procedures independently. Decisions regarding this training will be made according to a formalized review process, with the actual duration of training that will vary with each individual trainee. As a general rule, each trainee will perform and interpret at least 40 studies under supervision and will then perform and interpret an additional 40 studies independently with appropriate overview. As a general guideline, each trainee should perform at least 30 native kidney studies with interpretation, at least 5 native kidney biopsy guidance studies, at least 5 urinary bladder studies with interpretation, and, (for programs requesting accreditation in renal transplant studies) at least 15 renal transplant studies with interpretation.[7]

In order to achieve the above requirement for facility accreditation, an ongoing evaluation program must be in place. A formal evaluation process must be performed at the conclusion of training documenting competency and documenting the ability of trainees to perform renal ultrasonography skills independently. Each facility requesting accreditation must perform a sufficient number of studies to allow adequate exposure to the spectrum of renal pathology. At least 300 renal ultrasonography procedures are recommended annually with a minimum of 60 renal transplant studies for those facilities requesting accreditation in renal transplant ultrasonography.

Reports of each procedure should be generated and placed in the patient's permanent record. These reports must be stored along with the original images at the training center. Each trainee should receive documentation of the number of and type of procedures performed. The facility must have a means of generating reports and maintaining records of all studies performed, including the findings and interpretation of each study with identification of the trainee performing the study. This may be done electronically or through a paper-based system. All electronic records shall have an appropriate back-up mechanism in place.

Quality assurance

An ongoing quality assurance mechanism is an absolute requirement for program accreditation. A systematic method to assess and improve the performance and interpretation of sonograms must be in place. At a minimum, a mechanism to ensure that inadequate or inconclusive studies are repeated on a timely basis must be in place. Documentation on the quality of the ultrasound examinations and their interpretation must be present, with a mechanism for documentation of the quality of these studies should be developed. There must be a protocol to follow up on abnormal findings both for the accuracy of the interpretation and the appropriate clinical follow-up. This may involve additional or alternate imaging as appropriate. Ideally, a computerized database should be developed to assist in these requirements.

Application for accreditation and site visit

All programs requesting accreditation will require a site visit after the above criteria are documented, but not before 6 months after the program is initiated. This site visit will be performed by a representative of the ASDIN Accreditation Subcommittee. The visitor will review the program with attention to the above requirements and submit a report to the Subcommittee. Next, a recommendation may be made to the ASDIN on the basis of the entire application for accreditation. Once a program achieves accreditation, this shall remain in place for 5 years at which time the training facility may request re-accreditation.

▶ Accreditation for Peritoneal Dialysis Catheter Placement

Peritoneal dialysis is a useful modality for the treatment of end-stage renal disease. Therefore, placement of a catheter and the recognition and treatment of PD catheter problems are necessary skills. As part of its mission statement, the American Society of Diagnostic and Interventional Nephrology recognized the need for training in this area. The accreditation of training facilities in PD catheter insertion and management has emerged as an area of emphasis.[5]

Requirements

As with other ASDIN approved training programs, a facility that trains practitioners in PD catheter placement and management must have adequate funding, an appropriate facility, adequate equipment, a sufficient number of procedures to allow appropriate experience during the training process, and the ability to provide ongoing assessment of the trainee. An active quality assurance program and the ability to assess outcomes of procedures are essential. There must be a sufficient didactic program with accessible training materials.[8]

No specific technique for peritoneal dialysis catheter insertion is mandated, but a facility must have at least two physicians that can perform the procedure by the same technique and who meet the certification criteria set by the American Society for Diagnostic and Interventional Nephrology to apply for accreditation as a training center. This faculty must be committed to the modality of Peritoneal Dialysis and must have a history of placing no less than 50 catheters by the technique that will be taught to the trainees. Each procedure performed must be accompanied by a detailed report that will become part of the patient's permanent record. Each trainee should receive records of the procedures performed with documentation of the outcomes. Maintaining a computerized database is not mandated but is highly recommended.

Ongoing quality assurance is necessary. This should include evaluation of medical necessity, quality, costs, and appropriate solutions to identified problems. Practice guidelines should be developed and monitored. Outcome data should be collected and analyzed on an ongoing basis.

A formalized certification process for each trainee should be established. This should include a minimum of two practice placements, observation of two procedures, and the supervised performance of six procedures followed by a formalized system of monitoring for the first 10 catheter placements of each trainee.[8]

Application for accreditation and site visit

A facility requesting accreditation in Peritoneal Catheter Placement will, after submitting the necessary application materials undergo a site visit by a representative of the Accreditation Subcommittee of the American Society of Diagnostic and Interventional Nephrology. This may not occur until after the program at that center has been in existence for a minimum of 6 months. After submitting the site visit report to the Subcommittee, a recommendation may be made to ASDIN regarding the accreditation. Once a facility achieves accreditation, this shall remain in effect for 3 years after which time a reapplication may be submitted.

INDIVIDUAL CERTIFICATION IN INTERVENTIONAL NEPHROLOGY PROCEDURES

Certification is defined as "a process in which an individual, an institution, or an educational program is evaluated and recognized as meeting certain predetermined standards. Certification is usually made by a nongovernmental agency."[9] Once a practitioner is appropriately trained in an area of diagnostic or interventional nephrology, a level of expertise is desirable for each aspect of care. ASDIN has established certification criteria in the areas of sonography of the kidneys and urinary bladder, insertion of peritoneal dialysis catheters, and endovascular procedures on AV fistulas and grafts and placement of chronic central venous catheters for dialysis.[4] The purpose of certification is to ensure that the standards met are those necessary for safe and ethical practice of the profession or service."[9] This means that "an individual physician has met specified requirements for the performance of a particular procedure."[10]

▶ Process of Individual Certification

A prerequisite for any type of ASDIN certification is that the physician first be Board Certified in Nephrology, Radiology, or Surgery with documentation of ongoing practice in intervention. Certification by the American Society of Diagnostic and Interventional Nephrology involves a three-step process.

1. First, the application is submitted and reviewed by the ASDIN office to ensure that it is complete with

all the necessary documentation. If any information is missing, the applicant is notified and given the opportunity to provide this data.

2. Once the application is complete, the materials are forwarded to the Certification Committee for review and a decision is made regarding the certification of the applicant.

3. Finally, this decision is returned to the ASDIN office for processing and the individual applicant is notified of the decision.[7,8,11]

▶ Criteria for Individual Certification

A physician may apply for certification in the areas of tunneled hemodialysis catheter procedures (insertion, removal, and exchange) as a stand-alone entity or in conjunction with other hemodialysis vascular access procedures (angiography, angioplasty, and thrombolysis/thrombectomy), endovascular stent placement, obliteration of accessory veins and subcutaneous port placement. Each of these areas may be requested upon application. Endovascular stents, obliteration of accessory veins, and placement of subcutaneous ports are considered to be more advanced procedures that are pursued in conjunction with or as an addendum to endovascular procedures.[11] Performance of only five procedures is required for certification in these.

The applicant must provide evidence of formalized training or documentation of sufficient experience in those procedures as an initial basis for certification. Alternately, an applicant may request certification if they have practiced Interventional Nephrology for a minimum of 1 year.

Tunneled catheter procedure certification

For tunneled catheters, one must demonstrate proficiency and experience in catheter removal, catheter insertion, and catheter exchange. Formal training should include a defined curriculum at a qualified facility including didactic training in anatomy and the skills required for these catheter procedures. That training should then include placement of 25 nontunneled catheters and 10 tunneled catheters under the supervision of a qualified interventionalist using an established mechanism to evaluate the trainee during this period. The applicant is then asked to submit 10 reports of tunneled catheter placement as the primary operator. Finally, the applicant must provide peer references. If the physician did a formalized training program, at least one of the references must be from that applicant's trainer. At least one reference should have personal knowledge of the satisfactory performance of at least 25 tunneled catheter placements (not exchanges). Those pursuing certification in the placement of subcutaneous ports must submit documentation of five cases under supervision and provide three case reports as the primary operator.[11]

Hemodialysis and vascular access procedure certification

Hemodialysis vascular access procedures include angiography, angioplasty, and thrombolysis/thrombectomy. An applicant may also request certification in the more advanced techniques of endovascular stent placement, obliteration of accessory veins, and subcutaneous port placement. As with other areas of ASDIN certification, the applicant must provide evidence of formalized training or documentation of sufficient experience in those procedures. Formalized training must include a defined didactic curriculum that includes anatomy, physical examination of the vascular access, radiation safety, appropriate use of imaging equipment, and the basic tools and equipment used in interventional nephrology. The formalized program should also include training in surveillance techniques and monitoring of the vascular access, the safe use of sedation and analgesia, the safe performance of angioplasty of the dialysis access, the performance of thrombolysis/thrombectomy of the dialysis vascular access, and the diagnosis and management of complications when using endovascular techniques. Physicians pursuing certification in the use of endovascular stents or in the obliteration of accessory drainage veins should also be trained in the indications for, performance of and treating the complications of these entities.[11]

The applicant for certification must document the performance of 25 angiographies of the dialysis access (including both grafts and fistulae), 25 angioplasties of the hemodialysis access (including grafts and fistulae), and 25 thrombolysis/thrombectomy cases (including both AV grafts and fistulae). Records documenting the performance (as the primary operator) of 10 AVG angiograms, 10 AVG angioplasties, 10 AVG thrombolysis/thrombectomy procedures, 10 AVF angiograms, 10 AVF angioplasties, and 10 AVF thrombolysis/thrombectomy cases must be submitted. Peer references must be submitted including at least one from a person familiar with the applicant's training and at least one peer with direct knowledge of 25 angiograms, 25 angioplasties, and 25 thrombolysis/thrombectomy cases performed by the applicant.[11]

Peritoneal catheter placement certification

To be certified by ASDIN in this area of intervention, an applicant must demonstrate not only adequate training and experience but also document satisfactory outcomes. The applicant should become adept at one of the accepted techniques for catheter insertion. There is no requirement that the operator use one insertion modality over another. As with any other interventional skill, one must begin with the development of intellectual knowledge by observing the procedure and becoming familiar with the literature in the field. Next, there is a need to practice the technique using models or animals prior to the supervised placement of catheters into patients.[8]

The stated goal of the American Society of Diagnostic and Interventional Nephrology is that each operator desiring certification in PD catheter placement should develop the appropriate dexterity and judgment needed to perform the procedure.[8] Whether the catheter is inserted using a "blind" technique with a needle, guidewire, dilator, and split sheath, using a surgical technique with open dissection, using fluoroscopic guidance,[12] using a peritoneoscope,[13] or using a laparoscopic method, the operator should become familiar with their own capabilities, preferences, and limitations. Certification of an applicant will be based upon training, experience, and expertise in one or more of these insertion methods.

All physicians applying for certification must be certified by the American Board of Internal Medicine in Nephrology and must complete a program of study using either written or audio visual materials related to the procedure.[14,15] The trainee should then spend a minimum of 2 hours practicing the procedure using standard adult Tenckhoff catheters and the equipment normally used in the placement procedure. At least two catheter insertions should be performed in a Dummy Tummy model, an anesthetized dog or pig [in a program certified by an ACUC committee, or in a human cadaver (in a properly certified program)[8]].

The apprentice should then observe the placement of at least two peritoneal catheters in actual patents performed by physician trainers. To qualify for certification, the next step is the insertion of six peritoneal catheters with physician trainers skilled (ideally certified) in the procedure. These catheter placements should be performed within a 1-year period to allow an appropriate training experience and to allow for an adequate evaluation by those trainers. The apprentice is required to maintain a log including the time and date of all placement procedures and must record the outcome of each insertion procedure including catheter function and any problems (including flow failures, infection, and pericatheter leaks) at 1 week and 4 weeks.

Once a physician has accumulated enough experience as required above, the trainers should confirm that the applicant has achieved this goal and that the applicant has gained the appropriate knowledge and skills required for PD catheter placement. While peritoneal catheter placement success is one measure of ability, the applicant should not be penalized for placement failure in a high-risk patient such as those with obesity or preexisting adhesions. The training physician must assess the overall knowledge, experience, judgment, and skill of the apprentice evaluation and must consider any particular issues in performing the procedure including the occurrence of any complications. The applicant must provide a letter of documentation regarding the fulfillment of all of the requirements using the forms provided in the application. This should also be accompanied by the actual case records of peritoneal catheter placement in six patients.[8]

Diagnostic renal ultrasonography certification

A practitioner desiring certification in this area of nephrology must be able to demonstrate an adequate knowledge base as well as sufficient training and experience in both the performance of and the interpretation of studies of the kidney and urinary bladder. Achieving this level of expertise can be accomplished through a formalized training program or the documentation of experience.[5]

Trainees must have a working knowledge of ultrasound physics as it pertains to the performance and interpretation of sonograms. They must have a thorough understanding of the sonographic appearance of both normal renal anatomy with normal anatomic variants as well as the sonographic appearance of renal pathology. Therefore, an extensive background in the clinical presentation of and the natural history of renal disorders is necessary. There must be a thorough understanding of renal pathology with relevant laboratory findings. The ability to perform and interpret urinalysis is a mandatory requirement for certification. To develop this necessary background, the applicant will have generally completed at least 1 year of nephrology training in an accredited postgraduate program as well as specific training in ultrasonography.[7]

Specific training may be done through an accredited ultrasound program and entails a 6-week program devoted to the modality. Alternatively, nephrologists who have completed their postgraduate training may pursue program consisting of a minimum of 50 hours of formal Continuing Medical Education (CME)-accredited instruction that includes both the necessary didactic and hands-on training. This alternative approach must include a minimum of 3 hours devoted to ultrasound physics and instrumentation, 4 hours of instruction in basic ultrasound interpretation and extensive experience performing and interpreting sonography of the native kidney, bladder, and the transplanted kidney.[7]

The criteria for certification set forth by the American Society of Diagnostic and Interventional Nephrology require that the applicant interpret a minimum of 125 studies of which 80 must be supervised within an accredited renal ultrasonography program. These studies must include transplanted kidneys and the urinary bladder. If a training program is not accredited by ASDIN, that program must meet the ASDIN criteria for accreditation at the time of the supervision. Of the 80 supervised studies, at least 40 must be new studies in which the applicant participates in both the performance and the interpretation of the studies and must include the use of ultrasonic guidance for percutaneous renal biopsy. The remainder of the interpretations by the trainee may be previous ultrasounds presented as "unknowns" to be completely interpreted by the trainee. The remaining required experience (45 studies) must be performed and interpreted by the applicant in either a supervised or unsupervised setting. All unsupervised studies (but not more than 20) must be submitted for review with documented follow-up consisting of a CT scan, MR scan, pyelography, or another ultrasound performed and interpreted by an accredited ultrasound practice.[7]

In order to be certain that the applicant has sufficient exposure to a variety of renal anatomy and pathology, the trainee must submit unsupervised studies performed and interpreted after all formal training that consist of the list below. These may be studies done on patients with known abnormalities submitted for the purposes of the application rather than formal studies on patients with unknown disease. The required studies must include: normal kidneys (one study), chronic renal disease (two studies), cysts (two studies), hydronephrosis (two studies), nephrolithiasis (two studies), guidance for percutaneous renal biopsy (one study); renal allograft (at least two studies that must identify the ureter, psoas muscle, peritoneum, real vein, iliac or external iliac vein, and bladder), and measurement of the urinary bladder volume (one study).

Some applicants may elect to pursue certification to the performance and interpretation of sonograms limited to renal transplantation. The overall requirements are the same as those for general certification except that formal didactic training must include 1 hour devoted to the use of ultrasound in renal transplantation and formal hands-on training must be done at a site that is accredited for renal transplant sonography. Cases submitted for review must include at least two normal studies that identify (on at least one transverse and one longitudinal view) the renal allograft, the ureter, the psoas muscle, the peritoneum, the renal vein, the iliac or external iliac vein, and the bladder. The applicant must also submit one study used for ultrasonic guidance for a percutaneous transplant biopsy, three studies demonstrating a perirenal fluid collection, four studies demonstrating hydronephrosis, two studies documenting ureteric stents, and one study measuring the urinary bladder volume.

▶ Hemodialysis Vascular Access Procedure Recertification Criteria for Individuals

Currently, ASDIN has set recertification criteria for vascular access procedures only, and not for peritoneal dialysis catheter or renal ultrasonography.[16] To recertify, the applicants must be currently certified by ASDIN in HVA and actively doing interventional procedures and must be currently Board certified in Surgery, Radiology, or Nephrology. Recertification in HVA procedures will be granted for 5 years. Application can be made for recertification in HVA procedures in either "Broad Category" or "Hemodialysis Catheter Only Category." Each applicant must provide verification that a minimum number of procedures have been performed by the applicant in the past 12 months. Additionally, they must provide documentation of 7 hours of CME in vascular medicine, hemodialysis access, or interventional procedures obtained within the past 3 years. Documentation of current CQI (continuous quality improvement) must also be provided in the past 12 months. A review of personal complication rates for

interventional procedures or minutes of CQI meetings are examples of data that would satisfy this requirement.

THE ASDIN GOVERNANCE FOR ACCREDITATION AND CERTIFICATION

There is a formal process and policy structure set by the American Society of Diagnostic and Interventional Nephrology for accreditation and certification. The established standards have been described above. There is a defined committee, the Credentials Committee, which is composed of at least five members of ASDIN who are appointed by the organization's president on an annual basis. The stated policy for the committee's composition is to have representation from all the major areas of interventional nephrology as adopted by ASDIN. The committee is responsible for the development of those criteria used for certification and recertification of physicians in Diagnostic and Interventional Nephrology, for the development of those criteria for accreditation and reaccreditation, for the establishment of those procedures and policies by which adequate review of applicants for certifications or accreditation is pursued, for the review of the credentials of all physician applicants or program applicants and to subsequently make recommendations to the council of ASDIN in compliance with the bylaws and policies and procedures of ASDIN. The committee is also responsible to make reports to and to advise the Council on matters relating to certification and accreditation. The Council may also refer reports, inquiries, or problems to the committee for review and report. Finally, the committee is required to formulate and periodically review as necessary a Credentials Policy and Procedure Manual to contain all the policies and procedures governing the functions, duties, responsibilities, and procedures of the Credentials Committee.[5]

Meetings of The Credentials committee are held as necessary when called by the committee chair or the president of ASDIN. Of necessity, a permanent record of meetings and business of the committee is maintained. The Credentials Committee may meet in person or telephonically. The committee has a chair and vice chair appointed by the President of ASDIN. In addition, the Credentials Committee may create subcommittees composed of at least three members with expertise in that area for which the subcommittee has been created.[5]

POTENTIAL FUTURE AREAS OF ACCREDITATION AND CERTIFICATION

▶ AV Fistula Creation and Procedures

A patient's vascular access is of vital importance. Many feel that the arteriovenous fistula is the vascular access of choice.[17–21] Since the original description of this surgery was described in 1966,[22] the creation of an AV fistula has been performed by a number of practitioners. In the United States, the majority of fistula creations have been performed by surgeons. More recently, interventional nephrologists in the United States have begun creating fistulae[23] with good outcomes.[24–26] There have not been any accepted standards or certification in this area whether performed by vascular surgeons or interventional nephrologists. Outcomes from these surgeries are variable, and some feel that AV fistula creation should have a defined basis of training and that a level of expertise is vital. Therefore, accreditation of a training program by the American Society of Diagnostic and Interventional Nephrology could make sense. In addition, certification of AV fistula creators by ASDIN could ensure a minimal standard of care and improve the outcomes of the procedure and ultimately the prevalence of fistulae in the United States.

▶ Renal Artery Evaluation and Therapy

Much controversy exists regarding the optimal treatment of renal arterial disease.[27–29] However, imaging of the renal artery still plays a major clinical role.[30] Therefore, the need for adequate training in the performance of appropriate renal artery imaging, interpretation, and intervention is a potential challenge that could be met by the establishment of accreditation of facilities by ASDIN. This could aid in the development of a more standardized approach to the renal artery disease by the practitioners. An obvious next step would then be the development of certification criteria for those performing both the diagnostic evaluation and the endovascular treatment of renal artery disease. The American Society of Diagnostic and Interventional Nephrology is well situated to pursue this.

▶ Formal Subspecialty Certification

Despite a large amount of interest, from young nephrologists in particular, interventional nephrology remains without a dedicated subspecialty certification. Although there is interest in moving toward certification by the American Board of Medical Specialties, at present the volume of interventional nephrologists is low to justify the process and the costs involved in such certification. In future, as the number of practitioners will increase, it is quite likely that a subspecialty fellowship program and certification will be enacted.

REFERENCES

1. Vlăsceanu L, Grünberg L, Pârlea D. Quality *Assurance and Accreditation: A Glossary of Basic Terms and Definitions* (Papers on Higher Education, ISBN 92-9069-178-6. Bucharest, UNESCO-CEPES. 2004.
2. ASDIN, Personal Communication. August 23, 2010.
3. Niyyar VD, Work J. Interventional nephrology: Core Curriculum 2009. *Am J Kid Dis.* 2009;54:169–182.
4. ASDIN Mission Statement. Available at: http://www.ASDIN.org. Accessed April 24, 2011.
5. ASDIN Credentials Committee Policy and Procedure Manual. Available at: http://www.ASDIN.org. Accessed April 24, 2011.
6. O'Neill WC Renal ultrasonography: a procedure for nephrologists. *Am J Kidney Dis.* 1997;30:579–584.
7. ASDIN Application for Accreditation in Training Program in Renal Ultrasound. Available at: http://asdin.org/associations/9795/files/RUSApplicationforApprovalofTrainingProgram3-1-05.pdf. Accessed April 24, 2011.
8. ASDIN Application for Accreditation in Training Program in Interventional Nephrology Procedures (Placement of peritoneal dialysis catheters). Available at: http://asdin.org/associations/9795/files/2004ApplicationforApprovalOfTrainingProgram_peritoneal_dial_cath1-14-04.pdf. Accessed April 24, 2011.
9. Mosby's Medical Dictionary, 8th edition. © 2009, Elsevier.
10. ASDIN Website. Available at: http://www.ASDIN.org/displaycommon.cfm?an=1&subarticlebr=2. Accessed April 24, 2011.
11. ASDIN Application for certification in Hemodialysis Vascular Access Procedures (6/17/2010). Available at: http://asdin.org/associations/9795/files/HVA%20Application%20061710.pdf. Accessed April 24, 2010.
12. Abreo K, Bharat S, Maya I. Fluoroscopic Placement of Peritoneal Dialysis Catheters in ASDIN Core Curriculum for Peritoneal Dialysis Procedures. CreateSpace, January 2011.
13. Packer J, Mishler R. Peritoneoscopic Placement of Peritoneal Dialysis Catheters in ASDIN Core Curriculum for Peritoneal Dialysis Procedures. CreateSpace, January 2011.
14. Ash S. Guidelines for training, certification, and accreditation in placement of permanent tunneled and cuffed peritoneal dialysis catheters. *Semin Dial.* 2002;15:440–442.
15. Ash SR. Who should place peritoneal catheters? A nephrologist's view. *Nephrol News Issues.* 1993;7:33–34.
16. Hemodialysis Vascular Access Procedure Recertification Criteria. Available at: http://asdin.org/displaycommon.cfm?an=1&subarticlenbr=123. Accessed April 24, 2011.
17. Fistula First: *National Vascular Access Improvement Initiative,* July, 2003.
18. Nasser GM, Ayus JC. Infectious complications of the hemodialysis access. *Kidney Int.* 2001;60:1–13.
19. Dhingra RK, Young EW, Hulbert-Shearon TE, Leavey SF, Port FK. Type of vascular access and mortality in US hemodialysis patients. *Kidney Int.* 2001;60:1443–1451.
20. Woods JD, Turenne MN, Strawderman RL, Young EW, Hirth RA, Port FK, et al. Vascular access survival among incident hemodialysis patients in the United States. *Am J Kidney Dis.* 1997;30:50–57.
21. Allon M, Robbin ML. Increasing arteriovenous fistulas in hemodialysis patients: problems and solutions. *Kidney Int.* 2002;62:1109–1124.
22. Brescia MJ, Cimino JE, Appel K, Hurwich BJ. Chronic hemodialysis using venopuncture and a surgically created arteriovenous fistula. *N Engl J Med.* 1966;275:1089–1092.
23. Sreenarasimhaiah V, Ravani P. Arteriovenous fistula surgery: an American perspective from Italy. *Semin Dial.* 2005;18:6.
24. Packer, J. Fistula creation by interventional nephrologists, the next generation. *Semin in Dial.* 2008;21:107.
25. Packer J, Wang S, Mishler R. *Unconventional Fistula Creation. Is KDOQI Misleading?.* Poster Presentation 6th Annual ASDIN Scientific Meeting, Orlando, FL. February 19–21, 2010.

26. Mishler R, Yevzlin AS. Outcomes of arteriovenous fistulae created by a U.S. interventional nephrologist. *Semin in Dial.* 2010;23:224–228.

27. Dworkin LD, Jamerson KA. Case against angioplasty and stenting of atherosclerotic renal artery stenosis. *Circulation.* 2007;115:271–276.

28. Balk E, Raman G, Chung M, Ip S, Tatsioni A, Alonso A, Chew P, Gilbert SJ, Lau J. Effectiveness of management strategies for renal artery stenosis: a systematic review. *Ann Intern Med.* 2006;145:901.

29. Levin A, Linas SL, Luft FC, Chapman AB, Textor SC. Controversies in renal artery stenosis: A review by the American Society of Nephrology Advisory Group on Hypertension. *Am J Nephrol.* 2007;27:212–220.

30. Yevzlin A. Renal artery stenosis: An Interventional Nephrologist's Perspective. Presented at the 6th Annual ASDIN Scientific Meeting, Orlando, FL. Feb 19–21, 2010.

SECTION III
Principles of Practice and Techniques

10

BASIC ANATOMY FOR DIALYSIS VASCULAR ACCESS

GERALD A. BEATHARD

BASIC ANATOMY FOR DIALYSIS VASCULAR ACCESS

A basic knowledge of vascular anatomy especially that of the arm, thorax, and thigh is essential to the interventionalist managing dialysis vascular access problems. Detailed knowledge of both normal anatomy and its commonly occurring variants is critical. When passing a guidewire under fluoroscopic guidance, one must be able to recognize the vessel that is being entered. At times guidewires enter an area where it has not been possible to visualize the vessel prior to passage. It is also important to be able to recognize if the guidewire is following the expected course of a known vessel, if it is not, there may be a problem.

DEFINITIONS AND CONVENTIONS

The following definitions and conventions are provided to present a consistent set of terms that will be used throughout this chapter:

Downstream—flow in the normal direction within that vessel, also antegrade.

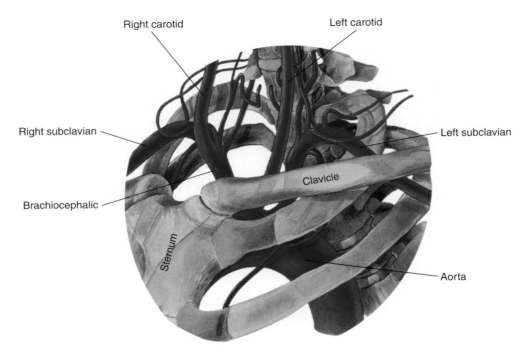

Figure 10-1. Arterial branches of the aortic arch.

Upstream—flow in the opposite direction of normal within that vessel, also retrograde.

Collateral—a secondary route of blood flow because of obstruction in the primary pathway, generally indicative of pathology, ie, downstream obstruction.

Proximal—the more central aspect of any vessel will be referred to as its proximal aspect, also central.

Distal—the more peripheral aspect of any vessel will be referred to as its distal aspect, also distal.

Central vessels—as related to the upper extremity, those vessels that lay within the bony thorax, starting with the subclavian; as related to the lower extremity, those vessels that lay within the bony pelvis, starting at the inguinal ligament.

Peripheral vessels—as related to the upper extremity, those vessels that lay peripheral to the bony thorax starting with the axillary; as related to the lower extremity, those vessels that lay peripheral to the bony pelvis, starting at the inguinal ligament.

VASCULAR ANATOMY RELATED TO UPPER EXTREMITY—ARTERIAL

▶ Central Arteries of Thorax

Thoracic aorta

The major vessel in the central group of arteries is the **thoracic aorta**. The initial part of the aorta, the **ascending aorta**, rises out of the left ventricle. The aorta then arches back over the right pulmonary artery. As it descends, it is situated on the left of the vertebral column; it approaches the median line as it descends; and, at its termination, it lies directly in front of the column. Three vessels come out of the aortic arch, the **brachiocephalic artery**, the **left common carotid artery**, and the **left subclavian artery** (Figure 10-1).

To the right of the thoracic aorta and running parallel and partially behind it is the **superior vena cava**. As discussed below, the **left brachiocephalic vein** crosses over the midline anterior to the vessels of the **aortic arch** and normally lies somewhat superior to the arch (Figure 10-1). As patients age, the aortic arch (entire aorta) and its branches may become somewhat ectatic and eventually begin to compress the **left brachiocephalic vein** because of is close proximity.

Brachiocephalic artery

The **brachiocephalic artery** is the first branch of the **aortic arch**, and soon after it emerges, the **brachiocephalic artery** divides into the **right common carotid artery** and the **right subclavian artery** (Figure 10-1). There is no brachiocephalic artery for the left side of the body. The **left common carotid** and the **left subclavian artery**, come directly off the **aortic arch** (Figure 10-1). However, there are two brachiocephalic veins as will be discussed later.

The **brachiocephalic artery** arises, on a level with the upper border of the second right costal cartilage, from the commencement of the arch of the aorta, on a plane anterior to the origin of the left carotid; it ascends obliquely upward, backward, and to the right to the level

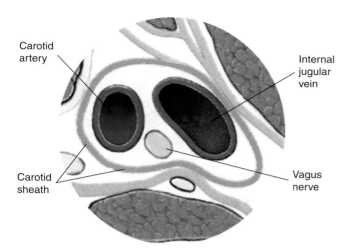

Figure 10-2. Structures of the carotid sheath.

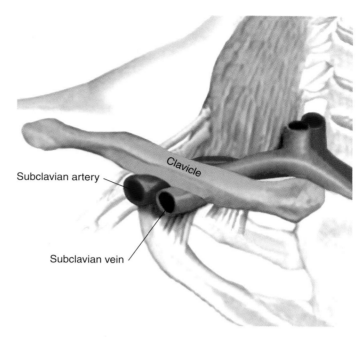

Figure 10-3. Relationship of subclavian with clavicle.

of the upper border of the right sternoclavicular articulation, where it divides into the **right common carotid** and **right subclavian arteries**. It usually gives off no branches.

Common carotid artery

The **common carotid artery** is a paired structure (Figure 10-1). The left and right common carotid arteries follow the same course with the exception of their origin. The **right common carotid** originates in the neck from the brachiocephalic trunk. The **left common carotid** arises from the aortic arch in the thoracic region. The cervical portions of the common carotids resemble each other so closely that one description will apply to both.

Each vessel passes obliquely upward, from behind the sternoclavicular joint to the level of the upper border of the thyroid cartilage, where it divides. The **common carotid artery** is contained in a sheath known as the **carotid sheath** (Figure 10-2), which is derived from the **deep cervical fascia** and encloses also the **internal jugular vein** and **vagus nerve**, the vein lying lateral to the artery, and the nerve between the artery and vein, on a plane posterior to both. On opening the sheath, each of these three structures is seen to have a separate fibrous investment.

At approximately the level of the **fourth cervical vertebra**, the **common carotid** artery bifurcates into an **internal carotid artery** and an **external carotid artery**.

Subclavian artery

On the left side of the body, the **subclavian artery** comes directly off the arch of **aorta**. On the right side of the body, the **subclavian artery** arises from the relatively short **brachiocephalic artery** when it bifurcates into the **subclavian** and the **right common carotid artery**.

From its origin, the **subclavian artery** travels laterally, passing between anterior and middle scalene muscles,

with the anterior scalene on its anterior side and the middle scalene on its posterior. This is in contrast to the **subclavian vein**, which travels anterior to the scalenus anterior. As the **subclavian artery** crosses the border of the first rib, it becomes the **axillary artery**.

It ascends a little above the clavicle, the extent to which it does so varying in different cases. Below and behind the artery is the pleura, which separates it from the apex of the lung. The terminal part of the artery lies behind the clavicle (Figure 10-3). The **subclavian vein** is in front of and at a slightly lower level than the artery. Behind, it lies on the lowest trunk of the **brachial plexus**, which intervenes between it and the middle scalene muscle. Below, it rests on the upper surface of the first rib.

▶ Peripheral Arteries of the Upper Extremity

Axillary artery

The **axillary artery** extends from the lateral border of the first rib to the lower border of the teres major muscle. Because the lower limiting landmark is not visible by X-ray, the junction between it and the **brachial artery** cannot be accurately defined radiologically. The **axillary artery** is continuous with the subclavian above and with the brachial below (Figure 10-4). It passes through the axillary fossa and is accompanied by the **axillary vein** along its length. In the axilla, it is surrounded by the **brachial plexus**. The distal third of the axillary artery is relatively superficial, being covered only by the skin and the superficial and deep fascia.

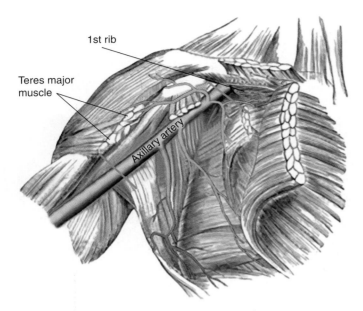

Figure 10-4. Axillary artery (between green lines).

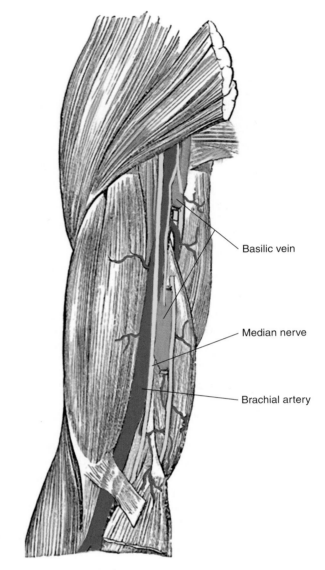

Figure 10-5. Brachial artery.

Brachial artery

The **brachial artery** is the continuation of the axillary artery beyond the lower margin of **teres major** muscle. It continues down the ventral surface of the arm until it reaches a point slightly below the center of the crease at the bend of the elbow (Figure 10-5). At this point, the brachial artery divides into the **radial artery** (lateral) and the **ulnar artery** (medial), which run down the forearm. In some individuals, the bifurcation occurs much higher and the **ulnar** and **radial arteries** extend through the upper arm.

The **brachial artery** is at first medial to the humerus, but as it passes down the arm it gradually passes in front of the bone. At the bend of the elbow, it generally lies midway between the two epicondyles of the humerus.

The **brachial artery** is closely related to the **median nerve** (Figure 10-5). In the upper arm, the **median nerve** is immediately lateral to the **brachial artery**. Distally, the **median nerve** crosses the medial side of the **brachial artery** and lies somewhat anterior to the elbow joint. The **brachial artery** is closely related to the **brachial veins** (Figure 10-6). These are paired veins, one on either side of the artery.

Accessory brachial artery—This is a variant in arterial anatomy that can cause confusion when the brachial artery is used for the creation of a dialysis access. This artery originates above the elbow level from the upper third of the **brachial artery**. It crosses anterior to the **median nerve** to rejoin the brachial artery proximal to the elbow, before its division into **ulnar** and **radial arteries** (Figure 10-7).

The incidence of this variation has been reported to be about 0.52% of patients or 1 in every 200 cases.[1] On dissection, it can be distinguished from the true **brachial** artery by its relationship with the **median nerve**. The **accessory brachial artery** crosses anterior to the median nerve. The normal **brachial artery** is crossed anteriorly by the nerve (ie, it lies posterior). As can be seen in Figure 10-7, the nerve actually lies between the two vessels.

Ulnar artery

The **ulnar artery** is the larger of the two terminal branches of the brachial (Figure 10-8). It terminates in the **palmar arches**, which join with the branches of the **radial artery**. Along its course, it is accompanied by similarly named veins, the **ulnar veins**, one of either side of the artery. The **ulnar artery**, the larger of the two terminal branches of the **brachial**, generally begins a little below the bend of the elbow, and, passing obliquely downward, reaches the ulnar side of the forearm at a point about midway

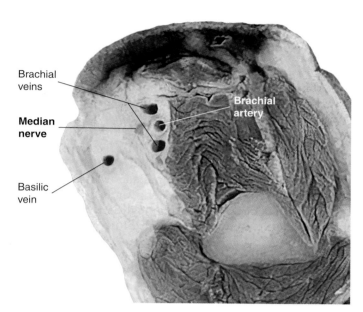

Figure 10-6. Cross-sectional anatomy of the left upper arm at the mid-humerus level (medial on left).

between the elbow and the wrist. It then runs along the ulnar border to the wrist.

At the wrist, the **ulnar artery** crosses the **transverse carpal ligament** on the radial side of the **pisiform bone**, and immediately beyond this bone divides into two branches. These branches enter into the formation of the **superficial** palmar arch and **deep palmar arch** in conjunction with the **radial artery** (Figure 10-9).

Radial artery

The **radial artery** arises from the bifurcation of the **brachial artery** at the elbow (Figure 10-8). It runs distally on the anterior part of the forearm. The **radial artery** runs, at first curving laterally, along the radial side of the forearm as far as the **styloid process**, then curving over the lateral and back part of the wrist it passes through the **anatomical snuff box**. When it enters the hand, it becomes the **deep palmar arch**, which joins with the deep branch of the **ulnar artery**. Along its course, the radial artery is accompanied by similarly named paired veins, the **radial veins**. These lie on either side of the artery.

Superficial palmar branch of the radial artery—The **superficial palmar branch of the radial artery** arises from the **radial artery**, just where this vessel is about to wind around the lateral side of the wrist. Running forward, it passes through, occasionally over, the **thenar muscles**, which it supplies, and sometimes anastomoses with the terminal portion of the **ulnar artery**, completing the **superficial palmar arch**. (Figure 10-9).

This vessel varies considerably in size: usually it is very small, and ends in the muscles of the thumb; sometimes it is as large as the continuation of the radial artery itself.

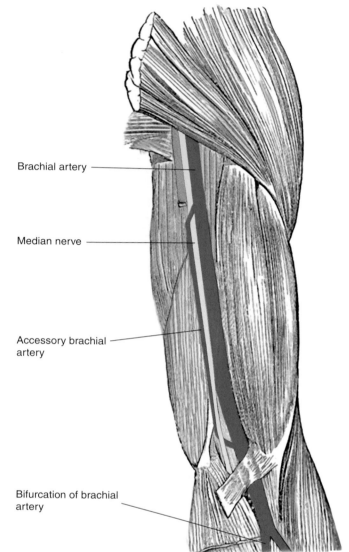

Figure 10-7. Accessory brachial artery.

Its exact point of origin from the radial artery is also somewhat variable. This can be important in cases when the proposed treatment for a radial based access steal is occlusion of the distal radial. If the occlusion is downstream from this vessel's origin, ischemia to the thenar muscles may result.

Palmar arches

There are two **palmar arches**, a **superficial arch** and a deep arch. Both represent communications between the **distal ulnar** and **radial arteries**.

Superficial palmar arch—The **superficial palmar arch** is formed predominantly by the ulnar artery, with a contribution from the **superficial palmar branch** of the **radial artery**. However, in some individuals, the contribution from the **radial artery** may be absent or very small. The

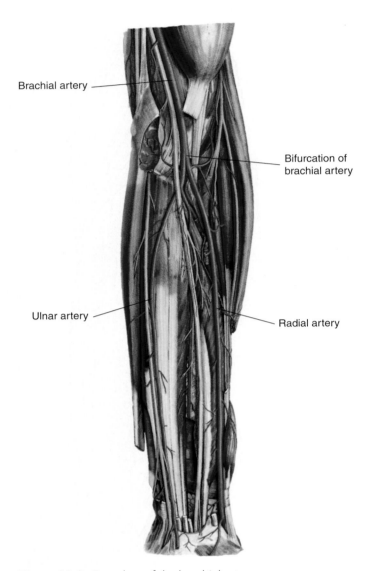

Brachial artery

Bifurcation of brachial artery

Ulnar artery

Radial artery

Figure 10-8. Branches of the brachial artery.

superficial palmar arch is more distal than the deep palmar arch. If one fully extends the thumb, the superficial palmar arch would lie approximately at the level of a line drawn from the distal border of the thumb horizontally across the palm. Three **common palmar digital arteries** arise from the arch, proceeding down on the second, third, and fourth **lumbrical muscles**, respectively. Near the level of the metacarpophalangeal joints, each **common palmar digital artery** divides into two **proper palmar digital arteries** (Figure 10-9).

Deep palmar arch—The **deep palmar arch (deep volar arch)** is an arterial network found in the palm. It is usually formed mainly from the terminal part of the **radial artery**, with the **ulnar artery** contributing via its **deep palmar branch**.

The deep palmar arch lies upon the bases of the metacarpal bones. The **superficial palmar arch** is more distally located than the **deep palmar arch**. The deep palmar arch is about a finger width proximal to the **superficial arch**, just distal to the heads of the **metacarpal bones**. From the deep palmar arch emerge **palmar metacarpal arteries** (Figure 10-9).

Palmar arch variants—The **superficial palmar arch** is most easily classified into two categories: complete or incomplete.[2] An arch is considered to be complete if an anastomosis is found between the vessels constituting it. An incomplete arch has an absence of a communication or anastomosis between the vessels constituting the arch (Figure 10-10). An incomplete superficial arch is seen in approximately 15%. The **deep palmar arch** is less variable.

An incomplete arch can be a problem with instrumentation of the radial artery. Additionally, evaluation of the patency of the arch using Doppler or a pulse oximeter can give misleading results.

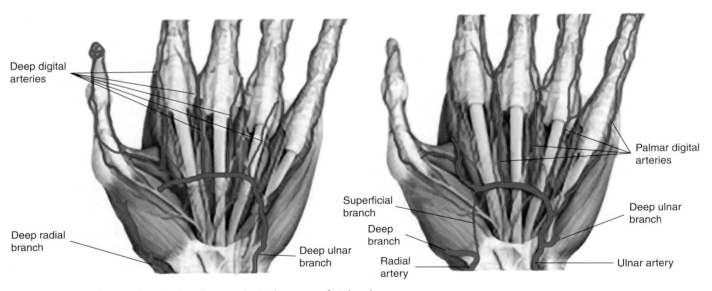

Deep digital arteries

Deep radial branch

Deep ulnar branch

Palmar digital arteries

Superficial branch

Deep branch

Radial artery

Deep ulnar branch

Ulnar artery

Figure 10-9. Palmar arches. Left—deep arch. Right—superficial arch.

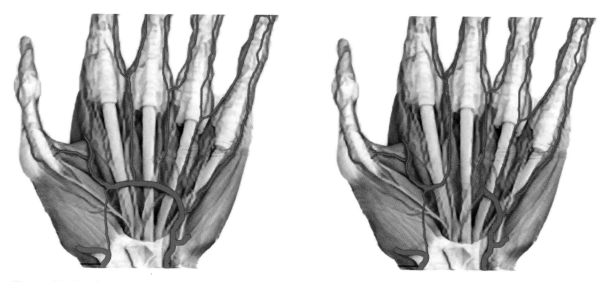

Figure 10-10. Comparison between complete (left) and incomplete (right) superficial palmar arches.

VASCULAR ANATOMY RELATED TO UPPER EXTREMITY—VENOUS

▶ Peripheral Veins of the Upper Extremity

There are two sets **peripheral veins** in the arm—the **superficial veins** and the **deep veins**. The superficial veins are the most important for dialysis vascular access considerations. These veins are contained in the subcutaneous tissue and the deep fascia. They do not accompany arteries. The deep veins do accompany the arteries and have the same relationships to adjacent structures as do those vessels. They are named for the accompanying artery (Figure 10-11). The superficial and the deep veins communicate at frequent intervals. These communications offer the opportunity for the formation of collaterals in the case of downstream obstruction.

Deep veins

These deep veins are also referred to as **vena comitans**, which is Latin for accompanying vein. Deep veins are paired, with one of the pair lying on either side of their accompanying artery and in close proximity to it. Because of valves allowing only forward flow within the vein, the pulsations of the artery actually aid venous return. There are frequent communications between these paired veins that cross the artery. Because they are generally found in pairs, they are often referred to by their plural form: **venae comitantes**.

Superficial veins of the upper extremity

The superficial veins of the arm begin in two irregular plexuses (Figure 10-12), one in the palm (**volar venous**

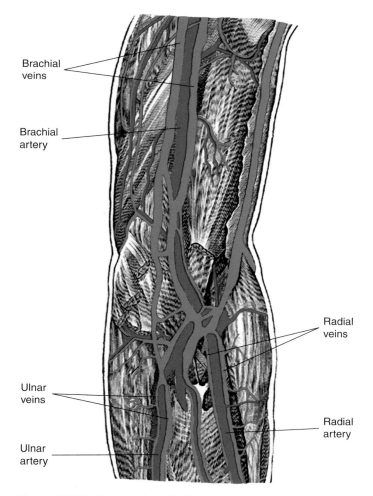

Figure 10-11. Deep veins of left arm.

Brachial veins

Brachial artery

Radial veins

Ulnar veins

Radial artery

Ulnar artery

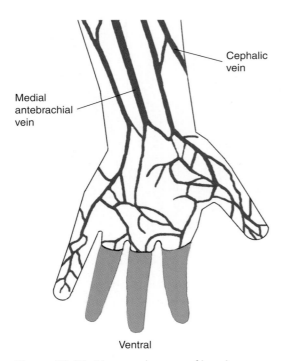

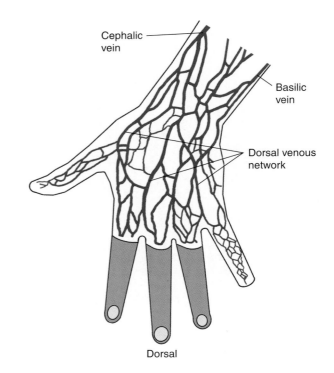

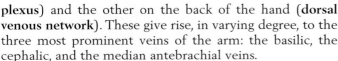

Figure 10-12. Venous plexuses of hand.

plexus) and the other on the back of the hand (**dorsal venous network**). These give rise, in varying degree, to the three most prominent veins of the arm: the basilic, the cephalic, and the median antebrachial veins.

Basilic vein—The **basilic vein** arises on the back of the hand on the medial (ulnar) side by a coalescing of the **dorsal venous network** (Figures 10-12 and 10-13). From there, it curves around the ulnar or medial side of the forearm. It generally lies on posterior–medial or the medial aspect of the forearm in the subcutaneous fat and other fasciae that lie superficial to the muscles of the upper extremity. Because of this, it is usually visible through the skin. The layout of superficial veins in the forearm is highly variable from person to person, and there are generally a variety of other unnamed superficial veins that the basilic vein communicates with in the forearm (**accessory veins**). The major vein is designated as the **basilic**. The remaining veins are referred to as **accessory veins**.

The **basilic vein** curves around the medial side of the forearm as it approaches the elbow to lie on the volar surface just distal to the elbow. It crosses the elbow anterior to the medial epicondyle of the humerus and enters the upper arm. In the upper arm, the **basilic vein** lies in **the median bicipital sulcus**. It extends up about one-third of the sulcus where it then pierces the **brachial fascia** (Figures 10-14). In the proximal third of the upper arm, near the axilla, the **basilic vein** typically joins with the **brachial venous system** to form the **axillary vein**. During its course in the upper arm, it makes several venous communications with the **brachial veins**.

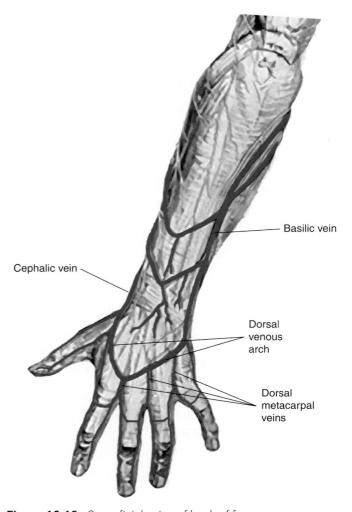

Figure 10-13. Superficial veins of back of forearm.

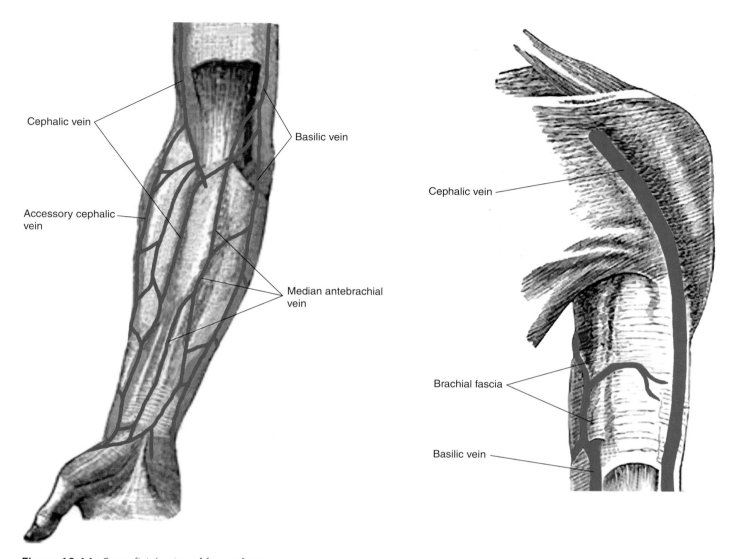

Figure 10-14. Superficial veins of front of arm.

There are variations in the anatomy of the **brachial vein**. In about one-third of the cases, the **basilic vein** joins with the **brachial venous system** in the middle or lower third of the upper arm. In some of these, the **brachial veins** are paired and come together in the upper third of the arm to form the **axillary vein**. In other instances, there is only a single unpaired **brachial vein** above the level of convergence with the **basilic vein**. This single vein is continuous with the **axillary vein** proximally.

Cephalic vein—The **cephalic vein** begins on the back of the hand on the radial side. It curves around the radial border of the forearm (Figures 10-12 and 10-14). It generally comes to lie on the ventral surface of the forearm, a short distance above the wrist. As was the case with the basilic, if there are several veins present, the major one is designated as the cephalic. The remaining veins are referred to as **accessory veins** (Figure 10-14). Although variable, one of these is constant enough to be named the **accessory cephalic vein** (Figure 10-14). The **cephalic vein** passes over the ventral

surface of the elbow where it connects with the **median antecubital vein** (Figure 10-14), which joins it to the **basilic vein**. It lies in the **lateral bicipital** sulcus just above the elbow (Figure 10-14). In the upper arm, the cephalic vein comes to lie in the groove (**deltopectoral grove**) between the **deltoid** and the **pectoralis major** muscles. Just below the clavicle, it turns to run deeper to empty into the axillary vein just before that vein becomes the **subclavian** (Figure 10-15). This region is referred to as the cephalic arch.

Cephalic arch—The **cephalic arch** is an anatomical area that is very problematic in dialysis vascular access. Some of the difficult encountered is undoubtedly related to its anatomy. As the proximal portion of this vein approaches its final destination, it creates a swan-neck type of curve (Figure 10-15) and passes though the **clavipectoral fascia**. This is a dense membrane occupying the interval between the **pectoralis minor** muscle and the **subclavian vessels**. It lies over the **axillary vessels** and nerves. It is pierced by the **cephalic vein, thoracoacromial artery** and

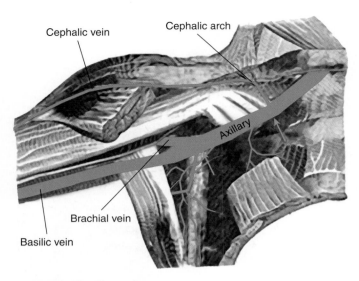

Figure 10-15. The axillary vein.

vein, and **lateral pectoral nerve**. The density of this fascial membrane and the fact that it is accompanied by other structures of significant size as it passes though the foramen may prove problematic when this vein is called upon to dilate with the increased flow associated with a functioning dialysis access.

Median antebrachial vein—The **median antebrachial vein** drains the venous plexus on the volar surface of the hand (Figure 10-14). It ascends on the ulnar side of the front of the forearm and ends in the **basilic vein** or in

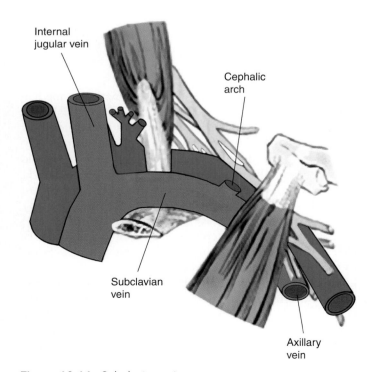

Figure 10-16. Subclavian vein.

the **median antecubital vein**; in a small proportion of cases, it divides into two branches, one of which joins the **basilic**, the other the **cephalic**, below the elbow. Because it is generally not quite as prominently visible as the **basilic** and **cephalic veins**, it is often ignored by the venipuncturist. This makes it a good candidate for vascular access creation. As with the other superficial veins, it has perforating branches that communicate with the **deep veins**. Additionally, it lies immediately over the proximal **radial artery**. These anatomical relationships make the creation of a fistula a simple process by simply connecting a perforating vein to the adjacent artery.

Axillary vein—The **axillary vein** is formed by the union of the **basilic vein** and the **brachial veins** (Figure 10-15). Anatomically it begins at the inferior border of the **teres major muscle**; however, this landmark is not visible radiographically. This makes the designation of the axillary somewhat arbitrary if viewed fluoroscopically. It accompanies the **axillary artery** through the axillary fossa, lying to its medial side and on a slightly anterior plane. At the lateral border of the first rib, it becomes the **subclavian vein**. This is the point at which the axillary is joined by the **cephalic arch** (Figure 10-15).

▶ **Central Veins of Thorax**

The veins that lie within the bony thorax are the subclavian vein, the brachiocephalic vein, and the superior vena cava. The **internal jugular vein** and the **external jugular vein** are not, strictly speaking, central veins. However, their place within this classification is not important. They are generally thought of as central veins.

Subclavian vein

The **subclavian vein** is a direct continuation of the **axillary vein** and runs from the outer border of the first rib to the medial border of **anterior scalene muscle** (Figure 10-16). From here, it joins with the **internal jugular vein** to form the **brachiocephalic vein**. When examining a venous angiogram, the identifying landmarks for the subclavian vein (Figure 10-16) are its junction with the **cephalic arch** (distally) and its junction with the **internal jugular vein** (proximally). The **subclavian vein** follows the course of the **subclavian artery** and is separated from it posteriorly by the insertion of **anterior scalene muscle**. The **subclavian vein** passes anterior to the **scalenus anterior**. The vein passes behind the clavicle as it courses centrally. It is in front of and at a slightly lower level than the **subclavian artery** (Figure 10-3).

The **external jugular vein** joins the **subclavian vein** at about the mid-point of the clavicle. This junction is lateral to or in front of the **scalenus anterior**. The **thoracic duct** drains into the left **subclavian vein**, near its junction with the left **internal jugular vein**. The much smaller **right lymphatic duct** drains its lymph into the junction of the right **internal jugular vein**, and the right **subclavian vein**.

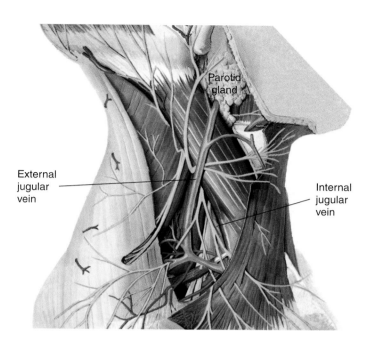

Figure 10-17. External jugular vein.

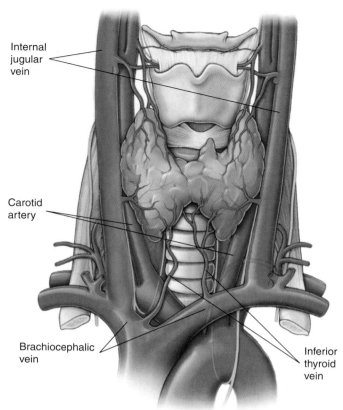

Figure 10-18. Internal jugular vein.

External jugular vein

The **external jugular vein** receives the greater part of the blood from the exterior of the cranium and the deep parts of the face (Figure 10-17). It commences in the substance of the **parotid gland**, on a level with the **angle of the mandible**, and runs perpendicularly down the neck (Figure 10-17), in the direction of a line drawn from the angle of the mandible to the middle of the clavicle at the posterior border of the **sternocleidomastoid muscle**.

In its course, the **external jugular vein** crosses the sternocleidomastoideus obliquely, perforates the deep fascia, and ends in the **subclavian vein** lateral to or in front of the **scalenus anterior muscle**. The vein is covered by the **platysma**, the superficial fascia, and the integument.

The **external jugular vein** varies considerably in size, bearing an inverse proportion to the other veins of the neck, it is occasionally double. It is provided with two pairs of **valves**, the lower pair being placed at its entrance into the **subclavian vein**, the upper in most cases about 4 cm above the **clavicle**. The portion of vein between the two sets of valves is often dilated, and is termed the sinus. These valves do not prevent the regurgitation of blood or the passage of a radiocontrast injection from below upward.

Internal jugular vein

The **internal jugular vein** begins in the posterior compartment of the **jugular foramen**, at the base of the skull. At its origin, it is somewhat dilated, and this dilatation is called the superior bulb. The **internal jugular vein** runs down the side of the neck in a vertical direction (Figure 10-18), being at one end lateral to the **internal**

carotid artery, and then lateral to the **common carotid** and slightly more superficial in its normal configuration. However, there is significant variability[3] in the relationship of the position of the internal jugular vein to the carotid artery (Figure 10-19). At the root of the neck, it

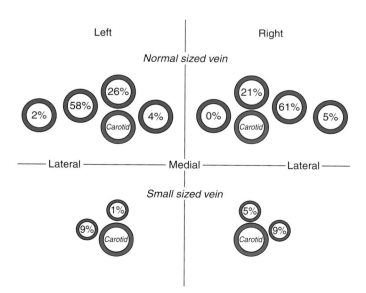

Figure 10-19. Variability in internal jugular vein in population of 104 ESRD patients.[3]

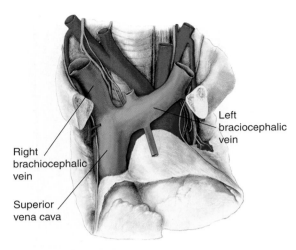

Figure 10-20. Brachiocephalic veins.

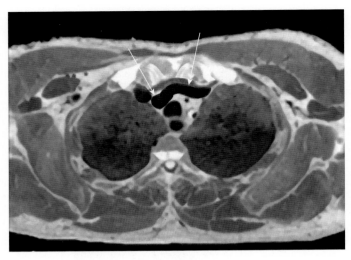

Figure 10-21. Cross-sectional anatomy through course of left brachiocephalic. The anteriorly directed curve that the vessel makes is evident is this sequence (arrows).

unites with the **subclavian vein** at a point a little lateral to the sternoclavicular articulation to form the **brachiocephalic vein** (Figure 10-18); a little above its termination is a second dilatation, the **inferior bulb**. The **vagus nerve** descends between and behind the jugular vein and the carotid artery in the carotid sheath (Figure 10-2).

At the root of the neck, the **right internal jugular vein** is a little distance from the **common carotid artery**, and crosses the first part of the **subclavian artery**, while the **left internal jugular vein** usually overlaps the **common carotid artery**. The left vein is generally smaller than the right, and each contains a pair of **valves**, which are placed about 2.5 cm above the termination of the vessel.

Brachiocephalic veins

The **brachiocephalic veins** are two large trunks, placed one on either side of the root of the neck (Figure 10-20), and formed by the union of the **internal jugular** and **subclavian veins** of the corresponding side. Except for these features they are totally different in their relationships.

Right brachiocephalic vein—The **right brachiocephalic vein** is a short vessel, about 2.5 cm in length, which begins behind the sternal end of the clavicle. It passes almost vertically downward. If a vertical line were to be drawn through the long axis of the **right internal jugular vein** and the **right brachiocephalic vein**, it would extend on downward through the **superior vena cava** to the **right atrium**.

It joins with the **left brachiocephalic vein** just below the cartilage of the first rib, close to the right border of the sternum, to form the **superior vena cava**. It lies in front and to the right of the **brachiocephalic artery**. On its right side is the pleura, which is interposed between it and the apex of the lung. If this vein is perforated laterally, bleeding into the pleural space will result.

Left brachiocephalic vein—The **left brachiocephalic vein** is about 6 cm in length. It begins behind the sternal end

of the **clavicle** and runs obliquely downward and to the right behind the upper half of the **manubrium** to the sternal end of the first **right costal cartilage**, where it unites with the **right brachiocephalic vein** to form the **superior vena cava**. Behind it are the three large arteries, **brachiocephalic, left common carotid**, and **left subclavian**, arising from the **aortic arch**, together with the **vagus and phrenic nerves**.

If a line were to be drawn from the **left internal jugular vein** through the **left brachiocephalic vein** and on through the **superior vena cava** to the **right atrium**, it would be characterized by a series of three curves. Two of these are in the vertical plane as the course transitions from the **left internal jugular** to the **superior vena cava**. These are easily appreciated in the usual radiological view. The third curve is not; however, this lies in the horizontal plane and is created by the **left brachiocephalic vein** crossing over the anatomical structures of the midline (Figure 10-21).

The **left brachiocephalic vein** receives the **left superior intercostal vein**. This is the vein that drains the upper **intercostal veins** on the left. When there is central vein obstruction central to the insertion of this vein into the **left brachiocephalic**, it becomes one possible route for collateral flow. In these instances it can enlarge considerably.

Superior vena cava

The **superior vena cava** drains the blood from the upper half of the body. It measures about 7 cm in length, and is formed by the junction of the two **brachiocephalic veins** (Figures 10-20 and 10-22). It begins immediately below the cartilage of the **right first rib** close to the **sternum** and, descending vertically behind the first and second intercostal spaces, ends in the upper part of the **right**

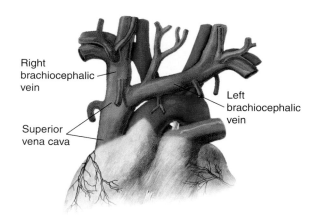

Figure 10-22. Superior vena cava.

atrium. The lower half of the vessel is within the **pericardium**. Just before it pierces the **pericardium**, it receives the **azygos vein**.

The location of junction between the **superior vena cava** and the **right atrium** is of importance to those dealing with dialysis vascular access. When a dialysis catheter is being used, it is recommended that the tip be located at or slightly below this junction. Unfortunately, this anatomical structure is not apparent with the usual fluoroscopic examination; it must be estimated by viewing the composite of structures that create the lateral **cardiac silhouette**. A good estimate of the location can be obtained by moving down the lateral cardiac silhouette approximately one-third.

Left sided superior vena cava—**A persistent** left superior vena cava **has been observed in 0.3–0.5% of the general population. This is a congenital anomaly.** During embryological development, two short transverse veins, the **common cardinal veins (ducts of Cuvier)**, appear (Figure 10-23). These are two short transverse veins that open, one on either side, into the **sinus venosus**. Each of these ducts receives an ascending and descending vein. The ascending veins are called right and left **posterior cardinal veins**. The descending veins are called right and left **anterior cardinal veins**. During morphogenesis, the **sinus venosus** becomes the **coronary sinus**. The upper portion of the left anterior cardinal vein becomes the internal jugular. The lower portion is comparable to the right-sided structure that becomes the superior vena cava. Normally, this obliterates in late embryonic or early fetal life (Figure 10-23). Failure of obliteration results in persistent **left superior vena cava**.

The persistent **left superior vena cava** may be connected to the **coronary sinus** or to the **left atrium**. In cases of connection to the **coronary sinus**, this sinus is enlarged and opens into the **right atrium**. These patients

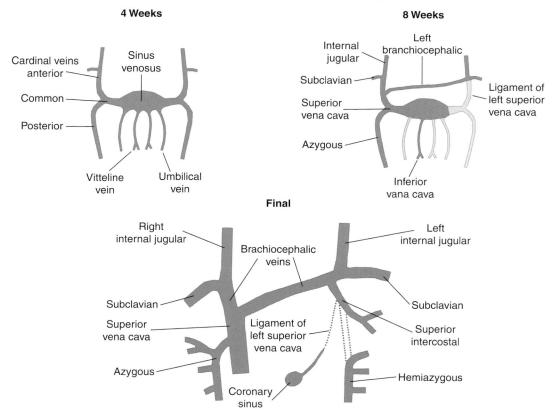

Figure 10-23. Morphogenesis of central veins of thorax.

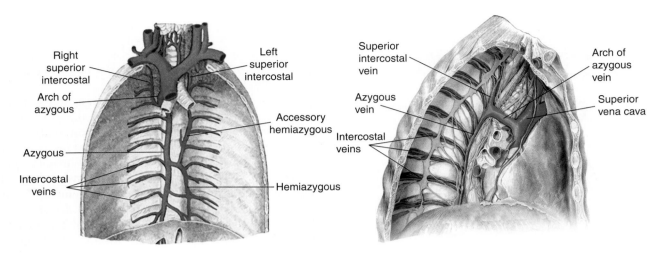

Figure 10-24. Azygos system.

are asymptomatic. The most common variation, present in 82.2% of reports, is the presence of both a left- and right-sided **superior vena cava**. In 8% of cases, the coronary sinus is absent and the vein drains into the left atrium. This is generally associated with a right-to-left shunt and cyanosis. It is commonly accompanied by an atrial septal defect, arrhythmias, and other cardiac malformations. Other variants include the presence or absence of the **left brachiocephalic vein**. Occasionally, the right **superior vena cava** is missing.

Azygos system

The **azygos system** of veins (Figure 10-24) is considered to be the **azygos vein**, along with its left-sided counterparts, the **hemiazygos vein** and the **accessory hemiazygos vein**. If obstruction of the central veins occurs, the **azygos and hemiazygos veins** are one of the principal routes for collateral flow of blood from the upper extremities back to the heart. They represent a possible connection between the **superior and inferior venæ cavæ**, and with the **common iliac veins** by the **ascending lumbar veins** as well as many of the tributaries of the inferior vena cava.

Azygos vein—The **azygos vein** (Figure 10-24) begins opposite the first or second lumbar vertebra. It enters the thorax through the aortic hiatus in the diaphragm, and passes along the right side of the vertebral column to the fourth thoracic vertebra, where it arches forward over the root of the right lung (**arch of the azygos**) and ends in the superior vena cava, just before that vessel pierces the pericardium. As a rare anatomical variation, the **arch of the azygos** (Figure 10-24) can be displaced laterally, thereby creating a pleural septum separating an azygos lobe from the upper lobe of the right lung.

The **azygos vein** receives the **right subcostal and intercostal veins**, the upper three or four of these latter opening by a common stem, the right **superior intercostal vein**. It receives the **hemiazygos veins** and often the **accessory hemiazygos vein**.

Hemiazygos vein—The **hemiazygos vein** (Figure 10-24) begins in the **left ascending lumbar** or **renal vein**. It enters the thorax, through the **left crus of the diaphragm**, and, ascending on the left side of the vertebral column, as high as the **ninth thoracic vertebra**, passes across the column, behind the **aorta, esophagus,** and **thoracic duct**, to end in the **azygos vein**. It receives the lower four or five **intercostal veins** and the **left subcostal vein**, and some **esophageal** and **mediastinal veins**.

Accessory hemiazygos vein—The **Accessory hemiazygos vein** (Figure 10-24) descends on the left side of the vertebral column, and varies inversely in size with the **left superior intercostal vein** (which drains into the **left brachiocephalic vein**). It receives veins from the three or four intercostal spaces between the **left superior intercostal vein** and the highest tributary of the **hemiazygos**. It either crosses the body of the **eighth thoracic vertebra** to join the **azygos vein** or ends in the **hemiazygos**. When this vein is small, or altogether wanting, the **left superior intercostal vein** may extend as low as the fifth or sixth intercostal space.

VASCULAR ANATOMY RELATED TO LOWER EXTREMITY—ARTERIAL

▶ Central Arteries of the Abdomen and Pelvis

Abdominal aorta

The **abdominal aorta** begins at the level of the **diaphragm**, crossing it via the **aortic hiatus** at the vertebral level of **T12**. It travels down the posterior wall of the abdomen in front of the vertebral column. It thus follows the curvature of the lumbar vertebrae, that is, convex anteriorly. The peak of this convexity is at the level of the third lumbar vertebra.

The **abdominal aorta** runs parallel to the **inferior vena cava**, which is located just to its right and becomes smaller in diameter as it gives off branches. The **abdominal aorta**

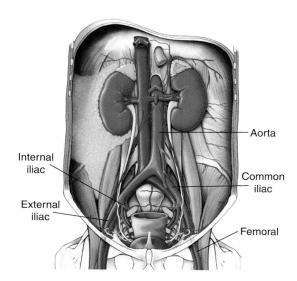

Figure 10-25. Abdominal aorta and iliac arteries.

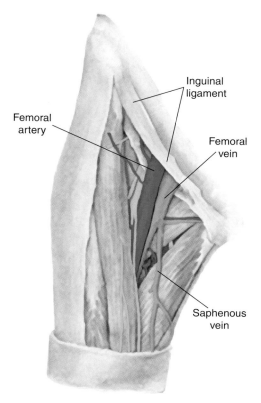

Figure 10-26. Femoral triangle.

bifurcates at the level of the **fourth lumbar vertebra**. It bifurcates to give rise to the **right and left common iliac arteries**.

Iliac arteries

The **common iliac arteries** (Figure 10-25) are two large arteries that originate from the **aortic bifurcation** at the level of the **fourth lumbar vertebra**. These vessels along with all of their branches exist as paired structures, one on the left side and one on the right. The **common iliac arteries** run inferolaterally, along the medial border of the **psoas muscles** to their bifurcation at the pelvic brim, in front of the **sacroiliac joints**. They bifurcate into the **external iliac artery and internal iliac artery** (also referred to as the **hypogastric artery**) opposite the lumbosacral articulation. The **external iliac artery** continues along the brim of the pelvis to the lower extremity. It terminates by becoming the **femoral artery**.

▶ Peripheral Arteries of Lower Extremity

Femoral artery

The **femoral artery** is a continuation of **external iliac artery** where it enters the **femoral triangle** at the mid inguinal point behind the **inguinal ligament**. The point of distinction between the **external iliac artery** and the **femoral artery** is the **inguinal ligament**. The artery leaves the **femoral triangle** (Figure 10-26) through the apex beneath the sartorius muscle. It enters the **popliteal fossa** where it becomes the **popliteal artery**.

Other arteries of the lower extremity

We will not discuss the other arteries of the lower extremity because of their lack of significant relevance to dialysis vascular access.

VASCULAR ANATOMY RELATED TO LOWER EXTREMITY—VENOUS

▶ Peripheral Veins of Lower Extremity

Femoral vein

The **femoral vein** is a continuation of the **popliteal vein**. It extends from a level just above the knee to the inguinal ligament where it accompanies the **femoral artery** in the **femoral sheath**. As the vein passes under the **inguinal ligament**, it lies medial to the **femoral artery** (Figure 10-27). The femoral vein becomes the **external iliac vein** after passing under the **inguinal ligament**.

Other veins of the lower extremity

We will not discuss the other veins of the lower extremity because of their lack of significant relevance to dialysis vascular access.

▶ Central Veins of Pelvis

Iliac veins

The **external iliac veins** (Figures 10-25 and 10-27) originate at the inferior margin of the **inguinal ligaments**. From there they continue around the rim of the pelvis to join with the **internal iliac veins** (also referred to as the **hypogastric veins**) opposite the lumbosacral articulation to form the **common iliac veins**. The **right and left common iliac**

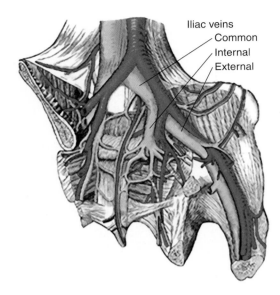

Figure 10-27. Iliac veins.

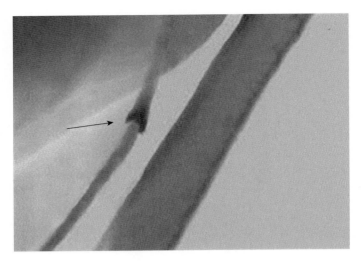

Figure 10-28. Venous valve.

veins converge and join to form the **inferior vena cava** at the level of the upper border of the **fifth lumbar vertebra**.

Inferior vena cava

The **inferior vena cava** is formed by the joining of the left and right **common iliac veins** and brings blood into the **right atrium** of the **heart**. It is retroperitoneal and runs alongside of the **vertebral column** on its right side. It enters the right atrium at the lower right, back side of the **heart**. Although it is not a main route for drainage, it has anastomoses with the **azygos system**.

▶ Venous Valves

The venous circulation is a low-pressure system. There is no head of pressure to force blood flow as in the arterial circulation. Many small veins in the peripheral circulation collapse when their lumens are not filled with blood; their appearance when a retrograde radiocontrast injection is made with proximal venous occlusion can cause confusion. A great deal of the circulation in the peripheral veins is due to muscle contraction and a series of valves. These structures are one-way flaps, a pair of delicate leaflets that prevent blood from flowing backward. The site in the vein where the valve is located generally appears slightly dilated (Figure 10-28).

Although there are certain locations where a venous valve is commonly seen, such as the proximal cephalic (Figure 10-29), their precise distribution is somewhat variable. In the upper extremities, all of the peripheral and central veins have valves until the innominate veins. These veins do not posses valves nor does the superior vena cava. In the lower extremity, valves are commonly seen up through the external iliac veins. The common iliac may or may not have valves.

With ultrasound, the leaflets of the valve can often be seen to flutter open and then close with a sudden motion. When an arteriovenous access is created and the vein is exposed to the high pressure of arterial blood, these delicate leaflets are plastered up against the vein wall permanently.

▶ Collateral Veins

When the normal vein develops an obstructive lesion, the pressure within the vein begins to rise. An elevated venous pressure predisposes to the development of new or collateral veins. It is important that this phenomenon be recognized. Firstly, they serve as a hallmark or signal that an obstructive lesion is present. This is generally obvious; occasionally, however, it is not. When collateral veins are seen, you can assume that an obstructive lesion is present. Secondly, these are abnormal vessels. They tend to be more fragile than the normal ones. Collateral veins are easily ruptured.

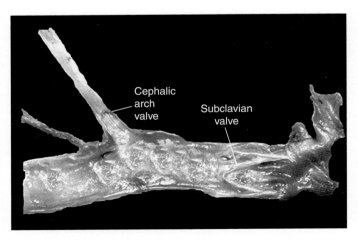

Figure 10-29. Subclavian and cephalic valves. (Courtesy of Dr. Kaveh Kian.)

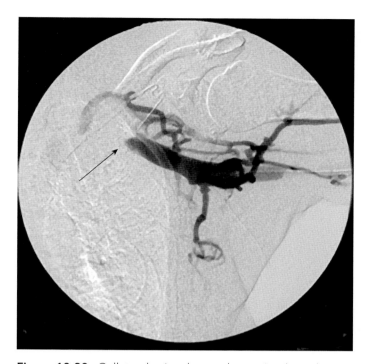

Figure 10-30. Collateral veins due to obstruction (arrow).

There are a several features that distinguish collateral veins from normal ones (Figure 10-30). Generally, when collateral veins form they are multiple. This is not always the case, but it is a valid general rule. Collateral veins bypass an area of obstruction; in doing so, they tend to deviate from the usual course of the normal vein. This is one of the primary reasons that it is important to be able to recognize normal venous pathways and locations. These anomalous veins tend to be more tortuous than normal. Their course is more random and they tend to come off of the main channel at odd angles.

REFERENCES

1. Rodriquea-Niedenfuhr M, Vazquez T, Nearn L, Ferreira B, Parkin I, Sanudo JR. Variations of the arterial pattern in the upper limb revisited: a morphological and statistical study, with a review of the literature. *J Anat.* 2001;199:547–566.
2. Gellman H, Botte MJ, Shankwiler J, Gelberman RH. Arterial patterns of the deep and superficial palmar arches. *Clin Orthop Related Res.* 2001;383:41–46.
3. Lin BS, Kong CW, Tarng DC, Huang TP, Tang GJ. Anatomical variation of the internal jugular vein and its impact on temporary haemodialysis vascular access: an ultrasonographic survey in uraemic patients. *Nephrol Dial Transplant.* 1998;13:134–138.

RADIOLOGICAL ANATOMY ATLAS

Figure 10B-1 – Aortic arch

1. Aortic arch
2. Brachiocephalic artery
3. Right subclavian artery
4. Right carotid artery
5. Left carotid artery
6. Left subclavian artery

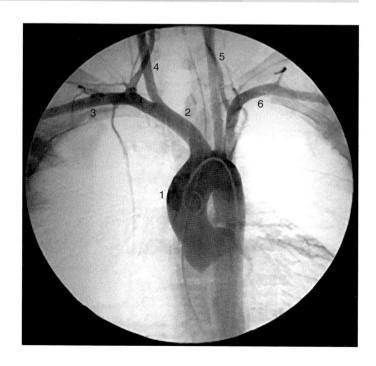

Figure 10B-2 – Branches of brachial artery

1. Brachial artery
2. Bifurcation
3. Ulnar artery
4. Radial artery

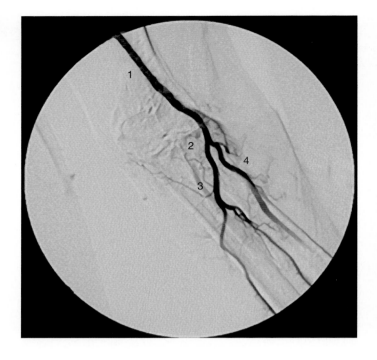

Figure 10B-3 – High bifurcation

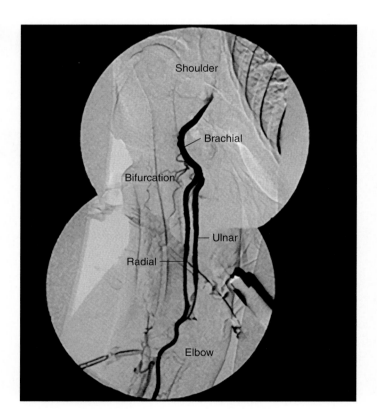

Figure 10B-4 – Accessory brachial artery

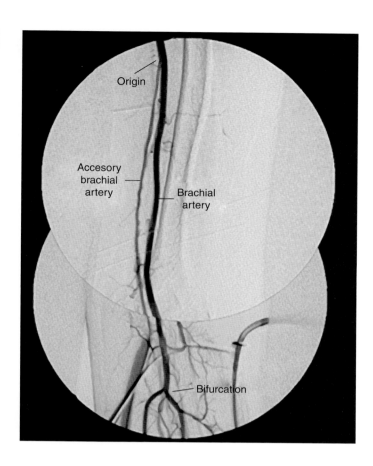

Figure 10B-5 – Superficial palmar arch

1. Ulnar artery
2. Volar interosseous artery
3. Radial artery
4. Palmar arch

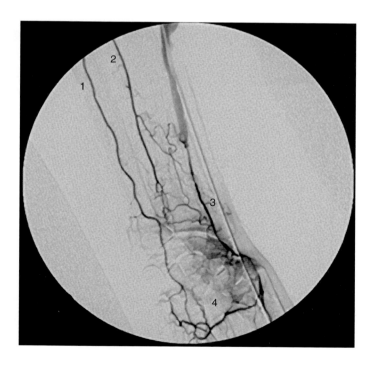

Figure 10B-6 – Superficial palmar arch

1. Ulnar artery
2. Radial artery
3. Palmar arch

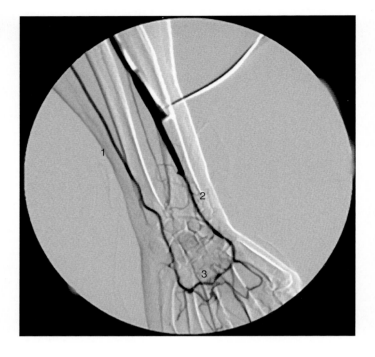

Figure 10B-7 – Radial artery and veins (ultrasound)

1. Radial vein
2. Radial vein
3. Radial artery

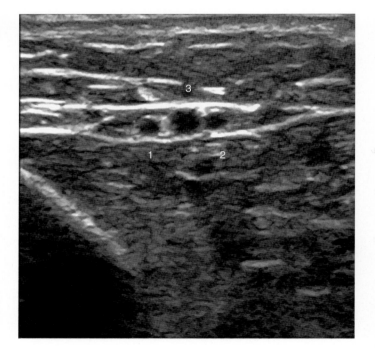

Figure 10B-8 – Brachial artery and veins

1. Ulnar vein
2. Ulnar vein
3. Ulnar artery

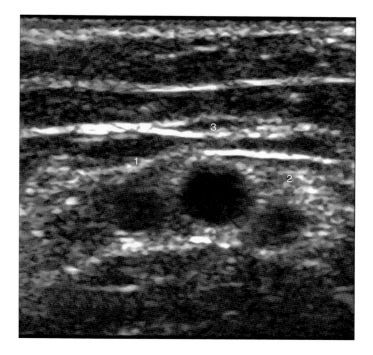

Figure 10B-9 – Forearm cephalic vein

1. Cephalic vein

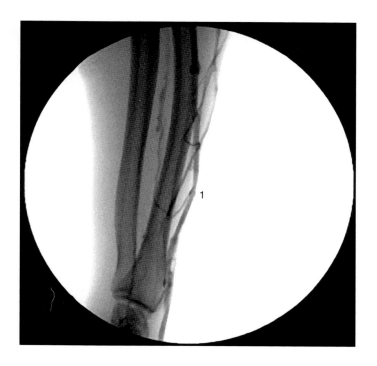

Figure 10B-10 – Superficial veins at elbow

1. Basilic vein
2. Cephalic vein
3. Median cubital vein

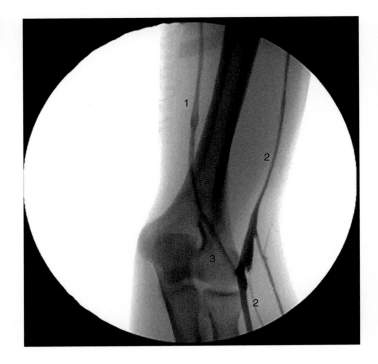

Figure 10B-11 – Upper cephalic vein

1. Cephalic arch
2. Cephalic vein

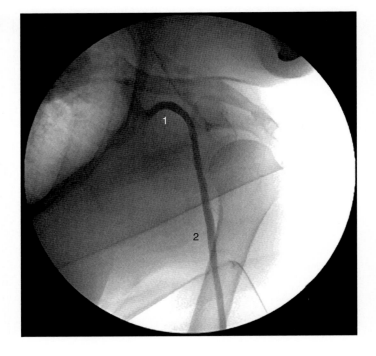

Figure 10B-12 – Upper basilic vein

1. Basilic vein
2. Venous valve
3. Axillary vein

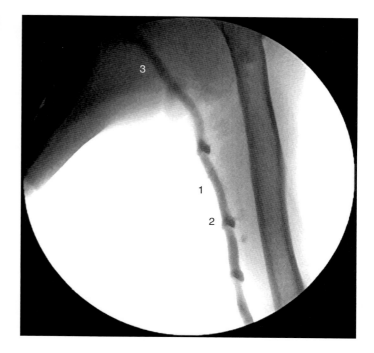

Figure 10B-13 – Cephalic arch with a valve

1. Cephalic vein
2. Cephalic arch (with valve)
3. Axillary vein
4. Subclavian vein
5. Brachiocephalic vein

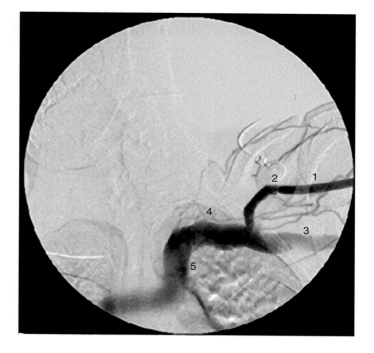

Figure 10B-14 – Double cephalic arch

1. Normal cephalic arch
2. Duplicate cephalic arch
3. Subclavian vein (bridged by second arch)
4. Brachiocephalic vein

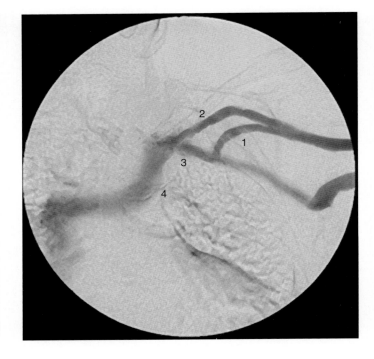

Figure 10B-15 – Central veins of left side

1. Subclavian vein
2. Internal jugular vein (stub)
3. Brachiocephalic vein

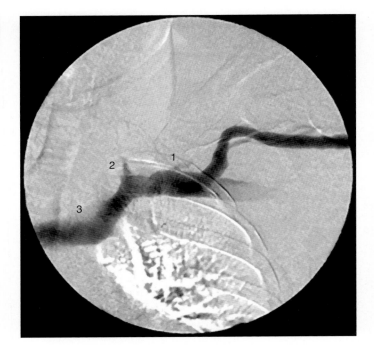

Figure 10B-16 – Central veins of the right side

1. Brachiocephalic vein
2. Subclavian vein
3. Internal jugular vein (stub)

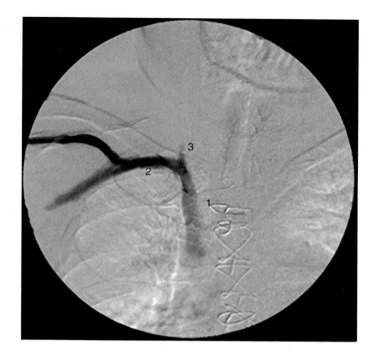

Figure 10B-17 – Dilated azygos vein (central vein obstruction)

1. Opening into the azygos arch
2. Azygos vein

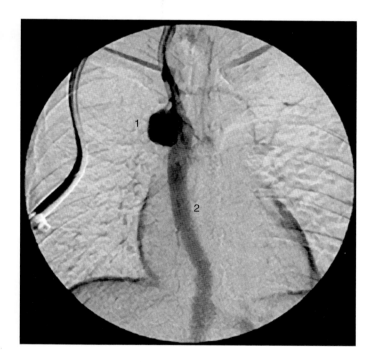

Figure 10B-18 – Azygos vein (lateral view)

1. Azygos arch
2. Azygos vein (dilated)
3. Superior vena cava
4. Catheter

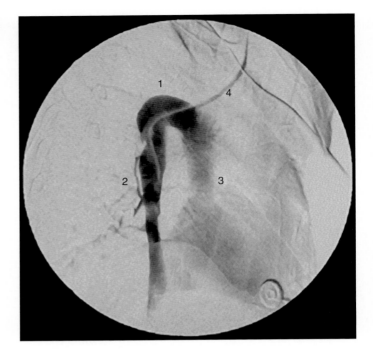

Figure 10B-19 – Left side of the azygos system (dilated from central vein obstruction)

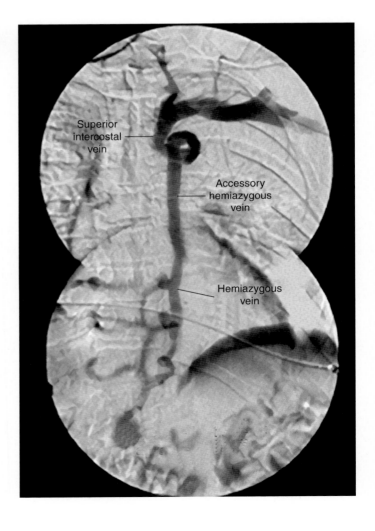

Figure 10B-20 – Left superior intercostal vein

1. Left superior intercostal vein
2. Left brachiocephalic vein

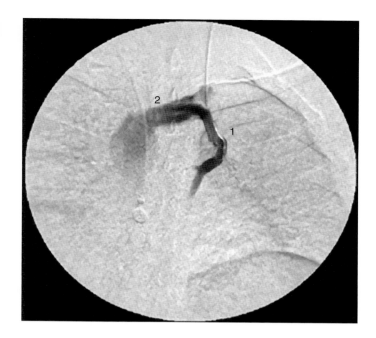

Figure 10B-21 – Superior vena cava

1. Right brachiocephalic vein
2. Left brachiocephalic vein. Superior vena cava
3. Superior vena caval–atrial junction
4. Right atrium
5. Right ventricle

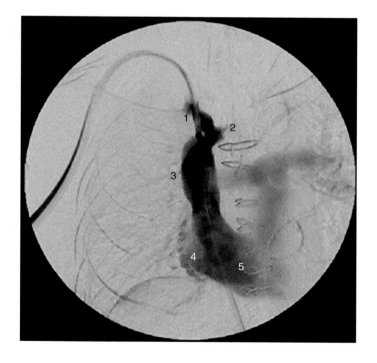

Figure 10B-22 – Left-sided superior vena cava

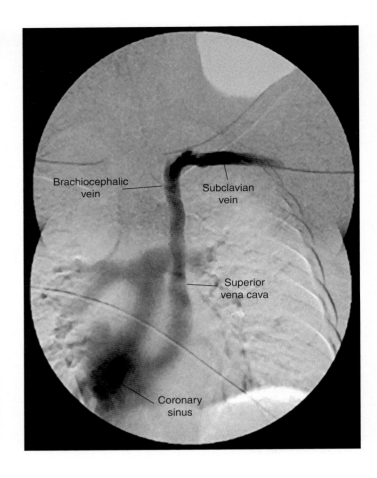

Figure 10B-23 – Iliac arteries

1. Aorta

2. Common iliac

3. Internal iliac

4. External iliac

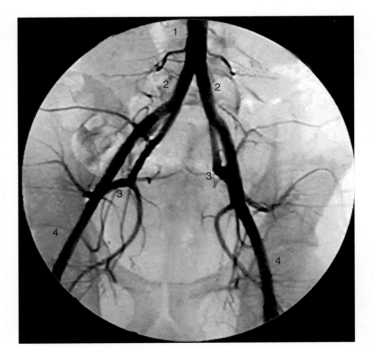

VASCULAR MAPPING

LOAY SALMAN & ARIF ASIF

1. Understand the importance of vascular mapping.
2. Understand the role of physical examination in vascular mapping.
3. Understand the role of ultrasound vascular mapping.
4. Understand the role of venography in vascular mapping.
5. Understand the limitations of each mapping technique and their advantages.

INTRODUCTION

Vascular access is needed for patients with end-stage renal disease who choose to receive hemodialysis. While there are multiple options of vascular accesses, arteriovenous fistulae (AVFs) continue to be the preferred types of vascular access when compared to arteriovenous grafts and tunneled hemodialysis catheters or a hemodialysis reliable outflow (HeRO) device. Once established, arteriovenous fistulae require the least number of procedures per year and have better patency rates, morbidity, and mortality profile relative to all other access modalities.[1-5] Both the National Kidney Foundation-Kidney Dialysis Outcomes Quality Initiative (NKF-KDOQI) for vascular access and the National Vascular Access Improvement Initiative (Fistula First) recommend an AVF as the preferred type of access for patients on hemodialysis.[6,7]

In order to achieve a functional, permanent access, it is critical to formulate a vascular access creation plan. This requires an understanding of each patient's unique anatomy. Thus, vessel mapping can be understood to mean any technique that leads to the acquisition of knowledge about a patient's inflow and outflow anatomy as they relate to arteriovenous access creation. Many reports have highlighted the various aspects of vessel mapping.[1-26] Indeed, preoperative mapping leads to a marked increase in placement of arteriovenous fistulae and a reduction in the use of tunneled hemodialysis catheters.[8-11]

Vascular mapping not only enables the operator to identify suitable vessels (veins and arteries) for the access creation but also helps with access creation in an orderly fashion (ie, operator will use the forearm vessels first in case both forearm and upper arm veins and arteries were available). If this order of creation is used it will maximize future options for an access creation. As of September 2010, the national fistulae rate is approximately 56.8%. While we have made much progress, we still fall somewhat short of the target of 66% set by the Fistula First Breakthrough Initiative.[7] If applied appropriately, mapping is one strategy that could potentially help in achieving this target.

VASCULAR MAPPING TECHNIQUES

▶ History and Physical Examination

Like any medical evaluation, this technique starts with obtaining a detailed history. In this regards, the emphasis is placed on investigating any previous history of central venous catheters, temporary dialysis catheters, or tunneled dialysis catheters. Past history of any hospitalization for a major event (such as trauma) including admission to an intensive care unit must raise the possibility of a central line placement. While patients may or may not remember the central line placement, they often remember such hospital admissions. The inspection and examination of any possible scar on the chest is of paramount importance. Special attention needs to be given to the presence of cardiac rhythm devices, as these equipments are associated with central venous stenosis. Physical examination should also include evaluation for the presence or absence of swelling of the arm, shoulder, chest, breast, and face in addition to the presence of collateral veins.

Physical examination is a simple evaluation that can be easily performed in the office. Both venous and arterial vessels can be evaluated using this technique. In simple terms, veins are evaluated by inspection following a tourniquet placement at the upper part of the arm. Venous evaluation involves measuring the diameter of the vein, length of potential cannulation segment, and the presence of any tortuousity. Arterial evaluation can start by recording blood pressure in both arms to detect any differences between the two arms. The normal difference is less than 10 mm Hg. A difference of 10–20 mm Hg should be considered marginal and a difference of blood pressure that exceeds 20 mm Hg should be considered abnormal and suggest the presence of a subclavian artery stenosis on the side of the lower pressure.[12] Arterial pulse evaluation can be undertaken at various levels (axillary, brachial, radial, and ulnar). Attention should be paid to normal, diminished, or absent pulses. The Allen test can be performed for further evaluation of the arterial system in both upper extremities. The purpose of the Allen test is to evaluate ulnar artery, radial artery, and their supply to the palmar arch and therefore the hand. The Allen test when performed appropriately can be reliable in 95–100% of the cases.[13–15]

A modified version of the Allen test is also used.[16] This test can be performed by having patient clinch the hand, occlude radial and ulnar arteries, and then raise the hand up (this will help to drain blood from the hand). At this point, the hand can be lowered (while maintaining pressure on both arteries) and patient can be asked to open this hand next to the opposite open hand. This will enable the investigator to compare the color of both hands. The occlusive pressure over the ulnar artery can be released. The return of hand color would indicate the patent ulnar artery. This test can now be repeated by releasing the pressure over the radial artery instead to check radial artery's patency. The normal Allen test indicates patent arteries. The same test can also be performed by using pulse oximetry before, during, and after the arterial pressure. The pulse oximetry probe is placed on the patient's index finger. The loss of the pulse oximeter waveform and oxygen saturation reading after arterial pressure is an objective indication that compression is adequate. Subsequent return of a pulse, oxygen saturation reading, and the waveform following the release of the ulnar artery indicate adequate ulnar circulation (normal test). The test can then be repeated with for radial artery evaluation.[16]

▶ Ultrasound Evaluation

Ultrasound is a simple tool that can be used to evaluate veins and arteries. It is inexpensive and accurate. It does not involve needle sticks or the use of iodine dye. It allows for an objective evaluation of both the arterial and venous systems. The Doppler analysis provides a functional

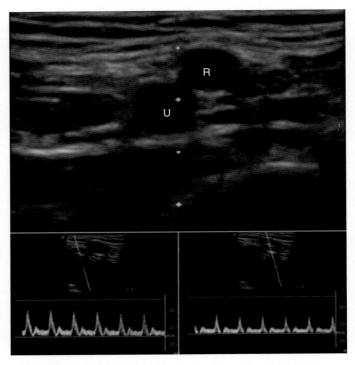

Figure 11-1. Ultrasound examination demonstrating high bifurcation of the brachial artery (R = radial artery, U = ulnar artery) (upper panel). The distance between each white dot is 0.5 cm shown in the upper panel. Lower panel demonstrates Doppler examination revealing flow (waveform) through both arteries.

assessment of venous and arterial vasculature. Ultrasound can also determine which artery has the optimal inflow for a successful AVF creation.[17] This tool can also detect major variations in the arteries of the upper extremity (Figure 11-1).

Many investigators have demonstrated a marked improvement in fistula placement with the use of this mapping technique.[8–10] Allon et al[10] documented a significant increase in arteriovenous fistula creation when preoperative vascular mapping using ultrasonography was employed compared with the traditional physical examination approach (preoperative physical examination = 34% vs preoperative sonographic vascular mapping = 64%; $p < 0.001$). Another study also demonstrated a significant improvement in arteriovenous fistulae creation (from 14% to 63%), reduction in graft placement (from 62% to 30%), and reduction in the use of tunneled hemodialysis catheters (from 24% to 7%) when preoperative mapping of the arteries and veins was performed using duplex Doppler ultrasonography.[8]

Preoperative ultrasound examination has also been used in the evaluation and subsequent function of the fistula. Malovrh[18] used duplex ultrasonography to examine forearm arteries and veins before creating AVFs in 116 consecutive patients. In this study, various parameters, including feeding-artery internal diameter, resistance index, blood flow before and after reactive hyperemia, and internal diameter of the vein before and after proximal vein compression, were obtained before AVF creation. The AVF primary patency rate (successful creation of AVFs) was 80.2%, mean values for feeding-artery internal diameter were 0.26 cm, resistance index at reactive hyperemia was 0.50, and blood flow was 54.5 mL/min in this group. This group's feeding-artery internal diameter increased by 59.3% after proximal vein compression. In the group with failed AVFs (19.8%), mean feeding-artery internal diameter was 0.16 cm, resistance index at reactive hyperemia was 0.70, and blood flow was 24.1 mL/min. In this group, feeding-artery internal diameter increased by only 12.4% after proximal vein compression. The investigator also found that the feeding artery blood flow of 300 mL/min was achieved in the group that had an feeding-artery internal diameter greater than 0.16 cm in less than 1 week compared with 3 to 8 weeks later when feeding-artery internal diameter was less than 0.16 cm ($p < 0.01$). Similarly, the group with an resistance index at reactive hyperemia before surgery of 0.7 or greater took 3 to 8 weeks to show a blood flow of 300 mL/min, whereas the group with an resistance index at reactive hyperemia less than 0.7 achieved a feeding-artery blood flow of 300 mL/min in less than a week ($p < 0.01$). The investigator concluded that duplex ultrasonography helps identify the optimal location for successful creation of vascular access and the time necessary for its development.

In summary, the preoperative arterial diameter equal to or exceeding 1.6 mm and the venous diameter of 2.5 mm at the anastomosis in the hands of a skilled surgeon are required for fistula creation. Optimal fistula depth needs to be not more than 5 mm from the skin. The depth can be measured accurately by ultrasound. In addition, anomalies of the arteries of the upper extremities can be easily discerned with ultrasonography and a better plan for fistula creation could be adopted (Figure 11-1).[26] While ultrasonography is a valuable mapping tool, the lack of direct visualization of the central veins is a major limitation of this technique. With a great majority of patients initiating dialysis with a central venous catheter such an evaluation is of critical importance. In the presence of a pre-existing central venous stenosis or occlusion, there is a high likelihood of the development of edema following access creation.

▶ Venography

Vessel mapping can also be performed by using radiocontrast material. For the most part, this method evaluates the venous system; however, the arterial system can also be evaluated using this technique. Contrast venous mapping can be achieved by cannulating a peripheral vein on the dorsum of the hand. A small amount (10–20 mL) of low-osmolar contrast medium is diluted with 10–20 mL of normal saline and injected through the cannula. Fluoroscopy is performed using the pulse (15 pulse per second) and road map feature (15 frames per second). Images are recorded and analyzed from the wrist veins all the way to the right atrium (Figure 11-2). The criteria used to determine suitability of veins include vein diameter of at least 2.5 mm, the absence of stenosis within the vein, a straight cannulation

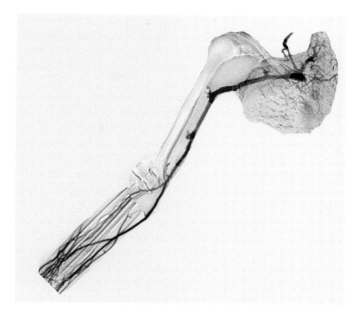

Figure 11-2. Venography can directly visualize the peripheral as well as the central veins. Notice the central venous occlusion (arrow) and the presence of collaterals. A tunneled dialysis catheter is seen traversing the right internal jugular vein. Extremity ultrasound performed in this patient would have demonstrated adequate veins for fistula creation.

segment of 8–10 cm long, continuity with central patent veins, and the absence of central venous stenosis.

This technique allows for direct visualization of the peripheral as well as the central veins. Patency of the vein and stenotic lesions with their characteristics and extension can all be directly observed. In contrast to the above-cited ultrasound studies, a recent analysis[11] prospectively identified hemodialysis patients who were consigned to long-term hemodialysis treatment by means of tunneled hemodialysis catheters.[11] Venography was performed to investigate the presence of veins suitable for an AVF creation. In this study, patients denied having been offered vessel mapping in the past. They also refuted receiving education regarding vascular access types, their advantages and disadvantages, associated complications, morbidity, and mortality. Of the 86 catheter-consigned patients agreeing to undergo venography, 82 patients (95%) were found to have patent veins that were suitable for arteriovenous access placement. Only four patients (5%) were found not to have the veins adequate for placement of an arteriovenous access and therefore were truly dependent on tunneled catheters for hemodialysis therapy. It is noteworthy that 97% of patients with no prior arteriovenous accesses (64/66) had suitable veins and that 90% of patients with previously failed arteriovenous accesses (18/20) had adequate veins—all basilic veins in the latter case (forearm + arm, $n = 2$; arm, $n = 16$). Out of the 82 patients with suitable veins for a fistula creation, 10 refused surgery. The remaining 72 received an arteriovenous access successfully (AVF = 68; grafts = 4). All four patients with a graft had a basilic vein suitable for AVF creation; however, the decision to place a graft was based on findings at the time of surgery. Angiography was not used to evaluate arteries in this study. Instead, a simple physical examination was employed to accomplish this task.

There have not been any randomized prospective studies comparing venography and vascular ultrasound mapping techniques to establish the superiority of one preoperative imaging evaluation over the other. However, using a combination of preoperative noninvasive (Doppler ultrasound) and invasive (venography and arteriography) techniques would be ideal to perform a complete vessel mapping in relatively simple outpatient settings. Huber et al[19] determined optimal configuration for an AVF as (criteria: vein >3 mm, no arterial inflow stenosis, no venous outflow stenosis) using DU. In this study, the unilateral arteriography/venography was performed to confirm the choice. A total of 139 new access procedures were performed in 131 patients. The noninvasive imaging showed that 83% of the patients were candidates for AVF, with a mean of 2.7 ± 2.1 possible configurations. Invasive imaging was abnormal in 38% with forearm arterial disease being more common than central vein stenosis leading to a change in the operative plan in 19%. An AVF was created in 90% of the cases (brachiobasilic > brachiocephalic > radiocephalic > radiobasilic). The AVF matured sufficiently for cannulation in 84% with adequate follow up. These fistulae were suitable for cannulation with a mean of 3.4 ± 1.8 months. On an intention to treat basis, an AVF sufficient for cannulation developed in 71% of the 139 cases. This study, by using multivariate analysis, predicted that female gender (odds ratio [OR] = 9.7; 95% confidence interval [95% CI], 2.2–43.5) and the radiocephalic AVFs (OR = 4.6; 95% CI, 1.1–18.6) were independent predictors of early fistula failure.

It is important to mention that a recent retrospective analysis did investigate the role of venography and ultrasound on AVF rates separately and in combination.[24] In this study, incident Medicare end-stage renal disease patient claims from the State of Florida were used to identify vessel mapping and CPT codes were used to identify the mapping techniques. This study used Chi-square statistics and logistic regression to ascertain the association of types of vessel mapping and AVF rates. After controlling for age, body mass index, gender, and race, venography ($n = 154$) resulted in significant higher AVF rates (51.30%) compared to ultrasound ($n = 4846$) (33.97%) ($p = 0.001$). A combination of the two mapping techniques ($n = 262$) did not increase AVF rates (49.24%) above and beyond what was achieved by venography (51.30%) alone ($p = 0.07$). The results of the study suggested that venography resulted in higher AVF rates compared to ultrasound. However, these results might not be causal and possibly related to the small number of surgeons or differences in the reasons for use of the two techniques. Finally, surgical expertise can have a major impact on fistula placement despite the availability of vessel mapping. In one study,[25] fistulae placement occurred

in 98% of the patients ($n = 40$) in the hands of a surgeon at a community medial center versus 71% of the patients ($n = 35$) by a surgeon working at an academic teaching medical center ($p = 0.001$). Demographic characteristics were similar except that patients referred to the community surgeon were older (52.7 ± 16.2 years vs 45.4 ± 13.7 years; $p = 0.04$) and tended to have more previously failed accesses (50% vs 29%; $p = 0.06$) and black race (65% vs 43%; $p = 0.055$) including a history of previously failed accesses (50% for surgeon I and 29% for surgeon II; $p = 0.06$). Similarly, there was no significant difference in the size of vessels between the patients operated on by the two surgeons. Characteristics predictive of fistula placement over an arteriovenous graft were surgeon selection (odds ratio [OR] = 19.52; $p = 0.01$).[25]

A major advantage of venography is direct visualization of the central veins as compared to the indirect assessment provided by Doppler evaluation. On the other hand, ultrasound offers the advantage of noninvasive arterial evaluation (along with functional assessment of the vessels) and no exposure to contrast material. Contrast venography may be of particular importance in obese patients, whose veins are deep beneath adipose tissue, and which are, therefore, not as easily visualized with ultrasound. A recent study of 18,020 patients investigated the role of vessel mapping according the body mass index (BMI).[23] Patients were categorized into underweight (<18.5), normal (18.5–24.9), overweight (25–29.9), and obese (>30) categories as per World Health Organization and National heart, Lung and Blood Institute BMI classification. Significantly increased AVFs rates were observed across all ranges of BMI when preoperative VM was performed. When VM was performed, the AVF rates for underweight, normal, overweight and obese patients were 28.4%, 35.4%, 36.0%, 35.1%, respectively. These differences were not statistically significant. However, these values were significantly higher for patients with similar BMI without vessel mapping (underweight = 18.7%, normal = 25.4, overweight = 27.1%, obese = 29.7%). In this study, the adjusted odds ratio for AVF was 1.46 (95% CI, 1.36–1.56) in favor of vessel mapping.[23] For these reasons, NKF-KDOQI guidelines for vascular access and the Fistula First also recommend the performance of vascular mapping before vascular access surgery whether it is creation of the first access or configuration of a new access following the failure of a pre-existing access.[6,7]

RISK OF CONTRAST-INDUCED NEPHROPATHY

Contrast material carries the risk of acute renal failure in patients with chronic kidney disease and can lead to deterioration of the residual kidney function in dialysis patients. However, recent data have emphasized that the use of low dose (10–20 mL) of low-osmolar contrast agent may be safer in patients with stages 4 and 5 CKD.[20,21] A recent prospective study reported on the safety of radiocontrast medium in CKD stages 4 and 5 patients.[20] In this investigation, 25 consecutive patients (CKD stages 4 and 5) undergoing venography for fistula creation were enrolled. Radiocontrast-induced nephropathy was defined as a 20% decrease in the estimated glomerular filtration rate (eGFR) from the baseline value at 48 hours after contrast administration. Venography was performed by using 10–20 cm of low-osmolar contrast medium. Complete sets of pre- and post-procedure GFRs were available in 21 patients. At 48 hours, there were no differences between the pre- and post-procedure GFRs. At 4 weeks of follow up, only one patient required dialysis owing to the development of flu-like syndrome and ensuing volume depletion. Subsequently, Kian et al[22] also reported on the incidence of radiocontrast-induced nephropathy in 34 CKD stage 4 patients undergoing salvage procedures for nonmaturing fistulae. Radiocontrast-induced nephropathy was defined as a 25% increase in serum creatinine from the baseline value. Serum creatinine was obtained pre-contrast administration and 2- and 7 day postcontrast administration. In this study, the mean contrast volume was 7.8 mL per procedure. The incidence of acute renal failure was 4.6% at 1 week. All values returned to baseline within 2 weeks. None of the patients required acute dialysis.

The use of small amount contrast material (less than 20 cc) of low-osmolar or iso-osmolar contrast material may minimize the risk of kidney injury. Although the above-mentioned reports are encouraging, caution must be exercised and examination undertaken on a case-by-case basis. Large-scale studies with a longer follow-up are needed to conclusively establish the safety of low-dose contrast administration in the development of acute renal failure.

CONCLUSION

A functioning arteriovenous fistula is the preferred access for hemodialysis. It is associated with a better profile in regards to patency, longevity, maintenance procedure requirement, morbidity, and mortality. All available evidence supports the conclusion that vessel mapping results in an increase in arteriovenous fistula creation. Because of these facts, preoperative vessel mapping in patients requiring new vascular access or patients with failing pre-existing vascular access is strongly recommended.

REFERENCES

1. Ascher, E, Gade, P, Hingorani, A, et al. Changes in the practice of angioaccess surgery: impact of dialysis outcome and quality initiative recommendations. *J Vasc Surg.* 2000;31:84.
2. Dixon, BS, Novak, L, Fangman, J. Hemodialysis vascular access survival: upper-arm native arteriovenous fistula. *Am J Kidney Dis.* 2002;39:92.
3. Dhingra RK, Young EW, Hulbert-Shearon TE, et al. Type of vascular access and mortality in U.S. hemodialysis patients. *Kidney Int.* October 2001;60(4):1443–1451.
4. Polkinghorne KR, McDonald SP, Atkins RC, et al. Vascular access and all-cause mortality: a propensity score analysis. *J Am Soc Nephrol.* February 2004;15(2):477–486.
5. Woods, JD, Port, FK. The impact of vascular access for haemodialysis on patient morbidity and mortality. *Nephrol Dial Transplant.* 1997;12:657.
6. Available at: http://www.kidney.org/professionals/kdoqi/pdf/12-50-0210_JAG_DCP_Guidelines-VA_Oct06_SectionC_ofC.pdf. Accessed December, 2011.
7. Available at: http://www.fistulafirst.org/. Accessed December, 2011.
8. Silva MB Jr, Hobson RW 2nd, Pappas PJ, et al. A strategy for increasing use of autogenous hemodialysis access procedures: impact of preoperative noninvasive evaluation. *J Vasc Surg.* 1998;27:302–307.
9. Robbin ML, Gallichio MH, Deierhoi MH, et al. Use vascular mapping before hemodialysis access placement. *Radiology.* 2000;217:83–88.
10. Allon M, Lockhart ME, Lilly RZ, et al. Effect of preoperative sonographic mapping on vascular access outcomes in hemodialysis patients. *Kidney Int.* 2001;60:2013–2020.
11. Asif A, Cherla G, Merrill D, et al. Conversion of tunneled hemodialysis consigned patients to arteriovenous fistula. *Kidney Int.* 2005;67:2399–2406.
12. www. Uptodate.com (Creating an arteriovenous fistula for hemodialysis, Author: Gerald A Beathard, MD, PhD, Section Editor: Jeffrey S Berns, MD, Deputy Editor: Theodore W Post, MD).
13. Agrifoglio M, Dainese L, Pasotti S, et al. Preoperative assessment of the radial artery for coronary artery bypass grafting: is the clinical Allen test adequate? *Ann Thorac Surg.* February 2005;79(2):570–572.
14. Hirai M, Kawai S. False positive and negative results in Allen test. *J Cardiovasc Surg (Torino).* May–June 1980;21(3):353–360.
15. Kamienski RW, Barnes RW. Critique of the Allen test for continuity of the palmar arch assessed by Doppler ultrasound. *Surg Gynecol Obstet.* June 1976;142(6):861–864.
16. Paul BZ, Feeney CM. Combining the modified Allen's test and pulse oximetry for evaluating ulnar collateral circulation to the hand for radial artery catheterization of the ED patient. *California J Emerg Med.* 2003;4:89.
17. Malovrh M. The role of sonography in the planning of arteriovenous fistulas for hemodialysis. *Semin Dial.* 2003;16:299–303.
18. Malovrh M. Native arteriovenous fistula: preoperative evaluation. *Am J Kidney Dis.* 2002;39:1218–1225.
19. Huber TS, Ozaki CK, Flynn TC, et al. Prospective validation of an algorithm to maximize native arteriovenous fistulae for chronic hemodialysis access. *J Vasc Surg.* 2002;36:452–459.
20. Asif A, Cherla G, Merrill D, et al. Venous mapping using venography and the risk of radiocontrast-induced nephropathy. *Semin Dial.* 2005;18:239–242.
21. Fitzgerald JT, Schanzer A, Chin AI, et al. Outcomes of upper arm arteriovenous fistulas for maintenance hemodialysis access. *Arch Surg.* 2004;139:201–208.
22. Kian K, Wyatt C, Schon D, et al. Safety of low-dose radiocontrast for interventional AV fistula salvage in stage 4 chronic kidney disease patients. *Kidney Int.* 2006;69:1444–1449.

23. Deuzimar Kulawik, Jifeng Ma, Jeffrey J. Sands et al. Improving AVF rates in obese patients: the role of vessel mapping. *J Am Soc Nephrol.* 2010;21:250.

24. Kulawik D, Mayo KM, Ma J, et al. Venography or ultrasound: which mapping technique is superior? *J Am Soc Nephrol.* 2010;21:242A.

25. Choi KL, Salman L, Krishnamurthy G, et al. Impact of surgeon selection on access placement and survival following preoperative mapping in the "Fistula First" era. *Semin Dial.* July–August 2008;21(4):341–345.

26. Kian K, Shapiro JA, Salman L, et al. High brachial artery bifurcation: clinical considerations and practical implications for an arteriovenous access. *Semin Dial.* Sep. 19, 2011 (Epub ahead of print).

12

VASCULAR ACCESS FOR HEMODIALYSIS: TYPES, CHARACTERISTICS, AND EPIDEMIOLOGY

ANIL K. AGARWAL

LEARNING OBJECTIVES

1. Describe types of vascular access for hemodialysis.
2. Explain characteristis of different types of vascular access.
3. Explore factors influencing creation and failure of vascular access.
4. Discuss epidemiology of vascular access.

INTRODUCTION

Vascular access is central to the performance of hemodialysis (HD). An ideal vascular access would have many attributes. It would be easy to create, readily available, and easily accessible. Further, it would provide adequate dialysis and require little maintenance by remaining free of mechanical and infectious complications. None of the current forms of vascular access have nearly all of these characteristics and the quest for a perfect access remains unquenched.

▶ Types of Vascular Access

Initial vascular access involved arterial cut downs but was unsustainable for long-term dialysis due to the loss of access sites. Arteriovenous (AV) shunt was pioneered by Belding Scribner in 1960.[1] Scribner shunt became popular as a preferred vascular access for maintenance HD, but fell out of favor due to high rates of infection and thrombosis. Cimino fistula, the precursor of current forms of AV access, was devised in 1966.[2] Although AV fistula (AVF), with its various modifications, is the favorite choice for vascular access, this form of access continues to have maturation issues. AV graft (AVG) was developed later as an option for those with inadequate veins for creation

of AVF. AVG is fraught with issues related to thrombosis and infection requiring high level of maintenance care and need for monitoring and surveillance. Dialysis catheters are the mainstay of access when impending kidney failure necessitates instant access to circulation. Catheters have high rates of infectious and noninfectious complications including thrombosis, venous stenosis, biofilm development and fibrin sheath formation.

At present, there are several options for vascular access that must be individualized for a patient requiring dialysis based on the urgency and the suitability in a particular clinical situation (Table 12-1). The AV accesses can be created at different anatomical locations and in different configurations, observing the general principle that the preferred site for an AV access is a nondominant upper extremity—starting distally and then moving proximally as the distal sites are exhausted (Figure 12-1).[3] For example, a preferred initial site would be wrist (radiocephalic) access, moving on to upper arm (brachiocephalic or brachiobasilic). It is often possible to use other veins that may be available at any of these sites. Other sites that have been commonly used include femoral–femoral, iliofemoral, and axilloaxillary anastomosis. In desperate cases, arterio-arterial anastomosis can also be done.

TABLE 12–1

Vascular Access Types (In Order of Preference)

Arteriovenous Fistula
  Primary AV fistula
  Transposed AV fistula
  Secondary AV fistula
Arteriovenous grafts
Hybrid access
Dialysis catheters

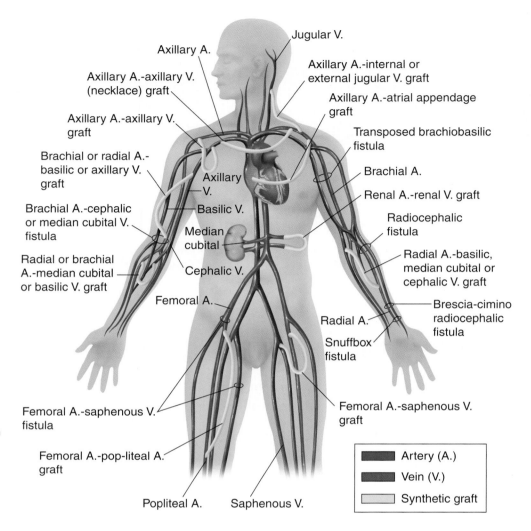

Figure 12-1. Sites and configurations of arteriovenous accesses. The figure displays a variety of anatomical sites and possible opportunities to create an arteriovenous access. Only a few of these sites are used routinely. (From Paulson WD, Ram SJ, Zibari GB. Vascular access: anatomy, examination, management. *Semin Nephrol.* 2002;22:183–194).

AV fistula

Radiocephalic native AV fistula was initially described in 1966 (Figure 12-2).[2,4] The surgical technique of creating a radiocephalic AVF has undergone continual modifications to make it possible to create and function in different circumstances as well as to reduce the likelihood of venous hypertension. Radiocephalic AVF has the advantage of providing high patency rates, low infection rates, and low rates of arterial steal, while preserving proximal sites. Due to a high incidence of poor cephalic veins in patients reaching end-stage renal disease (ESRD), these fistula do have a high early failure rate due to difficulty in maturation, patency of AVF requires selection of an adequate vein (at least 1.5–2 mm or even larger in diameter, flushes, and dilates well), adequate artery, and use of adjuvant heparin during the perioperative period.

Brachiocephalic AVF provides great blood flow, patency, and low infection rates, but is associated with higher rates of arterial steal (compared to the radiocephalic AVF) and higher likelihood of nerve injury (Figure 12-3A).[4] There may be more swelling and pain at this site immediately after its creation.

Transposed brachiobasilic AVF is more challenging and time consuming during creation and requires significant surgical training and experience (Figure 12-3B).[4] It can be created using a one- or a two-stage surgical procedure. Transposition is done to superficialize the basilic vein and place it more laterally in the arm for easy access for cannulation.

AV grafts

AVGs are created using a synthetic conduit in place of native vein, usually due to the lack of a suitable vein. A variety of AVG material is available, most commonly polytetrafluoroethylene (PTFE) and polyurethane. Other innovative conduits including cryopreserved artery or vein, bovine carotid artery, and long saphenous vein or human umbilical vein have also been used.

AVG can be placed in in various anatomic locations and in different configurations that may be straight, curved, or in the shape of a loop (Figures 12-1 and 12-4A–C).[4] AVG must provide enough length and ease of cannulation for dialysis. The AVG have the advantage of multiple possible insertion sites even in patients with often unsuitable

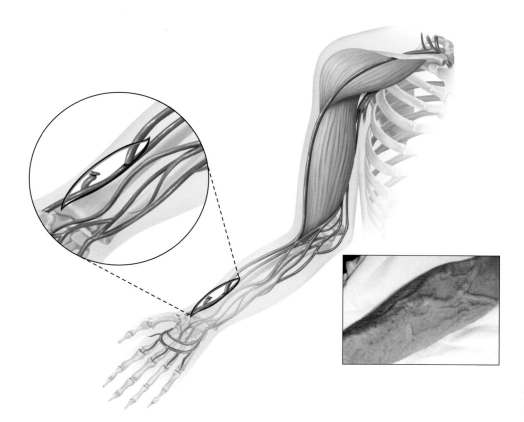

Figure 12-2. Radiocephalic AV fistula (Brescia-Cimino). (Reproduced with permission from Ref. [4].)

veins for AVF creation. AVGs have a short maturation time of usually 2 weeks, which is enough to allow incorporation of graft material into the surrounding tissues. AVGs are easy to cannulate and allow sufficient area for cannulation. Although AVGs have a lower primary patency rate than a fistula, maturation failure is much less common than AVG. AVG can provide better patency with better surveillance and are relatively easy to declot or to revise in case of failure. Longer AVG patency, however, requires higher rate of intervention due to the occurrence of stenosis, thrombosis, and pseudoaneurysm formation. Infections in AVG are more common than AVF, but much less than catheters. There is a higher rate of arterial steal in upper arm location. Occasionally, iatrogenic graft to vein fistula (GVF) can also form due to accidental cannulation of graft through and overlapping vein.[5]

Dialysis catheters

Dialysis catheters are placed in central veins or right atrium to provide free flow of blood for performance of dialysis. Catheters provide instant access to circulation, ease of insertion or removal as outpatient, and freedom from pain during cannulation for the patients (unlike AV accesses which require cannulation with a needle). These attributes often make these accesses the preferred choice for patients. However, catheters have serious shortcomings, including inadequate blood flow

over a long period of time due to thrombosis and fibrin sheath formation resulting in inadequate dialysis. There is several-fold higher rate of infection of the catheter compared to AV access, and noninfectious complications including venous stenosis occur commonly jeopardizing the extremity for future AV access. It is also impractical to swim or take shower with an indwelling catheter due to the risk of introducing infection. Many sites are available in upper and lower trunk veins for catheter insertion. In desperate cases, translumbar or transhepatic catheters have been used to provide at least a temporary bridge for dialysis.[6]

Other accesses

Entirely subcutaneous dialysis ports have been used in place of dialysis catheters, but are not widely adapted due to high rates of infection and central venous complications similar to those caused by catheters. A novel hybrid access has recently become available that, in essence, combines an AV graft that is connected to a catheter within the subcutaneous plain providing central venous outflow akin to a catheter. The subcutaneous nature of this access avoids creation of an exit site that decreases risk of infection while avoiding a typical catheter placement and may provide rescue for those with marginal venous system and no possibility of accommodating AVF or AVG.[7]

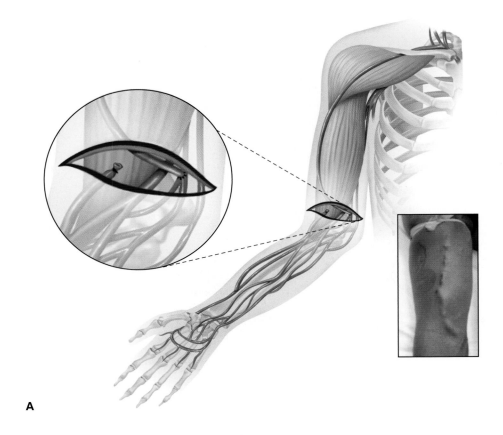

A

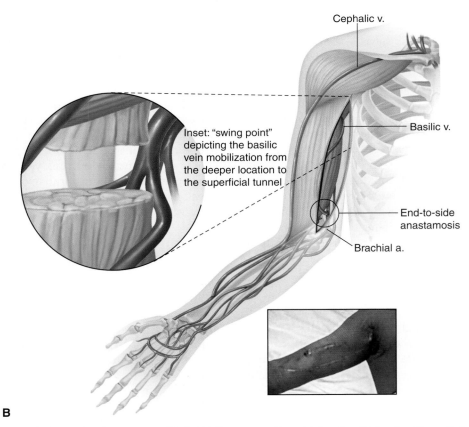

Cephalic v.

Inset: "swing point" depicting the basilic vein mobilization from the deeper location to the superficial tunnel

Basilic v.

End-to-side anastamosis

Brachial a.

B

Figure 12-3. (**A**) Brachiocephalic AV fistula. (From Ref. [4]). (**B**) Transposed brachiobasilic AV fistula. (From Ref. [4]).

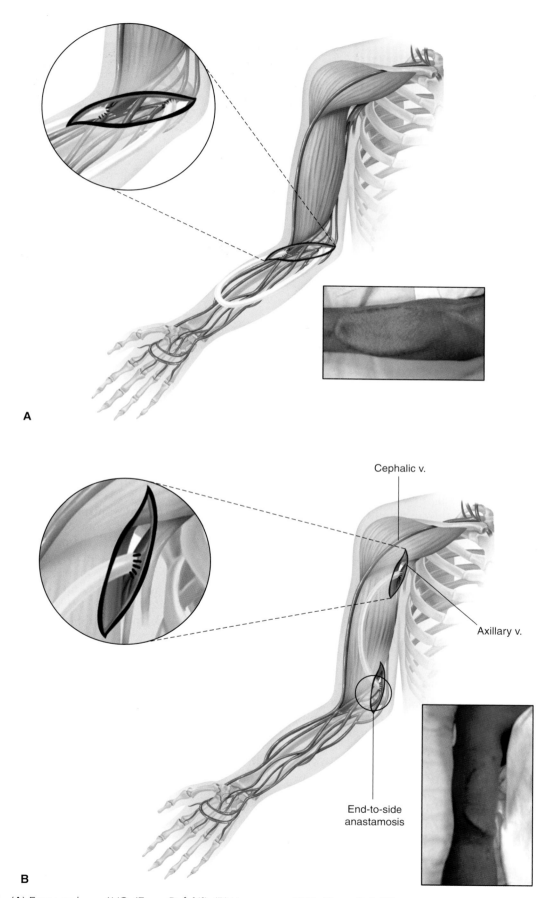

A

Cephalic v.

Axillary v.

End-to-side
anastamosis

B

Figure 12-4. (**A**) Forearm loop AVG. (From Ref. [4]). (**B**) Upper arm AVG. (From Ref. [4]).

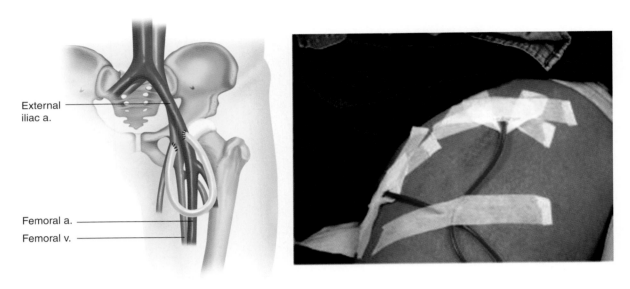

C

Figure 12-4. *(continued)* **(C)**. Thigh AVG using femoral vessels. (From Ref. [4]).

▶ Access Characteristics

AVF: Failure of maturation

Failure of maturation of newly created AVF is reported to range from 18% to 60% in multiple studies, requiring multiple interventions and unwanted prolonged catheter exposure.[8,9] A number of factors can influence placement, successful use, and survival of AVF. It is only intuitive that the intensity of surgical training and experience would influence the type of vascular access created and its survival. A study from the United Kingdom examined consecutive radiocephalic AVF created between 2002 and 2005, comparing primary and secondary patency rates of those created by senior surgeons ($n = 153$) to those created by junior surgeons ($n = 42$).[10] Primary and secondary patency rates at 22 months of follow up were 89% and 93%, respectively, in first group, and 74% and 81%, respectively, in the second group. These were significantly different. Prospective data from 12 countries showed that AVF success can be predicted by number of fistulae placed during training and degree of emphasis on VA creation during surgical training.[11] These studies indicate that a careful surgeon selection is important when planning vascular access.

Aside from the surgical technique of AVF creation, many molecular mechanisms may impact failure of AV access by causing thrombosis or endothelial dysfunction. Endothelial dysfunction may cause vascular smooth muscle cell (VSMC) migration and aggravate venous neointimal hyperplasia in an AVF to predispose vascular thrombosis. Upregulation of monocyte chemoattractant protein 1 (MCP-1) can potentiate chemotaxis of monocytes/macrophages, activation and migration of endothelial cells, promote proliferation and migration

of smooth muscle cells, induction of tissue factor and other procoagulant effects. In the venous segment of a murine model of AVF, MCP-1 increase was accompanied by an increased activity of the transcription factors NFκβ and activator protein-1. MCP-1 deficiency was associated with an increased fistula patency at 6 weeks with a decreased venous wall thickness and an increased luminal area.[12] AVF patency has also been associated with specific genotype polymorphisms of TGF-β1.[13] Similar associations have also been reported with methylene tetrahydrofolate reductase and heme oxygenase-1 polymorphisms as well.[14,15] Matrix metalloproteinases (MMPs) can degrade the extracellular matrix and contribute to AVF stenosis. A comparison of Chinese HD patients with or without AVF failure revealed that specific genotypes of MMP-1, MMP-3, and MMP-9 with lower transcriptional activity were associated with higher frequencies of AVF failure, thought to be due to accumulation of extracellular matrix causing stenosis.[16] Levels of Fetuin A, a protein secreted by hepatocytes and a potent inhibitor of vascular calcification, were measured in a prospective observational study of 238 prevalent HD patients.[17] Fetuin A deficiency was associated with a higher risk of loss of AV access (AVF and AVG) patency.

If the molecular mechanisms contribute to endothelial dysfunction and AVF failure, structural and physiologic characteristics of blood vessels must be associated with vascular access failure as well. A study of 225 hemodialysis patients in Taiwan showed that the ankle brachial index <0.9 was associated with vascular access failure.[18] Other factors influencing access failure in this study included the presence of AVG, high serum triglyceride level and high serum parathyroid hormone level. It is possible that uremic milieu itself might influence maturation of AVF. A recent study of femoral arteriovenous fistula in rats with or without CKD showed shrinking of media and increased vascular calcification in rats with CKD.[19] Arterial dilatation was also significantly impaired in rats with CKD. Indeed, there is clinical evidence demonstrating advanced process of neointimal hyperplasia in patients with CKD even prior to AVF creation.[20]

Failure of maturation is often attributed to many demographic factors and comorbidities. However, recent data does not support that notion.[21] During a 28 month period, 205 patients (69%) had primary AVF attempted as their primary access, with 64% success rate and no impact of comorbidity. A risk estimation equation for failure of maturation of AVF has also been proposed that provides a scoring system based on the age, race, presence, or the absence of coronary artery disease and peripheral vascular disease.[22] Although this equation was validated externally within the study, it was not found to be as predictive of failure of maturation in another study when applied to 346,291 incident HD patients from June 2005 to December 2008. The equation categorized 66% of these patients into low to moderate risk for AVF failure. However, hemodialysis was started using AVF in 13.8% of low risk patients, 13.3% of moderate risk patients, 13.2% of high risk patients, and 11.4% of very high risk patients.[23] The risk score was better correlated in the subgroup of patients under nephrology care for >12 months. However, the highest risk group had an AVF success rate only 10% lower than the low risk group, suggesting that AVF should be attempted irrespective of the risk score.

Nonsurgical interventions to improve maturation of AVF

To improve maturation and to prevent early thrombosis of AVF after creation, many small trials have evaluated use of aspirin, sulfinpyrazone, and ticlopidine, with inconclusive results. Recently, Dialysis Access Consortium (DAC) conducted a double blind, placebo-controlled, randomized trial comparing Clopidogrel started within 1 day of AVF creation (300 mg loading, followed by 75 mg daily for 6 weeks, $n = 441$) to placebo ($n = 436$) at US centers.[9] The patients were followed for 150–180 days after creation or 30 days after initiation of HD, whichever occurred later. Fistula thrombosis, primary outcome of the trial, occurred in 12.2% of participants in the active group, compared to 19.5% in placebo group, (RR 0.63). There was a high rate of the secondary outcome of failure to become suitable for HD in the two groups (67.5% vs 65.4%; relative risk, 1.04), with no significant difference between two groups. The results suggest that while early patency is essential for maturation of AVF, it is not the only factor for the AVF to become suitable for use. For example, other factors that may affect suitability for HD include arterial inflow, patency of outflow vein, vascular function, surgical technique, and configuration of AVF. The higher than expected rate of failure to become suitable for HD probably also, at least in part, reflects liberal creation of AVF in marginal patients due to emphasis on AVF creation. A randomized trial of fish oil and aspirin on fistula outcomes is ongoing in Australia.[24]

AVF: Postmaturation patency

There are many factors that may be associated with failure of AVF after its maturation and use. In a study of 831 HD patients in Southern Alberta Renal Program in Canada from January 2005 to June 2008, 10% of AVF failed within 6 months of first use.[25] A multivariate analysis showed that the odds ratio (OR) for loss of primary patency within first 6 months were independently associated with older age (>65%, OR 3.6), history of diabetes (OR 2.3), history of smoking (OR 4.3), forearm fistula (OR 4.0) and low initial intra-access blood flow (<500 mL/min, OR 29). Thus, poor initial flow in AVF may predict poor survival of AVF. Use of vasoactive drugs has been studied to look for fistula outcomes related to secondary patency. Recent data from 2815 incident patients enrolled in DOPPS study suggest that consistent aspirin use may be associated with lower risk of final AVF failure.[26] Treatment with angiotensin-converting enzyme inhibitors was associated with significantly better secondary fistula patency (RR, 0.56; $P = 0.010$).[27]

High hemoglobin and hematocrit have been thought to increase the risk of vascular access thrombosis in a number of studies examining effects of higher target hemoglobin in CKD.[28] In a Spanish study of prevalent dialysis patients, there was no such detrimental effect of higher hemoglobin.[29] In this study, a protective effect of ACE inhibitors and angiotensin receptor blockers was noted and the presence of diabetes, age >65 years, and iPTH >400 pg/mL were associated with worse vascular access survival. The route of epoetin administration has been noted to impact access thrombosis in a single study with higher rates of thrombosis with subcutaneous compared to the intravenous route.[30] Morbidity-and-Mortality Anemia Renal (MAR) Study, a prospective, multicenter cohort study followed 1710 patients over a year.[31] There was a higher risk of access-related events with low hemoglobin in patients with AVF, being even higher with AVG and catheter. The likelihood of remaining free of vascular access events at 12 month was 0.727 (baseline hb <10.0 g/dL), 0.801 (10.01 to 11.0 g/dL), 0.814 (11.01 to 12.0 g/dL), and 0.833 (>12.0 g/dL). Those with resistant anemia had a higher likelihood of vascular event. It is possible that the risk of vascular events was imparted by the higher dose of ESA used to correct anemia in such cases, rather than by the hb level itself.

▶ Cannulation Practices and AVF outcomes

Timing of cannulation is an important factor for successful use of AVF. This practice varies widely among different countries and optimal time to cannulation has not achieved a consensus. KDOQI Guidelines suggest using AVF no earlier than 1 month, and preferably after 2–3 months, with lesser success for earlier cannulation.[32] Data from the DOPPS study involving both incident and prevalent patients (n = 2154 for AVF) suggest that early cannulation is not a risk factor for AVF or AVG failure.[33] This data was based on a cross-section of prevalent patients who received a new access and the facility practice pattern of first cannulation, rather than on cannulation time of individual patients. Among incident patients, early cannulation was associated with late referral to nephrologist.[34] Also, there was no significant difference in outcomes of AVF if cannulated 15–28 days versus 43–84 days after creation. Cannulation times differed in different countries— < 2 months after placement in 36% of the United States, 79% of European, and 98% of Japanese facilities. As compared to the reference group of first cannulation at 1–2 months, the RR of fistula failure was 0.72 with first cannulation at < 4 weeks (P = 0.08), 0.91 at 2–3 months (P = 0.43), and 0.87 at > 3 months (P = 0.31). From the same DOPPS database, individual patient data from a smaller sample (n = 894) suggested worse outcomes if cannulated within 2 weeks of creation.[35]

In an Italian multicenter study of incident patients with AVF, there was a 94% increased risk of primary failure in those cannulated earlier than 1 month, and a 111% increased risk of final failure in those cannulated earlier than 2 weeks. The same study also found late referral (within 3 months of dialysis initiation), the presence of cardiovascular disease, and use of catheter at the start of dialysis to be additional predictors of failure.[36] Late referral to nephrologist is a well-known factor that has implications for overall care, morbidity, and mortality of CKD patients, not just vascular access outcomes.

Technique of cannulation may also influence fistula use and complications. The buttonhole technique requires cannulation of the same sites in AVF, and creates a track that allows consistent cannulation with less pain and less likelihood of bleeding or infiltration, especially when a short length of AVF is available to use the rotating (rope-ladder) technique. While many AVFs become available for use if buttonhole technique is used, recent observational data have raised concern for a higher incidence of infectious events, which can be mitigated by proper training.[37,38]

▶ AVG: Patency issues

Characteristics of AVG material may influence outcomes of access. The polyurethane urea (PUU) grafts have self-sealing property, which can allow cannulation immediately after its placement. A randomized, prospective, controlled, multicenter study enrolling 142 patients found PUU grafts with better hemostasis and ability to cannulate early, with similar 12 month primary and secondary patency.[39] Externally supported grafts have also been designed to enhance incompressibility and resistance to kinking to improve the patency of AVG. In a retrospective observational study including 990 patients using external supported AVG were

compared to 3412 nonsupported AVG. The patency rates of eternally supported AVG were superior.[40] This characteristic of supported graft will need further support from randomized-controlled trials.

Thigh grafts are generally considered after upper arm accesses have been abandoned. Femoral grafts placed in HD patients, once they have exhausted all arm access sites, can add significantly to patients' time on dialysis. In one study reporting results of 85 thigh graft recipients, thigh grafts had a low primary failure rate of 3%, survived longer than arm grafts and mature fistulas and had lower thrombosis rates.[41] Thus, prior to committing a patient to catheter-based access, a thigh graft must be considered.

Cannulation time for an AVG is generally shorter and K/DOQI guidelines suggested that PTFE AVGs should have at least 14 days, and preferably 3–6 weeks of maturation time. In the DOPPS study, 2730 grafts were studied.[33] AVGs were usually accessed during first 2–4 weeks (62% of US, 61% of European, and 42% of Japanese facilities). Less grafts failed in Europe than in the United States (RR 0.69). The RR of graft failure in reference to first cannulation at 2–3 weeks was 0.84 with first cannulation at < 2 weeks (P = 0.11), 0.94 with first cannulation at 3–4 weeks (P = 0.48), and 0.93 with first cannulation at > 4 weeks (P = 0.48). As mentioned earlier, these data are facility level data, not individual data. This suggests that there is no significant difference in outcomes with cannulation of AVG between 2 and 4 weeks.

Vasoactive drugs are commonly used in patients with ESRD and may influence maturation or survival of vascular access. An earlier small randomized clinical trial had suggested that dipyridamole, with or without aspirin, reduced graft thrombosis.[42] Early data from DOPPS regarding effect of drugs on VA showed that treatment with calcium channel blockers was associated with improved primary graft patency (RR for failure, 0.86; P = 0.034) and aspirin therapy was associated with better secondary graft patency (RR for failure, 0.70; P < 0.001).[27] Treatment with warfarin showed worse primary graft patency (RR, 1.33; P = 0.037) in this study. A randomized double-blind, placebo-controlled trial of aspirin with clopidogrel reported a 19% reduction in the hazard ratio for loss of primary unassisted graft patency, but the trial was stopped early because of increased risk of bleeding.[43] A dialysis access consortium (DAC) Aggrenox prevention of access stenosis trial evaluated the impact of administration of 200 mg extended release dipyridamole and 25 mg aspirin on patency of newly placed AVG in 649 patients.[44] At 1 year, patients receiving active treatment had an absolute risk reduction of 5% (primary patency of 28% in the combination group vs 23% in the placebo group) and adjusted relative risk reduction of 18% for loss of primary unassisted patency. The median cumulative graft patency was 22.5 months in the placebo group and was not significantly different in the active treatment group. The clinical benefit of the treatment was to prolong primary patency of AVG by 6 weeks only. The study also did not pursue postintervention impact of this treatment. At this time, due to the marginal benefit of therapy, an increase in cost does not justify routine use of these agents for improvement of AVG patency.

Dialysis patients frequently skip dialysis sessions and the incidence has noted to be 1–10% in different series.[45] A retrospective study examined 142 patients undergoing 15,692 HD sessions over 1 year, missing 1602 HD sessions (~10%).[46] Of the 78 patients who met the inclusion criteria, 50 patients (~64%) missed at least one HD session. Patients using AVF did not have significant impact of missing dialysis sessions on AVF patency; however, patients using AVG had 9.48 times risk of access thrombosis and 2.9 times higher incidence rate of intervention. It is plausible that missing access surveillance and not receiving anticoagulant dose normally received during dialysis resulted in this high risk of access-related complication.

▶ AVF versus AVG: Comparing Outcomes

It is challenging to compare outcomes of AVG and AVF. The mechanism of venous hyperplasia and rate of failure differ between these two accesses. Even though the statistical models involving Cox regression and similar methods are commonly used for survival analysis, these methods are semiparametric because they only estimate covariate coefficients and provide risk ratios, but do not measure instantaneous risk. As the hazard of failure is the highest soon after the placement of access, there is a gradual decline

in the risk with time, the rate of which varies between AVF and AVG. A study of survival modeling using semiparametric and parametric methods showed that the AVG had slower decline of hazard for failure than the AVF with shorter median survival time (8.4 vs 38.3 months).[47] The hazard of failure for AVG becomes proportional to that of AVF only at 3 months after placement with the hazard ratio of 3.2. Further, the primary failure rate is much less (~10%) for AVG.[44]

Primary reasons for failure of AV access are thrombosis and infection, which are also the predominant operative factors in resource utilization and expense. In a Canadian cohort of 347 HD patients, there was a 71% lower risk of thrombosis in AVF as compared to AVG.[48] Analysis of Medicare data also revealed that the risk of thrombosis of AVF was much lower as compared to graft.[49] The patency rates for AV grafts vary among studies and AVF, despite a high rate of failure of maturation, have better survival than AVG, even in the United States where AVF survival is not as good as in Europe.[34] A mature AVF has better cumulative survival than AVG. But, when failure to mature is included, cumulative survival of AVF and AVG become similar (Figure 12-5A).[50] The secondary patency of AVG ranges from 40% to 87% at 3 years with most centers reporting 3 year secondary patency around 50%. It is important to mention that improved secondary patency rates for AVG are only achieved at expense of three- to sixfold greater reintervention rates (Figure 12-5B).[50] The

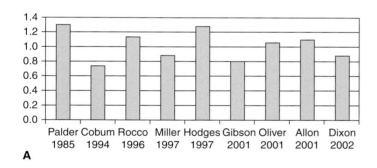

A

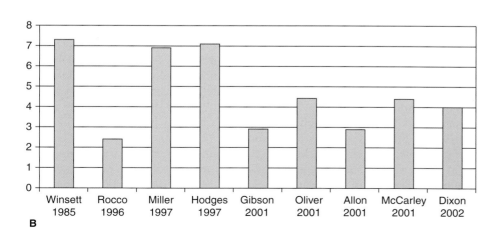

B

Figure 12-5. (**A**) Cumulative survival of graft/fistula at 1 year, from access creation to permanent failure, regardless of number of interventions required to maintain access patency). Bars represent ratio of cumulative survival in grafts *versus* fistulas reported in different large series. Note that the ratio is approximately 1.0, indicating comparable cumulative survival of grafts and fistulas. (From Ref. [15]). (**B**) Revision rate of access (graft/fistula) per year. Revisions include elective angioplasty, thrombectomy, and surgical revision. Bars represent ratio of revision rate in grafts *versus* fistulas reported in different large series. Note that all of the ratios are >1, with a median ratio of 3 to 4:1, indicating a much higher revision rate in grafts than in fistulas. (Data from Ref. [15]).

occurrence of thrombosis decreases survival of both AVF and AVG. However, the secondary patency of AVG after an episode of thrombosis is generally much worse than that of AVF and is reported as only 30–63% at 3 months and 11–34% at 6 months.[51,52]

In a previously failed forearm fistula, usual next access is an upper arm AVF or AVG. In an observational study of such upper arm AVF ($n = 59$) and AVG ($n = 51$), the primary failure was higher for AVF than AVG requiring more interventions to achieve successful use.[53] However, once the AVF was mature, it had longer survival than AVG and required less number of interventions to maintain long-term patency.

Intervention for AV access failure

Aggressive intervention has been used as a strategy to salvage AVF that do not mature.[54] Appropriate size of balloon and optimum level of pressure used for angioplasty are not yet established. There is concern that even though these measures may salvage a significant number of fistulae, the resulting endothelial damage may also promote proliferative changes leading to recurrent stenosis.[55] A recent retrospective study of 173 HD patients from two academic centers receiving new AVF revealed that 44% patients required one (31%) or more (13%) intervention to achieve suitability for dialysis.[56] Cumulative access survival to permanent failure in patients requiring two or more, one or no intervention was 68%, 78%, and 92%, respectively, at 1 year and 57%, 71%, and 85%, respectively, at 2 years and 42%, 57%, and 75%, respectively, at 3 years. There were 3.51 ± 2.2, 1.37 ± 0.31, and 0.76 ± 0.1 interventions per year in respective groups. Thus, the survival is poor in AVF and is achieved at a high rate of intervention in AVF requiring intervention to attain maturation. Due to study limitations, it cannot be inferred whether the interventions were simply marker of poor vessels or were causally associated with outcome.

▶ Guidelines, Goals, and Public Policy

The Dialysis Outcomes Quality Initiative (DOQI) guidelines were the first formal guidelines published by the National Kidney Foundation in 1997 to provide specific recommendations for focus issues for hemodialysis patients that included vascular access guidelines which were updated in 2000 and again in 2006.[57] Primary AVF was recommended as the access of choice with recommendations to place AVF in at least 50% of all new ESRD patients electing to receive HD. The guidelines also recommended that 40% of prevalent HD patients should have native A-V fistulae and fewer than 10% of chronic maintenance HD patients be maintained on catheters as their permanent chronic dialysis access. This goal of prevalent AVF was achieved in 2005 in the United States as a common goal of the "Fistula First" initiative that was implemented in 2003. The goal was reset to 66%, which is yet to be achieved.

The Fistula First breakthrough initiative (FFBI) was implemented by the Centers of Medicare and Medicaid (CMMS) in 2003 (first as National Vascular Access Improvement Initiative or NVAII) in partnership with ESRD networks to improve fistula prevalence and reduce catheter rates. A number of "Change Concepts" were developed to identify the barriers in using AVF and provided strategies to overcome those barriers (fistulafirst. org). The model clearly identifies the nephrologist as the leader for this initiative, directing the hospital, surgeon, and the patient in this endeavor. As a consequence of the momentum provided by this initiative, the rate of increase in fistula prevalence nearly doubled (from 2% per year to 4% per year) and the AVF prevalence has increased from 32.2% in July 2003 to 57.8% in February 2011. The current goal of Fistula First (66% AVF in prevalent patients) is getting closer with some of the ESRD networks already at the goal. As expected, the AVG use has significantly decreased from 40.1% to 19.9% during this period of time. There was an initial concern that the prevalent catheter use had increased due to a high AVF placement rates. However, the data show a steady decrease in catheter rates from 26.9% to 22.3% in 2011.[58] A catheter last strategy has also been incorporated to reduce catheter use to <10%.

Aside from the guidelines and national initiatives, other systematic efforts to reduce catheter rates have shown satisfying results. In a hemodialysis Catheter Reduction Collaborative that was implemented in 166 volunteer facilities managed by Fresenius Medical Care, catheter rates were reduced by 5% over a period of 8 months.[59] The attributes of the program included accountability of physicians, surgeon selection and referral, team focus, education, and use of a checklist. Thus, improving processes, logistics, and communication seem to be crucial in achieving this goal. Further, the RightStart Program for incident patients at Fresenius Medical Care facilities provided prompt medical management and self-management education, resulting in greater reduction of catheters (32%) versus the nonintervention group (27%) at day 120 among other outcomes.[60] Many other initiatives have focused on processes that can lead to improving vascular access outcomes. These include CKD focus of quality improvement organizations, inclusion of AVF in the quality assessment and performance improvement (QAPI) measures in Conditions for Coverage for dialysis facilities, as well as revision of relative value units (RVU) to improve reimbursement for AVF creation and decrease for AVG creation.[61] CMS also convened a clinical technical expert panel in 2010 to recommend measures to decrease vascular access-related infections. The panel recommended removing financial and regulatory barriers to timely placement and revision of hemodialysis fistulas and the concurrent avoidance of catheter use.[62] The measures suggested by the panel include earlier disbursement of Medicare benefits to uninsured patients needing AVF placement and changes to the current physician and hospital reimbursement for AVF placement.

Despite these efforts, several important hurdles in achieving vascular access goals remain. Poor awareness of risks of catheters, lack of uniform financial support of early creation of AVF by the states or hospitals, and less aggressive intervention for AVF maturation failure do not allow early creation and incident use of AVF. As the CKD epidemic spreads, it will be immensely important to identify CKD early so that appropriate referral to nephrologist can be made. Late referral to nephrologists is a common cause of poor vascular access choice at the time of initiation of dialysis. Providing only catastrophic coverage for dialysis in the absence of a defined strategy for preventive care is likely to make the situation worse.[63]

▶ Practice Pattern and Vascular Access Utilization

The multinational Dialysis Outcomes and Practice Patterns Study (DOPPS) has captured trends in the use of vascular access in a number of countries.[64] It is comforting to note that with the recent emphasis on AVF use in the United States, the three different phases of DOPPS have documented a progressive increase in the use of AVF in the United States. The use of AVF has remained stable or has slightly declined in most other countries. The factors that result in the lower prevalence of AVF in the DOPPS study include countries with greater prevalence of diabetes, facilities with longer time from referral to access surgery evaluation, from evaluation to creation of access, and from access creation until first AVF cannulation. There is a significant variation in the practice pattern for median time to referral for access creation among countries, ranging from 5 to 6 days in Italy, Japan, and Germany to 40–43 days in the UK and Canada. This practice correlates well with the significant variation in use of different accesses in incident and prevalent patients among counties participating in DOPPS.

Timing of creation of AVF and AVG is important in determining use of VA in prevalent HD patients. KDOQI recommends creation of AVF when either creatinine clearance is <25 mL/min, creatinine is >4 mg/dL, or initiation of HD is expected within 1 year.[32] Unfortunately, patients are frequently referred late for creation of AVF resulting in initiation of HD with a catheter. Initiation of HD with a catheter has been shown to be associated with adverse consequences. Multiple studies have shown that earlier nephrology referral prior to initiation of dialysis is associated with higher use of AVF.[34,36,64] An analysis of several Canadian administrative databases compared "early" creation of AVF or AVG (at least 4 months before initiation of HD, $n = 1240$), "just prior creations" (between 4 months and 1 month before initiation of HD, $n = 997$), and late creation (<1 month before initiation of HD and after initiation of HD, $n = 3687$).[65] Relative risk of sepsis with early creation was 0.57 as compared to late creation. There was a 41% increased risk of sepsis with catheter. Catheter use and sepsis were independently associated with increased mortality.

Routine preoperative physical examination and ultrasound vascular mapping have been shown to improve AVF outcomes including an increase in AVF placement rates.[66] Anatomical parameters such as vein diameter are considered important for creation of a successful AVF.[67] KDOQI guidelines recommend use of routine ultrasound mapping for all patients.[68] A recent randomized trial of 208 patients with newly created AVF showed lower immediate failure rate of forearm AVF in the ultrasound group in comparison to no ultrasound group (4% vs 11%) and among failed AVF, less thrombosis (38% vs 67%).[69] Assisted survival of AVF was also better in the ultrasound group (80% vs 65%). The number of patients requiring preoperative ultrasound to prevent one AVF failure was 12.

Type of insurance coverage seems to influence placement of AVF. In a study looking at the patients in Department of Defense and Veterans Affairs, those who received predialysis nephrology care were 10 times more likely to have a functioning AVF at initiation of dialysis in comparison to patients in United States Renal Data System (USRDS) database covered by other insurances including Medicare.[70] While the study shows that the universal coverage in this system was beneficial, the incident AVF rate in this study was much less than that in Europe. Exposure to nephrology care early has been shown to improve outcomes including better vascular access. The USRDS data indicates that incident patients with no pre-ESRD care had the highest rates of catheter use although nearly half of those receiving pre ESRD nephrology care for over 12 months still used a catheter at initial dialysis.[71] Even with similar rates of nephrology care >4 months prior to initiation of hemodialysis (about 65%), the incident use of AVF remains poor in the United States. Thus, it is important for the nephrologists to refer patients for AVF creation early. Other practices that may impact the incident use include delayed cannulation and higher prescribed blood flow rate in the United States.[35] It has also been suggested that lower nurse to patient ratio in the United States as compared to Europe may also impact attention to the care of AVF.[72] Further, practices specific to centers are also responsible for types of prevalent accesses and changes in those practices can influence outcomes. In the CIMINO initiative in the Netherlands multicenter, guideline-based intervention was able to increase the number of prevalent AVF.[73] It is a common experience that the presence of a dedicated vascular access nurse coordinator can improve AVF rates while decreasing catheter rates.[74]

Selection of a well-trained surgeon to create vascular access is an important factor in creation of successful AVF, as previously noted. Fistula First initiative suggested "change concepts" that would influence surgeon selection based on outcomes, willingness, and timeliness of providing access services. Based on this, outcomes of 75 patients undergoing access surgery by two high volume, dedicated vascular access surgeons and academic medical center were compared at a center in the United States.[75] Despite having older patients and those with history of previously failed accesses, dedicated surgeons placed fistulae in 98% (vs 71%) with 6 month and 1 year access survival rates were 82% and 58%, respectively (vs 82% and 47%). This study emphasizes that surgeon selection and willingness to place fistula as a part of planned strategy can increase placement and survival of AVF.

Demographics of dialysis patients impact type of vascular access. Females, older patients, those with greater body mass index, diabetes mellitus, and peripheral vascular disease are less likely to use AVF. Clinical Performance Measures (CPM) Project also analyzed the CMMS Medical Evidence form 2728 in incident patients during 1999–2003.[76] Female gender, ischemic heart disease, lack of obesity, factors indicative of poor pre-ESRD care, and successive year of dialysis initiation predicted CVC use at the time of initiation of HD. Perhaps either the nonobese subjects were in poor health to consider AVF or AVG, or the obese patients were not considered a candidate for AVF and were relegated to AVG that decreased the likelihood of CVC placement. Among prevalent patients using catheters, cuffed catheters are more commonly (80–95%) used than noncuffed catheters. Long-term exposure to catheter, even in those with a maturing AVF and AVG, leads to complications and poor survival of patients.[77] Examination of recent access trends in Canadian incident and prevalent patients has shown a significant increase in use of catheters, with a simultaneous increase in mortality.[78] This apparently reflects a change in practice pattern, with significant geographic variation. Similar data has also emerged out of the DOPPS II study.[79] The risk of increase in mortality with increasing use of catheters calls for a change in such practice. Disparity in vascular access care has also been observed within the United States. There is a high degree of variability among dialysis networks regarding use of vascular access type.[80] Such discrepancy has been noted even within a single metropolitan area.[81]

At present, there is no evidence that a higher or lower access flow contributes to mortality.[82] Also, the DOPPS study showed that the facility median blood flow was not associated with access failure.[33]

▶ Type of Vascular Access and Outcomes

Vascular access influences various biochemical and patient-related outcomes and choice of vascular access in an important aspect of predialysis care. Not only the AVF is associated with higher hemoglobin, albumin, and adequacy of dialysis, the cost of dialysis, first 90-day mortality, infections, and hospitalization rates are the lowest in patients using AVF. In the DOPPS-II study involving over 28,000 patients in 322 dialysis facilities, there was a 32% increase in adjusted relative risk of death of those using catheter and a 15% increase in those using graft as compared to those using an AVF.[83] Similar results have been shown in other studies as well.[84–86] Although it has been suggested that other covariates within these studies may have resulted in such differences in outcomes associated with catheters, there is evidence of a direct role of catheters in causing infection and inflammation that may explain poor outcomes. For example, extensive case mix adjustment in the DOPPS study was able to explain only a portion of the difference in the mortality risk between the United States and Europe; adjustment for pattern of vascular access was able to abrogate almost all of this risk and was also shown to account for almost 30% of excess risk in comparison to Japan (Figure 12-6).[87] Further, catheters have been associated with five to seven times higher risk of all-cause hospitalization, hospitalization due to any infection or vascular access related hospitalization as compared to use of AVF.[88]

First impressions: Initial vascular access and outcomes

Use of a particular type of access at initiation of HD can impart survival advantage. The Choices for Healthy Outcomes in Caring for ESRD (CHOICE) study enrolled 616 incident dialysis patients with 1084 accesses during the course of 3 years after initiation of HD.[89] The annual mortality rates were 11.7% for AVF, 14.2% for AVG, and 16.1% for CVC. As compared to AVF, hazard of death for AVG was 1.2. The hazard ratio for CVC was 1.5, with further

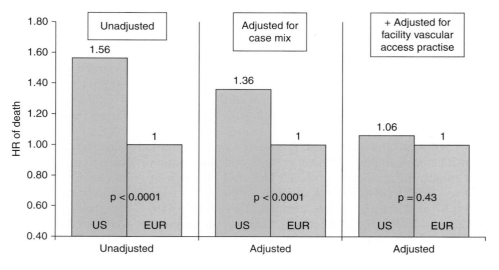

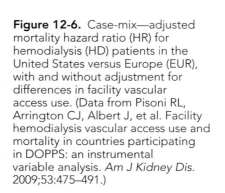

Figure 12-6. Case-mix—adjusted mortality hazard ratio (HR) for hemodialysis (HD) patients in the United States versus Europe (EUR), with and without adjustment for differences in facility vascular access use. (Data from Pisoni RL, Arrington CJ, Albert J, et al. Facility hemodialysis vascular access use and mortality in countries participating in DOPPS: an instrumental variable analysis. *Am J Kidney Dis.* 2009;53:475–491.)

worsening in men. Similarly, an analysis of Medicare data that included patients 67 year or older showed that those who started dialysis with an AVF had a lower mortality risk than those starting with an AVG or a catheter.[90] In fact, the majority of the difference in mortality risk in first 1–2 years of PD and HD can be attributed to the use of catheters. A comparison of survival of 7412 patients starting PD in Canada from 2001 to 2008 showed similar 1 year mortality of 6663 patients who started HD with an AVF or AVG, but 24,437 patients starting HD with a catheter had 80% higher mortality at 1 year.[91]

AVF has consistently been shown to be associated with better outcomes in numerous other studies. Analysis of the database from the Dialysis Mortality and Morbidity study Wave 2 found a significant correlation between initial access and septicemia or bacteremia with a hazard ratio of 1.95 for permanent catheters, 1.76 for temporary catheters, 1.05 for AVG, and 0.96 for PD catheters as compared to AVF.[92] Septicemia or bacteremia was associated with an increased risk of subsequent death (HR 2.33), myocardial infarction (HR 1.78), heart failure (HR 1.64), peripheral vascular disease (HR 1.64), and stroke (HR 2.04). As microinflammation can lead to high incidence of cardiovascular disease, it is plausible that septicemia or bacteremia related to vascular access can potentiate this mechanism.

Dialysis Mortality and Morbidity study Wave 2 data also compared patient-reported health status and quality of life scores among VA type at the time of initiation of HD ($n = 1563$) and found greater physical activity and energy, better emotional and social well-being, fewer symptoms, less effect of dialysis, and burden of kidney disease, and better sleep in patients using AVF as compared to those using CVC. Measures of cognition and sexual function were not different.[93]

Vascular calcification has been noted to be an independent predictor of mortality in CKD. Vascular access calcification in a cohort of 212 patients detected by plain X-ray in two dimensions also turned out to be a predictor of mortality.[94] Male gender, diabetes mellitus, and vintage on dialysis were independent predictors for access calcification. Intact PTH, serum high sensitivity CRP, serum fetuin A, and undercarboxylated matrix Gla protein were not significantly different in those with and without access calcification. Authors suggested that access calcification can be used as a prognostic marker in HD patients.

Initial access seems to be important in determining the survival of access as well; those starting with a permanent access fare better than those starting with a catheter (Figure 12-7A and B).[34] Taking these data into account, AVF is considered the access of choice.

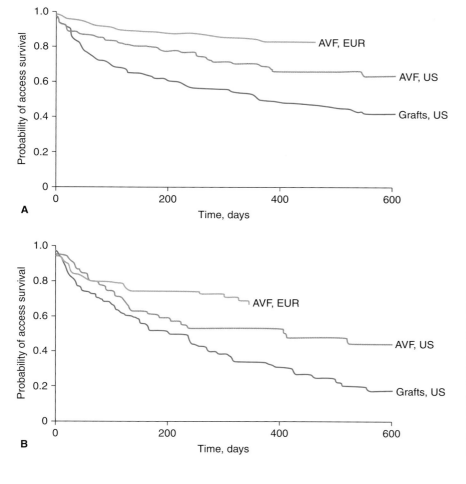

Figure 12-7. (**A**) Survival of AVF and AVG in the United States and Europe in incident patients starting dialysis with an arteriovenous access. ($N = 430$ for Europe and 428 for the United States). Survival of AVG could not be estimated due to small number in Europe. (From Ref. [34]). (**B**) Survival of AVF and AVG in the United States and Europe in incident patients starting dialysis with a temporary access. ($N = 430$ for Europe and 428 for the United States). Survival of AVG could not be estimated due to small number in Europe. (From Ref. [34]).

Catheters and outcomes

Although use of catheters for dialysis is frequently necessary, the data above show that this type of access is associated with higher risk of infection, thrombosis, poor adequacy, higher hospitalizations, and higher mortality. Significant evidence indicates an increased mortality and an increased number of infections associated with use of catheters for dialysis.[95] Data from the USRDS Morbidity and Mortality Study Wave 1 showed that in 5507 randomly selected diabetic patients with ESRD the relative mortality risk was higher with catheter (RR 1.54) and AVG (RR 1.41) as compared to AVF.[84] In nondiabetic individuals, this risk was higher with CVC (1.70) and lesser with AVG (1.08). This study also showed higher infection-related deaths for CVC (RR 2.30) and AVG (RR 2.47) in DM patients and CVC (RR 1.83) in non-DM patients. Death risk was also higher for cardiac causes in CVC patients as compared to AVF in both DM and non-DM groups. This may be related to ongoing inflammation that may be a trigger for accelerated atherosclerosis. In another retrospective cohort of 7497 prevalent patients on dialysis, there was higher mortality in those dialyzed with a catheter as compared to those dialyzed with AVG or AVF, with a higher rate of death from infection.[85] The adjusted odds ratio was 1.4 for all-cause death and 3.0 for infection-related death in those using catheters. Contrary to the misconception that AVF commonly lead to heart failure, AVF use has been linked to lower rates of cardiovascular death as compared to catheters.[96] This rather unintuitive phenomenon may be due to increased inflammation from infected and non-infected catheters.[97] It is also a common knowledge that the patients using catheter require higher erythropoietin dosage to achieve hemoglobin in target range. These findings have implications for use of catheters, even though the data is associative. Interestingly, spurious hyperphosphatemia may occur if alteplase (or heparin) is used as lock solution and an adequate aliquot of blood is not discarded before sample collection.[98]

Change of vascular access and outcomes

It is clear from the data mentioned above that there is a differential impact of type of vascular access on patient and access outcomes. Consequently, it is not surprising that a subsequent change in type of vascular access can also influence outcomes. The mortality according to type of vascular access used over a year and according to change in vascular access was examined in the hemodialysis study.[99] Those using a catheter during the whole year had a significantly higher mortality than those using an AV access (RR 3.43). The relative risk decreased to 1.37 in those switching from catheter to AV access. In a prospective observational study of 79,545 patients, the impact of change in vascular access type during the first 4 months of 2007 led to a change in mortality during next 8 months of 2007.[100] Compared with patients who continued using a catheter, those who converted to either a graft or fistula had a mortality hazard ratio of 0.69. Those who converted to a catheter from graft or fistula had an increase in the mortality hazard ratio to 2.12, with similar trends in incident patients. On the other hand, those who converted to grafts or fistulas from catheter had an adjusted hazard ratio of 0.69 for hospitalization, which was similar to the adjusted hazard ratio of 0.71 for fistulas. Patients changing to catheters had an adjusted hazard ratio for hospitalization of 1.22.[101] It should be noted that these studies are observational and do not suggest causality. The possibility that those who switched from AVF and AVG to catheters were inherently sicker, leading to worse outcomes, and vice versa cannot be ruled out.

▶ Economics of Vascular Access

The vascular access-related costs exceed $1 billion annually in the United States. The annual cost to maintain vascular access was shown to be the lowest for those patients starting HD with an AVF.[102] The overall cost was about five times higher for maintenance of catheters and eight times higher for maintenance of AVG. A study of 239 consecutive incident HD patients in Canada showed the mean annual cost of all vascular access care to be Canadian $6890.[103] The mean cost of access care per patient-year at risk for maintaining a catheter exclusively, attempting an arteriovenous fistula, or attempting a graft was $9180, $7989, and $11,685, respectively ($P = 0.01$). Thus, it is evident that vascular access care is responsible for a significant proportion of health care costs in the first year of HD. According to the USRDS report 2010, per person per year access expenditure is $8683 for AVG, $6402 for catheter, and $3480 for AVF.[71] The costs increased 7–17% in 2008 for hemodialysis patients and fell by 32% for the peritoneal dialysis catheter. The overall patient expenditure also differed significantly associated with type of access- per person per year total expenditure was $90,110 with catheter, $79,337 with AVG, and $64,701 with AVF. It is clear from these data that not only there is a significant difference in costs of establishing and maintaining different type of vascular access, overall care, cost, and outcome of a HD patient can be influenced by the type of access.

There remain concerns about comparison of costs related to different vascular access. In one study, analogous Markov models were created for AVF and AVG that were placed at the time of initiation of dialysis.[104] Probable outcomes, transition probabilities, utilities, and costs based on published studies were considered. Survival, quality-adjusted survival, and costs among incident patients were compared after attempted placement of AVF or AVG. The overall survival of AVF was slightly but significantly better (2.6 months) than AVG and so was quality-adjusted survival (3.6 quality adjusted life months). The incremental cost-effectiveness ratio for AVF relative to AVG was $446 per quality-adjusted life year saved. The benefit in this conceptual model was smaller than expected based on current evidence and may be due to a high incidence of maturation failure. Thus, it may be helpful to prospectively identify patients at high risk for AVF maturation failure. Although predictive risk equations have been attempted, these have not proved to be accurate in prediction.

▶ Vascular Access in Elderly and Adolescents

Analysis of Medicare data shows that the risk of thrombosis of AVF was much lower as compared to graft.[49] The advantage was higher in younger patients and was less, though maintained, in older patients. The relative risk (RR) of failure of AVF as compared to AVG changed with age, being 67% lower at 40 years, 54% lower at 50 years, and 24% lower at 65 years of age. The number of older patients starting HD has increased over the years. Due to the guidelines emphasizing use of AVF, a significant number of these patients receive AVF, despite a high risk of failure of maturation. A study of incident HD patients ($n = 444$), which included 196 patients over 65 years of age, found the cumulative survival of AVF at one year and five year to be 75.1% and 64.7%, respectively.[105] In comparison, those under 65 years had AVF survival of 79.7% and 71.4% at similar time intervals. The relative risk of failure of AVF was 1.7 in the older group. Intervention rates were no different in the two groups. The study suggests that age should not be the primary limiting factor when considering candidacy for AVF placement. A retrospective cohort study in Department of Veteran Affairs showed that older patients with CKD were less likely to receive VA, but were also less likely to start dialysis.[106] It was estimated if all patients had been referred for VA surgery at the beginning of the study the ratio of unnecessary to necessary procedures at the end of the study would have been 5:1 for patients aged 85–100 years, as opposed to 0.5:1 for those aged 18–44 years. The study results suggest that a commonsense approach should be used in certain cases. It is reasonable to individualize the approach since there may be diminishing return in the case of very old. However, it can be argued that a similar approach should be followed in all patients, not just the elderly. Also, the study was observational, likely flawed due to bias by indication, and did not take into account high mortality associated with catheters.[107] Yet another study suggested consideration of AVG in patients over 70 years of age based on lower cumulative fistula survival at 12 months and poor patient survival.[108]

In adolescents, vascular catheters are the predominant type of vascular access. In a retrospective cohort study of pediatric patients aged 12 to <18 years ($n = 418$) receiving in-center HD, in 2000 ESRD Clinical Performance Measures Project, 58% had vascular catheter and remaining had an AV access.[109] Adjusted relative risk for hospitalization for any cause was 4.74 and 2.72 for hospitalization as a result of infection in patients with catheter as compared to those with AV access. The results indicate high morbidity associated with catheter use in pediatric patients on dialysis. However, a recent report of 29 children and infants in Israel indicated that a catheter infection rate of only 1 in 5 years was achieved with median catheter survival time of 310 days for children and 211 days in infants.[110]

▶ Vascular Access in Immunocompromised

The number of patients with human immunodeficiency virus (HIV) requiring dialysis is increasing. Immune deficiency and frequent history of IV drug abuse result in higher incidence of access infections and may lead to poor access survival as compared to HIV negative patients.[111] In a small population of HIV-positive dialysis patients ($n = 15$), the overall 1 year AVG survival (41% vs 65%), thrombosis-free graft survival (17% vs 62%), and infection-free graft survival (61% vs 88%) were inferior to those in HIV-negative controls.[112] Primary failure rates and cumulative AVF survival were not different between two groups. Since AVF outcomes were similar and AVG outcomes were significantly worse, authors recommended that AVF should be the access of choice in patients with HIV. In a retrospective cohort study of 40 HIV-positive patients, the incidence of tunneled cuffed catheter-related bacteremia and exit site infections were not different although the risk of gram-negative bacteremia and fungemia was higher.[113]

▶ Vascular Access in Frequent Dialysis

Daily HD is becoming more popular, and promises high levels of clearance and better outcomes. There has been a concern that frequent use of VA can lead to access failure. An observational study of a small number of patients, however, showed that there was better AVF survival as compared to AVG or catheter, albeit with more complaints related to pain and redness around the fistula site.[114] No significant difference in the VA outcomes was detected in an Italian study comparing outcomes of access in the daily HD program versus the usual schedule of HD.[115] The gross incidence of vascular access failure was 1.3 per 100 patient months in the daily HD group and 1.2 per 100 patient months in the nondaily HD group. More recently, the Frequent Hemodialysis Network (FHN) Daily Trial compared 120 patients receiving traditional three times a week in-center dialysis with 125 patients receiving six times a week in-center dialysis for 1 year.[116] The trial reported more frequent interventions (hazard ratio 1.71) related to vascular access, including time to first intervention and need for multiple intervention in the more frequent hemodialysis group although the difference was not statistically significant. It cannot be inferred whether or not the higher number of interventions was related to more frequent surveillance as the number of access failures was, in fact, less in the more frequent dialysis group.

▶ Future of Vascular Access

The reimbursement for dialysis has changed significantly since January 1, 2011. The implementation of a prospective payment system (also known as bundling) has changed practices which are not only going to change use of various dialysis-related drugs, but also use of modalities of dialysis and types of vascular access. Catheters are associated with higher infection rate, antibiotics, and amount of ESA and loss of dialysis revenues due to higher hospitalization rate. The cost of taking care of a patient using a catheter is nearly $20,000 higher than the cost of a patient with AVF.[71] This provides yet another reason to use arteriovenous access than a catheter for dialysis. It is expected that the incident dialysis catheter rate will decrease as the focus now shifts to the "catheter last" approach. Approaches to improving quality by using special programs are also likely to result in better access outcomes. For example, the Right Start program for incident hemodialysis programs focuses on patient education, evaluation, and intervention in all areas of dialysis process including attention to catheter reduction. Indeed, in an initial program involving 4308 patients, there was 32% reduction in catheter use as compared to 24% in 4308 patients in control group on day 120 while reducing death risk by 34% during the same period of time.[60]

There has also been an interest from interventional nephrologists in placement of AVF. High rates of successful AVF maturation have been reported and may help in achievement of FF goals.[117] Improvements in technology for creating, using, and maintaining a vascular access are in progress. As these become available, improvement in vascular access outcomes are likely.

REFERENCES

1. Quinton W, Dillard D, Scribner BH. Cannulation of blood vessels for prolonged hemodialysis. *Trans Am Soc Artif Intern Organs.* 1960;6:104–113.
2. Brescia MJ, Cimino JE, Appel K, Hurwich BJ. Chronic hemodialysis using venipuncture and a surgically created arteriovenous fistula. *N Engl J Med.* 1966;275:1089–1092.
3. Cortez AJ, Paulson WD, Schwab SJ. Vascular access as a determinant of adequacy of hemodialysis. *Semin Nephrol.* 2005;25;96–101.
4. Vachharajani T. In, Atlas of Vascular Access. Available at: http://www.fistulafirst.org/LinkClick.aspx?fileticket=7w_juc-gK1w%3D&tabid=39. Accessed May 12, 2011.
5. Haddad NJ, Vachharajani TJ, Van Cleef S, et al. Iatrogenic graft to vein fistula (GVF) formation associated with synthetic arteriovenous grafts. *Semin Dial.* 2010;23: 643–647.
6. Power A, Singh S, Ashby D, et al. Translumbar central venous catheters for long term haemodialysis. *Nephrol Dial Transplant.* 2010;25:1588–1595.
7. Nassar GM. Long-term performance of the hemodialysis reliable outflow (HeRO) device: the 56-month follow-up of the first clinical trial patient. *Semin Dial.* 2010;23:229–232.
8. Allon M, Robbin ML. Increasing arteriovenous fistulas in hemodialysis patients: problems and solutions. *Kidney Int.* 2002;62:1109–1124.
9. Dember LM, Beck GJ, Allon M, et al. For the Dialysis Access Consortium Study Group. Effect of clopidogrel on early failure of arteriovenous fistulas for hemodialysis: a randomized controlled trial. *JAMA.* 2008;299:2164–2171.
10. Fassiadis N, Morsey M, Siva M, Marsh JE, Makanjuola AD, Chemla ES. Does the surgeon's experience impact on radiocephalic fistula patency rates? *Semin Dial.* 2007;20:455–457.
11. Saran R, Elder SJ, Goodkin DA, Akiba T, Ethier J, Rayner HC, Saito A, Young EW, Gillespie BW, Merion RM, Pisoni RL. Enhanced training in vascular access creation predicts arteriovenous fistula placement and patency in hemodialysis patients: results from the Dialysis Outcomes and Practice Patterns Study. *Ann Surg.* 2008;247: 885–891.
12. Juncos JP, Grande JP, Kang L, et al. MCP-1 contributes to arteriovenous fistula failure. *J Am Soc Nephrol.* 2011;22: 43–48.
13. Heine GH, Ulrich C, Sester U, et al. Transforming growth factor beta 1 genotype polymorphisms determine AVF fistula patency in hemodialysis patients. *Kidney Int.* 2003;64:1101–1107.
14. Fukasawa M, Matsushita K, Kamiyama M, et al. The methylenetetrahydrofolate reductase C677T point mutation is a risk factor for vascular access thrombosis in hemodialysis patients. *Am J Kidney Dis.* 2003;41: 637–642.
15. Lin CC, Yang WC, Lin SJ, et al. Length polymorphism in heme oxygenase-1 is associated with arteriovenous fistula patency in hemodialysis patients. *Kidney Int.* 2006;69;165–172.
16. Lin CC, Yang WC, Chung MY, et al. Functional polymorphisms in matrix metalloproteinases-1, -3 and -9 are associated with arteriovenous fistula patency in hemodialysis patients. *Clin J Am Soc Nephrol.* 2010;5:1805–1814.
17. Chen HY, Chiu YL, Chuang YF, et al. Association of low serum Fetuin A levels with poor arteriovenous access patency in patients undergoing maintenance hemodialysis. *Am J Kidney Dis.* 2010;56:710–727.
18. Chen SC, Chang JM, Hwang SJ, et al. Significant correlation between ankle-brachial index and vascular access failure in hemodialysis patients. *Clin J Am Soc Nephrol.* 2009;4:128–134.
19. Langer S, Kokozidou M, Heiss C, et al. Chronic kidney disease aggravates arteriovenous fistula damage in rats. *Kidney Int.* 2010;78:1312–1321.
20. Lee T, Chauhan V, Krishnamoorthy M, et al. Severe venous neointimal hyperplasia prior to dialysis access surgery. *Nephrol Dial Transplant.* 2011;26(7): 2264–2270.
21. Wang W, Murphy B, Yilmaz S, Tonelli M, MacRae J, Manns BJ. Comorbidities do not influence primary fistula success in incident hemodialysis patients: a prospective study. *Clin J Am Soc Nephrol.* 2008;3:78–84.
22. Lok CE, Allon M, Moist L, et al. Risk equation in determining unsuccessful cannulation events and failure to maturation in arteriovenous fistulas (Reduce FTM I). *J Am Soc Nephrol.* 2006;17:3204–3212.
23. Wish JB. Fistula first: myth vs. fact. *Nephrol News Issues.* 2010;24(4):36,39–41.
24. Irish A, Dogra G, Mori T, et al. Preventing AVF thrombosis:the rationale and design of the omega-3 fatty acids (Fish Oils) and Aspirin in Vascular access Outcomes in REnal disease (FAVOURED) study. *BMC Nephrology.* 2009;10:1.

25. Monroy-Cuadros M, Yilmaz S, Salazar-Banuelos A, Doig C. Risk factors associated with patency loss of hemodialysis vascular access within 6 months. *Clin J Am Soc Nephrol.* 2010;5:1787–1792.

26. Hasegawa T, Elder SJ, Bragg-Gresham JL, Pisoni RL, Yamazaki S, Akizawa T, Jadoul M, Hugh RC, Port FK, Fukuhara S. Consistent aspirin use associated with improved arteriovenous fistula survival among incident hemodialysis patients in the Dialysis Outcomes and Practice Patterns Study. *Clin J Am Soc Nephrol.* 2008;3:1373–1378.

27. Saran R, Dykstra DM, Wolfe RA, et al. Association between vascular access failure and the use of specific drugs: The Dialysis Outcomes and Practice Patterns Study (DOPPS). *Am J Kidney Dis.* 2002;40:1255–1263.

28. Besarab A, Bolton WK, Browne JK, Egrie JC, Nissenson AR, Okamoto DM, Schwab SJ, Goodkin DA. The effects of normal as compared with low hematocrit values in patients with cardiac disease who are receiving haemodialysis and epoetin. *N Engl J Med.* 1998;339:584–590.

29. Garrancho JM, Kirchgessner J, Arranz M, Klinkner G, Rentero R, Ayala JA, Marcelli D. Haemoglobin level and vascular access survival in haemodialysis patients. *Nephrol Dial Transplant.* 2005;20:2453–2457.

30. Lee YK, Koo JR, Kim JK, et al. Effect of route of EPO administration on hemodialysis arteriovenous vascular access failure: a randomized controlled trial. *Am J Kidney Dis.* 2009;53:815–822.

31. Portole's J, Lopez-Gomez JM, Gruss E, Aljama P, for the MAR study group. Course of vascular access and relationship with treatment of anemia. *Clin J Am Soc Nephrol.* 2007;2:1163–1169.

32. National Kidney Foundation. K/DOQI Clinical Practice Guidelines for Vascular Access: 2000. *Am J Kidney Dis.* 2001;37 (suppl 1):S137–S181.

33. Saran R, Dykstra DM, Pisoni RL, Akiba T, Akizawa T, Canaud B, Chen K, Piera L, Saito A, Young EW. Timing of first cannulation and vascular access failure in haemodialysis: an analysis of practice patterns at dialysis facilities in the DOPPS. *Nephrol Dial Transplant.* 2004;19:2334–2340.

34. Pisoni RL, Young EW, Dykstra DM, Greenwood RN, Hecking E, Gillespie B, Wolfe RA, Goodkin DA, Held PJ. Vascular access use in Europe and the United States: results from the DOPPS. *Kidney Int.* 2002;61:305–316.

35. Rayner HC, Pisoni RL, Gillespie BM Goodkin DA, Akiba T, Akizawa T, Saito A, Young EW, Port FK. Creation, cannulation and survival of arterio-venous fistulae—data from the Dialysis Outcomes and Practice Patterns Study (DOPPS). *Kidney Int.* 2003;63:323–330.

36. Ravani P, Brunori G, Mandolfo S, Cancarini G, Imbasciati E, Marcelli D, Malberti F. Cardiovascular comorbidity and late referral impact arteriovenous fistula survival: a prospective multicenter study. *J Am Soc Nephrol.* 2004;15:204–209.

37. Labriola L, Crott R, Desmet C, et al. Infectious complications following conversion to buttonhole cannulation of native arteriovenous fistulas: a quality improvement report. *Am J Kidney Dis.* 2011;57:442–448.

38. Nasrallah GE, Cuerden M, Wong JH, et al. Staphylococcus aureus bacteraemia and buttonhole cannulation: long-term safety and efficacy of mupirocin prophylaxis. *Clin J Am Soc Nephrol.* 2010;5:1047–1053.

39. Glickman M. Multicenter evaluation of a polyurethaneurea vascular access graft as compared with the expanded polytetrafluoroethylene vascular access graft in hemodialysis applications. *J Vascular Surg.* 2001;34:465–473.

40. Hung YN, Ko PJ, Ng YY, et al. The longevity of arteriovenous graft for hemodialysis patients—externally supported or nonsupported. *Clin J Am Soc Nephrol.* 2010;5:1029–1035.

41. Ram SJ, Sachdeva BA, Caldito GC, et al. Thigh grafts contribute significantly to patients' time on dialysis. *Clin J Am Soc Nephrol.* 2010;5:1229–1234.

42. Sreedhara R, Himmelfarb J, Lazarus JM, et al. Anti-platelet therapy in graft thrombosis: results of a prospective, randomized, double-blind study. *Kidney Int.* 1994;45:1477–1483.

43. Kaufman JS, O'Connor TZ, Zhang JH, et al. Randomized controlled trial of clopidogrel plus aspirin to prevent hemodialysis access graft thrombosis. *J Am Soc Nephrol.* 2013;14:2313–2321.

44. Dixon BS, Beck GJ, Vazquez MA, et al. Effect of dipyridamole plus aspirin on hemodialysis grant patency. *NEJM.* 2009;360:2191–2201.

45. Saran R, Bragg-Gresham JL, Rayner HC, et al. Nonadherence in hemodialysis: associations with mortality, hospitalization, and practice patterns in the DOPPS. *Kidney Int.* 2003;64:254–262.

46. Shah R, Bhatt UY, Van Cleef S, et al. Vascular Access Thrombosis and Interventions in Patients Missing Hemodialysis Sessions. *Clinical Nephrology.* 2011;76:435–439.

47. Ravani P, Parfrey P, MacRae J, et al. Modeling survival of arteriovenous accesses for hemodialysis: semiparametric versus parametric methods. *Clin J Am Soc Nephrol.* 2010;5:1243–1248.

48. Churchill DN, Taylor DW, Cook RJ, LaPlante P, Barre P, Cartier P, Fay WP, Goldstein MB, Jindal K, Mandin H. Canadian Hemodialysis Morbidity Study. *Am J Kidney Dis.* 1992;19:214–234.

49. Woods JD, Turenne MN, Strawderman RL, Young EW, Hirth RA, Port FK, Held PJ. Vascular access survival among incident hemodialysis patients in the United States. *Am J Kidney Dis.* 1997;30:50–57.

50. Allon M. Current management of vascular access. *Clin J Am Soc Nephrol.* 2007;2:786–800.

51. Lilly RZ, Carlton D, Barker J, et al. Clinical predictors of AV graft patency following radiologic intervention in hemodialysis patients. *Am J Kidney Dis.* 2001;37:945–953.

52. Turmel-Rodrigues L, Pengloan J, Baudin S, et al. Treatment of stenosis and thrombosis in haemodialysis fistulas and grafts by interventional radiology. *Nephrol Dial Transplant.* 2000;15:2029–2036.

53. Lee T, Barker J, Allon M. Comparison of survival of upper arm arteriovenous fistulas and grafts after failed forearm fistulas. *J Am Soc Nephrol.* 2007;18:1936–1941.

54. Beathard GA, Arnold P, Jackson J, et al. Aggressive treatment of early fistula failure. *Kidney Int.* 2003;64:1487–1494.

55. Chang CJ, Ko PJ, Hsu LA, et al. Highly increased cell proliferation activity in the restenotic hemodialysis vascular access after percutaneous transluminal angioplasty: implication in prevention of restenosis. *Am J Kidney Dis.* 2004;43:74–84.

56. Lee T, Ullah A, Allon M, et al. Decreased cumulative access survival in arteriovenous fistulas requiring interventions to promote maturation. *Clin J Am Soc Nephrol.* 2011;6:575–581.

57. Clinical Practice Guidelines and Clinical Practice Recommendations. 2006 Updates. Available at: http://www.kidney.org/professionals/KDOQI/guideline_upHD_PD_VA/index.htm. Accessed May 14, 2011.

58. Available at: http://www.fistulafirst.org/AboutFistulaFirst/FFBIData.aspx. Accessed May 7, 2011.

59. Available at: http://www.kidneycarequality.com/PDF/catheter_reduction_care_bundle.pdf. Accessed May 14, 2011.

60. Wingard RL, Chan KE, Lazarus JM, et al. The "Right" of passage: surviving the first year of dialysis. *Clin J Am Soc Nephrol.* 2009;4:S114–S120.

61. Amedia CA, Bolton WK, Cordray T, et al. Vascular access for HD: aligning payment with quality. *Semin Dial.* 2011;24:37–40.

62. Allon M, Dinwiddie L, Lacson E, et al. Medicare reimbursement policies and hemodialysis vascular access outcomes: a need for change. *J Am Soc Nephrol.* 2011;22:426–430.

63. Schwab SJ, Brown KD. Immature public policy for vascular access. *J Am Soc Nephrol.* 2010;21:1409–1421.

64. Ethier J, Mendelssohn DC, Elder SJ, Hasegawa T, Akizawa T, Akiba T, Canaud BJ, Pisoni RL. Vascular access use and outcomes: an international perspective: results from the Dialysis Outcomes and Practice Patterns Study. *Nephrol Dial Transplant.* 2008;23:3219–3226.

65. Oliver MJ, Rothwell DM, Fung K, Hux JE, Lok CE. Late creation of vascular access for hemodialysis and increased risk of sepsis. *J Am Soc Nephrol.* 2004;15:1936–1942.

66. Silva MB, Hobson RW, Pappas PJ, et al. A strategy for increasing use of autogenous hemodialysis access procedures: impact of preoperative noninvasive evaluation. *J Vasc Surg.* 1998;27:307–308.

67. Lauvao LS, Ihnat DM, Goshima KR, et al. Vein diameter is the major predictor of fistula maturation. *J Vasc Surg.* 2009;49:1499–1504.

68. National Kidney Foundation Kidney Disease Outcomes Quality Initiative: 2006 update vascular access. Guideline 2: selection and placement of hemodialysis access. *Am J Kidney Dis.* 2006;48 (suppl 1):s192–s200.

69. Ferring M, Claridge M, Smith SA, et al. Routine preoperative vascular ultrasound improves patency and use of arteriovenous fistulas for hemodialysis: a randomized trial. *Clin J Am Soc Nephrol.* 2011;5:2236–2244.

70. Hurst FP, Abbott KC, Raj D, Krishan M, Palant CE, Agadoa LY, Jindal RM. Arteriovenous fistulas among incident hemodialysis patients in Department of Defense and Veterans Affairs facilities. *J Am Soc Nephrol.* 2010;21:1571–1577.

71. U.S. Renal Data System, USRDS 2010 Annual Data Report: Atlas of Chronic Kidney Disease and End-Stage Renal Disease in the United States, National Institutes of Health, National Institute of Diabetes and Digestive and Kidney Diseases, Bethesda, MD, 2010. Available at: http://www.usrds.org/atlas.htm. Accessed May 14, 2011.

72. Allon M. Fistula First: recent progress and ongoing challenges. *Am J Kidney Dis.* 2011;57:3–6.

73. Huijbregts HJTAM, Bots ML, Moll FL, Blankestijn PJ, and on behalf of the CIMINO members. Accelerated increase of arteriovenous fistula use in haemodialysis centres: results of the multicentre CIMINO initiative. *Nephrol Dial Transplant.* 2007;22:2595–2600.

74. Polkinghorne KR, Seneviratne M, Kerr PG. Effect of a vascular access nurse coordinator to reduce central venous catheter use in incident hemodialysis patients: a quality improvement report. *Am J Kidney Dis.* 2008;53:99–106.

75. Cho KL, Salman L, Krishnamurthy G, Mercado C, Merrill D, Thomas I, Artikov S, Contreras G, Khan RAH, Warda A and Asif A. Impact of surgeon selection on access placement and survival following preoperative mapping in the "Fistula First" era. *Semin Dial.* 2008;21:341–345.

76. Wasse H, Speckman RA, Frankenfield DL, Rocco MV, McClellan WM. Predictors of central venous catheter use at the initiation of hemodialysis. *Semin Dial.* 2008;21:346–351.

77. Danese MD, Liu Z, Griffiths RI, Dylan M, Yu HT, Dubois R, Nissenson AR. Catheter use is high even among hemodialysis patients with a fistula or graft. *Kidney Int.* 2006;70:1482–1485.

78. Moist LM, Trpeski L, Na Y, Lok CE. Increased hemodialysis catheter use in Canada and associated mortality risk: data from the Canadian Organ Replacement Registry 2001–2004. *Clin J Am Soc Nephrol.* 2008;3:1726–1732.

79. Mendelssohn DC, Ethier J, Elder SJ, Saran R, Port FK, Pisoni RL. Haemodialysis vascular access problems in Canada: results from the Dialysis Outcomes and Practice Patterns Study (DOPPS II). *Nephrol Dial Transplant.* 2006;21:721–728.

80. Hirth RA, Turenne MN, Woods JD, et al. Predictors of type of vascular access in hemodialysis patients. *JAMA.* 1996;276:1303–1307.

81. Allon M, Ornt D, Schwab S, et al. Factors associated with the prevalence of AV fistulas in hemodialysis patients in the HEMO study. *Kidney Int.* 2000;58:2178–2185.

82. Al-Ghonaim M, Manns BJ, Hirsch DJ, Gao Z, Tonelli M, for the Alberta Kidney Disease Network. Relation between access blood flow and mortality in chronic hemodialysis patients. *Clin J Am Soc Nephrol.* 2008;3:387–391.

83. Pisoni RL, Arrington CJ, Albert JM, et al. Facility hemodialysis vascular access use and mortality in countries participating in DOPPS: an instrumental variable analysis. *Am J Kidney Dis.* 2009;53:475–491.

84. Dhingra RK, Young EW, Hulbert-Shearon TE, Leavey SF, Port FK. Type of vascular access and mortality in US hemodialysis patients. *Kidney Int.* 2001;60:1443–1451.

85. Pastan S, Soucie JM, McClellan WM. Vascular access and increased risk of death among hemodialysis patients. *Kidney Int.* 2002;62:620–626.

86. Polkinghorne KR, McDonald SP, Atkins RC, et al. Vascular access and all-cause mortality: a propensity score analysis. *J Am Soc Nephrol.* 2004;15:477–486.

87. Goodkin DA, Pisoni RL, Locatelli F, et al. Hemodialysis vascular access training and practices are key to improved access outcomes. *Am J Kidney Dis.* 2010;56: 1032–1042.

88. Combe C, Pisoni RL, Port FK, et al. Dialysis outcomes and practice patterns study (DOPPS): data on the use of central venous catheters in chronic hemodialysis. *Nephrologie.* 2001;22:379–384.

89. Astor BC, Eustace JA, Powe NR, Klag MJ, Fink NE, Coresh J, for the CHOICE study. Type of vascular access and survival among incident hemodialysis patients: the Choices for Healthy Outcomes in Caring for ESRD (CHOICE) Study. *J Am Soc Nephrol.* 2005;16:1449–1455.

90. Xue JL, Dahl D, Ebben JP, Collins AJ. The association of initial hemodialysis access type with mortality outcomes in elderly Medicare ESRD patients. *Am J Kidney Dis.* 2003;42:1013–1019.

91. Perl J, Wald R, McFarlane P, Bargman JM, Vonesh E, Na Y, Jassal SV, Moist L. Hemodialysis vascular access modifies the association between dialysis modality and survival. *J Am Soc Nephrol.* 2011;22;31:174–184.

92. Ishani A, Collins AJ, Herzog CA, Foley RN. Septicemia, access and cardiovascular disease in dialysis patients: the USRDS Wave 2 Study. *Kidney Int.* 2005;68: 311–318.

93. Wasse H, Kutner N, Zhang R, Huang Y. Association of initial hemodialysis vascular access with patient-reported health status and quality of life. *Clin J Am Soc Nephrol.* 2007;2:708–714.

94. Schlieper G, Kruger T, Djuric Z Damjanovic T, Markovic N, Schurgers LJ, Brandenburg VM, Westenfeld R, Dimkovic S, Ketteler M, Grootendorst DC, Dekker FW, Floege J, Dimkovic N. Vascular access calcification predicts mortality in hemodialysis patients. *Kidney Int.* 2008;74:1582–1587.

95. Feldman HI, Korbin S, Wasserstein A. Hemodialysis vascular access morbidity. *J Am Soc Nephrol.* 1996;7:523–535.

96. Wasse H, Speckman RA, McClellan WM. Arteriovenous fistula use is associated with lower cardiovascular mortality compared with catheter use among ESRD patients. *Semin Dial.* 2008;21:483–489.

97. Goldstein SL, Ikizler TA, Zappitelli M, et al. Non-infected hemodialysis catheters are associated with increased inflammation compared to arteriovenous fistulas. *Kidney Int.* 2009;76:1063–1069.

98. Schiller B, Virk B, Blair M, et al. Spurious hyperphosphatemia in patients on hemodialysis with catheters. *Am J Kidney Dis.* 2008;52: 617–620.

99. Allon M, Daugirdas J, Depner TA, Greene T, Ornt D, Schwab SJ. Effect of change in vascular access on patient mortality in hemodialysis patients. *Am J Kidney Dis.* 2006;47:469–477.

100. Lacson E, Want W, Lazarus JM, et al. Change in vascular access and mortality in maintenance hemodialysis patients. *Am J Kidney Dis.* 2009;54:912–921.

101. Lacson E, Wang W, Lazarus MJ, et al. Change in vascular access and hospitalization risk in long-term hemodialysis patients. *Clin J Am Soc Nephrol.* 2010;5: 1996–2003.

102. Lee H, Manns B, Taub K, Ghali WA, Dean S, Johnson D, Donaldson C. Cost analysis of ongoing care of patients with end stage renal disease: the impact of dialysis modality and dialysis access. *Am J Kidney Dis.* 2002;40:611–622.

103. Manns B, Tonelli M, Yilmaz S, Lee H, Laupland K, Klarenbach S, Radkevich V, Murphy B. Establishment and maintenance of vascular access in incident hemodialysis patients: a prospective cost analysis. *J Am Soc Nephrol.* 2005;16:201–209.

104. Xue H, Lacson E, Wang W, et al. Choice of vascular access among incident hemodialysis patients: a decision and cost-utility analysis. *Clin J Am Soc Nephrol.* 2010;5: 2289–2296.

105. Lok CE, Oliver MJ, Su J, Bhola C, Hannigan N, Jassal SV. Arteriovenous fistula outcomes in the era of the elderly dialysis population. *Kidney Int.* 2005;67: 2462–2469.

106. O'Hare AM, Bertenthal D, Walter LC, Garg AX, Covinsky K, Kaufman JS, Rodriguez RA, Allon M. When to refer patients with chronic kidney disease for vascular access surgery: should age be a consideration? *Kidney Int.* 2007;71,555–561.

107. Saran R, Mehta K. Commentary. *Nat Clin Pract Nephrol.* 2007;3:417.

108. Richardson AI, Leake A, Schmieder GC, et al. Should fistulas really be first in the elderly patient? *J Vasc Access.* 2009;199–202.

109. Fadrowski JJ, Hwang W, Frankenfield DL, Fivush BA, Neu AM, Furth SL. Clinical course associated with vascular access type in a national cohort of adolescents who receive hemodialysis: findings from the Clinical Performance Measures and US Renal Data System Projects. *Clin J Am Soc Nephrol.* 2006;1:987–992.

110. Eisenstein I, Tarabeih M, Magen D, et al. Low infection rates and prolonged survival times of hemodialysis catheters in infants and children. *Clin J Am Soc Nephrol.* 2011;6:793–798.

111. Curi MA, Pappas PJ, Silva MB, Patel S, Padberg FT, Jamil Z, Duran WN, Hobson RW. Hemodialysis access: influence of the human immunodeficiency viruszon patency and infection. *J Vasc Surg.* 1999;29: 608–616.

112. Mitchell D, Krishnasami Z, Young CJ, Allon M. Arteriovenous access outcomes in haemodialysis patients with HIV infection. *Nephrol Dial Transplant.* 2007;22:465–470.

113. Mokrzycki MH, Schroppel B, von Gersdorff G, Rush H, Zdunek MP, Feingold R. Tunneled-cuffed catheter associated infections in hemodialysis patients who are seropositive for the human immunodeficiency virus. *J Am Soc Nephrol.* 2000;11:2122–2127.

114. Kjellstrand CM, Blagg CR, Twardowski ZJ, et al. Blood access and daily hemodialysis: clinical experience

and review of the literature. *ASAIO J.* 2003;49: 645–649.

115. Piccoli GB, Bermond F, Mezza E, Burdese M, Fop F, Mangiarotti G, Pacitti A, Maffei S, Martina G, Jeantet A, Segoloni GP, Piccoli G. Vascular access survival and morbidity on daily dialysis: a comparative analysis of home and limited care haemodialysis. *Nephrol Dial Transplant.* 2004;19:2084–2094.

116. The FHN Group. In-center hemodialysis six times per week versus three times per week. *N Engl J Med.* 2010;363:2287–2300.

117. Mishler R, Yevzlin AS. Outcomes of arteriovenous fistulae created by a US interventional nephrologist. *Semin Dial.* 2010;23:224–228.

13

VASCULAR ACCESS MONITORING AND SURVEILLANCE

ANATOLE BESARAB, JARIATUL KARIM, & STAN FRINAK

LEARNING OBJECTIVES

1. Be able to define monitoring, surveillance, and diagnostic testing as it relates to dialysis vascular access.

2. Describe the importance of basic physical examination in the management of dialysis vascular access.

3. Describe the value of measuring recirculation as a surveillance tool for detecting venous stenosis.

4. Describe the technique currently favored for assessing static venous pressure as a surveillance tool for detecting venous stenosis.

5. Describe the basic technique used to measure access flow (Q_a) in the dialysis clinic.

6. Compare and contrast flow and pressure in an arteriovenous fistula with that in a synthetic graft.

7. Discuss the variables that act together to determine access flow (Q_a), particularly in autologous fistulae (artery to vein ratio) as a function of increasing degrees of venous stenosis.

8. Describe the pit falls inherent in using an isolated 25% to 30% decrease in flow measurement as an indicator for referral for angioplasty.

9. Contrast the value of a single measurement of flow or static venous pressure with the value of serial measures in the detecting of dialysis access dysfunction.

10. Contrast the above with serial measurements combined with clinical evaluation (physical examination).

11. Describe differences in the value of different surveillance methods based upon the location of the lesion.

12. Describe the relationship between rate of flow decrease (%) as detected by serial flow measurements and the absolute flow in the access in predisposing to a thrombotic event.

13. Describe the criteria that should be fulfilled before a dialysis vascular access is subjected to angioplasty treatment.

14. Discuss the importance of cohort size in conducting a randomized controlled study on dialysis access dysfunction.

15. Describe the effects that have been reported in the medical literature of instituting a surveillance program on thrombosis rates.

INTRODUCTION

More than 85% of the patients receive renal replacement therapy in the United States via hemodialysis (HD).[1] Adequate care of HD patients is inseparable from the problems of creating and maintaining the patency of vascular access. Chronic life-sustaining hemodialysis requires a durable access to the circulatory system to feed the extracorporeal circuit.[2] The ideal permanent vascular access should (a) provide longevity of use with minimal complication rate from infection and thrombosis and (b) supply high blood flow rates to deliver the prescribed dialysis dose. Currently, the arteriovenous autologous fistula (AVF) and arteriovenous graft (AVG) are considered to be permanent accesses, whereas tunneled cuffed catheters (TCC) are used as a transitional access. Delivery of optimal HD requires a well-functioning vascular access with a nominal blood flow rate of approximately 400–500 mL/min without access recirculation. Failure of access function limits the delivered dose of dialysis and has tremendous biological and economical health consequences. It has been estimated that vascular access procedures and complications account for over 15–20% of hospitalizations of dialysis patients and cost over $1 billion annually in the USA.[3,4] In an effort to improve vascular access outcomes, the National Kidney Foundation published the Dialysis Outcome Quality Initiative (DOQI) guidelines in 1997, 2001, and 2006[2] which describe approved techniques for maintaining access function.

Patients entering dialysis programs today tend to be older and to more commonly have diabetes. Aging of the population and the diabetes epidemic are associated with multiple comorbid conditions in such patients.[5] Older age, diabetes, and cardiovascular diseases are also associated with poor quality of the arteries and veins which make the construction of distal fistulas more challenging. A major problem with the AVF is the high frequency of primary failure, either due to early thrombosis or lack of maturation. Placing AVFs in more patients as recommended by the Fistula First Initiative (FFI)[6] has resulted in increased incidence of primary failure. Indeed, this risk was around 10–20% in former studies,[7] whereas it has been reported to be from two to five times higher in more recent series.[3] Programs that adopted the Center for Medicare Medicaid Services (CMS) FFI found an increasing fraction of such fistulas not maturing to a point permitting successful cannulation and hemodialysis.[8–11] Fistula placement tends to be less successful in these patients when measured as maturation, short- and long-term patency rates, ease of cannulation, and further assistance/intervention to prevent and treat complications. As a result, predictive models/scoring systems have been developed to aid in decision making[12] as to when an AVF is appropriate and when some other form of access such as AVG should be considered. The reader is reminded that the economic and functional superiority of AVF over AVG measured as 1 year primary (intervention-free or unassisted) and secondary (assisted) fistula survival probabilities is seen only after exclusion of early events but not when early events are included in the analyses.[13,14]

Access maturation durations (period from construction to ability to repeatedly cannulate the access with two needles) for AVF and AVG differ. In general, AVF seldom mature before 4–6 weeks and at times may take several months. On the other hand, AVG can be cannulated within several days with the newer composite graft materials or after 2–3 weeks with the more traditional PTFE materials. Of course, tunneled cuffed catheters can be used immediately after insertion. Once repeated cannulation of an AVF or an AVG is demonstrated, maintenance of patency requires the integrated implementation of monitoring and surveillance.

SCOPE OF THE PROBLEM OF MAINTAINING ACCESS PATENCY

Adequate vascular access function is the most important components determining the success or failure of hemodialytic therapy.[15] Access problems are frequently a daily occurrence in busy dialysis units. Low blood flow rates (Q_b) and loss of patency limit dialysis delivery, extend treatment times and result in under dialysis leading to increased morbidity and mortality.[16] Maintenance of adequate flow is the chief means of assuring delivery of "prescribed dialysis dose." Permanent mature accesses routinely deliver 400–550 mL/min. A Q_b value of 300 mL/min provides a minimally effective dialysis dose within a 3.5–5 h dialysis session in individuals weighing 60–100 kg. A Q_b value below this recommended level necessitates increased treatment time to provide adequate dialysis. Both patients and staff avoid prolonging treatment time as it often leads to early sign-off by patients and to conflicts between patient and physician as to the necessity of increased treatment time. All too often, the loss of access patency requires use of TCCs to bridge the interval until the access can be salvaged or a new one established. The leading cause of loss of vascular access patency is thrombosis which greatly increases health care spending.[3,17] Currently, CMS mandates that both monitoring and surveillance be performed on both arteriovenous AVF and grafts (AVG) under the Conditions of Coverage[18] as part of its focus on diagnosis and early intervention of vascular access problems as a means toward controlling costs.

SURVEILLANCE AND MONITORING: DEFINITIONS

Many medical and nursing practitioners use the two terms of monitoring and surveillance interchangeably. NKF KDOQI guidelines 2 are explicit in their definitions and are adopted by CMS. The goal of both monitoring and surveillance is the detection of an anatomically severe stenosis within the access, which is *physiologically significant and likely to result over time in thrombosis*. The detection of a stenotic lesion, however, is only the first step in the diagnostic algorithm and therapeutic process. Ultimately, the stenosis must be treated and if possible recurrence prevented. For the latter, diagnostic testing by angiography is usually needed.

The following *definitions* will be used throughout this dissertation.

▶ Monitoring

Monitoring (M) includes not only the physical examination (inspection, palpation, and auscultation) of the vascular access to detect physical signs that suggest the presence of dysfunction[19] but also all of the following:

- documentation of prolonged bleeding after needle withdrawal
- inadequate delivery of dialysis
- documented recirculation
- elevated dynamic venous pressures (DVP) [definition varies among centers]
- other clinical clues.

All of the above are paid for in the capitated or bundled rate for hemodialysis treatments.

For patients with maturing access not yet on dialysis, monitoring begins with the surgical construction of the access.

▶ Surveillance

Surveillance (S) refers to the periodic evaluation of the vascular access by means of specialized tests that involve special instrumentation. Such tests include access flow, access resistance or conductance, intra-access pressure, and direct measurement of access recirculation.

Measurements such as URR or Kt/V measure the effect of inadequate access function on the delivery of dialysis and are more properly catalogued under "monitoring." In grafts, these latter indicators are poor indicators of access dysfunction or presence of hemodynamically significant stenosis.[20] By contrast, in AVF that remains patent at much lower flows, sequential measurements of these values may indicate the presence of correctible stenosis.[21] Doppler duplex ultrasound (DDU) is unique among the surveillance tests since it is able to not only measure access flow but also visualize and quantify the severity of any stenosis present.[22]

Surveillance tests require additional time and effort from staff and in some circumstances the use of dedicated technicians or nurses to yield consistent results. There is no separate reimbursement for the costs of these tests by CMS.

▶ Diagnostic Testing

Diagnostic Testing refers to *specialized* testing that is prompted by some abnormality or other medical indication specifically undertaken to diagnose the cause of the vascular access dysfunction. The current gold standard is angiography but DDU can be used for this function as well.[23] In most cases, the individual is sent to a radiologic center where contrast visualization occurs.[24] In some cases, intra-access angioscopy and ultrasound can be performed.[25] Magnetic resonance angiography (MRA) can also be used to characterize the anatomic presence of stenosis[26–28] as well as to quantitate flow.[29] However, this technique is not cost-effective in most clinical settings.

These tests are usually paid for separately at the time of the study or intervention.

It is important to emphasize that *surveillance* and *monitoring* are complementary. The ultimate goal of "Evidence-based medicine is the integration of best research evidence with clinical expertise and patient values" as formulated by Sackett in 1996.[30] A screening surveillance exam to detect stenosis is not intended to be definitive and the sole reason for performing an intervention. The testing procedure should have a high degree of sensitivity (to avoid missing cases that can be salvaged), but the sensitivity should be measured against the "costs" of the event toward which it is directed and the availability of alternatives.

Clinical judgment is needed to interpret the data from surveillance tests. Not all stenoses are progressive enough to produce worsening abnormalities in access flow or intra-access pressure over time. Stable lesions should not be treated. The goal is to detect significant lesions before they become intractable and unmanageable and produce thrombosis. Thrombosis has effects on many levels. For the patient, it disrupts his/her life producing inconvenience, frustration, and discomfort. At the dialysis facility level, it disrupts treatment schedule, utilizes staff time and results in staff frustration, and leads to loss of revenue from missed or incomplete treatments. At the health care level, thrombosis increases hospitalization, is a major cause of access loss, and increases costs. It of course may result in increased catheter use, contributing significantly to morbidity and mortality.

Regular assessment of clinical parameters of the AVF (including physical examination) and dialysis adequacy must be combined with surveillance using specific hemodynamic assessments of flow, resistance, or intra-access pressure assessments. Within each dialysis center, these data should be tabulated and tracked as part of a Quality Assurance/Continuous Quality Improvement program. Best results are obtained when a multidisciplinary relationship among access surgeons, nephrologists, nurses, and interventional radiologists (vascular access team or VAT) is developed. Whatever the VAT's size and composition, its most important functions are: (1) to work proactively to ensure that the patient's access is ready when needed for dialysis and (2) thereafter to assure delivery of adequate dialysis dose by maintaining access function and patency.

SYSTEM DYSFUNCTION IN ACCESS EVALUATION IN DIALYSIS CLINICS

In the United States, basic skills of physical examination are frequently only superficially taught to the front line staff responsible for cannulation of the patient. Few centers actually have a certification process to assess the skill level and proficiency of the staff in performing assessments of the access through physical examination. It has been our experience that nurses do not perform better in this area than dialysis technicians. In the real world, our average nurse/technician frequently cannot tell the difference between an AVF and an AVG by physical exam alone and knows very little of what happens to an access from treatment to treatment unless it affects his/her ability to dialyze the patient that day. Enlarging aneurysms are too often cannulated without any consideration of the risks of bleeding or rupture. In most cases, patients are cannulated if a pulse is felt whether it is normal to have a pulse or not, as in the body of an AVF where a pulse is definitely an abnormal finding. The clinical assessment performed by staff emphasizes the performance of a clinical check list (Table 13-1) that can be entered into a computer.

This clinical assessment focuses on missed treatments, treatment length reductions from access clotting or blood flow problems, and dialysis duration. These events are

TABLE 13–1

Illustrative Check List for Clinical Access Evaluation

Patient Name:_____

Condition Present	Yes	No
Treatment initiated	○	○
Dialysis duration, achieved	○	○
Extremity swelling	○	○
Difficult cannulation	○	○
Prolonged bleeding after needle removal	○	○
Decrease in Kt/V (online) or URR (from monthly)	○	○
Able to achieve prescribed blood pump flow	○	○
Vascular "steal" symptoms or pain	○	○
Signs or symptoms of infection	○	○
Signs or symptoms of infiltration	○	○
Aneurysm formation	○	○
Other	○	○
Analyzed by physician/access coordinator	○	○

important but may not be the result of access dysfunction. More germane are assessments for swelling of the extremity ipsilateral to the access, cannulation difficulties, and events of prolonged bleeding, infection or infiltration, and aneurysm formation. Certainly, the presence of the latter is sufficient reason to refer patients for access dysfunction, yet frequently they are not.

To the clinical check list (Table 13-1), many centers are now adding results from new online technology, especially methodologies that are built in as "elective" modules, for measuring online clearance, access recirculation, and access blood flow measurements. Like other aspects, the information is only useful if the staff understand the values and the importance of trends in the measured parameter over time.

Particularly frustrating are occurrences of "pulling clot" after access cannulation. Many patients are directly referred to an access center by the clinical staff with a diagnosis of "clotted access" in the hope of a rapid declotting procedure (and avoidance of a catheter) and rescheduling of the patients for dialysis later the same day. All too often, the access is found to be "patent" by physical exam or angiography. Many of our staff interpret the "pulling of clot" from a miscannulation of the access as proof of access thrombosis. Referral for unnecessary angiography is totally avoidable by a proper physical exam demonstrating a palpable pulse or thrill depending on the case. Unfortunately, in many of these false positive referrals, an angiograph is performed and, because of their frequency, "anatomical" stenosis by angiography is found but whose physiologic significance is unknown. Pull back pressures to define hemodynamically significant lesions or actual flow measurements at the time of the procedure are infrequently done at most access centers during evaluation and only degree of stenosis is then used as a criterion for intervention. As a result, "hemodynamically insignificant stenoses" are dilated needlessly because they are merely "there" in accesses that are performing well.

There is no doubt that monitoring alone that includes properly conducted periodic physical exams of permanent accesses along with good trending of clinical problems over time works quite well. The positive predictive value (PPV) of clinical monitoring performed by properly trained and skilled dialysis personnel in detecting a functionally significant lesion may be as high as 70–80%.[19,31–33] It would be difficult to demonstrate an improvement in outcomes with surveillance compared to monitoring by performing a randomized clinical trial (RCT) using either flow or pressure technology if the positive predictive value of a surveillance test in a RCT only improves PPV to 85–90%. Sample sizes in excess of 500–600 subjects assigned to two groups would be needed. Also in a properly conducted RTC defining exactly what constitutes a successful angioplasty has to be explicitly defined. This is discussed later.

We believe that both monitoring and some form of surveillance should be performed in dialysis centers because with modern staffing patterns for the past 20 years, consistent access evaluations are not performed. Even when staff is taught to perform access evaluation, their performance is erratic and frequently not performed at all in the hectic world of dialysis at "put on and take off time." This circumstance puts our patients at risk for access failure and other complications. Long-term cross-over studies do demonstrate that adding surveillance to "everyday" monitoring as practiced in the typical dialysis unit lowers thrombosis rates.[34] We recently demonstrated that thrombosis event rates could be improved by using a surveillance process added to "clinical" monitoring using the elements in Table 13-1, Surveillance when practiced intelligently using repeated measurements and physiologic principles reduces thrombosis[35] without increasing false positive rates or increasing percutaneous transluminal angioplasty (PTA) rates. Similarly, Tessitore and co-worker[33] recently demonstrated that fistula stenosis could be detected and located during dialysis with a moderate to excellent accuracy using physical exam and a combination of flow (to detect inflow lesions) and derived static venous pressure (to detect outflow stenosis).

Thrombosis is a major event; it can be a life-changing event. It needs to be avoided. We know that stenosis is related to thrombosis, but is generally not the proximate cause. We can treat stenosis pre-emptively with PTA. It is the only option that has been proposed that appears to have any effect on thrombosis rate.

THE MONITORING/ SURVEILLANCE (M/S) PROCESS

Monitoring (the use of physical examination) is an integral process in the evaluation of all permanent accesses but especially so for AVF.[36] It must be carried out not only in those patients on hemodialysis but also in those with CKD stages 4–5 in whom an AVF has been created in preparation for dialysis. The techniques can be taught to renal trainees.[37] Many nonmaturing AVF can be salvaged using percutaneous treatments that include PTA and obliteration of competing venous collateral vessels.[38–41] Best results are obtained when patients with nonmaturing native fistulas are identified within 1–3 months of creation, permitting referral of patients for fistulography and percutaneous salvage.[42] If the physical examination does not clearly indicate the cause for nonmaturation, both Duplex ultrasound[22] (with or without color) or contrast fistulography (using dilute low volume injection, usually less than 10 mL) can be performed without risk of precipitating renal failure in patients with advanced CK[43,44] not yet on dialysis.

MATURATION OF PERMANENT ACCESSES

In order to detect access maturation problems, the examiner must have a good sense of the normal changes in flow and pressure over time within the differing accesses as they "mature." Lomonte et al[45] used duplex Doppler ultrasonography to document the changes in blood flow rate in the brachial artery following construction and maturation of a radiocephalic wrist AVF in 18 incident uremic patients. Seventeen of these matured. The internal diameter and blood flow rate of the brachial artery (Q_{BA}) at baseline were 4.3 ± 0.7 mm and 56.1 ± 19.2 mL/min. Q_{BA} increased to 438 ± 86 mL/min at day 7, 720 ± 133 mL/min (median 750 mL/min, range 480–890 mL/min) at day 28, and 998 ± 260 mL/min at 258 ± 63 days after AVF construction. In the one AVF with maturation failure, the flow was only 88 mL/min at day 28. Thus, within the 7 days, on average, a maturing AVF attains 50% of its maximum flow increasing to 75% at 30 days and thereafter slowly maturing over months to flows of a L/min.

Berman et al[46] have expanded the maturation studies to elbow level AVF as well. During a 12 month period, 70 autologous AVFs were created: 41 antecubital brachiocephalic, 21 radiocephalic, and 8 basilic vein transpositions. As expected for the USA population, renal failure resulted from diabetes in 78% and hypertension in 19%. Patients whose AVFs were patent, but required a secondary procedure to achieve a functional access, were considered maturation failures. There was a significant difference between the maximal intraoperative flow rates between those accesses that matured and those that did not, 574 ± 103 mL/min versus 217 ± 36 mL/min; $p < 0.05$. Age and gender were not factors in this study. Receiver operator curve (ROC) analysis suggested a threshold intraoperative value of 140 mL/min for radiocephalic and 308 mL/min for brachiocephalic AVFs to predict maturation to a functional access.

The conclusions from these two studies are important in our approach to monitoring and surveillance. Firstly, flow measurements obtained at the time of autologous AVF construction can identify fistulas that are unlikely to mature and therefore require immediate revision or abandonment which will ultimately expedite the establishment of a useful access in the HD patient. Secondly, if flow measurements are not available, physical examination or Doppler US flow measurements can predict maturation failure by

4 weeks postconstruction. Thus, all patients should have a follow-up at 4 weeks. This interval is shorter than the currently recommended interval of 6–8 weeks to begin assessment for maturation. Since the brachial artery flow is relatively easy to measure compared to that of the fistula itself, this measure may be helpful in determining which AVFs will probably fail. This screening should aid clinical assessment, thus allowing sound judgment of the level of maturation of an AVF and of its outcome.

Similar techniques of measuring brachial artery flow to assess the relationship of Q_{BA} to intra-access pressure[47] have been performed. Much less data is available for AVGs. In general, AVGs have higher initial blood flows than forearm AVF or elbow level AVF.[48] They are also deemed to mature more quickly since there is no vascular wall that has to remodel.[49] Autogenous AVFs with flow rates below 320 mL/min and polytetrafluoroethylene (PTFE) grafts with flow rates below 400 mL/min had significantly worse primary and secondary patency rates compared to their higher flow counterparts irrespective of anatomical site of construction. PTFE grafts with flow rates at or below 400 mL/min required more interventions and failed sooner (median time, 0.5 ± 4.7 months) than grafts with flow rates above 400 mL/min (median time, 1.6 ± 5.0 months; $P = 0.003$). The pressure flow profile may vary between arterial tapered and nontapered AVG; pressure drop at the arterial anastomosis of the tapered graft is up to three times higher compared to the straight graft.[50] Mathematical modeling of a 4 mm tapered compared to a conventional 6 mm graft shows a decrease in flow of 28–50% depending on the length of the taper.[51] Tapering of the graft also increases the risk of hemolysis and leukocyte activation in in vitro models.[52] Both effects are prothrombotic.

▶ Surgical Aspects

With the high nonmaturation rate of AVF that exists,[11,53] surgical technique should also be reviewed. In a multicenter clinical trial, anastomosis created with nonpenetrating interrupted vascular clips showed significant improvement in primary, assisted primary, and secondary patencies not only of AVF but of AVG also.[54,55] In addition, both charge and payment calculations indicated financial benefit with the use of vascular clips compared to traditional sutures.

VASCULAR ACCESS TEAMS

Once an AVF has been constructed and the patient is receiving maintenance hemodialysis, the responsibility for monitoring and surveillance transfers to the dialysis center. All too often, the responsibility is placed into the hands of one individual. It is not feasible for any one individual to manage all aspects of access care. The only successful programs that we are aware of have all developed multidisciplinary teams with a designated VA coordinator.[56,57]

In a properly managed program, asymptomatic but functionally significant stenoses in AVF are detected through a systematic M/S program, referred for study, intervened upon, and checked to verify that the hemodynamics or functional abnormality has "improved." A functionally significant stenosis is currently defined as a reduction greater than 50% of normal vessel diameter that is accompanied by a hemodynamic or clinical abnormality.[2] *Note that the presence of stenosis alone is not sufficient to define access dysfunction.* Detected stenoses must be accompanied by either clinical or hemodynamic abnormalities that interfere with the delivery of dialysis, produce patient symptoms, impede AVF maturation, or are likely to produce thrombosis within several months.

In those in whom the AVF is already being used for HD, the development of abnormal recirculation values, elevated intra-access pressures, decreased blood flow, swollen extremity, unexplained reduction in Kt/V, or elevated negative arterial prepump pressures that prevent an increase in the delivered blood flow to acceptable levels heralds the development of a functionally important stenosis.[58] Prospective M/S should provide the ability to prolong the use of an AVF, allow salvage of an existing AVF, or promote sequential vascular access through planning, coordination of effort, and elective corrective intervention rather than urgent procedures or replacement.[35,59]

SURVEILLANCE

The KDOQI vascular access Work Group developed explicit guidelines regarding which surveillance tests should be used to evaluate a given access type and when and how to intervene to reduce thrombosis and under dialysis.[2] A number of surveillance methods can be used with AVF: sequential access flow, sequential static pressures, recirculation measurements, physical examination, and of course combinations. According to the Clinical Performance Project of the CMS, the dynamic pressure test is still overwhelmingly used in AVF[60] without correction for the effect of needle gauge.[61] This surveillance technique has no place in AVF surveillance.[2]

The basic tenet of vascular access monitoring and surveillance is that stenosis, single or multiple, develops over variable intervals in the great majority of AVF and if detected and corrected, maturation can be promoted, under-dialysis minimized or avoided, and thrombosis avoided or reduced. The rationale for M/S depends on the "dysfunction" hypothesis: AVF stenosis reduces access flow and alters pressure profiles. An inflow stenosis either prevents maturation of the AVF or in an established AVF produces dysfunction, impairing the delivery of adequate dialysis and often precedes thrombosis. The usefulness of flow or pressure surveillance critically depends on the accuracy of the measurements themselves. Unfortunately, both access flow and pressure vary in patients during and more importantly between dialysis sessions. Variations arise from needle rotation for cannulation and changes in hemodynamics among dialysis sessions.[62] A single measurement of either flow or pressure is in general an inaccurate predictor of the presence of stenosis. The *only rational means to detect an evolving*

lesion is to perform analysis using multiple repetitive measurements correlated with clinical findings so that appropriate rather than inappropriate referrals are made. Currently, there is very little quality assurance of "success" of an intervention other than anatomical evidence at the time of the procedure. At most centers, intra-access pressures or flow measurements at the time of intervention are not performed and periprocedural assessment is usually unavailable to be correlated with prediction of secondary access patency.

▶ Intra-Access Hemodynamics and Physiology

Interpretation of any M/S technique is crucially dependent on some knowledge of the parameters that reflect "best function" of the AVF with respect to intra-access flow and pressure profile. The pressure-drop across the entire AVF system is set by the mean arterial pressure (MAP) less central venous pressure (see Figure 13-1). The useable access flow, Q_A, resulting from this driving force in turn depends on many variables: site of anastomosis (the arterial diameter is larger proximally), presence or absence of disease in the feeding artery, extent of arterial remodeling, the patient's ability to augment cardiac output in response to the fistula, health of the vein, and its ability to dilate and remodel, and the presence of tributaries. The actual flow achieved within the AVF will thus be determined by many factors; however, day-to-day changes in MAP will directly influence the flow.[47,62] Development of stenosis in the AVF circuit will either limit the initial flow increase during maturation or after maturation lead to a progressive decrease in Q_A. Intra-access pressure will usually not increase unless there is a downstream stenosis (as from a cephalic arch or central vein stenosis).[21]

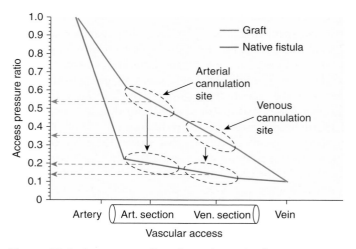

Figure 13-1. Pressure profiles along the path of an arteriovenous access for hemodialysis based on data from pullback measurements made at the time of angiography.[101] All intra-access pressures are normalized to the contra lateral arm mean arterial pressure. Note the difference in dissipation of the pressures between AVF and AVG. The ovals indicate the ratios expected at arterial and venous cannulation sites that are lower in AVF than AVG.

It is important to emphasize that the quality and physical dimensions of the artery and vein will determine the initial AVF or AVG flow. If the artery is healthy, the flow capacity of the AVF will be determined by the characteristics of the vein used in access construction. Too small a vein will limit the flow. In general, arteries at more distal sites have less capacity to deliver flow than more proximal sites. Forearm radiocephalic AVFs have flows 0.6–1.0 L/min, whereas elbow level fistulas have flows of 1–2 L/min.[63–65] Grafts at the elbow have flows similar to those of AVF constructed at the same site. Some AVF develop flow >3 L/min and are associated with cardiac decompensation.[66] Use of calcified or atherosclerotic arteries yields lower Q_A than those unaffected by such processes. Unfortunately, arterial disease is not uncommon; access inflow stenosis occurs in one third[67] of the graft cases referred to interventional facilities with clinical evidence of venous stenosis or thrombosis.[68] This high rate is due to the aging of the population and the progressive calcification of arteries that occurs in many patients prior to and over years of dialysis.

► Effect of Arterial Disease on Hemodynamics

A recent study from Spain[69] found a significant frequency of arterial disease in AVF during longitudinal observation of 102 patients, mean age 63.0 ± 13.0 years, mean time on HD 31.4 ± 44.0 months; 15.5% with diabetes. Q_A was measured every 4 months for 4 years using the delta-hematocrit method[64,70] in 116 vascular accesses (AVF 81%) with a mean access use of 28.2 ± 52.9 months. Angiography showed stenosis >50% in 40 of 43 accesses referred for evaluation. The new observation was the finding of stenosis in the feeding radial artery in 30.5% with a mean degree of stenosis of 83.5 ± 15.8%. These arterial lesions frequently co-existed with those in the rest of the fistula circuit. These patients tended to be older (67.5 ± 11.5 years), their AVF of longer vintage (48.9 ± 76.7 months). Diabetes did not appear to be a factor. Thus, the incidence of feeding arterial stenosis in AVF may be as high as in grafts. The functional results of elective surgery in radial artery stenosis were worse compared to vein stenosis.

Although the above study focused on the radial artery, arterial stenosis can occur upstream as well. Duijim et al[71] examined 66 AVF and found arterial inflow lesions in 10 AVF of which 7 were radiocephalic and 3 were brachiocephalic. Arterial lesions were located in the subclavian artery in five cases, axillary artery in one case, and radial artery in four cases. They recommend that radiologic evaluation comprises assessment of the complete arterial inflow not just that in immediate proximity to the anastomoses. This might require additional techniques in addition to retrograde angiography at the time of initial evaluation. In a follow up study of 116 dysfunctional hemodialysis fistulae and 50 grafts, digital subtraction angiography (DSA) demonstrated 247 significant stenoses: 30 located in the arterial inflow (12.1%), 128 at the AV anastomosis and arterial-graft region (51.8%), and 89 in the venous

outflow (36.0%), respectively.[72] Retrograde DSA depicted the complete vascular tree in 162 patients (97.6%). Eight (4.8%), 55 (33.1%), and 33 (19.9%) patients demonstrated stenoses in only inflow, access region, or outflow, respectively. Stenoses in two or three vascular territories were present in 53 (31.9%) and 7 (4.2%) patients, respectively.

The above studies indicate that multiple lesions are common in the territory of a vascular access and that the physiologic effects produced will depend on whether there are one simple lesion, inflow or outflow, or mixed (inflow and outflow) and whether these lesions develop independently over time or concurrently. In grafts, the influence of the arterial diameter relative to the venous diameter at which the two anastomoses are made has an enormous effect on access flow. The relationship between Q_A and stenosis is a reverse sigmoid: as stenosis progresses, Q_A initially remains relatively unchanged but then rapidly decreases as illustrated in Figure 13-2. A narrower artery increases flow resistance, causing a longer delay followed by a more rapid reduction in Q.[73]

► Methods of Surveillance

The relationship between Q_A and intra-access pressure in an AV fistula as a stenosis develops depends on the location of lesions. As stated previously, Q_A is determined by the pressure-drop across the entire fistula system, which is the mean arterial pressure (MAP) less central venous pressure (Figure 13-1) divided by the resistance. Note that, although the two profiles of pressure differ between an AVG and an

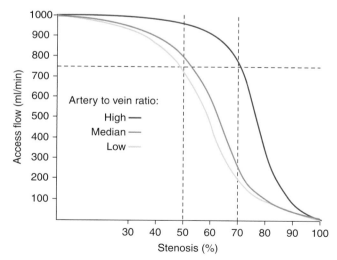

Figure 13-2. Effect of the ratio of artery diameter to vein on the changes in flow with degree of stenosis. Data based on Refs. [73] and [75]. Relatively small changes in flow occur as stenosis increased in grafts with median and high artery/vein ratios. In grafts with low artery to vein ratio, there is almost no change up to stenosis of 65% by diameter. Note how rapidly flow changes with stenosis thereafter in all grafts. Therefore, flow measurements taken early are not helpful but should be done frequently as stenosis advances beyond 50%D. Clinically, in a given patient, there is no way to know what the rate of progression is and at what point a 50% stenosis might be reached.

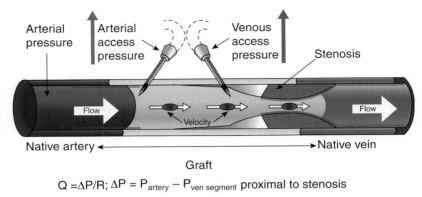

Figure 13-3. Hemodynamic relationship inside a flowing tube that is an arteriovenous access. Cannulation needles are shown. MAP drop from the arterial to venous end of the access.

$$Q = \Delta P / R; \ \Delta P = P_{artery} - P_{vein}$$

In the presence of a growing stenosis, flow must decrease and linear velocity of flow increase. An outflow stenosis will elevate the pressures compared to normal at both the arterial and venous needles.

AVF, the overall gradient is identical.[74] If an outflow stenosis develops and increases resistance, pressure will increase and flow decrease (Figure 13-3). The only difference between an AVG and an AVF is the presence of collaterals in the latter which can dissipate some of the increase in pressure build-up from a downstream stenosis. The increase in pressure will affect the postneedle bleeding time and may contribute to aneurismal dilatation and development of recirculation during a dialysis treatment. Since the stenotic process progresses variably with time, its detection requires sequential measurements of flow or pressure or both to detect a threshold at which action should be taken. The frequency of measurements depends on the rate of progression. With an inflow stenosis, venous pressures within an AVF usually do not change or decrease.[21] However, such inflow lesions are usually easily detected by physical examination since they occur in the first several centimeters distal to the anastomosis. In an AVF, this is manifested as the lack of "augmentation on physical examination," in a graft by a weak pulse in the arterial segment. Paradoxically, a higher basal intra-access pressure can occasionally be observed in an AVF in the absence of stenosis when the flow delivered by a healthy artery is in excess of the venous system's initial capacitance to accommodate to the flow.

Because of all of the above confounders (site of stenosis, anatomical variables, systemic changes in hemodynamics), there is little, if any, correlation between a single measurement of flow and intra-access pressure[47] whether in an AVF of AVG. Because of the variation in artery to vein size, mathematical models predict that measurements should be made frequently in order to detect changes in access function.[73] When the inflow artery is relatively narrow, the intra-access pressure increase may be initially delayed followed by a more rapid increase as critical stenosis is reach[75] leaving little time to detect the lesion if surveillance is carried out relatively infrequently.

AVF and AVG differ in their baseline hemodynamic profiles as one progressed from the artery into the vein and then centrally. In AVF, without inflow stenosis, the pressure in the early portion of the body of the fistula falls to less than 30% of MAP. As a fistula matures over many weeks to months, this pressure profile is maintained as the vein dilates and remodels its wall. A pulse is never felt in the body of the AVF. The pulse should not extend beyond the anastomosis; only a thrill should be felt. In contrast, AVG have their maximum flow within a month of construction. The intra-access profile of an AVG differs from that of AVF. In the absence of stenosis, depending on the presence of an arterial taper or not, the early segment of the graft has a pressure 30–65% of the MAP in the brachial artery, being lowest in tapered grafts. Thus, a pulse is usually present in the early segment of an untapered graft if the patient has a MAP > 60 mm Hg. However, the pulse is usually lost in the more distal venous cannulation segments. In tapered grafts, the pulse may be lost throughout.

As a stenosis develops, its effect on hemodynamics will depend on its location (inflow, body, or outflow) and its rate of development. As an outflow stenosis develops, whether in AVF or AVG, there is temporal progressive decrease in flow (accompanied by an increased intra-access pressure or resistance to flow). Thus, serial repeated measurements of pressure or flow within each patient's access correlated with findings of routine physical examination are more valuable in detecting a stenosis than any isolated measurements of absolute intra-access pressure, normalized ratio, or access flow. It is our opinion that the criterion that uses an "isolated" decrease in Q_A of ~25–30%[76] from some "preceding value" leads to too many interventional referrals and performance of some angioplasties that are not needed, resulting in an increased risk to the patient. As Figure 13-3 clearly shows, flow may decrease by less than 25% as a stenosis develops initially up to 50% restriction of the diameter of the vein. Thereafter, depending on the arterial to venous ratio, flow may either fall rapidly by 50% or by only 15% as a stenosis increases from 50% to 70%. As a result, infrequent measurements may fail to detect a hemodynamic stenosis. This is particularly the case in AVG, where stenosis can evolve within weeks to a few months.

Our own experience indicates that access flow measurements performed alone (without clinical correlation with physical findings) at greater than monthly intervals provide insufficient data on the "stability of flow" to make timely decisions in AVG. Analyses of bi-monthly data and statistical analysis of trends allows detection of a true progressive reduction of flow that can affect the delivery of dialysis dose. Because stenosis evolves more slowly in AVF, flow measurements can be a useful adjunct.[23,33]

▶ Dynamic Venous Pressure: DO NOT USE

The utility of DVP at flows of 150–225 mL/min to predict the presence of stenosis or the occurrence of thrombosis is quite limited.[77] Measuring venous pressure is the least expensive method of surveillance for stenosis.[78] There are, however, no direct studies of its sensitivity or specificity to detect hemodynamically significant stenosis in any permanent access, and the method is not currently recommended as a surveillance technique.[2] At best, it could detect pure outflow lesions. False negative results are obtained in the presence of any inflow problem, which as stated previously are not uncommon (up to 10–30%), even in AVG. More importantly, DVP is crucially dependent on the needle gauge and length of the metallic portion within the dialysis needle. The length of the needle shaft varies among manufactures as does the wall thickness of the needle shaft. Dialysis centers usually do not revalidate their procedures every time a cost-based decision is made to change the needles used.

▶ Recirculation

Measurement of access recirculation using the recommended urea-based method (Table CPG 4-6),[2] or one of the nonurea methods,[79–82] or online clearance should be conducted if the prescribed Kt/V is consistently not delivered in a patient who is using a native fistula. Online clearance where the expected clearance is lower than expected for the prescribed blood flow may be superior to urea-based methods that are prone to methodological errors of proper sample collection. Online clearance provides information almost instantaneously. In interpreting such online clearance values, the individual must have data on the expected clearance that should be achieved by the dialyzer under the given conditions of blood and dialysate flow rate through the system. Since very few clinical dialysis staff actually know such information, interpretation must be made by the treating physicians or advanced clinical nurse practitioners. However, in our experience, recirculation using blood urea methods is a late predictor of permanent access dysfunction and is less sensitive and less specific for detecting low flow access dysfunction unless performed frequently. Its usefulness is better in AVF than AVG.[20,21] Flow in AV fistulae, unlike AV grafts, can decrease to a level less than the prescribed blood pump flow (i.e., less

than 300 to 500 mL/min), while still maintaining access patency.[83,84] In contrast, AVG frequently clot while their intra-access flow is 600 mL/min or more, a value above most prescribed blood pump flows for dialysis, precluding the development of recirculation in most cases. In our experience, an increase in recirculation >5% was found in over 30% of AVF evaluated for dysfunction but less than 5% in AVG.[20,21]

▶ Access Flow, Doppler Ultrasound, and Static Intra-Access Pressures

By contrast to DVP and recirculation, flow measurements by a variety of techniques,[2,59,64,70] DDU (Duplex Doppler Ultrasound) assessment for stenosis,[85–87] and static pressure measurements (direct or indirect)[35,88] can detect hemodynamically significant stenosis in vascular accesses. Although the location of stenosis in fistulas (inflow) favors Q_A over some form of static pressure measurement, no direct comparisons have been made of the two techniques using DDU anatomical imaging or contrast angiography to determine the accuracy of the techniques in permanent accesses for detection of functionally important stenosis. Regular ultrasonographic screening alone has been shown to prolong graft patency if timely interventions are performed.[89]

All flow measurements are based on the principle of induced recirculation where the arterial and venous bloodlines are reversed as shown in Figure 13-4. A signal is engendered either by the infusion of a substance (saline, glucose), change in ultrafiltration rate (change in Hct), or addition of sodium (change in conductance) in the venous return line.[64] This mixes with the incoming arterial blood at the needle site, changing the magnitude of the signal. This modified signal is then sensed at the arterial detector. As shown in Figure 13-4, the ratio of the area under the curve multiplied by the arterial blood pump flow (which must be measured accurately) yields the access blood flow. Of all the methods, only DUS (Dilution Ultrasound) provides an independent accurate measure of blood pump blood flow. All others depend on adequate calibration by the biomed technicians. Unfortunately, such maintenance is done at 3-month periods and blood pump flow can drift significantly from the calibrated setting in between preventive maintenance operations. Because of the increasing difference between actual blood flow and the displayed blood pump flow on the machine at higher prepump pressure, most flow measurements are done at blood pump flows of 200–300 mL/min and not the prescribed blood flows of 350–500 mL/min. Flow measurements performed by DUS (Transonic[90]) and other techniques[2,64,70,91] can be done online during dialysis, providing rapid feedback. The same applies for static pressures.[88] Flow and pressure techniques can be combined to provide even more hemodynamic information.[92] Online access flow measurements[93] using conductivity are available but require further improvements in accuracy and reliability as well as the determination of the optimal frequency of measurement to be most effective.

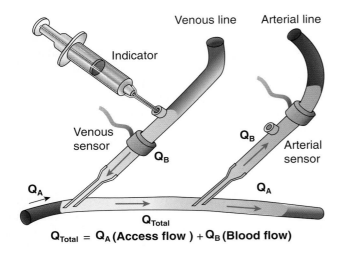

$$Q_{Total} = Q_A \text{ (Access flow)} + Q_B \text{ (Blood flow)}$$

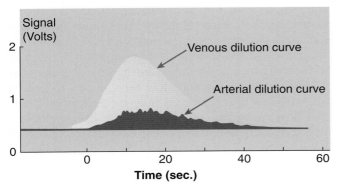

Figure 13-4. Principles of access flow measurement through induced recirculation. Top panel shows a segment of access that is cannulated with needles. A signal that can be measured is generated in many ways (see the text). Note that the venous needle is upstream of the arterial needle through deliberate reversal of the bloodlines. Blood that has gone through the dialyzer and contains the "signal indicator" now returns into the access and mixes with arterial blood diluting the indicator. This is deliberately induced recirculation (R).

In the case of the injection of a saline indicator (as shown by the syringe) using the ultrasound dilution method, the signal is the change in velocity of sound through blood and saline and measured as the time–area under the curve (AUC) that is detected by independent sensors on the arterial and venous lines. Access flow (Q_A) can be determined because blood pump flow (Q_{bpf}) is accurately measured using the same ultrasound transducers. The ratio of the arterial flow to the total flow is given by the formula $R = Q_{bpf}/(Q_{bpf} + Q_A)$. Since all of the indicators are injected into the venous line, the ratio of the arterial and venous dilution curves is also R. Solving the equation for R to determine Q_A yields the equation:

$$Q_A = Q_{bpf} [1/R - 1].$$

The effect of making a Q_A measurement during a dialysis treatment on delivered dialysis must be considered since in most methods, the blood pump flow rate is reduced from its prescribed level to 200–300 mL/min. During the interval of measurement, effective dialysis is reduced.

DUS measurements[90] can be made in only a few minutes producing virtually no effect on Kt/V. The delta-hematocrit method[70] reduces effective treatment for up to 8–10 minutes. Conductivity-based online clearance methods take the most time, 20 minutes or more, and have the greatest effect on reducing Kt/V delivered during the session. Due to the pace of dialysis between shifts, few extensions of treatment are provided as compensation for the low flows needed during flow measurements. All flow methods described above also need a device that can reverse the blood lines safely, near instantaneously, and sterilely. These are an add-on expense.

The recent study by Tessitore et al[33] clearly indicates that the best test to detect a given stenosis depends on its location. Flow may be better for inflow, but derived venous static pressure is better for outflow lesions. Since many accesses have coexistence of both types of lesions, it is imperative that one does not marry a technique but thinks of the process. When angiography is done, it is equally important that the hemodynamic significance of each lesion be evaluated prior to doing "blind" angioplasty. In grafts especially, the physiological (as opposed to anatomical) significance of a stenosis may not be evaluable until the dominant lesion is repaired.[94] In grafts, measurement of flow prior to referral for angiography shows the absence of any correlation between the intragraft blood flow and the location, length, or number of stenosis and only a moderate inverse correlation between the intragraft blood flow and the degree of stenosis ($P = 0.08$).[95] These observations support the modeling studies performed by Paulson and co-workers indicating that flow measurements need to be performed frequently in order to provide meaningful predictive value when to intervene[73,75] and not on some absolute value of flow or change in flow.[76]

The Current K/DOQI Work-Group feels that there is insufficient literature evidence to prefer one surveillance technique over another.[2] DDU studies are predictive of access stenosis and the likelihood for failure[96]; however, the frequency of measurement is limited by expense and operator skill.[97] DDU may be useful in AVF despite its increased cost.[87,98] Variation in the internal software used for calculating Doppler flow measurements by different manufacturers has until now prevented standardization and exchange of data among investigators. Among the more recent techniques, magnetic resonance flow has been found to be accurate but expensive.[99,100] Neither DDU flow nor magnetic resonance can be performed during dialysis sessions. The latter is more often used to plan surgery.[28] Finally, CT angiography produces excellent images of stenosis[71] but is impractical for routine use and does not provide physiological data.

Static venous dialysis pressure is a well-established technique for detecting physiologically significant stenosis in AVG[34,35] and is able to reduce graft thrombosis by almost 70%. It is currently unknown whether the method is less or more predictive of thrombosis and access failure than direct flow measurements in AVF. However, in our experience, combining sequential static measurements with prepump pressures to assess for changes in adequacy of inflow appears as effective[35] as other published observations using flow measurements. In the context of proper needle position, an elevated negative arterial prepump pressure that prevents increasing the blood flow rate to the prescribed level is predictive of arterial inflow stenosis in an AVF.

Measurement of static intra-access pressures has evolved over time. The original methodology used inline pressure transducers identical to those used in intensive care units with accurate output to an electronic device.[34,101] The expense of the inline transducers mandated a conversion to the use of the pressure transducers already available on a standard dialysis delivery machine. In a research setting, the correlations of static pressures measured using the machine pressure transducers with the values obtained from an inline pressure transducer was excellent.[102] However, this required careful calibration of the transducers and accurate setting of the zero values, which could not be readily accomplished in the real world producing the junk in–junk out phenomenon. As a result, we evolved a computerized method using the dynamic pressure readings taken many times during any dialysis session and extracting from it the static pressure when factoring out the contributions of chair height, blood pump flow, and hematocrit.[103] Because of the frequency of measurements within a given session and then sequentially with each session, inaccuracies from calibration and zero offset could be factored out and time trends developed. A static pressure to MAP ratio could then be used to assess a hemodynamic change within the access. Use of the original static pressure ratio was reported to reduce thrombosis in graft rate in 1995[34] and 1997.[104] The evolved computerized method[103] (available as VascAlert®) continues to achieve the same results in AVG and AVF 14 years later.[35]

Figure 13-5 is an illustrative example of the current method. In the top panel, the changes in pressure ratio are depicted. Increasing pressure without pre-emptive intervention was followed by a thrombosis. Because a thrombectomy followed by a PTA does not correct the underlying propensity to recurrence of stenosis, pressures subsequently increased. However, a timely PTA prevents another thrombosis. In some patients, repeated PTAs have kept AVG going for years. Recurrence of stenosis is not automatic after PTA as illustrated in the bottom panel. What leads to this biological difference among patients in response to the known injurious effects of PTA is unknown.

Figure 13-6 is an illustrative example of data from a patient with an AVF. The top panel depicts a well-functioning AVF. Note the spontaneous variation in pressures, but over time there is no trend for progressive elevation in pressures. By contrast, as shown in the bottom panel, the AVF in this patient showed multiple increases in pressures that required multiple interventions to maintain function and patency.

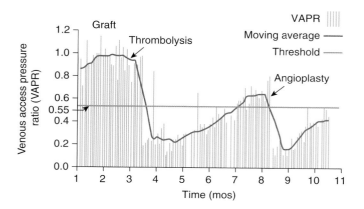

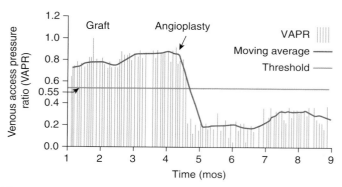

Figure 13-5. Representative data for two patients having an AVG (see the text). In the upper panel, a patient has a prolonged increase in the derived static venous ration and refuses intervention. Thrombosis results—after thrombectomy and PTA, which restores intra-access pressure to normal limits, pressures progressively increase. Pre-emptive PRA restores function and prevents a subsequent thrombosis. Note, however, that since PTA does not cure the underlying formation of neointimal hyperplasia, the stenosis recurs. The lower panel shows that recurrence is not invariable after PTA. In this illustrative case, intra-access pressures returned to normal and persisted for months. This patient's stenotic lesion redeveloped 19 months later (data not shown).

ROLE OF MONITORING

Monitoring is, as summarized in Table 13-1, a crucial part of any M/S program of AVF and enhances an organized surveillance program to detect access dysfunction. Specific findings predictive of venous stenosis include edema of the access extremity, prolonged bleeding postvenipuncture (in the absence of excessive anticoagulation), and changes in the physical characteristics of the thrill in the AVF.[19] An AVF that does not "collapse" or become less distended on arm elevation is likely to be harboring an outflow stenosis. Physical examination (augmentation test) is a useful screening tool to exclude low flow (<450 mL/min). Attention also has to be paid to the ratio of blood pump flow to prepump negative pressure. Normally, this ratio is >1.6 mL min/mm Hg. A progressively decreasing value may reflect inflow problems in the AVF. Our experience

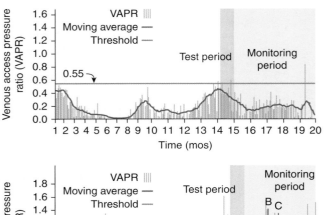

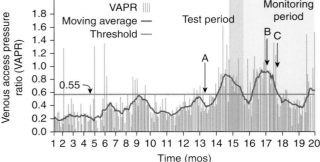

Figure 13-6. Representative data for two patients having AVF. The top panel shows a normally functioning AVF.

is that this ratio is less useful in AVG since grafts can fail while their flow is in excess of routinely prescribed blood flows. To use this test correctly, one should set the pre-pump pressure consistently to the same values, for instance between −200 and −250 mm Hg, and trend the blood flow achieved.

EVALUATION OF NONMATURATION OF AVF

In native AVF, inadequate flow prevents maturation. It is invariably due to a lesion at the arteriovenous anastomosis or within the vein 2–6 cm from the anastomosis. Nonmaturation increases reliance of hemodialysis patients on grafts and catheters, exposing them to associated higher complication risks. A meta-analysis of 33 articles addressing this issue examined both clinical and pre- and postoperative risks for nonmaturation. Patients with preoperative clinical risk factors had excess nonmaturation risks of 21% (CI, 11–30%) and a relative risk of 1. Patients with preoperative hemodynamic risk factors had a similar average estimated excess risk of 24% (CI, 15–33%) and a relative risk of 1.7. The worse outlook was in patients with hemodynamic risk factors present shortly after operation whose excess nonmaturation risk was 50% (95% CI, 42–58%) and a relative risk of 4.3 (95% CI, 3.4–5.5).[53] In established forearm AVF, inflow lesions tend to dominate outflow lesions.[68] By contrast, with elbow-level brachiocephalic AVF or transposed brachiobasilic AVF, outflow lesions are more frequent either in the cephalic arc[105] or at swing segments in transposed veins.[106]

TABLE 13–2

A Thrombosed Vascular Access is a Major Problem

For the dialysis staff
- Assist the patient in coping
- Arrange for transportation
- Interface between patient and physicians
- Rearrange dialysis schedule

For the nephrologist
- Console unhappy patient and family
- Arrange for logistics to resolve AVF failure

For the patient
- Cope with discomfort, pain anxiety, fear
- Delay of dialysis
- Concern about K^+ and fluid overlead
- Schedule disruption
- Decreased quality of life

ISSUES IN SURVEILLANCE/MONITORING

The usefulness of M/S depends on accurate prediction of AVF dysfunction so that problems producing under dialysis are corrected expeditiously and anatomical stenosis intervened upon within a reasonable interval of time. A dysfunctional access is a very real concern to patients since almost 60% of patients cite thrombosis of the access as one of the most feared problems associated with hemodialysis, ranking it second only to pain.[107] As summarized in Table 13-2, loss of access patency affects the treating staff as well. A body of evidence indicates that prospective M/S to detect stenosis reduces the rate of access failure and/or thrombosis in grafts through performance of more interventional procedures.[108–113] However, in a number of studies, the total number of events (thrombosis or elective PTA) does not change.[34,104,114] Since thrombosis is much more time-consuming and expensive to do, it makes sense to intervene before thrombosis can occur. Whether PTA or stent[115] is the preferred approach is addressed elsewhere. As demonstrated by Lilly et al,[116] the subsequent patency of a thrombosed graft is much shorter than one electively intervened upon by PTA. When an access is lost, the patient must receive dialysis using catheters increasing his risk for mortality and morbidity. It is crucially important that the stenotic lesion be adequately treated. Lilly et al[116] also demonstrated that duration of patency was inversely related to the degree of residual and the static venous pressure at the end of procedure. Similarly, Schwab et al[76] reported that restoration of access flow by the PTA intervention is more important than "procedural" success by degree of stenosis in predicting secondary access patency. In general, it is believed that intervention in AVF appears to more durable than in AVG but there are no good comparative studies.

▶ Flow Criteria for Intervention

Criteria are needed to determine the optimal time for referral for elective PTA of a suspected stenosis within a vascular access. Although there is general agreement that Q_A identifies stenosis in patients with native vessel AV fistulae (AVF), the threshold for intervention is debated. Practice guidelines recommend performing angiography when Q_A is <500 mL/min in AVF. This value was supported by Tonelli et al[117] who constructed receiver-operating characteristic curves examining the relationship between different threshold values of Q_A and stenosis in 340 patients with AVF. The area under the curve for the composite definition of stenosis was 0.86. The small gain in sensitivity associated with a <600 mL/min threshold was outweighed by a reduced specificity compared with <500 mL/min. Q_A measurements seemed to predict stenosis or incipient access failure equally well in groups defined by diabetic status, gender, and AVF location. Somewhat higher thresholds were found by an Italian study[23] in a group of 120 patients who all underwent fistulography, 54 of whom were found to have a stenosis of 50% by diameter. Q_A < 700–1000 mL/min and/or a reduction in Q_A > 25% were found to be optimal predictors for stenosis (91% efficiency) and a Q_A < 300 mL/min for incipient thrombosis for wrist AVF. A higher value of 1000 mL/min was noted for stenosis detection in fistulas constructed in the mid forearm. In their study, correction for systemic blood pressure did not improve performance, similar to the findings in the Canadian study.[109] A change in flow did, however, increase the sensitivity of Q_A in predicting the presence of stenosis. Note that, flows of 600–1000 mL/min in AVF may be associated with the presence of stenosis, but at these flow intervention might not be necessary as the access can still deliver adequate flow and still have a low risk for subsequent thrombosis (see Figure 13-7).

Another study followed 52 randomly selected patients whose accesses were followed for 4 years clinically, in whom Q_A measurements were made only annually, and intervention prohibited unless the AVF failed due to thrombosis or failed to deliver adequate dialysis.[81] All failures were due to thrombosis. ROC analysis revealed Q_A of <700 mL/min as the best predictor of failure over a *period of years*, sensitivity

89% but specificity only 69%. Four year actuarial survival was 74% in those with Q_A > 700 and only 21% in those with flow <700 mL/min. It should be noted that of the 24 AVF that remained patent throughout 4 years, 5 had Q_A consistently less than <500 mL/min. Thus, a single Q_A threshold for angiography in all patients is too simplistic in our opinion. The optimal threshold may vary by patient subgroup and the best function ever attained by the AVF. This is supported by a retrospective study of 294 incident and prevalent hemodialysis patients treated at a single institution, all of whom had a functioning AVF during the study period.[118] Q_A was measured bimonthly using ultrasound dilution; a total of 4084 Q_A measurements were made. Univariate analysis found that younger patient age, nondiabetic status, higher SBP, DBP, MAP (all at the time of Q_A measurement), upper arm AVF location, and overweight status (BMI ≥ 25) were significantly associated with Q_A. SBP was more strongly associated with Q_A than DBP or MAP. In a multivariate model, SBP, overweight status, and diabetic status were independently associated with Q_A. The strong association between SBP and Q_A suggests that adjusting Q_A for SBP may improve the specificity of access screening.

One study that used the ultrafiltration method which changes hematocrit as the indicator signal[70] also established the value of Q_A surveillance in AVF; the positive predictive value, negative predictive value, sensitivity, and specificity of this Q_A method for detecting VA stenosis were 84.2%, 93.5%, 84.2%, and 93.5%, respectively.[119] However, a study from Australia found less benefit of Q_A surveillance[120]; 67 and 68 patients were assigned to the control (usual treatment) and Q_A surveillance groups, respectively. The area under the receiver operating characteristic curve demonstrated, at best, a moderate prediction of (>50%) AVF stenosis (0.78, 95% CI, 0.63–0.94). Thus, unlike the Canadian and Italian groups, these clinicians felt that the addition of AVF Q_A monitoring to clinical screening for AVF stenosis resulted in a nonsignificant doubling in the detection of angiographically significant AVF stenosis. What produces these differences among populations is unclear, but I speculate that the clinical ability of dialysis staff to evaluate AVF might be crucial. In the USA, where the clinical skills are lacking, Q_A surveillance could make a huge difference.

Our own studies using flow to follow AVF and grafts[121] indicate that the probability of a permanent access event, a need for thrombectomy or a pre-emptive PTA to restore function, over a follow-up period of 3 months was a function of not only the absolute flow but also the rate of decrease of such flow as illustrated in Figure 13-7. An accurate measurement of the rate of change required five to six flow measurements performed weekly in the preceding 2 months. As shown in Figure 13-7 for grafts, if the current flow was 800 mL/min and flow was decreasing by 30 mL/min/month (by regression analysis), the probability of an event within the next 3 months was 0.12 (12%) and if flow was decreasing by 70 mL/min/month the probability of an event was 0.56 (56%). By comparison, if the

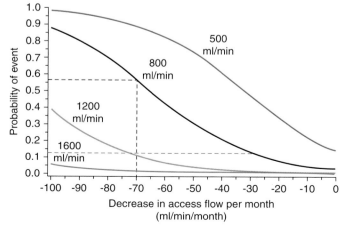

Figure 13-7. Probability of graft thrombosis.

current flow was 1200 mL/min and flow was decreasing by 70 mL/min/month, the probability of an event decreased to only 0.11 (11%). Note that, even a marginal graft with a flow of 500 mL/min and barely able to deliver 400 mL/min blood flow to the dialyzer without recirculation has a probability less than 25% of needing intervention if the flow is not decreasing over time. Similar curves were developed for AVF. Exactly when to intervene is thus still unclear; more definitive studies are needed. The level of probability at which elective PTA should be done to prevent thrombosis has not been rigorously studied.

▶ Static Pressure Ratio Criteria for Intervention

The original technique developed in the mid-1990s used the ratio of systolic intra-access pressure to arterial systolic pressure since the correlations with degree of stenosis were higher using systolic pressures than using diastolic or mean arterial pressure ratios.[34,101] Over time the pressure ratio changed to 0.45 using readings from the machine transducers (under no flow state) and to 0.55 in the currently used method.[35] The latter has been in use now for a decade.[103]

▶ Accuracy of Flow Measurements

Accuracy of measurement is important in surveillance. Several studies have assessed the degree of variability of Q_A among and within dialysis sessions. Polkinhorne et al[122] measured Q_A and MAP multiple times (30, 60, 120, 210, and 240 minutes) during three consecutive dialysis treatments. They noted a significant reduction in Q_A and MAP throughout the dialysis treatment with Q_A decreasing by 5% and 10% in the middle and last third of the treatment compared to the first third. Q_A could be as much as -30.6% from baseline during the last hour of dialysis. MAP influenced Q_A more in radiocephalic ($r^2 = 0.55$) than in brachiocephalic fistulae ($r^2 = 0.06$). Similar results were found by Huisman et al[123] who measured access flow predialysis using DDU and flow during dialysis using DDU on two successive treatments in 24 accesses of which 11 were brachiocephalic and 10 were radiocephalic. Although the mean value was unchanged, the mean coefficient of variation (CV) was large at 16.4%. Within session, CV was smaller at 7% . Variation was larger between sessions if the needle orientation was altered in a direction. The data suggested higher variance at higher flows, usually associated with elbow level AVF. We have previously demonstrated that variations in hydration, MAP, and hematocrit from week to week can alter cardiac output and therefore the access flow by as much as 30%.[62]

VALUE OF MONITORING/SURVEILLANCE

The need to add surveillance to monitoring has been vigorously debated.[24,125] In 1993, Dr. Harold Feldman using data we had gathered for publication[34] calculated that a cohort size of 572 would be necessary to demonstrate an increase

in average "in use access age" from 2 to 3 years. As stated previously, outcome should not focus on only prolongation of access survival. The more important outcome to the patient is a reduction in thrombosis rate. Unfortunately, as with access survival, cohort size statistical estimates by Dr. E. Peterson at Henry Ford Health System (using two different designs/models) indicated that >500 patients would be needed to demonstrate a 50% reduction in thrombosis rate based on data we recently published.[35] Even a very simple prepost model to "examine longitudinal differences in thrombosis rates" (before and after the introduction of surveillance) through the use of a generalized estimating equation (GEE) (negative binomial regression model with total person-years of follow-up for an interval) yields a value greater than the sample size of the population that was reported in most published RCT to date. A decrease in thrombosis rate from 13% to 6.8 % of patients per 6 month period yields a sample size of 438 subjects if there would be a 7%% mortality rate and 20% drop-out rate per 6 month period using a significance level of 0.05 and a power of 0.8. This is the simplest of designs using a prepost comparison of 6 months each (no surveillance vs surveillance in all patients in the two 6 month periods).

Yet not a single RCT on the influence of surveillance has had even 200 subjects and some were as small as 30–50 allocated to two to three groups.[126–130] All of the studies can be criticized on many levels including small sample size, lack of data on important confounders (control of which is impossible with sample sizes under 400), and whether the intervention produced the desired improvement in physiologic function. Success of the PTA only occurs if the procedure restores both the anatomical and clinical/physiological parameters used to detect the stenosis in the first place into acceptable limits. In a properly conducted RTC, defining exactly what constitutes a successful angioplasty is crucial. Dilatation of a stenotic lesion with an angioplasty balloon must also have a lasting beneficial effect. Without satisfying these two components, the angioplasty may actually cause harm. Therefore, in any planned future RCT, the adequacy of the intervention must be assessed by either pressure[94,116] and/or flow measurement[76,95] during the procedure before and after the PTA. Durability requires frequent measurements after the intervention procedure.

Valuable and often conflicting observations were frequently obtained within the same cited studies[127,129] and important follow-up reports using data from the same cohorts.[131,132] Many other available studies did demonstrate a benefit of duplex ultrasound[89] and access blood flow[133] on access patency. Is it premature to say that evidence (mostly from RCTs) does not show a beneficial effect or that observational studies of benefit from surveillance have been improperly designed and interpreted. However, the sample size estimates discussed previously for the design of an interventional trial are in keeping with recent RCT performed under the auspices of the NIH. As an example, the two NIH studies on the efficacy of pharmaceutical intervention on survival of accesses, Persantine in graft[11] and Plavix in AVF,[134] both required an initial sample size estimate of nearly 1000 patients to see a 20% difference in time to loss of patency.

From the perspective of the patient, the focus on whether AV access patency is maintained longer or not by M/S is inappropriate. We believe that *prevention of thrombosis without prolongation of overall longevity is by itself a worthy outcome*. The objective of access M/S is the early recognition of dysfunction in order to be able to correct the stenosis by angioplasty or surgery. A retrospective analysis of an incident cohort of 88 hemodialysis patients demonstrated a 24% primary access failure rate due to complications.[135] A total of 2.43 inpatient days and 1.05 outpatient encounters per patient year at risk were directly attributed to such access complications. Improvement in access patency can only come from better treatments of the lesions found. Pharmacological, cellular, and molecular engineering approaches are needed for preventing or producing regression of the lesion of neointimal hyperplasia.[136] The importance of the latter is that each intervention carries an increased risk for the patient. To minimize the number of such procedures, we need to minimize false positive results from our M/S and prolong the interval between procedures through therapies that can modify the neointimal process that leads to recurrence.

We believe that the dismally low and late positive predictive value of "clinical monitoring" as practiced in the typical dialysis unit requires the addition of surveillance as mandated by the CMS conditions of coverage,[18] if we are to effect nationally successful lowering of thrombosis rates. There is a plethora of "non-RCT" data demonstrating reduction in thrombosis rates after "surveillance" is added to clinical monitoring.[15,33–35,62,111,114,137–141] All achieved a twofold reduction in thrombosis rates through surveillance as shown in Figure 13-8. Specifically, Sands et al[138] showed a 6.5-fold reduction in thrombosis rates from 1.25 to 0.19 events per patient year at risk (Duplex ultrasound imaging), and McCarley et al[114] showed a 4.4-fold reduction from 0.71 to 0.16 (access flow). Both Hoeben et al[92] Glazer et al[141] achieved a twofold reduction in thrombosis events, from 0.32 to 0.17 (using flow methodology).

In 1995, Besarab et al reported a threefold reduction in thrombosis rate from 0.51 to 0.17[34] (using static pressure) duplicated 16 years later by Zasuwa et al (using derived static pressure).[35] It appears that the surveillance technique may not be as important as doing some form of surveillance that is effective. Last year, we performed a large pilot to introduce surveillance into 10 dialysis centers. The baseline clot rate was above 40%. During the 5 months of the pilot, this rate dropped to 12% with a false positive rate of only 4% (J Kennedy, personal communication), which should mitigate fears of unnecessary interventions from too many false positive results.

If "clinical monitoring" as practiced does not work, it puts our patients at risk. To reiterate, *surveillance when practiced intelligently using repeated measurements and physiologic principles reduces clots without increasing false positive diagnostic rates and therefore PTA rates*. We believe that the confluence of patient issues, best medical evidence, and clinical expertise mandate the continued ability to study the issue scientifically. We know that stenosis is related to thrombosis but is generally not the proximate cause and we have methods to detect stenosis with a high degree of sensitivity if our staff does not use clinical skills, even when taught. We can treat stenosis with PTA and such treatment is still the only option that has been proposed that appears to have any effect on thrombosis rate. The technique of PTA is too complex to describe here.

Several studies have been performed evaluating Q_A surveillance and AVF outcomes. Results of prospective surveillance in native fistulas in Spain with measurements made 4 months apart have been positive. The AVF thrombosis rate in 50 patients followed with Q_A surveillance was lower, 2/50 or 4%, than in 94 patients not followed with flow measurements, 6/94 or 17% ($P = 0.024$).[142] Similarly, a study by Tessitore et al[143] evaluated the effect of PTA on functioning AVF survival. In a prospective-controlled open trial, they evaluated whether prophylactic PTA of stenosis not associated with access dysfunction improved survival in native, virgin, radiocephalic forearm AVF. Sixty-two patients with stenotic, functioning AVF (able to provide adequate dialysis) were enrolled in the study: 30 control and 32 to prophylactic PTA. Kaplan–Meier analysis showed that PTA significantly ($P = 0.012$) improved AVF functional failure-free survival rates with a fourfold increase in median survival and a 2.87-fold decrease in risk of failure. The Cox proportional hazard model identified PTA as the only variable associated with outcome ($P = 0.012$). PTA induced an increase in Q_A by 323 (236 to 445) mL/min ($P < 0.001$), suggesting that improved AVF survival resulted from increased Q_A. Prophylactic PTA was also associated with a halving of the risk of hospitalization, central venous catheterization, and thrombectomy ($P < 0.05$).

A follow-up study by the same group reported on their 5 year randomized, controlled, open trial of blood flow surveillance and pre-emptive repair of subclinical stenoses (angioplasty alone or/and open surgery) with standard monitoring and intervention based upon clinical criteria

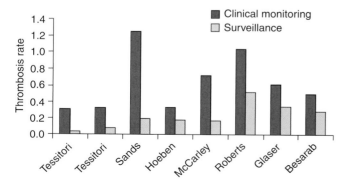

Figure 13-8. Representative results from observational trials of surveillance on access thrombosis rates.

alone.[133] Surveillance with blood pump flow (Q_b) monitoring during dialysis sessions and quarterly Q_A or recirculation measurements identified 79 AVF with angiographically proven, anatomically significant (>50%D) stenosis that were then randomized to either a control group (intervention done in response to a decline in the delivered dialysis dose or thrombosis; $n = 36$) or to a pre-emptive treatment group ($n = 43$). Kaplan–Meier analysis showed that the pre-emptive treatment reduced failure rate ($P = 0.003$) and the Cox hazard model identified treatment ($P = 0.009$) and higher baseline Q_A ($P = 0.001$) as the only variables associated with favorable outcome. Access survival was significantly higher in pre-emptively treated than in control AVF ($P = 0.050$). This study provides evidence that active blood flow surveillance and pre-emptive repair of subclinical stenosis reduce the thrombosis rate and prolong the functional life of mature forearm AVF and that $Q_A > 350$ mL/min prior to intervention portends a superior outcome with pre-emptive action in AVF.

An important aspect of the care is the degree of improvement in flow and the durability of the increase in Q_A following intervention. As found by Tessitore et al,[143] higher postintervention Q_A was the only variable associated with improved access longevity ($P = 0.044$). In the study by Roca et al,[142] elective intervention was successful in 88% of treated accesses (15/17) with mean Q_A increasing from 563.8 ± 115.4 mL/min just before intervention to 975.7 ± 351.8 mL/min just after intervention. The latter did not differ from the highest recorded mean Q_A before intervention, 877.7 ± 415.4 mL ($p = 0.25$). Access thrombosis during the follow-up period (354.4 ± 293.1 days) occurred in 3 of 17. Five accesses restenosed and two of them (40%) underwent reintervention by surgery.

A closer examination of changes in access flow was carried out by van der Linden and co-workers.[144] Q_A in AVF increased from 304 ± 24 to 638 ± 51 as degrees of stenosis was decreased from 72 ± 5 to $23 \pm 7\%$. Q_A values before PTA and the increase in Q_A postintervention correlated with long-term outcomes whereas angiographic results did not. The data from this study as well as that of the literature suggest that there is an optimal timing for PTA and we need more studies on this aspect. Similarly, Murray et al[145] found that AVG post-PTA that achieved a blood flow >1000 mL/min required fewer repeat interventions and had longer assisted patency than those which had flow <1000 mL/min. These studies confirm that procedural success should be measured functionally and not anatomically.[76,94,95,116]

Trerotola et al[146] collected prospectively data for 102 PTA procedures (66 prophylactic PTA procedures and 36 PTA procedures performed during access thrombectomy). Outcomes data other than residual stenosis were not collected, but the endpoint for all interventions was a thrill in the access. A total of 230 lesions were treated. Only two (1%) could not be successfully treated with PTA despite the use of "ultra high" pressure. Overall, 55% of lesions required pressures greater than 15 atm to efface the waist. More lesions in AVF than in grafts (20% vs. 9%) required very high pressure (>20 atm) to efface the waist ($P = 0.02$). Residual stenosis was positively correlated with severity of initial stenosis and negatively correlated with duration of inflation. Thus conventional angioplasty balloons are often inadequate for the treatment of most hemodialysis access stenosis, pressures >15 atm are commonly needed for PTA in hemodialysis access, and importantly very high pressures >20 atm are often needed in native fistulas.

The overall conclusion from the above studies is that prophylactic PTA of stenosis in functioning forearm AV access improves access survival and decreases access-related morbidity. This conclusion is supported by a meta-analysis of RCTs performed by Tonelli et al.[147] They also strongly support the surveillance program for early detection of stenosis. However, the urge to intervene with PTA to prevent thrombosis must be balanced by the observations that PTA almost invariably triggers repeated need for the same procedure. The optimal care of such patients requires individualization and not rigid application of protocols. Practice Guidelines need to be improved by incorporating recommendations that are specific to the patient.[148]

A main controversy that has arisen is whether Q_A-surveillance produces benefits in terms of cost and which methodology to use. Lok et al[109] concluded that the functional information provided by low flows was predictive of thrombosis, whereas stenosis detection alone was poorly predictive of incipient thrombosis. Mann et al[149] collected cost data on all ($n = 239$) incident patients between July 1, 1999 and November 1, 2001. During the first year, 18.4% of all admissions were for vascular access-related complications. As expected, AVF had the lowest total cost, but in all cases vascular access care consumed a significant portion of the health care costs in the first year of dialysis. Several studies have examined the trade-offs of vascular access flow surveillance. Winjen et al[150] noted that access-related costs during a 3 year period of surveillance tended to be lower than during the preceding 3 year period without monitoring; an increase in angioplasty interventions was offset by decreased hospitalization for thrombectomy. However, the benefit was seen with grafts and not AVF as grafts are more prone to stenosis and thrombosis. The results echo those from a half decade ago by McCarley et al.[114] The authors also noted significant improvement in catheter placement and in missed out-patient treatments, a result previously reported by Dossabhoy et al.[132]

Finally, Tonelli et al[151] examined the cost-effectiveness of performing angiography in AVF when Q_A is < 500 mL/min even though Q_A threshold of <750 mL/min is more sensitive for stenosis. Notably, screening strategies did not reduce expected access-related costs under any clinically plausible scenario. The cost to prevent one episode of AVF failure appeared to be approximately $8000–$10,000 over 5 years for both screening strategies, compared with no screening. However, the analysis also pointed out that Q_A surveillance might be worthwhile if reduced exposure to central catheters produces morbidity or mortality benefit or a change in quality of life for the patient. Obviously, if the vascular access assessment cost could be reduced by design or labor components, surveillance might become cost-effective even from the health purchaser point of view.

Perhaps the use of more than one modality needs to be evaluated. Some advocate the use of Doppler Duplex ultrasound imaging in addition to dilutional flow methods alone to guide PTA.[85] The DDU procedure is a known effective method for the diagnosis of vascular access stenosis[89] and according to Bacchini et al,[85] it could improve stenosis screening by avoiding the risks of exposure to ionizing radiation in those without stenosis but low flow and of adverse reactions to contrast media.

CONCLUSION

A lasting and properly functioning vascular access is pivotal in improving quality of life for patients on maintenance hemodialysis and reducing the cost of healthcare for end-stage renal disease. AVG thrombosis is a common cause of a long-term loss with only 42–60% remaining patent at 3 years even with interventions.[152] Arteriovenous fistulae (AVF) have a high incidence of early maturation failures, particularly if they are radio-cephalic AVFs. The body of evidence suggests that detection of stenosis and prevention of thrombosis in vascular accesses is valuable. Evidence from the DOPPS study suggests that with intervention, grafts perhaps function much longer and almost as good as AVF.[153] These can be detected by processes using monitoring and surveillance techniques but requires an integrated effort from a vascular access team. We have the tools for identification of patients in whom stenosis is present and is progressing. We need to refine our criteria for when to intervene. Till we do, however, when a test indicates the likely presence of a functionally significant stenosis, venography or fistulography should be used to definitively establish the presence of and the degree of the stenosis. In most cases, angioplasty should be performed if the stenosis is greater than 50% by diameter. Stenotic lesions should not be repaired merely because they are present. Surveillance is of significant value because at a minimum, it fosters the ability to salvage vascular access sites through planning, coordination of effort, and elective corrective intervention, rather than urgent procedures or replacement. We need therapies that prevent the development of neointimal hyperplasia both after initial construction and after elective or therapeutic PTA.[136,154] There is an urgent need for large randomized control trials looking at homogeneous patients with newly fashioned hemodialysis vascular access, suitably identified with monitoring and surveillance to predict vascular access at risk of thrombosis. This would help guide future interventions appropriately in both AVG and AVF.

REFERENCES

1. US Renal Data System. *USRDS 2010 Annual Data Report*. Atlas of chronic kidney disease and end-stage renal disease in the United States. Available at: http://www.usrds.org/atlas.htm (2010) Precis & Chapter 10 Reference tables.

2. NKF-K/DOQI Clinical Practice Guidelines for Vascular Access: *Update 2006. Am J Kidney Dis.* 2006;48(suppl 1):S176–S276.

3. Sehgal AR, Dor A, Tsai AC, et al. Morbidity and cost implications of inadequate hemodialysis. *Am J Kidney Dis.* 2001;37:1223–1231.

4. Allon M, Robbin ML. Increasing arteriovenous fistulas in hemodialysis patients: problems and solutions. *Kidney Int.* 2002;62(4):1109–1124.

5. US Renal Data System. *USRDS 2010 Annual Data Report.* Atlas of chronic kidney disease and end-stage renal disease in the United States. Available at: http://www.usrds.org/atlas.htm (2010). Chapter 5: Morbidity and mortality.

6. Available at: http://www.fistulafirst.org/.

7. Kinnaert P, Vereerstraeten P, Toussaint C, et al. Nine years' experience with internal arteriovenous fistulas for haemodialysis: a study of some factors influencing the results. *Br J Surg.* 1977;64:242–246.

8. Miller PE, Tolwani A, Luscy CP, et al. Predictors of adequacy of arteriovenous fistulas in hemodialysis patients. *Kidney Int.* 1999;56:275–280.

9. Miller CD, Robbin ML, Allon M. Gender differences in outcomes of arteriovenous fistulas in hemodialysis patients. *Kidney Int.* 2003;63:346–352.

10. Rodriguez JA, Armadans L, Ferrer E, et al. The function of permanent vascular access. *Nephrol Dial Transplant.* 2000;15:402–408.

11. Dember LM, Beck GJ, Allon M, et al. Effect of clopidogrel on early failure of arteriovenous fistulas for hemodialysis: a randomized controlled trial. *JAMA.* May 2008;14;299(18):2164–2171.

12. Lok CE, Allon M, Moist L,et al. Risk equation determining unsuccessful cannulation events and failure to maturation in arteriovenous fistulas (REDUCE FTM I). *J Am Soc Nephrol* 2006;17:3204–3212.

13. Oliver MJ, McCann RL, Indridason OS, et al. Comparison of transposed brachiobasilic fistulas to upper arm grafts and brachiocephalic fistulas. *Kidney Int.* 2001;60:1532–1539.

14. Allon M, Lockhart ME, Lilly RZ, et al. Effect of preoperative sonographic mapping on vascular access outcomes in hemodialysis patients. *Kidney Int.* 2001;60:2013–2020.

15. Besarab A. Access monitoring is worthwhile and valuable. *Blood Purif.* 2006;24:77–84.

16. Hakim RM, Breyer J, Ismail N, et al. Effects of dose of dialysis on morbidity and mortality. *Am J Kidney Dis.* 1994;23:661–619.

17. Rocco MV, Bleyer AJ, Burkart JM. Utilization of inpatient and outpatient resources for the management of hemodialysis access complications. *Am J Kidney Dis.* 1996;28:250–256.

18. Medicare and Medicaid Programs: Conditions for Coverage for End-Stage Renal Disease Facilities; Final Rule: Rules and Regulations, Part II, Department of Health and Human Services, *Federal Register.* 2008;73, April 15.

19. Beathard G. Physical examination: the forgotten tool. In: Gray JR, Sands JJ eds. *Dialysis Access: A Multidisciplinary Approach.* Philadelphia, PA: Lippincott, Williams & Williams; 2002:111–118.

20. Besarab A, Lubkowski T, Frinak S, et al. Detecting vascular access dysfunction. *ASAIO J.* 1997;43:M539–M543.

21. Besarab A, Lubkowski T, Frinak S. et al. Detection of strictures and vascular outlet stenoses in vascular accesses: which test is best? *ASAIO J.* 1997;43:M543–M547.

22. Schwartz C, Mitterbauer C, Boczula M, et al. Flow monitoring: performance characteristics of ultrasound dilution versus color Doppler ultrasound compared with fistulography. *Am J Kidney Dis.* 2003;42:539–545.

23. Tessitore N, Bedogna V, Gammaro L, et al. Diagnostic accuracy of ultrasound dilution access blood flow measurements in detecting stenosis and predicting thrombosis in native forearem ateriovenous fistulae for hemodialysis. *Am J Kidney Dis.* 2003;42:331–341.

24. Beathard GA, Litchfield T. Functions of a dedicated vascular access facility promoting AVF use. *Nephrol. News Issues.* 2004;11:44–48.

25. Arbab-Zadeh A, Mehta RL, Zeigler TW, et al. Hemodialysis access assessment with intravascular ultrasound. *Am J Kidney Dis.* 2002;39:813–823.

26. Froger CL, Duijm LE, Liem YS, et al. Stenosis detection with MR angiography and digital subtraction angiography in dysfunctional hemodialysis access fistulas and grafts. *Radiology.* 2005;234(1):284–291.

27. Smits JH, Bos C, Elgersma OE, et al. Hemodialysis access imaging: comparison of flow-interrupted contrast-enhanced MR angiography and digital subtraction angiography. *Radiology.* December 2002;225(3):829–834.

28. Han KM, Duijm LE, Thelissen GR, et al. Failing hemodialysis access grafts: evaluation of complete vascular tree with 3D contrast-enhanced MR angiography with high spatial resolution: initial results in 10 patients. *Radiology.* 2003;227(2):601–605.

29. Bakker CJ, Bosman PJ, Boereboom FT, et al. Measuring flow in hemodialysis grafts by non-triggered 2DPC magnetic resonance angiography. *Kidney Int.* March 1996;49(3):903–905.

30. Sackett D, Rosenbarg W, Gary JA, et al. Evidence based medicine: what it is and what it isn't. *Br Med J.* 1996;312:71.

31. Asif A, Leon C, Orozco-Vargas LC, et al. Accuracy of physical examination in the detection of arteriovenous fistula stenosis. *Clin J Am Soc Nephrol.* November 2007;2(6):1191–1194. Epub 2007 Oct 10.

32. Leon C, Orozco-Vargas LC, Krishnamurthy G, et al. Accuracy of physical examination in the detection of arteriovenous graft stenosis. *Semin Dial.* January–February 2008;21(1):85–88.

33. Tessitore N, Bedogna V, Melilli E, et al. In search of an optimal bedside screening program for arteriovenous fistula stenosis. *Clin J Am Soc Nephrol.* April 2011;6(4):819–826. Epub 2011 March 31.

34. Besarab A, Sullivan KL, Ross R, et al. The Utility of intra-access monitoring in detecting and correcting venous outlet stenoses prior to thrombosis. *Kidney Int.* 1995;47:1364–1373.

35. Zasuwa G, Frinak S, Besarab A, et al. Vascular access surveillance reduces vascular access thrombosis rate. *Semin Dial.* September–October 2010;23(5):527–535.

36. www.network13.org/QI/.../07-Beathard *Physical Exam Paper Final 12-3-03.doc.*

37. Leon C, Asif A. Physical examination of arteriovenous fistulae by a renal fellow: does it compare favorably to an experienced interventionalist? *Semin Dial.* November–December 2008;21(6):557–560. Epub 2008 August 28.

38. Beathard GA, Settle SM, Shields MW. Salvage of the nonfunctioning arteriovenous fistula. *Am J Kidney Dis.* 1999;33:910–916.

39. Turmel-Rodrigues L, Mouton A, Birmele B, et al. Salvage of immature forearm fistulas for haemodialysis by interventional radiology. *Nephrol Dial Transplant.* 2001;16:2365–2371.

40. Faiyaz R, Abreo K, Zaman F, et al. Salvage of poorly developed arteriovenous fistulae with percutaneous ligation of accessory veins. *Am J Kidney Dis.* 2002;39:824–827.

41. Beathard GA, Arnold P, Jackson J, et al. Aggressive treatment of early fistula failure. *Kidney Int.* 2003;64: 1487–1494.

42. Clark TWI, Cohen RA, Kwak A, et al. Salvage of nonmaturing native fistulas by using angioplasty. *Radiology.* 2006;242:286–292.

43. Kian K, Wyatt C, Schon D, et al. Safety of low-dose radiocontrast for interventional AV fistula salvage in stage 4 chronic kidney disease patients. *Kidney Int.* April 2006;69(8):1444–1449.

44. Asif A, Cherla G, Merrill D, et al. Venous mapping using venography and the risk of radiocontrast-induced nephropathy. *Semin Dial.* 2005;18:239–242.

45. Lomonte C, Casucci F, Antonelli M, et al. Is there a place for duplex screening of the brachial artery in the maturation of arteriovenous fistulas? *Semin Dial.* 2005;18:243–246.

46. Berman SS, Mendoza B, Westerband A, et al. Predicting arteriovenous fistula maturation with intraoperative blood flow measurements. *J Vasc Access.* October–December 2008;9(4):241–247.

47. Besarab A, Ross R, Al-Adel F, et al. The relation of intra-access pressure to flow (abstract). *J Am Soc Nephrol.* 1995;7:483.

48. Johnson CP, Zhu YR, Matt C, et al. Prognostic value of intraoperative blood flow measurements in vascular access surgery. *Surgery.* October 1998;124(4):729–737; discussion 737–738.

49. Akoh JA. Prosthetic arteriovenous grafts for hemodialysis. *J Vasc Access.* July–September 2009;10(3):137–147.

50. Van Tricht I, De Wachter D, Tordoir J, et al. Hemodynamics in a compliant hydraulic in vitro model of straight versus tapered PTFE arteriovenous graft. *J Surg Res.* February 2004;116(2):297–304.

51. Krueger U, Huhle A, Krys K, et al. Effect of tapered grafts on hemodynamics and flow rate in dialysis access grafts. *Artif Organs.* July 2004;28(7):623–628.

52. Van Tricht I, De Wachter D, Tordoir J, et al. Comparison of the hemodynamics in 6 mm and 4–7 mm hemodialysis grafts by means of CFD. *J Biomech.* 2006;39(2):226–236.

53. Voormolen EH, Jahrome AK, Bartels LW, et al. Nonmaturation of arm arteriovenous fistulas for hemodialysis access: a systematic review of risk factors and results of early treatment. *J Vasc Surg.* May 2009;49(5):1325–1336.

54. Schild AF, Pruett CS, Newman MI, et al. The utility of the VCS clip for creation of vascular access for hemodialysis: long-term results and intraoperative benefits. *Cardiovasc Surg.* 2001;9:526–530.

55. Shenoy S, Woodward RS. Economic impact of the beneficial effect of changing vascular anastomotic technique in hemodialysis access. *Vasc Endovascular Surg.* 2005;39:437–443.

56. Allon M, Bailey R, Ballard R, et al. A multidisciplinary approach to hemodialysis access: prospective evaluation. *Kidney Int.* February 1998;53(2):473–479.

57. Pfdederer TA, Darras FS, Welsch K, et al. How to organize hemodialysis vascular access quality assurance efforts into a cohesive whole for better patient outcomes. *Contem Dial Nephrol.* 2001;1:18–21.

58. Aruny JE, Lewis CA, Cardella JF, et al. Quality improvement guidelines for percutaneous management of the thrombosed or dysfunctional dialysis access. *J Vasc Interv Radiol.* 2003;14:S247–S253.

59. Besarab A. Advances in end-stage renal diseases 2000. Access monitoring methods. *Blood Purif.* 2000;18: 255–259.

60. Department of Health and Human Services Centers for Medicare and Medicaid Services. Adult in-center hemodialysis patients-vascular access. *2003 Annual Report ESRD Clinical Performance Measures Project.* 2003;30.

61. Schwab SJ, Raymond JR, Saeed M, et al. Prevention of hemodialysis fistula thrombosis. Early detection of venous stenoses. *Kidney Int.* 1989;36:707–711.

62. Besarab A, Lubkowski T, Vu A, et al. Effects of systemic hemodynamics on flow within vascular accesses used for hemodialysis. *ASAIO J.* 2001;47:501–506.

63. Begin V, Ethier J, Dumont M, et al. Prospective evaluation of the intra-access flow of recently created native arteriovenous fistulae. *Am J Kidney Dis.* December 2002; 40(6):1277–1282.

64. Leypoldt JK. Diagnostic methods for vascular access: access flow measurements. *Contrib Nephrol.* 2002;(137):31–7. Review.

65. Back MR, Maynard M, Winkler A, et al. Expected flow parameters within hemodialysis access and selection for remedial intervention of nonmaturing conduits. *Vasc Endovascular Surg.* April–May 2008;42(2):150–158. Epub 2008 February 14.

66. Dikow R, Schwenger V, Zeier M, et al. Do AV fistulas contribute to cardiac mortality in hemodialysis patients? *Semin Dial.* January–February 2002;15(1):14–17.

67. Kanterman RY, Vesely TM, Pilgram TK, et al. Dialysis access grafts: anatomic location of venous stenosis and results of angioplasty. *Radiology.* 1995;195:135–139.

68. Asif A, Gadalean FN, Merrill D, et al. Inflow stenosis in arteriovenous fistulas and grafts: a multicenter, prospective study. *Kidney Int.* May 2005;67(5):1986–1992.

69. Poch E, Martinez X, Rodrigo JA, et al. Prevalence and functional profile of unsuspected radial artery stenosis in native radiocephalic fistula dysfunction. Diagnosis by vascular access flow monitoring using Delta-H method. *Nefrologia.* 2006;26:581–586 [Article in Spanish].

70. Lopot F, Nejedly B, Sulkova S, et al. Comparison of different techniques of hemodialysis vascular access flow evaluation. *Int J Artif Organs.* 2003;26:1056–1063.

71. Duijim LEM, Liem YS, van der Rijt RHH, et al. Inflow stenosis in dysfunctional hemodialysis access fistulae and grafts. *Am J Kidney Dis.* 2006;48:98–105.

72. Duijm LE, Overbosch EH, Liem YS, et al. Retrograde catheterization of haemodialysis fistulae and grafts: angiographic depiction of the entire vascular access tree and stenosis treatment. *Nephrol Dial Transplant.* February 2009;24(2):539–547. Epub 2008 September 18.

73. White JJ, Ram SJ, Jones SA, et al. Influence of luminal diameters on flow surveillance of hemodialysis grafts: insights from a mathematical model. *Clin J Am Soc Nephrol.* September 2006;1(5):972–978. Epub 2006 July 26.

74. Sullivan K, Besarab A. Strategies for maintaining dialysis access patency. In Cope C, ed. *Current Techniques in Interventional Radiology.* chap 11, 2nd ed. Philadelphia, PA: Current Medicine; 1995:125–131.

75. White JJ, Jones SA, Ram SJ, et al. Mathematical model demonstrates influence of luminal diameters on venous pressure surveillance. *Clin J Am Soc Nephrol.* July 2007;2(4):681–687. Epub 2007 June 6.

76. Schwab SJ, Oliver MJ, Suhocki P, et al. Hemodialysis arteriovenous access: detection of stenosis and response to treatment by vascular access blood flow. *Kidney Int.* 2001;59(1):358–362.

77. Smits JH, van der Linden J, Hagen EC, et al. Graft surveillance: venous pressure, access flow, or the combination? *Kidney Int.* 2001;59:1551–1558.

78. Beathard GA. The treatment of vascular access graft dysfunction: a nephrologist's view and experience. *Adv Ren Replace Ther.* 1994;1:131–147.

79. Alloatti S, Molino A, Bonfant G, et al. Measurement of vascular access recirculation unaffected by cardiopulmonary recirculation: evaluation of an ultrasound method. *Nephron.* January 1999;81(1):25–30.

80. Brancaccio D, Tessitore N, Carpani P, et al. Potassium-based dilutional method to measure hemodialysis access recirculation. *Int J Artif Organs.* 2001 September;24(9):606–13. Review.

81. Basile C, Ruggieri G, Vernaglione L, et al. A comparison of methods for the measurement of hemodialysis access recirculation. *J Nephrol.* 2003;16:908–913.

82. Bosticardo GM, Morellini V, Schillaci E, et al. Two-operator glucose infusion test (GIT2) for vascular access recirculation measurement during hemodialysis. *J Vasc Access.* January–March 2010;11(1):38–40.

83. Besarab A, Ross R, Al-Aljel F, et al. The relation of brachial artery flow to access flow (abstract). *J Am Soc Nephrol.* 1995;7:483A.

84. Besarab A, Sherman RA. The relationship of recirculation to access blood type. *Am J Kidney Dis.* 1997;29:223–229.

85. Bacchini G, Cappello A, La Milia V, et al. Color Doppler ultrasonography imaging to guide transluminal angioplasty of venous stenosis. *Kidney Int.* October 2000;58(4): 1810–1813.

86. Gadallah MF, Paulson WD, Vickers B, et al. Accuracy of Doppler ultrasound in diagnosing anatomic stenosis of hemodialysis arteriovenous access as compared with fistulography. *Am J Kidney Dis.* 1998;32:273–277.

87. Malik J, Slavikova M, Malikova H, et al. Many clinically silent access stenoses can be identified by ultrasonography. *J Nephrol.* November–December 2002;15(6):661–665.

88. Frinak S, Zasuwa G, Dunfee T, et al. Dynamic venous access pressure ratio test for hemodialysis access monitoring. *Am J Kidney Dis.* October 2002;40(4): 760–768.

89. Malik J, Slavikova M, Svobodova J, et al. Regular ultrasonographic screening significantly prolongs patency of PTFE grafts. *Kidney Int.* April 2005;67(4):1554–1558.

90. Krivitski N, Gantela S. Access blood flow: debate continues. *Semin Dial.* 2001;14:460–461.

91. Department of Health and Human Services Centers for Medicare and Medicaid Services. Adult in-center

hemodialysis patients- vascular access. *2003 Annual Report ESRD Clinical Performance Measures Project,* 2003;30.

92. Hoeben H, Abu-Alfa AK, Reilly RF, et al. Vascular access surveillance: evaluation of combining dynamic venous pressure and vascular access blood flow measurements. *Am J Nephrol.* 2003;23:403–408.

93. Mercadal L, Challier E, Cluzel P, et al. Detection of vascular access stenosis by measurement of access blood flow from ionic dialysance. *Blood Purif.* 2002;20:177–181.

94. Asif A, Besarab A, Gadalean F, et al. Utility of static pressure ratio recording during angioplasty of arteriovenous graft stenosis. *Semin Dial.* 2006;19(6): 551–556.

95. Amin MZ, Vesely TM, Pilgram T. Correlation of intragraft blood flow with characteristics of stenoses found during diagnostic fistulography. *J Vasc Interv Radiol.* June 2004;15(6):589–593.

96. Finlay DE, Longley DG, Foshager MC, et al. Duplex and color Doppler sonography of hemodialysis arteriovenous fistulas and grafts. *Radiographics.* 1993;13:983–989.

97. Kirschbaum B, Compton A. Study of vascular access blood flow by angiodynography. *Am J Kidney Dis.* 1995;25: 22–25.

98. Grogan J, Castilla M, Lozanski L, et al. Frequency of critical stenosis in primary arteriovenous fistulae before hemodialysis access: should duplex ultrasound surveillance be the standard of care? *J Vasc Surg.* June 2005;41(6):1000–1006.

99. Han KM, Duijm LE, Thelissen GR, Cuypers et al. Failing hemodialysis access grafts: evaluation of complete vascular tree with 3D contrast-enhanced MR angiography with high spatial resolution: initial results in 10 patients. *Radiology.* 2003;227(2):601–605.

100. Duijm LE, Liem YS, van der Rijt RH, et al. Inflow stenoses in dysfunctional hemodialysis access fistulae and grafts. *Am J Kidney Dis.* July 2006;48(1):98–105.

101. Sullivan KL, Besarab A, Dorrell S, et al. The relationship between dialysis graft pressure & stenosis. *Invest. Radiology.* 1992;27:352–355.

102. Besarab A, Frinak S, Sherman RA, et al. Simplified measurement of intra-access pressure. *J Am Soc Nephrol.* 1998;9:284–289.

103. Frinak S, Zasuwa G, Dunfee T, et al. Computerized measurement of intra-access pressure. *Am J Kidney Dis.* 2002;40:760–768.

104. Sullivan KL, Besarab A. Hemodynamic screening and early percutaneous intervention reduce hemodialysis access thrombosis and increase graft longevity. *J Vasc Interv Radiol.* 1997;8:163–170.

105. Kian K, Asif A. Cephalic arch stenosis. *Semin Dial.* January–February 2008;21(1):78–82.

106. Badero OJ, Salifu MO, Wasse H, et al. Frequency of swing-segment stenosis in referred dialysis patients with angiographically documented lesions. *Am J Kidney Dis.* January 2008;51(1):93–98.

107. Bay WH, Van Cleef S, Owens M. The hemodialysis access: preferences and concerns of patients, dialysis nurses and technicians, and physicians. *Am J Nephrol.* 1998;18: 379–383.

108. Schwab SJ, Raymond JR, Saeed M. Prevention of hemodialysis fistula thrombosis. Early detection of venous stenoses. *Kidney Int.* 1989;36:707–711.

109. Lok CE, Bhola C, Croxford R, et al. Reducing vascular access morbidity: a comparative trial of two vascular access monitoring strategies. *Nephrol Dial Transplant.* June 2003;18(6):1174–1180.

110. Cayco AV, Abu-Alfa AK, Mahnensmith RL, et al. Reduction in arteriovenous graft impairment: results of a vascular access surveillance protocol. *Am J Kidney Dis.* 1998;32(2):302–308.

111. Sands JJ, Miranda CL. Prolongation of hemodialysis access survival with elective revision. *Clin Nephrol.* November 1995;44(5):329–333.

112. Safa AA, Valji K, Roberts AC, et al. Detection and treatment of dysfunctional hemodialysis access grafts: Effects of a surveillance program on graft patency and the incidence of thrombosis. *Radiology.* 1996;199: 653–657.

113. Beathard GA. Percutaneous therapy of vascular access dysfunction: optimal management of access stenosis and thrombosis. *Semin Dial.* 1994;7:165–167.

114. McCarley P, Wingard RL, Shyr Y, et al. Vascular access blood flow monitoring reduces access morbidity and costs. *Kidney Int.* 2001;60:1164–1172.

115. Maya ID, Allon M. Outcomes of thrombosed arteriovenous grafts: comparison of stents vs angioplasty. *Kidney Int.* March 2006;69(5):934–937.

116. Lilly. RZ, Carlton D, Barker J, et al. Predictors of arteriovenous graft patency after radiologic intervention in hemodialysis patients. *Am J Kidney Dis.* 2001;37: 945–953.

117. Tonelli M, Jhangri GS, Hirsch DJ, et al. Best threshold for diagnosis of stenosis or thrombosis within six months of access flow measurement in arteriovenous fistulae. *J Am Soc Nephrol.* 2003;14:3264–3269.

118. Tonelli M, Hirsch DJ, Chan CT, et al. Factors associated with access blood flow in native vessel arteriovenous fistulae. *Nephrol Dial Transplant.* 2004;19:2559–2563.

119. Roca-Tey R, Samon Guasch R, Ibrik O, et al. Vascular access surveillance with blood flow monitoring: a prospective study with 65 patients. *Nefrologia.* 2004; 24:246–252.

120. Polkinghorne KR, Lau KK, Saunder A, et al. Does monthly native arteriovenous fistula blood-flow surveillance detect significant stenosis—a randomized controlled trial. *Nephrol Dial Transplant.* 2006;21:2498–2506.

121. Besarab A, Lubkowski T, Ahsan M, et al. Access flow (QA) as a predictor of access dysfunction. *J Am Soc Nephrol.* 1999;11:202A.

122. Polkinhorne Kr, Atkins RC, Kerr PG. Native arteriovenous fistula flow and resistance during hemodialysis. *Am J Kidney Dis.* 2003;41:132–139.

123. Huisman RM, van Dijk M, de Bruin C, et al. Within-session and between-session variability of hemodialysis shunt flow measurements. *Nephrol Dial Transplant.* 2005;20:2842–2847.

124. Abreo K, Allon M, Asif A, et al. Is there a need to mandate access surveillance in the dialysis clinic? *Nephrol. News & Issues,* 2010;24:30–34.

125. Besarab A, Beathard G, Schon D. Is there a need to mandate vascular access surveillance in the dialysis clinic (Reply). *Nephrolgy. News & Issues,* July 2010;24:11–12.

126. Ram SJ, Work J, Caldito GC, et al. A randomized controlled trial of blood flow and stenosis surveillance of hemodialysis grafts. *Kidney Int.* 2003;64:272–280.

127. Moist LM, Churchhill DN, House AA, et al. Regular monitoring of access flow compared with monitoring of venous pressure fails to improve graft survival. *J Am Soc Nephrol.* 2003;14:2645.

128. Lumsden AB, MacDonald MJ, Kikeri D, et al. Prophylactic balloon angioplasty fails to prolong the patency of expanded polytetrafluoroethylene arteriovenous grafts: results of a prospective randomized study. *J Vasc Surg.* 1997;26:382.

129. Dember LM, Holmberg EF, Kaufman JS. Randomized controlled trial of prophylactic repair of hemodialysis arteriovenous graft stenosis. *Kidney Int.* 2004;66:390.

130. Robbin ML, Oser RF, Heudebert GR, et al. Randomized comparison of ultrasound surveillance and clinical monitoring on arteriovenous graft outcomes. *Kidney Int.* 2006;69:730.

131. Martin LG, MacDonald MJ, Kikeri D, et al. Prophylactic angioplasty reduces thrombosis in virgin ePTFE arteriovenous dialysis grafts with greater than 50% stenosis: subset analysis of a prospectively randomized study. *J Vasc Interv Radiol.* 1999;10:389.

132. Dossabhoy NR, Ram SJ, Nassar R, et al. Stenosis surveillance of hemodialysis grafts by duplex ultrasound reduces hospitalizations and cost of care. *Semin Dial.* 2005;18:550–557.

133. Tessitore N, Lipari G, Poli A, et al. Can blood flow surveillance and pre-emptive repair of subclinical stenosis prolong the useful life of arteriovenous fistulae? A randomized controlled study. *Nephrol Dial Transplant.* 2004;19:2325–2333.

134. Dixon BS, Beck GJ, Vazquez MA, et al. Effect of dipyridamole plus aspirin on hemodialysis graft patency. *N Engl J Med.* 2009;360:2191–2201.

135. Schwab SJ. Assessing the adequacy of vascular access and its relationship to patient out-come. *Am J Kidney Dis.* 1994;24:316–320.

136. Lee T, Roy-Chaudhury P. Advances and new frontiers in the pathophysiology of venous neointimal hyperplasia and dialysis access stenosis. *Adv Chronic Kidney Dis.* September 2009;16(5):329–338.

137. Tessitore N, Bedogna V, Poli A, et al. Adding access blood flow surveillance to clinical monitoring reduces thrombosis rates and costs, and improves fistula patency in the short term: a controlled cohort study. *Nephrol Dial Transplant.* November 2008;23(11):3578–3584.

138. Sands JJ, Jabyac PA, Miranda CL, et al. Intervention based on monthly monitoring decreases hemodialysis access thrombosis. *ASAIO J.* May–June 1999;45(3):147–150.

139. Hoeben H, Abu-Alfa AK, Reilly RF, et al. Vascular access surveillance: evaluation of combining dynamic venous pressure and vascular access blood flow measurements. *Am J Nephrol.* November–December;2003;23(6):403–408. Epub 2003 October 17.

140. Roberts AB, Kahn MB, Bradford S, et al. Graft surveillance and angioplasty prolongs dialysis graft patency. *J Am Coll Surg.* 1996 November 1996;183(5):486–492.

141. Glazer S, Diesto J, Crooks P, et al. Going beyond the kidney disease outcomes quality initiative: hemodialysis access experience at Kaiser Permanente Southern California. *Ann Vasc Surg.* 2006;20:75–82.

142. Roca-Tey R, Samon R, Ibrik O, et al. Functional vascular access evaluation after elective intervention for stenosis. *J Vasc Access.* 2006;7:29–34.

143. Tessitore N, Mansueto G, Bedogna V, et al. A prospective controlled trial on effect of percutaneous transluminal angioplasty on functioning arteriovenous fistulae survival. *J Am Soc Nephrol.* 2003;14:1623–1627.

144. Van der Linden J, Smitts JH, Assink JH, et al. Short- and long-term functional effect of percutaneous transluminal angioplasty in hemodialysis vascular access. *J Am Soc Nephrol.* 2002;13:715–720.

145. Murray BM, Herman A, Mepani B, et al. Access flow after angioplasty predicts subsequent arteriovenour graft survival. *J Vasc Interv Radiol.* 2006;17:303–308.

146. Trerotola SO, Kwak A, Clark TW, et al. Prospective study of balloon inflation pressures and other technical aspects of hemodialysis access angioplasty. *J Vasc Interv Radiol.* 2005;16:1613–1618.

147. Tonelli M, James N, Wiebe N, et al. Ultrasound Monitoring to detect access stenosis In hemodialysis patients. *Am J Kidney Dis.* 2008;51:630–640.

148. Owens DK. Improving practice guidelines with patient specific recommendations. *Ann Int Med.* 2011;154:638–639.

149. Mann B, Tonelli M, Yilmaz S, et al. Establishment and maintenance of vascular access in incident hemodialysis patients: a prospective cost analysis. *J Am Soc Nephrol.* 2005;16:201–209.

150. Wijnen E, Planken N, Keuter X, et al. Impact of a quality improvement programme based on vascular access flow monitoring on costs, access occlusion and access failure. *Nephrol Dial Transplant.* 2006;21:3514–3519.

151. Tonelli M, Klaarenbach S, Jindal K, et al. Economic implications of screening strategies in arteriovenous fistulae. *Kidney Int.* 2006;69:2219–2226.

152. Schwab S, Harrington J, Singh A, et al. Vascular access for hemodilaysis. *Kidney Int.* 1999;55:2078–2090.

153. Pisoni RL, Young EW, Dykstra DM, et al. Vascular access use in Europe and the United States: results from the DOPPS. *Kidney Int.* 2002;61:305–316.

154. Roy-Chaudhury P, Sukhatme VP, Cheung AK. Hemodialysis vascular access dysfunction: a cellular and molecular viewpoint. *J Am Soc Nephrol.* 2006;17:1112–1127.

PHYSICAL EXAMINATION OF THE HEMODIALYSIS ACCESS

GERALD A. BEATHARD

INTRODUCTION

Physical examination is basic to all fields of medicine, but has almost become a lost art. In many disciplines of medicine, it has been largely abandoned in favor of more elaborate and costly technical approaches to diagnosis. However, physical examination is easily performed, inexpensive to apply, and provides a high level of accuracy[1-8] in the evaluation of the arteriovenous fistula (AVF). While not quite as sensitive, it also serves reasonably well in evaluating an arteriovenous graft (AVG). Additionally, the basic principles are easily and quickly easily learned.[9] To the interventionalist working in this area, physical examination is an indispensible skill.

TABLE 14–1

Three Parameters used in Physical Examination of Dialysis Access

Parameter	Normal	Stenosis
Pulse	Soft	Increased intensity
	Easily compressible	Forceful
Thrill	Diffuse	Localized to site
	Soft	Accentuated
	Continuous	Systolic only
	Machinery-like	Turbulent
Bruit	Diffuse	Localized to site
	Continuous	Discontinuous
	Systolic and diastolic	Systolic only
	Low pitched	High pitched

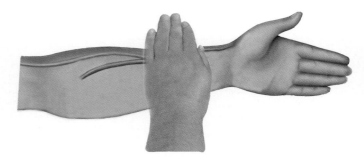

Figure 14-2. Feeling thrill with palm of hand. Normally, there is a soft, continuous background thrill palpable over course of access. This is best felt at the arterial anastomosis. Both systolic and diastolic components should be appreciated.

BASICS OF PHYSICAL EXAMINATION

There are three aspects of physical examination of the hemodialysis access that are important and need to be understood—pulse, thrill, and bruit (Table 14-1).

▶ Pulse

In general there should be very little pulse in an arteriovenous access. It should be soft and compressible. However, if there is an increase in downstream resistance as occurs with a stenotic lesion, a definite pulse will develop. The intensity of this pulse will be directly proportional to the severity of the stenosis. For this reason, a pulse in an access should be considered an adverse finding. The pulse may be best appreciated using the fingers (Figure 14-1).

▶ Thrill

A thrill is a palpable vibration. It is related to flow. There are two types of thrill that may be felt when examining an access—a diffuse thrill and a localized accentuated thrill. With flow in an arteriovenous access, either an AVF or an AVG, there will be a soft, continuous background thrill palpable over the course of the access. This is most obvious at the venous anastomosis. Its presence signifies flow and in that sense is a positive finding. If there is an area of

turbulent flow within the access or its drainage, one can detect a localized accentuated thrill in that area. This is generally very localized. Its presence should be considered an adverse finding. Normally, the thrill has a systolic and a diastolic component. As a stenotic lesion develops with progressively increasing resistance to flow, the thrill begins to lose its diastolic component. The thrill may be best evaluated by using the palm of the hand (Figure 14-2).

▶ Bruit

The bruit is the auditory manifestation of a thrill, often referred to as a "buzz." As with the thrill, a soft background bruit can be heard over a functioning access (Figure 14-3). Normally, this also has both a systolic and diastolic component. As with the thrill, increasing resistance from a stenotic lesion will result in the progressive loss of the diastolic component. Normally, this also bruit has a rather low pitch, actually a soft rumbling, machinery-like sound. With increasing resistance from a downstream stenosis, the pitch becomes progressively higher in pitch as the severity of the lesion increases. With severe downstream stenosis, the bruit may become almost whistling in quality and heard only in systole.

When examining an access to evaluate the pulse, thrill, or bruit, one has to be careful not to create artifact by compressing the access with the examining hand or fingers.

BASIC MANEUVERS

There are two basic maneuvers that can be used to great advantage in the initial evaluation of an arteriovenous AVF. These are elevation of the access arm and the assessment of pulse augmentation.

▶ Arm Elevation

When the patient's access arm is dependent, the AVF is generally distended somewhat due to the effects of gravity. If the arm is elevated to a level above that of the heart, the normal access will collapse (Figure 14-4). Even if the patient has a large "mega-fistula," it will at least become flaccid. However, if a venous stenosis is present, that portion of the AVF distal to the lesion will remain distended

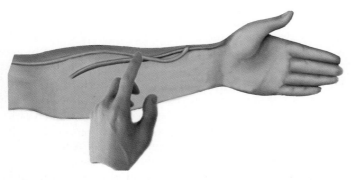

Figure 14-1. Feeling pulse with finger tips. Normally, there should be very little pulse in an arteriovenous access. It should be soft and compressible.

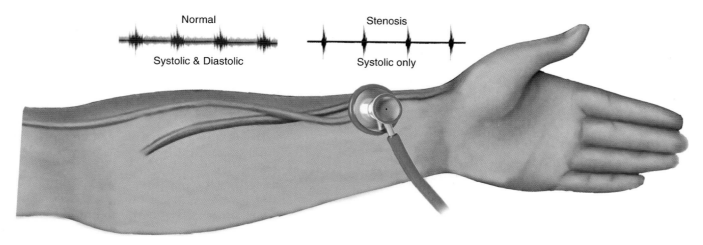

Figure 14-3. Listening to the bruit. This is best heard over the arterial anastomosis. Normally, a low pitched rumbling sound, both systolic and diastolic. With stenosis, pitch increases, systolic only.

while the proximal portion collapses. Because of this phenomenon, this test offers an excellent preliminary evaluation of access outflow. If the patient's arm is elevated and the entire AVF collapses, one can conclude with a reasonable degree of confidence that the outflow of the access is normal. If the maneuver results in an adverse finding, then further evaluation is indicated to more accurately define the problem. Unfortunately, this maneuver does not work with an AVG because of the higher level of pressure that characterizes this type of access.

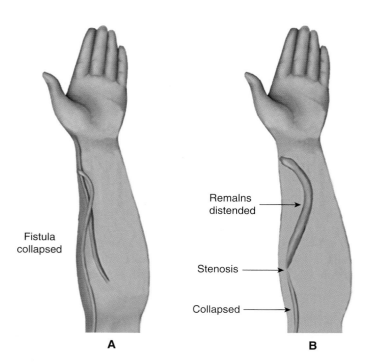

Figure 14-4. Access arm elevation. (**A**) With a normal outflow, the fistula will collapse when the arm is elevated. (**B**) With stenosis, the portion of the fistula peripheral to the lesion will stay distended. That portion central to the site will collapse normally.

▶ Pulse Augmentation

The normal arteriovenous access is relatively soft and easily compressible. This is especially true for an AVF. If one first assesses the intensity of the pulse within a normal access and then occludes the access completely some distance from the arterial anastomosis, the pulse intensity between these two points will be augmented (Figure 14-5). The degree of this increase in pulse intensity is directly proportional to the quality of the access inflow. This makes this maneuver an excellent means of making a preliminary evaluation of access inflow. If there are problems anywhere within the arterial system from the anastomosis upward, it will affect the degree to which the pulse is augmented. While this works better for AVF evaluation, it also serves reasonably well in the evaluation of an AVG. It only takes minimal experience with this evaluation for one to begin to recognize what is normal and what is abnormal and to arrive at a reasonable quantification using a scale of 1 to 10.

If the pulse within the access happens to already be increased due to the presence of a downstream venous stenosis, the test is still useful. If the hyperpulsatile access

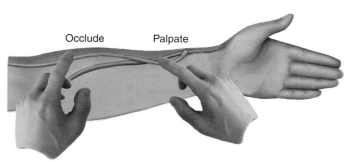

Figure 14-5. Pulse augmentation. When a normal access is occluded at some point distant from the arterial anastomosis, the pulse between that site and the anastomosis will be augmented reflecting the quality of the inflow.

does not augment with occlusion, it suggests that the stenosis is essentially equivalent to complete obstruction. If it augments 50%, then it suggests 50% occlusion for the stenosis. The pulse intensity within the hyperpulsatile access can still be taken as a gauge for the quality of the inflow.

10 SECOND FISTULA EXAMINATION

By combining these two basic maneuvers, one can conduct a reasonably good evaluation of a patient's AVF by simply raising the arm to see if it collapses and then occluding it to check augmentation. This allows one to check both the inflow and the outflow very quickly. If either of these is abnormal, then addition examination is indicated. Unfortunately, this 10 second evaluation cannot be accomplished while the patient is on dialysis.

SPECIFIC EXAMINATIONS

There are a variety of conditions and situations in which physical examination of the patient's vasculature relative to an arteriovenous hemodialysis access may be used to advantage (Table 14-2). In general, the same information can be obtained whether the patient has an AVF or an AVG. However, physical examination techniques are much more sensitive when the access being examined is an AVF. The following discussion related to both types of access except where a specific point unique to one or the other is specifically mentioned.

▶ Evaluation Prior to Access Placement

Evaluation of the new end-stage renal disease (ESRD) patient in preparation for the placement of a peripheral arteriovenous access is extremely important. Proper patient selection will materially enhance the opportunity to place an AVF. A great deal of useful information relative to access placement can be gleaned from a careful physical examination. Examination of both the arterial and venous systems is important.

TABLE 14–2
Specific Examinations
Evaluation prior to access placement
Evaluation post access placement (evaluation of nonmaturation)
Evaluation of the mature access
Detection of arterial stenosis
Detection of venous stenosis
Evaluation of the access for infection
Evaluation aneurysms and pseudoaneurysms
Evaluation of ischemia
Detection of direction of flow
Detection of recirculation

▶ Arterial Evaluation

In relation to the arterial system, two issues are important. Firstly, the vessel must be capable of delivering blood flow at a rate adequate to support dialysis and secondly, the utilization of the vessel for the creation of an access must not jeopardize the viability of the digits and hand. Arterial narrowing and calcification are relatively common in ESRD patients, especially those that are diabetic and hypertensive. This problem can usually be diagnosed before the patient is sent for surgery.

A significant amount of data can be obtained by physical examination relative to the adequacy of arterial inflow for the creation of an AVF. There are four evaluations (Table 14-3) that are important. Three of these lend themselves to physical examination—pulse examination, segmental blood pressure measurement, and the Allen test.

Pulse examination

The axillary, brachial, radial, and ulnar pulses should be examined in both upper extremities.[10] A vascular Doppler is often very useful for this purpose. The quality of these pulses should be scored as either normal, diminished or absent. This can be graded as normal: 2+, intermediate: 1+, or absent: 0.

Simultaneous blood pressures

Differences in systolic blood pressure between the two arms should be should be reported and graded.[10] It is important that these two readings be taken within minutes of each other since blood pressure can change over the period of a few minutes when the patient is anxious. A difference of less than 10 mm Hg should be considered as normal. A difference of 10 to 20 mm Hg is considered marginal and over 20 as problematic. A difference of 20 mm Hg or greater in systolic blood pressure is suggestive of subclavian artery stenosis in the low pressure arm.

Modified Allen test

The modified Allen test (Table 14-4) is used to determine competence of the palmar arch. (Referred to as modified because the original Allen test only checked for patency of the radial artery, the test as commonly done adds the ulnar.) Use of a pulse oximeter (Figure 14-6) makes the test more objective and has been reported to increase its sensitivity. With a patent palmar arch, pulsation should be present during occlusion of either the radial or ulnar artery.[11] If

TABLE 14–3
Arterial Evaluation for AVF
Pulse examination
Differential blood pressures
Patent palmar arch
Arterial size

TABLE 14-4

The Modified Allen Test

1. Position the patient so that they are facing you with their arm extended with the palm turned upward. Do not hyper-extend the wrist or fingers.
2. Compress both the radial and ulnar arteries at the wrist.
3. With the arteries compressed firmly, instruct the patient to create a fist repetitively in order to cause the palm to blanch.
4. When the patient's hand is blanched, release the compression of the ulnar artery and watch the palm to determine if it becomes pink. Then release all compression.
5. Repeat steps 2–4 for the radial artery.

Interpretation—when color returns to the blanched palm upon release of the arterial compression, it indicates arterial patency and reflects upon adequacy of flow. Interpretation:

    < 5 seconds—negative test
    5 to 10 seconds—intermediate
    > 10 seconds—positive test

Prolonged recovery after release of the artery with the other artery still occluded is a positive test for insufficiency of that vessel. In other words, prolonged recovery after release of the radial artery with the ulnar occluded indicates that the radial artery has a problem.

the ulnar artery is occluded, a radial-based AVF should be avoided because of risk of ischemia. If the radial artery is occluded, it is not available for access creation. The test can be complicated by the fact that there is a significant number of cases in which a incomplete palmar arch occurs as a normal variant.[12]

Proper positioning of the hand for this examination is important.[11] It is important to avoid hyperextension of the wrist and fingers. This has been shown to result in incomplete capillary refilling of the hand in many patients.

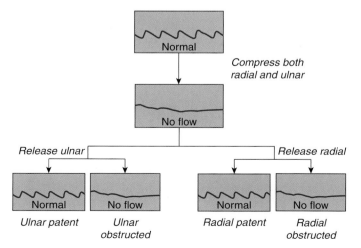

Figure 14-6. Pulse oximeter used to perform modifier Allen teat.

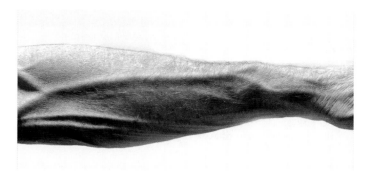

Figure 14-7. Vein mapping by physical examination.

If the results are abnormal, an incomplete palmar arch can usually be suspected by checking the results with the sensory for the pulse oximeter placed alternatively on the index and the little finger and comparing the results.

Arterial size

In order to complete the arterial evaluation, the arterial anatomy must be imaged in order to determine if it is suitable.

▶ Venous Evaluation

Venous anatomy is extremely important for access creation, either an AVF or an AVG. Most problems incurred with access creation are actually venous problems rather than arterial. The primary goal when evaluating any patient for a dialysis vascular access should be the identification of a venous anatomy conducive to the creation of an AVF. This is best done by vein mapping.

In some patients, this can be done adequately by physical examination (Figure 14-7). It is essential that the patient be evaluated with outflow obstruction so as to dilate the veins of the arm adequately for evaluation. This is best done using a blood pressure cuff inflated to a pressure about 5 mmHg above diastolic pressure. This should be left in place for periods of no more than 5 minutes at a time. While this provides excellent information in many patients, most surgeons will want a more detailed evaluation performed using color flow Doppler ultrasound or angiography prior to surgery. Optimum features on venogram (Table 14-5) for the creation of an AVF are a luminal diameter at the point of anastomosis of 2.5 mm or greater, a straight segment of vein, absence of obstruction, and continuity with the proximal central veins.[13]

TABLE 14-5

Venous Requirements for AVF

Luminal diameter 2.5 mm or greater at anastomosis point
Absence of obstruction
Straight segment for cannulation
Within 1 cm of surface
Continuity with proximal central veins

TABLE 14–6

Categories of Lesions Causing Failure of AVF Maturation

Inflow problems—stenosis or inadequate
    Feeding artery
    Arterial anastomosis
    Juxta-anastomosis
    Combination
Problems with body of AVF
    Accessory vein
    Stenosis
Outflow problems—stenosis or inadequate vein

EVALUATION POST ACCESS PLACEMENT

If a newly placed AVF is going to develop to the point that it is functional, it will be obvious by 4 to 6 weeks. Those that do not develop will, in most instances, have a definable lesion. These lesions can generally be easily diagnosed by physical examination. Once detected in this manner, the next step is imaging for more specific characterization followed by treatment to salvage the access. Failure to mature can be treated with a high expectation of success.

The lesions that result in the failure of a newly placed AVF to mature can be categorized into three broad categories—inflow problems, problems with the body of the AVF, and outflow problems (Table 14-6).

▶ Inflow Problems

The arteriovenous access should be thought of as a circuit that begins and ends with the heart. Lesions anywhere on the arterial side of this circuit can cause failure of the AVF to mature. These lesions can be thought of as being within the feeding artery, the arterial anastomosis, and the juxta-anastomotic portion of the AVF (not actually part of the arterial circuit). It should be possible to avoid problems with the feeding artery with good preaccess evaluation (vascular mapping); however, since this may not be done or not done well, these lesions can account for AVF failure to mature.

A problem with the feeding artery or the anastomosis can be detected by assessing the pulse augmentation (Figure 14-2). If the pulse augments less than one would consider to be optimum, it points the diagnostic finger in this direction. Juxta-anastomotic stenosis is a unique acquired problem. This is the most common pathology that is seen in AVFs that fail to mature.[14–16]

Juxta-anastomotic stenosis

Juxta-anastomotic stenosis is defined as stenosis that occurs within that portion of the AVF that is immediately adjacent to the arterial anastomosis (Figure 14-8). It seldom extends for more than 2 to 3 cm. The effect of the lesion is to obstruct AVF inflow. Since it occurs early, it results in failure to mature.

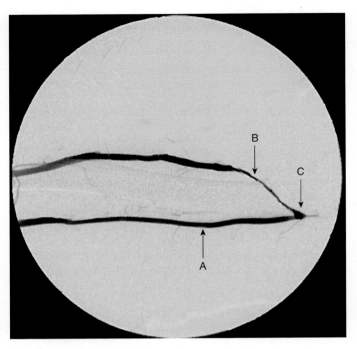

Figure 14-8. Angiogram of juxta-anastomotic stenosis. (**A**) Radial artery. (**B**) Stenotic segment of fistula. (**C**) Arterial anastomosis.

This lesion can be easily diagnosed by palpation of the anastomosis and distal vein.[4,6] Normally, a very prominent thrill is present at the anastomosis (Figure 14-9). In the absence of abnormalities, the pulse is soft and easily compressible. With juxta-anastomotic stenosis, a very forceful

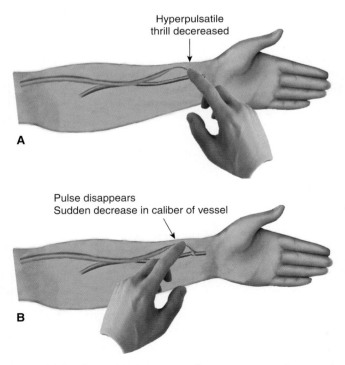

Figure 14-9. Physical examination of juxta-anastomotic stenosis. (**A**) Examing the anastomosis. (**B**) Examing the juxta-anastomotic region.

pulse is felt at the anastomosis. The thrill, which is normally continuous, is present only in systole. In some instances (severe lesion), it may be very short and even difficult to detect. As one moves up the vein from the anastomosis with the palpating finger (Figure 14-9), the pulse goes away rather abruptly as the site of stenosis is encountered. Above this level, the pulse is very weak and may be difficult to detect. The stenosis itself can frequently be felt as an abrupt diminution in the size of the vein, almost like a shelf. Once these typical physical findings are detected, the cause for poor AVF development becomes obvious.

▶ Problems with Body of AVF

The body of the AVF is that portion of the vein that is considered the zone available for cannulation. Stenosis can occur in this area. Generally, these lesions can be avoided by good preplacement evaluation (vascular mapping). Unfortunately, even with best efforts, old sites of venipuncture can cause unanticipated problems. These lesions can be easily diagnosed using the parameters described in Table 14-1. Accessory veins represent a unique problem.

Accessory veins

The occurrence of accessory veins is essentially limited to the forearm. Since most of the AVFs involve the cephalic vein, they are generally branches of the cephalic and as such represent normal anatomy. It should be emphasized that with downstream stenosis, collateral veins can appear and can be confused with this entity. However, collaterals are pathological and the presence of the stenotic lesion should alert the examiner to their etiology. Although most accessory veins cause no problems, a large one in conjunction with a marginal AVF can result in failure to develop. Physical examination will allow one to detect their presence[6] and will also shed some light on their significance.

Frequently, the side branch is visible (Figure 14-10). If not, it can be detected by palpating the AVF. Normally, the thrill that is palpable over the arterial anastomosis disappears when the downstream AVF is manually occluded. This causes flow to stop, no flow—no thrill. If it does not disappear, an outflow channel (accessory vein) is present below the point of occlusion. Palpation of the AVF below the occlusion point will generally reveal the location of the accessory vein by the presence of a thrill over its trunk. As long as

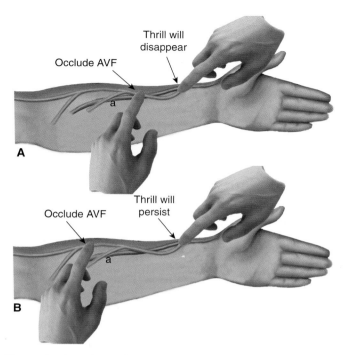

Figure 14-11. Physical examination of accessory vein. (**A**) Occluding fistula distal to accessory vein. (**B**) Occluding fistula proximal to accessory vein. (a) Accessory vein.

the main channel can be identified for occlusion, the entire length of the vein can be evaluated by moving the point of AVF occlusion progressively upward (Figure 14-11).

Once an accessory vein is detected, one is faced with determining its significance. It should be kept in mind that not all of these side branches are problematic. The first issue is whether this is an AVF that has failed to mature. If this is the case, then there is a reason; it could be the accessory vein. A determination of size is important. If the vein is one-fourth the size of the AVF or more it is more likely to be problematic (the principles of Poiseuille's law are not applicable—these veins open into a field of veins). Determine if the flow in the AVF appears to be augmented with manual occlusion of the side branch (use of a vascular Doppler is helpful). If it is easily visible or if it has a strong thrill, it is more likely to be significant.

▶ Outflow Problems

As is the case with the body of the AVF, stenosis can occur in the draining veins. Most of these lesions can be easily diagnosed using the parameters described in Table 14-1. This is not necessarily the case with central venous lesions. These lesions will be discussed below under the evaluation of the mature AVF.

▶ Algorithm for Systemic Evaluation

While a single lesion is frequently observed accounting for failure of AVF maturation, a significant percentage of cases will have combinations of lesions.[16] This can lead to confusion due to a confluence of compounding variables, but it

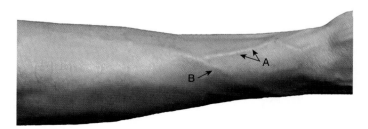

Figure 14-10. Accessory vein. (**A**) Radial-cephalic AVF. (**B**) Accessory vein.

TABLE 14–7
Step 1—Basic Information of Importance

How long since it was created?
Where is it located?
What type of fistula is it?
Use history
    Has it been used?
    Have there been problems with use?
    Has patient noticed a change?

TABLE 14–8
Step 2—Examination of Anastomosis

Feel for thrill
    Indicator of flow
    Strong—good flow
    Weak—poor flow
    Systolic and diastolic—good flow
Feel for pulse
    Indicator of downstream resistance
    Soft—low resistance, no stenosis
    Hard—high resistance, stenosis present

also dictates the need for doing a systematic evaluation of each of these cases in order to assure completeness. The following algorithm has been suggested for this purpose.[17]

Step 1—basic information

Begin the evaluation of the AVF by gathering pertinent information (Table 14-7). At times, AVF development is so poor that its presence is not even apparent upon first examination. It is helpful to know when the access was created, where it is located, and exactly what type of AVF it is supposed to be. Different types of AVF have a predilection for different types of lesions (site of lesion). The most common lesion associated with a radial-cephalic AVF is juxta-anastomotic stenosis, with a brachial-cephalic AVF it is cephalic arch stenosis and with a brachial-basilic fistula it is "swing-point" stenosis where the position of the vein begins to swing laterally (Figure 14-12). Additionally, it is helpful to know if it has ever been used and if so, what sorts of problems were encountered. Often the patient will have noticed a change that will be helpful in making the assessment.

Step 2—examine the anastomosis

The next step to follow is to perform a detailed physical examination, starting with the anastomosis (Table 14-8). There are two components of this examination, (1) the thrill which is an indicator of flow and (2) the pulse which is an indicator of downstream resistance (presence of stenosis).

Normally, the thrill should be relatively strong and have both systolic and diastolic components. With the decreased flow, the strength of the thrill diminishes. With downstream stenosis (resistance), flow may occur only during systole. In this instance, there will only be a systolic thrill. The pulse should be very soft (without manual occlusion). If the pulse is forceful, it suggests a downstream stenosis or obstruction. The intensity of the hyper-pulsatility is proportional to the severity of the stenosis. Check specifically for juxta-anastomotic stenosis as described above.

Problems such as juxta-anastomotic stenosis and downstream stenosis or occlusion should be detectable from this examination. If there is no thrill or pulse, then the AVF is completely dead and detection of specific pathology will not be possible. The prognosis for the early AVF failure with such a finding at this time post-AVF creation is poor.

Step 3—examine the body of the AVF

Examination of the anastomosis should be followed by a detailed examination of the body of the AVF (Table 14-9). In doing this, it is especially helpful to know what type of AVF the patient is supposed to have. In some instances, the AVF is not palpable except at the anastomosis. Normally, the pulse should be soft and compressible. With downstream stenosis, it will be hyperpulsatile in proportion to the degree of stenosis. The factors that determine an AVF's usability relate to diameter and flow. This can generally be evaluated adequately by physical examination.

Check for the presence of an accessory vein as described above. In addition to this anomaly, problems that should be discoverable at this time include an AVF that is too deep, stenosis, and occlusion of the downstream portion of

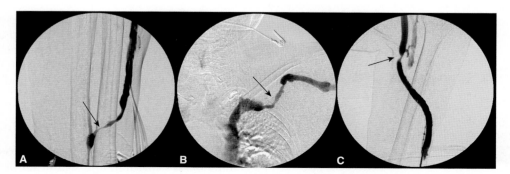

Figure 14-12. Sites of predilection for stenosis by fistula type. (**A**) Radial-cephalic AVF with juxta-anastomotic stenosis. (**B**) Brachial-cephalic AVF with cephalic arch stenosis. (**C**) Brachial; basilic SAVF with swing-point stenosis.

TABLE 14–9
Step 3—Examination of Body of Fistula

Over what extent is fistula visible?
  Does it seem to disappear?
What is fistula's diameter?
  Is it large enough to be readily cannulated?
What is its depth?
  Is it there but too deep?
Is fistula pulse palpable?
  Soft—normal
  Hyperpulsatile—downstream stenosis
Check for accessory vein
  Is one present?
  Are multiple accessory veins present?

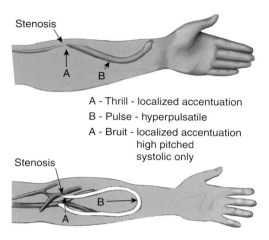

A - Thrill - localized accentuation
B - Pulse - hyperpulsatile
A - Bruit - localized accentuation
        high pitched
        systolic only

Figure 14-13. Physical examination of access with severe venous stenosis.

the AVF. It is important to remember that with early AVF failure, accessory veins may be multiple and that more than one anomaly may be present.[16]

Step 4—assess pulse augmentation

Assess pulse augmentation (Table 14-10) is directly proportional to the arterial inflow pressure. Assessment of the pulse without manual occlusion reflects the status of the outflow (is it hyperpulsatile?); with manual occlusion, the test reflects the status of the inflow. Remember that there is a reciprocal relationship between the degree of augmentation and the degree of downstream stenosis. If it is already hyperpulsatile, it cannot increase further.

This evaluation should detect problems such as anastomotic stenosis, stenosis of the feeding artery, and any problem related to the arterial portion of the circuit that will affect arterial inflow.

▶ Evaluation of the Mature Access

Problems can occur with the mature access. Prospective detection of these adverse events allows early treatment thus avoiding missed treatments and emergent situations. Physical examination can play a major role in the detection of these problems. The most common complications associated with an established access are venous and arterial stenosis, thrombosis, ischemia, aneurysm, and pseudoaneurysm formation and infection.

TABLE 14–10
Step 4—Check Pulse Augmentation

Strength of pulse without occlusion—outflow
Strength of pulse with occlusion—inflow
If pulse is normal
  Augmentation is indicative of inflow
If pulse is hyperpulsatile (indicative of stenosis)
  Degree of augmentation can be used to gauge degree of
    stenosis
  No augmentation—indicates very severe stenosis
  Moderate augmentation—moderate stenosis

▶ Detection of Arterial Stenosis

Diabetes is a common cause of end-stage renal disease and as the dialysis population ages, the occurrence of acquired arterial lesions that adversely affect access function can occur. The detection of inflow (arterial) stenosis by physical examination using pulse augmentation has been described above in relationship to the evaluation of the AVF that fails to mature. The same principles apply to the mature access.

▶ Detection of Venous Stenosis

As was pointed out earlier, significant venous stenosis causes hemodynamic changes within the access. These changes result in abnormalities that can be easily detected by physical examination (Figure 14-13). Unfortunately, venous stenosis is such a common occurrence that many nephrologists do not recognize these changes as being abnormal. A strong pulse or a vigorous thrill is often misinterpreted as evidence of a good access with excellent flow rather than as a sign of a pathological lesion. A properly functioning access has a soft easily compressible pulse. A localized thrill is palpable (without compression) only at the arterial anastomosis. The normal bruit is low-pitched and continuous with both systolic and diastolic components (Table 14-1).

Narrowing within the blood flow channel causes turbulence. Turbulent blood flow results in a palpable localized thrill. The greater the turbulence, the stronger the thrill. Both the turbulence and the thrill are localized to the site of the stenotic lesion. By palpating over the venous anastomosis and the course of the veins that drain the access, a stenotic site can be identified by detecting the associated thrill. These abnormal thrills are frequently not continuous. As the stenosis becomes more severe and the resistance increases, it will eventually exceed the diastolic pressure. Then the thrill will only be systolic. As resistance continues to increase, the access eventually becomes thrombosed.

The examiner should also listen to the access with a stethoscope paying attention to both the auditory frequency (pitch) and the duration of the bruit. As the degree of stenosis increases, the velocity of flow increases and the pitch of the bruit rises. As the resistance to flow increases, the duration of the diastolic component decreases. An estimate of the severity of the lesion can be made from the presence and duration of the diastolic component of the bruit. With severe stenosis, the bruit is high pitched and only a systolic component is audible.

The entire length of the veins draining the access should be examined with the stethoscope. Normally, it is difficult to hear a bruit in the upper arm unless there is some degree of compression of the vein. If a bruit is heard, it is of low pitch and decreases in pitch as one moves up the arm. Because there is turbulence in an area of stenosis, a localized bruit or a localized increase in the pitch of the bruit develops suggesting narrowing. Continuing to listen high into the upper arm or even into the axilla or subclavian area may sometimes reveal a venous stenosis at that point as a localized bruit or increase in the pitch of a bruit. The degree to which all of these changes occur is dependent upon the severity of the stenotic lesion.

Thrombosis is, in most instances, the end point of the process. There are no particular physical findings that are unique for thrombosis other than what would be expected—a silent access.

Central venous stenosis

While the findings that have been described for venous stenosis are classic, when the lesion occurs within the central veins, physically unique findings are generally observed. The access is generally not as pulsatile as one expects to see with a more peripheral lesion. The greater distance, along with the elastic nature of the veins serves to dampen the pulse. Often, especially in thin chested individuals, a thrill can be felt over the anterior chest just below the clavicle and a localized bruit is frequently evident. The classic appearance of a patient with a significant central venous stenosis is ipsilateral arm edema. At times, this can be massive (Figure 14-14). However, not all patients have this finding.[18,19] Additionally, subcutaneous collateral veins over the arm and chest are frequently evident.

▶ Evaluation of the Access for Infection

Infection of an arteriovenous hemodialysis access is a serious problem. It has been reported to account for 20% of all dialysis access complications.[20] It is the second leading cause of AVG loss and, although he infection rate for AVFs is approximately one-tenth of AVGs,[21,22] it is still a major concern. The great majority of access infections can be easily recognized by physical examination.

Most infections associated with an AVF are actually perivascular cellulitis recognized by localized erythema, swelling, and tenderness on physical examination. Occasionally, infection-associated anatomic abnormalities such as aneurysms, perigraft hematomas, or an abscess from infected needle puncture sites may be observed. These

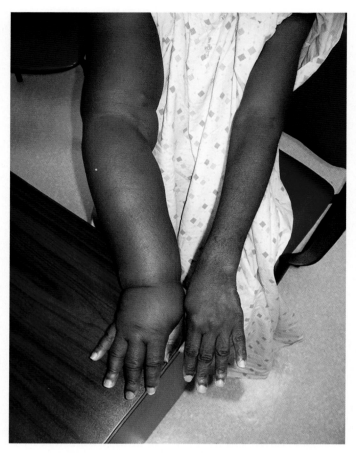

Figure 14-14. Central vein stenosis in a patient with left arm arteriovenous access. Note marked difference in size of arms.

lesions are frequently associated with purulent drainage and may be fluctuant to palpation.

Infection associated with an AVG may be either superficial or deep. Superficial infections do not involve the AVG itself. These are generally related to a cannulation site (Figure 14-15). On physical examination, they are recognized as small pustular lesions with minimal or no inflammation, swelling, or pain. They are not fluctuant.

Deep infections are recognized on physical examination by the classic combination of signs of infectious inflammation—erythema, swelling, tenderness, and purulence (Figure 14-16). The erythema is generally localized and spreads outwardly in a circumferential manner so that it extends beyond the skin immediately overlying the AVG. Swelling of some degree is often seen and on occasion is also fluctuant. Tenderness is frequent; pain may be present, but is variable. The area generally feels warm, but this is not a very reliable sign because the skin overlying a flowing AVG is always warmer than normal.

This appearance needs to be distinguished from what is actually a dermal flare. This is occasionally seen immediately following AVG placement. It is characterized by a bright red flare that is restricted to the skin immediately overlying the AVG (Figure 14-17). Typically, it is generalized to the entire course of the AVG. With a loop

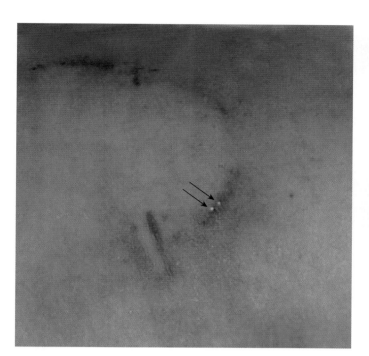

Figure 14-15. Superficial infection. Small pustules at cannulation sites (arrows).

AVG, this erythematous flare does not spread to the skin lying within the loop, only the immediate course of the AVG itself. There is generally little to no swelling, it is not fluctuant, and there is frequently no pain other than some postsurgery discomfort. This is felt to be a dermal reaction related to the AVG being tunneled more superficially than usual.

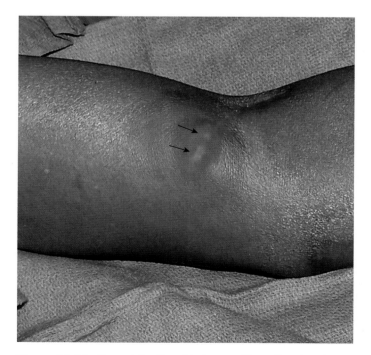

Figure 14-16. Deep infection. Notice swelling, discoloration, pustules (arrows).

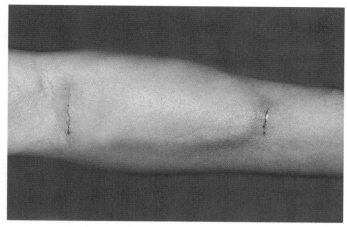

Figure 14-17. Dermal flare following AVG placement. Erythema follows entire course of the graft. Notice recent surgical incisions.

▶ **Evaluation Aneurysms and Pseudoaneurysms**

An arteriovenous hemodialysis access, either an AVF or an AVG, can develop an area of bulging. In the case of an AVF, this generally represents a true aneurysm (includes all layers of the vessel); in the case of an AVG, these areas generally represent pseudoaneurysms (false aneurysms, disruption of the layers of the wall). These anomalies are common and can lead to serious problems. They need to be detected early and, if present they need to be monitored for adverse changes in the overlying skin. Both of these activities are best accomplished by physical examination.

With the passage of time, blood flow in an AVF increases and with this the diameter of the AVF also increases. However, it does this in a diffuse fashion. This is normal for an AVF and is not seen with AVGs. If a localized area of bulging appears with either type of access, it suggests that two problems have occurred. Firstly, the wall of the access has been weakened. This is generally due to poor cannulation practices and segmental over-utilization. Secondly, it suggest that there is an increase in downstream resistance (venous stenosis) causing a commensurate increase in intraluminal pressure. As this process progresses, the resulting bulge in the access can become problematic to the point of being life-threatening. If an access is examined on a regular basis, this problem can be detected early and progression can be prevented.

Once either an aneurysm or a pseudoaneurysm has developed, there should be concern for the development of the complications associated with these lesions. The most severe adverse event that can occur is rupture. These anomalies should be monitored by physical examination at the time of each dialysis treatment. Changes in its size should be noted, a rapidly enlarging bulge should be a sign for immediate concern. The overlying skin should be examined for evidence of marked thinning, ulceration, or spontaneous bleeding (Figure 14-18). In addition to thinning, depigmentation and tightening of the overlying skin

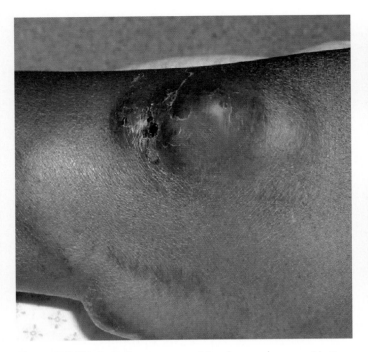

Figure 14-18. Pseudoaneurysm with adverse changes. Notice depigmentation, thinning of skin, and ulceration.

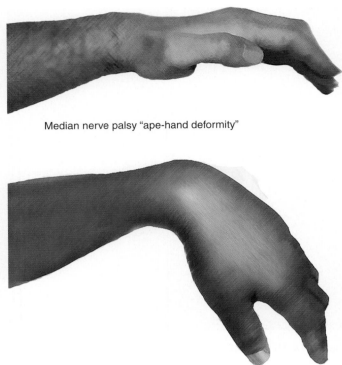

Median nerve palsy "ape-hand deformity"

Radial nerve palsy "wrist drop"

Figure 14-19. Typical nerve palsies resulting from ischemic monomelic neuropathy.

can occur. If the skin is tissue paper thin and if you cannot pinch the skin between your index finger and thumb, it has advanced to a dangerous degree and early attention to the problem should be sought.

▶ Evaluation of Ischemia

Two distinct clinical variants of hand ischemia are recognized following the placement of an access: ischemic monomelic neuropathy (IMN), where change is confined to the nerves of the hand sparing other tissues,[23,24] and dialysis access-associated steal syndrome (DASS), in which ischemic changes affect all tissues of the affected area to a varying degree of severity. Both of these have characteristic findings on physical examination.

Ischemic monomelic neuropathy

IMN is an underrecognized ischemic complication of vascular access creation related to nerve ischemia or infarction.[24,25] This syndrome generally occurs immediately after access placement. In the typical case, the patient complains of profound weakness of the hand immediately postoperatively, and frequently there is associated severe pain and paraesthesia. Physical examination is characterized by weakness in the distal muscle groups (Figure 14-19) and a sensory defect characterized by reduced or absent responses to pinprick and vibration. These findings may be located in the distribution of the median, ulnar, or radial nerves and may affect any or all three of these. Typically, no appearance of ischemia of the other tissues of the hand is present. The hand appears warm and well perfused and the pulses are normal or at least comparable to the opposite side.

Dialysis access associated steal syndrome

Because the resistance to flow is lower in the access than in the distal arterial run off, the access receives not only antegrade blood flow from the feeding artery, but also "steals" blood retrograde from the hand via the palmar arch. The majority of forearm as well as proximal arteriovenous accesses have steal, but it is usually clinically silent and asymptomatic.[26] This is referred to as physiologic steal. However, in some cases steal can be associated with symptoms of ischemia. This symptomatic steal occurs in patients who are unable to develop collaterals or direct flow to offset steal in the presence of local or diffuse arteriopathy proximal or distal to the angioaccess.[27,28] This situation has come to be referred to as dialysis associated steal syndrome or DASS. Predisposing risk factors include female sex, age >60 years, diabetes, peripheral artery disease, multiple previous access procedures on the same arm and the use of the brachial artery as the donor vessel.[29]

DASS symptoms generally appear immediately following AV graft placement,[30] but this is not always true. Some have divided cases into those that occur early (<30 days) or late (>30 days). It has been observed that symptoms that occur acutely are often self-limiting and resolve with observation.[31] In contrast, symptoms with a late onset (>30 days) are frequently progressive and tend not to resolve with conservative treatment several months or even years after the creation of the access. At times, steal can occur after an angioplasty due to the increased flow and the decreased resistance that occurs after that procedure.

The patient generally first presents with complaints of hand pain. A physical examination of these cases is important because there are several entities that can cause hand pain in the dialysis patient. Commonly encountered symptoms include cold hand, numbness, and hand pain on and/or off dialysis. Lowering of BP and provocation of peripheral vasoconstriction have been used to explain the development of pain during dialysis [203]. Physical findings in patients with DASS are somewhat variable depending upon the severity of the problem and the pre-existing status of the peripheral circulation. In most instances, it is very helpful to compare the affected side to the opposite normal or relatively normal side.

There are three types of changes that should be examined for. Firstly, the generally appearance and feel of the hand should be evaluated. In the mildest cases, the affected hand is pale or cyanotic in appearance and feels cold. In order to be confident in attributing these changes to DASS, it is important to compare the affected side to the opposite normal or relatively normal side. Secondly, there are often changes in the radial pulse, it is diminished or absent. Again, it is helpful to make comparisons with the opposite extremity. Occlusion of the access may be found to either increase the strength of a previously weak radial pulse or result in the appearance of a previously absent pulse. Using a Doppler to listen to the bruit over the vessel frequently aids in this examination. The sound is significantly augmented when the AVG is occluded. Thirdly, advanced cases reveal trophic changes that are characterized by the development of ischemic ulcers and dry gangrene of one or more digits (Figure 14-20).

▶ Detection of Direction of Flow

Most arteriovenous accesses are created with a standard configuration; however, occasionally it is necessary to deviate from the usual pattern of placement in order to accomplish the task. This is especially true for AVGs.

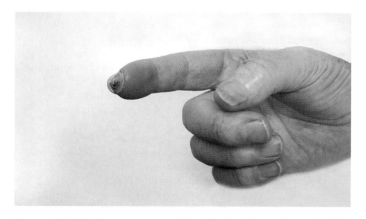

Figure 14-20. Dry gangrene of tip of index finger due to DASS.

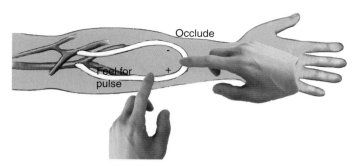

Figure 14-21. Detection of direction of blood flow in a loop graft.

When this occurs, the orientation of the dialysis needles must correspond to the direction of blood flow or gross recirculation will result. In order to avoid this occurrence, the direction of blood flow should be determined and documented for each patient in the dialysis facility. This can be accomplished easily by occluding the AVG with the tip of the finger and palpating on each side of the occlusion point for a pulse (Figure 14-21). The side without a pulse is the downstream (venous) side of the AVG. The upstream (arterial) pulse will increase in intensity during the occlusion. While it is easier to accomplish this when the patient is not on dialysis, the maneuver can generally be adequately performed with needles in place if they are not placed too closely together.

▶ Detection of Recirculation

Recirculation occurs when the blood flow of the access falls below the rate demanded by the blood pump. This results in varying degrees of reversal of flow between the needles depending upon the severity of the problem. There are two problems that can result in recirculation—poor inflow and obstructed outflow. If the degree of recirculation is more than minimal, it can frequently be detected by physical examination. To perform this maneuver, simply occlude the access between the two needles during dialysis and observe the venous and arterial pressure gauges (Figure 14-22).

A hard object such as a closed hemostat seems to work more efficiently that a finger in affecting occlusion (Figure 14-16). With a normal access, very little or no change should be seen in either the venous or arterial pressure readings. If recirculation is secondary to outflow obstruction (venous stenosis), the pressure will rise in the venous return because the lower resistance, recirculation route has been occluded. As pressure limits are exceeded, the alarm will sound and the blood pump will stop. This will happen very quickly. The arterial pressure may become slightly more negative as the pressure head generated by the venous side is no longer transmitted through the occluded site in the AVG. If recirculation is due to poor inflow (arterial stenosis or insufficiency), the major pressure change observed will be a drop (become more negative) as the blood pump demands more blood

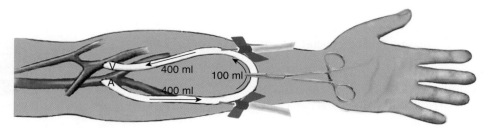

Figure 14-22. Testing for recirculation. In this example, the access is capable of delivering only 400 mL of blood flow (because of either venous or arterial problems). However, the pump is running at 500 mL. This creates a 100 mL recirculation circuit. The graft is being occluded between the needles with a pair of hemostats. In this instance, one of the alarms will go off, depending upon where the problem is located.

than is available with the recirculation route occluded. In this instance the arterial alarm will sound, again, this will happen very quickly. In this instance, the venous pressure may change very little. If the needles are too close together, this examination is not be possible. This maneuver can also be used to detect reversed placement of needles, the most common cause of recirculation.

REFERENCES

1. Beathard G. Physical examination of AV grafts. *Semin Dial.* 1992;5:74.
2. Trerotola SO, Scheel PJ Jr., Powe NR, et al. Screening for dialysis access graft malfunction: comparison of physical examination with US. *J Vasc Interv Radiol.* 1996;7:15.
3. Safa AA, Valji K, Roberts AC, et al. Detection and treatment of dysfunctional hemodialysis access grafts: effect of a surveillance program on graft patency and the incidence of thrombosis. *Radiology.* 1996;199:653.
4. Beathard G. Physical examination of the dialysis vascular access. *Semin Dial.* 1998;11:231.
5. Migliacci R, Selli ML, Falcinelli F, et al. Assessment of occlusion of the vascular access in patients on chronic hemodialysis: comparison of physical examination with continuous-wave Doppler ultrasound. STOP Investigators. Shunt Thrombotic Occlusion Prevention with Picotamide. *Nephron.* 1999;82:7.
6. Beathard G. *Physical Examination: The Forgotten Tool.* Philadelphia: Lippincott Williams & Wilkins; 2002.
7. Asif A, Leon C, Orozco-Vargas LC, et al. Accuracy of physical examination in the detection of arteriovenous fistula stenosis. *Clin J Am Soc Nephrol.* 2007;2:1191.
8. Leon C, Orozco-Vargas LC, Krishnamurthy G, et al. Accuracy of physical examination in the detection of arteriovenous graft stenosis. *Semin Dial.* 2008;21:85.
9. Leon C, Asif A. Physical examination of arteriovenous fistulae by a renal fellow: does it compare favorably to an experienced interventionalist? *Semin Dial.* 2008;21:557.
10. Sidaway AN, Gray R, Besarab A, et al. Recommended standards for reports dealing with arteriovenous hemodialysis accesses. *J Vasc Surg.* 2002;35:603.
11. Kamienski RW, Barnes RW. Critique of the Allen test for continuity of the palmar arch assessed by Doppler ultrasound. *Surg Gynecol Obstet.* 1976;142:861.
12. Gellman H, Botte MJ, Shankwiler J, Gelberman RH. Arterial patterns of the deep and superficial palmar arches. *Clin Orthop Relat Res.* 2001:41.
13. Silva MB Jr., Hobson RW, 2nd, Pappas PJ, et al. A strategy for increasing use of autogenous hemodialysis access procedures: impact of preoperative noninvasive evaluation. *J Vasc Surg.* 1998;27:302.
14. Romero A, Polo JR, Garcia Morato E, et al. Salvage of angioaccess after late thrombosis of radiocephalic fistulas for hemodialysis. *Int Surg.* 1986;71:122.
15. Beathard GA, Settle SM, Shields MW. Salvage of the nonfunctioning arteriovenous fistula. *Am J Kidney Dis.* 1999;33:910.
16. Beathard GA, Arnold P, Jackson J, Litchfield T. Aggressive treatment of early fistula failure. *Kidney Int.* 2003;64:1487.
17. Beathard GA. An algorithm for the physical examination of early fistula failure. *Semin Dial.* 2005;18:331.
18. Schwab SJ, Quarles LD, Middleton JP, et al. Hemodialysis-associated subclavian vein stenosis. *Kidney Int.* 1988;33:1156.
19. Beathard GA. Percutaneous transvenous angioplasty in the treatment of vascular access stenosis. *Kidney Int.* 1992;42:1390.
20. Butterly DW. A quality improvement program for hemodialysis vascular access. *Adv Ren Replace Ther.* 1994;1:163.
21. Albers FJ. Causes of hemodialysis access failure. *Adv Ren Replace Ther.* 1994;1:107.
22. Beathard G, ed. *Complications of Vascular Access.* New York: Dekker; 2000.
23. Miles AM. Vascular steal syndrome and ischaemic monomelic neuropathy: two variants of upper limb ischaemia after haemodialysis vascular access surgery. *Nephrol Dial Transplant.* 1999;14:297.
24. Miles AM. Upper limb ischemia after vascular access surgery: differential diagnosis and management. *Semin Dial.* 2000;13:312.
25. Hye RJ, Wolf YG. Ischemic monomelic neuropathy: an under-recognized complication of hemodialysis access. *Ann Vasc Surg.* 1994;8:578.
26. Duncan H, Ferguson L, Faris I. Incidence of the radial steal syndrome in patients with Brescia fistula for hemodialysis: its clinical significance. *J Vasc Surg.* 1986;4:144.
27. DeCaprio JD, Valentine RJ, Kakish HB, et al. Steal syndrome complicating hemodialysis access. *Cardiovasc Surg.* 1997;5:648.

28. Morsy AH, Kulbaski M, Chen C, et al. Incidence and characteristics of patients with hand ischemia after a hemodialysis access procedure. *J Surg Res*. 1998;74:8.

29. Goff CD, Sato DT, Bloch PH, et al. Steal syndrome complicating hemodialysis access procedures: can it be predicted? *Ann Vasc Surg*. 2000;14:138.

30. Lazarides MK, Staramos DN, Kopadis G, et al. Onset of arterial 'steal' following proximal angioaccess: immediate and delayed types. *Nephrol Dial Transplant*. 2003;18:2387.

31. Wixon CL, Hughes JD, Mills JL. Understanding strategies for the treatment of ischemic steal syndrome after hemodialysis access. *J Am Coll Surg*. 2000;191:301.

15

EARLY AND LATE FISTULA FAILURE

GERALD A. BEATHARD

INTRODUCTION

The native arteriovenous fistula (AVF) comes the closest to being an ideal vascular access when compared to what is currently available. Although it does not meet all the criteria that one would list, when the criteria are weighted according to clinical consequence, the AVF is definitely the superior access.[1-11] Although the AVF is associated with fewer complications than are seen with other types of vascular access, they do occur and they should be dealt with effectively.

The vascular access used for hemodialysis should be thought of as a complete arteriovenous circuit (Figure 15-1). It is convenient to think of this circuit as being composed of three parts (not counting the heart)—the inflow or feeding arteries, the vascular access itself which is cannulated for hemodialysis treatments, and the outflow or draining veins. This circuit begins with the heart and ends back at the heart. Access flow can be adversely affected by problems that occur anywhere within this complete circuit including the heart.

The major complications that are seen in conjunction with arteriovenous fistulas may be categorized under the headings of early failure, late failure, excessive flow leading to congestive heart failure, steal syndrome, aneurysm formation, and infection (Table 15-1). The purpose of this discussion is to review early and late AVF failure; both can have multiple causes.

GENERAL

Unfortunately there is not a standard definition for early fistula failure. In fact the designation is not even standardized. Different reports have used the terms early failure, failure to mature, and primary failure to mean basically the same thing. Additionally, there is an obvious difference

Vascular access circuit

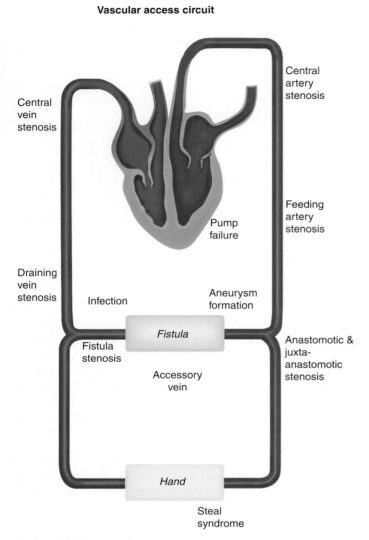

Figure 15-1. Vascular access circuit.

TABLE 15–2
Requirements for a Successful AVF

- Blood flow adequate to support dialysis
- Maturation adequate to allow for repetitive cannulation
- Within 1 cm of the skin surface (preferably 0.5 cm)
- Relatively straight segment available for cannulation
- Anatomical location that is accessible

low blood flow (unlike a synthetic graft), the flow in the fistula only has to be marginally greater than the demands of the blood pump. Less flow can result in recirculation unless the dialysis prescription is modified. This generally means a flow in the range of 600–700 mL/min will be adequate. However, fistulas with low flow may not develop adequate for use since the primary stimulus for fistula development is flow.[12] In a study of radial-cephalic fistula maturation in 43 patients,[13] fistula function was evaluated postoperatively by clinical examination and noninvasively measured AVF blood flow. The blood flow in functioning AVFs was significantly higher compared to nonfunctioning AVFs at 1 (754 vs 440 cc/min), 7 (799 vs 524 cc/min), and 42 days (946 vs 532 cc/min) postoperatively.

Secondly, the AVF must be adequately matured to allow for repetitive cannulation, hopefully without undue frustration on the part of the dialysis facility staff or the patient. In general, two variables are required for AVF maturation. Firstly, the AVF should have adequate blood flow to support dialysis as mentioned above; second, it should have enough size to allow for successful repetitive cannulation. Although flow and size may appear as two separate parameters, they are intricately related. The single most important determinant of AVF size development is the response of both the feeding artery and the draining vein to the increase in shear stress that occurs after the creation of an arteriovenous anastomosis mediated by flow.[14–19] When the vein is connected to an artery, both are subjected to a high blood-flow environment. The venous wall undergoes remodeling as a result of increased circumferential stress due to higher shear forces. Similar changes occur in the artery. Pressure does not play an appreciable role in this normal developmental sequence.[14]

Thirdly, the fistula must be within 1 cm (preferably 0.5 cm) of the skin surface in order for it to be reliably cannulated with a dialysis needle of the length that is commonly available. Additionally, the nurse has to be able to feel it. A fistula that is mature but too deep is a problem. The solution for deep veins that are used to create an AVF is transposition. The vein can be dissected free and tunneled in a more superficial position.

Fourthly, the AVF must have a relatively straight segment available for cannulation. At a minimum, this must be several centimeters long (6 cm or more). The dialysis needle must be threaded into the vein in order to be stable. Attempts at threading a needle into a tortuous fistula are often met with disaster.

between a mature fistula and a successful fistula, that is, one that can be used repetitively as a dialysis access.

For an AVF to be successful it must be usable. This means that several characteristics must be present (Table 15-2). Firstly, it must have blood flow adequate to support dialysis. In order to be used as a dialysis access, an AVF must be able to sustain the blood flow that is demanded by the dialysis prescription. Since an AVF can stay patent with a relatively

TABLE 15–1
Major Complications of Fistulas

- Early failure
- Late Failure
- Excessive flow
- Steal syndrome
- Aneurysm formation
- Infection

Lastly, the AVF must be created in an anatomical location that is accessible with the patient in a sitting position. A fistula that is on the back of the arm or under the arm is not easily used. The ideal location is on the volar surface of the forearm, the lateral surface of the upper arm, or, in the case of a brachial-basilic fistula, the anterior surface of the upper arm.

EARLY FAILURE

▶ Definition

For the purposes of our discussion here we shall define early failure as an AVF that is never usable for dialysis or that fails within 3 months of use.[20] This may also be referred to as primary failure or failure to develop. The emphasis here is on maturation. The distinction between early and late failure is made because there are certain unique lesions that are seen in the early category. Unfortunately, these unique lesions are also major causes of late failure because they were not diagnosed and corrected during the early period.

The causes of early failure can be thought of in terms of either inflow or outflow problems (Table 15-3). Both of these overlap anatomically with the body of the AVF itself. It is important to realize that most of the potential problems of both types can be obviated by proper patient evaluation prior to an attempt at access creation.

▶ Incidence

Early failure has always been a problem. However, as efforts have been intensified to create more AVFs, it appears that the incidence of early failure has increased. Although the definitions have varied, studies of 20–25 years ago observed early failure rates in the range of 10–25%.[3] In more recent reports, the incidence has been higher, in the range of 20–60%.[2,3,21–29]

▶ Predisposing Factors

The reasons for this high incidence of early failure are not totally clear. However, one must realize that the population at risk has changed over the years. When the radiocephalic

TABLE 15–3
Causes of Early Fistula Failure

Inflow problems
Pre-existing arterial anomalies
   Anatomically small
   Atherosclerotic disease
Acquired
   Juxta-anastomotic stenosis
Outflow problems
Pre-existing venous anomalies
Anatomically small
Fibrotic vein (stenotic)
Accessory veins (side branches)

fistula first was described in 1966 by Cimino and Brescia,[30] the patients' average age was 43 years, almost all had chronic glomerulonephritis, and blood flows used for dialysis were 250–300 mL/min. The early fistula failure rate was in the range of 10%. Today's dialysis patients are different—they are much older (>70 years), three-quarters of them have five or more comorbidities, with 90% having cardiovascular disease and 50% having diabetes.[31,32] In addition, the average blood pump speed is much higher: 350–450 mL/min. It is not surprising that achieving functional fistulas in today's population is frequently a challenge.

Part of the problem appears to be related to differences in surgical expertise.[33–36] In addition, being female,[24,28,29,37–40] African-American,[41] elderly,[40,42] having greater body mass index ($\geq$ 35 kg/m^2),[43] diabetes,[28,44] peripheral vascular disease,[28] or coronary artery disease,[28] has an effect on early fistula development.

There are a variety of fistula configurations that can be created; however, the three most commonly used are the radial-cephalic, the brachial-cephalic, and the brachial-basilic transposition fistulas. These are not equal in their propensity to be associated with early failure. The early failure rate for the brachial-basilic transposed fistula has been reported to be the lowest, followed by the brachial-cephalic and then the radial cephalic with the highest rate.[45–52] The early failure rate for brachial-basilic transposition fistulas has been reported to be in the range of 0–21% in various series.[45–49] When compared to brachial-cephalic fistulas in the same series, brachial-basilic transpositions have had an early failure rate of 0% versus 27%,[47] 21% versus 32%,[49] and 18% versus 38%.[46] Radial-cephalic fistula failure rates of over 60% have been reported.[53] What early failure rate actually means is somewhat of a problem; there is no standard definition. For this reason, one cannot readily compare the rates reported by different studies.

▶ Associated Lesions

Most investigators agree that 100% of AVFs that present with failure to mature have an anatomical problem of some type (Table 15-3).[20,54–58] Multiple problems are frequently seen; in one report of 100 cases 34% had more than one lesion present.[20] In another, multiple derangements were observed in 85 of 123 cases (71.4%).[55] The lesions that have been identified in cases of early AVF failure fall into two categories—those that existed prior to the creation of the access (Figures 15-2 and 15-3A) and those that are acquired and the result of the surgical procedure itself (Figure 15-3B). In the first category are lesions and anatomy that should have been detected and addressed (or avoided) by good preoperative vascular mapping; however, because this is not universally done, they are seen. In series that have been reported, stenosis of the feeding artery has been reported in 4–6%, proximal venous stenosis in 4–59%, and central venous stenosis in 2.6–9% of cases.[20,54,55,59–62] These are all pathological lesions. The wide variations seen are perhaps related to the variability in preoperative evaluation applied to these cases (case selection).

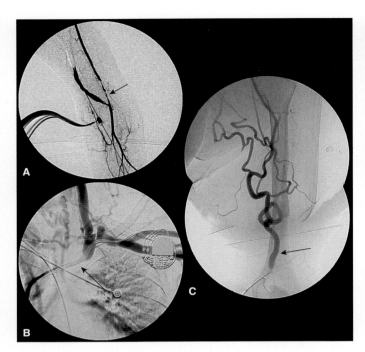

Figure 15-2. Lesions (arrows) present before creation of fistula. (**A**) Brachial artery stenosis; (**B**) brachiocephalic stenosis; (**C**) cephalic vein obstruction. All of these could be avoided.

Another type of pre-existing problem that can affect AVF development and maturation is the presence of accessory veins.[20,55,58–60,63,64] These are side branches of the forearm veins used for the construction of a fistula. Accessory veins (Figure 15-3A) represent normal anatomy and as such, they should not be erroneously referred to as collateral veins, which are pathological and related to downstream stenosis. Unfortunately, the distinction between the two is not always clear; stenosis can make a normally present accessory vein larger and more prominent. Basically, if a downstream stenosis is present, the side branch should be assumed to be related to it and therefore represent a collateral vein until proven otherwise. The incidence of accessory veins has been reported to be 4–78%.[20,55,58–60,64] This marked variability probably represents differences in case selection. When all early failure cases are systematically evaluated, an incidence in the lower portion of this range can be anticipated. It should be mentioned that this is almost exclusively a problem with forearm AVFs. The upper arm superficial veins do not normally have any significant side branches.

Acquired lesions are thought to be a result of the surgical procedure. Stenosis of the venous segment immediately adjacent to the arterial anastomosis (first 3–5 cm), referred to as juxta-anastomotic stenosis (Figure 15-3B), has been reported in 27%–68% of cases studied.[20,54,55,58–62] It is difficult to evaluate the arterial anastomosis in absolute terms because it is an artificially created orifice. However, it has become a common practice to compare the diameter of the orifice to the adjacent normal feeding artery and if it is less than 50% to consider it as stenotic.[65]

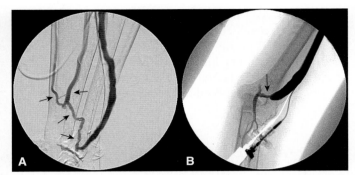

Figure 15-3. (**A**) Accessory vein (arrows); (**B**) Juxta-anastomotic stenosis.

Although it is not always clear as to whether this criterion was applied, the incidence of anastomotic stenosis has been reported to range from 38% to 47%.[20,55,59] In the majority of cases, this has been associated with part of the juxta-anastomotic lesion, but in some cases it is definitely separate.

▶ **Early Failure Evaluation**

A thorough evaluation of a new AVF 4–6 weeks after creation should be considered mandatory in order to detect problems as early as possible.[66,67] The maturation of a newly created AVF, if it is going to happen, should be apparent at this time. Waiting exposes the patient to one of two risks: (1) if the patient has already started dialysis they are exposed to the risks of continued dialysis with a catheter, or (2) if the patient has not yet initiated dialysis, they are exposed to the risks of beginning dialysis with a catheter. When one considers the potential complications commensurate with catheter use, either of these possibilities should be avoided if possible.

Physical examination

Evaluation of the newly created AVF at this 4–6-week period should be directed toward answering one simple question—"can the access be repetitively cannulated?" Robbin, et al[29] found that the determination of both AVF diameter and AVF flow was very valuable in predicting the chances that a newly created AVF would be adequate. However, of considerable interest was the fact that in this study, an experienced dialysis nurse had 80% accuracy in predicting the ultimate utility of an AVF for dialysis. In other words an experienced, knowledgeable person can simply examine the AVF and predict with a high degree of confidence its utility as a dialysis access. This examination will naturally take into account the diameter, depth, and length of the access that can be cannulated, but a subjective evaluation is adequate—if it can be cannulated and if this can be done repetitively. If the AVF does not appear to be developing adequately for eventual use as a dialysis access, more detailed physical examination of the access will, in most instances, reveal the cause of the arrested maturation.[68,69] Physical examination has been shown to be very accurate in assessing a fistula and is not difficult to learn.[70–72]

The evaluation of a recently created fistula is facilitated by following a standard algorithm (Figure 15-4).[69] Lesions are often multiple, a fact that should encourage a thorough systematic examination even after an obvious abnormality has been detected. Abnormalities that might be detected at each step are listed in Figure 15-4.

Step 1—Basic information. In order to understand the fistula that is failing to develop, one must start with some basic information. This helps to define the problem and will immediately start raising possibilities for the dysfunction. Firstly, how long has it been since the fistula was created? A fistula that is only 4-weeks old but looks as though it has been in place for a year or more could be the victim of proximal stenosis. Knowing the type of fistula is helpful.

Secondly, there are certain lesions that are more common with certain types of fistulas; this is especially true for the "swing point" stenoses.[73,74] Third, the fistula's "use history" can be very important, if attempts have been made to use the fistula. Was the problem difficulty with cannulation, was the flow inadequate—these are important clues to the problem.

Step 2—Examine the anastomosis. Feel for a thrill and a pulse. If there is no thrill or pulse, the fistula may be "dead." It may not be possible to resuscitate a completely dead fistula. Before concluding that function is totally absent, one should listen with a Doppler device.

The palm of the hand is thought to be more sensitive in feeling a thrill. The thrill corresponds to flow, the stronger the thrill the better the flow. It is helpful to listen to the bruit (the auditory manifestation of flow) to determine the character of the diastolic component. Overall, the

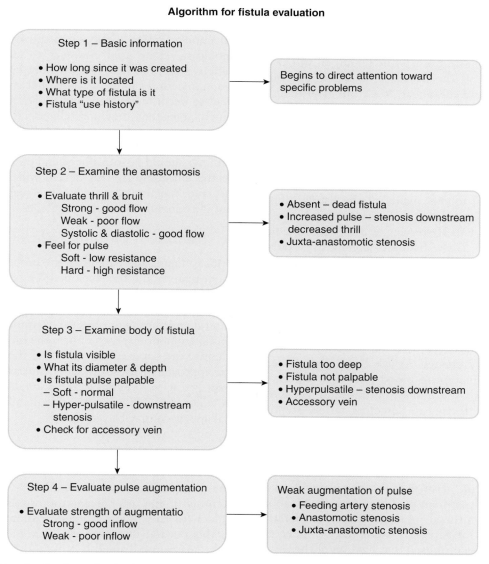

Figure 15-4. Algorithm for fistula evaluation.

bruit should have a low rumbling pitch with a prominent diastolic component. The diastolic, occurring at a lower pressure, will disappear first when a lesion is present downstream resulting in increased resistance. Additionally, the pitch will become higher.

The pulse should be soft and compressible. A strong thrusting pulse indicates the presence of a downstream problem creating increased resistance. In a general sense a thrill may be thought of a "good," indicating flow. A pulse may be thought of as "bad," indicating a downstream obstruction. Check for the presence of a juxta-anastomotic stenosis. In the presence of this lesion, the anastomosis will be hyperpulsatile and the thrill will be weak (systolic only) or absent.

Step 3—Check the body of the fistula. Firstly, inspect the fistula to determine if it is visible and if so for what length. Assess its apparent diameter and depth to determine if it has the potential for being cannulated repetitively. Secondly, feel for a pulse being careful in doing so not to compress the vein and create a spurious one. The fistula should be soft and compressible. A strong pulse is an indication of downstream obstruction to some degree. Thirdly, check for an accessory vein. This can be done by manually occluding the fistula at progressively increasing intervals from the anastomosis while feeling of the anastomosis for a thrill. If the fistula is occluded, stopping flow, the thrill should disappear. If a thrill is present in the face of occlusion, there is a side branch between the point of compression and the anastomosis or the previous point of compression.

Step 4—Check pulse augmentation. If the fistula is manually occluded, the pulse distal to that point will be augmented (increased). The degree of this augmentation is directly proportional to the quality of the fistula inflow. With experience, the result of this maneuver can be quantitated on a scale of 1 to 10, serving as a very useful guide to inflow evaluation. If the fistula is already hyperpulsatile (an indication of outflow stenosis), the change in pulse produced by manual occlusion is reflective of the degree of the occlusion (stenosis) causing the hyperpulsatility.

Ultrasound evaluation

Doppler ultrasound has been used to predict the ultimate maturation of newly created AVFs.[29,75-78] This has been based upon determination of blood flow and evaluation of vessel diameters. Additionally, ultrasound has been shown to be very effective in detecting inflow stenosis in dysfunctional fistulas.[79] However, ultrasound is also very useful in further defining problems that have been detected by physical examination. Basically, there is no need for doing ultrasound unless the physical examination reveals a problem.[70] However, it is very valuable as an aid in developing a treatment plan for a case that is about to undergo interventional management. Preoperative assessment looking for accessory veins has been recommended.[64] It has been proposed that ligation of these vessels during initial AVF creation could potentially reduce nonmaturation rates.

Angiographic evaluation

Accurate diagnosis and localization of problems that have contributed to the failure of a newly created AVF to mature is primarily dependent upon angiography. Since many of these patients have not yet begun dialysis and virtually all have significant residual renal function, concern has been expressed related to the renal toxicity of radiocontrast. However, studies have shown that the volume of radiocontrast used for such evaluations in early AVF failure does not cause problems.[80,81] Some investigators have preferentially used an arterial approach to the angiographic evaluation of the failed AVF[54,61] and others have relied primarily upon a venous approach[20,55,58-60] amply demonstrating that an arterial cannulation is not necessary. In some cases, however, it is not possible to palpate a segment of the vein adequate for introduction of a needle making an arterial approach necessary.[59]

When a venous approach has been utilized, the arterial anastomosis and the juxta-anastomotic portion of the AVF can be easily demonstrated by simply occluding the downstream AVF and performing a retrograde radiocontrast injection to reflux the dye into the artery. This technique should never be used, however, to identify and evaluate venous side branches. The pressure created by the retrograde injection can cause veins that are not normally evident to become apparent and cause small veins to appear much larger than they normally are. If it is not possible to demonstrate the region of the AVF being evaluated with an antegrade, unobstructed radiocontrast injection, then a catheter should be introduced and passed retrograde down to the anastomosis. This device will allow for an unobstructed injection to visualize the suspect anatomy without introducing obfuscating artifacts.

▶ Treatment of Early Failure

Prior to taking the patient to the procedure room, a treatment plan should be developed. The individuality of each case precludes the use of a standard algorithm for management. The development of a plan should begin with a careful and thorough physical examination.[82] The goals of this examination are to confirm the presence of a problem, identify the nature and location of the problem, and plan the approach. In most instances, the case can be adequately managed with a venous cannulation; however, in instances in which the AVF cannot be adequately palpated, an arterial approach may be required.[59]

Juxta-anastomosis stenosis management

The most common location for stenosis is the juxta-anastomotic segment of the AVF.[20,54,55,58-62] Additionally, stenosis of the arterial anastomosis is frequently associated with this lesion. Three variations may be observed in this portion of the access—juxta-anastomotic stenosis only, anastomotic stenosis only, and a combination of the two. Regardless of its precise nature, management of these lesions is best approached with a retrograde cannulation.

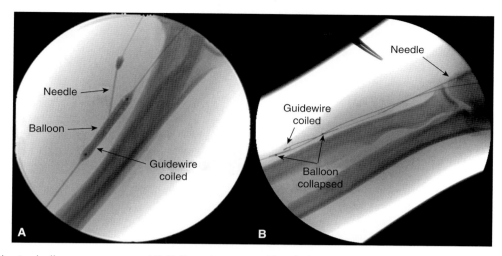

Figure 15-5. Guidewire-balloon entrapment. (**A**) Balloon in proximal fistula has been cannulated and micro-guidewire has been introduced. (**B**) Cannulated balloon is being withdrawn, pulling micro-guidewire with it.

In some cases, the segment of AVF that is palpable is too short to allow for a retrograde cannulation. In this instance, either an arterial approach or a technique that is referred to as balloon-guidewire entrapment[83] may be used.

Balloon-guidewire entrapment. This technique (Figure 15-5) is accomplished in the forearm by first cannulating the lower segment of the AVF in an antegrade direction. A standard guidewire is passed upward and an angioplasty balloon, generally a 4 × 6, is inserted and advanced to a level just below the elbow. The balloon is inflated with only enough pressure to obtain full dilatation. A site over the upper portion of the balloon is anesthetized and then cannulated using a Micropuncture needle (Cook, Bloomington, IN). When the balloon is entered, the clear liquid used to fill the balloon will start escaping from the needle hub indicating that cannulation has been accomplished. The micro-guidewire is then passed into the balloon where it becomes coiled. The balloon along with the entrapped guidewire is then slowly withdrawn bringing the guidewire into the lower portion of the AVF. Then by holding the guidewire secure and continuing to withdraw, the balloon can be extracted leaving the guidewire behind. The dilator can then be inserted at the cannulation site to secure the access.

Angioplasty. Once the AVF has been cannulated in the desired manner, an angiogram should be done to evaluate and accurately localize the lesion (Figure 15-6). This can be easily accomplished by occluding the upper AVF and performing a retrograde injection to reflux radiocontrast

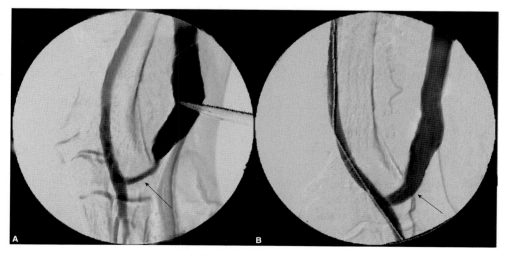

Figure 15-6. Juxta-anastomotic stenosis. (**A**) Lesion. (**B**) Post-treatment.

into the feeding artery. This should allow identification of all of the pertinent structures. For a lesion to qualify as significant enough to warrant treatment, it should be 50% stenotic or greater.[84] Stenosis is judged by a comparison with the adjacent normal AVF. In order to judge the size of the anastomosis, its diameter should be compared with the diameter of the adjacent normal artery.[65]

The first step in treating a juxta-anastomotic or anastomotic lesion is to pass a guidewire across the anastomosis and into the artery far enough to allow optimal positioning of the angioplasty balloon. Due to the angle of the vein to the artery at the anastomosis and the fact that the area is stenotic, difficulty may be encountered in passing the guidewire. Cannulation of the artery across the anastomosis may be facilitated by the use of a vascular guiding catheter. In some instances, it is possible to safely and effectively treat the lesion that is present with the guidewire passing downward in an antegrade direction. However, in many cases it is better to have it pass up the artery. Making this turn is difficult at times. The use of a 5-French Rosch Inferior Mesenteric (RIM) catheter may facilitate the process. A 25-cm catheter is available and is especially useful in these types of cases (AngioDynamics, Queensbury, NY).

While the use of single angioplasty balloon is possible for a juxta-anastomotic lesion that does not involve the anastomosis, when the anastomosis is also affected two sizes of balloon are often necessary. If the angioplasty balloon crosses the anastomosis to lie within the artery, it should be sized to match the diameter of the artery. In most instances a 4-mm balloon will be found to be appropriate for a radial artery and a 6-mm for a brachial artery, but individual variations exist and should be followed. When treating the lesion within the AVF itself, oversizing the balloon 20–30% is appropriate. Care should be taken to avoid allowing this larger (generally) balloon to enter the anastomosis and adjacent artery.

Following dilatation, a post-treatment angiogram (Figure 15-6) should be performed to assess the result and check for complications. While upstream occlusion and a retrograde injection of radiocontrast are permissible for the pretreatment evaluation, this should not be done post-treatment. To be effective, angioplasty physically damages (tears) the vessel. The pressure created with a retrograde injection following a successful angioplasty can result in venous rupture and extravasation.[85] This unfortunate complication can be avoided by passing a vascular catheter over the guidewire into the artery immediately adjacent to the anastomosis and using this to inject the radiocontrast.

Proximal vein stenosis management

Management of stenosis in the vein proximal to the anastomosis (excluding the juxta-anastomotic variety) is generally more easily accomplished (Figure 15-7). The same process as described above should be followed. The major difference is that these lesions can, in most instances, be treated with an antegrade cannulation. The major problem that is

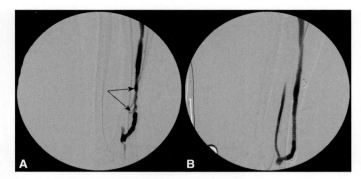

Figure 15-7. Fistula stenosis (arrows). (**A**) Pre-treatment. (**B**) Post-treatment.

encountered relates to the development of collaterals. At times the anatomy presented by the lesion is so complex because of multiple collaterals as to require considerable time and effort to determine the location and status of the normal vein. A careful comparison of the physical examination findings and the appearance of the angiogram is often very illuminating.

The first step is to pass a guidewire. If the guidewire goes up following the expected path of the normal vein, it is very helpful, especially if it passes up into the central veins. This may occur at times even when the vascular structure through which it passes is not opacified by the radiocontrast. When this occurs, the passage of a vascular catheter (5-French straight) followed by injections of radiocontrast through the catheter as it is slowly withdrawn is often very helpful in assuring that the path of the guidewire is indeed the normal vessel.

Once the guidewire is up and its proper location has been assured, an angioplasty balloon can be introduced. The balloon should be oversized for the normal portion of the vein by 20–30%. Some of the lesions that are encountered may be resistant to dilatation and require an ultra-high pressure balloon.[55,84,86] One study[86] found that 20% of lesions in native AVFs required balloon inflation pressures that exceeded 20 atmospheres. Once the stenosis has been resolved, the anatomy observed on angiography should become considerably simplified as the collaterals observed initially frequently disappear.

In cases in which the main lumen of the AVF is totally obstructed, dilatation of a collateral vein may suffice to salvage the access.[87] This must be done with care because collateral veins are frequently thin-walled and more easily ruptured than normal vessels. Additionally, multiple treatment sessions with increasing balloon sizes may be necessary to arrive at a satisfactory conclusion.

In some instances, it is not possible or perhaps even wise to do all that needs to be done for the lesions, the pathology and anomalies associated with early fistula failure in a single procedure.[55,60] At times spasm accompanies almost any intervention that is undertaken. In these cases, one loses the ability to judge what is happening. There are even cases in which the fistula looks worse after treatment than it did before the procedure began because of the induction of venous spasm. Staging the overall intervention that is planned over more than one encounter is a useful approach. Interval evaluation is a valuable tool in judging the effect of what has been done and determining what still needs to be addressed. A clinical evaluation of the access 2–3 weeks following treatment to determine the effect of the therapy and assess the need for further treatment should be done in all cases.

In cases where the overall treatment of the problem is staged over two or more sessions, the question arises as to how one measures primary patency. It does not seem reasonable for this parameter of effectiveness and success to be determined for each stage of the staged treatment. Basically, the procedure is not complete until all stages of the procedure have been completed. This is when the time used to determine the duration of primary patency should begin.

Small-diameter veins are often a limiting factor for the successful creation of AVFs. In an attempt to address this problem, primary balloon angioplasty (PBA) has been used at the time of fistula creation surgery to enlarge the vein. In one report,[88] 62 PBAs were performed in 55 patients just before AVF creation using 2.5–4-mm angioplasty balloons. This was then followed using a technique referred to as sequential balloon angioplasty maturation (BAM). This was used to salvage failed fistulas, expedite maturation, and improve the patency of AVFs after PBA. BAM was performed in 53 of the 62 cases at 2, 4, and 6 weeks after the initial procedure (PBAQ and surgery). Successful outcome was defined as the functional ability to use the fistula for hemodialysis without surgical revision. Forty-seven (85.4%) of the 55 cases were successful.

Arterial stenosis management

Under the heading of arterial stenosis, one must consider two lesions: anastomotic stenosis and feeding artery stenosis. The former is the more common and its management has already been discussed in association with juxta-anastomotic stenosis. Arterial stenosis affecting the feeding artery at a point removed from the anastomosis is seen in 4–6%.

This inflow problem can be easily treated in most cases by a retrograde venous cannulation. It is only the occasional case that actually requires an arterial approach. As mentioned above, with a venous approach, it is essential that the guidewire pass retrograde up the artery in order to reach the lesion. This passage may also be difficult to achieve, the guidewire may have to be manipulated in order to cross the anastomosis and enter the artery. In this instance, 5-French RIM catheter may facilitate the process.

The choice of angioplasty balloon size should be governed by the diameter of the normal artery adjacent to the lesion being treated. While the vein tolerates and often requires high pressure, this should be avoided in arterial dilatations. In general, pressures greater than 10–12 atmospheres should not be exceeded. It must be kept in mind

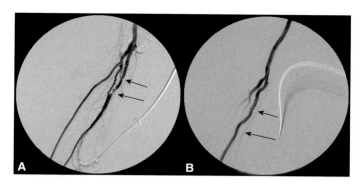

Figure 15-8. Arterial stenosis (radial artery). (**A**) Lesion (arrows). (**B**) Post-treatment.

that the artery has a vital function and its damage could jeopardize the viability of digits or the hand. A post-treatment angiogram is often facilitated by using a vascular catheter that is passed over the guidewire that has been left in place following the angioplasty. In fact a vascular catheter can be extended all the way to the aortic arch to evaluate the entire arterial inflow if such is indicated[84] and has been recommended by some in cases with obvious inflow problems.[57]

Stenotic lesions detected within the feeding arteries associated with early fistula failure can be treated successfully with angioplasty (Figure 15-8). In one study[89] the success rate for such lesions was 91% with a 1-year primary patency of 83%.

Accessory vein obliteration

The treatment of side branches is said to be controversial by those who do not treat them (and may not even recognize their existence). However, most investigators reporting series dealing with the nonmaturing fistula have treated them.[20,55,58–60,63,64] When side branches are observed on the angiogram of an AVF which has failed to mature, the first step is to determine if they are accessory or collateral veins. This is done by first determining if a downstream stenosis is present. If such is the case, then this lesion should always receive priority and be treated first to see if this will resolve the situation. The resistance with increased intraluminal pressure created by a stenotic lesion will not only cause the appearance of collateral veins, but will also cause accessory veins to be larger than they actually will be when normal pressures are restored.

If there is no stenosis downstream from the side branch in question, or after the stenosis has been resolved if one is present, the next step is to decide the significance of the observed vessel. The mere presence of an accessory vein is not an adequate indication for its treatment. Small side branches are frequently encountered and are of no consequence. Additionally, there should be concern only if there is fistula dysfunction that can be attributed to the accessory vein. Such a structure in a fistula that is functioning well may be an advantage, offering an additional area for cannulation. Significance in the dysfunctional fistula should be judged by three criteria: size, flow, and changes that occur with manual occlusion. Unfortunately, there have been no clinical trials to provide guidance in this matter. The judgments made are somewhat subjective, but should be based upon sound reasoning. All three factors—size, flow, and changes that occur with manual occlusion—should be considered.

Changes that occur with manual compression of the side branch are often best evaluated using a vascular Doppler and comparing the sound over the AVF above the accessory vein with and without compression of the structure in question. Flow can be determined using Doppler ultrasound with and without downstream compression. It can also be judged subjectively by comparing flow in the accessory and the main AVF side-by-side with a small bolus of radiocontrast. While this is subjective, it does add weight to a decision to obliterate when other factors are also supportive. One study [64] found that preoperatively detected accessory veins, with a diameter >70% of the cephalic vein diameter, had a sensitivity, specificity, positive predictive value, and negative predictive value 80%, 100%, 100%, and 91% for prediction of radial-cephalic nonmaturation. However, this was based upon a rather small cohort of patients (4 of 10 nonmaturing AVFs). We have used 25% of the diameter of the AVF as an indicator of possible significance.

It seems reasonable that Poiseuille's law would be a good guide in determining the significance of an accessory vein. This would suggest that if the ratio between the diameter of the side branch and the main trunk of the fistula was 1:4, the flow would be 1:256, 1:3 would be 1:81, and 1:2 would be 1:16. However, this is not true; Poiseuille's law does not apply here. The assumptions of the equation are that the flow is laminar viscous and incompressible and that the flow is through a rigid circular cross-section that is substantially longer than its diameter. None of these assumptions hold for the accessory vein. Basically, one is left with the need for making a subjective judgment based upon size, flow, and changes that occur with manual occlusion in a dysfunctional fistula.

Accessory vein treatment modalities. There are three modalities that may be used to obliterate an accessory vein: percutaneous ligation, surgical ligation, and the placement of an embolization coil. All three, when used appropriately, are successful.

Percutaneous ligation—If the accessory vein is easily visible or readily palpable, it can be ligated percutaneously (Figure 15-9).[63] This is done by simply anesthetizing the skin over the vein, close to the body of the fistula, and placing a suture through the intact skin and around the side branch. A double stitch is generally used. It is important that the stitch be tied tight enough to totally occlude the vein. If there is only minimal flow, it will not work. The stitch is typically left in place for about 10 days and then removed.

Surgical ligation—Once the accessory vein is accurately located, a small incision can be made close to the body of

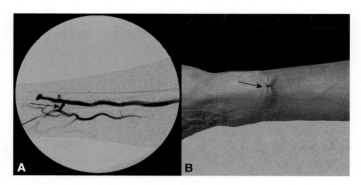

Figure 15-9. Percutaneous ligation. (**A**) Accessory vein (arrow). (**B**) Ligation (arrow).

the fistula.[58] The side branch is then isolated and ligated (Figure 15-10). The vein will frequently undergo spasm when it is manipulated. For this reason, it is often advantageous to either pass a guidewire up the vein or insert a 5-French catheter into it to aid in its localization.

Embolization coil—An accessory vein can be very effectively obliterated using an embolization coil.[20] The vein must first be selectively catheterized. This process can often be greatly facilitated by using a Cobrita catheter (AngioDynamics, Queensbury, NY). This is like a Cobra catheter, except it is one-third the size. The coil is inserted through the catheter using a guidewire. These coils come in a variety of sizes. It is best to select a coil that is slightly larger than the vein so that it will be less likely to migrate. Once the coil has been placed, it takes a few minutes for flow to cease and the vein to become thrombosed (Figure 15-11).

▶ **Results of Treatment of Early Failure**

The results gained by the treatment of nonmaturing AVFs have been variable. Nevertheless, when compared with the alternative of abandonment, one is forced to conclude that the results are extraordinarily good. It is very possible that the outcome variations in reported series are due to variations in the populations studied.

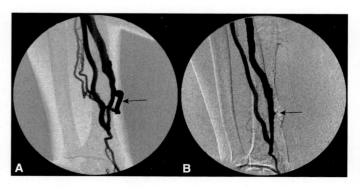

Figure 15-10. Surgical ligation. (**A**) Accessory vein (arrow). (**B**) After ligation (arrow).

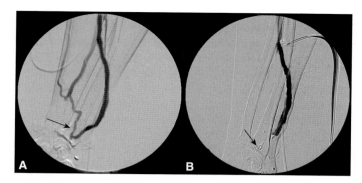

Figure 15-11. Embolization coil. (**A**) Accessory vein (arrow). (**B**) Coil in place (arrow).

Prescreening of cases may have led to case selection favoring a successful outcome. The degree to which this was done is not clear in most reports.

Primary patency rates ranging from 72% to 84% at 3 months and 26% to 75% at 1 year have been reported. Secondary patency rates of 79–82% and 68–82% have been documented for 3 months and 1 year follow-ups.[20,54,55,58–62] One series[55] reported that follow-up in their cohort of treated cases showed a total adverse event rate of 0.38/access-year which included a thrombosis rate of 0.12/access-year and an AVF loss rate of 0.04/access-year.

In an analysis[90] of data from 23 dialysis facilities over a 3-year period regarding the functionality of an AVF at initial puncture following construction, failure occurred in 7.6% of 5007 cases. However, there was a wide distribution of failure cases among these facilities ranging from 0.8% to 23.6%. In the data collected, many methods were used to salvage the failed accesses. The salvage rate was 70%.

▶ **Prevention of Early Failure**

In view of the high early failure rates that have been reported, it is not at all clear that it is possible to totally prevent this complication. There is a prevailing opinion that vascular mapping should be considered mandatory in all patients in whom a dialysis vascular access is planned.[2,51,91,92] The earliest report to show strong support for this approach[51] demonstrated a marked increase in the percentage of AVFs placed (14–63%) and an equally impressive decrease in early failure rates (from 38% to 8.3%). Not all studies have demonstrated this degree of benefit, however. In some, the incidence of early failure has not improved and in some has actually increased with vascular mapping.[27,91] The reasons for this are not clear.

Choice of surgeon is very important.[8,33–35,93,94] The algorithm that appears to have the best chance of decreasing the incidence of early failure while increasing the prevalence of fistulas is that which has been emphasized by Fistula First.[94] Especially the idea of starting early, doing vascular mapping, careful selection of a surgeon, evaluation of all newly created fistulas at 4 weeks, and an aggressive program of salvage for early failures.

LATE FAILURE

▶ **Definition**

Late fistula failure is defined as failure that occurs after a period of normal usage. The primary causes of late failure are venous stenosis and acquired arterial lesions. These lesions are manifest as pathological changes in the fistula from increased pressure, and decreased flow leading to inadequate dialysis and eventually thrombosis. The same type of lesions that are seen in association with early failure may be seen here. Whether these were there initially and failed to cause problems earlier or they developed (or progressed) over time as the AVF was being used is not clear.[58]

▶ **Venous Stenosis**

Fortunately, venous stenosis does not occur in AVFs with the same degree of frequency as is seen with synthetic grafts. Nevertheless it is the most common cause of late fistula loss.[54,93] For this reason it is important that each dialysis facility have in place an organized program for the prospective diagnosis of venous stenosis.[94] This program should consist of weekly monitoring (done by physical examination) and regular surveillance (done using specific tests).

The site of stenoses varies with the site of the AVF arteriovenous anastomosis: in distal radiocephalic AVFs, virtually all stenoses were found in the inflow region (anastomotic and juxta-anastomotic), while outflow lesions were found almost exclusively in mid-forearm and elbow/upper arm AVF.[65,96,97] Unlike the case with grafts, venous stenosis associated with the AVF generally develops more centrally at areas of vein bifurcation, pressure points, swing points, and in association with venous valves.[58,73,74] The development of collateral veins is frequent and often preserves flow in the access.

The treatment of venous stenosis in AVFs presents no unique problems when compared with lesions seen in association with AV grafts. Prospective treatment of stenosis before thrombosis can occur is important and will materially prolong access survival. Percutaneous angioplasty has come to be the treatment of choice for these lesions with greater than 95% success rate.[98,99] Long-term primary patency rates (Figure 15-12) have been in the range of 84–92% at 3 months, 57–77% at 6 months, and 35–69% at 1 year.[95,98] Lesions associated with upper arm fistulas have not fared quite as well as those in the forearm. These numbers are comparable to those seen for the treatment of venous stenosis associated with grafts.

▶ **Arterial Stenosis**

In a report dealing with a cohort of 101 dysfunctional AVF cases,[65] 8% were found to have lesions in the feeding artery and 21% had stenosis of the arterial anastomosis. There was a higher incidence of inflow stenosis for forearm as compared to upper arm AVFs. Others[54,93] have

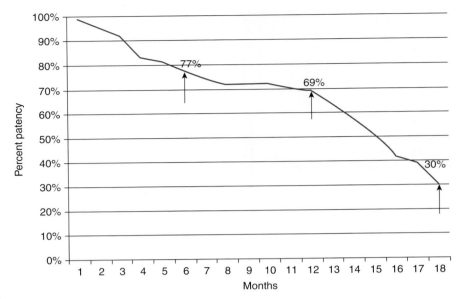

Figure 15-12. Primary patency for treatment of venous stenosis in fistulas (n = 478).[95]

reported the incidence of arterial stenosis in these cases at 6–18%. These lesions can lead to decreased blood flow in the access leading to inadequate dialysis. The treatment of feeding artery lesions presents no unique problems when compared with arterial stenosis seen in association with AV grafts. The management of anastomotic and juxta-anastomotic lesions is as described above in association with early failure.

▶ Thrombosed Fistula

Although AVFs are much less prone to develop problems that are synthetic grafts, they certainly do experience dysfunction. The thrombosis rate for AVFs is reported to be approximately one-sixth that for a graft.[99] Even though there were early reports of the successful treatment of thrombosed AVFs,[56] most AVFs that clotted were abandoned until only a few years ago.

Nature of fistula thrombosis

Just as is the case with a synthetic graft, when blood flow in an AVF slows, either because of a venous stenosis causing increased resistance to flow or because of an arterial inflow problem, it can eventually thrombose. However, unlike the typical, monotonous picture generally presented by clotted grafts, thrombosed AVFs can vary considerably, so much so that they almost have to be considered individually.[100] It is clear that a standard treatment algorithm will not suffice. This is due to the fact that an AVF behaves quite differently from a graft. Firstly, it can tolerate much lower blood flow rates without clotting. Because of this an AVF clots later in the progression of a lesion that slows blood flow. The lesion has longer to develop and therefore may be much more severe than is seen with a graft. Secondly, an AVF can develop collaterals that allow for a continuation of blood flow even after the lesion in the main body of the AVF has become totally obstructive. Severely stenotic lesions and a proliferation of collaterals frequently result in a very complex and complicated picture being presented to the interventionalist when an angiogram is finally performed.

From a clinical perspective, when an AVF no longer has detectable flow in the dialysis facility, it is generally labeled as a thrombosed AVF. In actual fact, many of these, if not most, actually contain no thrombus. They simply have flow that is so diminished that it is no longer detectable or there is complete obstruction of the main channel and all the flow (diminished) is going through collaterals. This is not to say that the AVF diagnosed clinically as being thrombosed never has thrombus. The amount of clot, when clot is present, varies considerably.[100] In fact the thrombus load in some cases can be quite large. This is more likely to be seen in the upper arm AVFs and in what has come to be referred to as a "mega-fistula," that is, one that is markedly dilated, tortuous, with multiple aneurysms.

A synthetic graft is relatively inert. When it clots there is no significant reaction between the access and the thrombus. This is not the case with an AVF. The thrombus in this type of access is inflammatory.[101] It reacts with the wall of the AVF, becomes attached, and begins to undergo organization. This can also complicate efforts directed toward treatment and removal of the thrombus. It is also pertinent in considering how long one can wait to treat a thrombosed AVF.

Lesions associated with fistula thrombosis

Essentially 100% of all thrombosed AVFs have associated pathological anatomy.[54] Essentially all the lesions that described above may be seen in association with

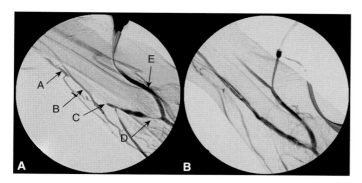

Figure 15-13. Thrombosed brachial-cephalic fistula. (**A**) Upper cephalic vein. (**B**) Collateral. (**C**) Total obstruction. (**D**) Juxta-anastomotic stenosis. (**E**) Brachial artery.

thrombosis. Because thrombosis is a late occurrence, the lesions tend to be severe and total obstruction is not unusual (Figures 15-13 and 15-14).

▶ Thrombosed Fistula Salvage

A variety of techniques have been used to treat the thrombosed AVF[56,100,102–108] with no obvious best choice. It is important to adapt the technique used to the situation found when the thrombosed AVF is evaluated.[100] The case that is referred to the interventionalist bearing a diagnosis of "thrombosed AVF," but is found to have no thrombus present, should not be considered a thrombectomy. These cases only need treatment of the stenotic lesion(s). At the other extreme is the well-developed chronic AVF that

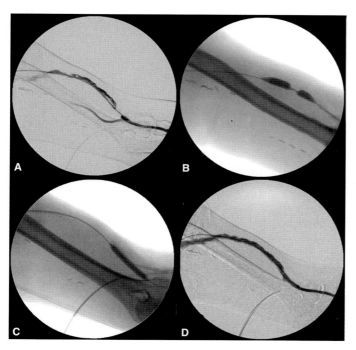

Figure 15-14. Thrombosed brachial-basilic fistula. (**A**) Thrombosed fistula (minimal thrombus). (**B**) Lesion. (**C**) Balloon effacement. (**D**) Final result with flow.

actually has the general basic characteristics of a graft and may be declotted using the same basic technique that one uses to treat a graft (see Chapter 16).

Contraindications to the procedure

There are absolute and relative contraindications to performing this procedure.

Infection. Infection is an absolute contraindication. This is not seen with the frequency that is the case for synthetic grafts, but it can occur. If the access is infected it will contain a variable amount of infectious material. This will be released into the circulation if an endovascular thrombectomy is attempted and have potentially disastrous results.

Right to left shunt. As is the case with performing a thrombectomy procedure on a synthetic graft, a known right-to-left cardiac shunt should be regarded as an absolute contraindication to an endovascular thrombectomy. Embolization of thrombus fragments associated with any type of thrombectomy is not uncommon[109–112] and paradoxical embolization can occur.[113]

Chronic occlusion. Thrombus within an AVF is mildly inflammatory. As a result it becomes attached to the wall of the vessel and begins to organize very early. Therefore, if one delays in treating an AVF that is thrombosed, the chances for success become increasingly compromised. Nevertheless, one should not hesitate to evaluate a thrombosed fistula no matter how long it has been nonfunctional as long as there is still a pulse or a thrill present. The ASVF, being a native vein, develops multiple collaterals and flow can persist even though the main channel has become totally occluded. In some instances, it is possible to salvage the access by utilizing one of the larger collaterals. On the other hand if the AVF is totally dead, having neither a pulse nor a thrill, it is unlikely that one's efforts will be rewarded if more than a few days have passed.

Excessive clot load. Some AVFs become much dilated and diffusely aneurysmal. These "mega-fistulas" can contain a very large clot load when they thrombose. Some can have over 200 mL of thrombus. They can be treated, but it is a time-consuming and a dangerous procedure. With any type of thrombectomy treatment modality, there is the risk of embolization as has been mentioned. In these cases, the embolus can be large enough to be life-threatening. There is also the question as to whether such an AVF should be salvaged. The wisdom of treating such a case by endovascular means should be seriously questioned.

Accessing the AVF

Cannulation of the fistula must be accomplished in such a manner as to allow access to both the venous and arterial circulations in most but not all cases. This can be determined only after the procedure begins. Nevertheless, the dialysis access should be thought of as a circuit that starts and ends at the heart. Problems may occur anywhere within this circuit and will need to be evaluated for possible therapy.

The entire venous drainage up through the superior vena cava needs to be evaluated routinely as does the arterial anastomosis and the adjacent feeding artery. Cannulation of the dysfunctional fistula is often facilitated by the use of a Micropuncture needle (Cook, Bloomington, IN).

Thrombectomy procedures

Each case that presents should be individualized. Knowing what is going to be required starts with a thorough physical examination of the dysfunctional AVF. This needs to identify the location and the type of AVF, the optimum cannulation site(s), and the basic plan of attack. Then once the patient is on the procedure table and the access has been cannulated according to the plan, a decision as to the most optimal technique for the thrombectomy can be completed from an examination of the anatomy and thrombus volume that is found.

Thrombectomy procedure for AVF with minimal thrombosis. There are some cases that when examined are found to have very minimal or no thrombus present. These can generally be handled in the following manner:

1. Do a careful physical examination of the dysfunctional fistula. Try to determine the location of the problem and plan your approach. In some cases it will be best to cannulate close to the anastomosis with the needle pointing downstream (antegrade) as in Figure 15-9A. In other instances, the case will be best managed with a high cannulation and the needle pointing upstream (retrograde). Remember that not all cases can be handled with a single cannulation.

2. Cannulate the fistula according to the plan developed from your physical examination. Cannulate with a micropuncture needle.

3. Perform an angiogram (Figure 15-14A) in order to identify the pathology and determine if significant thrombus is present. (It is important that the angiogram be done very carefully. It is possible to push clots back into the artery. It should be done slowly watching for any evidence of retrograde flow that, if seen, is a sure indication for stopping.) If there is a significant amount of clot, use of tPA may be indicated. In most instances, very little or no thrombus will be evident. The usual problem is venous stenosis, which may be very severe. At times it is difficult to unravel the relationships because of numerous collaterals.

4. Attempt to pass a guidewire through the dilator of the micropuncture set. If the cannulation is antegrade, attempt to pass the guidewire up to the upper arm. If it is retrograde, attempt to pass the guidewire downward to the anastomosis. You will need to go both directions before the procedure is over.

5. Once the guidewire is positioned, insert a 6-French sheath.

6. Pass a 5-French vascular catheter up to the level of the central veins and perform an angiogram.

7. Administer 5000 units of heparin and the sedation/analgesia medication that is to be used. This has to be done in such a manner that it gets into the circulation.

8. Then pull the catheter back to the level of the fistula and perform an angiogram as you do so to evaluate the draining veins.

9. Select the appropriate size angioplasty balloon and dilate the lesion (Figures 15-14B, C).

10. Recheck the angiogram to evaluate the result (Figure 15-14D). Often this is all that is necessary. If additional work is required, it will be apparent from the angiogram.

11. At some point in the procedure, the opportune time will vary, check the feeding artery and the arterial anastomosis by performing an angiogram via a 5-French catheter passed across the anastomosis.

12. Obtain hemostasis.

Thrombolysis procedure for AVF thrombosis using tPA. In some cases there is significant thrombus present. In these cases, incorporate tPA into the procedure. This procedure is described for a radial-cephalic AVF. If the AVF is in the upper arm, appropriate modifications will obviously need to be made.

1. Do a careful physical examination of the dysfunctional fistula. Try to determine the location of the problem and plan your approach. In most cases the thrombus will be in the lower fistula; this is best approached from above with a retrograde or upstream cannulation.

2. Cannulate the fistula according to the plan developed from your physical examination. Cannulate using a micropuncture needle.

3. Perform an angiogram in order to identify the pathology that is present and determine the amount and location of the thrombus. (It is important that the angiogram be done very carefully. It is possible to push clots back into the artery. It should be done slowly watching for any evidence of retrograde flow that, if seen, is a sure indication for stopping.)

4. Administer 5000 units of heparin and the sedation/analgesia medication that is to be used. This has to be done in such a manner that it gets into the circulation.

5. Attempt to pass a guidewire through the dilator of the micropuncture set. If the cannulation is antegrade, attempt to pass the guidewire up to the upper arm. If it is retrograde, attempt to pass the guidewire downward to the anastomosis.

6. Once the guidewire is positioned, insert a 6-French sheath.

7. Place a tourniquet slightly below the elbow. Adjust it so that it is tight. This is important to arrest flow and hold the lytic agent stationary long enough to allow it to act.

8. Instill the tPA. In most cases 2 mg (Cathflo®, Genentech, Inc., San Francisco, CA) diluted with 2–5 cc saline will be adequate. How this is done will depend on where the thrombus is located in relationship to the sheath. It may be possible to inject it directly through the sheath. Often it is best done through a 5-French straight catheter. The catheter should be positioned adjacent to the thrombus.

9. Manually massage the fistula along its entire length starting at the arterial anastomosis to macerate the clot and mix in the tPA. Within minutes you should begin to feel a pulse in the fistula above the thrombus.

10. Treat any stenotic lesions that are present.

11. Perform a final angiogram.

12. At some point in the procedure, the opportune time will vary, check the feeding artery and the arterial anastomosis by performing an angiogram via a 5-French catheter passed across the anastomosis. Also check the venous drainage up through the central veins.

13. Obtain hemostasis.

Thrombolysis procedure for AVF thrombosis using thromboaspiration. In cases where a larger amount of thrombus is present, a thromboaspiration using one or two (crossed) sheaths may be advantageous (Figure 15-15).

1. Do a careful physical examination of the dysfunctional fistula. Try to determine the location of the problem and plan your approach.

2. Cannulate the fistula according to the plan developed from your physical examination. Cannulate using a micropuncture needle.

3. Perform an angiogram in order to identify the pathology that is present and determine the amount and location of the thrombus (Figure 15-15A). (It is important that the angiogram be done very carefully. It is possible to push clots back into the artery. It should be done slowly watching for any evidence of retrograde flow that, if seen, is a sure indication for stopping.)

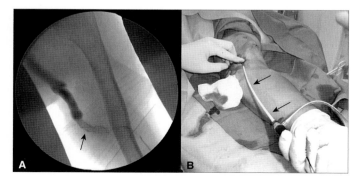

Figure 15-15. Thromboaspiration of an AVF. (**A**) Agiogram of AVF showing thrombus (arrow). (**B**) Use of 25 cm 9F sheath (arrows) to aspirate thrombus.

4. Administer 5000 units of heparin and the sedation/analgesia medication that is to be used. This has to be done in such a manner that it gets into the circulation.

5. Attempt to pass a guidewire through the dilator of the micropuncture set. If the cannulation is antegrade, attempt to pass the guidewire up to the upper arm. If it is retrograde, attempt to pass the guidewire downward to the anastomosis. You will need to go both directions in some cases. In others in may be possible to access all the thrombus for aspiration from a single cannulation.

6. Once a guidewire is in place insert a 7–9-French Brite-tip Sheath™ (Cordis, Bridgewater, NJ) over the guidewire (Figure 15-15B).

7. Remove the dilator, but leave it on the guidewire. Attach a 30–50-cc syringe to the side arm of the sheath and aspirate clot as you move in and out along the fistula. When the sheath becomes occluded with clot, remove it and flush. Then reinsert it using the dilator that has been kept in readiness on the guidewire. You may have to go both directions depending upon the distribution of the clot that is present.

8. Once the fistula is clear of thrombus, treat any stenosis that is present.

9. Perform a final angiogram.

10. At some point in the procedure, the opportune time will vary, check the feeding artery and the arterial anastomosis by performing an angiogram via a 5-French catheter passed across the anastomosis. Also check the venous drainage up through the central veins.

11. Obtain hemostasis.

▶ Initial Success of AVF Thrombectomy

Initial success in the reported treatment of thrombosed AVFs has ranged from 88% to 100%.[103–108] Primary patency rates ranging from 20% to 56% at 6 months and 27% to 40% at 1 year have been reported (Figure 15-16). Secondary patency rates of 54–83% and 51–80% have been documented for 6 month and 1 year follow-ups, respectively.[54,56,100,102–104] This data is significantly better than that reported for the treatment of thrombosed synthetic grafts.[114]

AVFs can have very large clot volumes in some instances. This is especially true for the large dilated aneurysmal AVF, at times referred to as a "mega-fistula." Some of these can have over 200 mL of thrombus. The wisdom of treating such a case by endovascular means should be seriously questioned. There is a significant risk of pulmonary embolism that may be associated with disastrous results.

Surgical therapy for the thrombosed AVF has also been advocated.[13,93,115–117] Success rates ranging from 70% to 90% have been documented. Primary patency rates ranging from 51% to 84% at 6 months and in the range of 75% at 1 year have been reported. Secondary patency rates of

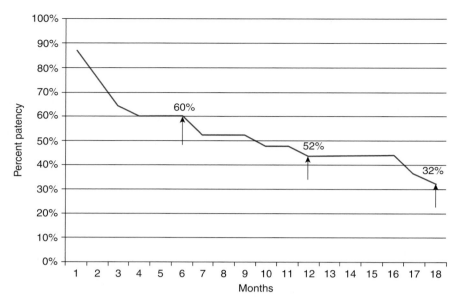

Figure 15-16. Figure 15-12 – Primary patency for thrombectomy in fistulas (n = 218).[95]

69–88% and in the range of 77% have been documented for 6 month and 1-year follow-ups, respectively. When these data are compared with that obtained with endovascular therapy, it is apparent that no significant difference exists for these two modalities.

► Complications

It is important to establish a systematic method to continuously assess and improve patient outcomes through an ongoing assessment of important aspects of the procedures performed based on quality, cost, and outcome. The best way to handle this is a good quality assurance program. Data is essential. Monitoring complication rates is essential to this effort. The primary complications of endovascular thrombectomy are the same as those listed for venous angioplasty (see Chapter 17) in addition to a unique complication—peripheral arterial embolization. This adverse event occurs with a much lower frequency than is seen with thrombectomy of synthetic grafts (which is itself low). The reason for this is not totally clear but is thought to be related to the inflammatory nature of the thrombus in an AVF and the fact that it becomes attached to the vessel wall relatively early.

In a report that included a series of 228 fistula thrombectomy cases,[106] there were only three major complications. All were related to vein rupture. Two were grade 2 hematomas, which were salvaged. One access was lost due to a grade 3 hematoma. There were no instances of arterial embolization.

► Surgical Therapy for Thrombosed AVF

Surgical therapy for the thrombosed AVF has also been advocated.[13,93,115–117] Success rates ranging from 70% to 90% have been documented. Primary patency rates ranging

from 51% to 84% at 6 months and in the range of 75% at 1 year have been reported. Secondary patency rates of 69–88% and in the range of 77% have been documented for 6 month and 1-year follow-ups, respectively. When these data are compared with that obtained with endovascular therapy it is apparent that no significant difference exists for these two modalities.

REFERENCES

1. Feldman HI, Kobrin S, Wasserstein A. Hemodialysis vascular access morbidity. *J Am Soc Nephrol.* 1996;7:523.
2. Ascher E, Gade P, Hingorani A, et al. Changes in the practice of angioaccess surgery: impact of dialysis outcome and quality initiative recommendations. *J Vasc Surg.* 2000;31:84.
3. Allon M, Robbin ML. Increasing arteriovenous fistulas in hemodialysis patients: problems and solutions. *Kidney Int.* 2002;62:1109.
4. Dixon BS, Novak L, Fangman J. Hemodialysis vascular access survival: upper-arm native arteriovenous fistula. *Am J Kidney Dis* 2002;39:92.
5. Anel RL, Yevzlin AS, Ivanovich P. Vascular access and patient outcomes in hemodialysis: questions answered in recent literature. *Artif Organs.* 2003;27:237.
6. Huber TS, Carter JW, Carter RL, Seeger JM. Patency of autogenous and polytetrafluoroethylene upper extremity arteriovenous hemodialysis accesses: a systematic review. *J Vasc Surg.* 2003;38:1005.
7. Pisoni RL. Vascular access use and outcomes: results from the DOPPS. *Contrib Nephrol.* 2002;13:252–264.
8. Pisoni RL, Young EW, Dykstra DM, et al. Vascular access use in Europe and the United States: results from the DOPPS. *Kidney Int.* 2002;61:305.
9. Ethier J, Mendelssohn DC, Elder SJ, et al. Vascular access use and outcomes: an international perspective from the

Dialysis Outcomes and Practice Patterns Study. *Nephrol Dial Transplant.* 2008;23:3219.

10. Ethier JH, Lindsay RM, Barre PE, et al. Clinical practice guidelines for vascular access. Canadian Society of Nephrology. *J Am Soc Nephrol.* 1999;10(suppl 13):S297.

11. Bradbury BD, Chen F, Furniss A, et al. Conversion of vascular access type among incident hemodialysis patients: description and association with mortality. *Am J Kidney Dis.* 2009;53:804.

12. Asif A, Roy-Chaudhury P, Beathard GA. Early arteriovenous fistula failure: a logical proposal for when and how to intervene. *Clin J Am Soc Nephrol.* 2006;1:332.

13. Tordoir JH, Rooyens P, Dammers R, et al. Prospective evaluation of failure modes in autogenous radiocephalic wrist access for haemodialysis. *Nephrol Dial Transplant.* 2003;18:378.

14. Corpataux JM, Haesler E, Silacci P, et al. Low-pressure environment and remodelling of the forearm vein in Brescia-Cimino haemodialysis access. *Nephrol Dial Transplant.* 2002;17:1057.

15. Kamiya A, Togawa T. Adaptive regulation of wall shear stress to flow change in the canine carotid artery. *Am J Physiol.* 1980;239:H14.

16. Zarins CK, Zatina MA, Giddens DP, et al. Shear stress regulation of artery lumen diameter in experimental atherogenesis. *J Vasc Surg.* 1987;5:413.

17. Ballermann BJ, Dardik A, Eng E, Liu A. Shear stress and the endothelium. *Kidney Int Suppl.* 1998;67:S100.

18. Paszkowiak JJ, Dardik A. Arterial wall shear stress: observations from the bench to the bedside. *Vasc Endovascular Surg.* 2003;37:47.

19. Papaioannou TG, Stefanadis C. Vascular wall shear stress: basic principles and methods. *Hellenic J Cardiol.* 2005;46:9.

20. Beathard GA, Arnold P, Jackson J, Litchfield T. Aggressive treatment of early fistula failure. *Kidney Int.* 2003;64:1487.

21. Dember LM, Beck GJ, Allon M, et al. Effect of clopidogrel on early failure of arteriovenous fistulas for hemodialysis: a randomized controlled trial. *JAMA* 2008;299:2164.

22. Hodges TC, Fillinger MF, Zwolak RM, et al. Longitudinal comparison of dialysis access methods: risk factors for failure. *J Vasc Surg.* 1997;26:1009.

23. Kalman PG, Pope M, Bhola C, et al. A practical approach to vascular access for hemodialysis and predictors of success. *J Vasc Surg.* 1999;30:727.

24. Huber TS, Ozaki CK, Flynn TC, et al. Prospective validation of an algorithm to maximize native arteriovenous fistulae for chronic hemodialysis access. *J Vasc Surg.* 2002;36:452.

25. Lok CE, Oliver MJ. Overcoming barriers to arteriovenous fistula creation and use. *Semin Dial.* 2003;16:189.

26. Ernandez T, Saudan P, Berney T, et al. Risk factors for early failure of native arteriovenous fistulas. *Nephron Clin Pract.* 2005;101:c39.

27. Patel ST, Hughes J, Mills JL, Sr. Failure of arteriovenous fistula maturation: an unintended consequence of exceeding dialysis outcome quality Initiative guidelines for hemodialysis access. *J Vasc Surg.* 2003;38:439.

28. Lok CE, Allon M, Moist L, et al. Risk equation determining unsuccessful cannulation events and failure to maturation in arteriovenous fistulas (REDUCE FTM I). *J Am Soc Nephrol.* 2006;17:3204.

29. Robbin ML, Chamberlain NE, Lockhart ME, et al. Hemodialysis arteriovenous fistula maturity: US evaluation. *Radiology.* 2002;225:59.

30. Brescia MJ, Cimino JE, Appel K, Hurwich BJ. Chronic hemodialysis using venipuncture and a surgically created arteriovenous fistula. *N Engl J Med.* 1966;275:1089.

31. Mendelssohn DC, Ethier J, Elder SJ, et al. Haemodialysis vascular access problems in Canada: results from the Dialysis Outcomes and Practice Patterns Study (DOPPS II). *Nephrol Dial Transplant.* 2006;21:721.

32. Woods JD, Turenne MN, Strawderman RL, et al. Vascular access survival among incident hemodialysis patients in the United States. *Am J Kidney Dis.* 1997;30:50.

33. O'Hare AM, Dudley RA, Hynes DM, et al. Impact of surgeon and surgical center characteristics on choice of permanent vascular access. *Kidney Int.* 2003;64:681.

34. Choi KL, Salman L, Krishnamurthy G, et al. Impact of surgeon selection on access placement and survival following preoperative mapping in the "Fistula First" era. *Semin Dial.* 2008;21:341.

35. Saran R, Elder SJ, Goodkin DA, et al. Enhanced training in vascular access creation predicts arteriovenous fistula placement and patency in hemodialysis patients: results from the Dialysis Outcomes and Practice Patterns Study. *Ann Surg.* 2008;247:885.

36. He C, Charoenkul V, Kahn T, et al. Impact of the surgeon on the prevalence of arteriovenous fistulas. *ASAIO J.* 2002;48:39.

37. Marcus RJ, Marcus DA, Sureshkumar KK, et al. Gender differences in vascular access in hemodialysis patients in the United States: developing strategies for improving access outcome. *Gend Med.* 2007;4:193.

38. Kinnaert P, Vereerstraeten P, Toussaint C, Van Geertruyden J. Nine years' experience with internal arteriovenous fistulas for haemodialysis: a study of some factors influencing the results. *Br J Surg.* 1977;64:242.

39. Thomsen MB, Deurell SI, Elfstrom J, Alm A. What causes the failures in surgically constructed arteriovenous fistulas? *Acta Chir Scand.* 1983;149:371.

40. Peterson WJ, Barker J, Allon M. Disparities in fistula maturation persist despite preoperative vascular mapping. *Clin J Am Soc Nephrol.* 2008;3:437.

41. Obialo CI, Tagoe AT, Martin PC, Asche-Crowe PE. Adequacy and survival of autogenous arteriovenous fistula in African American hemodialysis patients. *ASAIO J.* 2003;49:435.

42. Lazarides MK, Georgiadis GS, Antoniou GA, Staramos DN. A meta-analysis of dialysis access outcome in elderly patients. *J Vasc Surg.* 2007;45:420.

43. Chan MR, Young HN, Becker YT, Yevzlin AS. Obesity as a predictor of vascular access outcomes: analysis of the USRDS DMMS Wave II study. *Semin Dial.* 2008; 21:274.

44. Goldfarb-Rumyantzev AS, Rout P. Characteristics of elderly patients with diabetes and end-stage renal disease. *Semin Dial.* 2010;23:185.

45. Chemla ES, Morsy MA. Is basilic vein transposition a real alternative to an arteriovenous bypass graft? A prospective study. *Semin Dial.* 2008;21:352.

46. Maya ID, O'Neal JC, Young CJ, et al. Outcomes of brachiocephalic fistulas, transposed brachiobasilic fistulas, and upper arm grafts. *Clin J Am Soc Nephrol.* 2009;4:86.

47. Hakaim AG, Nalbandian M, Scott T. Superior maturation and patency of primary brachiocephalic and transposed basilic vein arteriovenous fistulae in patients with diabetes. *J Vasc Surg*. 1998;27:154.

48. Moossavi S, Tuttle AB, Vachharajani TJ, et al. Long-term outcomes of transposed basilic vein arteriovenous fistulae. *Hemodial Int*. 2008;12:80.

49. Oliver MJ, McCann RL, Indridason OS, et al. Comparison of transposed brachiobasilic fistulas to upper arm grafts and brachiocephalic fistulas. *Kidney Int*. 2001;60:1532.

50. Silva MB, Jr., Hobson RW, 2nd, Pappas PJ, et al. Vein transposition in the forearm for autogenous hemodialysis access. *J Vasc Surg*. 1997;26:981.

51. Silva MB, Jr., Hobson RW, 2nd, Pappas PJ, et al. A strategy for increasing use of autogenous hemodialysis access procedures: impact of preoperative noninvasive evaluation. *J Vasc Surg*. 1998;27:302.

52. Ascher E, Hingorani A, Yorkovich W. *Techniques and Outcome after Brachiocephalic and Brachiobasilic Arteriovenous Fistula Creation*, New York: Lippincott, Williams & Wilkins, 2002.

53. Moncef G. Surgical revision of failing or thrombosed native arteriovenous fistulas: a single center experience. *Saudi J Kidney Dis Transpl*. 2010;21:258.

54. Turmel-Rodrigues L, Mouton A, Birmele B, et al. Salvage of immature forearm fistulas for haemodialysis by interventional radiology. *Nephrol Dial Transplant*. 2001;16:2365.

55. Nassar GM, Nguyen B, Rhee E, Achkar K. Endovascular treatment of the "failing to mature" arteriovenous fistula. *Clin J Am Soc Nephrol*. 2006;1:275.

56. Poulain F, Raynaud A, Bourquelot P, et al. Local thrombolysis and thromboaspiration in the treatment of acutely thrombosed arteriovenous hemodialysis fistulas. *Cardiovasc Intervent Radiol* 1991;14:98.

57. Duijm LE, Liem YS, van der Rijt RH, et al. Inflow stenoses in dysfunctional hemodialysis access fistulae and grafts. *Am J Kidney Dis*. 2006;48:98.

58. Beathard GA, Settle SM, Shields MW. Salvage of the nonfunctioning arteriovenous fistula. *Am J Kidney Dis*. 1999;33:910.

59. Clark TW, Cohen RA, Kwak A, et al. Salvage of nonmaturing native fistulas by using angioplasty. *Radiology*. 2007;242:286.

60. Falk A. Maintenance and salvage of arteriovenous fistulas. *J Vasc Interv Radiol*. 2006;17:807.

61. Manninen HI, Kaukanen E, Makinen K, Karhapaa P. Endovascular salvage of nonmaturing autogenous hemodialysis fistulas: comparison with endovascular therapy of failing mature fistulas. *J Vasc Interv Radiol*. 2008;19:870.

62. Shin SW, Do YS, Choo SW, et al. Salvage of immature arteriovenous fistulas with percutaneous transluminal angioplasty. *Cardiovasc Intervent Radiol*. 2005;28:434.

63. Faiyaz R, Abreo K, Zaman F, et al. Salvage of poorly developed arteriovenous fistulae with percutaneous ligation of accessory veins. *Am J Kidney Dis*. 2002; 39:824.

64. Planken RN, Duijm LE, Kessels AG, et al. Accessory veins and radial-cephalic arteriovenous fistula non-maturation: a prospective analysis using contrast-enhanced magnetic resonance angiography. *J Vasc Access*. 2007;8:281.

65. Asif A, Gadalean FN, Merrill D, et al. Inflow stenosis in arteriovenous fistulas and grafts: a multicenter, prospective study. *Kidney Int*. 2005;67:1986.

66. CMS: National Vascular Access Improvement Initiative.

67. NKF-K/DOQI Clinical Practice Guidelines For Vascular Access. Clinical Practice Guideline 5. Treatment of AVF complications 5.1.2 A program should be in place to detect early access dysfunction.

68. Malovrh M. Non-matured arteriovenous fistulae for haemodialysis: diagnosis, endovascular and surgical treatment. *Bosn J Basic Med Sci*. 2010;10(suppl 1):S13.

69. Beathard GA. An algorithm for the physical examination of early fistula failure. *Semin Dial*. 2005;18:331.

70. Migliacci R, Selli ML, Falcinelli F, et al. Assessment of occlusion of the vascular access in patients on chronic hemodialysis: comparison of physical examination with continuous-wave Doppler ultrasound. STOP Investigators. Shunt Thrombotic Occlusion Prevention with Picotamide. *Nephron*. 1999;82:7.

71. Leon C, Asif A. Physical examination of arteriovenous fistulae by a renal fellow: does it compare favorably to an experienced interventionalist? *Semin Dial*. 2008;21:557.

72. Leon C, Orozco-Vargas LC, Krishnamurthy G, et al. Accuracy of physical examination in the detection of arteriovenous graft stenosis. *Semin Dial*. 2008;21:85.

73. Falk A, Teodorescu V, Lou WY, et al. Treatment of "swing point stenoses" in hemodialysis arteriovenous fistulae. *Clin Nephrol*. 2003;60:35.

74. Badero OJ, Salifu MO, Wasse H, Work J. Frequency of swing-segment stenosis in referred dialysis patients with angiographically documented lesions. *Am J Kidney Dis*. 2008;51:93.

75. Wong V, Ward R, Taylor J, et al. Factors associated with early failure of arteriovenous fistulae for haemodialysis access. *Eur J Vasc Endovasc Surg*. 1996;12:207.

76. Seyahi N, Altiparmak MR, Tascilar K, et al. Ultrasonographic maturation of native arteriovenous fistulae: a follow-up study. *Ren Fail*. 2007;29:481.

77. Back MR, Maynard M, Winkler A, Bandyk DF. Expected flow parameters within hemodialysis access and selection for remedial intervention of nonmaturing conduits. *Vasc Endovascular Surg*. 2008;42:150.

78. Berman SS, Mendoza B, Westerband A, Quick RC. Predicting arteriovenous fistula maturation with intraoperative blood flow measurements. *J Vasc Access*. 2008;9:241.

79. Salman L, Ladino M, Alex M, et al. Accuracy of ultrasound in the detection of inflow stenosis of arteriovenous fistulae: results of a prospective study. *Semin Dial*. 2010;23:117.

80. Asif A, Cherla G, Merrill D, et al. Venous mapping using venography and the risk of radiocontrast-induced nephropathy. *Semin Dial*. 2005;18:239.

81. Kian K, Wyatt C, Schon D, et al. Safety of low-dose radiocontrast for interventional AV fistula salvage in stage 4 chronic kidney disease patients. *Kidney Int*. 2006;69:1444.

82. Beathard G. Physical examination of the dialysis vascular access. *Semin Dial*. 1998;11:231.

83. Chen MC, Chang SC, Weng MJ, et al. Use of angioplasty balloon-assisted Seldinger technique for complicated small vessel catheterization. *J Vasc Interv Radiol*. 2006;17:2011.

84. Duijm LE, van der Rijt RH, Cuypers PW, et al. Outpatient treatment of arterial inflow stenoses of dysfunctional hemodialysis access fistulas by retrograde venous access puncture and catheterization. *J Vasc Surg*. 2008;47:591.

85. Salman L, Asif A, Beathard GA. Retrograde angiography and the risk of arteriovenous fistula perforation. *Semin Dial*. 2009;22:698.

86. Trerotola SO, Kwak A, Clark TW, et al. Prospective study of balloon inflation pressures and other technical aspects of hemodialysis access angioplasty. *J Vasc Interv Radiol*. 2005;16:1613.

87. Ahmad I. Salvage of arteriovenous fistula by angioplasty of collateral veins establishing a new channel. *J Vasc Access*. 2007;8:123.

88. De Marco Garcia LP, Davila-Santini LR, Feng Q, et al. Primary balloon angioplasty plus balloon angioplasty maturation to upgrade small-caliber veins (<3 mm) for arteriovenous fistulas. *J Vasc Surg*. 2010;52:139.

89. Raynaud A, Novelli L, Bourquelot P, et al. Low-flow maturation failure of distal accesses: treatment by angioplasty of forearm arteries. *J Vasc Surg*. 2009;49:995.

90. Ohira S, Kon T, Imura T. Evaluation of primary failure in native AV-fistulae (early fistula failure). *Hemodial Int*. 2006;10:173.

91. Allon M, Lockhart ME, Lilly RZ, et al. Effect of preoperative sonographic mapping on vascular access outcomes in hemodialysis patients. *Kidney Int*. 2001;60:2013.

92. Gibson KD, Caps MT, Kohler TR, et al. Assessment of a policy to reduce placement of prosthetic hemodialysis access. *Kidney Int*. 2001;59:2335.

93. Romero A, Polo JR, Garcia Morato E, et al. Salvage of angioaccess after late thrombosis of radiocephalic fistulas for hemodialysis. *Int Surg*. 1986;71:122.

94. Fistula First. Change concept 4. http://fistulafirst.org/Professionals/FFBIChangeConcepts.aspx (accessed 1-10-2012).

95. Beathard G. Results of endovascular treatment of venous stenosis and thrombosis in fistulas. In: (unpublished data).

96. Bakran A, Mickley V, Passlick-Deetjen J. *Management of the Renal Patient: Clinical Algorithms on Vascular Access for Hemodialysis*, Lengerich, Berlin, Bremen, Miami, Riga, Viernheim, Wien, Zagreb: Pabst Science Publishers, 2003.

97. Schwarz C, Mitterbauer C, Boczula M, et al. Flow monitoring: performance characteristics of ultrasound dilution versus color Doppler ultrasound compared with fistulography. *Am J Kidney Dis*. 2003;42:539.

98. Turmel-Rodrigues L, Pengloan J, Baudin S, et al. Treatment of stenosis and thrombosis in haemodialysis fistulas and grafts by interventional radiology. *Nephrol Dial Transplant*. 2000;15:2029.

99. Beathard G. Complications of vascular access. In *Complications of Dialysis—Recognition and Management*, Lameire N, Mehta R (Eds), New York: Marcel Dekker, Inc., 2000:1.

100. Haage P, Vorwerk D, Wildberger JE, et al. Percutaneous treatment of thrombosed primary arteriovenous hemodialysis access fistulae. *Kidney Int*. 2000;57:1169.

101. Chang CJ, Ko YS, Ko PJ, et al. Thrombosed arteriovenous fistula for hemodialysis access is characterized by a marked inflammatory activity. *Kidney Int*. 2005;68:1312.

102. Jain G, Maya ID, Allon M. Outcomes of percutaneous mechanical thrombectomy of arteriovenous fistulas in hemodialysis patients. *Semin Dial*. 2008;21:581.

103. Schon D, Mishler R. Salvage of occluded autologous arteriovenous fistulae. *Am J Kidney Dis*. 2000;36:804.

104. Schon D, Mishler R. Pharmacomechanical thrombolysis of natural vein fistulas: reduced dose of TPA and long-term follow-up. *Semin Dial*. 2003;16:272.

105. Turmel-Rodrigues L, Pengloan J, Rodrigue H, et al. Treatment of failed native arteriovenous fistulae for hemodialysis by interventional radiology. *Kidney Int*. 2000;57:1124.

106. Beathard GA, Litchfield T. Effectiveness and safety of dialysis vascular access procedures performed by interventional nephrologists. *Kidney Int*. 2004;66:1622.

107. Huang HL, Chen CC, Chang SH, et al. Combination of duplex ultrasound-guided manual declotting and percutaneous transluminal angioplasty in thrombosed native dialysis fistulas. *Ren Fail*. 2005;27:713.

108. Shatsky JB, Berns JS, Clark TW, et al. Single-center experience with the Arrow-Trerotola Percutaneous Thrombectomy Device in the management of thrombosed native dialysis fistulas. *J Vasc Interv Radiol*. 2005;16:1605.

109. Schilling JJ, Eiser AR, Slifkin RF, et al. The role of thrombolysis in hemodialysis access occlusion. *Am J Kidney Dis*. 1987;10:92.

110. Beathard GA. Mechanical versus pharmacomechanical thrombolysis for the treatment of thrombosed dialysis access grafts. *Kidney Int*. 1994;45:1401.

111. Trerotola SO, Johnson MS, Shah H, et al. Incidence and management of arterial emboli from hemodialysis graft surgical thrombectomy. *J Vasc Interv Radiol*. 1997;8:557.

112. Kinney TB, Valji K, Rose SC, et al. Pulmonary embolism from pulse-spray pharmacomechanical thrombolysis of clotted hemodialysis grafts: urokinase versus heparinized saline. *J Vasc Interv Radiol*. 2000;11:1143.

113. Bentaarit B, Duval AM, Maraval A, et al. Paradoxical embolism following thromboaspiration of an arteriovenous fistula thrombosis: a case report. *J Med Case Reports*. 2010;4:345.

114. Beathard GA, Welch BR, Maidment HJ. Mechanical thrombolysis for the treatment of thrombosed hemodialysis access grafts. *Radiology*. 1996;200:711.

115. Palmer RM, Cull DL, Kalbaugh C, et al. Is surgical thrombectomy to salvage failed autogenous arteriovenous fistulae worthwhile? *Am Surg*. 2006;72:1231.

116. Ponikvar R. Surgical salvage of thrombosed arteriovenous fistulas and grafts. *Ther Apher Dial*. 2005;9:245.

117. Lipari G, Tessitore N, Poli A, et al. Outcomes of surgical revision of stenosed and thrombosed forearm arteriovenous fistulae for haemodialysis. *Nephrol Dial Transplant*. 2007;22:2605.

16

ARTERIOVENOUS GRAFT STENOSIS AND THROMBOSIS

GERALD A. BEATHARD

1. Discuss the means by which a vessel is judged to be stenotic.
2. Discuss the frequency of venous stenosis according to location.
3. Discuss the unique nature of the cephalic arch as it relates to venous stenosis.
4. Discuss the unique characteristics of central vein stenosis.
5. Discuss access inflow stenosis as it relates to the feeding artery, arterial anastomosis, and juxta-anastomotic portion of the access.
6. Discuss the frequency of thrombosis as it relates to a population of hemodialysis patients.
7. Discuss the causes of access thrombosis as it relates to anatomical lesions and precipitating causes.
8. Understand how monitoring and surveillance can be used to decrease the incidence of thrombosis in a population of hemodialysis patients.
9. Describe the nature of the thrombus that may be found within a thrombosed dialysis access graft as it relates to types and volume of thrombus.
10. Describe the requirements for treating a thrombosed graft whether the treatment be endovascular or surgical.
11. Discuss the relationship between planning for a secondary fistula and thrombosis of a dialysis access graft.
12. Discuss the treatment choices that are available for salvaging a thrombosed graft.
13. Discuss the contraindication to an endovascular thrombectomy procedure.
14. Discuss the considerations that are important in selecting cannulation sites for performing an endovascular thrombectomy.
15. Describe the details of performing a thrombectomy procedure using the thromboaspiration technique.
16. Describe the approach that one would take if it was not possible to pass a Fogarty catheter across the arterial anastomosis during thromboaspiration.
17. Describe the approach that one would take if it was not possible to restore flow to a dialysis access graft after a Fogarty catheter has been passed across the arterial anastomosis.
18. Discuss the implications and management of obtaining an intermittent pulse during the thromboaspiration procedure.
19. Describe the management of residual thrombus left after the thromboaspiration procedure.
20. Describe the problems created by the presence of a pseudoaneurysm in a thrombosed dialysis access graft.
21. Discuss the results that should be expected when performing thrombectomy procedures in a population of hemodialysis patients.
22. Discuss arterial embolization as a complication of endovascular thrombectomy as it relates to causes, diagnosis, significance, and management.

VENOUS STENOSIS

▶ Introduction

The most common complications associated with an arteriovenous graft (AVG) are venous stenosis and thrombosis. In most cases these two problems share the relationship of disease and symptom. The reported 1-year primary patency rate for AVGs is 40–50%, with a 2-year patency rate of approximately 25%.[1,2] Eight-five to 90% of all cases of graft thrombosis are associated with an anatomical lesion.[3]

The histology of venous stenosis has been well characterized as aggressive neointimal hyperplasia in both AV grafts and fistulas.[4-6] This lesion is characterized by (a) the presence of smooth muscle cells, (b) an abundance of extracellular matrix, (c) neovascularization within the neointima and adventitia, (d) a macrophage layer lining the perigraft region, and (e) an increased expression of mediators and cytokines such as TGF-β, PDGF, and endothelin within the media, neointima, and adventitia.[5,7] The net result of this process is a progressively enlarging pannus-like lesion that encroaches upon the lumen of the vessel causing a progressive increase in resistance and a decrease in flow. Eventually thrombosis occurs.

Events that are believed to contribute to the pathogenesis of neointimal hyperplasia include[8] (1) surgical trauma at the time of AV surgery, (2) abnormal shear stress at the vein-graft anastomosis, (3) bioincompatibility of the AV graft, (4) vessel injury due to dialysis needle punctures, and (5) uremia resulting in endothelial dysfunction. Although there are multiple possible causes or contributing factors, it appears that there are certain sites for which the lesion has a predilection (Figure 16-1).

▶ Diagnosis of Stenosis

The likelihood of a significant stenotic lesion can generally be suspected using data gained from monitoring and surveillance (see Chapter 13). Its presence can often be diagnosed with reasonable assurance using basic principles of physical examination (see Chapter 14). However, the interventionalist needs to have an objective method for determining the presence and degree of stenosis prior to initiating treatment. Within the dialysis circuit, there are vessels of various sizes. There is often a size discrepancy between the graft and the vein at the point of anastomosis. While there are methods for accurately gauging the size of a vascular structure, an essential task for research studies, for routine purposes, stenosis is adequately determined by size comparisons. The observed lesion is judged by the adjacent presumably normal vein or graft.

▶ Location of Venous Stenosis

Stenosis occurs most frequently at the venous anastomosis, but may occur anywhere within the system composed of the graft, the anastomosis, and its draining veins, both peripheral and central. In a review of 2300 cases of venous stenosis[9] (Figure 16-1), the following distribution of lesions was found: venous anastomosis 60%, peripheral vein 37.1%, within the graft 38.4%, central veins 3.2%, and multiple locations 31.3%.

Intragraft stenosis

Stenosis within the graft is not uniformly distributed. In loop grafts, the changes occur primarily on the venous side of the loop (Figure 16-2). In straight grafts, the involvement generally spares the portion of the graft immediately adjacent to the arterial anastomosis.[10] The lesions that occur within the graft are not related to neointimal hyperplasia. Many of these lesions are the result of the deposition of fibrin, lipid, and cellular debris within the graft. Additionally, it is probable that defects in the graft from repetitive dialysis needle puncture allow for some tissue ingrowth. The percentage of venous stenosis lesions reported here has varied from one-third[10] to only 2%.[11] The reasons for the differences is not clear but may be related to differences in the age of the AVGs.

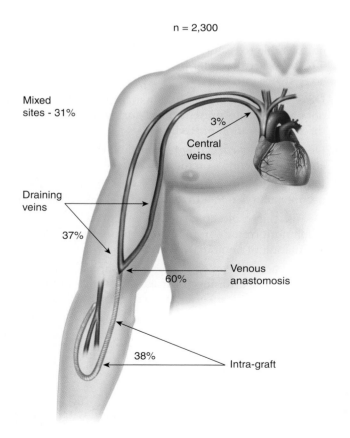

n = 2,300

Mixed sites - 31%

3%
Central veins

Draining veins

37%

60%

Venous anastomosis

38%

Intra-graft

Figure 16-1. Location of venous stenosis lesions (*n* = 2300).

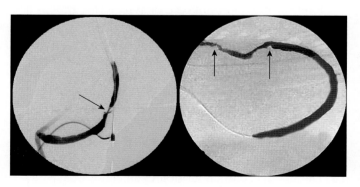

Figure 16-2. Intragraft stenosis (arrows).

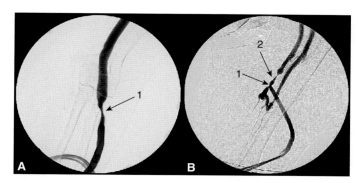

Figure 16-3. Anastomotic stenosis. (**A**) Lesion at anastomosis (1). (**B**) Lesion at anastomosis (1), and also in juxta-anastomotic portion of vein (2).

Venous anastomotic stenosis

The venous anastomosis is the most common site for stenosis to occur (Figure 16-3). This is generally the place when NH starts and is most active. The interface between the graft and the vein is commonly a site of turbulence. At least a part of this is thought to be due to the mismatch that occurs between the graft and the vein in size and configuration. This lesion may be associated with stenosis within the first portion of the vein (juxta-anastomotic) also. Approximately two-thirds of the venous stenosis lesions observed occur at the anastomosis.

Draining vein stenosis

In peripheral veins, stenosis may vary considerably in its location. There appears to be some predilection for lesions to occur in association with valves. Venous valves are associated with slight dilatations of the vein. With the increased pressure that occurs coincident with the establishment of flow from an AVG, the valve leaflets become continuously pressed against the vessel wall. It is possible that this creates turbulence and may play a role in the development of stenosis at that site. It was noted very early in the treatment

of these lesions that a significant number suggested the appearance of a stenotic valve (Figure 16-4) in that they were narrow, well-circumscribed and circumferential.[10] The lesion as described may actually represent the annulus of the valve that has become hypertrophied. These lesions are often very resistant to treatment. Lesions in the draining veins may consist of single or multiple short foci or long segments of the vein, at times in excess of 40 cm in length (Figure 16-5).[10]

Cephalic arch

The cephalic arch is particularly prone to the development of venous stenosis. It has been suggested that this is related to high blood flow rates through this unique vascular structure.[12] This area has been referred to as a "swing point"[13] in reference to the distinct angle that the vein makes before it joins the axillary to form the subclavian. This is an area with abnormal shear stress. Based upon studies performed with arteriovenous fistulas,[12,14,15] one would expect that the incidence of cephalic arch stenosis would be less in cases where all are a portion of the drainage from the access was routed through the basilic vein. By avoiding the cephalic arch in this manner, blood flow through that structure is reduced.

Central venous stenosis

The introduction of any foreign indwelling object into the central veins can lead to the development of central venous stenosis. The most common causative factor is the central venous catheter. In general, the frequency of central venous stenosis is directly proportional to the frequency of dialysis catheter usage. However, lesions do occur in the central veins in the absence of this etiology. Peripherally inserted central venous catheters[16,17] and transvenous leads associated with cardiac rhythm devices[18–26] are especially problematic.

Stenosis can involve the subclavian, brachiocephalic, superior vena cava or a combination when the upper

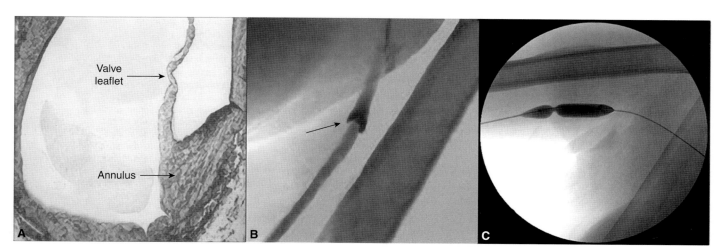

Figure 16-4. Venous valve. (**A**) Histology of valve. (**B**) Radiograph appearance of valve (arrow). (**C**) Radiographic appearance of lesion suspicious for being a stenotic valve.

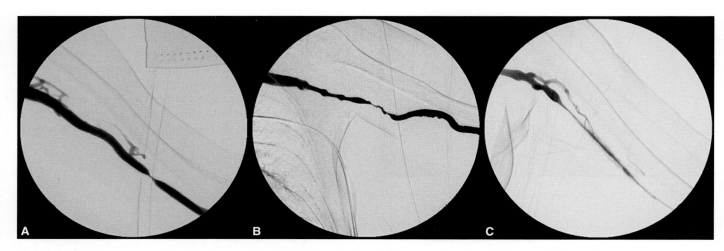

Figure 16-5. Venous stenosis affecting basilic vein. (**A**) Short lesion. (**B**) Intermediate length lesion. (**C**) Long lesion.

extremity is affected (Figure 16-6). In the lower extremity, both the iliac and the inferior vena cava or a combination can become stenotic. Not only can these lesions adversely affect the dialysis access, but they can also eventually become very symptomatic due to venous obstruction (see Chapter 32).

ARTERIAL STENOSIS

▶ Introduction

The dialysis vascular access should be thought of a complete circuit starting and ending with the heart. The venous side represents only one-half of the circuit, while the other half is arterial. Lesions in this region adversely affect inflow. These may be within any of the arteries that ultimately lead to the access or they can affect the arterial anastomosis, which is considered to be the arterial component of the access itself. Frequently these two types of lesions are reported together with juxta-anasto-

motic lesions as inflow stenosis. Reports of inflow stenosis in general have been in the range of 14–42%.[27–29] These lesions are easily treatable with angioplasty.[28,30,31]

A study of 40 patients with synthetic grafts reported that 11 cases (28%) had 13 arterial inflow lesions.[27] Ten of the lesions were at the arterial anastomosis, with two having stenoses in the brachial artery in addition. One patient had a single stenosis in the brachial artery. In another report,[28] a review of 122 dysfunctional arteriovenous grafts found inflow stenosis in 36 (29%) cases. These 36 cases involved 47 stenotic lesions. The distribution of these 47 lesions was 8 arterial (6.6% of total cases), 29 artery-graft anastomosis (23.8% of total cases), and 10 juxta-anastomotic (8.2% of total cases). Several cases had a lesion in more than one site.

▶ Feeding Artery Stenosis

Stenosis can occur in any of the arteries that ultimately lead to the access (Figure 16-7). These lesions result in

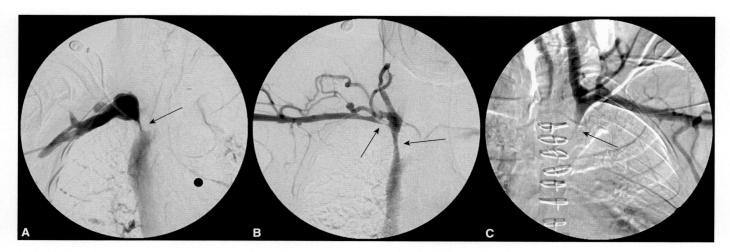

Figure 16-6. Central vein stenosis. (**A**) Right brachiocephalic lesion (arrow). (**B**) Combination of right subclavian and brachiocephalic (arrows). (**C**) Left brachiocephalic lesion (arrow).

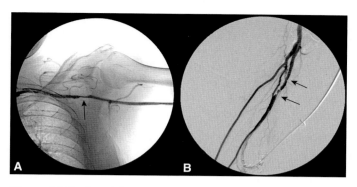

Figure 16-7. Arterial stenosis. (**A**) Lesion in axillary artery (arrow), (**B**) Lesion in radial artery (arrows).

a decrease in blood flow and pressure to the access and additionally, to the extremity beyond the arterial anastomosis. The criteria used for the diagnosis of stenosis are generally based upon a comparison with the adjacent vessel.[10,11,27,28,32,33] If it is less than 50% of the normal caliber, the lesion is classified as stenotic.

When the feeding artery is affected, the patient can develop ischemic problems in the distal extremity—hand and digits. In an evaluation of 12 patients with symptoms of steal syndrome, one report[34] documented arterial stenotic lesions in 10 of the cases (83%). Treatment of these lesions resulted in resolution of the ischemic syndrome.

▶ Arterial Anastomosis Stenosis

Arterial anastomotic stenosis is stenosis occurring at the junction of the artery with the synthetic graft material. While lesions in this area are not as commonly seen as is the case for the venous anastomosis, they do regularly occur as stated above. This type of stenosis can take one of several forms. It can involve just the anastomosis itself, the artery adjacent to the anastomosis, or both (Figure 16-8). The net effect of this lesion is poor blood flow in the access. Defining arterial anastomotic stenosis is difficult. This junction is artificially created and lacks an optimal standard. Its size is based upon the surgeon's judgment and

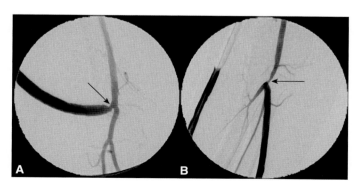

Figure 16-8. Arterial anastomosis stenosis. (**A**) Lesion is at anastomosis (arrow). (**B**) Lesion is in artery adjacent to anastomosis (arrow); note the collateral between the lesion and the graft.

is often smaller than the adjacent vessel. In addition, there is always a major drop in pressure across this site. The generally accepted criteria are based upon a comparison with the adjacent normal artery in the same manner as for the diagnosis of arterial stenosis. If the anastomosis is less than 50% the size of the adjacent normal artery, it is classified as stenotic.

THROMBOSIS

▶ Introduction

Thrombosis is the end result of venous stenosis in most instances. This is the most common complication associated with a synthetic dialysis access graft. It is generally 85–90%, associated with an anatomical lesion and 85% of graft loss occurs in conjunction with an episode of thrombosis.[3]

▶ Frequency of Thrombosis

To appreciate its frequency, one has to go back to a time when essentially no monitoring or surveillance was being done. Reports of that period indicated that the frequency of this event at that time was about 1–1.5 per patient per year.[3] However, this does not give a realistic picture because not all grafts thrombose with the same degree of frequency. In one study[35] a population of approximately 700 patients receiving dialysis via a synthetic graft was evaluated to determine the frequency of thrombosis over a period of 12 months for two consecutive years (Figure 16-9). Then overall thrombosis rate was approximately 1 per patient per year; however, it was found that in each of these two periods, only one-third of the cases actually experienced a thrombotic episode. Within this group, 40% had a single

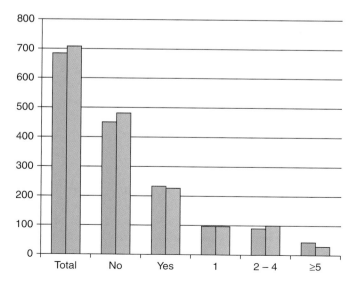

Figure 16-9. Frequency of thrombosis. Total: total number of cases, No: cases with no thrombosis, Yes: cases with at least one episode, 1: single episode, 2–4: two to four episodes, ≥5: five or more episodes.

episode, 40% had two to four episodes, and 20% had five or more. Some within this later group had more than 10 occurrences of graft thrombosis within the year. This suggests that there are individual differences that materially affect the frequency of this complication for certain patients.

Causes of Thrombosis

More than a century ago, Rudolph Virchow identified a triad of factors responsible for vascular thrombosis as vessel injury, alteration in blood flow, and changes in the coagulability of the blood. This is true for the clotting of a synthetic graft. Of all cases of graft thrombosis 85–90% are associated with an anatomical lesion,[3] neointimal hyperplasia leading to venous stenosis as stated above. These lesions cause progressively increasing resistance and a concomitant decrease in blood flow. However, access thrombosis can occur without anatomic abnormalities,[2,36] and there are other causes of decreased flow such as hypotension, hypovolemia, and excessive pressure to obtain hemostasis at the end of dialysis.[37] In addition, the patent may have a hypercoagulable state resulting or at least contributing to thrombosis of the access.[38,39]

The factors that relate to graft thrombosis in the dialysis patient can be divided into predisposing causes and precipitating causes. The basic predisposing cause in most instances is anatomical. The importance of this can be appreciated by noting the decrease in thrombosis rates that occur when venous stenosis is prospectively treated.[40–46] These lesions develop slowly and can exist for varying periods of time without thrombosis occurring. Nevertheless, the graft is predisposed to the event and when one of the precipitating events occurs, it happens.

The precipitating causes include hypotension, hypovolemia, and excessive pressure to obtain hemostasis at the end of dialysis. Over aggressive use of antihypertensive medications is a recurrent cause of graft thrombosis. A common scenario is the patient who takes his/her medications after dialysis to avoid blood pressure drops during the treatment, but leaves the dialysis clinic with a normal or low blood pressure. They go home, take their medication, lie down for a nap, and wake up with a thrombosed graft. Marked bradycardia is an occasional precipitating cause of recurrent thrombosis.

Prevention of Thrombosis

Monitoring and surveillance on a routine basis has been recommended as a strategy for decreasing the incidence of thrombosis through the prospective diagnosis of venous stenosis.[40–46] Population studies confirm that this is effective. Even when there is an apparent anatomical explanation for loss of patency within the graft, contributing factors should be sought with each thrombotic episode. Appropriately addressing the precipitating factor may be more effective prophylactically than treatment of the anatomical predisposing cause.

Although a variety of hypercoagulable states (thrombophilias) have been reported to cause graft thrombosis,[47–58] general screening for defects is not very cost effective due to their relatively low frequency. Therefore, the routine testing of dialysis patients for these disorders is not recommended. However, in a patient with frequent unexplained thrombosis, it may be worthwhile.

Nature of the Thrombus

The occluded graft contains two types of thrombus: a firm arterial plug and a variable amount of soft thrombus (Figure 16-10). Most of the clot is of the latter type. This is poorly organized red thrombus that is friable and disintegrates easily. The arterial plug consists of a firm, laminated, organizing thrombus that is found just downstream (antegrade) from the arterial anastomosis. This thrombus has a concave surface and forms a plug that is firmly attached to the wall of the graft at the point of maximum turbulence from the arterial inflow. It has been reported to be present (discoverable) in up to 73% of cases[59] treated percutaneously and has been reported to be resistant to enzyme lysis.[59,60]

The volume of actual clot that is present within a graft is frequently overestimated. If one calculates the maximum clot volume that is possible (Table 16-1), it is found to be rather small.

It has been determined from surgical specimens that the total clot volume for grafts measuring 30 to more than 50 cm (mean = 42 cm) averages only 3.2 mL in volume; this includes the arterial plug.[61] Some grafts have pseudoaneurysms. These anomalous structures are frequently lined with laminated, organized thrombus. In a patient with large pseudoaneurysms that are very firm, the clot load within the thrombosed graft may be quite large.

Treatment of Arteriovenous Graft Thrombosis

The management of access thrombosis should incorporate certain essential elements for which there should be no compromise (Table 16-2). Treatment must be timely, not delayed, and central venous catheters should be avoided. Angiography to detect venous stenotic lesions should be considered mandatory. Venous stenosis must be corrected and all abnormal hemodynamic parameters present prior to thrombosis should return to normal.[62] Although the procedure can be easily performed in the inpatient or outpatient setting, routine hospitalization for management of graft thrombosis should be avoided.

The goals in promulgating these principles are several: patient welfare, patient comfort, best medical practices (evidence based), and economy. The necessity for their promulgation is based upon the fact that they have not been followed in many locales in the past. Additionally, if a thrombosed graft is not addressed in a timely manner, it will, in most instances, become more difficult and eventually impossible to open. There are anecdotal cases where a graft has been opened after a prolonged period,[63,64] even several

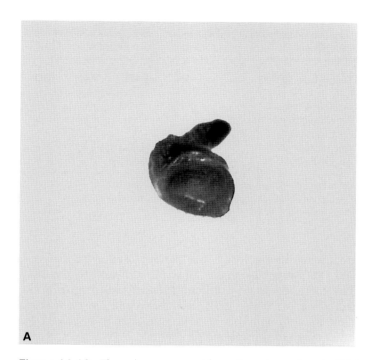
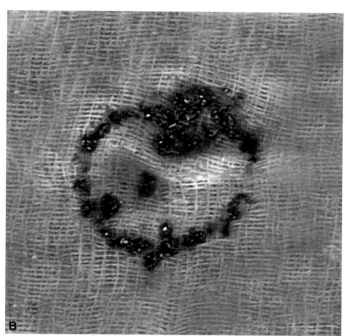

Figure 16-10. Thrombus removed from thrombosed graft. (**A**) Arterial plug, notice concave surface. (**B**) Clot fragments from thrombosed graft.

years; however, these are unusual cases and the successful results reported are not to be expected in routine cases. In general once a graft has been left untreated for more than a week, it becomes increasingly more difficult to open.

Additionally, every thrombosed access case should be evaluated for a secondary arteriovenous fistula, that is, a fistula created using upper arm veins that have become dilated because of the presence of the graft.[65] The algorithm that should be followed is shown in Figure 16-11. With the first episode of graft dysfunction, either stenosis or thrombosis, the patient should have a salvage procedure and should also have vascular mapping to evaluate the prospects for a secondary fistula. Most of the necessary information for mapping is actually obtained in the routine conduct of the procedure. With the second episode, unless the time interval is especially long, the case should be referred for conversion to a fistula. If this is not possible, then surgical revision should be considered if the problem is anatomical.

▶ Treatment Choices

There are two choices for the treatment of the thrombosed graft: surgical and endovascular. Endovascular therapy fits the strategy described above very well and has come to be regarded as the standard in many localities. In a study that compared 237 cases treated with endovascular thrombectomy with 229 receiving surgical therapy, percutaneous management gave results equivalent to surgical thrombectomy with revision and superior to simple thrombectomy.[35] However, either modality is acceptable as long as the basic principles outlined above (Table 16-2) can be adhered to.

▶ Endovascular Thrombectomy

Endovascular therapy may be divided into two general categories: enzyme-mediated thrombolysis and endovascular thrombectomy using mechanical means (Tables 16-3 and 16-4).

TABLE 16–1
Considerations on Clot Volume in a Graft
Assume a graft of 40 cm with an average diameter of 7 mm Graft volume = (Vol = $L \times \pi R^2$) or 40 cm × (3.14) × (0.35 × 0.35) cm = 15.4 cc
If a solid clot forms in a 15.4 cc graft in a patient with a hematocrit of 35%, then:
Maximum possible clot volume is 15.4 cc × 0.35 = 5.4 cc This would be the maximum possible unless the clot extends outside of the graft.

TABLE 16–2
Requirements for Treating Thrombosed Dialysis Access Graft
• Treatment must be timely • Central venous catheters should be avoided • Angiography to detect venous stenotic lesions is mandatory • Venous stenosis must be corrected • Abnormal hemodynamic parameters should return to normal • Cases should be handled as outpatients • Routine hospitalization must be avoided • Every case must be evaluated for a secondary native fistula

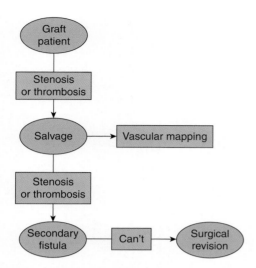

Figure 16-11. Algorithm for management of recurrent thrombosis.

TABLE 16–4

Comparison of Techniques for Endovascular Therapy

Technique	PT	PMT	TA	MD
Lytic enzyme	+++	++	−−	−−
Mechanical maceration	−−	++	++	++
Clot removal	−	−	++	++
Angiography	−	++	++	++
Angioplasty	−	++	++	++

Abbreviations: PT, pharmacological thrombolysis; PMT, pharmacomechanical thrombolysis; TA, thromboaspiration; MD, mechanical device.

During its history, three different fibrinolytic enzymes have been use to lyse thrombus occluding the dialysis access: streptokinase, urokinase, and tissue plasminogen activator (tPA). Streptokinase has been associated with an erratic response, drug resistance, and allergic reactions.[66] Urokinase was removed from the market for a period of time during which tPA was the only lytic agent available. Now that it is once more available, it is used very little because tPA appears to have definite advantages.[59,60,67]

Based upon the mechanism used and the overall procedure applied to the thrombosed access graft, the endovascular treatment of the thrombosed graft can be divided into four general categories. The general features characteristic of each of these is shown in Table 16-4. Enzyme-mediated thrombolysis can be divided into two categories: pharmacological and pharmacomechanical. Mechanical thrombolysis can be divided into a type that uses a mechanical device and one which relies primary on clot maceration and aspiration (thromboaspiration). The attributes of each of these are discussed below.

Pharmacological thrombolysis (PT)

This refers to thrombus dissolution using only the effects of a fibrinolytic enzyme. The enzyme is infused over a prolonged period of time. This is associated with poor results, a high complication rate, a prolonged period of

TABLE 16–3

Endovascular Treatment of Thrombosed Dialysis Access Grafts

- Enzyme lysis
  - Pharmacological thrombolysis
  - Pharmacomechanical thrombolysis
- Mechanical methods
  - Thromboaspiration (mechanical thrombolysis)
  - Mechanical devices

treatment during which the patient cannot be dialyzed, and the patient generally must be admitted to the ICU. This method was very difficult (dangerous) to apply in the treatment of dialysis graft thrombosis and has been abandoned[66] although this general approach is still used for other types of thrombotic problems.

A variant of this technique referred to as "lyse and wait" is widely used.[68,69] According to this technique, lytic agent is injected into the thrombosed graft through an angiocatheter needle. It is then allowed to dwell for a period of time that ranges from a few minutes to over an hour. It is stated that during this period, there is a return of the pulse within the graft in many cases. The patient is then taken into the procedure room for the remainder of the treatment that ranges from only an angioplasty to treat an anatomical lesion to the completion of the thrombectomy procedure. In either instance, the final procedure required is deemed to be easier than it would have been without the use of the thrombolytic agent.[70]

Pharmacomechanical thrombolysis (PMT)

This technique combines angiography, angioplasty, and thrombolysis. The clot is macerated and enzyme is administered directly into the clot, generally using a pulse-spray catheter.[59] The technique can be accomplished quickly, and is safe and effective. It does have the added expense of the enzyme and is no more effective than the less expensive mechanical methods.[66] It has also been largely abandoned in the treatment of dialysis vascular access.

Thromboaspiration (TA)

This technique has been referred to as mechanical thrombolysis in the past. It also combines the procedures of angiography, angioplasty, and thrombolysis. Since it uses no enzyme, it is better referred to as endovascular thrombectomy or thromboaspiration.[71] As currently performed the clot is macerated, extracted using a Fogarty catheter, and aspirated through a sheath. The technique is safe, effective, can be quickly accomplished, and is the least expensive of any of the techniques. In two large series reported using this technique, one consisting of 1176 cases[71] and the other 4671 cases[72]; the success rates were 95.5% and 93%, respectively.

Thrombectomy with a mechanical device (MD)

The most prolific development in the approach to the thrombosed graft has been the appearance of mechanical devices that are used to treat thrombosed dialysis access grafts (and fistulae) through a combination of fragmentation, homogenization, dissolution, and aspiration. Several types of devices have been tested and used clinically.[73] These vary in complexity of design, mechanism of action, and costs. Currently, these devices have been shown to be safe, effective, and can quickly accomplish the thrombectomy task. However, their use adds an additional $450 to $600 to the cost of the procedure.

Which technique is best?

With this variety of techniques available to use, the question as to which is best often arises. The answer to this question from a strictly medical view point is it does not matter (as long as you do not use the original PT approach). Judged based upon the important principles of safety, effectiveness, and efficiency, they are all equal. It appears that as long as one accomplishes the critical components of the thrombectomy procedure—angiography to identify pathological anatomy, clot removal, and angioplasty to treat pathological anatomy—the actual technique used is unimportant. The techniques do differ based upon economic factors. Thromboaspiration is the least costly and for that reason is the author's choice.

▶ Thrombectomy Procedure

As stated above there are multiple techniques available to safely, effectively, and efficiently perform a thrombectomy on a dialysis access graft. We will discuss thromboaspiration in detail. Many of the basic principles listed will apply to any technique that might be used.

Contraindications to the procedure

There are absolute and relative contraindications to performing this procedure.

Infection Infection is an absolute contraindication. If the access is infected, it will contain a variable amount of infectious material. This will be released into the circulation if an endovascular thrombectomy is attempted and have potentially disastrous results. Occasionally a graft is infected and it is not obvious by external examination. In this instance, purulent material may be obtained with cannulation, a sure indication for immediately discontinuing the procedure. If the patient begins to have signs or symptoms suggestive of septicemia such as chills, fever, or a drop in blood pressure during the procedure, the possibility (probability) of an infected graft should be entertained and further management should be done accordingly.

Some patients will develop a dermal reaction following the placement of a graft (Figure 16-12). This is

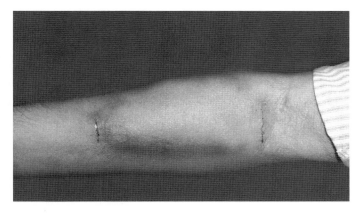

Figure 16-12. Dermal flare: notice the recent incisions and diffuse nature of discoloration following entire course of graft.

manifest as diffuse redness following the entire course of the graft tunnel. Since this dermal flare reaction has many of the features associated with infection, it can lead to confusion. Its diffuse distribution, time of occurrence, and absence of evidence of suppuration will add in distinguishing it.

Right-to-left shunt A known right-to-left cardiac shunt should also be regarded as an absolute contraindication to an endovascular thrombectomy. Embolization of thrombus fragments associated with any type of thrombectomy is not uncommon.[74–78] In one study, postoperative angiograms were obtained following surgical thrombectomy. Emboli were following in 12% of 67 cases.[77] Approximately 20% of the "normal" population has a probe-patent foramen ovate. This means that if, at autopsy, a probe is used to explore the foramen ovale, it is found to be open. These individuals do not have right-to-left shunts normally. They are at risk for its development, however. If the patient develops severe pulmonary hypertension, shunting from right to left can occur. The high incidence of pulmonary hypertension in the dialysis patient[79] place them at risk of developing paradoxical emboli with an endovascular thrombectomy technique for a thrombosed graft and this has been reported.[80] Unfortunately, the risk is probably about the same for surgical therapy.

Chronic occlusion Chronic occlusion and a large clot load should be considered as relative contraindications. As stated above, there are instances in which a chronically occluded graft has been opened[63,64]; however, these instances are very uncommon. In general if a graft has been occluded for several weeks, attempts at salvage should be discouraged. Also as previously stated, the clot load in a thrombosed graft is normally quite small, less than 5 cc. In cases where there are large or multiple pseudoaneurysms, however, the clot load may be very large (Figure 16-13). In these instances, judgment is required as to the safety of an attempt at graft salvage. There are two issues: if it is safe and if it is appropriate. A large embolus resulting from an attempt at clot removal could be dangerous to the

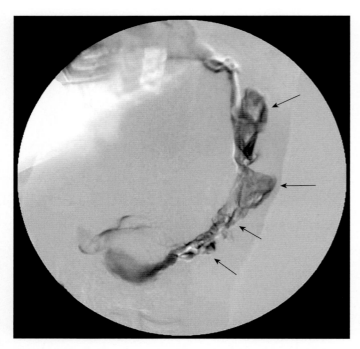

Figure 16-13. Upper arm thrombosed graft with large clot load.

patient.[76] Additionally, the patient with such a graft might be better served by graft revision.

Important considerations

Before beginning the procedure, there are several important considerations that need to be taken into consideration.

Accessing the graft Cannulation of the graft must be accomplished in such a manner as to allow access to both the venous and arterial circulations (Figure 16-14). The dialysis access should be thought of as a circuit that starts and ends at the heart. Problems may occur anywhere within this circuit and will need to be evaluated for possible therapy. The entire venous drainage up through the superior vena cava needs to be evaluated routinely and management of the arterial plug just inside (graft side) the arterial anastomosis is critical to the success of the procedure.

The total thrombectomy procedure generally involves angioplasty as well. As in simple balloon angioplasty, it is preferable to have a straight section of graft for insertion of the balloon catheter. In instances in which there is some resistance to the passage of the catheter tip across a stenosis, the presence of a curved length of catheter will cause it to buckle with forward pressure. This dampens the forward force that you are applying and can interfere with a successful catheter placement.

There should be enough space between the venous and arterial access sites to allow one to work between the two in clearing the graft of thrombi. A space of four finger-breaths (10 cm) is generally adequate.

Use of a sheath Either one or two sheaths can be used for the thromboaspiration procedure. As originally described, only was inserted in the arterial access position; however, many operators prefer two. The difference is unimportant as long as one takes care that they do not overlap. It is possible that overlapping sheaths can obstruct the graft during the procedure causing problems with restoration of flow. A

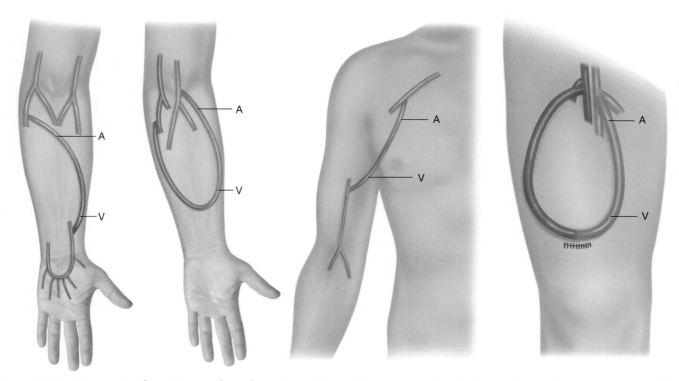

Figure 16-14. Access sites for various graft configurations. (**A**) arterial access site (needle directed toward arterial anastomosis) (**B**) Venous access site (needle directed toward venous anastomosis).

sheath is essential at the arterial access. This sheath serves dual purposes during the procedure. It is used to insert the Fogarty catheter to remove the arterial plug and it serves to aspirate the clot fragments. For this reason, it should be no smaller than 7 French. It is also helpful if this sheath has a removal cap. This allows for easy clearing of the sheath should it become occluded during clot aspiration.

Choice of a guidewire One only needs to use a basic guidewire. A guidewire with marked flexibility may not pass easily through a thrombosed graft. The same guidewire is used several times during the course of the treatment; only one guidewire is generally needed.

Embolectomy catheter The Fogarty embolectomy catheter is optimal for the removal of clot from the graft. The balloon on this catheter is very compliant, it adapts to the size and configuration of the available space as it is pulled through graft lumen. A noncompliant balloon does not work well for this purpose. The 4 French size is optimal. It is possible to obtain an embolectomy balloon catheter that can be inserted over a guidewire; however, the Fogarty works just as well and is much less expensive.

Postprocedure arteriogram It is common practice to manually occlude a graft and do a retrograde radiocontrast injection to visualize the arterial anastomosis and adjacent artery. This should never be done in the case of a thrombosed graft. There are always thrombi present that can be swept back into the artery with a retrograde injection. The angiogram should always be done using a vascular catheter that is passed over a guidewire into the artery.

Details of the procedure It is useful to think of the thromboaspiration procedure as consisting of five basic steps (Table 16-5): (1) venous access, medications, and angiogram; (2) arterial access and thrombectomy; (3) angioplasty of stenotic lesions; (4) evaluation of flow with aim to optimize; and (5) hemostasis. If a problem is encountered on any of these steps, you should solve it before moving on to the next step.

Step 1: Venous access, medications, and angiogram
End point of step 1: completion of task

1. Select a site just above the apex of the loop on the venous side or just above the arterial anastomosis in a straight graft (Figure 16-14), infiltrate with lidocaine.

TABLE 16–5

Treatment Modalities for Emboli

- Percutaneous: mechanical
  - Balloon catheter embolectomy
  - Catheter thromboaspiration
  - Back-bleeding
- Percutaneous: pharmacological
  - Thrombolysis
- Surgical embolectomy

2. Cannulate the graft with the needle pointing toward the venous anastomosis.
3. Pass the guidewire up to the level of the central veins. (If two sheaths are desired, the first sheath should be inserted.)
4. Insert a 5-French straight vascular catheter over guidewire and pass up to the lateral edge of the ribs. This is to give enough room to visualize all the central veins in the next step.
5. Remove the guidewire and inject radiocontrast to visualize the central veins. Document any pathology that is present.
6. Inject medications: heparin and sedation/analgesia medication.
7. Inject radiocontrast as the catheter is pulled back to visual the peripheral vein down to the level of the venous anastomosis. Document any pathology that is present. Reinsert the guidewire.
8. Remove the catheter and replace it with a 6 French dilator. (If a sheath has not been used). Remove the guidewire to use on the next step.

Step 2: Arterial access and thrombectomy
End point of step 2: presence of pulse between cannulation sites

1. Select a site that is approximately 4 cm from the venous anastomosis (Figure 16-14), infiltrate with lidocaine.
2. Cannulate the graft with the needle pointing toward the arterial anastomosis.
3. Insert guidewire pass far enough to allow for insertion of sheath.
4. Insert a 7-French sheath and remove guidewire and dilator.
5. Insert a 4-French Fogarty catheter through the sheath up to and across the arterial anastomosis. Do not go more than 1 or 2 cm into the artery.
6. Inflate the balloon of the Fogarty and gently pull it across the arterial anastomosis.
7. Use the Fogarty to sweep the entire graft. Inflate the balloon and pull it toward you using just enough pressure to create a resistance that you can feel, but still allow it to move forward.
8. Have your assistant apply suction to the sheath with a 20- or 30-cc syringe during this procedure to aspirate clot fragments.
9. Repeat steps 7 and 8 several times. If the side arm of the sheath becomes occluded, remove the cap (be careful where you put it) and go directly into the sheath with the Fogarty. Your assistant cannot aspirate with the cap removed. However, after each pull of the Fogarty, they should flush the sheath with a few cubic centimeters of saline to clear the hub. Continue this action until blood flows freely from the sheath. Then replace the cap.

10. Palpate the entire length of the graft after each sweep with the Fogarty to determine if a pulse is being obtained and where the pulse can be felt. Clear the graft up to a level above the venous cannulation site, between the two sites. This should be confirmed by the presence of a pulse between the two cannulation sites.

Step 3: Angioplasty of stenotic lesions
End point of step 3: flow in graft

1. Insert the guidewire through the dilator (or sheath) at the venous cannulation site and pass it up to the level of the central veins.
2. Insert the appropriate sized angioplasty balloon catheter over the guidewire and dilate any stenotic lesions that have been identified in the peripheral draining veins.
3. Lastly, dilate the venous anastomosis and venous side of graft.
4. Remove the angioplasty balloon catheter from the graft, leaving the guidewire in place.
5. Reinsert the dilator into the venous cannulation site (if a sheath was not used).
6. Inject a small puff of contrast through the sheath to check flow. At this point all you need to know is that there is flow. This is done with a small puff of contrast—you need to be able to see both the front and the end of the column of dye in order to judge its movement and detect flow. If there is no flow, immediately stop in the injection and determine the location of the occlusion, additional work with the Fogarty may be needed (or an angioplasty balloon). Do not remove the guidewire parked in the venous site until you see that there is flow without complication.

Step 4: Evaluation of flow with aim to optimize
End point of step 4: optimization of flow in graft

The point of this step is to answer the question "what can be done to improve flow?" The evaluation starts at the feeding artery and progresses antegrade. If a problem is encountered, stop and deal with it before moving on. The goal is flow optimization.

1. Pass the guidewire through the sheath and across the arterial anastomosis.
2. Pass the 5-French straight catheter over the guidewire up to a level so that its tip is slightly beyond the arterial anastomosis. Do not do a retrograde injection; small clots always remain, only inject through a catheter.
3. Remove the guidewire and inject with radiocontrast to visualize the feeding artery, arterial anastomosis, and adjacent graft. By carefully positioning the fluoroscopy machine, the entire loop of the graft can generally be visualized with one injection.
4. If a problem (stenosis or residual clot) is observed it should be dealt with before moving on.
5. After this process is complete, perform a final complete angiogram to check the graft, venous anastomosis, and any area that was treated with the angioplasty balloon for documentation.

Step 5: Hemostasis
End point of step 5: completion of task

Hemostasis can be obtained either by manual compression by suture. Suturing can be done only if one can be sure that the suture will be removed in a timely manner. If left in place for a prolonged period it can result in skin necrosis and the result can be disastrous.

1. Place a figure of eight stitch with 3–0 Ethilon or Prolene at each cannulation site. This should be done by placing stitch and then tightening and tying as the device at the access site is removed.
2. Cover the site with an adhesive dressing.
3. Remove sutures at 24 hours.

or

1. Apply manual compression as the device at the access site is removed. This is facilitated by the use of an adhesive, collagen coated, compression dressing (Tip-Stop, Cobe, Gambro Hospal Co.).

Management of problems

As with any procedure, problems may be encountered. It is important to be able to resolve this and continue with the treatment in order to be successful.

Inability to get Fogarty across arterial anastomosis
When passing the Fogarty catheter, it is important that it should not be forced. If resistance is met, try again with a twisting motion. Use only moderate pressure. If still it does not pass, remove it and insert the guidewire. Pass the tip of the guidewire across the arterial anastomosis. Insert an appropriately sized angioplasty balloon catheter and pass it across the problem site. Dilate the anastomosis. The fact that the Fogarty would not pass generally indicates anatomical pathology. Once the area is dilated, the Fogarty should pass with ease. The Fogarty is more effective than an angioplasty balloon in removing clot and should be used at this point.

Inability to restore inflow
The point at which a pulse is restored to the graft during the thrombectomy procedure varies. However, it should always appear after the Fogarty is pulled across the arterial anastomosis. There are occasional cases in which this does not occur. In this instance, the process should be repeated several times. If there is still no pulse, remove the Fogarty and insert the guidewire. Pass the guidewire across the arterial anastomosis; use the guidewire to place a 5-French straight catheter so that its tip is just inside the anastomosis. Inject contrast to visualize the site and determine the cause of the difficulty. There are several possibilities. In some instances the exact site of the arterial anastomosis has been miscalculated. In other instances, there may be thrombus extending up into the feeding artery, the presence of an anatomical lesion, or the

presence of a residual clot that is resistant to removal. Once the apparent cause of the problem is identified, corrective action can be taken.

The pulse is intermittent Once a good pulse is obtained, it should be persistent. Rarely, one will encounter a case in which a good pulse is obtained, but then disappears. Redoing the Fogarty catheter causes it to appear again, but then it disappears. This suggests that a flap valve has been created that allows for an intermittent return of flow. This can occur in at least two types of situation. Firstly, it could be the pseudoendothelial lining of the graft that has come loose and is intermittently obstructing flow. When a graft is placed, it begins to develop a lining that eventually becomes firmly attached. If the graft is relatively recent, within the first few months of creation, this lining may come loose and obstruct flow, acting as a flap valve. Secondly, layers of thrombus can form within pseudoaneurysms. Since this material is in contact with tissue rather than graft material, it can become attached and as such may be somewhat resistant to removal. This can create a flap-valve resulting in intermittent flow during the thrombectomy procedure. This problem is generally best resolved by using the Arrow-Trerotola thrombectomy device (Arrow International, Inc., Reading, PA). This mechanical device has a spinning basket (Figure 16-15) that makes surface contact within the graft, macerating thrombus as it removes it from its attachment.

Residual thrombus present at end of procedure At the end of the procedure when the final venogram is performed, residual thrombus may be noted within the graft (Figure 16-2a). This residual material falls into two categories. Firstly, it may lose thrombus that has gotten caught, or at least was not removed by the process used. This is most often seen in relation to the sheath at the arterial access site. Secondly, it may be chronic attached thrombus that is resistant to removal. Residual thrombus should be eliminated because of concerns that it could promote recurrent graft thrombosis.

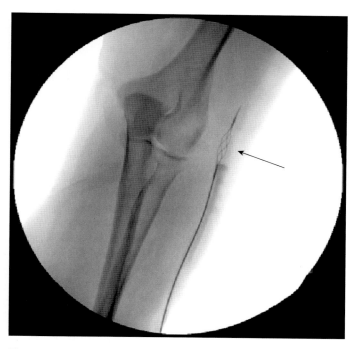

Figure 16-15. Arrow-Trerotola device. Basket (arrow) makes surface contact with the wall of the graft.

The first approach should be a very simple one that is referred to as "polishing" (Figure 16-16). This is done by using the Fogarty catheter in an antegrade fashion from the venous cannulation site (this requires a sheath). Inflate the balloon just enough to fill the graft, but not so much that you cannot move in forward. Once inflated, move the Fogarty catheter forward within the graft. Deflate the balloon to retract, then inflate and repeat the forward motion. This will serve to dislodge the clot fragments that will then be swept away. Move up and down the graft. If the residual clot appears to be caught upon the arterial access sheath, perform the polishing maneuver with the sheath removed after a guidewire has been inserted to save the site.

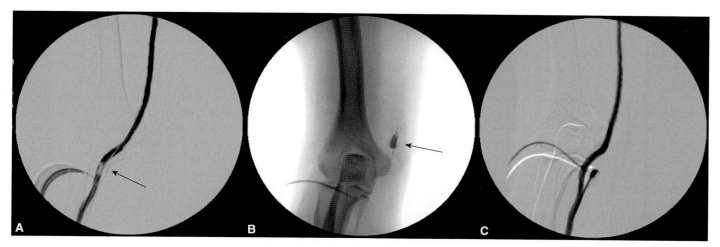

Figure 16-16. Removal of residual clot by polishing. (**A**) Residual clot caught on sheath (arrow), (**B**) Fogarty catheter balloon (arrow) used antegrade for removal, (**C**) final result.

Dealing with pseudoaneurysms Pseudoaneurysms can be a problem. At the least they cause difficulty with the passage of the guidewire. In some instances they present a problem that cannot be resolved using endovascular techniques and need to be referred to surgery. Pseudoaneurysms vary according to two variables: size and the nature of the thrombus they contain.

The thrombus contained within the pseudoaneurysm ranges from soft, no different from what is in the remainder of the graft, to firm, laminated, and adherent clot. This later variant is chronic thrombus that has undoubtedly accumulated over time. The nature of the clot contained within the structure can sometimes be appreciated by its firmness to palpation before you start the case. A pseudoaneurysm that is soft will generally cause no problems; one that is hard may be difficult.

Small pseudoaneurysms generally cause no problems. The larger the anomalous structure, the more likely it is to cause difficulty. This is in part because of its size, but is also in part because it is more likely to contain the chronic type of thrombus material. The basic approach to cleaning out a pseudoaneurysm is to use the Fogarty balloon in combination with manual compression of the dilated structure. The pseudoaneurysm should be pressed down onto the Fogarty as firmly as possible. After several passes, you will be able to feel that it has become soft and compressible. If residual clot is present, it will be obvious when radiocontrast is injected after flow is achieved. If a residual is seen, further work with the Fogarty is required. The basic guiding principle is that when doing a thrombectomy, all pseudoaneurysms that are present must be completely cleared of thrombus.

If all of the clot cannot be removed after multiple passes using manual compression onto the Fogarty, consider using an Arrow-Trerotola thrombectomy device (Figure 16-17). This should be used in combination with manual compression of the pseudoaneurysm onto the spinning device. Multiple passes should be performed. The result can often be felt, but can be easily demonstrated with a puff of radiocontrast.

Remember that it takes two problems to create a pseudoaneurysm: a defect in the graft and a stenosis to increase the intragraft pressure. In doing the thrombectomy, care must be given to elimination of the associated stenosis. If this is not relieved completely, the pseudoaneurysm will continue to grow. In all instances remember that some cases need to be dealt with by surgical revision. If this is obvious before you start, it may be best to not do the case, refer it on to the surgeon.

Expected results of thrombectomy procedure

A successful thrombectomy is defined as the ability to use the access for one dialysis.[81] This definition takes into account the fact that the thrombectomy procedure may not be able to adequately address the precipitating causes of the event even though the graft was opened and cleared of thrombus. The immediate success rate should be 85% or greater according to the NKF/KDOQI Practice Guidelines.[81]

Long-term primary patency rates for thrombectomy are not as good as for angioplasty (Figure 16-18). For this reason every effort should be made to prevent thrombosis by the prospective diagnosis and treatment of venous stenosis. Every dialysis facility should maintain a database to monitor outcome results. Primary (unassisted) patency goals for the treatment of the thrombosed dialysis access graft for percutaneous thrombolysis with angioplasty should be at least 40% at 3 months.[81] Since surgical revision results in a loss of vein and extension of the access up the arm, it is held to a higher standard. Surgical thrombectomy and revision should result in a 50% primary patency at 6 months and 40% at 1 year.[81]

Complications of thrombectomy

It is important to establish a systematic method to continuously assess and improve patient outcomes through an ongoing assessment of important aspects of the procedures

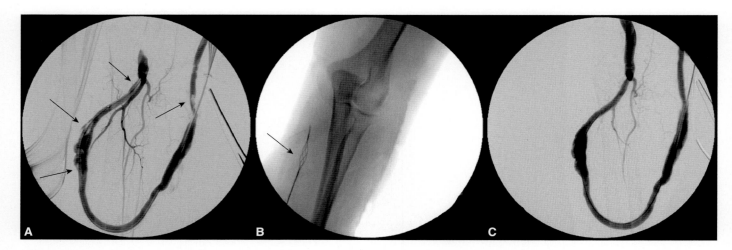

Figure 16-17. Using Arrow Trerotola to remove residual clot. (**A**) Multiple areas with residual (arrows), (**B**) Arrow Trerotola device (arrow), (**C**) final result.

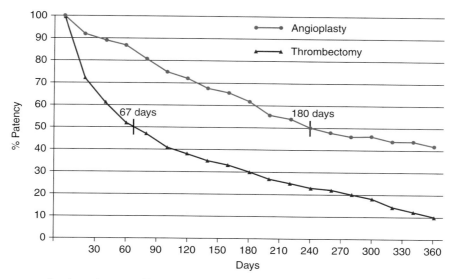

Figure 16-18. Primary patency for thrombectomy[71] versus angioplasty.[10] Notice the difference in median (50%) patency.

performed based on quality, cost, and outcome. The best way to handle this is a good quality assurance program. Data is essential. Monitoring complication rates is essential to this effort. The primary complications of endovascular thrombectomy are the same as those listed for venous angioplasty (see Chapter 17) in addition to a unique complication, peripheral arterial embolization.[33]

Arterial embolization As stated above the occluded synthetic graft contains two types of thrombus: a firm arterial plug and a variable amount of soft thrombus. Any of this thrombotic material has the potential for giving rise to an embolus; however, it is usually the arterial plug that is involved, or at least a piece of it, that gives rise to a symptomatic situation. Residual thrombi are present following an endovascular thrombectomy even after the graft is flowing.[82] Overinjection (injection of saline or radiocontrast into the graft in an amount that exceeds the graft volume) will promote this occurrence, especially if there is an upstream obstruction. Just the passage of a catheter or guidewire across the arterial anastomosis can result in this complication.

Most arterial emboli are asymptomatic and are recognized only radiographically. These do not require treatment.[77] Symptomatic emboli are not common but must be treated in a timely fashion in order to prevent permanent sequelae. In a series of 1176 cases of thrombosed grafts treated by endovascular means, only four cases of symptomatic arterial emboli were seen.[71] In another series of 4671 graft thrombectomies, only 18 cases (0.38% incidence) of arterial embolization were seen.[72] In both the series, the thrombectomy was performed using the thromboaspiration technique. Although the frequency is relatively low, it is higher than is associated with fistula thrombectomy.[72] Although the reasons for this are not clear, it should be noted that the thrombus present in a fistula is mildly inflammatory and tends to become attached to the vessel wall.

Since most emboli are recognized only if they are symptomatic, they tend to be larger and as such lodge in the upper portion of the arterial tree downstream from the arterial anastomosis. This means that in a brachial artery associated access, the embolus generally stops just before the bifurcation. However, the offending thrombotic material can move more distally into much smaller arterial branches. These emboli are less likely to be symptomatic and are therefore more likely to go undetected.

The symptoms are those of hand ischemia (Figure 16-19). The hand, especially the fingers, turns cold and takes on a

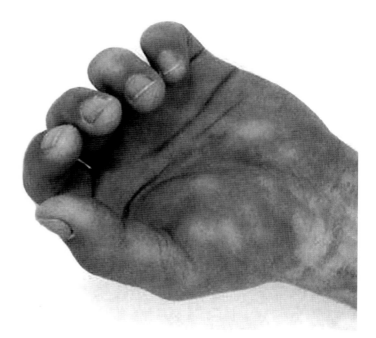

Figure 16-19. Ischemic hand from embolus to brachial artery during thrombectomy procedure. Note the mottled discoloration and blanching of finger tips.

bluish discoloration that becomes mottled. These symptoms generally come with the sudden onset of pain. In evaluating a patient's hand for a suspected embolus, it is important to compare it with the opposite hand. If both are cold and mottled, it is not likely that the hand in question reflects an acute problem. The pulses at the wrist are generally absent or considerably diminished—a change that can be appreciated only if the patient was carefully evaluated prior to having the thrombectomy procedure. A Doppler signal is generally present over the arteries at the wrist, although frequently diminished. If nothing is detected with Doppler examination, the urgency for immediate treatment to avoid tissue damage is even greater.

Treatment of symptomatic arterial emboli Symptomatic emboli must be treated in a timely fashion in order to prevent permanent sequelae. Treatment is urgent and directed at restoring flow to the ischemic hand as quickly as possible in order to relieve the patient's pain and preserve hand function by avoiding secondary muscle ischemia and necrosis. Outcomes and prognosis largely depend on the rapid diagnosis and initiation of appropriate and effective therapy.[83]

Several techniques have been described for the treatment (removal) of an arterial embolus that occurs during the process of doing a thrombectomy upon a dialysis access graft (Table 16-5). These can be divided into percutaneous and surgical. The percutaneous category can be further subdivided into mechanical and pharmacological approaches.

Balloon catheter embolectomy This technique involves the use of an embolectomy catheter.[63] Because of the anatomy involved, it generally requires that a catheter that can be passed over a guidewire be used. A standard angioplasty balloon works well in most instances although there are embolectomy balloon catheters that can be passed over a guidewire that that can be utilized. The procedure is as follows:

1. Document the presence and location of the embolus angiographically (Figure 16-20).

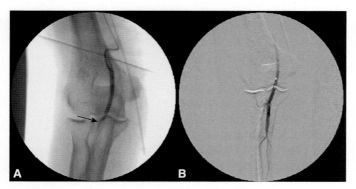

Figure 16-20. Brachial artery embolus. (**A**) Angiogram showing site of blockage (arrow), (**B**) angiographic appearance after removal of thrombus.

2. Pass a guidewire (a hydrophilic guidewire has a potential advantage) past the blockage.

3. Insert an angioplasty balloon catheter; one that has not been used has an advantage since it will have a lower profile.

4. Once the balloon is beyond the level of the embolus, inflate and pull back to retrieve the clot. The clot will be pulled back into the graft.

5. Document the final appearance of the vessel angiographically (Figure 16-20).

Catheter thromboaspiration This technique is based on using a large caliber catheter to aspirate the embolus, or at least capture the embolus using suction applied via a catheter.[84] The technique is performed as follows:

1. Document the presence and location of the embolus angiographically.

2. Pass a guidewire beyond the clot fragment and insert a 7- or 8-French catheter.

3. Position the catheter just above the embolus and in contact with it.

4. Apply strong manual aspiration pressure using a 50-mL Luer-Lok syringe attached to the catheter as it is slowly withdrawn.

5. Check the aspirate to see if the clot has been removed.

6. Repeat the angiogram with a small volume of radiocontrast to document the result.

Back-bleeding This technique is dependent on the fact that, except in the face of severe peripheral artery disease, when the distal brachial artery is occluded, there is enough blood flow to the distal extremity through other vessels to still provide distal perfusion. The success of this procedure is dependent upon the presence of this persistent perfusion causing blood to flow retrograde in the artery below the arterial anastomosis. This flow continues retrograde up the occluded artery and pushes the clot upward and into the graft relieving the obstruction.[85] The technique is performed as follows:

1. Document the presence and location of the embolus angiographically.

2. Occlude the distal brachial artery central to the anastomosis using a balloon Fogarty catheter or an angioplasty balloon.

3. Instruct the patient to exercise their hand vigorously for approximately 1 minute.

4. This increases blood flow to the hand and enhances the back flow up the artery.

5. After the occluding balloon has been deflated, perform an arteriogram to document the result.

If this fails to work the first time, repeat the procedure before abandoning the attempt.

Thrombolysis The technique that is used to treat an embolus in this situation is referred to as selective regional intra-arterial infusion. The occluded arterial segment is selectively catheterized using a vascular catheter. The catheter shaft is then positioned just proximal to the embolus and the lytic agent is infused. tPA is the agent generally used which is a very effective fibrinolytic agent and has the additional advantage of an extremely short half-life (5.0 ± 1.8 minutes). Since this technique takes a longer period of time to effect, it is usually reserved as a back-up in the event of failure of one or more of the other percutaneous techniques.

Additionally, the cases are more likely to be referred to the hospital for the procedure; this involves additional delay in obtaining resolution.

The arterial plug is frequently the clot that results in an embolus and it is somewhat resistant to fibrinolysis. The reasons for this are not totally clear. It is a dense fibrin plug and it has been shown that clots composed of dense fibrin networks have reduced permeability to the lytic agent making them more resistant to lysis; whether this applies in this situation is not known.

Surgical embolectomy A surgical thrombectomy generally consists of opening the exposed artery and extracting the clot with an embolectomy balloon. If a patient with an embolus is referred for surgery, an angiogram to document the exact position of the clot should be performed and sent with the patient. Surgical removal is facilitated considerably by localizing the exact site of the embolus prior to beginning. Clot resistance plus the fact that thrombolysis is not rapid has led some to feel that prompt surgical treatment may have an advantage. This is especially true in cases of severe ischemia requiring emergent reperfusion.

REFERENCES

1. Hodges TC, Fillinger MF, Zwolak RM, Walsh DB, Bech F, Cronenwett JL. Longitudinal comparison of dialysis access methods: risk factors for failure. *J Vasc Surg.* 1997;26: 1009–1019.
2. Schwab SJ, Harrington JT, Singh A, Roher R, Shohaib SA, Perrone RD, Meyer K, Beasley D. Vascular access for hemodialysis. *Kidney Int.* 1999;55:2078–2090.
3. Beathard G. *Complications of Vascular Access.* New York: Marcel Dekker, Inc., 2000.
4. Roy-Chaudhury P, Arend L, Zhang J, Krishnamoorthy M, Wang Y, Banerjee R, Samaha A, Munda R. Neointimal hyperplasia in early arteriovenous fistula failure. *Am J Kidney Dis.* 2007;50:782–790.
5. Roy-Chaudhury P, Kelly BS, Miller MA, Reaves A, Armstrong J, Nanayakkara N, Heffelfinger SC. Venous neointimal hyperplasia in polytetrafluoroethylene dialysis grafts. *Kidney Int.* 2001;59:2325–2334.
6. Wang Y, Krishnamoorthy M, Banerjee R, Zhang J, Rudich S, Holland C, Arend L, Roy-Chaudhury P. Venous stenosis in a pig arteriovenous fistula model—anatomy, mechanisms and cellular phenotypes. *Nephrol Dial Transplant.* 2008;23: 525–533.

7. Weiss MF, Scivittaro V, Anderson JM. Oxidative stress and increased expression of growth factors in lesions of failed hemodialysis access. *Am J Kidney Dis.* 2001;37:970–980.
8. Roy-Chaudhury P, Sukhatme VP, Cheung AK. Hemodialysis vascular access dysfunction: a cellular and molecular viewpoint. *J Am Soc Nephrol.* 2006;17:1112–1127.
9. Beathard GA. Angioplasty for arteriovenous grafts and fistulae. *Semin Nephrol.* 2002;22:202–210.
10. Beathard GA. Percutaneous transvenous angioplasty in the treatment of vascular access stenosis. *Kidney Int.* 1992;42:1390–1397.
11. Kanterman RY, Vesely TM, Pilgram TK, Guy BW, Windus DW, Picus D. Dialysis access grafts: anatomic location of venous stenosis and results of angioplasty. *Radiology.* 1995;195:135–139.
12. Jaberi A, Schwartz D, Marticorena R, Dacouris N, Prabhudesai V, McFarlane P, Donnelly S. Risk factors for the development of cephalic arch stenosis. *J Vasc Access.* 2007;8:287–295.
13. Falk A, Teodorescu V, Lou WY, Uribarri J, Vassalotti JA. Treatment of "swing point stenoses" in hemodialysis arteriovenous fistulae. *Clin Nephrol.* 2003;60:35–41.
14. Rajan DK, Clark TW, Patel NK, Stavropoulos SW, Simons ME. Prevalence and treatment of cephalic arch stenosis in dysfunctional autogenous hemodialysis fistulas. *J Vasc Interv Radiol.* 2003;14:567–573.
15. Hammes M, Funaki B, Coe FL. Cephalic arch stenosis in patients with fistula access for hemodialysis: relationship to diabetes and thrombosis. *Hemodial Int.* 2008;12:85–89.
16. Gonsalves CF, Eschelman DJ, Sullivan KL, DuBois N, Bonn J. Incidence of central vein stenosis and occlusion following upper extremity PICC and port placement. *Cardiovasc Intervent Radiol.* 2003;26:123–127.
17. Allen AW, Megargell JL, Brown DB, Lynch FC, Singh H, Singh Y, Waybill PN. Venous thrombosis associated with the placement of peripherally inserted central catheters. *J Vasc Interv Radiol.* 2000;11:1309–1314.
18. Asif A, Salman LH, Lopera GG, Carrillo RG. The dilemma of transvenous cardiac rhythm devices in hemodialysis patients: time to consider the epicardial approach? *Kidney Int.* 2011;79:1267–69.
19. Korzets A, Chagnac A, Ori Y, Katz M, Zevin D. Subclavian vein stenosis, permanent cardiac pacemakers and the haemodialysed patient. *Nephron.* 1991;58:103–105.
20. Deighan CJ, McLaughlin KJ, Simpson K, Jones JM. Unsuspected subclavian vein stenosis resulting from a permanent pacing wire. *Nephrol Dial Transplant.* 1996;11:2333–2334.
21. Sticherling C, Chough SP, Baker RL, Wasmer K, Oral H, Tada H, Horwood L, Kim MH, Pelosi F, Michaud GF, Strickberger SA, Morady F, Knight BP. Prevalence of central venous occlusion in patients with chronic defibrillator leads. *Am Heart J.* 2001;141:813–816.
22. Da Costa SS, Scalabrini Neto A, Costa R, Caldas JG, Martinelli Filho M. Incidence and risk factors of upper extremity deep vein lesions after permanent transvenous pacemaker implant: a 6-month follow-up prospective study. *Pacing Clin Electrophysiol.* 2002;25:1301–1306.
23. Teruya TH, Abou-Zamzam AM, Jr., Limm W, Wong L. Symptomatic subclavian vein stenosis and occlusion in hemodialysis patients with transvenous pacemakers. *Ann Vasc Surg.* 2003;17:526–529.

24. Lickfett L, Bitzen A, Arepally A, Nasir K, Wolpert C, Jeong KM, Krause U, Schimpf R, Lewalter T, Calkins H, Jung W, Luderitz B. Incidence of venous obstruction following insertion of an implantable cardioverter defibrillator. A study of systematic contrast venography on patients presenting for their first elective ICD generator replacement. *Europace.* 2004;6:25–31.

25. Tourret J, Cluzel P, Tostivint I, Barrou B, Deray G, Bagnis CI. Central venous stenosis as a complication of ipsilateral haemodialysis fistula and pacemaker. *Nephrol Dial Transplant.* 2005;20:997–1001.

26. Riezebos RK, Schroeder-Tanka J, de Voogt WG. Occlusion of the proximal subclavian vein complicating pacemaker lead implantation. *Europace.* 2006;8:42–43.

27. Khan FA, Vesely TM. Arterial problems associated with dysfunctional hemodialysis grafts: evaluation of patients at high risk for arterial disease. *J Vasc Interv Radiol.* 2002;13:1109–1114.

28. Asif A, Gadalean FN, Merrill D, Cherla G, Cipleu CD, Epstein DL, Roth D. Inflow stenosis in arteriovenous fistulas and grafts: a multicenter, prospective study. *Kidney Int.* 2005;67:1986–1992.

29. Duijm LE, Liem YS, van der Rijt RH, Nobrega FJ, van den Bosch HC, Douwes-Draaijer P, Cuypers PW, Tielbeek AV. Inflow stenoses in dysfunctional hemodialysis access fistulae and grafts. *Am J Kidney Dis.* 2006;48:98–105.

30. Samaha A, Salman L, Asif A. Arterial angioplasty to treat hand ischemia in a radial-cephalic fistula. *Semin Dial.* 2009;22:561–563.

31. Salman L, Maya ID, Asif A. Current concepts in the pathophysiology and management of arteriovenous access-induced hand ischemia. *Adv Chronic Kidney Dis.* 2009;16:371–377.

32. Gray RJ. Percutaneous intervention for permanent hemodialysis access: a review. *J Vasc Interv Radiol.* 1997;8:313–327.

33. Beathard GA. Management of complications of endovascular dialysis access procedures. *Semin Dial.* 2003;16:309–313.

34. Asif A, Leon C, Merrill D, Bhimani B, Ellis R, Ladino M, Gadalean FN. Arterial steal syndrome: a modest proposal for an old paradigm. *Am J Kidney Dis.* 2006;48:88–97.

35. Beathard GA. Thrombolysis versus surgery for the treatment of thrombosed dialysis access grafts. *J Am Soc Nephrol.* 1995;6:1619–1624.

36. Beathard GA, Marston WA. Endovascular management of thrombosed dialysis access grafts. *Am J Kidney Dis.* 1998;32:172–175.

37. Windus DW. Permanent vascular access: a nephrologist's view. *Am J Kidney Dis.* 1993;21:457–471.

38. Smits JH, van der Linden J, Blankestijn PJ, Rabelink TJ. Coagulation and haemodialysis access thrombosis. *Nephrol Dial Transplant.* 2000;15:1755–1760.

39. Knoll GA, Wells PS, Young D, Perkins SL, Pilkey RM, Clinch JJ, Rodger MA. Thrombophilia and the risk for hemodialysis vascular access thrombosis. *J Am Soc Nephrol.* 2005;16:1108–1114.

40. Besarab A, Sullivan KL, Ross RP, Moritz MJ. Utility of intra-access pressure monitoring in detecting and correcting venous outlet stenoses prior to thrombosis. *Kidney Int.* 1995;47:1364–1373.

41. Neyra NR, Ikizler TA, May RE, Himmelfarb J, Schulman G, Shyr Y, Hakim RM. Change in access blood flow over time predicts vascular access thrombosis. *Kidney Int.* 1998;54:1714–1719.

42. McCarley P, Wingard RL, Shyr Y, Pettus W, Hakim RM, Ikizler TA. Vascular access blood flow monitoring reduces access morbidity and costs. *Kidney Int.* 2001;60:1164–1172.

43. Schwab SJ, Oliver MJ, Suhocki P, McCann R. Hemodialysis arteriovenous access: detection of stenosis and response to treatment by vascular access blood flow. *Kidney Int.* 2001;59:358–362.

44. Hoeben H, Abu-Alfa AK, Reilly RF, Aruny JE, Bouman K, Perazella MA. Vascular access surveillance: evaluation of combining dynamic venous pressure and vascular access blood flow measurements. *Am J Nephrol.* 2003;23:403–408.

45. Maoz D, Reinitz R, Rimon U, Knecht A, Badayev L, Holtzman E, Schneiderman J. Hemodialysis graft flow surveillance with prompt corrective interventions improves access long-term patency. *Clin Nephrol.* 2009;71:43–49.

46. Zasuwa G, Frinak S, Besarab A, Peterson E, Yee J. Automated intravascular access pressure surveillance reduces thrombosis rates. *Semin Dial.* 2010;23:527–535.

47. Fodinger M, Mannhalter C, Pabinger I, Koizar D, Rintelen C, Horl WH, Sunder-Plassmann G. Resistance to activated protein C (APC): mutation at Arg506 of coagulation factor V and vascular access thrombosis in haemodialysis patients. *Nephrol Dial Transplant.* 1996;11:668–672.

48. Hernandez E, Praga M, Alamo C, Araque A, Morales JM, Alcazar JM, Ruilope LM, Rodicio JL. Lipoprotein(a) and vascular access survival in patients on chronic hemodialysis. *Nephron.* 1996;72:145–149.

49. LeSar CJ, Merrick HW, Smith MR. Thrombotic complications resulting from hypercoagulable states in chronic hemodialysis vascular access. *J Am Coll Surg.* 1999;189:73–79; discussion 79–81.

50. Shemin D, Lapane KL, Bausserman L, Kanaan E, Kahn S, Dworkin L, Bostom AG. Plasma total homocysteine and hemodialysis access thrombosis: a prospective study. *J Am Soc Nephrol.* 1999;10:1095–1099.

51. Valeri A, Joseph R, Radhakrishnan J. A large prospective survey of anti-cardiolipin antibodies in chronic hemodialysis patients. *Clin Nephrol.* 1999;51:116–121.

52. Adler S, Szczech L, Qureshi A, Bollu R, Thomas-John R. IgM anticardiolipin antibodies are associated with stenosis of vascular access in hemodialysis patients but do not predict thrombosis. *Clin Nephrol.* 2001;56:428–434.

53. Atac B, Yakupoglu U, Ozbek N, Ozdemir FN, Bilgin N. Role of genetic mutations in vascular access thrombosis among hemodialysis patients waiting for renal transplantation. *Transplant Proc.* 2002;34:2030–2032.

54. Palomo I, Pereira J, Alarcon M, Vasquez M, Pierangeli S. Vascular access thrombosis is not related to presence of antiphospholipid antibodies in patients on chronic hemodialysis. *Nephron.* 2002;92:957–958.

55. Hojs R, Gorenjak M, Ekart R, Dvorsak B, Pecovnik-Balon B. Homocysteine and vascular access thrombosis in hemodialysis patients. *Ren Fail.* 2002;24:215–222.

56. Nampoory MR, Das KC, Johny KV, Al-Hilali N, Abraham M, Easow S, Saed T, Al-Muzeirei IA, Sugathan TN, Al Mousawi M. Hypercoagulability, a serious problem in patients with ESRD on maintenance hemodialysis, and its correction after kidney transplantation. *Am J Kidney Dis.* 2003;42:797–805.

57. O'Shea SI, Lawson JH, Reddan D, Murphy M, Ortel TL. Hypercoagulable states and antithrombotic strategies

in recurrent vascular access site thrombosis. *J Vasc Surg.* 2003;38:541–548.

58. Fukasawa M, Matsushita K, Kamiyama M, Mikami Y, Araki I, Yamagata Z, Takeda M. The methylentetrahydrofolate reductase C677T point mutation is a risk factor for vascular access thrombosis in hemodialysis patients. *Am J Kidney Dis.* 2003;41:637–642.

59. Valji K, Bookstein JJ, Roberts AC, Oglevie SB, Pittman C, O'Neill MP. Pulse-spray pharmacomechanical thrombolysis of thrombosed hemodialysis access grafts: long-term experience and comparison of original and current techniques. *AJR Am J Roentgenol.* 1995;164:1495–1500; discussion 1501–1493.

60. Kumpe DA, Cohen MA. Angioplasty/thrombolytic treatment of failing and failed hemodialysis access sites: comparison with surgical treatment. *Prog Cardiovasc Dis.* 1992;34:263–278.

61. Winkler TA, Trerotola SO, Davidson DD, Milgrom ML. Study of thrombus from thrombosed hemodialysis access grafts. *Radiology.* 1995;197:461–465.

62. NKF-K/DOQI Clinical Practice Guidelines For Vascular Access: update 2006. Clinical Practice Guideline 6: treatment of arteriovenous graft complications, 6.7 treatment of thrombosis and associated stenosis.

63. Beathard GA. Successful treatment of the chronically thrombosed dialysis access graft: resuscitation of dead grafts. *Semin Dial.* 2006;19:417–420.

64. Weng MJ, Chen MC, Chi WC, Liu YC, Liang HL, Pan HB. Endovascular revascularization of chronically thrombosed arteriovenous fistulas and grafts for hemodialysis: a retrospective study in 15 patients with 18 access sites. *Cardiovasc Intervent Radiol.* 2010;11:373–377.

65. NKF-K/DOQI Clinical Practice Guidelines for Vascular Access 2006. Clinical Practice Guideline 2: Selection and placement of hemodialysis access, 2.1 the order of preference for placement of fistulae, 2.1.4 Patients should be considered for construction of a primary fistula after failure of every dialysis AV access.

66. Beathard GA. *Options for Restoration of Thrombosed Vascular Access: Thrombolysis.* Oxford: Oxford University Press, 2000.

67. May RE, Himmelfarb J, Yenicesu M, Knights S, Ikizler TA, Schulman G, Hernanz-Schulman M, Shyr Y, Hakim RM. Predictive measures of vascular access thrombosis: a prospective study. *Kidney Int.* 1997;52:1656–1662.

68. Cynamon J, Lakritz PS, Wahl SI, Bakal CW, Sprayregen S. Hemodialysis graft declotting: description of the "lyse and wait" technique. *J Vasc Interv Radiol.* 1997;8:825–829.

69. Cynamon J, Pierpont CE. Thrombolysis for the treatment of thrombosed hemodialysis access grafts. *Rev Cardiovasc Med.* 2002;3(suppl 2):S84–S91.

70. Vogel PM, Bansal V, Marshall MW. Thrombosed hemodialysis grafts: lyse and wait with tissue plasminogen activator or urokinase compared to mechanical thrombolysis with the Arrow-Trerotola Percutaneous Thrombolytic Device. *J Vasc Interv Radiol.* 2001;12:1157–1165.

71. Beathard GA, Welch BR, Maidment HJ. Mechanical thrombolysis for the treatment of thrombosed hemodialysis access grafts. *Radiology.* 1996;200:711–716.

72. Beathard GA, Litchfield T. Effectiveness and safety of dialysis vascular access procedures performed by interventional nephrologists. *Kidney Int.* 2004;66:1622–1632.

73. Vesely TM. Mechanical thrombectomy devices to treat thrombosed hemodialysis grafts. *Tech Vasc Interv Radiol.* 2003;6:35–41.

74. Schilling JJ, Eiser AR, Slifkin RF, Whitney JT, Neff MS. The role of thrombolysis in hemodialysis access occlusion. *Am J Kidney Dis.* 1987;10:92–97.

75. Beathard GA. Mechanical versus pharmacomechanical thrombolysis for the treatment of thrombosed dialysis access grafts. *Kidney Int.* 1994;45:1401–1406.

76. Swan TL, Smyth SH, Ruffenach SJ, Berman SS, Pond GD. Pulmonary embolism following hemodialysis access thrombolysis/thrombectomy. *J Vasc Interv Radiol.* 1995;6:683–686.

77. Trerotola SO, Johnson MS, Shah H, Namyslowski J, Filo RS. Incidence and management of arterial emboli from hemodialysis graft surgical thrombectomy. *J Vasc Interv Radiol.* 1997;8:557–562.

78. Kinney TB, Valji K, Rose SC, Yeung DD, Oglevie SB, Roberts AC, Ward DM. Pulmonary embolism from pulse-spray pharmacomechanical thrombolysis of clotted hemodialysis grafts: urokinase versus heparinized saline. *J Vasc Interv Radiol.* 2000;11:1143–1152.

79. Yigla M, Abassi Z, Reisner SA, Nakhoul F. Pulmonary hypertension in hemodialysis patients: an unrecognized threat. *Semin Dial.* 2006;19:353–357.

80. Briefel GR, Regan F, Petronis JD. Cerebral embolism after mechanical thrombolysis of a clotted hemodialysis access. *Am J Kidney Dis.* 1999;34:341–343.

81. NKF-K/DOQI Clinical Practice Guidelines for Vascular Access: update 2006. Clinical Practice Guideline 6: Treatment of arteriovenous graft complications, 6.7 treatment of thrombosis and associated stenosis.

82. Vesely TM, Hovsepian DM, Darcy MD, Brown DB, Pilgram TK. Angioscopic observations after percutaneous thrombectomy of thrombosed hemodialysis grafts. *J Vasc Interv Radiol.* 2000;11:971–977.

83. Rajan DK, Patel NH, Valji K, Cardella JF, Bakal C, Brown D, Brountzos E, Clark TW, Grassi C, Meranze S, Miller D, Neithamer C, Rholl K, Roberts A, Schwartzberg M, Swan T, Thorpe P, Towbin R, Sacks D. Quality improvement guidelines for percutaneous management of acute limb ischemia. *J Vasc Interv Radiol.* 2005;16:585–595.

84. Turmel-Rodrigues LA, Beyssen B, Raynaud A, Sapoval M. Thromboaspiration to treat inadvertent arterial emboli during dialysis graft declotting. *J Vasc Interv Radiol.* 1998;9:849–850.

85. Trerotola SO, Johnson MS, Shah H, Namyslowski J. Backbleeding technique for treatment of arterial emboli resulting from dialysis graft thrombolysis. *J Vasc Interv Radiol.* 1998;9:141–143.

VENOUS ANGIOPLASTY

GERALD A. BEATHARD

HISTORY OF ANGIOPLASTY

The first clinical dilation of blood vessels was described by Dotter and Judkins in 1964.[1] They used a coaxial catheter design, applying it to the femoral artery with mixed success.[2] This became known as the "Dotter technique." Variations on this approach included that first described by Staple[3] and later by van Andel[2] who used gradually tapered catheters. Latex balloons were tried, but met with little success because they were too compliant and had a tendency to inflate in the direction of least resistance. Only soft lesions could be dilated. In 1973, Porstmann[4] described a "caged balloon" catheter to get around this problem. Unfortunately, although it applied more force, it produced a lot of debris and a rough surface. In 1974, Gruntzig and Hopff[5] described a nonelastic balloon catheter and used it to treat coronary artery lesions.[6] This type of device, referred to as the "Gruntzig" catheter, eventually became the technique of choice.

In 1982, the first reports of applying this technique to the lesions observed in dysfunction dialysis vascular access were published.[7–9] These early reports were followed by further accounts demonstrating the success of this approach.[10–13] Since that time angioplasty has become the standard treatment for venous stenosis in both fistulae and grafts.

Percutaneous angioplasty is a general technique that can be used for the management of venous stenosis problems relating to both arteriovenous fistulae (AVF) and arteriovenous grafts (AVG).

This type of treatment of venous stenosis is an outpatient procedure that does not prohibit the immediate use of the access for dialysis. There is minimal to no blood loss, hospitalization is avoided, and there is rarely any postprocedure discomfort for the patient. Lesions in all locations within the venous system, both peripheral and central, can be easily, effectively, and safely treated. Its only disadvantages are that there are occasional lesions that do not respond to treatment; some lesions are elastic and the results obtained are not permanent.

VENOUS ANGIOPLASTY—GENERAL

Percutaneous angioplasty treatment of venous stenosis is an outpatient procedure, with the access immediately available for dialysis once the lesion is corrected. Lesions in all locations within the arteriovenous access and its draining veins, both peripheral and central, can be easily, effectively, and safely treated.

Direct fluoroscopic observation is necessary to perform angioplasty, with digital capability being very advantageous. Heparinization is unnecessary because of the high blood flow that is present within the access. During dilatation, flow is occluded for only short intermittent periods, and clotting of the access therefore rarely occurs. Because the procedure is potentially very painful, the patient requires adequate sedation/analgesia. Midazolam hydrochloride, alone or in combination with fentanyl, has been used to produce a state of relaxation for the 5–10 minutes required to perform the treatment.[14,15] Patients must be monitored very closely during this process. Since individual patient requirements for adequate sedation/analgesia vary considerably, the dosage must be carefully titrated.

▶ Preprocedure Evaluation

In addition to a general history and physical examination directed toward the risk of the procedure, a specific, detailed physical examination of the access and access arm

should be performed.[16] This examination is important for several reasons:

- Although the patient should have been sent for a valid reason, it is wise to be assured that a problem is actually present before initiating the procedure. A dysfunctional access should be obvious by physical examination.

- Evaluating the access preprocedure will help in planning the approach to the procedure; this is especially true for a patient with an AVF.

- It will serve as a comparison for evaluating the access after the procedure is complete.

- It is necessary for detecting the presence of a contraindication to the procedure.

▶ Cannulating the Access

When accessing an AVG or a mature AVF, a standard introducer needle works well and is perfectly adequate. However, when dealing with a dysfunctional fistula that is not well developed or has failed to mature, a Micropuncture® Introducer (Cook medical, Inc., Bloomington, IL) offers a definite advantage (Figure 17-1).

There are two points that determine the selection of the cannulation site. Firstly, you must be directed toward the stenotic lesion. A thorough pre-examination should indicate the location of the stenosis; based upon this an appropriate cannulation site can be selected. Secondly, unless the distance is relatively short, it is preferable to have a section of access for insertion of the balloon catheter that lies in a straight line with the vessel in which the lesion is located. In instances in which there is some resistance to the passage of the catheter tip across a stenosis, the presence of a curved length of catheter will cause it to buckle with forward pressure. This dampens the forward force that you are applying and can interfere with a successful catheter passage.

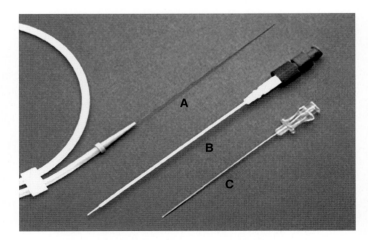

Figure 17-1. Micropuncture needle. (**A**) 0.018 Guidewire, (**B**) compound dilator (3 French inside of 5 French), (**C**) 21 gage needle.

Additionally, if large pseudoaneurysms are present, it may be advantageous to cannulate above these so as to avoid the problems of passing a guidewire through them. This presumes that the lesion is downstream from the bulging structures.

Selection of a Sheath

An intravascular sheath should always be used for this procedure. Medications may be required during the procedure and it is essential that the affected site be evaluated with radiocontrast after treatment, prior to removal of the guidewire. This can be most easily accomplished if an intravascular sheath is in place. The size of the sheath is determined by the diameter of the angioplasty balloon that is to be used. If it is too small, insertion and removal of the catheter will be difficult if not impossible. Catheter removal is the critical variable. After use, the balloon will be larger than when it was inserted. If one uses a larger sheath than is necessary, an unnecessarily large hole will be created in the graft. The manufacturer specifies the required sheath size on the label of the balloon catheter (Figure 17-2).

In general, a 6-French sheath is appropriate for standard catheters with balloons in the 8-mm diameter size (5 or 5.8 mm shaft). However, if a larger sized balloon is required, a larger sheath will be necessary. Some interventionalists prefer a 7-French sheath as their routine sheath to be sure that difficulty will not be encountered when removing the balloon after inflation and to avoid having to insert a second sheath in the event that a larger balloon is required. One must keep in mind that the size designation for a sheath refers to the inner diameter. The outer diameter is 1.5–2 French larger. A 7-French dilator actually results in a 9-French hole.

Balloon daimeter (Inflated)	8 MM
Balloon length	4 CM
Recommended introducer	6 F
French size (Catheter)	5 F
Catheter length (Usable)	75 CM
Recommended guidewire	.035 IN
Rated burst pressure	16 ATM

Figure 17-2. Angioplasty balloon label.

Passing the Guidewire

A guidewire should be passed through the sheath and advanced up to the level of the central veins. The inability to pass the guidewire precludes correction of the lesion with angioplasty. In cases where the vein is tortuous, guidewire manipulation may be required, which can be a considerable challenge. In most instances, a specialized guidewire is not needed when doing a simple angioplasty. A Newton (AngioDynamics, Queensbury, NY), Bentson (Cook Inc., Bloomington, IN), or similar guidewire works quite well and is relatively inexpensive. Only if difficulty is encountered should one resort to specialized types of guidewires which are more expensive.

Preprocedure Angiogram

An angiogram should be performed to evaluate the anatomy of the graft and its draining veins up through the superior vena cava. It is important that the entire circuit be evaluated since multiple lesions are seen in many cases, both AVG[13] and AVF.[17-21] All lesions should be documented for later reference. It is also important to evaluate the arterial portion of the circuit by looking at the arterial anastomosis, and adjacent feeding artery. This can be easily accomplished through a retrograde arteriogram performed by injecting radiocontrast while manually occluding the access downstream from the injection site. Additionally, one can occlude the access with the angioplasty balloon for this retrograde injection once the venous angioplasty, if one is to be done, has been accomplished.

Diagnosing Stenosis

The criteria used for the diagnosis of stenosis are based upon a comparison with the adjacent vessel or graft.[13,22-27] At the venous anastomosis, there is often a significant size discrepancy between the graft and the adjacent "normal" vein. In this instance, the comparison used for the diagnosis should be the graft.

The diagnosis of arterial anastomosis stenosis is difficult because there is a lack of a standardized definition. This is an artificially created orifice structure that lacks an optimal standard. Its size is based upon the surgeon's judgment and is generally smaller than the adjacent vessel. Some surgeons use a tapered graft that may resemble a stenosis. In addition, there is always a major drop in pressure across this site. Basically, the inflow of the graft is composed of three parts: the artery adjacent to the graft, the anastomosis, and the juxta-anastomotic access (2 cm downstream from the arterial anastomosis). Stenosis of the artery and the juxta-anastomotic access can be easily determined by a size comparison with the adjacent normal vessel or graft. The problem lies with a definition of what constitutes stenosis of the artificially created anastomotic orifice. To solve this issue, it has been suggested that anastomosis stenosis be defined by a size comparison with the adjacent normal artery.[28] If the difference is 50% or more, it should be classified as stenotic.

Lesion Selection

NKF-k/DOQI Practice Guidelines state that in order to qualify for angioplasty treatment a venous stenosis lesion should cause a greater than 50% decrease in the luminal diameter and be associated with clinical/physiological abnormalities.[29] In other words, the key indication for treatment is the presence of pathophysiology not abnormal anatomy. This is a very important distinction.

In most instances when a venous angioplasty treatment is being contemplated, it is because the patient has been referred to the treatment facility because of an abnormality that has been detected at the dialysis clinic. However, in the course of treating a lesion that has caused access dysfunction or during an evaluation associated with the treatment of a thrombotic episode, areas of vessel narrowing may be recognized. The question frequently arises as to whether this should be dilated. Although angioplasty of a hemodynamically significant stenosis associated with a nonthrombosed vascular access can maintain functionality and delay thrombosis, there is no convincing evidence that repair of an asymptomatic anatomic stenosis has any beneficial effect. Therefore, prophylactic treatment of a stenosis that fulfills the anatomic criteria (>50% diameter reduction), but is not associated with a hemodynamic, functional, or clinical abnormality, is not warranted and should not be performed.[30–33]

Asymptomatic lesions, even if there is greater than 50% narrowing, do not require treatment and are better managed by simple observation.[34] This was shown in a retrospective study of 35 patients in which the natural history of high grade (>50%) asymptomatic central venous stenosis and the outcome of treatment with percutaneous transluminal angioplasty were documented.[34] Differences in rate of lesion progression between treated and nontreated patients were tabulated. Twenty-eight percent of lesions were not treated, and the remainder was treated with angioplasty. No untreated lesion progressed to symptoms, stent placement, or additional stenosis. Eight percent of treated cases were followed by stenosis or symptom escalation; one patient developed arm swelling, four required stents, and four developed additional stenosis.

One should realize, however, that multiple lesions less than 50% can be additive. The key issue is pathophysiology. If there is low flow, there is a reason. In some instances it is the additive effect of lesions which of themselves individually, would not warrant treatment.

Pseudostenosis

Not everything that looks like a stenosis actually is. Venous spasm is probably the most common cause of "pseudostenosis"; however, external compression can also cause confusion.

Spasm

Venous spasm is a relatively common occurrence (Figure 17-3). Simply passing a guidewire can precipitate

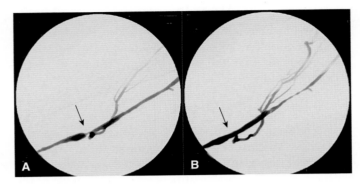

Figure 17-3. Venous spasm. (**A**) Prior to instrumentation, (**B**) immediately after showing spasm. Arrows indicate site of stenotic lesion.

spasm. It may be localized or it may be more generalized. It can be easily confused for a stenotic lesion if one is not careful. Attempts at dilatation may make it worse. At the least, attempted treatment exposes normal vein to the potential for endothelial damage from a needless exposure to the pressure of the angioplasty balloon. When a vein is first examined fluoroscopically, it is important to make a mental note of the location, appearance, and extent of all lesions that are present. After angioplasty, if a new lesion is recognized, it has to be spasm.

External compression

There are a variety of ways that a vein can be compressed by extrinsic pressure giving rise to the artifactual appearance of stenosis (Figure 17-4). In patients with an ectatic aorta, the left innominate vein can be compressed either by the aortic arch or by the vessels coming off of the arch. In very muscular dialysis patients, a muscle imprint can lead to an erroneous suspicion of stenosis of the axillary vein when the arm is adducted.[35] In very thin (cachectic) patients, the cephalic vein as it crosses the shoulder with the patient lying flat may look stenotic due to compression. Large breast or even a tight drape can also cause confusion at times. Although these situations do not usually have any hemodynamic consequence, extrinsic compression of the left innominate vein from an ectatic aorta can result in elevated venous pressure and collateral veins can develop.[36]

Angioplasty Balloon Selection

The basic technique of angioplasty as applied to the dialysis access and associated venous drainage system is dependent upon the use of a high-pressure angioplasty balloon catheter. These are molded to their inflated geometry from relatively noncompliant materials that retain their designed size and shape even under high pressure. They are thin-walled and exhibit high tensile strength. For angioplasty, balloons must have a controlled or repeatable size (diameter vs pressure) in order to ensure that the balloon will not continue to expand (low compliance) and damage

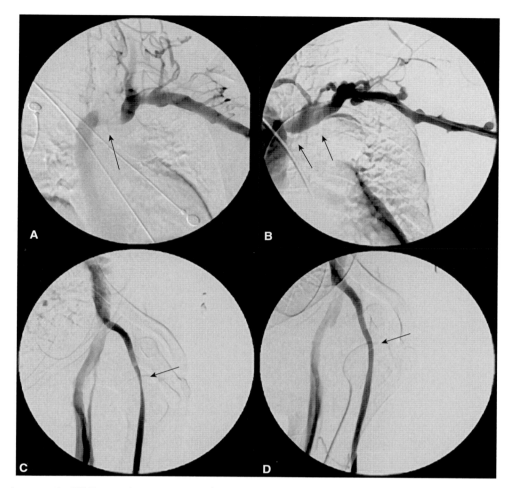

Figure 17-4. Pseudostenosis. (**A**) External compression due to aortic arch, (**B**) compression by brachiocephalic and carotid arteries, (**C**) thin patient lying down with arm on table, (**D**) same patient with arm elevated.

or rupture the artery after it opens the narrowing. Rated pressures for angioplasty balloons are typically in the range of 12–30 atmospheres (1 atm = 14.696 psi) depending on the size; the larger the diameter, the lower the rated pressure. High-pressure balloons with a manufacturer's assigned burst-pressure in the range of 30 have come to be referred to as "ultrahigh-pressure" balloons. These are in contrast to low-pressure balloons that are elastic, are very compliant (can stretch), and cannot be used to exert high pressure in medical applications. (The Fogarty balloon catheter is an example.) Use of ultrahigh-pressure balloons has markedly reduced the incidence of "resistant" lesions. In one study of 87 patients with venous stenosis treated with standard high-pressure balloons, 7 cases (8%) were resistant to dilatation. Using the newer ultrahigh-pressure design, 100% success was obtained in these cases.[37]

There are several reports of the use of a cutting angioplasty balloon (CAB) to treat resistant lesions.[38–44] Most of these reports are hampered by being retrospective, uncontrolled, or of such small size that meaningful conclusions are impossible. However, from these studies, it appears that CAB is generally safe; although, an increased incidence of

vein rupture has been reported.[45] The clinical results have been mixed. Whether or not it offers an advantage over other approaches remains to be demonstrated. Additional controlled, prospective studies based on a large cohort of patients are needed.

When considering which angioplasty balloon catheter to use, there are several considerations that should be taken into account.

Balloon size (diameter and length)

In performing angioplasty on venous lesions, the balloon should be 20–30% larger than the normal vessel judged by comparison with the vessel lumen adjacent to the lesion. The use of a smaller balloon will be met with decreased success (primary patency). The size of the balloon is registered as diameter, measured in millimeters, and length measured in centimeters, for example, an 8 × 4 balloon would be 8 mm in diameter and 4 cm in length (Figure 17-2). Unless the veins are of unusual size, a 7–8-mm diameter balloon will generally be appropriate for both the access and draining veins up to the subclavian (or at least the axillary) and a 12–14 mm balloon will be needed centrally; however, it is important to individual the size of the balloon used to that of the patient's vein. The length of the balloon used should be the shortest that is practical for the lesion being treated to avoid exposing normal vessel to the pressure trauma of the dilatation. This trauma can injure the endothelium and induce the development of a hyperplastic lesion.

Pressure rating

The package label lists the pressure rating for the angioplasty balloon (Figure 17-2). This rating indicates the amount of pressure that the balloon will tolerate before rupture within 95% confidence limits. Each manufacturer rates their balloons so that there is a safety margin of approximately 50%. This allows you to take a 16-atm rated balloon to 20 atm. The balloon selected should have at least a rating of at least 16–17 atm. In instances in which a lesion is recurrent and it is know that the last time it was treated an ultrahigh-pressure balloon was required, many interventionalist prefer to start with this type of balloon.

Balloon dilatation

Pressure in the range of 10 atm is routinely applied to dilate a venous stenotic lesion. If this is not successful, the pressure is increased incrementally up to the maximum that is tolerated by the particular angioplasty balloon that is being used. In a report[46] of 230 lesion treated in 138 cases, it was found that 55% of lesions required pressures greater than 15 atm. Excluding initial failures, 20% of lesions in native fistulas and 9% in grafts required very high pressure (>20 atm). High pressure was needed less frequently in PTA procedures performed in the setting of thrombectomy than in prophylactic PTA.

It is best to avoid rupturing the balloon. The balloon has been designed to simple come loose at one of its weld points and leak when it ruptures; however, it can tear circumferentially and fragment. This can be a problem requiring the retrieval of a piece of errant balloon material. With some balloon designs it is possible to tell when the balloon is about to break. The normally pointed ends of the balloon will round up like the ends of a sausage indicating an impending rupture.

Applying pressure to balloon   There are two approaches to the application of pressure to the angioplasty balloon: using a mechanical device or doing it manually (Figure 17-5). There are a variety of devices available to provide pressure for the inflation of the angioplasty balloon. These inflation devices are composed of three basic parts: the barrel, the plunger, and a pressure manometer. Overall, the inflation device has the general appearance of a modified syringe (some are). It has a locking mechanism so that the pressure can be maintained once it is generated. These devices work well, but are designed for one-time use creating what some consider an unnecessary expense.

Some interventionalists prefer to dilate the lesion manually using a syringe or a syringe assembly. This is a more economical approach. The amount of pressure applied depends upon the size of the syringe that is used; this is an inverse relationship. It has been shown that achievable inflation pressures are quite reproducible across multiple operators.[47] Actually, it is best to use two syringes—a 10 cc and a 3 cc—connected into an assembly with a three-way stopcock. (This must be a high-pressure stopcock and the syringes must be acrylic because of the high pressures required.) The 10 cc syringe is used to simply inflate the balloon, then the switch is turned, and pressure is applied with the 3 cc syringe. This requires much less pressure on the hand.

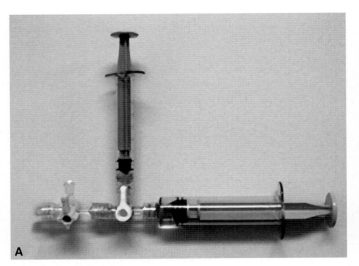

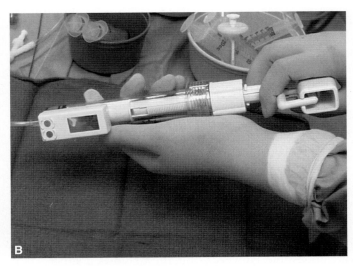

Figure 17-5. Inflation devices. (**A**) Syringe assembly using a 3 cc and a 100 cc syringe, (**B**) inflation device with digital pressure gage.

Maintaining pressure after dilatation Once the lesion has been dilated, the question arises as to how long pressure should be held. Most reports have listed inflation times in the range of 1–3 minutes.[22,37,48–50] Additionally, residual stenosis, which correlates with poor long-term outcome, has been reported to correlate negatively with duration of inflation.[37]

In a randomized controlled study the benefit of a 3-minute dilatation time was tested.[51] A total of 48 patients were enrolled: 27 patients (40 stenoses) randomly assigned to the 1-minute group and 21 (36 stenoses) to the 3-minute group. In this study, a mechanical inflation devise was used. Pressure of 18 atm was applied and held continuously for the stated time period. Technical success rates in the 1- and 3-minute inflation groups were 75% and 89%, respectively. Logistic regression analysis demonstrated that technical success was 4.7 times more likely in the 3- versus the 1-minute inflation group. The 1-, 3-, and 6-month postintervention patencies, however, were not significantly different between the two groups.

VENOUS ANGIOPLASTY—THE BASIC PROCEDURE

▶ Dilatation Sequence

The balloon is positioned across the previously identified stenosis; it is the inflated under direct fluoroscopic observation (Figure 17-6). At this time a definite defect in the balloon should be noted (dog-bone defect). With continued pressure, in the successful treatment, the defect disappears and there is total effacement of the balloon.

Steps of the procedure

The actual steps in the angioplasty procedure are as follows:

1. Select the appropriate site for cannulation. Anesthetize the skin with lidocaine. Insert the introducer needle and pass the guidewire. Advance the guidewire only as far as is necessary to secure it for sheath placement. If difficulty is encountered in passing the guidewire, do not attempt to manipulate it through the needle. Go ahead with the next step and then do your manipulations.

2. Pin (this means fix it so that it cannot move) the guidewire and remove the needle. Thread the dilator tip of the sheath over the guidewire and insert the sheath into the cannulation site. Advance the sheath 4–6 cm to minimize inadvertent removal later in the procedure.

3. Remove the dilator from the sheath. The guidewire can be left in place or removed which ever seems to be the most convenient.

4. Inject radiocontrast through the sidearm of the sheath to visualize the access and draining veins all the way through the superior vena cava. Make careful mental note (and document) of any stenotic lesions that are discovered. Manually occlude the graft above the tip of the sheath and make a retrograde injection to visualize the arterial anastomosis and adjacent artery. Take note of any lesions and make a subjective judgment of the quality of flow in the main artery.

5. Once you have seen that there is a lesion that will require treatment, prepare for the angioplasty.

6. Pass the guidewire so that the tip lies well above the most central lesion that is present.

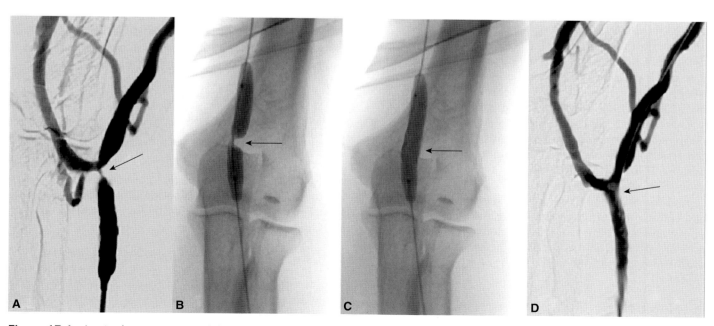

Figure 17-6. Angioplasty sequence. (**A**) Lesion, (**B**) balloon indentation, (**C**) full balloon effacement, (**D**) post-treatment anatomical result.

7. Administer the appropriate dose of sedation.

8. Insert the angioplasty balloon catheter over the guidewire.

9. Pass the balloon catheter up to the most central lesion. Position the balloon across the lesion.

10. Dilate the lesion. Hold pressure (use a stop-cock) for 3 minute once the lesion has dilated.

11. Deflate the balloon completely before moving it downstream to the next lesion. If there are no more lesions to be dilated, remove the deflated balloon. Be sure to pin the guidewire before removing the catheter so as to not lose the site.

12. Leave the guidewire across the treated site until you have been able to examine it for result and any complications.

13. Inject radiocontrast through the sidearm of the sheath to visualize the lesion. Determine the effectiveness of the treatment. Check for complications.

14. If all appears satisfactory, remove the guidewire.

15. Wait 10–15 minutes and recheck the result to determine if any recoil of the treated lesion has occurred.

16. Remove the sheath and obtain hemostasis.

▶ Dilating Multiple Lesions

When multiple lesions are present that require treatment with angioplasty, the sequence in which they are treated is of some importance. This is determined by two factors. Firstly, the major complication of consequence that can occur is venous rupture. The severity of the extravasation that can occur with this event is directly related to intra-access pressure. If the outflow is occluded, the situation will be worse than if it is open. Therefore, when dilating a series of lesions, always start with the one that is the most proximal (downstream).

Secondly, the angioplasty balloon will have a larger profile once it has been used. If a series of lesions is present, it is much easier to pull the balloon back into a stenosis than to advance the larger profile through a tight narrowing. This is another reason to start proximally.

This rationale breaks down somewhat when both a peripheral and a central lesion are present. Unless the central lesion is very tight, it is customary to start with the peripheral lesion(s) before addressing it. This is done to avoid having to transitioning the larger balloon used for central lesions through peripheral stenoses both going in and coming out. On the other hand if the central lesion is severe and is causing a significant increase in intravascular pressure peripherally, it would be better to start there to assure an open outflow in the event of a peripheral vessel rupture.

▶ Hemostasis

At the end of the procedure it is necessary to obtain hemostasis. The fact that the patient will not generally have received heparin is an advantage. Hemostasis can be obtained with manual compression or with a cutaneous suture.

Manual compression

As in the dialysis clinic, hemostasis can be obtained by manual compression. However, as in the dialysis clinic this may take time. It is generally desirable to use something to facilitate the process. The "tip stop" (Gambro-Hospal, Cambridgeshire, England) consists of an adhesive bandage with a small plastic button in its center. This button is covered with a layer of collagen. When applied to the site, the button applies pressure and the collagen promotes thrombosis. These bandages are relatively inexpensive and very effective in most cases. Using this device, hemostasis should be accomplished within 5–10 minutes even in a heparinized patient.

Cutaneous suture

This is an excellent approach for obtaining hemostasis. To do this a figure-of-eight or purse-string stitch is made using 3-O suture prior to removing the dilator or other device that is in the graft. The suture is then tied behind and beneath the device. The tie is tightened to control bleeding as the device is removed. The stitches should be removed 24–38 hours later when the patient goes for dialysis. Failure to do so can result in skin necrosis.

JUDGING THE SUCCESS OF BALLOON ANGIOPLASTY

The lesion of venous stenosis is resistant to dilatation at times and at times has a tendency to be elastic. In some patients, recoil can obviate the results of therapy within a relatively short period, at times in a matter of minutes to hours. Therefore it is important to have some type of criteria for judging the success of therapy. There are several parameters that can be used. In fact, all should be applied.

▶ Anatomic Criteria

NKF-K/DOQI Practice Guideline 8.4[52] states that no more than 30% residual stenosis should remain following angioplasty treatment. This should be judged by comparison with the adjacent normal vein. One would like to see less residual than this; however, this guide should be used as the minimum criteria. The goal should be the elimination of any residual (see discussion below) regardless of what the Guideline states.

▶ Clinical Criteria at the Procedure Table

The use of clinical criteria (physical examination) in the lab at the procedure table is also of importance. When there is significant venous stenosis, physical examination will reveal the presence of the abnormality.[16] The abnormalities evident in the presence of significant pathology should not be apparent in its absence. In practical terms, following successful balloon angioplasty one should feel a palpable continuous, soft thrill over the graft with a soft compressible pulse. This is evidence of success.

▶ Hemodynamic/Physiologic Criteria

According to NKF-K/DOQI Practice Guideline 6.4[29,53] a patient should not be sent for angioplasty unless there are hemodynamic or physiological abnormalities. These abnormal clinical parameters used to suspect the presence of stenosis should return to within acceptable limits following intervention. This should be considered the gold standard for judging success of an angioplasty treatment. The abnormalities that suggested the presence of the stenotic lesion prior to therapy should be reassessed as soon as practical following treatment. A failure of these indices to return to normal or near normal indicates treatment failure and the need for either repeat of alternative treatment.

MANAGEMENT OF SPECIFIC PROBLEMS

It is important that each interventionalist be able to recognize and appropriately deal with problems and complications that arise during the course and following an angioplasty procedure.

▶ Difficult Cannulation

Difficult graft cannulation can be extremely frustrating and time consuming. There are several aids that can be used to facilitate a successful cannulation

Using a dilator as a guide

If difficulty is encountered entering the graft at a point from which the purpose of the procedure can be accomplished, there is generally some point in the graft at which cannulation is more easily possible. A secondary site can be used to facilitate the cannulation of the primary or first site using a dilator as a guide.

1. Cannulate the secondary (easy) site with the introducer needle directed toward the primary (difficult) site.
2. Pass the guidewire into the graft in this direction and remove the needle.
3. Introduce a dilator into the graft over the guidewire. Pass the dilator until its tip is well beyond the selected site for the primary cannulation.
4. Perform the primary cannulation using the dilator as a target under fluoroscopy. You will be able to see the guidewire that will be protected from damage by the dilator. In addition, you will be able to feel the dilator with the tip of the introducer needle. By using direct visualization, you can guide the tip of the needle to where it touches the dilator. At that point, the needle is within the graft lumen and the guidewire should pass.

Though and through cannulation

Basically, this technique is useful only for the cannulation of a graft. Unlike the dilator-guide approach, this does not require a prior cannulation. It has the disadvantage of creating a needle hole in the backside of the graft, which can result in hematoma formation. However, this is a small price to pay if you have no other alternative.

1. Enter the graft with a very flat angle and go all the way through.
2. Torque the tip of the needle upward using your index finger as a fulcrum and slowly pull it backwards. As you do this, you should feel the needle pop into the lumen.
3. At that point, pass the guidewire.

Real-time cannulation using ultrasound

The lumen of the vascular structure that you are trying to cannulate should be visible with ultrasound. This makes real-time cannulation with ultrasound possible. This technique can be utilized successfully in many cases when cannulation is difficult. This technique is especially useful for cannulating a vein. A micropuncture needle may be found to be very useful in this endeavor.

Guidewire–balloon entrapment

Guidewire–balloon entrapment (Figure 17-7) is useful for the cannulation of a vein.[54] It requires that the access already have a prior cannulation with the ability to pass a guidewire in the direction of the desired site. It involves placing an angioplasty balloon at the selected site and perforating it with a micropuncture needle. It has the disadvantage of destroying an angioplasty balloon, but it is successful in accomplishing cannulation at the desired site.

1. Pass a guidewire beyond the desired site for cannulation of the vein that is causing the problem.
2. Pass an angioplasty balloon over the guidewire up to the desired site and inflate it softly with the usual radiocontrast mixture (Figure 17-7A). This should be just enough to fully inflate the balloon.
3. Under fluoroscopic visualization, perforate the inflated balloon with a micropuncture needle (Figure 17-7B). The site on the balloon selected for this should be relatively close to the end opposite the direction the guidewire is to be passed (if guidewire is to be passed down, perforate the upper end of balloon). When the needle enters the balloon, clear liquid will start to leak from the hub of the needle (contents of balloon).
4. Insert the microguidewire through the needle and into the balloon. Allow it to coil up. If you see that you have gone all the way through the balloon, do not worry; the balloon will still entrap the guidewire.
5. With the guidewire entrapped within the balloon, retract the balloon and remove it to pull the guidewire into the vein (Figure 17-7C). Allow the guidewire to enter the

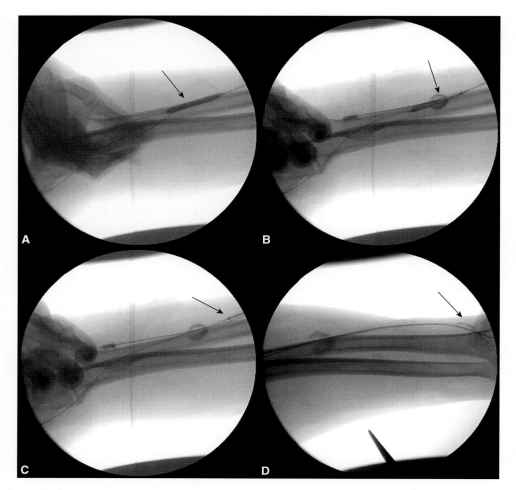

Figure 17-7. Guidewire-balloon entrapment. (**A**) Balloon (arrow) inflated with needle ready, (**B**) balloon perforated, note small extravasation (arrow), (**C**) balloon being retracted, arrow at dot marking distal end of balloon, (**D**) guidewire down, arrow indicates the coiled guidewire, note the extravasation marking the site of cannulation.

vein as the balloon is pulled downward, but do not lose the guidewire by allowing it to go too far.

6. Now with the guidewire in place (Figure 17-7D), insert the dilator over the guidewire and proceed with the procedure.

▶ Cannulating a Fistula: Special Considerations

In many cases, there are no real differences between the cannulation of a fistula and a graft. This is certainly true if it is a mature fistula. The only difference is that the fistula is more compressible and therefore one must exert a greater degree of caution to avoid passing all the way through the back wall. Unfortunately, when a patient with a fistula is sent to the lab for a study or a procedure it is because they have a problem. This problem may have caused changes in the fistula that cause it to be difficult to cannulate. In these cases the use of a micropuncture needle may facilitate the process. The small size of this needle facilitates difficult cannulations.

A fistula with poor flow or a poorly developed fistula is especially difficult to cannulate. Using manual compression above the cannulation site to engorge the vein will help. This occlusion of the vessel making cannulation easier to accomplish should always be done with fistulas.

▶ Inability to Pass Guidewire

There are times when the guidewire is difficult to pass; this is generally because the stenotic lesion is severe (even occluded) or the vein is very tortuous. The appropriate manner in which to approach this problem will depend upon the circumstance and a number of different variables; however, there are several choices. Firstly, make multiple attempts with the standard guidewire by repetitively advancing and withdrawing it. Simply by chance (trial and error) it may go across. If this does not succeed, remove the guidewire and create a slight J at the tip. (This presumes that one is using a basic stainless steel guidewire.) To do this, grasp the tip of the guidewire between your thumb and a hemostat. Pull the wire through your grasp.

This will bend the wire into a J. It requires some practice to do this and avoid overdoing it, creating a coil (pig-tail). Using the newly created J-tipped guidewire, repeat your attempt turning the guidewire so as to steer the J-tip in different directions.

A guiding catheter is frequently beneficial in this setting; the exact shape of the tip of the catheter will depend upon the individual situation. One of these types of catheters can be used not only to guide the guidewire, but also to stiffen it and prevent it from buckling. If this is not successful, a specialized steerable guidewire (with a J-tip) may solve the problem. Actually, the use of a specialized guidewire and the use of a guiding catheter rank about equally in their success rate; however, in general, the catheter is more economical. A torquing device should be used to maneuver the guidewire.

Regardless of the approach one selects to attempt to cross a difficult area, creating a road-map may be found to be helpful. Unfortunately, there are some situations in which the guidewire cannot be passed, but one should not give up too easily.

▶ Inability to Get Balloon Catheter to Track Over Guidewire

This is generally a problem only when there is a sharp curve that must be negotiated. A curve in the catheter tends to dampen the longitudinal force being applied to push it forward. This is made worse by the flexibility of the guidewire. First apply traction of the guidewire (be careful not to pull it back too far). This has the effect of stiffening it. This is done by slowly pulling back on the guidewire as an attempt is made to advance the catheter. Obviously, to do this safely, one must have an adequate length of guidewire extending beyond the catheter tip. If this is not effective, the best solution is to use a more rigid (stiffer) guidewire. A variety of these are available.

▶ Inability to Cross Stenotic Lesion

Occasionally, you will encounter a vein that is so stenotic that it will not permit the passage of the selected (the one of a size appropriate for the vein being treated) angioplasty balloon catheter. In these cases one must exert care in trying to force the catheter in order to avoid irreparable damage. There are two approaches that may work.

Using the selected balloon catheter

Since you already have a balloon in place, it is reasonable to first try to solve the problem using it. The tip of the balloon on the angioplasty catheter is tapered. Even though you cannot pass the catheter across the lesion, you may be able to get the tip into it. Wedge the catheter into the lesion forcefully and inflate. Do this repetitively. If the procedure is working, you will notice that the balloon is slowly advancing. Once the stenotic point is passed, the catheter should advance easily. There is a disadvantage to this technique. The balloon profile is significantly larger after it has been inflated. For this reason, if you are not successful, you are now trying to advance a larger device than before.

Using a smaller balloon catheter

If you cannot advance the regular angioplasty balloon catheter across the lesion, a smaller one may pass without difficulty. Try the smallest balloon diameter that you have. If it will pass, dilating the lesion to this size will generally permit passage of the selected angioplasty balloon. If the lesion is so tight that even the smallest balloon will not pass, try the same wedging technique described above with the smaller balloon. If still unsuccessful, send the patient for surgical revision.

▶ Dealing with Residual Stenosis

In spite of NKF-K/DOQI Practice Guideline 8.4s[29,52] definition of success, residual stenosis of any degree is a problem (Figure 17-8). In a prospective study of 330 angioplasty procedures designed to identify predictors of arteriovenous graft patency after radiological intervention, the median graft survival was found to be inversely related to the magnitude of residual stenosis.[55] With complete resolution, the primary patency was 6.9 months; by comparison, it was reduced to 4.6 months with residual stenosis. The goal of venous stenosis therapy should be no residual. There are basically two situations in which one is left with residual stenosis following angioplasty: a resistant lesion and an elastic lesion. In either instance, the result is less than optimum because complete dilatation has not been achieved. The approach to these two, however, is different.

Resistant lesion

Some lesions are extremely resistant to dilatation. When this occurs there are three courses of action that are available: more pressure, do something to weaken the lesion, or refer for surgical revision.

More pressure As stated above most angioplasty balloons are designed to allow for 16–20 atm of pressure. If one exceeds this, the balloon will rupture. One should continue to increase the pressure applied to a resistant lesion with the balloon that is in place until there is concern that rupture is imminent or it actually occurs. If this has not accomplished the desired effect, move to an ultrahigh-pressure balloon and apply maximum pressure with this device; it will tolerate more than 30 atm. With the advent of the ultrahigh-pressure balloon, it is possible to treat most, but not all, of these successfully.[37] If this is still unsuccessful move to an alternative approach, one of the other two that are listed.

Weaken the lesion It appears in some cases that multiple prolonged dilatations can weaken a resistant lesion to the point that it eventually gives way. However, there are techniques available that are specifically designed to weaken the integrity of a stenotic lesion. These involve cutting it in some manner. The use of a cutting balloon

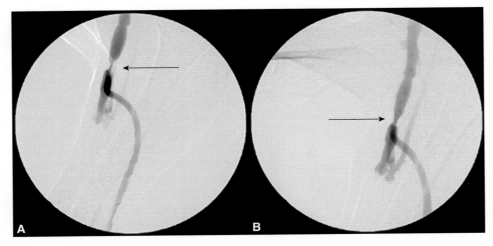

Figure 17-8. Residual stenosis. (**A**) Pretreatment lesion, (**B**) post-treatment showing significant residual.

has been advocated by some interventionalists for this problem[56]; however, there are techniques that may be equally as effective and are more economical.

Parallel guidewire This technique makes use of a second guidewire used as a cutting device.[57–59] A second guidewire is passed so that it lies parallel to the angioplasty balloon across the resistant lesion. The balloon is then dilated to maximal pressure causing the wire to cut into the lesion. In one series of 22 cases,[59] this technique was successful in all instances. In 18 of the cases, satisfactory results were obtained with a pressure lower than had been used for the initial unsuccessful angioplasty. In the remaining four cases, the technique was implemented several times using maximum dilatation pressures, changing the guidewire position before each additional inflation.

1. Once the resistant lesion has been detected by an inability to dilate it at maximum pressures, insert a second guidewire through the sheath and pass it to a level beyond the angioplasty balloon that should be centered over the resistant lesion.
2. Inflate the angioplasty balloon to maximum pressure with the second guidewire in place.
3. If unsuccessful in obtaining dilatation, shift the position of the guidewire and try again.

Needle perforation Needle perforation (Figure 17-9) involves damaging the integrity of the lesion using a 22-gauge needle. The site of the lesion is identified under fluoroscopy, infiltrated with xylocaine and then perforated multiple tiles in order to weaken it. Then dilatation with the angioplasty balloon is repeated.

1. Once the resistant lesion (Figure 17-9A) has been detected, localize it under fluoroscopy using a 21-gage needle (Figure 17-9B).

2. Retract the angioplasty balloon, leaving the guidewire in place to serve as a marker.
3. Infiltrate the lesion with lidocaine.
4. Insert the needle down to the lesion; it should be possible to feel it, and perforate it 20–30 times (do this without removing the needle).
5. Replace the angioplasty balloon and dilate the lesion again.

Elastic lesion

There are times when a lesion shows total effacement with the angioplasty balloon, only to recoil after it is deflated (Figure 17-10). If the problem is recoil due to elasticity of the vessel, the best solution is a larger balloon. A balloon 1 mm larger should be tried. Basically, for an angioplasty to be successful, something has to rip, tear, or break.[60] If it only stretches, there is a risk of recoil. Unfortunately, there is a risk to either higher pressure or larger balloon approach to residual stenosis. However, if the lesion is a problem, the problem must be addressed. It needs to be dealt with either by angioplasty or a surgical referral.

Elastic recoil is more likely to occur in central veins.[60,61] Part of this may be related to the unusually large size of the central vessels in hemodialysis patients; it is difficult to overdilate a vein of this size. In one study,[61] 30 patients with central venous stenosis were treated with angioplasty; 70% had 50% or greater improvement in the luminal diameter while 23% showed no improvement due to the presence of an elastic lesion. Subsequently, 81% of those with a successful result restenosed at an average of 7.6 months, while 100% of the elastic lesions occluded at an average of 2.9 months. In the same study, 10 patients underwent angioplasty and Wallstent placement; 5 of these were due to elastic lesions. They had four recurrences at a mean of 8.6 months. Four of the five

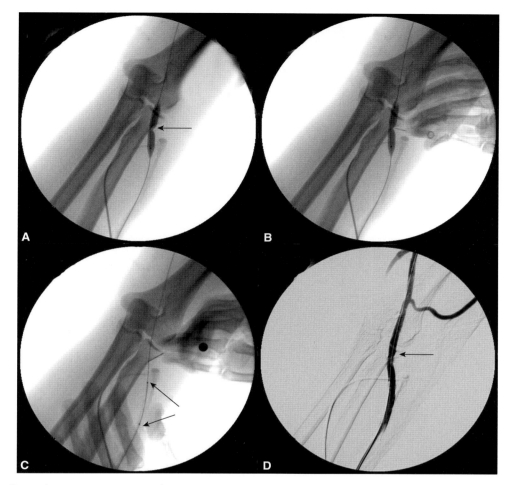

Figure 17-9. Needle perforation. (**A**) Resistant lesion (arrow), (**B**) localizing lesion under fluoroscopy, (**C**) position of deflated balloon (arrows) and perforation with 21 gage needle, (**D**) final result.

patients stented with nonelastic lesions had a reappearance of symptoms at a mean of 4.2 months.

INITIAL SUCCESS OF ANGIOPLASTY TREATMENT

NKF-K/DOQI Practice Guideline 8.4[52] defines a successful angioplasty by stating that the treated lesion should have less than 30% residual stenosis and the clinical/physiological parameters used to detect the stenosis should return to acceptable limits after the intervention. Using anatomical criteria, initial success rates for venous angioplasty have ranged from 80% to 98% for AVGs.[10,13,14,49,62–65] There are only a few small studies available that present data derived strictly from fistulas. These have reported an initial success rate ranging from 89.5% to 97%.[41, 66–71] The largest of these involved a series of 1561 cases, which had a 97% success rate.[71]

Reports have indicated that approximately 20–30% of patients fail to show an increase in blood flow after what had been judged to be a successful angioplasty based upon anatomical criteria.[72–74] The reasons for this hemodynamic failure are not clear, but are undoubtedly related to three possible factors: residual stenosis, elasticity, or a missed lesion.

VENOUS ANGIOPLASTY PATENCY RATES

NKF-K/DOQI Practice Guidelines state that the expected 6-month primary patency rate for the treatment of dialysis access graft dysfunction treated by percutaneous angioplasty should be at least 50%.[52] This should be regarded as a minimum criterion.

Long-term success rates are generally listed as either primary or unassisted rates (primary or unassisted patency refers to that period from the time the procedure is performed until a second procedure is required to maintain patency). Primary patency rates (Table 17-1) for angioplasty in grafts generally range from 41% to 76% at 6 months and 31–45% at 1 year.[10,13,14,22,31,49,55,62,75,76]

As with immediate outcomes, the treatment of central lesions is also associated with relatively poor long-term

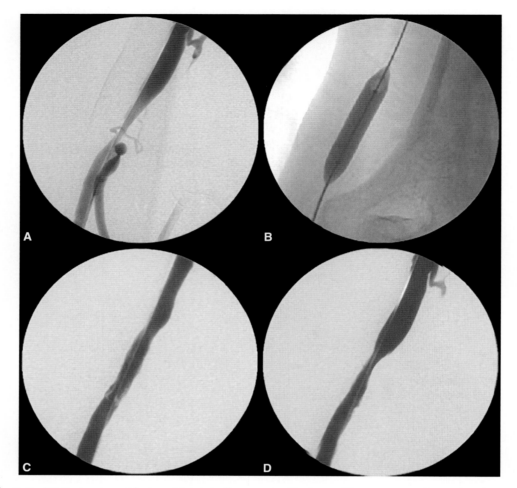

Figure 17-10. Elasticity. (**A**) Pretreatment lesion, (**B**) total effacement of balloon, (**C**) appearance immediately post-treatment, (**D**) appearance 10 minutes post-treatment.

success. Older studies have shown a primary patency in the range of 25% at 6 months.[13] However, more recent studies have had somewhat better results. In one report, hemodialysis patients that underwent successful endovascular treatment of central venous obstruction were retrospectively evaluated.[77] Angioplasty treatments for 101 were documented. Primary patency data showed a mean of 24.5 ± 1.7 months. Secondary patency had a mean of 31.4 ± 2.0 months with an average number of interventions per vein of 1.5 ± 1.0.

TABLE 17–1

Analysis of Dialysis Access Graft Patency

		Primary Patency				
Author	Cohort size	1 mo	2 mo	3 mo	6 mo	12 mo
Saeed	28				76%	
Beathard	536			91%	61%	38%
Beathard	30	100%	91%	85%	72%	17%
Mori	164			68%	42%	25%
Beathard	1120	87%	85%	77%	66%	44%
Kanterman	215				63%	41%
Longwitz	166				55%	47%
Vesely	167	76%		61%	36%	
Wu	35	97%		63%	43%	
Average	2311	86%	85%	78%	64%	41%

FREQUENT RECURRENCES

There is a tendency for venous stenosis problems to be recurrent,[13,22,78] making repeat therapy necessary. In one series, for example, it was found that once successfully performed, repeat angioplasty was required at a mean 5.8 month intervals in order to maintain graft flow at acceptable levels.[72]

The NKF-K/DOQI guidelines state that if repeat angioplasty is required more than twice within 3 months, the patient should be referred for surgical revision.[29] This recommendation has considerable validity. If a lesion is recurring at a frequent interval, elasticity of the lesion is often the cause and an alternative to what has been previously done should be sought. The alternatives are surgery or the placement of a stent.

▶ Use of Endoluminal Stent

A peripheral lesion that has failed balloon angioplasty may be considered an indication for the placement of a stent[29] (see Chapter 19).

▶ Surgical Revision

The efficacy of surgical treatment has been both lauded and questioned. In a surgical study conducted over a 2-year period, 101 operative procedures were performed on failed grafts.[79] All cases had previously been treated with percutaneous dilatation. The number of previous interventions ranged from one to five. Primary patency rates of the angioaccess grafts following surgical revision were 43%, 24%, and 12% at 30, 60, and 90 days, respectively. These surgical investigators concluded that surgical intervention did not significantly prolong the patency of angioaccess grafts that have previously failed percutaneous interventions. Nevertheless, in cases with frequent recurrences following what has appeared to be successful angioplasty treatment, an alternative must be sought. Ultimately, surgery may be the best choice.

COMPLICATIONS ASSOCIATED WITH VENOUS ANGIOPLASTY

As with any type of medical procedure, angioplasty can result in procedure-related complications; however, the complication rate that has been reported is low. Procedure-related complications are generally classified according to the reporting standards of the Society for Interventional Radiology.[80] According to this standard, all complications, including pulmonary and cardiac events that occur within 30 days following the procedure, are considered procedure related. Minor complications are those that require either no therapy or only nominal therapy and resolved without any adverse consequence. Major complications are defined as those that require an increase in the level of care, or result in hospitalization, permanent adverse sequelae, or death.

In a report of 3560 cases of dialysis access graft angioplasty performed by 29 interventional nephrologists in 11 different freestanding facilities, the overall complication rate was reported to be 1.15%[71]; of these, 1.04% were minor. The most frequent procedure-related complication seen in association with angioplasty that dictates the need for intervention is tearing of the vein or vein rupture.[31] In this series, the incidence of vein rupture was 0.9%. In another studies of over 1200 cases a 0.9% incidence[45] and a 2% incidence[25] of vein rupture was reported.

The clinical significance of vein rupture is variable, ranging from none to disaster for the access. The difference lies in the severity of the tear. The presence of this complicating event is heralded by the extravasation of contrast, blood, or both. Small extravasations are of no clinical significance. It is not unusual to observe a small ecchymosis over the treated site the day following therapy. There may be tenderness at the site as well. These are of no consequence. Nothing need be done except to reassure the patient. They need not be listed as a complication, although it is obvious that a small break has occurred.

Vein rupture with extravasation becomes more obvious when there is either the extravasation of contrast creating an image on fluoroscopy or the formation of an obvious hematoma. These occurrences should be listed as procedure-related complications; however, their clinical consequence may range from minimal to major. The amount of extravasated contrast associated with the hematoma may be minimal or absent.

▶ Categories of Procedure Related Complication

Complications directly related to angioplasty can be categorized as endothelial tear, venous rupture, and venous spasm.

Endothelial tear

When an angioplasty is success, it is generally because something broke or tore. Sometimes an endothelial tear is such that it can cause a problem by interfering with blood flow (Figure 17-11). This can generally be managed by placing the angioplasty balloon across the affected area, inflating it with a soft pressure, and leaving it for several minutes (3–5 minutes). This is frequently successful. If it is not and flow is still adversely affected, the placement of a stent should be considered.

Venous rupture

The most frequent procedure-related complication seen in association with angioplasty that dictates the need for intervention is tearing of the vein or vein rupture.[36] Although some investigators have reported an alarmingly high incidence of vein rupture in association with angioplasty treatment of autologous fistulae,[76] in our experience the occurrence has been relatively low. In a series of 5121 angioplasty procedures performed on dialysis access an

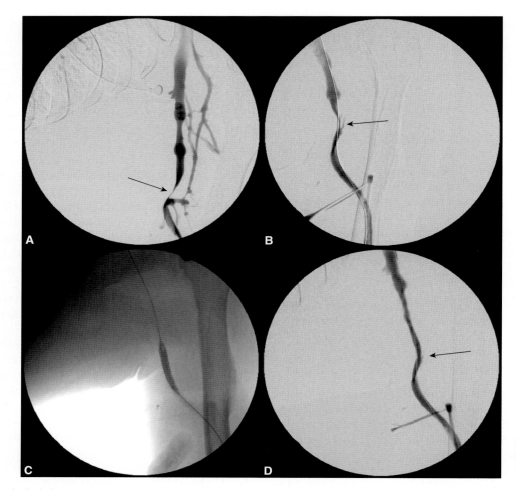

Figure 17-11. Endothelial tear. (**A**) Lesion prior to angioplasty, (**B**) endothelial tear (arrow) flow was slowed, (**C**) balloon tamponade, (**D**) appearance of region after 5 minutes of pressure with slowly inflated angioplasty balloon.

overall complication rate of 3.54% was seen. This series was composed of synthetic grafts—3560 cases with a 1.15% complication rate and autologous fistulae—1561 cases with a 4.48% complication rate. Seventy percent of these complications were vein rupture of some degree.[71]

Definitions and management The clinical significance of this complication is variable, ranging from none to disaster for the access. The difference lies in the severity of the tear. The presence of this complicating event is generally heralded by the extravasation of contrast, blood or both. Small extravasations are of no clinical significance. They need not be listed as a complication although it is obvious that a small break has occurred.

Vein rupture with extravasation becomes more obvious when there is the formation of an obvious hematoma. These occurrences should be tabulated as procedure-related complications; however, its clinical consequence may range from minimal to major. The amount of extravasated contrast associated with the hematoma may be minimal or absent. It is useful to use a classification system (Table 17-2) for extravasation based upon their clinical significance.[26,81,82]

TABLE 17–2
Extravasation Classification

Subclinical extravasation of contrast
    No associated hematoma[a]
    Only evident on fluoroscopy
Grade 1 hematoma
    Does not interfere with flow[a]
    Size variable
    Requires no therapy
    Stable[a]
Grade 2 hematoma
    Slows or stops flow[a]
    Size variable
    Therapy required
    Stable[a]
Grade 3 hematoma (vein disruption)
    Large extravasation or hematoma
    Size variable, generally large
    Continues to expand may be rapid[a]
    Pulsatile[a]

[a]Defining feature.

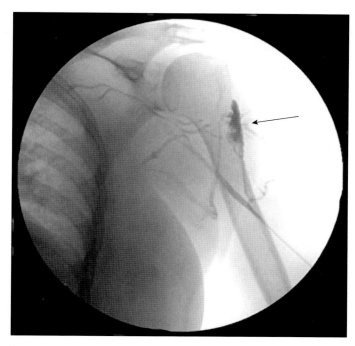

Figure 17-12. Subclinical extravasation of contrast. No clinical effect and no palpable hematoma.

Subclinical extravasation of contrast (SEC) Occasionally, during the course of an angioplasty procedure, a blush of contrast adjacent to the vein at the site of the dilatation is observed but there is no associated hematoma (Figure 17-12). As is the case with blood, this small extravasation is subclinical in that it is asymptomatic and only obvious on fluoroscopy. It takes on significance because it is immediately obvious on the fluoroscopic image. An SEC should be listed as a minor complication. It is of no clinical consequence. No treatment is required.

Grade 1 hematoma When a hematoma is noted, one must make two determinations: (1) if it is stable or continuing to enlarge, and (2) if it affects flow. A grade 1 hematoma (Figure 17-13) is stable, for example, not continuing to grow, and does not affect flow. If it is not stable, it will rapidly become a grade 2 or it may actually be a grade 3 hematoma. Although the grade 1 situation causes concern on the part of the operator and the patient, it is of no real consequence to the outcome of the procedure and requires no specific treatment. This is true regardless of its size. In general, a hematoma that remains stable over 30 minutes to an hour period will continue to behave in this manner as long as the downstream vascular drainage is patent. It does not require further observation. A grade 1 hematoma is a minor complication. In the large angioplasty series previously mentioned,[35] the incidence of a grade 1 hematoma in grafts was 0.76% (27 cases out of 3560) and with fistulas was 3.35% (53 cases out of 1561). This is generally the most frequent complication observed.

The patient with a grade 1 hematoma will have an ecchymosis and will need reassurance and may require symptomatic treatment measures.[36] Localized discomfort may be significant and may last for several days. Mild analgesics and a heating pad may be helpful. The resulting ecchymosis may be quite large, depending on the size of the hematoma.

Grade 2 hematoma If a hematoma is stable but affects flow it is classified as a grade 2 hematoma (Figure 17-14). This is not strictly dependent upon size. Most of these lesions stabilize very quickly after they form. If they do not, they will soon develop into a grade 3 extravasation. In these cases a tear has been created in the vein's wall that requires treatment. The grade 2 hematoma is classified as a major complication even if it is successfully treated. It is classified as a major complication if the access is lost. In the series mentioned previously,[35] the incidence of this complication was 0.11% in grafts (4 cases out of 3560) and 0.04% (6 cases out of 1561) with fistulas.

With this problem, it appears that the tear in the wall of the vessel with a flap that is being displaced into the

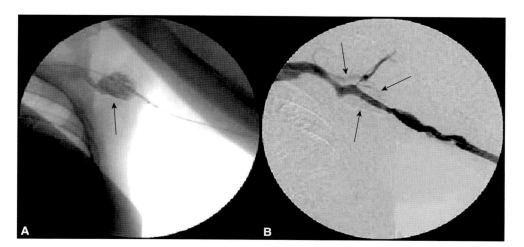

Figure 17-13. Grade 1 hematoma, note that even though sizable hematoma is present (arrows, **A** and **B**), flow is unaffected (B).

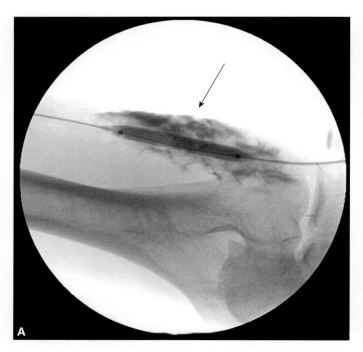 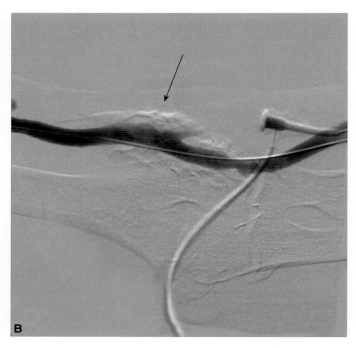

Figure 17-14. Grade 2 hematoma. (**A**) Balloon in place in an attempt to restore flow, arrow indicates the hematoma, (**B**) flow restored, note the shadow of the hematoma (arrow).

former lumen results in its obstruction. The goal of treatment is to press the flap outward in order to open the lumen and restore flow. If the lumen is opened with an angioplasty balloon, the pressure of the balloon will frequently stabilize the situation after a few minutes and allow for the restoration of flow.

This treatment requires that a guidewire be positioned across the lesion. For this reason, it is important that the guidewire should never be removed after an angioplasty until the treated lesion has been evaluated for complications. If the guidewire has not been retained, it is often difficult or impossible to replace it. With a guidewire in position, the first step is to determine the site of the tear. The tear is not actually visible; its location has to be estimated by deduction. Firstly, it is obviously in the region of the hematoma and secondly, it is most likely located in the region covered by the angioplasty balloon when pressure was applied to the stenotic lesion. This is not invariably true; movement of a guidewire or catheter can cause tears inadvertently during the procedure, but this is the place to start.

Once the location has been decided, the next step is to pass the angioplasty balloon over the guidewire and position it over the site of the tear (Figure 17-12A). If there is doubt, err on the upstream side (distal). Additional intraluminal obstruction downstream (proximal) from the lesion can make it worse. Use the same balloon that created the tear, unless it was grossly oversized to begin with. Once in position, the balloon should then be inflated with a low pressure; only the amount necessary to fully expand the balloon should be applied. The use of higher pressures may make the tear worse. Leave the inflated balloon in place for 4–5 minutes. This is done to plaster the torn endothelial surfaces against the wall and to displace the compressing hematoma.

Occlude the access using manual compression during the time of balloon inflation in order to avoid applying high pressure to the site of the rupture. If the balloon is not placed properly, the pressure of the access can make the situation worse while the balloon is inflated. After the required time, deflate the balloon and remove it gently. Check the site using a puff of radiocontrast to see if flow is now present. If flow appears normal or relatively so and the hematoma is stable, nothing further needs to be done (Figure 17-13B). It is important at this time that you should not do unnecessary manipulations in the area—accept a result that works although not perfect.

If flow continues to be significantly affected, consider inserting an endovascular stent.[83–85] If the hematoma is continuing to enlarge, you are probably dealing with a grade 3 rupture. It is critical to realize that if there is any downstream resistance (from a stenotic lesion that has not yet been treated), this must be relieved. The blood flow will follow the course of least resistance. If the downstream intravascular resistance is greater than the resistance of the perivascular tissue, extravasation will continue.

If the guidewire has been inadvertently removed prior to recognizing that one is dealing with a grade 2 hematoma, it may still be possible to salvage the situation. The goal is to get a guidewire back into position across the lesion; more specifically it is to accomplish this without making the situation worse in the process.

If the guidewire enters the tear in the vessel wall, it can enlarge it and enlarge the perivascular space into which the bleeding is occurring. This means that attempts to pass a guidewire must be done with great care. Unfortunately, many times the extravasated radiocontrast obscures the area making visualization difficult.

The first step in accomplishing the goal of passing the guidewire is the selection of which type of guidewire to use. The one at hand may not be the best choice. What is needed is the most atraumatic guidewire possible, one that will have the least tendency to cause additional damage. The Roadrunner guidewire fits this need the best. Its tip is very flexible and when it meets even a slight degree of resistance, it will buckle allowing passage with a very atraumatic leading edge. This guidewire should be used and it should be passed very carefully under direct observation. If there is any suggestion that it is going outside of the vein, stop immediately and torque the wire to redirect. If after several attempts there is no success, use a guiding catheter (hockey-stick—Kumpe or Berenstein) to direct the guidewire.

It is very helpful to know approximately where on the circumference of the vein the tear occurred. With this knowledge, the hockey-stick guiding catheter can be used to direct the guidewire away from the tear. Actually, it is frequently very easy to obtain this information. The extravasation is generally eccentric. Even if it appears to be diffuse, by turning the arm to obtain orthogonal views, it can be seen to be eccentric. The position of the extravasation relative to the vessel indicates the position of the tear. With the arm positioned so that you have the best view of the position of the extravasation, use the hockey-stick catheter to direct the guidewire away from the tear. If the guidewire is passed successfully, proceed with the procedure for management of a grade 2 hematoma as described above.

Grade 3 hematoma A grade 3 hematoma is an unstable hematoma (Figure 17-15). It is a catastrophic event resulting from a complete or near complete rupture (or dehiscence) of the vein. Hematoma formation generally occurs very rapidly. The size of the hematoma, however, is quite variable. It depends on how quickly the condition is recognized and controlled.

When a grade 3 hematoma occurs, there is a risk of losing the access. It is always classified as a major complication. The primary goal in the management of a grade 3 hematoma is to arrest a progressing process. This is critical to limit the size of the hematoma. The hematoma begins, expands rapidly, and is pulsatile. Arterial blood is being pumped directly into the tissue surrounding the area. Early recognition is critical, but not always easy. It can be diagnosed by palpating the area just dilated. A rapidly expanding, pulsatile hematoma will be evident. It may be painful.

As soon as the situation is recognized, the access should be manually occluded to arrest further extravasation.[26] A stent graft should be attempted and may be successful.[86, 87] If it is not, the graft should be thrombosed. To accomplish this, simply inflate the angioplasty balloon to a low pressure within the access below the site of rupture. This

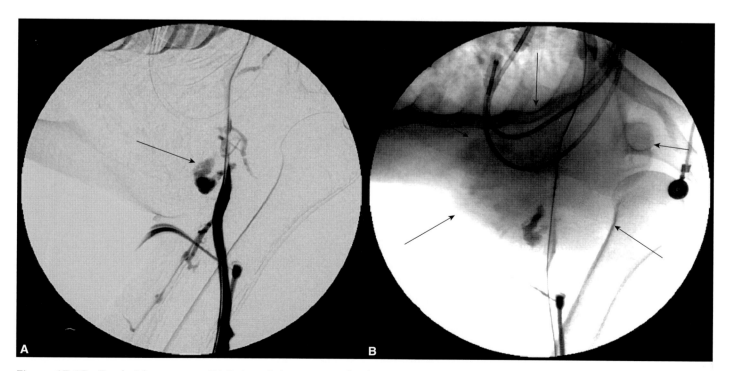

Figure 17-15. Grade 3 hematoma. (**A**) Only a slight amount of radiocontrast extravasation is noted (arrow), (**B**) very large hematoma with bleeding into chest wall and breast (arrows).

may need to be left overnight. Emergency surgery is not necessary; however, the patient will need a dialysis access for both the short and long term.

Venous spasm

Venous spasm can occur following instrumentation of a vein. This is generally of no consequence unless it is confused for a stenotic lesion. Rarely a patient may be encountered in whom it is a problem. It is important that the location of stenotic lesions be noted before beginning the angioplasty. If "new lesions" appear afterward, these are areas of spasm. One should not become confused and try to dilate these "new lesions"; it will do no good and can aggravate the situation. In a rare patient the spasm can be so severe as to cause a loss of flow and thrombosis of the access.

A successful treatment for severe venospasm is difficult. Further instrumentation may make it worse. Intravenous nitroglycerine has been reported to be beneficial. The dose to use is 100 μg. If this is not successful, it is best to heparinize the patient and wait it out. Spasm will go away over a period of 1 or 2 hours. If flow is not completely lost early and followed by thrombosis, the problem will resolve.

In order to minimize the chances for venous spasm, always use the least amount of instrumentation possible. Even the passage of a wire can precipitate spasm in susceptible patients.

BENEFITS OF PROSPECTIVE TREATMENT OF VENOUS STENOSIS

Prospective treatment (treatment prior to thrombosis) of venous stenosis requires some method for the prospective diagnosis of venous stenosis, that is, monitoring and surveillance. Advocates of prospective venous angioplasty base their view on studies that are nonrandomized for the most part. These studies have reported that PTA of a hemodynamically significant stenosis associated with a nonthrombosed AVG has been shown to prolong the useful life span and reduce the rate of thrombosis of the vascular access.[13,30–32,49,75,76,88–93]

In one study of 132 chronic hemodialysis patients in whom surveillance was done followed by an aggressive treatment program for venous stenosis, the overall benefits of the program were documented.[92] A marked decrease in AVG thrombosis, dialysis catheter usage, hospital day related to vascular access, and missed dialysis treatments was observed. As one would anticipate, the angioplasty rate rose significantly; however, the cost of treatment for thrombosis-related events decreased by 49%.

Another report involved a cohort of 101 patients.[94] Patients were randomly assigned to control, flow, or stenosis groups, and were followed for up to 28 months. Referral criteria were control group, and clinical criteria flow group, access flow < 600 mL/min, or clinical criteria

stenosis group, stenosis > 50% detected by ultrasound evaluation or clinical criteria. In the stenosis group, prospective angioplasty was found to reduce hospitalization rates and costs, reduce total cost of access-related care, and a trend of reduced dialysis catheter utilization rates.

There are also those that conclude that that the correction of prospectively detected stenosis with percutaneous transluminal angioplasty does not provide clear benefits. They base their view on studies that have been reported as randomized controlled studies.[95–99] However, all these studies can be criticized on several levels. Firstly, they are based upon small sample size and in general lack of data on important confounders, control of which is impossible with sample sizes under 400. Secondly, what constituted a successful angioplasty is often not included. It is known that many of these lesions are elastic; success of the treatment is dependent upon lasting anatomical changes that need to be documented.

An example of what can happen when a randomized study does not control for confounding variables is illustrated by a report of 64 patients identified to have a 50% stenosis by using ultrasound and confirmed by using angiography.[97] Prospective angioplasty was performed, but produced no change in 6-month or 12-month patency. Because of confounding issues, a subanalysis was performed on 21 "virgin" grafts with the cohort that had not previously clotted or required intervention.[89] In this group of cases, prospective angioplasty reduced the thrombosis rate from 0.44 to 0.10 episodes/patient-year at risk.

REFERENCES

1. Dotter CT, Judkins MP. Transluminal treatment of arteriosclerotic obstruction. Description of a new technique and a preliminary report of its application. *Circulation*. 1964;30:654–670.
2. van Andel G. *Percutaneous Transluminal Angioplasty: The Dotter Procedure*. Amsterdam: Excerpta Medica; 1976.
3. Staple TW. Modified catheter for percutaneous transluminal treatment of arteriosclerotic obstructions. *Radiology*. 1968;91:1041–1043.
4. Portsmann W. [A new corset balloon catheter for Dotter's transluminal recanilization with special reference to obliterations of the pelvic arteries]. *Radiol Diagn (Berl)*. 1973;14:239–244.
5. Gruntzig A, Hopff H. [Percutaneous recanalization after chronic arterial occlusion with a new dilator-catheter (modification of the Dotter technique) (author's transl)]. *Dtsch Med Wochenschr*. 1974;99:2502–2510.
6. Gruntzig A. Transluminal dilatation of coronary-artery stenosis. *Lancet*. 1978;1:263.
7. Glanz S, Bashist B, Gordon DH, Butt K, Adamsons R. Angiography of upper extremity access fistulas for dialysis. *Radiology*. 1982;143:45–52.
8. Gordon DH, Glanz S, Butt KM, Adamsons RJ, Koenig MA. Treatment of stenotic lesions in dialysis access fistulas and shunts by transluminal angioplasty. *Radiology*. 1982;143: 53–58.

9. Probst P, Mahler F, Krneta A, Descoeudres C. Percutaneous transluminal dilatation for restoration of angioaccess in chronic hemodialysis patients. *Cardiovasc Intervent Radiol.* 1982;5:257–259.

10. Glanz S, Gordon DH, Butt KM, Hong J, Lipkowitz GS. The role of percutaneous angioplasty in the management of chronic hemodialysis fistulas. *Ann Surg.* 1987;206:777–781.

11. Schwab SJ, Saeed M, Sussman SK, McCann RL, Stickel DL. Transluminal angioplasty of venous stenoses in polytetrafluoroethylene vascular access grafts. *Kidney Int.* 1987;32:395–398.

12. Newman GE, Saeed M, Himmelstein S, Cohan RH, Schwab SJ. Total central vein obstruction: resolution with angioplasty and fibrinolysis. *Kidney Int.* 1991;39: 761–764.

13. Beathard GA. Percutaneous transvenous angioplasty in the treatment of vascular access stenosis. *Kidney Int.* 1992;42:1390–1397.

14. Beathard GA. Angioplasty for arteriovenous grafts and fistulae. *Semin Nephrol.* 2002;22:202–210.

15. Beathard GA, Urbanes A, Litchfield T, Weinstein A. The risk of sedation/analgesia in hemodialysis patients undergoing interventional procedures. *Semin Dial.* 2011;24:97–103.

16. Beathard G. Physical examination of the dialysis vascular access. *Semin Dial.* 1998;11:231.

17. Turmel-Rodrigues L, Mouton A, Birmele B, Billaux L, Ammar N, Grezard O, Hauss S, Pengloan J. Salvage of immature forearm fistulas for haemodialysis by interventional radiology. *Nephrol Dial Transplant.* 2001;16:2365–2371.

18. Beathard GA, Arnold P, Jackson J, Litchfield T. Aggressive treatment of early fistula failure. *Kidney Int.* 2003;64: 1487–1494.

19. Falk A. Maintenance and salvage of arteriovenous fistulas. *J Vasc Interv Radiol.* 2006;17:807–813.

20. Nassar GM, Nguyen B, Rhee E, Achkar K. Endovascular treatment of the "failing to mature" arteriovenous fistula. *Clin J Am Soc Nephrol.* 2006;1:275–280.

21. Clark TW, Cohen RA, Kwak A, Markmann JF, Stavropoulos SW, Patel AA, Soulen MC, Mondschein JI, Kobrin S, Shlansky-Goldberg RD, Trerotola SO. Salvage of nonmaturing native fistulas by using angioplasty. *Radiology.* 2007;242:286–292.

22. Kanterman RY, Vesely TM, Pilgram TK, Guy BW, Windus DW, Picus D. Dialysis access grafts: anatomic location of venous stenosis and results of angioplasty. *Radiology.* 1995;195:135–139.

23. Gray RJ. Percutaneous intervention for permanent hemodialysis access: a review. *J Vasc Interv Radiol.* 1997;8:313–327.

24. Vesely T. Percutaneous transluminal angioplasty for the treatment of failing hemodialysis grafts and fistulae. *Semin Dial.* 1998;11:351.

25. Pappas JN, Vesely TM. Vascular rupture during angioplasty of hemodialysis raft-related stenoses. *J Vasc Access.* 2002;3:120–126.

26. Beathard GA. Management of complications of endovascular dialysis access procedures. *Semin Dial.* 2003;16:309–313.

27. Duijm LE, Liem YS, van der Rijt RH, Nobrega FJ, van den Bosch HC, Douwes-Draaijer P, Cuypers PW, Tielbeek AV. Inflow stenoses in dysfunctional hemodialysis access fistulae and grafts. *Am J Kidney Dis.* 2006;48:98–105.

28. Khan FA, Vesely TM. Arterial problems associated with dysfunctional hemodialysis grafts: evaluation of patients at high risk for arterial disease. *J Vasc Interv Radiol.* 2002;13:1109–1114.

29. NKF-K/DOQI Clinical Practice Guidelines For Vascular Access *Clinical Practice Guideline 6.4 Treatment of stenosis without thrombosis.*

30. Schwab SJ, Raymond JR, Saeed M, Newman GE, Dennis PA, Bollinger RR. Prevention of hemodialysis fistula thrombosis. Early detection of venous stenoses. *Kidney Int.* 1989;36:707–711.

31. Beathard GA. The treatment of vascular access graft dysfunction: a nephrologist's view and experience. *Adv Ren Replace Ther.* 1994;1:131–147.

32. Besarab A, Sullivan KL, Ross RP, Moritz MJ. Utility of intra-access pressure monitoring in detecting and correcting venous outlet stenoses prior to thrombosis. *Kidney Int.* 1995;47:1364–1373.

33. Tuka V, Slavikova M, Krupickova Z, Mokrejsova M, Chytilova E, Malik J. Short-term outcomes of borderline stenoses in vascular accesses with PTFE grafts. *Nephrol Dial Transplant.* 2009;24:3193–3197.

34. Levit RD, Cohen RM, Kwak A, Shlansky-Goldberg RD, Clark TW, Patel AA, Stavropoulos SW, Mondschein JI, Solomon JA, Tuite CM, Trerotola SO. Asymptomatic central venous stenosis in hemodialysis patients. *Radiology.* 2006;238:1051–1056.

35. Fabbian F, Bortot A, Galeotti R, Dall'Ara S, Galdi A, Bergami M, Catizone L. Pseudostenosis of axillary vein due to adduction of the upper limb. *J Vasc Access.* 2008;9:67–68.

36. Itkin M, Kraus MJ, Trerotola SO. Extrinsic compression of the left innominate vein in hemodialysis patients. *J Vasc Interv Radiol.* 2004;15:51–56.

37. Trerotola SO, Stavropoulos SW, Shlansky-Goldberg R, Tuite CM, Kobrin S, Rudnick MR. Hemodialysis-related venous stenosis: treatment with ultrahigh-pressure angioplasty balloons. *Radiology.* 2004;231:259–262.

38. Vesely TM, Siegel JB. Use of the peripheral cutting balloon to treat hemodialysis-related stenoses. *J Vasc Interv Radiol.* 2005;16:1593–1603.

39. Kariya S, Tanigawa N, Kojima H, Komemushi A, Shomura Y, Shiraishi T, Kawanaka T, Sawada S. Primary patency with cutting and conventional balloon angioplasty for different types of hemodialysis access stenosis. *Radiology.* 2007;243:578–587.

40. Heerwagen ST, Lonn L, Schroeder TV, Hansen MA. Cephalic arch stenosis in autogenous brachiocephalic hemodialysis fistulas: results of cutting balloon angioplasty. *J Vasc Access.* 2010;11:41–45.

41. Wu CC, Lin MC, Pu SY, Tsai KC, Wen SC. Comparison of cutting balloon versus high-pressure balloon angioplasty for resistant venous stenoses of native hemodialysis fistulas. *J Vasc Interv Radiol.* 2008;19:877–883.

42. Wu CC, Wen SC. Cutting balloon angioplasty for resistant venous stenoses of dialysis access: immediate and patency results. *Catheter Cardiovasc Interv.* 2008;71:250–254.

43. Guiu B, Loffroy R, Ben Salem D, Cercueil JP, Aho S, Mousson C, Krause D. Angioplasty of long venous stenoses in hemodialysis access: at last an indication for cutting balloon? *J Vasc Interv Radiol.* 2007;18:994–1000.

44. Peregrin JH, Rocek M. Results of a peripheral cutting balloon prospective multicenter European registry in

hemodialysis vascular access. *Cardiovasc Intervent Radiol.* 2007;30:212–215.

45. Bittl JA. Venous rupture during percutaneous treatment of hemodialysis fistulas and grafts. *Catheter Cardiovasc Interv.* 2009;74:1097–1101.

46. Trerotola SO, Kwak A, Clark TW, Mondschein JI, Patel AA, Soulen MC, Stavropoulos SW, Shlansky-Goldberg RD, Solomon JA, Tuite CM, Chittams JL. Prospective study of balloon inflation pressures and other technical aspects of hemodialysis access angioplasty. *J Vasc Interv Radiol.* 2005;16:1613–1618.

47. Foering K, Chittams JL, Trerotola SO. Percutaneous transluminal angioplasty balloon inflation with syringes: who needs an inflator? *J Vasc Interv Radiol.* 2009;20:629–633.

48. Turmel-Rodrigues L, Pengloan J, Blanchier D, Abaza M, Birmele B, Haillot O, Blanchard D. Insufficient dialysis shunts: improved long-term patency rates with close hemodynamic monitoring, repeated percutaneous balloon angioplasty, and stent placement. *Radiology.* 1993;187:273–278.

49. Safa AA, Valji K, Roberts AC, Ziegler TW, Hye RJ, Oglevie SB. Detection and treatment of dysfunctional hemodialysis access grafts: effect of a surveillance program on graft patency and the incidence of thrombosis. *Radiology.* 1996;199:653–657.

50. Tessitore N, Mansueto G, Bedogna V, Lipari G, Poli A, Gammaro L, Baggio E, Morana G, Loschiavo C, Laudon A, Oldrizzi L, Maschio G. A prospective controlled trial on effect of percutaneous transluminal angioplasty on functioning arteriovenous fistulae survival. *J Am Soc Nephrol.* 2003;14:1623–1627.

51. Forauer AR, Hoffer EK, Homa K. Dialysis access venous stenoses: treatment with balloon angioplasty—1- versus 3-minute inflation times. *Radiology.* 2008;249:375–381.

52. NKF-K/DOQI Clinical Practice Guidelines for Vascular Access. Clinical Practice Guideline 8.4 Efficacy of corrective intervention.

53. NKF-K/DOQI Clinical Practice Guidelines for Vascular Access, Clinical Practice Guideline 6.4. Treatment of stenosis without thrombosis.

54. Beathard GA. Fistula salvage by endovascular therapy. *Adv Chronic Kidney Dis.* 2009;16:339–351.

55. Lilly RZ, Carlton D, Barker J, Saddekni S, Hamrick K, Oser R, Westfall AO, Allon M. Predictors of arteriovenous graft patency after radiologic intervention in hemodialysis patients. *Am J Kidney Dis.* 2001;37:945–953.

56. Bittl JA, Feldman RL. Cutting balloon angioplasty for undilatable venous stenoses causing dialysis graft failure. *Catheter Cardiovasc Interv.* 2003;58:524–526.

57. Yamaya H, Horita Y, Nakazawa T, Taguchi T, Saitoh Y, Ichikawa I. Effectiveness of the parallel wire technique for stenotic hemodialysis fistulas. *J Jpn Soc Dial Ther.* 2000;33:127–131.

58. Kamikou T, Tsunoda T, Ikeda Y, Manjou T, Harada T. The efficacy of parallel wire technique for the dilatation of stenotic hemodialysis fistula. *Kidney Dialysis Access.* 2000;49:116–120.

59. Fukasawa M, Matsushita K, Araki I, Tanabe N, Takeda M. Self-reversed parallel wire balloon technique for dilating unyielding strictures in native dialysis fistulas (Letter to editor). *J Vasc Interv Radiol.* 2002;13:943–945.

60. Davidson CJ, Newman GE, Sheikh KH, Kisslo K, Stack RS, Schwab SJ. Mechanisms of angioplasty in hemodialysis fistula stenoses evaluated by intravascular ultrasound. *Kidney Int.* 1991;40:91–95.

61. Kovalik EC, Newman GE, Suhocki P, Knelson M, Schwab SJ. Correction of central venous stenoses: use of angioplasty and vascular Wallstents. *Kidney Int.* 1994;45:1177–1181.

62. Hunter DW, So SK. Dialysis access: radiographic evaluation and management. *Radiol Clin North Am.* 1987;25:249–260.

63. Burger H, Kluchert BA, Kootstra G, Kitslaar PJ, Ubbink DT. Survival of arteriovenous fistulas and shunts for haemodialysis. *Eur J Surg.* 1995;161:327–334.

64. Vesely T. Percutaneous transluminal angioplasty for the treatment of failing hemodialysis grafts and fistulae. *Semin Dial.* 1998;11:351.

65. Vesely TM. Endovascular intervention for the failing vascular access. *Adv Ren Replace Ther.* 2002;9:99–108.

66. Bohndorf K, Gunther RW, Vorwerk D, Gladziwa U, Kistler D, Sieberth HG. Technical aspects and results of percutaneous transluminal angioplasty in Brescia-Cimino dialysis fistulas. *Cardiovasc Intervent Radiol.* 1990;13:323–326.

67. Castellan L, Miotto D, Savastano S, Chiesura-Corona M, Pravato M, Feltrin GP. [The percutaneous transluminal angioplasty of Brescia-Cimino arteriovenous fistulae. An evaluation of the results]. *Radiol Med.* 1994;87:134–140.

68. Lay JP, Ashleigh RJ, Tranconi L, Ackrill P, Al-Khaffaf H. Result of angioplasty of brescia-cimino haemodialysis fistulae: medium-term follow-up. *Clin Radiol.* 1998;53:608–611.

69. Longwitz D, Pham TH, Heckemann RG, Hecking E. [Angioplasty in the stenosed hemodialysis shunt: experiences with 100 patients and 166 interventions]. *Rofo.* 1998;169:68–76.

70. Sugimoto K, Higashino T, Kuwata Y, Imanaka K, Hirota S, Sugimura K. Percutaneous transluminal angioplasty of malfunctioning Brescia-Cimino arteriovenous fistula: analysis of factors adversely affecting long-term patency. *Eur Radiol.* 2003;13:1615–1619.

71. Beathard GA, Litchfield T. Effectiveness and safety of dialysis vascular access procedures performed by interventional nephrologists. *Kidney Int.* 2004;66:1622–1632.

72. Schwab SJ, Oliver MJ, Suhocki P, McCann R. Hemodialysis arteriovenous access: detection of stenosis and response to treatment by vascular access blood flow. *Kidney Int.* 2001;59:358–362.

73. Ahya SN, Windus DW, Vesely TM. Flow in hemodialysis grafts after angioplasty: do radiologic criteria predict success? *Kidney Int.* 2001;59:1974–1978.

74. van der Linden J, Smits JH, Assink JH, Wolterbeek DW, Zijlstra JJ, de Jong GH, van den Dorpel MA, Blankestijn PJ. Short- and long-term functional effects of percutaneous transluminal angioplasty in hemodialysis vascular access. *J Am Soc Nephrol.* 2002;13:715–720.

75. Katz SG, Kohl RD. The percutaneous treatment of angioaccess graft complications. *Am J Surg.* 1995;170:238–242.

76. Turmel-Rodrigues L, Pengloan J, Baudin S, Testou D, Abaza M, Dahdah G, Mouton A, Blanchard D. Treatment of stenosis and thrombosis in haemodialysis fistulas and grafts by interventional radiology. *Nephrol Dial Transplant.* 2000;15:2029–2036.

77. Ozyer U, Harman A, Yildirim E, Aytekin C, Karakayali F, Boyvat F. Long-term results of angioplasty and stent placement for treatment of central venous obstruction in 126 hemodialysis patients: a 10-year single-center experience. *AJR Am J Roentgenol.* 2009;193:1672–1679.

78. Murray BM, Rajczak S, Ali B, Herman A, Mepani B. Assessment of access blood flow after preemptive angioplasty. *Am J Kidney Dis.* 2001;37:1029–1038.

79. Alexander J, Hood D, Rowe V, Kohl R, Weaver F, Katz S. Does surgical intervention significantly prolong the patency of failed angioaccess grafts previously treated with percutaneous techniques? *Ann Vasc Surg.* 2002;16: 197–200.

80. Sacks D, McClenny TE, Cardella JF, Lewis CA. Society of Interventional Radiology clinical practice guidelines. *J Vasc Interv Radiol.* 2003;14:S199–S202.

81. Beathard GA, Urbanes A, Litchfield T. The classification of procedure-related complications—a fresh approach. *Semin Dial.* 2006;19:527–534.

82. Vesely TM, Beathard G, Ash S, Hoggard J, Schon D. A position statement from the American Society of Diagnostic and Interventional Nephrology. *Semin Dial.* 2007;20:359–364.

83. Funaki B, Szymski GX, Leef JA, Rosenblum JD, Burke R, Hackworth CA. Wallstent deployment to salvage dialysis graft thrombolysis complicated by venous rupture: early and intermediate results. *AJR Am J Roentgenol.* 1997;169:1435–1437.

84. Rundback JH, Leonardo RF, Poplausky MR, Rozenblit G. Venous rupture complicating hemodialysis access angioplasty: percutaneous treatment and outcomes in seven patients. *AJR Am J Roentgenol.* 1998;171: 1081–1084.

85. Zaleski GX, Funaki B. Use of stents for angioplasty-induced venous rupture. *J Vasc Interv Radiol.* 1999;10:1135–1136.

86. Raynaud AC, Angel CY, Sapoval MR, Beyssen B, Pagny JY, Auguste M. Treatment of hemodialysis access rupture during PTA with Wallstent implantation. *J Vasc Interv Radiol.* 1998;9:437–442.

87. Sofocleous CT, Schur I, Koh E, Hinrichs C, Cooper SG, Welber A, Brountzos E, Kelekis D. Percutaneous treatment of complications occurring during hemodialysis graft recanalization. *Eur J Radiol.* 2003;47:237–246.

88. Besarab A, Dorrell S, Moritz M, Michael H, Sullivan K. Determinants of measured dialysis venous pressure and its relationship to true intra-access venous pressure. *ASAIO Trans.* 1991;37:M270–M271.

89. Martin LG, MacDonald MJ, Kikeri D, Cotsonis GA, Harker LA, Lumsden AB. Prophylactic angioplasty reduces thrombosis in virgin ePTFE arteriovenous dialysis grafts with greater than 50% stenosis: subset analysis of a prospectively randomized study. *J Vasc Interv Radiol.* 1999;10:389–396.

90. Tordoir JH, Hoeneveld H, Eikelboom BC, Kitslaar PJ. The correlation between clinical and duplex ultrasound parameters and the development of complications in arterio-venous fistulae for haemodialysis. *Eur J Vasc Surg.* 1990;4:179–184.

91. Maoz D, Reinitz R, Rimon U, Knecht A, Badayev L, Holtzman E, Schneiderman J. Hemodialysis graft flow surveillance with prompt corrective interventions improves access long-term patency. *Clin Nephrol.* 2009;71:43–49.

92. McCarley P, Wingard RL, Shyr Y, Pettus W, Hakim RM, Ikizler TA. Vascular access blood flow monitoring reduces access morbidity and costs. *Kidney Int.* 2001;60:1164–1172.

93. Zasuwa G, Frinak S, Besarab A, Peterson E, Yee J. Automated intravascular access pressure surveillance reduces thrombosis rates. *Semin Dial.* 2010;23:527–535.

94. Dossabhoy NR, Ram SJ, Nassar R, Work J, Eason JM, Paulson WD. Stenosis surveillance of hemodialysis grafts by duplex ultrasound reduces hospitalizations and cost of care. *Semin Dial.* 2005;18:550–557.

95. Ram SJ, Work J, Caldito GC, Eason JM, Pervez A, Paulson WD. A randomized controlled trial of blood flow and stenosis surveillance of hemodialysis grafts. *Kidney Int.* 2003;64:272–280.

96. Moist LM, Churchill DN, House AA, Millward SF, Elliott JE, Kribs SW, DeYoung WJ, Blythe L, Stitt LW, Lindsay RM. Regular monitoring of access flow compared with monitoring of venous pressure fails to improve graft survival. *J Am Soc Nephrol.* 2003;14:2645–2653.

97. Lumsden AB, MacDonald MJ, Kikeri D, Cotsonis GA, Harker LA, Martin LG. Prophylactic balloon angioplasty fails to prolong the patency of expanded polytetrafluoroethylene arteriovenous grafts: results of a prospective randomized study. *J Vasc Surg.* 1997;26: 382–390; discussion 390–392.

98. Dember LM, Holmberg EF, Kaufman JS. Randomized controlled trial of prophylactic repair of hemodialysis arteriovenous graft stenosis. *Kidney Int.* 2004;66:390–398.

99. Robbin ML, Oser RF, Lee JY, Heudebert GR, Mennemeyer ST, Allon M. Randomized comparison of ultrasound surveillance and clinical monitoring on arteriovenous graft outcomes. *Kidney Int.* 2006;69:730–735.

18

ARTERIAL INTERVENTION IN HEMODIALYSIS ACCESS AND CHRONIC KIDNEY DISEASE

ALEXANDER S. YEVZLIN

LEARNING OBJECTIVES

1. Understand the evolving role of interventional nephrology in the overall care of the general nephrology patient.
2. Describe arterial cannulation strategies.
3. Understand the epidemiology, techniques, and outcomes of upper extremity arterial intervention.
4. Understand the epidemiology, techniques, and outcomes of renal arterial intervention.
5. Understand the techniques required for successful stent deployment in the arterial system.
6. Describe arterial closure strategies.

INTRODUCTION

Interventional Nephrologists traditionally have focused on dialysis access. These procedures tend to be limited to interventions in the venous outflow tract or at the arterial anastomosis of arteriovenous fistulae (AVF) or arteriovenous grafts (AVG).[1] Recent scholarship has suggested that arterial disease is an important component of overall dialysis access care.[2-3] Interventional Nephrologists, consequently, have begun to broaden their focus to include arterial interventions *per se*. Examples of this increasing diversity of interventions include arterial inflow stenosis (eg, subclavian artery stenosis), peripheral vascular disease management (eg, distal hand ischemia syndrome), as well as the more traditional renal artery stenosis (RAS) intervention. Because the biology, techniques, and outcomes differ greatly between the fields of vascular access and cardiovascular medicine,[4] this chapter endeavors to bridge the knowledge gap for Interventional Nephrologists who are beginning to focus more than before on the arterial system.

ARTERIAL CANNULATION IN HEMODIALYSIS ACCESS INTERVENTION

Cannulation of a typical hemodialysis access case is achieved by inserting a catheter into the lumen of the AVF or AVG directly. There are several advantages to cannulating the venous outflow circuit in this fashion: (1) the AVF or AVG are repeatedly cannulated for hemodialysis and are, therefore, able to tolerate this process; (2) the AVF or AVG are relatively easy to cannulate given their superficial location and prominence; and (3) the potential complications of cannulation can be treated more easily due to their superficial location.

One situation that poses a challenge to this orthodoxy is severe stenosis or thrombosis of the outflow circuit (Figure 18-1). A severe lesion in the outflow tract may make it difficult to insert an adequately sized introducer safely. Even when an introducer can be inserted, there may not be adequate distance between the insertion point of the introducer and the lesion to allow for safe and effective intervention. When this sort of case is encountered, arterial access may be the safest option.

Another situation commonly encountered in access intervention is that of multiple lesions, with one lesion in the outflow circuit and another at the inflow anastomosis. Inflow stenosis has been reported to occur in up to 28% of patients referred for access dysfunction.[5-10] This observation implies that a second cannulation is required for intervention in almost one-third of dysfunctional access. More recent literature has established the prevalence of dysfunctional accesses with both an inflow and outflow lesion to be as high as 14%.[3] In this scenario, access to both inflow

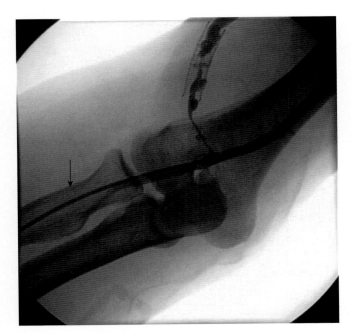

Figure 18-1. Severe stenosis of AVF preventing venous cannulation and introduction of sheath into AVF. Arterial cannulation was performed by introducing a 6-French catheter into the right radial artery (arrow).

and outflow lesions can be achieved with a single arterial cannulation.

A third clinical scenario that may argue for an arterial approach is the digital hypoperfusion ischemic syndrome (DHIS). Formerly called arterial steal syndrome, DHIS has been shown to occur in up to 20% of hemodialysis patients.[2,11–14] Several recent studies have suggested that arterial stenoses are present in 50% of dialysis patients with symptoms of hand ischemia or vascular access dysfunction.[15–21] Moreover, these lesions can occur anywhere within the arterial system, including the central arteries. Complete arteriography from the aortic arch to the vessels of the hand was recently performed in 13 hemodialysis (HD) patients with symptoms of peripheral ischemia to assess the presence of arterial stenosis.[15] In this provocative study, 62% of the patients who were referred for the evaluation of symptoms of steal syndrome demonstrated a significant arterial stenosis greater than 50%. To properly evaluate the arterial system, the standard occlusive retrograde arteriogram that Interventional Nephrologists tend to perform is not adequate. Therefore, if there is any suspicion of distal ischemia from a proximal arterial lesion, a thorough investigation of the entire arterial circuit is required.

The best cannulation approach to the clinical scenarios described above is to perform a single arterial cannulation that would provide access to both inflow and outflow lesions (Figure 18-2). One can approach from the classic femoral cannulation or from the radial artery in the retrograde direction. One advantage of the femoral approach is that the large femoral vessels afford the opportunity to insert large-diameter sheaths through which one can pass large-diameter angioplasty balloons. Another advantage of the femoral approach is that the entire arterial system can be imaged from the aortic arch to the periphery. This can be regarded as a disadvantage of the technique as well, since catheterization and angiography of the aortic arch can lead to embolic phenomena into the cerebral vasculature. If a peripheral (axillary, brachial, or radial) arterial lesion is suspected, we recommend cannulation via the radial or ulnar system in the wrist. If an arterial lesion is suspected in the central system (aortic arch, ostial subclavian, or subclavian), if the DHIS is suspected, or if there is an abnormal Allen test, then we recommend femoral artery cannulation.

ARTERIAL STENOSIS OF THE UPPER EXTREMITY

▶ Epidemiology

The most common peripheral artery lesion of the upper extremity is subclavian artery stenosis. Subclavian stenosis accounts for 15% of symptomatic extracranial cerebrovascular disease.[22] It is present in up to 7% of patients referred to noninvasive vascular laboratory for any reason.[23] The incidence may be even higher in patients with chronic kidney disease, especially those with arteriovenous fistulae or grafts. While atherosclerosis is the pathophysiology behind

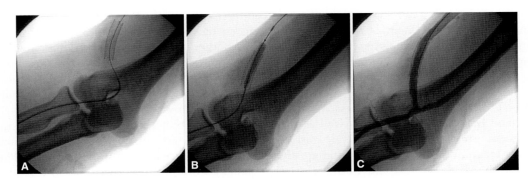

Figure 18-2. **(A)** JR4 catheter is used to selectively cannulate the 99% lesion from Figure 1-1 via the brachial artery and hydrophilic wire is inserted across the lesion. **(B)** Angioplasty balloon inflated in lesion. **(C)** Post-intervention arteriogram.

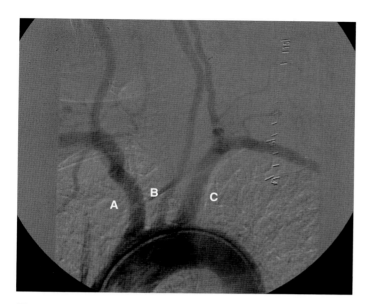

Figure 18-3. Type 1 aortic arch anatomy. (**A**) Right brachiocephalic trunk branching into the right subclavian and carotid arteries. (**B**) Left carotid artery. (**C**) Left subclavian artery.

most subclavian arterial disease, there is a differential diagnosis to consider when faced with a patient who exhibits concerning symptoms. It includes Takayasu arteritis, fibromuscular dysplasia, trauma, radiation, and thoracic outlet compression.

▶ Anatomy

An understanding of the symptoms of this disease is dependent on knowledge of the anatomy of the aortic arch. There are 3 major branches off the aortic arch. In most people they include from proximal to distal the (1) brachiocephalic trunk, which further branches into the right subclavian and right common carotid, (2) the left common carotid, and (3) the left subclavian artery (Figure 18-3). The vertebral arteries, which provide flow to the posterior cerebral circulation, arise from the ipsilateral subclavian artery. The internal mammary arteries also arise from their ipsilateral subclavian just distal to the vertebral arteries. The subclavian artery becomes the axillary artery as it leaves the thorax and continues as the brachial artery between the axilla and the elbow. The brachial artery gives off the deep brachial artery in its midportion, and then branches into the radial and ulnar arteries.[24] This branches provide flow to the palms and fingers.

▶ Clinical Presentation

The symptoms of subclavian artery disease and stenosis follow from this anatomy. The most common symptom is upper extremity claudication. Other less common symptoms include vertebrobasilar insufficiency (including the subclavian steal syndrome), angina pectoris if there is stenosis proximal to a left or right internal mammary graft to a coronary artery, and upper extremity embolic disease.

In patients with vascular access on the ipsilateral side of the arterial stenosis, signs and symptoms may also include poor flow through the access (subjectively, on physical exam, or via access monitoring), recurrent, frequent thrombosis of the access, and symptoms of distal ischemia (hand ulceration, numbness, motor dysfunction). As Nephrologists, we must be particularly cognizant of vascular disease outside of our access comfort zone (the AVF or AVG and anastomoses). This latter point has recently been highlighted by a study on patients with DHIS that showed that up to 14% of patients had isolated inflow stenosis proximal to the access as the cause of dysfunction.[21] Therefore, complete angiographic examination performed to evaluate digital ischemia should include the central arteries, in addition to the access site itself.

▶ Physical Examination

Traditionally, a difference in systolic blood pressure of at least 15 mm Hg between the upper extremities raises suspicion for stenosis of the subclavian artery ipsilateral to the extremity with the lower blood pressure.[25] Of course, this method of screening is not always possible for patients with existing HD fistulae or grafts. When performing the physical examination of the vascular access, which has been elegantly described in several recent studies,[26–28] one must pay close attention to the arterial system. Specifically, if poor inflow is detected by various observations and maneuvers, then one must endeavor to distinguish an anastomotic arterial lesion from a lesion in the more proximal arteries. This is particularly difficult to do on physical exam without the ability to perform blood pressure gradients, but it is not impossible. Anatomic locations where the arterial system is often palpable include the axilla, the elbow, and the wrist (using the Allen test in the case of the latter). A large difference in the pulse between these anatomic locations should raise suspicion of a peripheral artery lesion.

▶ Noninvasive Imaging

Computed tomography (CT) and magnetic resonance (MR) angiography are very sensitive diagnostic tools for stenosis of a major vessel off the aortic trunk. However, their use in the evaluation of patients with chronic kidney disease (CKD) of various stages may be limited by the necessity of using gadolinium-based contrast agents.[29] Further, the presence of some medical devices in the body may render images suboptimal or the test unsafe. It has been suggested that ultrasound is useful as a screening tool for subclavian stenosis.[30] There are 3 major ways of detecting subclavian stenosis by ultrasound. The first is by direct visualization of the lumen of the subclavian artery using 2-dimensional imaging in an effort to define a narrow segment. Employing color Doppler in this area will detect increased flow velocity through a hemodynamically significant stenosis.

A second method depends on a stenosis severity significant enough to cause a measurable decrease in flow velocity in the vessel distal to the stenosis. It has been proposed that this pressure gradient results in the Doppler equivalent to parvus et tardus in which the systolic peak velocity distal to the stenosis/occlusion is both reduced and delayed.[31] The loss of the normal triphasic waveform distal to the stenosis may further suggest hemodynamic compromise.

Finally, the third method uses the degree (if any) of subclavian steal physiology to determine the significance of stenosis. As the degree of subclavian stenosis increases, a dip in antegrade flow velocity occurs in the ipsilateral vertebral artery. Initially this dip appears early and briefly, but with increasing stenosis, this decrease in antegrade flow velocity becomes more prolonged and may even reverse late in systole or diastole.[30] True subclavian steal from severe or total occlusion of the subclavian artery results in complete reversal of flow in the ipsilateral vertebral artery away from the brain toward the affected arm at rest or with exercise of the upper extremity being evaluated.

Conceptually, the first two methods could be used to detect axillary and brachial stenosis, in addition to subclavian stenosis. The utility of the third, however, is limited to the level of the subclavian artery.

▶ Invasive Angiography

When symptoms, screening tests, or clinical suspicion dictate, invasive angiography is performed. The general indications for angiography and percutaneous treatment of subclavian stenosis have been outlined in previous publications.[25] Indications specific to HD patients are summarized in Table 18-1. Aspirin 325 mg should be administered prior to the diagnostic procedure for 24–48 hours. Typically, anticoagulation is unnecessary for basic diagnostic procedures. However, some operators will employ an anticoagulant strategy if the diagnostic procedure is prolonged or a great deal of catheter manipulation in the aortic arch is required. In these cases, unfractionated heparin (UFH) is the preferred anticoagulant, and is given as a single bolus of 70 units/kg. In these select cases, a direct thrombin inhibitor such as bivalirudin (Angiomax, The Medicines Company, Parsippany, NJ) is used if a contraindication to UFH exists. Of note, this agent requires dose reduction in patients with CKD, and its use for this indication would be off-label.

In procedures performed to evaluate the entire arterial inflow system to a hemodialysis access, arterial cannulation is performed with a 5- or 6-French sheath in the common femoral or radial artery. Next, using a pigtail catheter and power injector, angiography of the aortic arch in the left anterior oblique projection is performed with 20 mL of contrast over one second. This angiogram delineates the arch anatomy, and can be used as a roadmap for selective cannulation. The subclavian artery can be engaged in the antero-posterior (AP) projection with a Judkins right coronary catheter and a standard 0.035 J-tipped wire (Figure 18-4). Selective angiography can also be performed using this catheter, or it can be exchanged over an exchange-length 0.035-inch guidewire for a multipurpose catheter. If the axillary and brachial arteries are to be examined, a multipurpose catheter likely carries less potential for vessel trauma and is, therefore, preferred.

Imaging of the subclavian artery is best performed from the contralateral oblique projection. For example, the left

TABLE 18–1

Indications for Invasive Arterial Evaluation/Intervention

General Population[26]	Hemodialysis Population
Upper extremity (UE) claudication	To investigate or relieve obstruction prior to placement of vascular access for HD
Bilateral subclavian stenosis and need to assess blood pressure (BP) noninvasively	To evaluate/preserve inflow to the existing HD access
SC steal	To evaluate/treat upper extremity ischemia that occurs on the ipsilateral side of a vascular access
Coronary-SC steal	Any indication applicable to the general population
Left SC stenosis > 50% before coronary artery bypass graft (CABG) with planned left internal mammary artery (LIMA)	
Symptomatic common carotid stenosis	
Symptomatic vertebral artery stenosis	

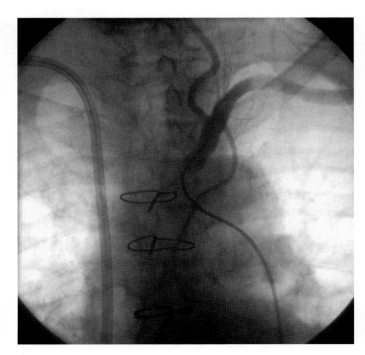

Figure 18-4. Catheter directed angiogram via femoral access and a JR4 catheter in the ostium of the left subclavian artery.

subclavian is best imaged in the straight right anterior oblique (RAO) projection. Digital subtraction angiography should be used if available with the patient holding his or her breath. Imaging of the axillary or brachial arteries can be achieved in the AP projection over the abducted and supine extremity being examined.

► Troubleshooting

When encountering difficulty passing a standard 0.035-inch J-tipped wire into the subclavian artery sufficiently distal to provide support for catheter advancement and selective angiography, a 0.035-inch Wholey Hi-Torque guidewire (Mallinckrodt, Hazelwood, MO) or angled Glidewire (Terumo, Somerset, NJ) may be employed through the same diagnostic catheter. If the exchanged wire also fails to advance, and/or intervention is being considered, upsizing the sheath and catheter system or switching to a guide catheter may provide the extra backup needed for wire advancement.

Alternatively, the system can be exchanged for a Shuttle Select delivery system (Cook Medical, Bloomington, IN). This system is a 6-French 90-cm hydrophilic sheath with an included dilator that can be inserted over a 0.035-inch wire in exchange for the 6-French 12-cm arterial sheath usually used to gain initial arterial access. It is advanced over the wire with its dilator in place proximal to the artery of interest. Then, the dilator is held in place, while the sheath is advanced under fluoroscopic guidance to the desired location. It is attached to a Tuohy-Borst adapter, which can be connected to a manifold. Through this adapter and sheath, a guide catheter can be advanced (telescoped) over the wire into the vessel of interest to provide extra support for advancement of the sheath. Once the sheath is in the desired position, the telescoped catheter is withdrawn, and selective angiography is performed through the sidearm of the sheath itself.

In some cases, specialized guide catheters such as a JB, Vitek, or Simmons (Cook Medical, Bloomington, IN) may provide superior backup for wire advancement. These are 5-French catheters and can be used alone, or as an extension of a 6-French Shuttle Select sheath. Ultimately, the shuttle sheath can be advanced over this type of guide if additional backup is needed.

The decision to use a standard guiding system versus the Shuttle Select System depends on multiple factors, but rests ultimately on the previous experiences of the operator. For the distal subclavian, axillary, or brachial arteries, a guide catheter through a standard sheath is our preferred approach with selective engagement of the subclavian ostium. In more proximal or ostial lesions, we use the Shuttle Select System just proximal to the subclavian ostium. If balloon angioplasty or stenting is to be performed, the latter of the two options allows for balloons/stents that can fit over 0.035-, 0.014-, and 0.018-inch wires, whereas the former guide-based approach is compatible only with 0.014- and 0.018-inch equipment.

► Percutaneous Intervention

Balloon angioplasty with an undersized balloon catheter followed by placement of an appropriately sized balloon-expandable stent is the current standard methodology for subclavian intervention.[32] Currently, all our patients are pretreated with 325 mg aspirin and 300 mg of clopidogrel. A bolus of intravenous UFH at 70–100 units/kg is given to obtain an activated clotting time (ACT) of 200–300 seconds. All patients who receive a stent should be treated for an extended period of time with the dual antiplatelet regimen consisting of lifelong daily aspirin 81–325 mg, and daily clopidogrel 75 mg for 3–6 months. Randomized controlled trials in support of this treatment strategy are lacking, but it would be difficult to justify and unlikely to significantly alter management.

Percutaneous intervention can be performed over 0.014-, 0.018-, or 0.035-inch wires. Generally, we use 0.035 wires to guide advancement of the guide or Shuttle Sheath (Cook Medical, Bloomington, IN) into the desired area of the target artery, and then switch to a 0.014-inch wire to cross the lesion and place angioplasty balloons and stents. Distal embolic protection devices (EPDs) are not usually employed. On average, the diameter of the subclavian arteries treated is 7 mm. Predilatation balloons range in diameter from 3 to 12 mm. The balloon-expandable stents range from 5 to 7 mm. Larger balloon diameters can be used over 0.035-inch guidewires. In general, we inflate an undersized predilatation balloon at nominal pressure in the area of stenosis or occlusion. If the balloon expands as predicted and post-balloon expansion angiography demonstrates reasonable patency of the target lesion, an appropriately sized balloon-expandable stent is deployed. Ideally, the stent expands fully if the predilatation balloon expands optimally. However, a residual stenosis may occur despite maximal inflation of the stent balloon. In these cases, we generally accept up to 30% residual angiographic stenosis. Sometimes a post-stent deployment, gradient is measured if adequate stent expansion is in question. If the gradient is significantly reduced, a suboptimal angiographic result may be preferable to repeated post-stent deployment balloon dilatations, as the latter approach may increase the risk of complications. The restenosis rate for stents placed in previously stenotic lesions would generally be low (3–11% at 17–60 months) if angiographic and hemodynamic success is confirmed.[32–34]

► Outcomes

Treatment of symptomatic subclavian artery stenosis can be surgical or percutaneous. Both offer excellent procedural success and long-term patency with the decrease in morbidity and mortality favoring the percutaneous approach as the primary treatment strategy in most cases. Most commonly, the left subclavian artery is the target of revascularization. A large series was reported in which the primary success rate approached 100% in patients with stenotic lesions.[35] Earlier, small studies had reported similarly excellent short- and long-term patency rates.[32] Complete occlusions have a lower likelihood of successful revascularization than do stenotic lesions. Amor et al described a patency rate of 53% for stenting of total occlusions.[35] Long-term results may also differ with the severity of the steal physiology caused by the culprit lesion. A recent study on 42 patients concluded that the presence of a complete steal syndrome might portend a higher risk of symptomatic subclavian restenosis over 5 years, when compared to those with lesser degrees of steal.[33]

▶ Possible Complications

Major complications resulting from this technique are uncommon, but could include death, stroke, TIA, and stent thrombosis. The sentinel paper on subclavian intervention reported a 0% event rate for any of these potential complications.[32] Minor complications are also rare (up to 5%), and include access site hematoma or pseudoaneurysm, peripheral emboli, and stent embolization.[32,34] Very little is known about the impact on the hemodialysis access of arterial intervention on the ipsilateral side. This represents an important avenue for future research.

▶ Hemostasis

Hemostasis after percutaneous intervention can be achieved using manual pressure or an approved vascular closure device. If the manual approach is used, the sheath is left in place until the ACT is <170. After the sheath is removed, manual pressure is held for 15 minutes. If bleeding continues, a FemoStop® HD Femoral Compression System (Radi Medical Systems, Inc., Wilmington, MA) can be employed. Typically, we use an appropriately sized Angioseal (St. Jude Medical, Inc., St. Paul, MN) or Perclose (Abbott Laboratories, Abbott Park, IL) device in the lab followed by 2 hours of bed rest if the groin anatomy is amenable (ie, no evidence of ipsilateral peripheral vascular disease and sheath placement in the common femoral artery above its bifurcation). If the radial artery is chosen for initial cannulation, closure can be achieved with the digital pressure described above or with a TR band (Terumo, Somerset, NJ), a radial pressure device that allows gradual reduction of pressure with syringe suction of air out of the occlusive balloon over the span of 60 minutes to achieve hemostasis.

RENAL ARTERY INTERVENTION

▶ Epidemiology

Atherosclerosis accounts for approximately 90% of all renovascular lesions.[36–38] In the Cardiovascular Health Study (CHS), the prevalence of significant (≥60%) RAS was detected by renal duplex sonography in 6.8% of subjects.[39] Renovascular disease was not correlated with ethnicity, but was independently associated with age, hyperlipidemia, and hypertension. In a series of 3987 patients

undergoing coronary angiography, aortography demonstrated ≥75% renal artery stenosis in 4.8% patients.[40] In 3.7% of patients, the renal arteries were affected bilaterally.[41] In patients with aortic aneurysms, aorto-occlusive or lower-extremity occlusive disease greater than 50% stenosis was present in more than 30% of patients.[42] The increased prevalence of RAS in patients with coronary or peripheral arterial disease reflects the systemic nature of atherosclerosis and the overlapping existence of the disease in multiple vascular beds.

Atherosclerotic RAS is a progressive disease. In a series of 295 kidneys followed by renal artery duplex scans, the 3-year cumulative incidence of renal artery disease progression stratified by initial degree of stenosis was 18%, 29%, and 49% for renal artery classified as normal, with <60% stenosis, and with ≥60% stenosis, respectively.[43] In this study, there were 9 occlusions, which occurred in patients who had ≥60% stenosis at the time of initial evaluation. Schreiber et al, however, have reported progression to total occlusion in 39% of patients with ≥75% stenosis at renal arteriography.[43] In the Dutch Renal Artery Stenosis Intervention Cooperative (DRASTIC) study, a randomized trial of medical therapy versus balloon angioplasty for the treatment of hypertension in RAS patients, progression to complete occlusion occurred in 16% of patients treated medically.[44]

In addition to the initial degree of stenosis, other factors associated with disease progression include diabetes mellitus and hypertension.[45]

▶ CKD Due to Chronic Ischemia

The term "ischemic nephropathy" refers to the deterioration of renal function that is thought to occur as a result of renovascular disease, and which may lead to end stage renal disease (ESRD) in 14% to 20% of affected patients.[46–47] The nature of ischemic nephropathy is complex and multifactorial. Since the main function of the kidney is filtration, renal blood flow is among the highest of all organs, and only 10% is necessary for this organ's metabolic needs.[48] Furthermore, the kidney is capable of autoregulating blood flow in the presence of renal artery stenosis of up to 75% diameter reduction and, in conditions of impaired perfusion, oxygen delivery can be maintained by the development of collaterals from the adrenal and lumbar arteries.[49]

Proposed pathways activated in chronic renal hypoperfusion, and which can lead to parenchymal injury and interstitial fibrosis involve the complex and inter-related effects of angiotensin II, nitric oxide (NO), endothelin, vasodilating and vasoconstrictive prostaglandins, and a variety of cytokines.[50] Angiotensin II maintains glomerular filtration pressure and glomerular filtration rate (GFR) by constricting the efferent arterioles, but its effects in the kidney also include local inflammatory responses, cell hypertrophy, and hyperplasia, which are mostly mediated by angiotensin 1 receptors.[50] Other Angiotensin II effects also include vascular smooth muscle proliferation, mesangial cell growth, platelet aggregation, activation of adhesion molecules and macrophages, induction of gene transcription for proto-oncogenes, and oxidation of low-density lipoproteins.[51,52]

These and other mechanisms, such as the generation of free oxygen radicals, interact with each other, eventually resulting in renal scarring even in the absence of "true" renal ischemia.[53] The complexity and variability of these interactions in different individuals are another factor that makes predictions on the recovery of kidney function after revascularization difficult, and explain why patients with impaired renal function before revascularization may have no significant increase in their GFR after percutaneous or surgical interventions.[54,55]

▶ Diagnostic Angiography

Contrast angiography remains the gold standard for diagnosis and the assessment of the severity of both atherosclerotic and fibrodysplastic RAS. The value of this diagnostic modality has been buoyed by the recently described association of nephrogenic systemic fibrosis (NSF) with MR contrast agents, such as are required for MR angiography.[56] Angiography, further, allows evaluation of the abdominal aorta, renal arteries, and branch vessels, the presence of accessory renal arteries, as well as cortical blood flow and renal dimensions. Moreover, pressure gradients across a renal artery stenosis can be obtained to evaluate its hemodynamic significance. Digital subtraction angiography (DSA) is now available in many institutions and, although its resolution is inferior to film, it permits the use of lower concentrations of iodinated contrast, as well as of alternative contrast agents such as CO_2.[57]

Typically, an abdominal aortogram is performed prior to selective catheterization of the renal artery, usually positioning a pigtail catheter at the lower edge of the first lumbar vertebra and power-injecting 15–20 mL of dye at 20 mL/second (Figure 18-5). The abdominal aortogram will provide information regarding the aorta itself, the position of the renal arteries, and the presence of accessory arteries as well as of aortic or renal artery calcification. In most instances, the aortogram provides adequate visualization of the renal arteries, but if optimal imaging or pressure gradient measurement is needed, selective catheterization becomes necessary. This can be achieved with a variety of different 4- to 6-French diagnostic catheters. Whatever catheter shape is used, the goal is to achieve selective cannulation of the renal artery without excessive catheter manipulation, especially when evaluating atherosclerotic RAS, since aortic atheromas are often adjacent or contiguous to the renal artery lesion and distal embolization can occur. In visualizing the renal arteries, it is important to recognize that they originate posteriorly from the aorta; therefore, it may be necessary to obtain ipsilateral oblique projections (15°–30°) to optimally outline the ostium and the proximal segments of the vessels. Furthermore, angiography should be performed long enough to image the renal cortex and assess renal size and perfusion.[58]

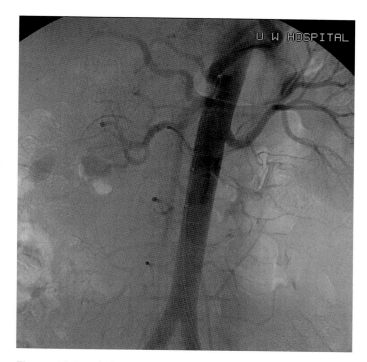

Figure 18-5. Abdominal aortogram.

The obvious disadvantages of catheter-based angiography are its invasiveness, the exposure of patients to ionizing radiation, and the use of nephrotoxic contrast. However, in patients with renal insufficiency, alternative contrasts such as CO_2 can be used. When compared to conventional angiography in the identification of RAS of more than 60%, CO_2 angiography with DSA has a sensitivity and a specificity of 83% and 99%, respectively.[59] In these patients, proper hydration and minimization of contrast load, and prophylaxis with sodium bicarbonate and/or acetylcysteine, are all strategies which may be adopted to minimize the incidence of nephrotoxicity.

▶ Percutaneous Intervention

Percutaneous therapy for renovascular disease has largely supplanted surgery; it is associated with a lower incidence of adverse events, equivalent outcome in terms of hypertension control, and lower cost compared to surgery.[60-62] The first description of balloon angioplasty for renovascular disease was provided by Gruntzig and colleagues in 1978.[63] Balloon angioplasty remains the treatment of choice in patients with uncontrolled hypertension and renovascular disease secondary to fibromuscular dysplasia (FMD).[64,65]

To date, there are three randomized controlled trials of balloon angioplasty compared to medical therapy in patients with atherosclerotic renovascular disease.[66,67] These trials are limited by small number of patients enrolled and frequent crossover from the medical to the percutaneous group. Probably the most widely cited publication is the DRASTIC trial, which randomized 106 patients with >50% stenosis and diastolic hypertension despite treatment with two antihypertensive medications to either balloon angioplasty or medical therapy.[16] Primary endpoints were systolic and diastolic blood pressures at 3 and 12 months. At three months, there was a statistically significant improvement in blood pressure control in the balloon angioplasty arm; one-year analysis, however, showed no difference in blood pressure control between the two groups. Importantly, 22 of the 50 patients in the medical therapy group had crossed over to the angioplasty arm for persistently difficult-to-control blood pressure, and patients in the angioplasty group required significantly fewer anti-hypertensive medications. The absence of any blood pressure difference at 12 months led the authors to conclude that angioplasty was of little benefit over medical therapy in treating hypertension and renal artery stenosis. Opponents of percutaneous therapy for renovascular disease have argued that this trial demonstrates the ineffectiveness of catheter-based therapy in these patients. With the high degree of crossover reported, however, a definite conclusion based upon its results is very difficult to draw.

Stenting has largely supplanted balloon angioplasty in the catheter-based treatment of renovascular disease. A randomized trial of stenting versus balloon angioplasty in 84 patients with ostial renovascular disease demonstrated improved procedural success and patency rates with stenting; however, there were no significant differences in hypertension (HTN) control or improvement in renal function.[68] Two meta-analyses have analyzed the success and durability of renal artery stenting.[69,70] Initial angiographic success rates were significantly improved compared to balloon angioplasty at 96–100% with no significant difference in complication rates. The ability of renal artery stenting to improve blood pressure control and renal function has been studied in multiple series. A meta-analysis demonstrated an overall HTN cure rate of 20% and improved HTN control in 49%, and improvement in renal function in 30% with stabilization of renal function in 38% of patients.[71] With similar complication rates and improved initial and long-term angiographic success, it is safe to say that renal artery stenting is the percutaneous treatment of choice in patients with renal artery stenosis.

Although not necessarily true in the past, modern procedural techniques for percutaneous renal intervention utilize much the same equipment as coronary interventions. The choice of guide catheter is determined by the angle with which the renal artery arises off the aorta. Most commonly, retrograde access via the femoral artery is used. A very sharp caudal angle of origin of the renal artery may however require an antegrade approach using the radial or brachial arteries to achieve optimal guide-catheter engagement. Interventions are usually performed using a 6- or 7-French system with commonly used guide catheters with shapes such as the Judkins-Right series, the "renal standard curve," "renal double curve," and "hockey stick." Engagement of the guide catheter can be performed directly or using a telescoping technique (see above section on arterial stenosis of the upper extremity for technique details).

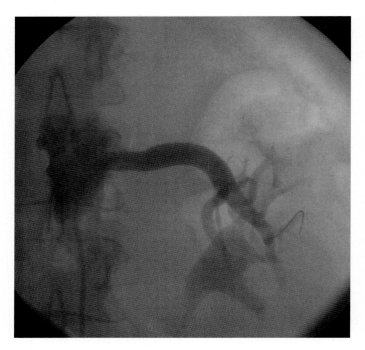

Figure 18-6. Visualization of the renal artery via subselective injection of contrast.

High-grade ostial lesions with concomitant aortic plaque can increase the risk for atheroembolism. The recently proposed "no-touch" technique attempts to minimize trauma to the vessel ostium, at least theoretically lessening the risk of atheroembolism to the renal parenchyma.[72] With this technique, a 0.035-inch "J-tip" guidewire is advanced just past the guide-catheter tip, to lean against the abdominal aorta above the renal artery, thus keeping the catheter away from the aortic wall. Once the guide catheter is directed toward the ostium of the renal artery visualization of the renal artery is obtained by subselective injection of contrast (Figure 18-6), a 0.014-inch guidewire is navigated past the target lesion into the distal renal vessel. The 0.035-inch guidewire is then withdrawn from the catheter, allowing it to gently slide into or adjacent to the ostium of the renal artery over the 0.014-inch wire. Pre-dilatation of the target lesion is especially recommended in aorto-ostial atherosclerotic lesions, and is typically performed with a balloon approximately 1 mm less than the measured diameter of the vessel.

The two balloon-expandable stents specifically approved by the Food and Drug Administration (FDA) for use in failed renal angioplasty are the Palmaz stent (Cordis Corporation) and the Double Strut stent (Medtronic Corporation), but the most frequently used stents have been approved for biliary tree interventions. In ostial lesions, after the stent is deployed, its proximal portion can be "flared" with a slightly oversized balloon protruding into the aorta. Stent placement should be confirmed in two views. Careful attention to contrast dye load is required, especially in patients at high risk for contrast nephropathy. As mentioned above, CO_2 can be used as alternative contrast agents at least during some parts of the intervention.

Adjuvant pharmacology before and after renal artery percutaneous intervention has not been systematically studied. Heparin to maintain an activated clotting time of 250–300 seconds is frequently used as the anticoagulant of choice during interventional procedures; most interventionalists are quite familiar with its use and it can be easily reversed with protamine. Patients are usually pre-treated with aspirin, which is continued indefinitely. The use of clopidogrel seems theoretically necessary following percutaneous intervention; however, there are no controlled studies exploring its use in the renal artery. Other possible intra-procedural anticoagulants such as glycoprotein 2B3A receptor antagonists and direct thrombin inhibitors such as bilvalrudin have not been formally studied in renal interventions.

► Possible Complications

Complications related to percutaneous intervention can be related to vascular access, guide catheter engagement, wiring of the artery, balloon and stent deployment, or contrast administration.

As with all percutaneous procedures, complications related to vascular access are the most frequent and include groin and retroperitoneal hematomas and bleeding, pseudoaneurysm, arterio-venous fistula, and infection. Atheroembolism to the kidney parenchyma, bowel, or lower extremities can occur and result in renal failure, bowel ischemia, or digital ischemia. Renal artery dissection is typically treated with stenting. Distal wire perforation should be treated with reversal of anticoagulation and coiling if necessary. Perforation should be treated with prolonged balloon inflation, reversal of anticoagulation, or possibly the deployment of a covered stent graft. In cases not responding to percutaneous treatment, surgery may be necessary. Rocha-Singh and others reported in-hospital adverse events in 4.5% of patients and 2-year adverse events in 19.7% with 14.4% of these being target lesion revascularization.[71]

Like coronary artery stenting, restenosis remains the Achille heel of renal artery stenting. Reported rates of restenosis range from 11% to 23% with 2 meta-analyses reporting rates of 16% and 17%.[73–76] Multiple studies have examined clinical and angiographic predictors of restenosis.[73,74] These studies have demonstrated that a larger minimum luminal diameter is the only factor consistently associated with a lower incidence of restenosis. In one series of 748 patients, a stent diameter ≤5 mm was associated with an odds ratio of 2.31 for target vessel revascularization as compared to those with a diameter >5 mm.[75] The type of stent can also have an impact on restenosis. Gold-coated stents are associated with a significantly increased rate of restenosis compared to stainless steel stents.[76] The treatment of restenosis remains somewhat controversial with very limited data. Described modalities for the treatment of restenosis include repeat balloon angioplasty, stenting, cutting balloon angioplasty, and vascular brachytherapy.[77–80] More recently, the use of drug-eluting stents for the treatment of in-stent restenosis has been described.[81,82]

Another possible complication of percutaneous renal intervention is distal embolization into the kidney parenchyma; this, along with the use of nephrotoxic contrast, could potentially be the cause for the deterioration in renal function sometimes observed after these interventions. One small series demonstrated that embolization after surgical revascularization of the renal arteries was associated with worse survival.[83] Atheroembolism related to aortic angiography has been reported and could have similar deleterious effects.[84] The true incidence, risk factors, and consequences of renal atheroemboli following renal angiography, however, remainunknown. Several studies have examined the utilization of distal protection devices in renal artery stenting in an attempt to prevent atheroembolism.[85,86] These series have examined the effects of distal balloon occlusion devices and filter wires, and have reported retrieval of debris in 65–100% of patients. The Cardiovascular Outcomes in Renal Atherosclerotic Lesions (CORAL) trial in patients with HTN and renal artery stenosis is currently enrolling and using embolic protection devices in all patients randomized to stenting, although the study will not have a control arm where distal protection is not used. There are potential complications and limitations associated with deployment of the currently available distal protection devices. For their use, a 2-cm landing zone is ideally required distal to the lesion, and although this is usually the case in the saphenous vein grafts for which the devices were developed, it may not be in short or bifurcating renal arteries.

Filters and occlusive balloons can also potentially cause distal vessel trauma, resulting in perforation or dissection; wire kinking and filter entrapment are also potential concerns in tortuous renal with unfavorable take-off from the aorta. Whether distal protection will become an integral part of percutaneous renal intervention remains a topic of active investigation; meanwhile, however, their use should be considered in patients with severe atherosclerosis of the abdominal aorta, baseline renal insufficiency, single functional kidney, and when the anatomy is suitable.

► Future Directions

Patient selection remains a very challenging part of renal revascularization, given the variable response in blood pressure control or kidney function. Several series have attempted to find clinical, laboratory, or angiographic predictors of improved blood pressure or renal outcomes.[87–89] Factors independently associated with improvement in renal function include higher baseline serum creatinine and left ventricular function.[129] These studies are by no means definitive, but rather highlight the ongoing quest for a test to identify patients who will benefit from renal revascularization.

CONCLUSION

The past decade has witnessed an evolution of the specialty of Nephrology in the United States to an interventional discipline. As the scope of Interventional Nephrology broadens, arterial procedures, both diagnostic and interventional, will more commonly fall under the purview of the specialty. Because the biology, techniques, and outcomes of arterial interventions differ vastly from the venous interventions more familiar to Interventional Nephrologists, the education of the specialty must evolve to include arterial interventions *per se*.

REFERENCES

1. Asif A, Merrill D, Briones P, Roth D, Beathard GA. Hemodialysis vascular access: percutaneous interventions by nephrologists. *Semin Dial*. 2004;17(6):528–534.

2. Leon C, Asif A. Arteriovenous access and hand pain: the distal hypoperfusion ischemic syndrome. *Clin J Am Soc Nephrol*. 2007;2(1):175–183.

3. Duijm LE, Liem YS, van der Rijt RH, et al. Inflow stenoses in dysfunctional hemodialysis access fistulae and grafts. *Am J Kidney Dis*. 2006;48(1):98–105.

4. Roy-Chaudhury P, Spergel LM, Besarab A, Asif A, Ravani P. Biology of arteriovenous fistula failure. *J Nephrol*. 2007;20(2):150–163.

5. Kanterman RY, Vesely TM, Pilgram TK, Guy BW, Windus DW, Picus D. Dialysis access grafts: anatomic location of venous stenosis and results of angioplasty. *Radiology*. 1995;195:135–139.

6. Beathard GA. Angioplasty for arteriovenous grafts and fistulae. *Semin Nephrol*. 2002;22:202–210.

7. Schwab SJ, Oliver MJ, Suhocki P, McCann R: Hemodialysis arteriovenous access: detection of stenosis and response to treatment by vascular access blood flow. *Kidney Int*. 2001;59:358–362.

8. Guerra A, Raynaud A, Beyssen B, Pagny J, Sapoval M, Angel C. Arterial percutaneous angioplasty in upper limbs with vascular access devices for haemodialysis. *Nephrol Dial Transplant*. 2002;17:843–851.

9. Khan FA, Vesely TM. Arterial problems associated with dysfunctional hemodialysis grafts: evaluation of patients at high risk for arterial disease. *J Vasc Interv Radiol*. 2002;13:1109–1114.

10. Asif A, Gadalean FN, Merrill D, et al. Inflow stenosis in arteriovenous fistulas and grafts: a multicenter, prospective study. *Kidney Int*. 2005;67:1986–1992.

11. Morsy A, Kulbaski M, Chen C, Isiklar H, Lumsden AB. Incidence and characteristics of patients with hand ischemia after a hemodialysis access procedure. *J Surg Res*. 1998;74:8–10.

12. Tordoir JHM, Dammers R, van der Sande FM: upper extremity ischemia and hemodialysis vascular access. *Eur J Vasc Endovasc Surg*. 2004;27:1–5.

13. Haimov M, Baez A, Neff M, Sliftin R. Complications of arteriovenous fistulae for hemodialysis. *Arch Surg*. 1975;110:708–712.

14. Rinnaert P, Struyvan J, Mathieu J. Intermittent claudication of the hand after creation of an arteriovenous fistula in the forearm. *Am J Surg*. 1980;139:838–843.

15. Valji K, Hye RJ, Roberts AC, Oglevie SB, Ziegler T, Bookstein JJ. Hand ischemia in patients with hemodialysis access grafts: angiographic diagnosis and treatment. *Radiology*. 1995;196:697–701.

16. Guerra A, Raynaud A, Beyssen B, Pagny JY, Sapoval M, Angel C. Arterial percutaneous angioplasty in upper limbs with vascular access devices for haemodialysis. *Nephrol Dial Transplant*. 2002;17:843–851.

17. Asif A, Leon C, Merrill D, et al. Arterial steal syndrome: a modest proposal for an old paradigm. *Am J Kidney Dis*. 2006;48:88–97.

18. Asif A, Gadalean FN, Merrill D, et al. Inflow stenosis in arteriovenous fistulas and grafts: a multicenter, prospective study. *Kidney Int*. 2005;67:1986–1992.

19. Khan FA, Vesely TM. Arterial problems associated with dysfunctional hemodialysis grafts: evaluation of patients at high risk for arterial disease. *J Vasc Interv Radiol*. 2002;13:1109–1114.

20. Lockhart ME, Robbin ML, McNamara MM, Allon M. Association of pelvic arterial calcification with arteriovenous thigh graft failure in haemodialysis patients. *Nephrol Dial Transplant*. 2004;9:2564–2569.

21. Duijm LEM, Liem YS, van der Rijt RHH, et al. Inflow stenosis in dysfunctional hemodialysis access fistulae and grafts. *Am J Kidney Dis*. 2006;48:98–105.

22. Cho L, Casserly IP, Wholey MH. Subclavian, brachiocephalic, and upper extremity. In: Casserly, IP, Sachar R, and Yadav JS, eds. *Manual of Peripheral Vascular Intervention*. Philadelphia: LWW; 2005 [chapter 8].

23. Shadman R, Criqui MH, Bundens WP, et al. Subclavian artery stenosis: prevalence, risk factors, and association with cardiovascular diseases. *JACC*. 2004;44(3):618–623.

24. Casserly IP, Kapadia SR. *The Handbook of Peripheral and Cerebrovascular Intervention*. London: Remedica Publishing; 2004.

25. Mahmud E, Cavedish J, Salami A. Current treatment of peripheral vascular disease. *JACC*. 2007;50(6): 473–490.

26. Asif A, Leon C, Orozco-Vargas LC, et al. Accuracy of physical examination in the detection of arteriovenous fistula stenosis. *Clin J Am Soc Nephrol*. 2007;2(6): 1191–1194.

27. Leon C, Asif A. Physical examination of arteriovenous fistulae by a renal fellow: does it compare favorably to an experienced interventionalist? *Semin Dial*. 2008;21(6):557–560.

28. Leon C, Orozco-Vargas LC, Krishnamurthy G, et al. Accuracy of physical examination in the detection of arteriovenous graft stenosis. *Semin Dial*. 2008;21(1): 85–88.

29. Sadowski EA, Bennett LK, Chan MR, et al. Nephrogenic systemic fibrosis: risk factors and incidence estimation. *Radiology*. 2007;243(1):148–157.

30. Vijay G, Kalaria VG, Jacob S, Irwin W, Schainfeld RM. Duplex ultrasonography of Vertebral and Subclavian Arteries. *J Am Soc Echocardiogr*. 2005;18: 1107–1111.

31. Duan YY, Yuan LJ, Ding K, Liu X, Lv FQ, Cao TS. "Tardus and Parvus" Phenomenon in upper limb arteries for identifying subclavian arterial stenosis. *Echocardiography: J CV Ultrasound Allied Tech*. 2008;25(5):504–512.

32. Hadjipetrou P, Cox S, Piemonte T, Eisehauer A. Percutaneous Revascularization of atherosclerotic obstruction of aortic arch vessels. *JACC*. 1999;33(5): 1238–1245.

33. Filippo F, Francesco M, Francesco R, et al. Percutaneous angioplasty and stenting of left subclavian artery lesions for the treatment of patients with concomitant vertebral and coronary subclavian steal syndrome. *Cardiovasc Intervent Radiol.* 2006;29:348–353.

34. De Vries JP, Jager LC, Van den Berg JC, et al. Durability of percutaneous transluminal angioplasty for obstructive lesions of proximal subclavian artery: long-term results. *J Vasc Surg.* 2005;41:19–23.

35. Amor M, Eid-Lidt G, Chati Z, Wilnetz JR. Endovascular Treatment of the subclavian artery: stent implantation with or without predilatation. *Cathet Cardiovasc Intervent.* 2004;63:364–370.

36. Safian RD, Textor SC. Renal-artery stenosis. *N Engl J Med.* 2001;344(6):431–442.

37. Hansen KJ, Edwards MS, Craven TE, et al. Prevalence of renovascular disease in the elderly: a population-based study. *J Vasc Surg.* 2002;36(3):443–451.

38. Conlon PJ, Little MA, Pieper K, Mark DB. Severity of renal vascular disease predicts mortality in patients undergoing coronary angiography. *Kidney Int.* 2001;60(4): 1490–1497.

39. Rihal CS, Textor SC, Breen JF, et al. Incidental renal artery stenosis among a prospective cohort of hypertensive patients undergoing coronary angiography. *Mayo Clin Proc.* 2002;77(4):309–316.

40. Olin JW, Melia M, Young JR, Graor RA, Risius B. Prevalence of atherosclerotic renal artery stenosis in patients with atherosclerosis elsewhere. *Am J Med.* 1990;88(1N):46N–51N.

41. Caps MT, Perissinotto C, Zierler RE, et al. Prospective study of atherosclerotic disease progression in the renal artery. *Circulation.* 1998;98(25):2866–2872.

42. Schreiber MJ, Pohl MA, Novick AC. The natural history of atherosclerotic and fibrous renal artery disease. *Urol Clin North Am.* 1984;11(3):383–392.

43. van Jaarsveld BC, Krijnen P, Pieterman H, et al. The effect of balloon angioplasty on hypertension in atherosclerotic renal-artery stenosis. Dutch Renal Artery Stenosis Intervention Cooperative Study Group. *N Engl J Med.* 2000;342(14):1007–1014.

44. Dean RH, Kieffer RW, Smith BM, et al. Renovascular hypertension: anatomic and renal function changes during drug therapy. *Arch Surg.* 1981;116(11):1408–1415.

45. Scoble JE, Maher ER, Hamilton G, Dick R, Sweny P, Moorhead JF. Atherosclerotic renovascular disease causing renal impairment: a case for treatment. *Clin Nephrol.* 1989;31(3):119–122.

46. Simon P, Benarbia S, Charasse C, et al. Ischemic renal diseases have become the most frequent causes of end stage renal disease in the elderly. *Arch Mal Coeur Vaiss.* 1998;91(8):1065–1068.

47. Epstein FH. Oxygen and renal metabolism. *Kidney Int.* 1997;51(2):381–385.

48. Yune HY, Klatte EC. Collateral circulation to an ischemic kidney. *Radiology.* 1976;119(3):539–546.

49. Kontogiannis J, Burns KD. Role of AT1 angiotensin II receptors in renal ischemic injury. *Am J Physiol.* 1998; 274(1 pt 2):F79–90.

50. Lerman L, Textor SC. Pathophysiology of ischemic nephropathy. *Urol Clin North Am.* 2001;28(4): 793–803, ix.

51. Matsusaka T, Hymes J, Ichikawa I. Angiotensin in progressive renal diseases: theory and practice. *J Am Soc Nephrol.* 1996;7(10):2025–2043.

52. Lerman LO, Nath KA, Rodriguez-Porcel M, et al. Increased oxidative stress in experimental renovascular hypertension. *Hypertension.* 2001;37(2 Part 2):541–546.

53. Garovic VD, Textor SC. Renovascular hypertension and ischemic nephropathy. *Circulation.* 2005;112(9):1362–1374.

54. Textor SC, Wilcox CS. Renal artery stenosis: a common, treatable cause of renal failure? *Annu Rev Med.* 2001;52:421–442.

55. Sadowski EA, Bennett LK, Chan MR, et al. Nephrogenic systemic fibrosis: risk factors and incidence estimation. *Radiology.* 2007;243(1):148–57.

56. Fisher JEO, Jeffrey W. Renal artery stenosis: clinical evaluation. In: Saunders E, ed. *Vascular Medicine.* Philadelphia: Elsevier; 2006:343.

57. Reginelli JPCCJ. Renal artery intervention. In: Wilkins LW, ed. *Peripheral Vascular Interventions.* Philadelphia: Williams & Wilkins Co; 2005:175.

58. Schreier DZ, Weaver FA, Frankhouse J, et al. A prospective study of carbon dioxide-digital subtraction vs standard contrast arteriography in the evaluation of the renal arteries. *Arch Surg.* 1996;131(5):503–507; discussion 507–508.

59. Hawkins IF Jr, Wilcox CS, Kerns SR, Sabatelli FW. CO2 digital angiography: a safer contrast agent for renal vascular imaging? *Am J Kidney Dis.* 1994;24(4):685–694.

60. Weibull H, Bergqvist D, Bergentz SE, Jonsson K, Hulthen L, Manhem P. Percutaneous transluminal renal angioplasty versus surgical reconstruction of atherosclerotic renal artery stenosis: a prospective randomized study. *J Vasc Surg.* 1993;18(5):841–850; discussion 842–850.

61. Xue F, Bettmann MA, Langdon DR, Wivell WA. Outcome and cost comparison of percutaneous transluminal renal angioplasty, renal arterial stent placement, and renal arterial bypass grafting. *Radiology.* 1999;212(2):378–384.

62. Bettmann MA, Dake MD, Hopkins LN, et al. Atherosclerotic vascular disease conference: Writing Group VI: revascularization. *Circulation.* 2004;109(21):2643–2650.

63. Gruntzig A, Kuhlmann U, Vetter W, Lutolf U, Meier B, Siegenthaler W. Treatment of renovascular hypertension with percutaneous transluminal dilatation of a renal-artery stenosis. *Lancet.* 1978;1(8068):801–802.

64. Tegtmeyer CJ, Elson J, Glass TA, et al. Percutaneous transluminal angioplasty: the treatment of choice for renovascular hypertension due to fibromuscular dysplasia. *Radiology.* 1982;143(3):631–637.

65. Sos TA, Pickering TG, Saddekni S, et al. The current role of renal angioplasty in the treatment of renovascular hypertension. *Urol Clin North Am.* 1984;11(3):503–513.

66. Webster J, Marshall F, Abdalla M, et al. Randomised comparison of percutaneous angioplasty vs continued medical therapy for hypertensive patients with atheromatous renal artery stenosis. Scottish and Newcastle Renal Artery Stenosis Collaborative Group. *J Hum Hypertens.* 1998;12(5):329–335.

67. Plouin PF, Chatellier G, Darne B, Raynaud A. Blood pressure outcome of angioplasty in atherosclerotic renal artery stenosis: a randomized trial. Essai Multicentrique Medicaments vs Angioplastie (EMMA) Study Group. *Hypertension.* 1998;31(3):823–829.

68. van de Ven PJ, Kaatee R, Beutler JJ, et al. Arterial stenting and balloon angioplasty in ostial atherosclerotic renovascular disease: a randomised trial. *Lancet*. 1999;353(9149):282–286.

69. Leertouwer TC, Gussenhoven EJ, Bosch JL, et al. Stent placement for renal arterial stenosis: where do we stand? A meta-analysis. Radiology. 2000;216(1):78–85.

70. Isles CG, Robertson S, Hill D. Management of renovascular disease: a review of renal artery stenting in ten studies. *Qjm*. 1999;92(3):159–167.

71. Rocha-Singh K, Jaff MR, Rosenfield K. Evaluation of the safety and effectiveness of renal artery stenting after unsuccessful balloon angioplasty: the ASPIRE-2 study. *J Am Coll Cardiol*. 2005;46(5):776–783.

72. Feldman RL, Wargovich TJ, Bittl JA. No-touch technique for reducing aortic wall trauma during renal artery stenting. *Cathet Cardiovasc Interv*. 1999;46(2): 245–248.

73. Vignali C, Bargellini I, Lazzereschi M, et al. Predictive factors of in-stent restenosis in renal artery stenting: a retrospective analysis. *Cardiovasc Intervent Radiol*. 2005;28(3):296–302.

74. Lederman RJ, Mendelsohn FO, Santos R, Phillips HR, Stack RS, Crowley JJ. Primary renal artery stenting: characteristics and outcomes after 363 procedures. *Am Heart J*. 2001;142(2):314–323.

75. Bates MC, Rashid M, Campbell JE, Stone PA, Broce M, Lavigne PS. Factors influencing the need for target vessel revascularization after renal artery stenting. *J Endovasc Ther*. 2006;13(5):569–577.

76. Nolan BW, Schermerhorn ML, Powell RJ, et al. Restenosis in gold-coated renal artery stents. *J Vasc Surg*. 2005;42(1): 40–46.

77. Stoeteknuel-Friedli S, Do DD, von Briel C, Triller J, Mahler F, Baumgartner I. Endovascular brachytherapy for prevention of recurrent renal in-stent restenosis. *J Endovasc Ther*. 2002;9(3):350–353.

78. Reilly JP, Ramee SR. Vascular brachytherapy in renal artery restenosis. *Curr Opin Cardiol*. 2004;19(4): 332–335.

79. Munneke GJ, Engelke C, Morgan RA, Belli AM. Cutting balloon angioplasty for resistant renal artery in-stent restenosis. *J Vasc Interv Radiol*. 2002;13(3):327–331.

80. Bax L, Mali WP, Van De Ven PJ, Beek FJ, Vos JA, Beutler JJ. Repeated intervention for in-stent restenosis of the renal arteries. *J Vasc Interv Radiol*. 2002;13(12):1219–1224.

81. Zeller T, Rastan A, Rothenpieler U, Muller C. Restenosis after stenting of atherosclerotic renal artery stenosis: is there a rationale for the use of drug-eluting stents? *Cathet Cardiovasc Interv*. 2006;68(1):125–130.

82. Kakkar AK, Fischi M, Narins CR. Drug-eluting stent implantation for treatment of recurrent renal artery in-stent restenosis. *Cathet Cardiovasc Interv*. 2006;68(1):118–122; discussion 123–114.

83. Krishnamurthi V, Novick AC, Myles JL. Atheroembolic renal disease: effect on morbidity and survival after revascularization for atherosclerotic renal artery stenosis. *J Urol*. 1999;161(4):1093–1096.

84. Scolari F, Tardanico R, Zani R, et al. Cholesterol crystal embolism: a recognizable cause of renal disease. *Am J Kidney Dis*. 2000;36(6):1089–1109.

85. Holden A, Hill A. Renal angioplasty and stenting with distal protection of the main renal artery in ischemic nephropathy: early experience. *J Vasc Surg*. 2003;38(5):962–968.

86. Henry M, Henry I, Klonaris C, et al. Renal angioplasty and stenting under protection: the way for the future? *Cathet Cardiovasc Interv*. 2003;60(3):299–312.

87. Zeller T, Frank U, Muller C, et al. Predictors of improved renal function after percutaneous stent-supported angioplasty of severe atherosclerotic ostial renal artery stenosis. *Circulation*. 2003;108(18):2244–2249.

88. Rocha-Singh KJ, Mishkel GJ, Katholi RE, Ligon RA, Armbruster JA, McShane KJ, Zeck KJ. Clinical predictors of improved long-term blood pressure control after successful stenting of hypertensive patients with obstructive renal artery atherosclerosis. *Cathet Cardiovasc Interv*. 1999;47(2):167–172.

89. Burket MW, Cooper CJ, Kennedy DJ, et al. Renal artery angioplasty and stent placement: predictors of a favorable outcome. *Am Heart J*. 2000;139(1 pt 1):64–71.

19

STENT PLACEMENT IN HEMODIALYSIS ACCESS

ALEXANDER S. YEVZLIN & ARIF ASIF

INTRODUCTION

The term "stent" traces its etymologic origin to the name (Charles Stent) of the inventor of a molding compound used in dentistry in 1856.[1] Today stents are known broadly as any structure that provides support for collapsible tissues. The concept of endovascular stent placement *per se* derived from the early experience of cardiologists performing percutaneous transluminal angioplasty (PTA). Although the artery would be dilated successfully using an angioplasty balloon, in a small percentage of cases, it collapsed shortly thereafter. This phenomenon came to be known as "elastic recoil" and necessitated emergency bypass graft surgery until the advent of the stent. It is in this clinical context that, in 1986, Puel and Sigwart deployed the first coronary stent.[2] In the modern era, this endoluminal scaffold functions to prevent vascular closure after PTA and reduces the incidence of vascular restenosis.[3] Coronary percutaneous intervention is currently the most common medical procedure in the world, due in no small part to the advent of endovascular stent placement.[3–5]

In contrast to the routine placement of stents in coronary and peripheral interventions, the role of stent placement in the management of hemodialysis access dysfunction remains controversial.[6–9] The concerns associated with use of intravascular stent are critically important as vascular access assumes a more central role in interventional nephrology. These management uncertainties are important because they can lead to underutilization and consequent loss of device-associated benefit, result in the overutilization of stents with a concomitant increase in device-associated complications in the absence of its undisputed benefit, and cause a tremendous increase in the cost of medical care. Recent information from United States Renal Data System (USRDS) has reported a marked increase in stent placement in hemodialysis access.[10] While the total number of access interventions increased from 52,380 to 98,148 (a 1.8-fold increase), the number of stent placements has increased from 3,792 to 8,514 (a 2.2-fold increase) (Table 19-1). Of note, the relative percentage growth of stent placement has outpaced that of angioplasty each year during the same time period (Figure 19-1).[10]

Early investigations assessing the potential benefit of stent placement have addressed the question "to stent or not to stent." More recent investigations have focused on a slightly more subtle question, attempting to define under what circumstances and in which patients stent placement may be useful. This chapter endeavors to familiarize interventional nephrologists with the current understanding of intravascular stent placement in the management of dialysis access stenosis. The use of stents in the peripheral and central vasculature is addressed and

TABLE 19–1		
Number of PTA and Stent Procedures Performed in the United States 1998–2005		
Year	Number of PTA Procedures	Number of Stent Procedures
1998	52,380	3,792
1999	66,235	4,953
2000	70,602	5,468
2001	82,550	6,518
2002	98,148	8,514
2003	111,825	10,801
2004	128,745	12,327
2005	139,024	15,260

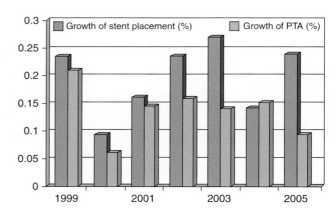

Figure 19-2. Relative growth of stent and PTA procedures 1999–2005.

the role of stents for the obliteration of aneurysms and ruptured vessels is discussed. Deployment techniques and strategies are also discussed. Finally, a perspective is offered on the biology of stent-endothelial interaction and future directions for research.

THE EARLY ERA OF STENT PLACEMENT

▶ Peripheral Venous Intervention

The insertion of an intravascular stent in a patient with dialysis access followed soon after coronary stent placement. Zollikofer et al[11] were the first to report stent deployment in the outflow track of an AVF or an AVG in 1988. In this seminal work, the authors reported successful stent placement in 4 patients. Subsequently, the same group published a study in which 7 patients received stents for 13 AVF outflow lesions.[12] The mean assisted patency rate was 9.7 months on follow-up angiography, although all patients were noted to have in-stent restenosis.

Based on these early studies, the 1990s witnessed several randomized trials of stent versus PTA (Figure 19-2). The outcomes evaluated in these studies include primary patency (time from access creation to first intervention) and assisted patency (time from access creation to final failure of the access, also referred to as secondary and overall patency).

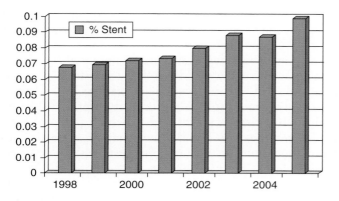

Figure 19-1. Stent placement increase (%) 1998–2005.

Quinn et al[13] in 87 patients, found the primary patency rates for PTA at 60, 180, and 360 days to be 55%, 31%, and 10%, respectively. For the stent group the primary patency rates were 36%, 27%, and 11% at 60, 180, and 360 days, respectively ($P = 0.6528$). Also, no difference was noted in secondary patency rates between the PTCA and stent groups.[13] Similarly, Beathard et al[12] evaluated 58 patients with 50% or greater stenosis who were randomly assigned to a stent or a PTA group. The results disclosed no significant difference in any parameter prior to treatment, in the response to intervention, or in the patency rates compared to the PTA group, with 90-, 180-, and 360-day survival of 85–92%, 72–82%, and 17–19% for stents and 79%, 64%, and 28% for PTA, respectively ($P > .07$).[14]

Another prospective randomized trial of 37 cases concluded that, despite significant added costs, there was no advantage to stent placement for recurrent AVG stenoses that were already adequately dilated with balloon angioplasty[13]. The primary patency rates for PTA at 30, 60, 180, and 360 days were 89%, 53%, 23%, and 7%, respectively. The primary patency rates for the stents at 30, 60, 180, and 360 days were 81%, 56%, 12%, and 0%, respectively. The secondary patency rates were 100%, 81%, and 47% for PTA, and 100%, 81%, 69%, and 60% for stents. The mean primary, primary assisted, and secondary patency for the PTA group was 137, 395, and 432 days, respectively, whereas for the stent group, these measures were 119, 327, and 431 days, respectively. The authors noted that the difference in patency rates between the 2 groups was not statistically significant.[15]

Multiple observational studies with no comparative group were also published.[16–25] Unfortunately, the observational nature of these investigations (the lack of comparison group) as well as the small sample size remains a fundamental limitation in applying these results to clinical practice. Some of the early studies evaluating the role of stents in the treatment of peripheral hemodialysis access lesions are presented (Table 19-2). On a more fundamental level, advances in stent technology render these early studies inapplicable to modern practice; there are new materials and techniques available today that have

TABLE 19-2

Investigations of the Role of Stent Placement in the Treatment of Peripheral Hemodialysis Access Lesions

Authors	Study Design	Year of Publication	Number of Cases	Primary Patency	Secondary Patency	Notes
Chan, MP	Retrospective	2007	211	91% vs 80% at 30 days, 69% vs 24% at 90 days, and 25% vs 3% at 180 for AVG	N/A	The primary assisted AVF patency did not differ significantly between the stent and angioplasty groups
Vesely, TM	Retrospective	2007	70	81%, 70%, and 54% at 1, 3, and 6 months for PTA; 96%, 93%, 87%, and 47% at 1, 3, 6, and 12 months for stent	89%, 82%, and 74% at 3, 6, and 12 months for stent	Multiple stent types
Naoum JJ	Observational (no control group)	2006	8	50% and 75%, and 25% and 75%, at 3 and 6 months	N/A	
Liang HL	Observational (no control group)	2006	23	At 3, 6, 12, and 24 months were 69% +/−9%, 88% +/−6%, 41% +/−10%, and 30% +/−10%	At 3, 6, and 12 months were 77% +/−10%, 12% +/−8%, and 61% +/−13%	
Maya ID	Retrospective	2006	48	Median survival, 85 vs 27 days, $P = 0.02$	Median survival, 1215 vs 46 days, $P = 0.049$	Thrombosed AVG only
Vogel PM	Prospective, non-randomized	2005	60	5.6 months after PTA and 8.2 months after stent treatment ($P = .050$)	N/A	
Sreenarasimhaiah VP	Observational (no control group)	2005	34	63% grafts functioning at 6 months	88% grafts functioning at 6 months	
Pan HB	Observational (no control group)	2005	12	3, 6, 12, and 24 months was 92% +/− 8%, 81% +/− 12%, 31% +/− 17%, and 31% +/− 17%	3 months was 92% +/− 8%, and 82% +/− 12% at 6, 12, and 24 months each	
Vogel PM	Retrospective	2004	19	Increased from 2.5 months to 10.6 months after placement of the SMART stent ($P = .0003$)	N/A	
Aytekin C	Observational (no control group)	2004	14	1-, 3-, 6-, and 12-month primary stent patency rates were 92.8%, 85.7%, 50%, and 14.3%	3-, 6-, 12-month, and 2-year assisted stent patency rates were 100%, 88.8%, 55.5%, and 33.3%	
Quinn SF	Observational (no control group)	2003	17	At 60, 180, and 360 days was 55% 39%, and 32%, respectively	At 60, 180, and 360 days was 70%, 40%, and 32%, respectively	
Kolakowski S Jr	Prospective, non-randomized	2003	61	3, 6, and 12 months (from stent placement) was 36.4%, 15.6%, and 0%, for forearm access 59.5%, 34.0%, and 17.0%, for upper arm access	40.9%, 40.9%, and 30.7% for forearm grafts 64.9%, 42.3%, and 19.7% for upper arm grafts	Distinguished between forearm and upper arm access

(continued)

TABLE 19–2

Investigations of the Role of Stent Placement in the Treatment of Peripheral Hemodialysis Access Lesions (continued)

Authors	Study Design	Year of Publication	Number of Cases	Primary Patency	Secondary Patency	Notes
Hatzimpaloglou A	Observational (no control group)	2002	15	Primary one-year and 2-year patency rate of 70%	N/A	
Lombardi JV	Retrospective	2002	52	37% vs 55% at 3 months, 25% vs 45% at 6 months, and 25% vs 15% at 12 months; $P = 0.37$	78% vs 59% at 3 months, 78% vs 48% at 6 months, and 54% vs 32% at 12 months; $P =$ NS	
Zaleski GX	Observational (no control group)	2001	19	36% at 6 months after stent placement, 12% at 12 months, and 12% at 18 months	91% at 6 months after stent placement, 71% at 12 months, and 47% at 18 months	
Oderich GS	Observational (no control group) Multicenter	2000	14	73%, 17%, and 17% at 3, 12, and 24 months, respectively	80%, 56%, and 35% at 3, 12, and 24 months, respectively	
Haage P	Observational (no control group)	1999	50	3-, 6-, 12-, and 24-month rates were 92%, 84%, 56%, and 28%, respectively	97% after 6 and 12 months, 89% after 24 months, and 81% after 36 and 48 months	
Funaki B	Observational (no control group)	1999	44	87% 60 days after the procedure, 51% 180 days after, 39% 1 year after, and 20% 2 years after	95% 60 days after the procedure, 92% 180 days after, 81% 1 year after, and 62% 2 years after	
Patel RI	Observational (no control group)	1998	26	3 and 6 months were 34% +/− 9% and 27% +/− 9%, respectively	77% +/− 8% at 3 months, 72% +/− 9% at 6 months, and 50% +/− 10% at 12 months	
Hoffer EK	Prospective, randomized	1997	37	Primary patency of 128 days and secondary patency of 431 days were similar for both groups	Secondary patency required a mean of 1.8 and 1.6 additional interventions for the PTA and stent groups, respectively	The adjunctive stent placement increased the cost of the procedure by 90%
Turmel-Rodrigues LA	Observational (no control group)	1997	52	PTFE grafts were 58% +/− 10% at 6 months and 23% +/− 10% at 1 year for native fistulas, 47% +/− 12% at 6 months and 20% +/− 18% at 1 year	PTFE grafts were 100% at 6 months and 88% +/− 8% at 1 year for native fistulas, 95% +/− 6% at 6 months and 79% +/− 14% at 1 year	Distinguished between AVG and AVF
Quin SF	Prospective, randomized	1995	87	PTA at 60, 180, and 360 days were 55%, 31%, and 10%, respectively, and for stents were 36%, 27%, and 11%, respectively ($P = .6528$)	PTA at 60, 180, and 360 days were 94%, 80%, and 71%, respectively, and for stents were 73%, 64%, and 64%, respectively ($P = .1677$)	
Beathard GA	Prospective, randomized	1993	58	100% at 30 days, 91% at 60 days, 85% at 90 days, 72% at 180 days, and 17% at 360 days	N/A	No difference between stent and PTA found
Antonucci F	Observational (no control group)	1992	13	N/A	Secondary patency 9.7 months	

essentially changed the landscape too thoroughly to base current clinical decisions on studies conducted in the past.

► Central Venous Intervention

The role of stent placement in the treatment of central venous stenosis (CVS) is widely regarded as less controversial than in the peripheral veins. (Table 19-3) The Society of Interventional Radiology (SIR) guidelines have indicated stent placement for central vein lesions.[26] Some investigators have even argued that central venous lesions represent a primary indication for stent placement due to the poor outcome usually found with balloon dilation alone.[27–28] The work of Beathard[29] supports this assertion. In his seminal study, lesions were classified by location and type. Central lesions had the worst secondary patency with only 28.9% of all lesions remaining patent at 180 days, compared with a secondary patency 61.3% for peripheral lesions treated with PTA alone (p < 0.01).

An earlier study from the 1990s evaluated the use of stents in 52 hemodialysis patients with 56 lesions.[30] Thirty-two lesions were in central veins and 24 were in peripheral veins. Stents were placed immediately after failed angioplasty in 39 patients. The primary patency rate was 46% at 6 months and 20% at 12 months. The assisted patency rate was 76% at 6 months and 33% at 12 months. In this study, the causes of recurrence included intimal hyperplasia in or near the stent, stent slippage, and stenosis in another part of the access circuit. Complications included 2 stent migrations due to central line placement and one stent-related pseudoaneurysm. Although in this study the outcomes were not reported separately for central versus peripheral lesions, the authors state that the patency rates were similar among the various lesion locations.

While intravascular stents have been inserted following failed angioplasty, Haage et al[31] in 1999, analyzed the effectiveness of stent placement as the primary treatment for central venous obstruction in hemodialysis patients. Fifty-seven stents were placed in 50 patients with access dysfunction and arm swelling due to CVS. The primary patency rates were 92%, 84%, 56%, and 28% at 3, 6, 12, and 24 months. Secondary patency was 97% at 6 and 12 months, 89% after 24 months, and 81% after 36 and 48 months. Seventy-three episodes of restenosis occurred during the duration of the study. Nineteen cases (26%) necessitated additional stent placement. Aytekin et al[32] evaluated the efficacy of stent placement for treating upper extremity CVS in 14 hemodialysis patients. The 1-, 3-, 6-, and 12-month primary patency rates were 92.8, 85.7, 50, and 14.3%, respectively. Repeat interventions, including percutaneous transluminal angioplasty and additional stent placement, were required in 9 patients (64%). The 3-, 6-, 12-month, and 2-year secondary patency rates were 100, 88.8, 55.5, and 33.3%, respectively. It is important to note that the investigators placed central vein stents as a primary treatment for central stenosis; there was no attempt at initial angioplasty.

THE MODERN ERA OF STENT PLACEMENT

► Innovations in Stent Design

Like many innovations in the field of percutaneous vascular intervention, the first study on an endovascular stent was reported by Charles Dotter in 1969.[33] Due the technological limitations of Dr. Dotter's time, further developments did not take place until the early 1980s, when Maas et al[34–36] started to experiment with a self-expanding "double helix spiral prosthesis." Using heat-treated metal bands of inert steel in the form of a double helix spiral, an expandable prosthesis of variable diameters up to 35 mm was constructed. In animal experiments the double helix spiral stents were completely endothelialized within 6 weeks, and intimal reaction was largely insignificant. These early stents were introduced clinically for the first time in 1982 in 2 patients with aortic aneurysms, but applications in the venous system were soon to follow.[37]

Endovascular stents used for arteriovenous dialysis access fall into 4 major categories.[38] These include balloon-expandable, self-expanding, covered, and drug-eluting stents. Balloon-expandable stents are mounted on a balloon and are deployed using balloon inflation. These stents can be crushed. Since many stents are placed in peripheral veins, these stents may not be suitable for this situation. However, they are particularly useful for highly elastic central venous stenosis where precise location is desired. Self-expanding stents come preloaded on a sheath and expand without a balloon. They can be made up of stainless steel or nitinol. Compared to stainless steel, nitinol stents do not shorten during placement. Nitinol is a nickel-titanium alloy with unique thermal recovery (commonly known as "smart metal") properties.[39–40] If nitinol wire is initially formed into a desired shape, and heated to 500°C, it will "memorize" that shape. When cooled, the wire will become soft again and can be deformed without changing the "memorized" shape. If the straightened wire is then warmed to its transition temperature (usually body temperature for most alloys of nickel-titanium), it resumes its initially formed shape. This concept "shape memory" is of particular importance in vascular access stenosis, since many of the lesions that need to be stented occur at the elbow or at tortuous intersections of veins.

Endovascular stents can also be covered with PTFE or Dacron (stent grafts or covered stents) and can be used in a variety of situations discussed below. Drug-eluting stents provide one possible means for delivering pharmacologic interventions to the site of stenosis. Indeed, an animal study indicated that sirolimus-eluting stents may provide short-term effectiveness in porcine arteriovenous grafts.[41]

Currently, clinicians have a great deal of variety to choose from when it comes to stent types, although most of the current designs are largely based on the initial concepts described above. The characteristics of various stent designs include the stent length, the stent diameter, the material composition of the wire mesh, the delivery system, and a host of more technical data. These features of

TABLE 19-3

Investigations of the Role of Stent Placement in the Treatment of Central Hemodialysis Access Lesions

Authors	Study Design	Year of Publication	Number of Central Lesions	Primary Patency	Secondary Patency	Notes
Bakken AM	Retrospective	2007	75	30-day rates of 76% for both groups and 12-month rates of 29% for PTA and 21% for stent ($P = .48$)	Secondary patency was also equivalent ($P = .08$), with a 30-day patency rate of 81% and 12-month rate of 73% for the PTA group, vs stent secondary patency rates of 84% at 30 days, and 46% at 12 months	
Rajan DK	Observational (no control group)	2007	6	83.3% (95% CI 0.5-1.2) at 3 months, and 66.7% at 6 and 12 months (0.2-1.1, 0.1-1.2)	Secondary patency was 100% at 12 months with 3 patients censored over that time period	
Rajan DK	Observational (no control group)	2007	89	In the fistula group the rates were 88.5% +/− 4.8%, 59.4% +/− 7.6%, and 46% +/− 7.9% at 3, 6, and 9 months, respectively. In the graft group, the rates were 78.1% +/− 7.3%, 40.7% +/− 9%, and 16% +/− 7.3%, respectively	N/A	
Maya ID	Observational (no control group)	2007	23	19% at 1 year	64% at 1 year	All stent had restenosis on follow-up venogram
Sprouse LR	Observational (no control group)	2004	32	N/A	Symptoms related to central stenosis were controlled for 6.5 months on average	
Aytekin C	Observational (no control group)	2004	14	1-, 3-, 6-, and 12-month primary stent patency rates were 92.8%, 85.7%, 50%, and 14.3%	3-, 6-, 12-month, and 2-year secondary patency rates were 100%, 88.8%, 55.5%, and 33.3%	
Chen CY	Observational (no control group)	2003	18	3, 6, 12, and 18 months were 100% and 89%, 73% and 68%, 49% and 42%, and 16% and 0%, respectively	100% after 3 months, 93% and 100% after 6 months, 85% and 91% after 12 months and, 68% and 72% after 24 months	

Author	Study type	Year	N	Outcome	Outcome	Comments
Hatzimpaloglou A	Observational (no control group)	2002	15	70% at 12 and 24 months	N/A	
Smayra T	Observational (no control group)	2001	9	56% at 1 year	75% at 1 year	
Haage P	Observational (no control group)	1999	50	3-, 6-, 12-, and 24-month were 92%, 84%, 56%, and 28%	97% after 6 and 12 months, 89% after 24 months, and 81% after 36 and 48 months	
Vesely TM	Observational (no control group)	1997	20	1 month, 3 months, 6 months, and 1 year: 90%, 67%, 42%, and 25%	At 3 months, 6 months, 1 year, and 2 years: 89%, 64%, 56%, and 22%	
Mickley V	Observational (no control group)	1997	15	1 year was 100%; 2 year was 85%	1 year was 70%; 2 year was 50%	
Lumsden AB	Observational (no control group)	1997	25	84% at 1 month, 42% at 6 months, and 17% at 1 year		
Vesely TM	Observational (no control group)	1997	20	1 month, 3 months, 6 months, and 1 year: 90%, 67%, 42%, and 25%	at 3 months, 6 months, 1 year, and 2 years: 89%, 64%, 56%, and 22%	
Mickley V	Observational (no control group)	1997	15	1 year was 100%; 2 year was 85%	1 year was 70%; 2 year was 50%	
Gray RJ	Observational (no control group)	1995	32	46% at 6 months and 20% at 12 months	76% at 6 months and 33% at 12 months	(1) Peripheral and central outcomes were mixed in the data reporting (2) Two central stents migrated after catheter placement
Beathard GA	Observational (no control group)	1992	24	N/A	70.4% at 1 month, 62.1% at 2 months, 48.6% at 3 months, and 28.9% at 4 months	
Matthews R	Case report	1992	2	N/A	N/A	

TABLE 19–4

Indications for Stent Placement

Peripheral vein stenosis
   Stents are useful in selected instances
      limited residual access sites
      surgically inaccessible lesions
      contraindication to surgery
   PTA fails
      greater than 30% residual stenosis
      more than 2 interventions required in 3-month period
Central vein stenosis
   Elastic central vein stenoses
   More than 2 interventions required in 3-month period

the stent are critical to proper delivery and function, and are summarized in Table 19-4. Most of the current stents used for the treatment of vascular access stenosis are bendable (they can be placed at the elbow joint), non-crushable (they will not permanently collapse under direct pressure),[42-44] covered and bare-metal, and can be cannulated for dialysis purposes.[45]

▶ Clinical Outcomes in the Modern Era of Stent Placement: Peripheral Lesions

The technological advances cited above (eg, novel alloys, delivery systems, etc), improvement in interventional techniques, and recognition of the limitations of the earlier studies have spurred some investigators to readdress stent deployment in the management of specific subsets of patients with access stenosis. In one such study, Maya et al evaluated whether graft patency following thrombectomy is improved by placement of a stent in the stenotic lesion.[46] Using a prospectively collected computerized vascular access database, the authors identified 14 patients with thrombosed AVGs treated with a stent at the venous anastomosis. The outcomes of these grafts were historically compared with those observed in 34 demographically matched control patients whose thrombosed AVGs were treated with PTA alone. The primary patency rate was greater for the stent group, with a median survival of 85 versus 27 days ($P = 0.02$). The secondary patency rate was also greater for the stent group, with a median survival of 1,215 versus 46 days ($P = 0.049$). The strength of this investigation is that the authors focused only on AVGs, that only the subset of patients with thrombosed accesses was analyzed, and that the location of the stenoses was restricted to the venous anastomosis.

Vogel et al followed their early work with a prospective study comparing nitinol stent placement with PTA.[47] A non-randomized study was conducted in 60 patients with AVG dysfunction. The indications for stent placement were similar to previous studies and included acute PTA failure, rapid restenosis, and vessel perforation. Thirty-five patients showed a response to PTA alone. The remainder received stents. Restenosis after intervention was less frequently observed in the stent group compared with angioplasty alone (7% vs 16%, $P = 0.001$). The primary graft patency was 5.6 months after PTA and 8.2 months after stent treatment ($P = 0.05$). Interestingly, the authors noted that the primary patency was similarly improved for stents placed across the level of the elbow joint.

Differences exist in patency rates between forearm and upper arm arteriovenous accesses. Kolakowski et al[48] performed a prospective, non-randomized study on 61 subjects comparing the use of stents in the forearm versus the upper arm. The primary patency rates at 3, 6, and 12 months in the forearm group were 36.4%, 15.6%, and 0%, respectively. This did not compare favorably with the 59.5%, 34.0%, and 17.0% primary patency rate observed for upper arm grafts ($P = 0.0307$). Secondary patency rates did not differ between the distal and proximal arm with rates of 40.9%, 40.9%, and 30.7%, over the above time interval, for forearm grafts, and 64.9%, 42.3%, and 19.7% for upper arm grafts ($P = $ NS). Although the latter investigation was an important contribution in that it was prospective and that it attempted to define the role of access location, it did not compare stent outcomes with angioplasty directly.

While patency of the access circuit is crucial, the patency of the stent *per se* (target lesion) may also be an important consideration. In one study, 70 subjects were retrospectively evaluated with stent placement.[49] The primary patency of the vascular access was 81%, 70%, and 54% at 1, 3, and 6 months, respectively. Secondary patency of the vascular access was 89%, 82%, and 74% at 3, 6, and 12 months, respectively. Interestingly, the primary patency of the stent *per se* was 96%, 93%, 87%, and 47% at 1, 3, 6, and 12 months. This investigation suggests that other areas of the access circuit are the likely culprits in its ultimate demise.

Whereas the aforementioned studies have primarily focused on the patency rates, a recent study included the assessment of post-stent access blood flow and urea reduction ratio (URR) determination.[50] In this retrospective study ($n = 211$), the primary assisted AVG patency was significantly longer for the stent group as compared to angioplasty, with a median survival of 138 versus 61 days, respectively ($P < 0.001$). The primary AVG patency for stent versus angioplasty was 91% versus 80% at 30 days, 69% versus 24% at 90 days, and 25% versus 3% at 180 days, respectively. The primary assisted AVF patency did not differ significantly between the stent and angioplasty groups. In patients dialyzing via AVF, multiple regression analysis revealed that stent placement was associated with improved after intervention peak blood flow (Qa), 1627.50 mL/min versus 911.00 mL/min ($P = 0.008$), change in Qa from before to after intervention, 643.54 mL/min versus 195.35 mL/min ($P = 0.012$), and change in URR from before to after intervention, 5.85% versus 0.733% ($P = 0.039$). All the stents in this study were uncovered, nitinol stents. Although limited by its retrospective design, these results suggest that stent placement in the modern era may be associated with improved AVG primary patency and improved AVF blood flow.

The same authors also examined the concerning issue of in-stent restenosis. Using a retrospective analysis of hemodialysis patients referred for access dysfunction during a 2-year period, 76 patients seen for follow-up angiography due to access dysfunction after stent placement were identified. The effect of in-stent restenosis versus de novo lesions in patients with previously placed endovascular stents was compared. Thirty-five (46.1%) patients had de novo lesions, while 41 (53.9%) had in-stent restenosis. In-stent restenosis was found to be the only factor associated with severity of luminal stenosis ($\beta = 0.35$, 95% CI 2.21 to 15.48, $P = 0.01$). The authors concluded that in-stent restenosis is associated with higher percent luminal diameter lesions compared to de novo lesions.[51]

▶ Clinical Outcomes in the Modern Era of Stent Placement: Central Lesions

In contrast to the relatively modest outcomes of the early era, a recent study achieved an enviable 70% primary patency at 2 years.[52] Fifteen stainless steel stents were implanted in 10 hemodialysis patients for the treatment of symptomatic CVS. Stent deployment functioned to relieve symptoms in all cases. Although limited by its small sample size, this was the first study to describe the outcomes of stent placement exclusively in central lesions.

Sprouse et al[53] similarly endeavored to determine the success of percutaneous therapy for relieving symptoms and maintaining central venous patency in hemodialysis patients with CVS. PTA or stent placement or both were performed as indicated in 32 lesions. PTA was followed by stent placement in 6 cases (19%). Patient symptoms were controlled for 6.5 months after the initial intervention. Recurrent edema led to additional PTA in 20 cases (63%). Fifty percent of the patients in the study with an AVF experienced recurrent symptoms after initial intervention and required access ligation. Importantly, the authors observed that complete resolution after the initial PTA was predictive of long-term success.

While stent placement can resolve symptoms of central venous stenosis, restenosis within a previously deployed stent is a commonly observed phenomenon. Maya and colleagues[54] recently investigated the primary and secondary patency of stent placement in cases of symptomatic CVS. Using a prospective vascular access database the authors retrospectively identified 23 patients who underwent stent placement due to residual stenosis following angioplasty. The median primary central vein patency was 138 days, with a 19% patency at 1 year. Recurrence of ipsilateral edema was due to in-stent restenosis in 100% of the cases. The median secondary central vein patency was 1036 days, with a 64% patency at 1 year. The authors concluded that stent deployment provides short-term relief of ipsilateral upper extremity edema due to CVS, but that long-term symptomatic relief can only be achieved with multiple subsequent interventions.

Distinct from the work of Maya and Sprouse,[53–54] which aims to define the role of stent placement in symptomatic central stenosis, the contemporary work of Levit et al[55] speaks to the issue of asymptomatic central lesions. In this study, 86 patients with asymptomatic CVS were identified upon referral for venogram. The authors excluded patients with arm swelling, multiple CVS, indwelling catheters, and already indwelling stents at the first encounter. The mean degree of CVS before intervention was 71% (range 50%–100%). No cases of untreated CVS progressed to symptoms. Meanwhile, mean progression was 0.21 percentage point per day in those patients whose asymptomatic CVS was treated with PTA ($P = .03$). Indeed, 80% of the interventions were followed by CVS escalation. The authors concluded that PTA of asymptomatic CVS greater than 50% in the setting of hemodialysis access maintenance procedures is associated with more rapid stenosis progression and escalation of lesions, compared with a non-treatment approach. These results, although very provocative, do not speak to the issue of stent placement *per se*; it is conceivable that stent placement in the intervention arm of the study would have demonstrated a better outcome than with angioplasty alone. Additionally, the small sample size and retrospective design of the study do not allow us to draw definitive conclusions.

Recently, investigators have endeavored to determine the difference in access patency for CVS between patients with AVF and those with AVG. Thirty-eight patients underwent 89 interventions (83 angioplasty procedures and 6 stent insertions). Technical and clinical success of the interventions was somewhat low at 93.3% and 94.4%, respectively. The primary patency rates at 3, 6, and 9 months in the AVF group were 88.5%, 59.4%, and 46%, respectively. In the AVG group, the rates were 78.1%, 40.7%, and 16%. With multivariate analysis, intervention patency remained significantly longer for fistulas ($P = 0.014$) and in patients who did not have a previous catheter ($P = 0.001$). Unfortunately, stent and angioplasty were not directly compared in this study.[56]

It is important to note that the use of stents in dialysis access stenosis, be it peripheral or central, has historically been an off-label use. However, a recent multi-center, randomized study that evaluated the role of a covered stent (FLAIR; Bard Peripheral, Tempe, Arizona) in the treatment of vein-graft anastomotic stenosis was the first to bring this device to approval by FDA.[57] A total of 227 patients were included in this study at 16 U.S. investigational sites. The safety and effectiveness of the covered stent compared to percutaneous balloon angioplasty were evaluated. Patients ($n = 97$) were randomized to the treatment (a covered stent [stent graft]) or balloon angioplasty procedure ($n = 93$). The results revealed that the treatment area primary patency at 6 months in the stent graft group was significantly higher than that found in the balloon angioplasty cohort (stent graft = 50.55%, angioplasty = 23.28%; $P < 0.001$). Importantly, this study also evaluated the primary patency of the entire access circuit. The access circuit primary patency ended when an intervention was performed anywhere within the circuit for stenosis or occlusion. A surgical intervention that excluded the index stenotic area from the access circuit also ended the access circuit primary patency. The results demonstrated that the primary patency for the access circuit at 6 months in the stent graft group was significantly higher than that found in the balloon angioplasty cohort (stent graft = 38.04%, angioplasty = 19.77%; $P < 0.001$).

This important contribution by Haskel et al has several limitations. Firstly, it was designed and statistically evaluated as a non-inferiority study.[57] As such, the authors' conclusion that stents are superior is not justified by the study methodology; the most that can be concluded in a non-inferiority study is that the investigational device is not inferior to the control. In addition, the critical outcome of assisted patency, which is listed as a secondary outcome in the trial (http://clinicaltrials.gov/), did not differ between the angioplasty and stent group. Despite these methodological limitations, the FDA has recently approved the use of this stent graft in the treatment of vein-graft anastomotic stenosis. This is the first and thus far the only stent graft that is approved by FDA for use in dialysis access.

INDICATIONS, DEPLOYMENT TECHNIQUES, AND OTHER CLINICAL CONSIDERATIONS

▶ Indications

Guideline 6 of the NKF-K/DOQI Clinical Practice Guidelines for Vascular Access defines the situations in which stent deployment should be considered.[58] The guideline states that patients with extremity edema that persists beyond 2 weeks after graft placement should undergo an imaging study (including dilute iodinated contrast) to evaluate patency of the central veins. The preferred treatment for central vein stenosis is percutaneous transluminal angioplasty (PTA). Stent placement should be considered in the following situations: if acute elastic recoil of the vein (50% stenosis) is present after angioplasty and if the stenosis recurs within a 3-month period. Furthermore, if angioplasty of the same lesion is required more than 2 times within a 3-month period, the patient should be considered for surgical revision if the patient is a good surgical candidate. If angioplasty fails, stents may be useful in the following situations: if the lesion is surgically inaccessible, if the patient has a contraindication to surgery, or if the angioplasty has induced vascular rupture.

The ability of a stent to provide rescue therapy in the events of angioplasty-induced vessel rupture has been recognized for a number of years outside the field of vascular access intervention.[59-60] This percutaneous rescue procedure is performed by keeping the guide wire across the intended lesion after the initial angioplasty is performed. If on the post-intervention angiogram extravasation of contrast is detected, then the operator can elect to exclude

the rupture by placement of a covered stent that opposes the walls of the vessel at the site of rupture. Alternatives to this form of therapy include surgical revision or ligation of the access.

The application of this technique to vascular access intervention was first rigorously described in 1997.[61] Funaki et al reported on 23 patients who were treated by covered stent placement after venous rupture attributed to balloon angioplasty during thrombectomy procedures. Twenty-one ruptures occurred in peripheral veins and 2 occurred in central veins. Stent placement allowed completion of the thrombectomy in all patients. Complications were limited to hematomas in 4 patients. The primary patency rate of the access was 52%, 26%, and 11% at 60, 180, and 360 days, respectively. The secondary patency rate was 74%, 65%, and 56% at 60, 180, and 360 days, respectively. A pseudoaneurysm developed 6 months after stent placement in one patient.

The following year, Raynaud et al[62] reported a larger series with similar results. Over a 5-year period, the authors performed over 2,000 angioplasty procedures. Vascular rupture occurred in 40 (1.7%) cases. Covered stents were deployed in 37 of these ruptures. Importantly, this was the first study to describe the technique in AVF rather than in AVG only. Stent placement stopped the bleeding immediately in 28 cases and after prolonged inflation within the stent in 4 cases. A second stent had to be deployed within the lumen of the first in one case of refractory bleeding. One hematoma was drained surgically and one access occluded on the second day post-stent placement. The primary patency of the accesses at 1 year was 48%. The 1-year secondary patency was 86%.

More recently, an interesting case was reported in which an endovascular stent was used to repair an iatrogenic superior vena caval injury that occurred in the setting of a catheter placement.[63] The perforation in the vena cava occurred at the confluence of the innominate veins when left subclavian catheter was being inserted. The covered stent was delivered through a femoral approach while the catheter was simultaneously removed to attenuate hemorrhage. This case report represents a novel, percutaneous approach to a problem that, in the past, would have required emergent surgery.

The placement of an intravascular stent can effectively treat angioplasty-induced vascular rupture. Complete vascular rupture is one situation where stent placement is warranted beyond any doubt.

The treatment options for vascular access pseudoaneurysms have traditionally consisted of surgical revision or ligation of the access. The stent grafts (covered stents) have a particularly useful role in the treatment of pseudoaneurysms. Recently, investigators have reported on the role of these stents in the percutaneous treatment of pseudoaneurysms.[64-65] The first report described 2 patients who presented with an expanding mass over their AVG.[64] The pseudoaneurysms were repaired in both cases by transluminally introducing a balloon-expandable stainless steel stent covered with PTFE material. The authors reported that after the procedure both AVGs were patent at 5 and 6 months, respectively. In the same year, Hausegger et al[65] reported three cases in which pseudoaneurysms were walled off by percutaneous insertion of a stainless steel, PTFE-covered stent. The authors reported a patency rate of the access as 8–9 months, but, interestingly, in 2 of the cases the stent was punctured repeatedly during follow-up and the aneurysms recurred.[65]

A more systematic evaluation of this percutaneous solution quickly followed. Najibi et al[66] reported a series of 10 patients with AVG or AVF pseudoaneurysms treated with covered stent placement to exclude the lesion. On initial follow-up, all patients had lost the palpable pseudoaneurysm pulsation. Moreover, the access remained patent in 9/10 patients. At 6 months, 7/10 patients had patent access and no further issues with pseudoaneurysms.[66] More recently, 11 patients had undergone endoluminal insertion of a covered stent to repair.[67] All 11 procedures were technically successful. The primary access patency rate reported in this study was 71% at 3 months and 20% at 6 months. While these studies demonstrated the exclusion of pseudoaneurysm, problems such as recurrence of the pseudoaneurysm and stent graft damage due to repeated cannulation continue to surround this approach.

Stent graft cannulation is a controversial area that deserves to be mentioned. To date, no study has conclusively established the safety of repeated cannulation of a stent graft. Some of the reports that have evaluated the role of stent grafts in the management of pseudoaneurysms have commented on the stent cannulation.[64–67] These analyses, however, were limited by retrospective study design and a very small sample size (3 to 11 patients). While cannulation of the stent graft was clearly possible, these studies have documented that repeated cannulation through the stent could cause damage to these devices.[64–67] Indeed, stent damage by repeated cannulation has been documented by many investigators.[64–67] It is for this reason that Vesely has clearly pointed out the inability of the current stent grafts to withstand repeated needle puncture and called for a new stent graft design for cannulation application specifically.[67] The broken stent struts observed by Vesely can potentially protrude through the skin and pose a threat of injury to the staff placing the patient on dialysis. Additionally, such a scenario also exposes the device to the development of infection. A recent report highlighted 2 cases where cannulation was performed though the stent. Both developed infection and required surgical removal of the access to combat infection.[67] Indeed, the safety of cannulation through covered stent used to treat pseudoaneurysm has not been conclusively established in a prospective fashion.

Dialysis staff responsible for cannulating the access through the stent might require a specific order by the nephrologist. In this context, it is prudent for the interventionalist to communicate with the renal physician regarding the stented area and cannulation guidance.

Dialysis staff should then be made aware of the stent and given specific instructions regarding cannulation to minimize infection and avoid injury. As an aside patient education regarding the position of the stent might be important for the following reason. It is conceivable that for an access procedure, the patient might end up in a center that did not perform the original stent. In this context, the new interventionalist might find himself/herself cannulating the stented area and encountering problems. Patient education regarding vascular access is then critical. The above-cited issues gain more importance as these devices are not approved for this purpose. It is important to note that the use of covered stents in the treatment of pseudoaneurysm presents an "off-label" use of these devices. While critically important, medico-legal ramifications of cannulation through a stent are unknown.

▶ **Deployment Techniques**

When choosing the stent to be deployed, several key features need to be considered. The first is the material of which the stent is composed. Today most stents are made of nitinol, which is described in detail above. Briefly, due to its "thermal memory," this material is widely regarded as superior to stainless steal in the modern era of stent placement. The next decision point is a covered (aka "stent graft") or uncovered ("bare metal") stent (Figure 19-3). There is a great deal of controversy concerning the advantages and disadvantages of covered versus uncovered stents with very little data to support either perspective. Anecdotally, it is believed that stent grafts are more likely to thrombose than bare metal stents and are in general less forgiving technically during placement. Bare metal stents, on the other hand, are more likely to fall victim to aggressive neointimal hyperplasia and may succumb faster to in-stent restenosis. A recent study found that in-stent restenosis is associated with higher percent luminal diameter lesions, while de novo lesions rather than in-stent restenosis are associated with higher risk of AVG access failure and reduced primary patency.[68] Using a prospectively collected, vascular access database, the authors identified 76 patients seen for follow-up angiography due to access dysfunction after stent

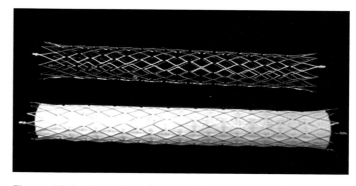

Figure 19-3. Examples of covered (stent graft) and uncovered stents.

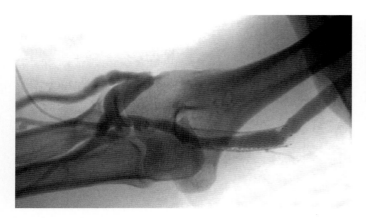

Figure 19-4. Stent placement, if not properly sized, may lead to turbulent flow and neointimal hyperplasia acceleration.

placement. The effect of in-stent restenosis versus de novo lesions in patients with previously placed endovascular stents were compared, with 35 (46.1%) patients having de novo lesions, while 41 (53.9%) had in-stent restenosis. In-stent restenosis was found to be the only factor associated with severity of luminal stenosis (beta = 0.35, 95% confidence interval 2.21-15.48, P = 0.01). However, in-stent restenosis was associated with increased primary patency among AVGs (hazards ratio 3.10; 95% confidence interval 1.35-7.10; P = 0.008). Primary patency of in-stent restenosis versus de novo lesions for AVGs were, respectively: 78% versus 94% at 1 month, 56% versus 42% at 3 months, and 33% versus 6% at 6 months. For arteriovenous fistulas, the difference in primary patency of in-stent versus de novo lesions was not statistically significant. Thus, the role of in-stent restenosis and neointimal hyperplasia in bare metal versus stent grafts remains undefined.

Another key factor in choosing a stent is stent size, with both length and diameter being critical considerations that actually influence one another (Figure 19-4). Stent length is typically chosen to flank the target lesion by 5–10 mm on each end. Stent diameter is typically chosen to exceed the natural diameter of the native vessel by 1 mm. Shortening of the stent upon deployment can be almost completely avoided if a stent graft of a diameter that is 1 mm greater than the lumen to be stented is chosen. In this case the compressed stent graft length is equivalent to the length of the expanded stent graft. Using the above guideline, the stent length stated on the product label is the minimum possible length of the expanded stent graft; in no case will the expanded length of the stent graft be shorter than this. Thus, the choice of stent diameter and length are dependent on one another.

Stents can be deployed as balloon-expandable or self-expanding devices. The advantage of balloon-expandable stents is that they tend not to jump as readily out of the lesion upon deployment. The disadvantage is that they typically require a larger-diameter introducer for placement than self-expanding stents. A recent publication was the first to describe a long-known technique that obviates the need for large sheath upsizing when placing a stent.[69] Caution must be taken when using this technique due to the inability of performing a confirmatory angiogram immediately prior to deployment.

There are several additional points to consider when deploying a stent of any variety. The delivery system must always be introduced, moved, and withdrawn over a suitable guide wire. Even though the radiopaque ends of most stents will appear as marker, it is advisable to confirm location in the lesion by obtaining angiographic confirmation of position prior to deployment. This is not possible if the stent is placed "bare back" as described above. During release of the stent graft, the entire length of the flexible delivery system should be kept as straight as possible to minimize "jumping" in the case of self-expanding stents. A slight tension on the handgrip is recommended to ensure that the catheter is straight. In the case of self-expanding stents, begin deployment slowly until the sheath has moved 1–2 cm proximally and thereby exposed the stent, then wait a few seconds to ensure secure "anchoring" of the distal stent end. Once anchored, the remainder of the stent graft can be released slowly. Oversizing of the stent graft of more than 2 mm relative to the normal lumen diameter be should be avoided.

The stent deployment procedure can be summarized as follows:

1. Place a suitable guide wire across the stricture (usually a .035 inch is required, but this depends on the nature of the stent and the lesion).

2. Insert the prepared delivery system over the guide wire to the location of the stricture.

3. Advance the stent graft across the stricture using the radiopaque stent graft ends to center the stent graft across the stricture. Some operators recommend advancing the delivery system past the stricture and then pulling back slightly on the entire system to attain correct positioning of the markers and to help ensure the delivery catheter is straight.

4. Confirm the exact position of the radiopaque markers on the stent graft ends with the lesion ends by direct angiography whenever possible immediately prior to deployment.

5. A slight back tension on the handgrip is recommended to ensure that the deployment system is stationary and straight and to diminish the probability of jumping in the case of self-expanding stents.

6. Pull back on the Y-injection-adapter slowly until it has moved 1–2 cm proximally, and then wait few seconds in order to ensure secure "anchoring" of the distal stent graft end. Once anchored, the remainder of the stent graft can be released slowly.

7. Full release of the stent graft is achieved by the pin and pull method or by deflation of the balloon, depending on stent type chosen.

8. Remove the flexible deployment system back over the guide wire. Keep the wire across the lesion until post-stent angiography confirms a desirable outcome.

9. Careful post dilatation of the stent graft may be desirable with a balloon equal in diameter to that of the stent graft.

Other Clinical Considerations

The ideal adjuvant medical treatment strategy for stent placement in hemodialysis access has yet to be rigorously defined. In the arterial system, patients typically receive 325 mg of aspirin and 300 mg of clopidogrel prior to intervention. A bolus of intravenous UFH at 70–100 U/kg is typically administered at the time of intervention to obtain an activated clotting time (ACT) of 200–300 seconds. All patients who receive an arterial stent are treated for an extended period of time with the dual antiplatelet regimen consisting of lifelong daily aspirin 81–325 mg, and daily clopidogrel 75 mg for 3–6 months.[70] However, it is difficult to translate these practices from the arterial to the venous side of the access.

In reality the vascular biology of the veins differs drastically from that of the arteries. Moreover, the pathology of the venous lesion (hyperplasia) is fundamentally distinct from the arterial lesion (atherosclerotic plaque rupture). Heparin can be used at the time of stent placement at doses of 50–70 U/kg if there is no contraindication to systemic anticoagulation. If there is a hypercoagulable state or if the stent is being placed into a vessel after thrombectomy, anticoagulation is encouraged. The use of anti-platelet agents cannot be recommended at this time for adjuvant medical therapy for stent placement in hemodialysis access.

The occasional complications associated with stent placement are important to recognize. These complications include shortening, migration, and fracture. Infectious complications are usually not evident until many days after the procedure. Verstandig et al[71] recently reported shortening and migration of covered stents after treatment of central venous stenoses in hemodialysis patients. In 70% of the cases there was significant stent shortening. All these cases required additional stents to be deployed in order to cover the target lesion. An additional 2 patients in this series experienced stent migration. Shortening tends to occur because, as a stainless steel stent is radially compressed, it becomes elongated.[72] Thus, when deployed, it becomes relatively foreshortened. The normal expansion and contraction of the central veins during respiration, when combined with the geometry of the stent, can lead to a sequence of shortening-lengthening-shortening of the stent. This sequence can lead to stent movement and migration.

Tsuji et al described stent fracture in the left brachiocephalic vein.[73] The authors described a hemodialysis patient with severe left arm edema on the side of his AVF. A brachiocephalic vein stenosis was initially treated with a self-expanding stent. Eight months after this initial procedure, a stent fracture was discovered. A second stent was deployed in the lumen of the previously placed fractured stent. This technique proved efficacious over the next 9 months, during which time the access remained patent. Similarly, a recent case report described fracture of 2 overlapping stents (9 × 80-mm and 9 × 60-mm).[74] After 6 months a fistulogram revealed stent fracture. Maleux et al[75] also reported a case of collapsed stent in the cephalic vein that led to thrombosis of a vascular access approximately one month after initial deployment.

Shortly after placement of an uncovered stent, the metallic struts are covered by endothelium. The stent can become infected, however, prior to full endothelialization.[76] Alternatively, if a covered stent is placed, endothelialization is delayed, and infection is a risk for a longer duration of time. One report describes a fatal outcome after a stent became infected.[77] Another report described a similar infectious event that was treated conservatively.[78] In the latter case, a Staph aureus infection was treated by local delivery of antibiotic into the infected stent. Nevertheless, most cases of stent infection require surgical removal of the stent. Another recent report describes the development of fever and positive blood cultures 3 weeks after stent placement.[79] A tagged white blood cell scan localized the infection to the stent. Due to the authors' conviction that the patient would not tolerate surgery, 6 weeks of systemic antibiotics was successful in effecting complete clinical resolution of the infection. Although this last report offers a more optimistic perspective, stent infection, however rare, is a life-threatening complication that requires aggressive intervention.

Infection related to a covered stent inserted in an arteriovenous access has also been reported recently.[80] Two diabetic patients with covered stent infection were described in this analysis. One patient was seen for left upper arm brachiocephalic graft dysfunction. An 8 × 40 mm stent graft was placed with excellent results. Two months later, the patient presented with signs of cellulitis at the area overlying the stent with strut wire palpable just under the skin. The staff had been cannulating through the stent. Antibiotic therapy was unsuccessful. Surgical intervention was performed to remove the stent and the arteriovenous graft. Another patient was seen for a dysfunctional right upper arm brachiocephalic fistula. An 8 × 60 mm stent graft was inserted with excellent results. The stented area was used for cannulation. The patient was admitted 5 months later with sepsis and signs of cellulitis of the skin overlying the cannulated area of the stent. The blood cultures revealed *Staphylococcus aureus*. Stent was surgically removed with loss of the access. The above-cited reports indicate that the stents can get infected particularly when they are used for cannulation. While stents are being used frequently to treat stenoses, cannulation through these devices can result infection and devastating consequences.

While the primary focus of the NKF/KDOQI guidelines as well as the National Vascular Access Improvement Initiative has been on fistula placement in incident hemodialysis patients,[81] the creation of secondary AVFs has recently

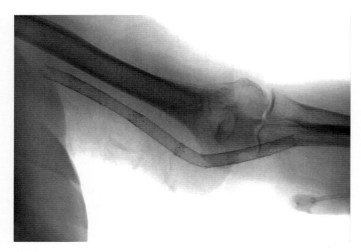

Figure 19-5. Multiple stents placed contiguously in the outflow vein ("stentula") prevent conversion to a secondary AVF.

come to be viewed as an important strategy to maximize the use of fistulas in prevalent hemodialysis patients.[82–83] A functional vascular access in the lower arm commonly results in dilatation of the veins in the upper arm. These dilated veins can then be used to create an AVF when the primary access starts to malfunction. What is more, the ability of these already mature veins to accept immediate cannulation obviates the need for the catheter bridge in many cases. If, on the other hand, there is a stent in the outflow vein that prevents the relatively easy creation of a secondary AVF, the matter becomes much more complex if not impossible (Figure 19-5).

The validity of a strategy to create secondary AVFs in patients with malfunctioning vascular accesses has been successfully demonstrated in a recent study.[84] In this analysis, 9 patients undergoing percutaneous interventions were evaluated for secondary AVF creation. All were found to have suitable vascular anatomy and had the AVF created. The secondary fistula was successful in all 9 patients with a mean follow-up of 4.8 +/− 1.4 months in post-AVG cases and 5.6 +/− 1.7 months in the post-AVF patients. Perhaps as important, it was possible to continue dialysis without the catheter bridge in 3/9 patients. Again, if there is a stent taking up "vascular real estate" in the upper arm, the methodology described above becomes extremely difficult. Indeed, a recent report described a scenario where multiple stents placed in the outflow tract of an access completely precluded subsequent creation of a secondary AVF.[85] It is, therefore, prudent to consider the creation of secondary fistula before the insertion of an intravascular stent where a secondary fistula is a real possibility.

CONCLUSION AND FUTURE DIRECTIONS

Despite the advances in knowledge described above, the role of stent placement in the management of hemodialysis access dysfunction remains controversial (see Table 19-4 for stent placement indications). It will remain so largely because the existing vascular access literature has attempted to address the question "to stent or not to stent," with limited success. The past few years have witnessed an evolution of the essential question to one of a more subtle nature: under what circumstances is the placement of a stent beneficial. Despite these recent advances, the issue of stent placement will remain controversial until large, multi-center, prospective, randomized, controlled trials are conducted. Until studies are published that correct for the type of access (eg, AVG or AVF), type of lesion (eg, inflow, outflow, or central), patient characteristics (eg, diabetic or not), and previous history of intervention, and take quality of delivered hemodialysis into account among a host of other variables that are believed to affect access outcomes, the hemodialysis access stent debate will be heard.

REFERENCES

1. Malvin RE. How a dentist's name became a synonym for a life-saving device: the story of Dr. Charles Stent. *J Hist Dent.* 2001;49(2):77–80.
2. Sigwart U, Puel J, Mirkovitch V, Joffre F, Kappenberger L. Intravascular stents to prevent occlusion and restenosis after transluminal angioplasty. *N Engl J Med.* 1987;316(12): 701–716.
3. Serruys PW, Kutryk MJB, Ong ATL. Coronary-artery stents. *N Engl J Med.* 2006;354:483–495.
4. Arjomand H, Turi Z, McCormick D, et al. Percutaneous coronary intervention: historical perspectives, current status, and future direction. *Am Heart J.* 2003;146:787–796.
5. Gruentzig AR, Senning A, Siegenthaler WE. Non-operative dilatation of coronary artery stenoses. Percutaneous transluminal coronary angioplasty. *N Engl J Med.* 1979;301:61–68.
6. Rasmussen RL, Feldman D, Beathard G, Rubin JE. Indications for stent placement in a dialysis access. *Semin Dial.* 2008;21(1):83–84.
7. Asif A, Leon C, Merrill D, Ellis R, Bhimani B, Pennell P. Optimal timing for secondary arteriovenous fistula creation: devastating effects of delaying conversion. *Semin Dial.* 2006;19(5):425–428.
8. Yevzlin AS, Maya ID, Asif A. Endovascular stents for dialysis access: under what circumstances do the data support their use? *Adv Chronic Kidney Dis.* 2009;16(5):352–359.
9. Yevzlin A, Asif A. Stent placement in hemodialysis access: historical lessons, the state of the art and future directions. *Clin J Am Soc Nephrol.* 2009;4(5):996–1008.
10. U.S. Renal Data System, USRDS 2006 Annual Data Report: Atlas of Chronic Kidney Disease and End-Stage Renal Disease in the United States, National Institutes of Health, National Institute of Diabetes and Digestive and Kidney Diseases, Bethesda, MD, 2007.
11. Zollikofer CL, Largiader I, Bruhlman W. Endovascular stenting of veins and grafts: preliminary clinical experience. *Radiology.* 1988;167:707–712.
12. Antonucci, F, Salomonowitz E, Stuckmann G, Stiefel M, Zollikofer CL. Placement of venous stents: clinical experience with a self-expanding prosthesis. *Radiology.* 1992;183:493.

13. Quinn SF, Schuman ES, Demlow TA, et al. Percutaneous transluminal angioplasty versus endovascular stent placement in the treatment of venous stenoses in patients undergoing hemodialysis: intermediate results, *J Vasc Interv Radiol.* 1995;6:851–855.

14. Beathard GA. Gianturco self-expanding stent in the treatment of stenosis in dialysis access grafts. *Kidney Int.* 1993;43:872–877.

15. Hoffer EK, Sultan S, Herskowitz MM, et al. Prospective randomized trial of a metallic intravascular stent in hemodialysis graft maintenance, *J Vasc Interv Radiol.* 1997;8:965–973.

16. Zaleski GX, Funaki B, Rosenblum J, et al. Metallic stents deployed in synthetic arteriovenous hemodialysis grafts, *Am J Roentgenol.* 2001;176:1515–1519.

17. Oderich GS, Treiman GS, Schneider P, Bhirangi K. Stent placement for treatment of central and peripheral venous obstruction: a long-term multi-institutional experience. *J Vasc Surg.* 2000;32(4):760–769.

18. Hatzimpaloglou A, Velissaris I, Gourasas I, Grekas D, Kiskinis D, Kaitzis D, Louridas G. Stenting of central venous stenoses and occlusions to maintain hemodialysis vascular access. *J Vasc Access.* 2002;3(1):10–13.

19. Quinn SF, Kim J, Sheley RC. Transluminally placed endovascular grafts for venous lesions in patients on hemodialysis. *Cardiovasc Intervent Radiol.* 2003;26(4):365–369.

20. Aytekin C, Boyvat F, Yağmurdur MC, Moray G, Haberal M. Endovascular stent placement in the treatment of upper extremity central venous obstruction in hemodialysis patients. *Eur J Radiol.* 2004;49(1):81–85.

21. Pan HB, Liang HL, Lin YH, Chung HM, Wu TH, Chen CY, Fang HC, Chen CK, Lai PH, Yang CF. Metallic stent placement for treating peripheral outflow lesions in native arteriovenous fistula hemodialysis patients after insufficient balloon dilatation. *Am J Roentgenol.* 2005;184(2):403–409.

22. Sreenarasimhaiah VP, Margassery SK, Martin KJ, Bander SJ. Salvage of thrombosed dialysis access grafts with venous anastomosis stents. *Kidney Int.* 2005;67(2):678–684.

23. Liang HL, Pan HB, Lin YH, Chen CY, Chung HM, Wu TH, Chou KJ, Lai PH, Yang CF. Metallic stent placement in hemodialysis graft patients after insufficient balloon dilation. *Korean J Radiol.* 2006;7(2):118–124.

24. Naoum JJ, Irwin C, Hunter GC. The use of covered nitinol stents to salvage dialysis grafts after multiple failures. *Vasc Endovascular Surg.* 2006;40(4):275–279.

25. Lombardi JV, Dougherty MJ, Veitia N, Somal J, Calligaro KD. A comparison of patch angioplasty and stenting for axillary venous stenoses of thrombosed hemodialysis grafts. *Vasc Endovascular Surg.* 2002;36(3):223–229.

26. Aruny JE. l. Quality Improvement Guidelines for Percutaneous Management of the Thrombosed or Dysfunctional Dialysis Access. *JVIR.* 2003;14(9):S247–S253.

27. Vorwerk D, Guenther RW, Mann H, et al. Venous stenosis and occlusion in hemodialysis shunts: followup results of stent placement in 65 patients. *Radiology.* 1995;195:140–146.

28. Aytekin C, Boyvat F, Yağmurdur MC, Moray G, Haberal M. Endovascular stent placement in the treatment of upper extremity central venous obstruction in hemodialysis patients. *Eur J Radiol.* 2004;49(1):81–85.

29. Beathard GA. Percutaneous transvenous angioplasty in the treatment of vascular access stenosis. *Kidney Int.* 1992;42(6):1390–1397.

30. Gray RJ, Horton KM, Dolmatch BL, et al. Use of Wallstents for hemodialysis access-related venous stenoses and occlusions untreatable with balloon angioplasty. *Radiology.* 1995;195:479–484.

31. Haage P, Vorwerk D, Piroth W, Schuermann K, Guenther RW. Treatment of hemodialysis-related central venous stenosis or occlusion: results of primary Wallstent placement and follow-up in 50 patients. *Radiology.* 1999;212(1):175–180.

32. Aytekin C, Boyvat F, Yağmurdur MC, Moray G, Haberal M. Endovascular stent placement in the treatment of upper extremity central venous obstruction in hemodialysis patients. *Eur J Radiol.* 2004;49(1):81–85.

33. Dotter CT. Transluminally placed coilspring endarterial tube grafts: Long-term patency in canine popliteal artery. *Invest Radiol.* 1969;4:327–332.

34. Maass D, Kropf L, Egloff L, Demierre D, Turma M. Senning A. Transluminal implantation of intravascular "double helix" spiral prostheses: technical and biological considerations. *ESAO Proc.* 1982;9:252–256.

35. Maass D, Demierre D, Deaton D, Largiadér F, Senning A. Transluminal implantation of self-adjusting expandable prostheses: principles, techniques, and results. *Prog Artif Org.*1983;9:979–987.

36. Maass D, Zollikofer CHL, Largiader F, Senning A. Radiological follow-up of transluminally inserted vascular endoprostheses: an experimental study using expanding spirals. *Radiology.* 1984;152:659–663.

37. Zollikofer CL, Antonucci F, Stuckmann G, Mattias P, Salomonowitz EK. Historical overview on the development and characteristics of stents and future outlooks. *Cardiovasc Intervent Radiol.* 1992; 15:272–278.

38. Beathard GA. Central vein stenosis associated with dialysis access. Uptodate: http://www.utdol.com/online/content/topic.do?topicKey=dialysis/32202&selectedTitle=9~150&source=search_result. Accessed online 11-24-09

39. Cragg A, Lurid G, Rysavy J, Castaneda F, Castaneda-Zuniga WR, Amplatz K. Non-surgical placement of arterial endoprostheses: a new technique using nitinol wire. *Radiology.* 1983;147:261–263.

40. Clark TWJ. Nitinol stents in hemodialysis access. *J Vasc Interv Radiol.* 2004;15:1037–1040.

41. Rotmans, JI, Pattynama, PM, Verhagen, HJ, et al. Sirolimus-eluting stents to abolish intimal hyperplasia and improve flow in porcine arteriovenous grafts: a 4-week follow-up study. *Circulation.* 2005;111:153.

42. Dyet JF, Watts WG, Ettles DF, Nicholson AA. Mechanical properties of metallic stents: how do these properties influence the choice of stent for specific lesions? *Cardiovasc Intervent Radiol.* 2000;23:47–54.

43. Shabalovskaya SA. On the nature of the biocompatibility and on medical applications of NiTi shape memory and superelastic alloys. *Biomed Mater Eng.* 1996;6:267–289.

44. Duda SH, Wiskirchen J, Tepe G, et al. Physical properties of endovascular stents: an experimental comparison. *J Vasc Interv Radiol.* 2000;11:645–654.

45. Rhodes ES, Silas AM. Dialysis needle puncture of Wallgrafts placed in polytetrafluoroethylene hemodialysis grafts. *JVIR.* 2005;16(8):1129–1134.

46. Maya ID, Allon M. Outcomes of thrombosed arteriovenous grafts: comparison of stents vs angioplasty. *Kidney Int.* 2006;69:934–937.

47. Vogel PM, Parise C. Comparison of SMART stent placement for arteriovenous graft salvage versus successful graft PTA. *J Vasc Interv Radiol.* 2005;16(12):1619–1626.

48. Kolakowski S Jr, Dougherty MJ, Calligaro KD. Salvaging prosthetic dialysis fistulas with stents: forearm versus upper arm grafts. *J Vasc Surg.* 2003;38(4):719–723.

49. Vesely T, Pilgram T, Amin MZ. Use of stents and stent grafts to salvage angioplasty failures in patients with hemodialysis grafts. *Semin Dialysis*, early online edition.

50. Chan MR, Bedi S, Sanchez RJ, Young HN, Becker YT, Kellerman PS, Yevzlin AS. Stent placement versus angioplasty improves patency of arteriovenous grafts and blood flow of arteriovenous fistulae. *Clin J Am Soc Nephrol.* 2008;3(3):699–705.

51. Chan MR, Young HN, Yevzlin AS. The effect of in-stent restenosis on hemodialysis access patency. *Hemodial Int.* 2009;13(3):250–256.

52. Hatzimpaloglou A, Velissaris I, Gourasas I, Grekas D, Kiskinis D, Kaitzis D, Louridas G.J. Stenting of central venous stenoses and occlusions to maintain hemodialysis vascular access. *Vasc Access.* 2002;3(1):10–13.

53. Sprouse LR 2nd, Lesar CJ, Meier GH 3rd, Parent FN, Demasi RJ, Gayle RG, Marcinzyck MJ, Glickman MH, Shah RM, McEnroe CS, Fogle MA, Stokes GK, Colonna JO. Percutaneous treatment of symptomatic central venous stenosis. *J Vasc Surg.* 2004;39(3):578–582.

54. Maya ID, Saddekni S, Allon M. Treatment of refractory central vein stenosis in hemodialysis patients with stents. *Semin Dial.* 2007;20(1):78–82.

55. Levit RD, Cohen RM, Kwak A, Shlansky-Goldberg RD, Clark TW, Patel AA, Stavropoulos SW, Mondschein JI, Solomon JA, Tuite CM, Trerotola SO. Asymptomatic central venous stenosis in hemodialysis patients. *Radiology.* 2006;238(3):1051–1056.

56. Rajan DK, Chennepragada SM, Lok CE, Beecroft JR, Tan KT, Hayeems E, Kachura JR, Sniderman KW, Simons ME. Patency of endovascular treatment for central venous stenosis: is there a difference between dialysis fistulas and grafts? *J Vasc Interv Radiol.* 2007;18(3):353–359.

57. http://www.fda.gov/cdrh/pdf6/p060002.html.

58. http://www.kidney.org/Professionals/kdoqi/guideline_upHD_PD_VA/va_intro.htm.

59. Oderich GS, Panneton JM, Hofer J, Bower TC, Cherry KJ Jr., Sullivan T, Noel AA, Kalra M, Gloviczki P. Iatrogenic operative injuries of abdominal and pelvic veins: a potentially lethal complication. *J Vasc Surg.* 2004;39; 931–936.

60. Asensio JA, Chahwan S, Hanpeter D, Demetriades D, Forno W, Gambaro E, Murray J, Velmahos G, Marengo J, Shoemaker WC, Berne TV. Operative management and outcome of 302 abdominal vascular injuries. *Am J Surg.* 2000;180; 528–533.

61. Funaki B, Szymski GX, Leef JA, Rosenblum JD, Burke R, Hackworth CA. Wallstent deployment to salvage dialysis graft thrombolysis complicated by venous rupture: early and intermediate results. *Am J Roentgenol.* 1997;169(5):1435–1437.

62. Raynaud AC, Angel CY, Sapoval MR, Beyssen B, Pagny JY, Auguste M.J Treatment of hemodialysis access rupture during PTA with Wallstent implantation. *Vasc Interv Radiol.* 1998;9(3):437–442.

63. Azizzadeh A, Pham MT, Estrera AL, Coogan SM, Safi HJ. Endovascular repair of an iatrogenic superior vena caval injury: a case report. *J Vasc Surg.* 2007;46(3):569–571.

64. Rabindranauth P, Shindelman L. Transluminal stent-graft repair for pseudoaneurysm of PTFE hemodialysis grafts. *J Endovasc Surg.* 1998;5(2):138–141.

65. Hausegger KA, Tiessenhausen K, Klimpfinger M, Raith J, Hauser H, Tauss J. Aneurysms of hemodialysis access grafts: treatment with covered stents: a report of three cases. *Cardiovasc Intervent Radiol.* 1998;21(4):334–337.

66. Najibi S, Bush RL, Terramani TT, Chaikof EL, Gunnoud AB, Lumsden AB, Weiss VJ. Covered stent exclusion of dialysis access pseudoaneurysms. *J Surg Res.* 2002; 106(1):15–19.

67. Vesely TM. Use of stent grafts to repair hemodialysis graft-related pseudoaneurysms. *J Vasc Interv Radiol.* 2005;16(10):1301–1307.

68. Chan MR, Young HN, Yevzlin AS. The effect of in-stent restenosis on hemodialysis access patency. *Hemodial Int.* 2009;13(3):250–256.

69. Yevzlin AS, Chan MR, Gimelli G, Maya ID. How I do it: endovascular stent deployment using a novel technique that obviates the need for introducer-sheath upsizing. *Semin Dial.* 2009;22(5):584–587.

70. Yevzlin AS, Schoenkerman AB, Gimelli G, Asif A. Arterial interventions in arteriovenous access and chronic kidney disease: a role for interventional nephrologists. *Semin Dial.* 2009;22(5):545–556.

71. Verstandig AG, Bloom AI, Sasson T, Haviv YS, Rubinger D. Shortening and migration of Wallstents after stenting of central venous stenoses in hemodialysis patients. *Cardiovasc Intervent Radiol.* 2003;26(1):58–64.

72. Gray RJ, Dolmatch BL, Horton KM, Romolo JL, Zarate AR. Migration of Palmaz stents following deployment for venous stenoses related to hemodialysis access. *J Vasc Interv Radiol.* 1994;5(1):117–120.

73. Tsuji T, Iijima R, Nakajima R, Yoshitama T, Hara H, Hara H, Tsunoda T, Nakamura M, Wada M, Yamamoto M, Shiba M. Stent fracture in the left brachiocephalic vein. *Cardiovasc Revasc Med.* 2007;8(2):103–106.

74. Brewster UC, Mojibian HR, Aruny JE, Perazella MA. Access stenosis and stent fracture. *Am J Kidney Dis.* 2006;47(3):A45, e35–e36.

75. Maleux G, Rousseau H, Otal P, Joffre F. Collapsed Palmaz stent after deployment for hemodialysis access-related venous stenosis. *J Vasc Interv Radiol.* 1998;9(1 Pt 1):169–171.

76. Thibodeaux LC, James KV, Lohr JM, Welling RE, Roberts WH. Infection of endovascular stents in a swine model. *Am J Surg.* 1996;172:151–154.

77. Bruneau L, Gaboury L. Infection with fatal outcome after endovascular metallic stent placement. *Radiology.* 1994;192:363–365.

78. Naddour F, Yount RD, Quintal RE. Successful conservative treatment of an infected central venous stent. *Cathet Cardiovasc Intervent.* 2000;51:196–198.

79. Guest SS, Kirsch CM, Baxter R, Sorooshian M, Young J. Infection of a subclavian venous stent in a hemodialysis patient. *Am J Kidney Dis.* 1995;26(2):377–380.

80. Gadalean F. Covered stent outcomes for arteriovenous hemodialysis access salvage. *J Am Soc Nephrol.* 2008;19:899A.

81. Beasley C, Rowland J, Spergel L: Fistula First: an update for renal providers. *Nephrol News Issues*. 2004;18:88–90.

82. Beathard GA: Interventionalist's role in identifying candidates for secondary fistulas. *Semin Dial*. 2004;17:233–236.

83. Asif A, Leon C, Merrill D, Ellis R, Bhimani B, Pennell P. Optimal timing for secondary arteriovenous fistula creation: devastating effects of delaying conversion. *Semin Dial*. 2006;19(5):425–428.

84. Asif A, Unger SW, Briones P, Merrill D, Cherla G, Lenz O, Roth D, Pennell P. Creation of secondary arteriovenous fistulas: maximizing fistulas in prevalent hemodialysis patients. *Semin Dial*. 2005;18(5):420–424.

85. Rasmussen RL, Feldman D, Beathard G, Rubin JE. Indications for stent placement in a dialysis access. *Semin Dial*. 2008;21(1):83–84.

20

ACCESSORY VEINS: RECOGNITION AND MANAGEMENT

ANIL K. AGARWAL & TUSHAR J. VACHHARAJANI

LEARNING OBJECTIVES

1. Define accessory veins and differentiate from collateral veins.
2. Explain pathophysiology and significance of accessory veins.
3. Discuss management of accessory veins.

INTRODUCTION

Accessory veins in an arteriovenous fistula (AVF) are the side branches that arise from the principal outflow vein of the AVF (Figure 20-1). These veins are usually part of normal anatomy and can dilate alongside the fistula due to increased blood flow after its creation. It is important to note that such a vein is considered an accessory vein only if there is no proximal stenosis in AVF at any point.

It should be emphasized that the side branches in presence of a proximal stenosis or occlusion are, in fact, collateral veins. Collateral veins develop to bypass the obstruction to flow and are able to drain either more proximal to it or to a different venous tract. It is not uncommon to find veins arising of distal AVF and initially considered accessory vein, only to find a more proximal stenosis, making it a collateral vein (Figure 20-2).

PREVALENCE

As well matured AVF are not studied routinely, the prevalence of accessory veins has only been reported in dysfunctional AVF. Thus, while accessory veins can occur in isolation, these are often seen in presence of other lesions causing poor maturation. For example, in an angiography series of 100 patients presenting for maturation failure, an accessory vein was found in 46% of the cases.[1] Another series of 119 patients with poorly maturing AVF reported the presence of accessory veins in 29.4% of the cases.[2] In most of these patients other lesions were also present, with isolated accessory veins present in only 3.4%. Management of these lesions resulted salvage of AVF in 83%.

Accessory veins are particularly noted to be prevalent in forearm cephalic AVF, although the location can vary.

PATHOPHYSIOLOGY

Although a large accessory vein can be problematic from many points of view and lead to failure of maturation, all accessory veins should not be considered pathological. Typically, when such a venous branch is greater than 25% of the diameter of AVF, it may steal enough blood away from the principal AVF outflow. Distribution of incoming blood flow among these branches reduces blood flow to the intended AVF vein and decreases the pressure required to dilate the vein. In a maturing AVF, these veins may provide enough competition with AVF outflow to cause its failure to mature. However, if there is a large enough inflow into the AVF, both veins may be able to mature. In this circumstance, this may be beneficial and provide a dual outflow for cannulation. However, often there are a number of relatively small accessory veins that not only are sufficiently large to cannulate, but also may criss-cross the AVF and accidentally punctured during cannulation causing infiltration, development of hematoma, and painful cannulation. These veins can also cause difficulty in cannulation by obscuring the main venous outflow and by making it difficult to judge the direction of AVF.

Collateral veins, often mistaken for an accessory vein, play an important role in maintaining flow and patency

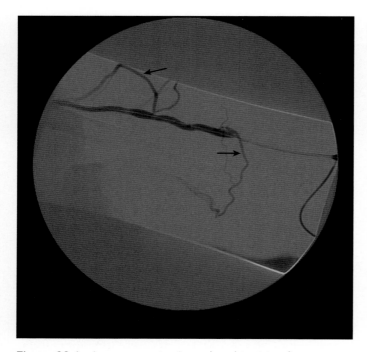

Figure 20-1. Accessory veins (arrowheads) arising from upper arm cephalic vein.

IDENTIFICATION OF ACCESSORY VEINS

Frequently, the accessory veins can be identified by simple inspection, palpation, and auscultation of these veins (Figure 20-3). These veins can become prominent if the main venous outflow is occluded and the thrill and bruit over these veins can become stronger. This, by itself, does not indicate that these accessory veins are significant. Contrarily, if compression of the accessory vein leads to significant enhancement of blood flow in a dysfunctional AVF, it indicates that the accessory vein is diverting a significant amount of blood flow and obliteration of this vein may help in improving the function of AVF. The diagnosis can be confirmed by angiography, especially utilizing an arteriogram of the inflow artery that identifies accessory veins arising close to the arteriovenous anastomosis. Attempts to perform a retrograde arteriogram can fail to show the arterial anastomosis if there are one or more accessory veins providing another outflow for the radiocontrast. At the same time, if these veins were not visualized on antegrade angiogram, these are unlikely to be pathological.

MANAGEMENT OF ACCESSORY VEINS

The presence of accessory veins is considered to be an important factor in non-maturing AVF, although this issue remains controversial.[1-5] As discussed above, the mere presence of accessory veins in a well-developed fistula is not always an indication to intervene. The accessory veins that do not prevent successful cannulation of the fistula should not be considered as pathological. In fact, these accessory veins in a well matured fistula can be considered as "insurance" for future patch venoplasty if a surgical revision is indicated. Intervention should only be considered if an accessory vein is considered as contributing to poor maturation or failure of AVF.

of the AVF. These veins are known to decrease in size or disappear altogether when angioplasty or stent placement is successful in relieving the stenosis. Unless causing difficulty in cannulation, these veins can be left unintervened and may prevent thrombosis of AVF when stenosis recurs.

Whether accessory veins cause immaturity of AVF remains controversial. In the absence of a randomized controlled trial and uniform reporting standards, dependence on observational data may lead to introduction of bias and incorrect conclusions.

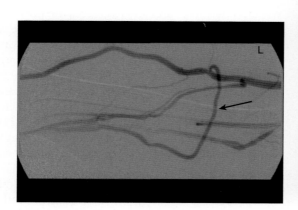

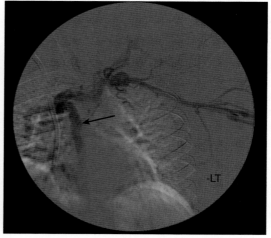

Figure 20-2. Appearance of side branches that appear to be accessory veins (arrowhead) on initial angiogram of upper arm AVF (right panel). However, in the right panel, central venogram displays near-occlusion of superior vena cava and a dilated azygous vein (arrowhead), making it obvious that these veins are collateral veins trying to bypass blood flow to other venous channels.

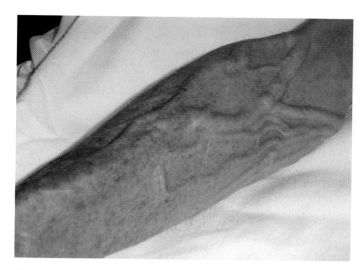

Figure 20-3. Accessory veins visible on physical examination.

The treatment of accessory vein depends on the presence or absence of proximal venous stenosis and its luminal size. Beathard et al[1] reported venous stenosis to be present in 78% of the 100 arteriovenous fistulae evaluated for immaturity. A significant accessory vein was found in 46 cases, of which only 12 had accessory vein as the only lesion identified on angiography. Significant proximal stenosis in the body of the fistula or in the central veins was identified in the remaining 34 cases with accessory veins. In this series, 100% success was obtained in obliterating these veins by various means including percutaneous ligation, venous cutdown, or coil insertion. With these aggressive procedures, 92% of the AVF were able to mature and were used for dialysis. In a prior study by Beathard et al, venous stenosis was present in 33.3% of cases evaluated for immaturity.[3]

In the presence of stenosis, the significance of accessory veins should be evaluated once the stenosis has been appropriately treated with angioplasty. As shown in (Figure 20-4), the right upper arm brachiocephalic fistula was evaluated for failing to mature and, on initial angiography, a significant proximal stenosis was noted with small accessory veins. The post-angioplasty angiogram performed 3 months later did not reveal any accessory veins and a well-developed brachiocephalic fistula (Figure 20-5). Thus, small accessory veins are best ignored and an active effort should be made to rule out stenosis.

Turmel-Rodrigues et al over a 6-year period treated 69 immature forearm fistulae and found stenosis in 100% of their cases. No accessory veins were ligated or embolized and using aggressive approach to locate and treat stenosis both on the arterial and venous sides achieved a 1-year primary and secondary patency rates of 39% and 79%, respectively.[4]

▶ Embolization or Ligation of Accessory Veins

An accessory vein is considered significant if it is large and diverts the blood flow away from the main body of

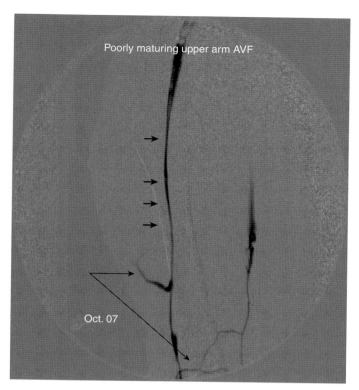

Figure 20-4. Small and extensive stenosis of the proximal cephalic vein in a brachiocephalic fistula (arrowheads). Small insignificant accessory veins are seen distal to the stenosis (arrows).

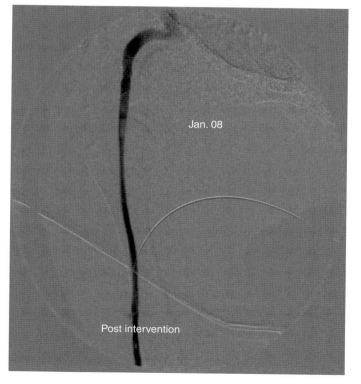

Figure 20-5. Well-developed brachiocephalic fistula with absent accessory veins 3 months later.

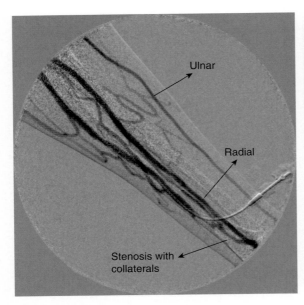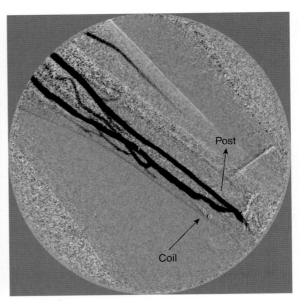

Figure 20-6. Multiple accessory veins identified in a radiocephalic fistula along with stenosis in the juxta-anastomotic region. Post-angioplasty and coil embolization angiography confirms the patent arterial anastomosis and obliterated accessory vein.

the fistula. It is of paramount importance to rule out any proximal venous stenosis and treat the stenosis if present, before considering definitive intervention of the accessory vein. The accessory vein can be obliterated either with surgical ligation or with coil embolization. The ultimate goal to obliterate the collateral veins is to augment the blood flow within the intended main outflow tract in anticipation of eventually being used for cannulation during dialysis.

Ligation of accessory veins has been shown to improve blood flow and maturation of AVF. This procedure can be easily performed in an intervention suite by placing a 3-0 nylon suture (Ethilon) around the vein close to its junction with the main trunk of the fistula without a skin incision as described by Faiyaz et al.[6] Seventeen arteriovenous fistulae with accessory veins were ligated without any skin incision resulting in 88% of arteriovenous fistulae maturing in 1.7 ± 1 month following the procedure. Open surgical ligation can be performed with a small skin incision to identify the accessory vein and ligating the vein with a non-absorbable suture. Post ligation, venography can be performed to confirm the success of the procedure.

Coil embolization is often utilized if the accessory vein is amenable for endovascular intervention and the operator expertise is available. Several different varieties of coils are available for embolization and the selection is generally based on the operator's preference and cost of the material. Typically, stainless steel coils have been used for this purpose and can be delivered through commonly used 4-5-French angiographic catheters. More expensive platinum coils are considered to be biocompatible and require small delivery catheters as compared to stainless steel coils. Occlusion of the accessory vein occurs as a result of coil-induced thrombosis rather than mechanical occlusion of the lumen by the coil.

Coil embolization requires identification of the accessory vein on angiography with selective placement of a guiding catheter inside the vein. The number of coils to be deployed is dependent on the size of the accessory vein. Generally, 2-3 coils are delivered into each accessory vein and a follow-up angiogram is performed to confirm the obliteration (Figure 20-6). There may be transient phlebitis after coiling. There is also a risk of coil migration.

▶ Collateral Vein Ligation During Initial Arteriovenous Fistula Creation

Ligation of accessory veins during initial fistula creation can potentially reduce the incidence of poor maturation. Planken et al used contrast enhanced magnetic resonance angiography to preoperatively evaluate vessel diameters, accessory veins, and presence or absence of stenosis in 15 consecutive radiocephalic fistulae. Ten of fifteen fistulae failed to mature at 2 months. The presence of large-caliber accessory vein was the only significant predictor of fistula non-maturation. Preoperatively detected accessory veins with a diameter of more than 70% of the diameter of the cephalic vein had a very high sensitivity and specificity of predicting radiocephalic fistula non-maturation. The authors concluded that preoperative assessment and ligation of large accessory veins can reduce the failure rate of radiocephalic fistula.[7] However, one has to be cautious about using gadolinium for contrast in patients with advanced kidney failure or in those with end-stage renal disease due to the risk of nephrogenic systemic fibrosis associated with this agent. Whether duplex ultrasound can provide such visualization of accessory veins prior to the creation of AV fistula remains to be seen.

In summary, accessory veins have to be properly identified by a combination of physical examination and angiography to differentiate from collateral veins. The significance of these veins in contributing to AVF immaturity or dysfunction should be carefully assessed, including a prior angioplasty of stenosis if present. Various methods of obliterating these side branches are available and can be used according to available equipment and expertise. Prospective trials of such findings and management are necessary to provide more evidence in this controversial area.

REFERENCES

1. Beathard GA, Arnold P, Jackson J, Litchfield T. Physician operators forum of RMS Lifeline. Aggressive treatment of early fistula failure. *Kidney Int.* 2003; 64:1487–1494.
2. Nassar GM, Nguyen B, Rhee E, Achkar K. Endovascular treatment of the "failing to mature" arteriovenous fistula. *Clin J Am Soc Nephrol.* 2006; 1(2):275–280.
3. Beathard GA, Settle SM, Shields MW: Salvage of the nonfunctioning arteriovenous fistula. *Am J Kidney Dis.* 1999;33(5):910–916.
4. Turmel-Rodrigues L, Mouton A, Birmele B, et al. Salvage of immature forearm fistulas for haemodialysis by interventional radiology. *Nephrol Dial Transplant.* 2001;16(12):2365–2371.
5. Malovrh M. Non-matured arteriovenous fistulae for haemodialysis: diagnosis, endovascular and surgical treatment. *Bosn J Basic Med Sci.* 10 (suppl 1):S13–S17.
6. Faiyaz R, Abreo K, Zaman F, Pervez A, Zibari G, Work J. Salvage of poorly developed arteriovenous fistulae with percutaneous ligation of accessory veins. *Am J Kidney Dis.* 2002;39(4):824–827.
7. Planken RN, Duijm LE, Kessels AG, et al. Accessory veins and radial-cephalic arteriovenous fistula non-maturation: a prospective analysis using contrast-enhanced magnetic resonance angiography. *J Vasc Access.* 2007;8(4):281–286.

21

PSEUDOANEURYSM AND ANEURYSM FORMATION

GERALD A. BEATHARD

INTRODUCTION

Arteriovenous dialysis access, either a polytetrafluoroethylene (PTFE) graft or a native fistula (AVF), may develop areas of bulging dilatation. Although these look very similar, they are in most cases quite different in structure. In the case of a PTFE graft, this is generally a pseudoaneurysm while with a fistula the anomalous site most often represents an aneurysm. The difference lies in the makeup of the structure's wall. An aneurysm ("true" aneurysm) is a pathological dilation of a vessel that involves all layers of the wall of the vessel. A pseudoaneurysm ("false" aneurysm) is characterized by actual disruption of the layers of its walls leading to a bulging anatomical defect.

PSEUDOANEURYSMS

The use of PTFE grafts for dialysis access is associated with complications. These occur much more frequently than with fistulas. The major complications that are seen are venous stenosis (including the venous anastomosis), arterial stenosis (including the arterial anastomosis), thrombosis, infection, ischemia, and pseudoaneurysm formation.[1]

▶ Etiology

Pseudoaneurysm deformities are not uncommon; they result from repeated puncturing of the graft at the same site ("one-site-itis" or segmental overutilization). The dialysis needle is somewhat unusual in its design. Firstly, it has a very thin wall in order to maximize the lumen diameter in comparison to the needle size. Secondly, it is very sharp. Both the tip and the bevel are sharp; this later feature is contributed to by the thinness of the needle's wall. When this device punctures the wall of the PTFE graft, it acts like a cookie-cutter, either removing a small plug or creating a flap. Other types of needles, even those of large gage, make a slit when they puncture the graft. This closes when the needle is removed.

Over time, the repetitive removal of material from the graft results in a loss of its structural integrity (Figure 21-1). This occurs earlier and is more accentuated if puncture sites are not rotated.[2-3] However, even with site rotation, the structural damage to the graft over a prolonged period will result in a defect. With long-term graft survival, this defect can be quite extensive and can be easily palpated. The incidence of pseudoaneurysm formation is much

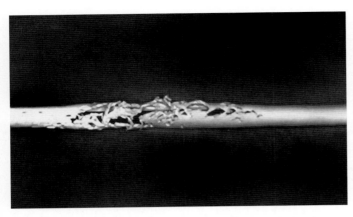

Figure 21-1. The result of repeated needle cannulation in the same general area is damage to the vascular graft. The importance of rotating puncture sites cannot be overstated. (Courtesy of W.L. Gore & Associates.)

lower than that of defects in the graft. Two concurrent events are required for the appearance of the dilatation that characterizes a pseudoaneurysm—a defect in the graft and increased intragraft pressure. The rapidity with which the dilatation progresses is directly related to the degree of elevation in intragraft pressure present. With very high levels, it can occur very quickly (Figure 21-2), at times, overnight.

The skin over the graft can become scarred, thinned, and avascular. In some cases this can lead to ulceration and spontaneous bleeding. Delorme et al[2] analyzed 52 surgically excised PTFE grafts used as vascular access in chronic hemodialysis patients. In that study, pseudoaneurysm formation at the site of repeated venipuncture was

the main cause of surgical removal of the graft more than 2 years after implantation. Histological evaluation revealed a perigraft fibrous tissue capsule directly above the areas where the graft was punctured. The microporous structure of the graft wall was disrupted. Occasionally, capillary formation was observed within the puncture sites. A layer of pseudointima was present on the luminal surface of the pseudoaneurysm.

The dilated segment, the pseudoaneurysm, adjacent to graft lumen of normal caliber (Figure 21-3), results in a relative increase in pressure (large diameter flowing into a small diameter) within the anomalous site that can cause further progression even if the more distal resistance is relieved. Once a pseudoaneurysm is formed, it does not regress even with treatment of the causative factor.

▶ **Complications**

The seriousness of a pseudoaneurysm lies in its associated complications, which are several.

▶ **Cosmetic Appearance**

Some patients are concerned about the cosmetic appearance of pseudoaneurysms that can obtain rather large size, several times the diameter of the graft. These are more obvious if on the forearm. At times, surgical repair is performed for this indication.

▶ **Difficult Cannulation**

If pseudoaneurysms are multiple and cover a large area of the PTFE graft, they can make it difficult to find a normal area to cannulate for dialysis. Cannulations should not be

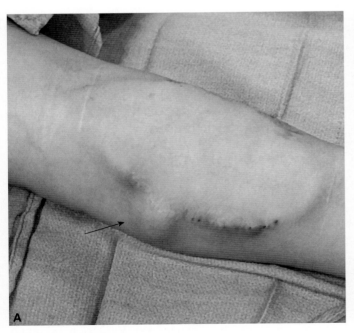

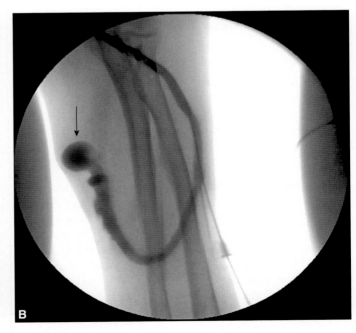

Figure 21-2. Appearance of early pseudoaneurysm. (**A**) Appearance of graft (arrow). (**B**) Appearance of angiogram (arrow). Note other smaller pseudoaneurysms on angiogram.

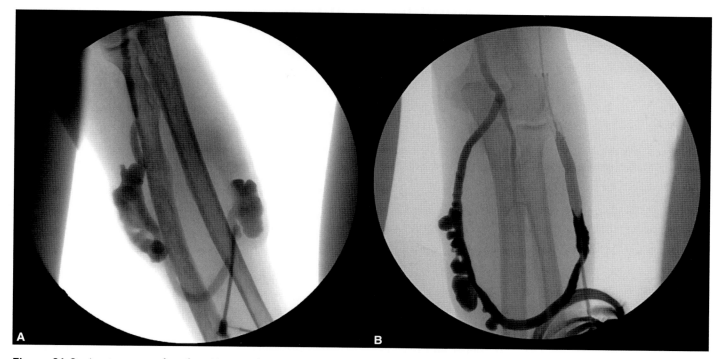

Figure 21-3. Angiograms of grafts with pseudoaneurysms. (**A**) Large structures in both arterial and venous cannulation sites. (**B**) Note multiple pseudoaneurysms on arterial side of graft.

made in the pseudoaneurysm itself. This can lead to prolonged bleeding post-dialysis. Additionally, a needle puncture in the thinned skin overlying the structure can further weaken the site and predispose to spontaneous bleeding or even rupture.

▶ Pain

At times, patients can experience pain in a pseudoaneurysm. This is more likely to occur with rapidly expanding dilatations. However, it can occur at other times as well.

▶ Clotting

In some instances, conditions are conducive to promote clotting within an expanded pseudoaneurysm. This can result in the laying down of successive layers of thrombotic material within the structure where they can become attached (Figure 21-4). This material promotes eventual clotting of the access. Removal of this chronic thrombus at the time of thrombectomy is at times difficult.

▶ Infection

Although not common, a pseudoaneurysm can become infected. Thinning of the overlying skin with progressive loss of vascular integrity predisposes to infection. Additionally, the fact that chronic thrombi can form within this dilated segment can predispose it to this event. When infection does occur, it can be more serious than the usual graft infection. In essence, the pseudoaneurysm becomes an abscess, often with infected thrombus that can metastasize.

▶ Rupture

Rupture is the most serious of the complications associated with a pseudoaneurysm. This occurs because of a combination of thinning of the skin and the high pressure within the structure. Often, the event is heralded by ulceration of the overlying skin and spontaneous bleeding. The fact that

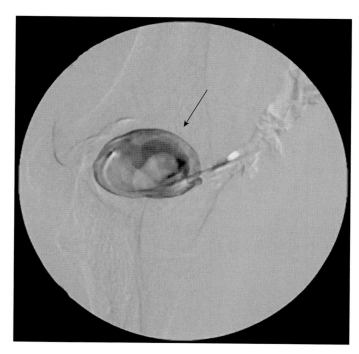

Figure 21-4. Large thrombus within pseudoaneurysm (arrow).

there is only skin and fibrous connective tissue overlying the pulsating mass predisposes the patient to this complication. When rupture occurs, it is a medical emergency. If not immediately controlled, exsanguination can occur.

▶ Prevention of Pseudoaneurysms

Understanding the etiology of a pseudoaneurysm is important in planning a strategy to prevent or at least limit their occurrence. It is important that cannulation sites be rotated ("rope–ladder" technique). Any limitation of this approach (segmental overutilization) will predispose the patient to the possibility of early graft disruption. If this is followed by the development of a downstream venous stenosis, a common occurrence with grafts, the development of a pulsating bulge indicating the beginning of a pseudoaneurysm will appear.

It is important that the patient's access be carefully examined at each dialysis. In addition, patients should be taught to do self-examinations. If a bulge in the graft begins to appear, the case should be evaluated for venous stenosis as a causative factor. This can generally be done by physical examination.[4-5] Pseudoaneurysm can appear and progress very rapidly in some cases. Early detection of these rapidly developing cases is important in order to prevent more serious complications.

▶ Evaluation of Pseudoaneurysms

The physical evaluation of a patient for the development of a pseudoaneurysm and the examination of any of these anomalous structures that have developed is important. In doing this, several features should be evaluated.[5]

▶ Size

The size of a pseudoaneurysm should be noted in order to provide a baseline for future evaluations. If the bulge is increasing, prompt action is important. This is especially true if the increase in size is rapid.

▶ Availability Cannulation Sites

Assess the availability of cannulation sites on the access. If the presence of a large or, more often, multiple pseudoaneurysms makes it difficult to cannulate the graft at dialysis (Figure 21-5), there will be a tendency for needles to be

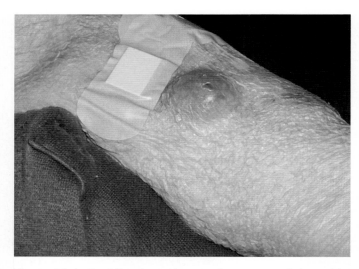

Figure 21-6. Rapidly advancing pseudoaneurysm, 3 days old.

introduced into the bulge itself. This can lead to problems such as prolonged bleeding post dialysis. Additionally, the skin over these anomalous structures is thin and often has poor vascularity. Needle punctures can lead to eventual rupture.

▶ Appearance of Skin

Evaluating the appearance of the skin overlying the pseudoaneurysm is extremely important. As the pseudoaneurysm enlarges, it can easily cause adverse skin changes. The skin can become depigmented and thin (Figure 21-6). As this progresses, the circulation of the skin can become compromised. Eventually ulceration and spontaneous bleeding may develop. When this is observed, the situation should be dealt with as an emergency.

▶ Indications for Treatment

With good cannulation practices and early recognition of problems, the need to repair pseudoaneurysms can be minimized. However, there are instances where elective repair may be advisable and there are situations in which emergency treatment is mandatory. It is important for the physician caring for a dialysis patient to be able to recognize these situations. The goal is 2-fold—arrest the development of the pseudoaneurysm and prevent its rupture. Indications for treatment are several.

▶ Spontaneous Bleeding

As the skin becomes increasingly thin, the pseudoaneurysm becomes more susceptible to spontaneous bleeding. This may be related to the ill-advised cannulation of the structure or to inadvertent trauma. When it is noted, it should be taken as a prelude to rupture and an indication for immediate surgical treatment.

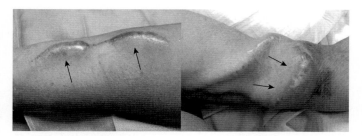

Figure 21-5. Large pseudoaneurysms limiting availability of cannulation sites (arrows).

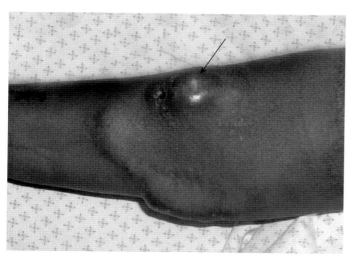

Figure 21-7. Ulceration of skin overlying pseudoaneurysm (arrows).

▶ Thinning of the Skin

As the pseudoaneurysm enlarges, thinning of the skin will eventually occur (Figure 21-7). In many instances this is progressive. The question arises as to what point in the progression the patient should be referred for treatment. This decision is generally based on somewhat subjective judgment. Things that tend to occur in addition to thinning are depigmentation and tightening of the overlying skin. If the skin is tissue paper thin and if you cannot pinch the skin between your index finger and thumb, it has advanced to a dangerous degree and early treatment should be sought.

▶ Ulceration

The pseudoaneurysm is covered only by a layer of thin skin, sometimes very thin, and fibrous connective tissue (Figure 21-8). If ulceration occurs, it means that the skin has lost its integrity and rupture is imminent. This should be taken as an indication for emergency surgical treatment.

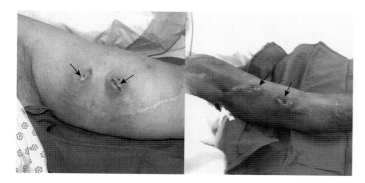

Figure 21-8. Note the thinning of skin and loss of pigmentation (arrow).

▶ Infection

Infection in a pseudoaneurysm is a definite indication for immediate treatment. This, like other graft infections, requires antibiotics and surgery. These cases may be complicated by metastatic septic emboli.

▶ Newly Developed Pseudoaneurysm

Patients should be evaluated at each dialysis treatment for the development of a bulge in their graft. If this is noted, it should be taken as evidence to suggest that there is outflow stenosis in addition to some degree of graft degeneration. These cases should be evaluated for venous stenosis and treated in order to arrest the process.

▶ Rapidly Advancing Pseudoaneurysm

Rapidly advancing pseudoaneurysms (Figure 21-6) are usually small and are more indicative of severe intra-graft hypertension due to outflow stenosis than degeneration of the graft. When these are observed, hopefully early, the patient needs to be evaluated for outflow stenosis at the earliest possible time. The offending stenotic lesion should be treated by either endovascular or surgical means.

▶ Limitation of Cannulation Sites

If it is difficult to find accessible unaffected sites or if the overall size of the mass of the pseudoaneurysm is such that cannulation is difficult, the patient should be sent for repair. Cannulation through the site should be discouraged.

▶ Unacceptable Cosmetic Appearance

Although unacceptable cosmetic appearance may be a reason for repair of the graft, it is not common. Not because it is an unacceptable indication, but because there are generally other indications that make treatment a medical necessity when a graft has progressed to the point of cosmetic unacceptability.

▶ Treatment of the Pseudoaneurysm

A pseudoaneurysm is treated most effectively by surgery. This generally consists of resection and segment interposition.[6-7] In recent years, there have been reports of cases treated with stent grafts.[8-14] This is an interesting approach to the problem; however, there are drawbacks. The treatment of a pseudoaneurysm with a stent-graft is not always successful.[14] When used for this purpose, the stent graft is frequently placed within the cannulation zone of the graft. Although cannulation can be performed successfully through the device, studies have shown that it can be damaged resulting in real or potential problems.[14-16] There is also a serious question as to the cost-effectiveness of a stent-graft versus surgery.

ANEURYSMS

Although a pseudoaneurysm can occur in a native vessel (false aneurysm), most of the bulges that are noted in association with a fistula are aneurysms. They represent a pathological dilatation of the vessel rather than a rupture of the layers of its wall. Most of these are fusiform in shape.

▶ Etiology

Aneurysms develop as a matter of course in many fistulas (AVF). They may take 1 of 2 forms—diffuse or localized. There is a tendency for blood flow in a fistula to increase with time, and with this augmented flow, the diameter of the fistula also increases in a diffuse fashion. However, it does not become aneurysmal unless there is a significant increase in the normally low blood pressure that characterizes this type of arteriovenous access. With the development of a significant downstream venous stenosis, pressure within the fistula increases and it begins to dilate diffusely distal to the lesion. This can happen rather quickly. If not detected and allowed to progress, the fistula can become diffusely aneurysmal (Figure 21-9). These are often referred to a "mega-fistula." Their occurrence is a sure indication of a lack of regular monitoring and surveillance. A mega-fistula associated with the cephalic vein in the upper arm is most often due to severe stenosis of the cephalic arch.

There are 3 options for cannulation: (A) the rope ladder pattern, (B) the area puncture pattern, and (C) the buttonhole pattern. In the rope ladder pattern, the punctures are regularly distributed along the entire length of the arterialized vein. This is the most desirable approach to repetitive cannulation. In contrast, with the area puncture technique, cannulations are restricted to a small area. With the buttonhole technique, punctures are always performed through the exactly identical spot. This procedure creates a track between the skin and AVF lumen. The integrity of the surrounding vessel wall is not disturbed. The area puncture pattern is the worst scenario, leading to segmental over utilization. This will eventually cause aneurysm formation due to disruption of wall integrity and a circumscribed dilation of the AVF (Figure 21-10). Such aneurysms are often a composite of true and false aneurysms, intact parts of the wall alternating with scar tissue. Thinning of the wall of the vein causes progressive enlargement of the aneurysm because wall stress increases progressively with increasing lumen diameter according to Laplace's law.

As is the case with pseudoaneurysms, as the aneurysm enlarges there is a tendency for the skin to become affected, although generally, because of the lower pressure, to a lesser degree. However, it can become scarred, thinned, and avascular, and occasionally, this can lead to ulceration and spontaneous bleeding (Figure 21-11). This is especially true if the aneurysm is cannulated.

▶ Complications

The natural history of an aneurysm is frequently benign. However, associated complications can occur and are the same as those associated with pseudoaneurysms. However,

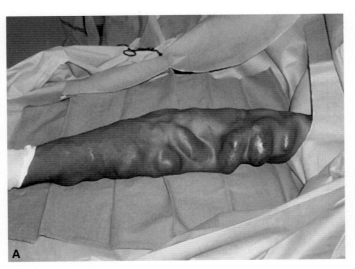

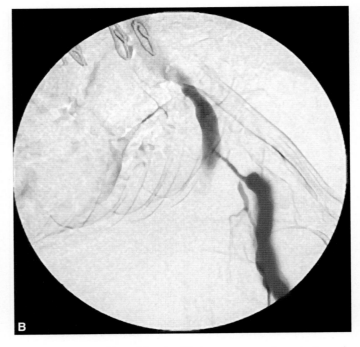

Figure 21-9. Mega fistula (diffusely aneurysmal fistula). **(A)** Patients arm with ectatic dilated fistula. **(B)** Appearance of cephalic arch with severe stenosis.

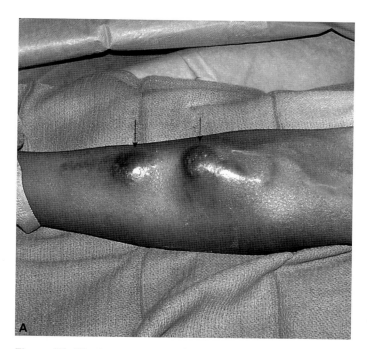

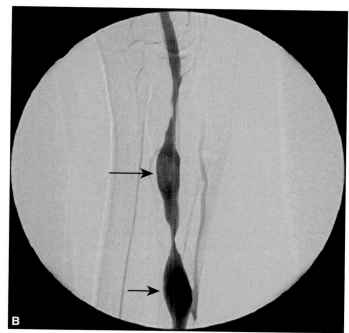

Figure 21-10. Aneurysms in radial-cephalic fistula (arrows). One is in arterial cannulation zone, the other in the venous. (**A**) Only sites available for cannulation. (**B**) Note fusiform shape. (2 separate cases).

serious complications such as rupture occur with less frequency than is seen with aneurysms. Aneurysms are most frequently seen in association with fistulae that have lower intra-access pressure than is seen in association with grafts; therefore, there is less of a tendency for rupture to occur.

▶ **Prevention of Aneurysms**

Aneurysms should be viewed as a preventable problem. Monitoring and surveillance to detect venous stenosis early, followed by prospective treatment, is important. Rotation of cannulation sites is also a valuable deterrent.

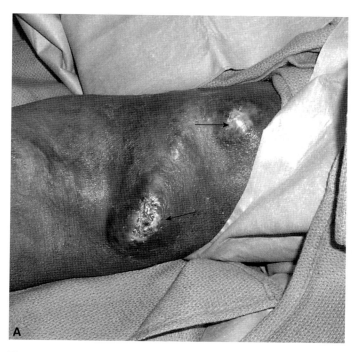

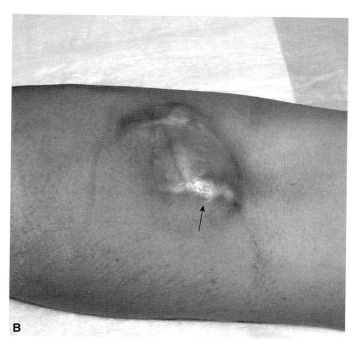

Figure 21-11. Skin complications associated with aneurysms. (**A**) Depigmentation and ulceration associated with cannulation of aneurysm (arrows). (**B**) Depigmentation and scarring (arrow).

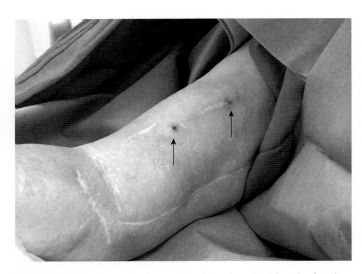

Figure 21-12. Buttonholes created in a brachial-basilic fistula.

There is often a tendency in the dialysis clinic for the same site to be used repetitively for ease of cannulation or patient comfort. This should be discouraged.

An alternative method has been proposed for use with fistula. This is the "constant-site" method of cannulation, or "buttonhole" technique[17-21] (Figure 21-12). With this method, cannulas are inserted at exactly the same spot at consecutive dialysis sessions, thus developing a channel in the arteriovenous fistula. This technique that promotes patient self-cannulation minimizes the tendency toward aneurysm formation.[22] However, it is associated with a definite increased risk of infection, the avoidance of which demands a strict adherence to proper technique.[22-23]

An additional feature that should be noted here is the fistula that develops too rapidly. In general, a fistula should be adequately developed for use within 4 to 6 weeks and will continue to enlarge slowly after this in association with increasing flow over time. However, a fistula that is unusually large at this time should be suspect. Instead of representing good development, it may be a reflection of an undetected stenosis downstream that, if allowed to continue, may ultimately lead to the formation of a mega-fistula.

▶ Complications, Evaluation, and Indications for Treatment of Aneurysms

The same principles discussed above for pseudoaneurysms should be followed with aneurysms. There is, as has been stated, less of a tendency for the more severe skin changes seen with pseudoaneurysms to occur here because the intra-access pressure is generally lower. As with the pseudoaneurysm, venipuncture should avoid the aneurysm. This is particularly true in patients whose skin layer overlying the aneurysm is thin and prone to infection—a sign of impending perforation.

In a study,[24] 23 patients with a mean age of 55-years were found to have 29 upper extremity aneurysms of the outflow vein on duplex ultrasound scan. Nine patients (39%) had radial-cephalic, 11 patients (48%) had brachial-cephalic, 2 patients (9%) had brachial-basilic, and 1 patient (4%) had radial-basilic AVFs. The average aneurysm size was 3.3 cm, and the mean time from fistula placement to treatment was 47.1 months. Four patients (17%) were asymptomatic and were repaired due to technical and mechanical problems with AVFs, including stenosis and lack of normal vein for cannulation, compromising continued use. Nineteen patients (83%) presented with symptoms, including pain (48%), skin changes (30%), venous hypertension (22%), steal syndrome (22%), and high output failure (9%). Four patients (17%) were found to have outflow vein stenosis, 2 patients (9%) had central venous stenosis, and 2 patients (9%) had central venous occlusion.

▶ Treatment of the Aneurysm

With the passage of time, flow in a fistula has a tendency to increase, and with this augmented flow, its diameter also increases and can eventually reach a point that could be considered diffusely aneurysmal. These changes are benign and do not require treatment.

When treatment is required, it may be either surgical or endovascular. At times, a combination of the 2 is the most appropriate solution.[25] Since this abnormal anatomy is so closely associated with venous stenosis, either in the adjacent section of vein or more distally as in cephalic arch stenosis, an endovascular approach is the first line of therapy. With monitoring and surveillance, these lesions can often be caught early. Treatment will arrest the further development of the aneurysmal dilatation. The therapy of choice for these stenoses is angioplasty. If elastic recoil occurs, angioplasty may need to be combined with stent insertion. The insertion of a stent graft in an area that is subject to cannulation should be avoided if possible. Recurrent stenoses should undergo surgery.

There are a series of surgical procedures available for the treatment of aneurysms. With smaller lesions, excision and primary veno-venous anastomosis may be possible. With larger aneurysms, partial resection of the wall of the structure with a plastic repair (reduction aneurysmoplasty) should be considered.[26-27] Since the fistula is a native vessel, collateral veins develop secondary to the associated stenosis in many cases. At times, these veins can be used in effecting a surgical repair. As a last resort, synthetic graft can be employed. This can be used in the manner of a patch graft after a portion of the redundant vein has been resected (aneurysmorrhaphy)[28] or the insertion of a short segment.[29] The latter approach has the adverse effect of predisposing the access to many of the complications of a synthetic graft. In all cases treated surgically, the contribution of venous stenosis to the development of the problem should be addressed. Angioplasty may be required.

ARTERIAL ANEURYSMS

Most aneurysmal dilatations associated with dialysis access are venous (fistula) or within a synthetic graft; however, rarely this anomaly can occur within the artery. In a series of 13 cases,[30] several interesting correlations were noted. Firstly, 12 of the 13 cases were male. Second, the aneurysms occurred late, after a mean of 40.3 months. Third, all of the problems occurred in association with a brachial-cephalic fistula. None were seen in association with other vascular accesses involving the brachial artery: basilic vein transpositions or brachial artery to axillary vein bypass grafts. Fourth, the majority of patients developed the aneurysm after the patient had received a renal transplant. Lastly, the majority were symptomatic with signs of related ischemia or thrombosis. However, none presented with rupture, including those with acute presentation over a short period.

In this small series of cases, all were treated successfully by surgical means. All cases had a patent brachial artery with complete relief of the presenting symptoms at a median follow-up of 16 months.

REFERENCES

1. Beathard G. *Complications of vascular access.* New York: Marcel Dekker, Inc.; 2000.
2. Delorme JM, Guidoin R, Canizales S, et al. Vascular access for hemodialysis: pathologic features of surgically excised ePTFE grafts. *Ann Vasc Surg.* 1992;6:517–524.
3. Charara J, Guidoin R, Gill F, Guzman R. Morphologic assessment of ePTFE graft wall damage following hemodialysis needle punctures. *J Appl Biomater.* 1990;1:279–287.
4. Beathard G. Physical examination of the dialysis vascular access. *Semin Dial.* 1998;11:231–236.
5. Beathard G. *Physical examination: the forgotten tool.* Philadelphia: Lippincott Williams & Wilkins; 2002.
6. Rizzuti RP, Hale JC, Burkart TE. Extended patency of expanded polytetrafluoroethylene grafts for vascular access using optimal configuration and revisions. *Surg Gynecol Obstet.* 1988;166:23–27.
7. Ballard JL, Bunt TJ, Malone JM. Major complications of angioaccess surgery. *Am J Surg.* 1992;164:229–232.
8. Sapoval MR, Turmel-Rodrigues LA, Raynaud AC, Bourquelot P, Rodrigue H, Gaux JC. Cragg covered stents in hemodialysis access: initial and midterm results. *J Vasc Interv Radiol* 1996;7:335–342.
9. Hausegger KA, Tiessenhausen K, Klimpfinger M, Raith J, Hauser H, Tauss J. Aneurysms of hemodialysis access grafts: treatment with covered stents: a report of three cases. *Cardiovasc Intervent Radiol.* 1998;21:334–337.
10. Rabindranauth P, Shindelman L. Transluminal stent-graft repair for pseudoaneurysm of PTFE hemodialysis grafts. *J Endovasc Surg.* 1998;5:138–141.
11. Najibi S, Bush RL, Terramani TT, et al. Covered stent exclusion of dialysis access pseudoaneurysms. *J Surg Res.* 2002;106:15–19.
12. Silas AM, Bettmann MA. Utility of covered stents for revision of aging failing synthetic hemodialysis grafts: a report of three cases. *Cardiovasc Intervent Radiol.* 2003;26:550–553.
13. Ryan JM, Dumbleton SA, Doherty J, Smith TP. Technical innovation. Using a covered stent (wallgraft) to treat pseudoaneurysms of dialysis grafts and fistulas. *AJR Am J Roentgenol.* 2003;180:1067–1071.
14. Vesely TM. Use of stent grafts to repair hemodialysis graft-related pseudoaneurysms. *J Vasc Interv Radiol.* 2005;16:1301–1307.
15. Gadalean F. Covered stent outcomes for arteriovenous hemodialysis access salvage. *J Am Soc Nephrol.* 2008;19:899A.
16. Asif A, Gadalean F, Eid N, Merrill D, Salman L. Stent graft infection and protrusion through the skin: clinical considerations and potential medico-legal ramifications. *Semin Dial.* 2010;23:540–542.
17. Kronung G. Plastic deformation of cimino fistula by repeated puncture. *Dial Transplant.* 1984;13:635–636.
18. Twardowski Z. Constant site (buttonhole) method of needle insertion for hemodialysis. *Dial Transplant.* 1995;24:559–576.
19. Peterson P. Fistula cannulation: the buttonhole technique. *Nephrol Nurs J.* 2002;29:195.
20. Toma S, Shinzato T, Fukui H, et al. A timesaving method to create a fixed puncture route for the buttonhole technique. *Nephrol Dial Transplant.* 2003;18:2118–2121.
21. Ball LK. The buttonhole technique for arteriovenous fistula cannulation. *Nephrol Nurs J.* 2006;33:299–304.
22. van Loon MM, Goovaerts T, Kessels AG, van der Sande FM, Tordoir JH. Buttonhole needling of haemodialysis arteriovenous fistulae results in less complications and interventions compared to the rope-ladder technique. *Nephrol Dial Transplant.* 2010;25:225–230.
23. Birchenough E, Moore C, Stevens K, Stewart S. Buttonhole cannulation in adult patients on hemodialysis: an increased risk of infection? *Nephrol Nurs J.* 2010;37:491–498, 555; quiz 499.
24. Pasklinsky G, Meisner RJ, Labropoulos N, et al. Management of true aneurysms of hemodialysis access fistulas. *J Vasc Surg.* 2011;53:1291–1297.
25. Georgiadis GS, Nikolopoulos E, Papanas N, Mourvati E, Panagoutsos S, Lazarides MK. A hybrid approach to salvage a failing long-standing autogenous aneurysmal fistula in a hemodialysis patient. *Int J Artif Organs.* 2010;33:819–823.
26. Pierce GE, Thomas JH, Fenton JR. Novel repair of venous aneurysms secondary to arteriovenous dialysis fistulae. *Vasc Endovascular Surg.* 2007;41:55–60.
27. Georgiadis GS, Lazarides MK, Panagoutsos SA, et al. Surgical revision of complicated false and true vascular access-related aneurysms. *J Vasc Surg.* 2008;47:1284–1291.
28. Berard X, Brizzi V, Mayeux S, et al. Salvage treatment for venous aneurysm complicating vascular access arteriovenous fistula: use of an exoprosthesis to reinforce the vein after aneurysmorrhaphy. *Eur J Vasc Endovasc Surg.* 2010;40:100–106.
29. Georgiadis GS, Lazarides MK, Lambidis CD, et al. Use of short PTFE segments (<6 cm) compares favorably with pure autologous repair in failing or thrombosed native arteriovenous fistulas. *J Vasc Surg.* 2005;41:76–81.
30. Chemia E, Nortley M, Morsy M. Brachial Artery Aneurysms Associated with Arteriovenous Access for Hemodialysis. *Semin Dial.* 2010;23:440–444.

22

HEART FAILURE AND LEFT VENTRICULAR HYPERTROPHY

CARLO BASILE, LUIGI VERNAGLIONE, & CARLO LOMONTE

1. Discuss the relationships between heart and kidney diseases.
2. Describe the pathophysiology of heart changes in patients affected by chronic kidney diseases.
3. Understand the key elements of left ventricular hypertrophy, left ventricular diastolic dysfunction, and heart failure in chronic kidney diseases.
4. Describe the hemodynamic effects determined by the opening of an arteriovenous access.
5. Describe the maturation and the long run of an arteriovenous fistula.
6. Discuss when an arteriovenous access must be considered to have an inappropriately high blood flow rate.
7. Discuss how an arteriovenous access should be modified because of an inappropriately high blood flow rate.

EPIDEMIOLOGICAL CONSIDERATIONS

There are many interactions between heart and kidney diseases. Either acute or chronic dysfunction of the heart or kidneys can induce acute or chronic dysfunction in the other organ. The clinical importance of this relationship is underscored by the following points.[1–2]

1. Mortality is increased in patients with heart failure (HF) associated with reduced glomerular filtration rate (GFR).
2. Patients affected by chronic kidney disease (CKD) have an increased risk of both atherosclerotic cardiovascular diseases (CVDs) and HF.
3. Cardiovascular disease (CVD) is responsible for up to 50% of deaths in patients affected by CKD.

Coronary artery disease, left ventricular hypertrophy (LVH), and HF are common in patients affected by CKD.[3–4] LVH appears to be directly related to a low GFR and length of time on dialysis.[5–6] Furthermore, LVH appears to be a strong predictor of progression to dialysis in non-diabetic CKD, especially in patients with less advanced renal dysfunction.[7] The presence of LVH is associated with increasing incidence of HF, ventricular arrhythmias, death following myocardial infarction, decreased left ventricular (LV) ejection fraction, and sudden cardiac death.[8–10]

Epidemiological understanding concerning the relationship between CKD and cardiovascular (CV) morbidity and mortality has increased considerably. It is well established that CVD is the leading cause of death in patients affected by CKD (Figure 22-1).[11–12] These patients, especially those at the end-stage of renal disease (ESRD), should be considered to be in the highest risk group for CV events.[12] Taking into account that the prevalence of early stages of CKD is about 100-fold greater than that of ESRD,[13] the majority of patients affected by CKD die before ever reaching ESRD. For the patient with a reduced GFR, the risk of a fatal CV event is much higher than their risk of advancing to ESRD.[14]

Even moderate lowering of kidney function is associated with a significant increase of CV risk, and the level of kidney function itself is an independent predictor of CV outcome and all-cause mortality.[15–16] The traditional CV risk factors, often present in patients with CKD, do not fully account for the incidence of CVD in CKD and treatment of these risk factors does not necessarily lead to better CV outcome.[17] Additionally, non-traditional CV risk factors have been identified in CKD patients, such as secondary hyperparathyroidism and anemia (Table 22-1).[18–21]

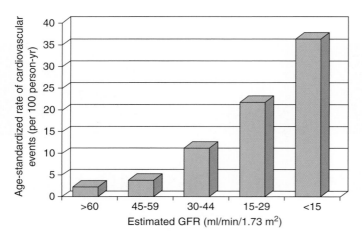

Figure 22-1. Age-standardized rates of cardiovascular events according to the estimated GFR among 1,120,295 ambulatory adults. (Data extracted from reference 4.)

Today, hypertension and diabetes are the primary causes of CKD.[22–23] Hypertension in itself represents a powerful risk factor for CVD in CKD and is almost invariably present in patients with renal failure. It should also be noted that renal failure is highly represented among hypertensive patients.[24–26] Sodium retention, sympathetic nervous system overdrive, and activation of the renin-angiotensin system have been considered the key mechanisms involved in the etiology of hypertension in cases of kidney disease.[27]

PATHOPHYSIOLOGY

► Left Ventricular Hypertrophy

LVH is the most frequent (present in 80%) cardiac abnormality diagnosed in patients starting hemodialysis (HD).[28–29] It is an independent and strong risk factor for CV morbidity and mortality in both the normal population[30] and ESRD patients.[31] In the ESRD population, LVH is principally due to an increased demand in the LV minute work resulting from volume/flow and pressure overload.[32] Two forms of LVH—eccentric and concentric—may be present and are relatively equivalent in prevalence in the dialysis population. Eccentric hypertrophy results from volume overload leading to cardiac myocyte dropout due to myocyte to arteriolar capillary mismatch. Concentric hypertrophy is typically the result of hypertension and increased afterload and is exacerbated by anemia, hyperparathyroidism, and high angiotensin II concentrations. In experimental renal failure, LVH has been shown to be associated with reduced capillary density and subsequent interstitial fibrosis.[33–34] This fibrosis is probably the reason for diastolic and eventually systolic dysfunction of the LV in LVH. While in the general population hypertension is the most frequent cause of LVH, in ESRD patients the correlation between LV mass and blood pressure is weak. Experimental and clinical studies have shown that hypertrophy develops even in normotensive ESRD subjects.[35]

LVH has been found in as many as 30–45% of patients with CKD who are not yet on dialysis, with a higher prevalence and more severe features in those with lower degrees of renal function.[3–4] Concentric LVH has been documented in 42% of patients at the start of dialysis[5] and in as many as 75% of patients who have been on HD for 10 years.[6] LVH is an important predictor of mortality in patients affected by CKD.[5,36–39] Its presence has been associated with more than 25 CV deaths/1000 patient-years. In incident HD patients, the relative mortality risk of LVH at 6, 12, and 24 months ranges between 29% and 61%.[39]

The pathogenesis of LVH in CKD is multifactorial; however, hypertension, alterations of fluid and electrolyte balance and anemia are identified as its major determinants.[37,40–43] From a hemodynamic point of view, LVH is an adaptive remodeling process induced by the increase in cardiac work following volume and/or pressure overload. Pressure overload due to hypertension leads to concentric hypertrophy, while volume overload, secondary to anemia, the presence of an arteriovenous fistula (AVF) or edema, leads to the development of eccentric hypertrophy.[40]

TABLE 22–1

Traditional, Non-Traditional, and "Uremia-Specific" Cardiovascular Risk Factors in CKD

Traditional Risk Factors	Nontraditional Risk Factors	"Uremia-specific" Risk Factors
Older age	Albuminuria	Anemia
Male gender	Carbamylation of proteins	Phosphate retention
Higher LDL cholesterol	Lipoprotein(a) and apolipoprotein(a) isoforms	Secondary hyperparathyroidism
Lower HDL cholesterol	Lipoprotein remnants	Vascular calcification
Diabetes mellitus	Sympathetic activation	Uremic toxins
Smoking	Oxidative stress	Hyperhomocysteinemia
Physical inactivity	Inflammation (C-reactive protein)	Extracellular fluid volume overload
Family history of cardiovascular diseases	Wasting	Electrolyte imbalance
LVH	Thrombogenic factors	
Insulin resistance	Sleep disturbances	
Hypertension	Altered nitric oxide/endothelin balance	

Frequently, patients with CKD present both patterns of LVH characterized by an increase in diameter and wall thickness. Among hemodynamic factors, another frequent feature of patients affected by CKD is an increased arterial stiffness, which has been associated with LVH as well as with CV mortality.[41–43]

In addition to hemodynamic factors, other factors such as an inappropriate activation of the renin-angiotensin-aldosterone system, oxidative stress, inflammation,[44–46] and the increased activation of collagen and muscle cell growth factors may have a relevant role in LV growth in CKD. It has been suggested that in cases of renal dysfunction, decreased clearance of some growth factors such as the carboxy-terminal propeptide of collagen type I or cardiotrophin-1, which are involved in the development of LVH in hypertensive heart disease,[47] could play a role. Further evidence indicates that sodium/potassium ATPase inhibitors may be involved in the pathogenesis of LVH in CKD.[48] Recently, some attention has been focused on fibroblast growth factor-23 (FGF-23). This is a recently discovered hormone, secreted by osteoblasts and osteocytes, which helps in maintaining normal serum phosphate concentrations in CKD by stimulating urinary phosphate excretion and decreasing dietary phosphorus absorption through inhibition of 1,25-dihydroxyvitamin D synthesis.[49] In CKD patients, an independent relationship between FGF-23 and LVH has been found.[50] It can be hypothesized that at the markedly elevated concentrations that FGF-23 reaches in CKD patients, it can non-selectively bind to FGF receptors normally activated by other factors, thus inducing enhanced fibrosis. In patients affected by CKD, increased myocardial fibrosis has been demonstrated either in post-mortem analysis or by means of endomyocardial biopsies.[51] Increased myocardial fibrosis presumably contributes to myocardial ischemia due to the reduction in capillary density and coronary reserve.[52] Recently, even subclinical renal damage has been found to be associated with impaired coronary flow reserve.[53] Impaired LV function leads to hemodynamic changes including reduced stroke volume and cardiac output (CO), arterial underfilling, elevated atrial pressures, and venous congestion.[54] These situations trigger compensatory neurohormonal adaptations including activation of the sympathetic nervous system and the renin-angiotensin-aldosterone system, increase in the release of vasopressin and endothelin-1, which promote salt and water retention coupled with systemic vasoconstriction. All these adaptations preserve the perfusion of vital organs (the brain and heart) by maintenance of systemic pressure via arterial vasoconstriction in other circulations, including the renal circulation, and by increasing myocardial contractility and heart rate. However, systemic vasoconstriction increases cardiac afterload with reduction of CO, which has a net effect of lowering renal perfusion. The negative impact of these adaptations is underlined by the slowing of disease progression and reduction in mortality with the administration of angiotensin inhibitors and beta-blockers in patients with HF due to systolic dysfunction.

▶ Left Ventricular Diastolic Dysfunction

LV diastolic dysfunction is very frequent among CKD patients and may be associated with the subsequent development of HF and its associated mortality.[55] It has been reported that in ESRD patients, diastolic function deteriorates in parallel with the progression of LVH.[56] LV diastolic dysfunction has been found in CKD patients affected by LVH not undergoing dialysis.[52] In patients affected by HF, the presence of CKD is associated with worse diastolic function, intra-cardiac conduction, and a poorer prognosis.[57] The negative impact on CV outcome seems to be stronger in patients with diastolic HF.[57] However, impairment of diastolic function in patients affected by CKD may occur very early, even in the absence of LVH.[58]

Although conventional mitral inflow assessment has become the main tool in assessing diastolic function in daily practice, preload dependency of flow patterns constitutes the major limitation of the technique to assess either ventricular relaxation or filling pressures separately.[59] An interesting feature of early mitral filling measured by tissue Doppler imaging is its relative preload independence. Consequently, early mitral filling remains reduced even in those stages of diastolic dysfunction characterized by increased preload compensation. Moreover, early mitral filling has been demonstrated to be inversely related to the degree of fibrosis in ischemic as well as in normal myocardial segments.[60]

▶ Heart Failure

HF is frequently associated with a reduction in GFR. The prevalence of moderate to severe kidney impairment (defined as a GFR < 60 mL/min per 1.73 m^2) is approximately 30–60% in patients affected by HF.[61–64] The following observations are illustrative of this relationship.

1. In 80,000 hospitalized and non-hospitalized patients affected by HF, moderate to severe kidney impairment (defined as an estimated GFR < 53 mL/min, a serum creatinine ≥ 1.5 mg/dL, or a serum cystatin C ≥ 1.56 mg/dL) has been described in 29% of patients.[61]

2. In the Acute Decompensated Heart Failure National Registry (ADHERE) database, approximately 30% of over 100,000 patients affected by HF requiring hospitalization had a diagnosis of CKD (defined as a serum creatinine >2.0 mg/dL).[64]

More than 50% of ESRD subjects treated by chronic HD die from CVD.[65] Congestive heart failure (CHF) is present in more than one-third of new dialysis patients[66] with an incidence of 71/1000 person-years. This figure is substantially greater than the incidence of acute coronary syndromes in ESRD (29/1000 person-years in US Renal data system (USRDS) Morbidity and Mortality Study Wave 2).[67] CHF contributes significantly to mortality and morbidity and also worsens the quality of life. For instance,

TABLE 22–2

Factors Leading to the Increase of Preload, Worsening of Myocardial Oxygen Supply, and the Increase or the Decrease of LV Afterload

	↑ Preload	↓ Cardiac Oxygen Supply	↑ Afterload	↓ Afterload
Anemia	+	+		+
Interdialysis volume overload	+		+	
Hypertension		+	+	
Increased arterial stiffness			+	
Vascular access	+			+
Sympathetic activation			+	
Endothelial dysfunction			+	
Ultrafiltration				+
Inflammation	+			
LVH		+		
Coronary artery and valvular disease		+		

the median overall survival of ESRD patients with CHF is reported to be 36 months compared with 62 months in patients without CHF.[68] Fewer than 15% of dialysis patients are living 3 years after hospitalization for CHF.[67]

By definition, CHF is a state in which the heart is unable to pump blood at a rate appropriate to the requirements of the metabolizing tissues or can do so only at an elevated filling pressure. CHF in ESRD patients differs from CHF states in subjects with preserved renal function in several ways. Interdialytic volume overload and vascular access (VA) flow are important issues and are specific for ESRD. Therefore, HD contributes *per se* to the development of CHF.

Mechanisms of congestive heart failure

Schematically, factors contributing to the development of CHF in ESRD include those increasing preload, those decreasing the myocardial perfusion or oxygenation of the LV, and those increasing LV afterload (Table 22-2). Among these, we will discuss very briefly the role of anemia, interdialytic volume overload, hypertension and arterial wall stiffness, and, more extensively, the role of VA.

Anemia Severe anemia is associated with LVH, LV dilatation, HF, and poorer all-cause and CV prognosis in patients affected by CKD and cardiac disease.[3,69–72] Each 1 g/dL decrease in hemoglobin has been associated with a 20–40% increase in likelihood of LV dilatation, de novo HF, recurrent HF, and mortality.[69] Moreover, patients affected by LVH present lower mean hemoglobin levels compared to those without initial LVH.[71]

Potential mechanisms for explaining the relationship between anemia and the development of LVH include effects of reduced oxygen delivery to the myocardium, perhaps leading to increased myocyte necrosis and apoptosis, anemia-related increased CO and reduced systemic vascular resistance, increased oxidative stress, and activation of the sympathetic nervous system.[73]

Effects of erythropoietin independent of those due to anemia correction may also play some role.[74] Erythropoietin receptors are present in cardiac tissue,[75] and erythropoietin administration reduces cellular damage and myocyte apoptosis, lowers infarct size and subsequent LV dilatation and functional decline.[76]

Anemia is a frequent condition even in milder stages of CKD, mainly due to a decreased synthesis of erythropoietin. Non-hemodynamic mechanisms of body adaptation to anemia include increased oxygen extraction in tissues, mediated by increased 2,3-diphosphoglycerate levels. Mechanisms of hemodynamic compensation of anemia are complex. There is a reduced afterload due to a decrease in systemic vascular resistance and increased preload due to an increase in venous return. This is accompanied by increased LV function attributed to increased sympathetic activity and inotropic factors. Increased LV performance can result from an increased preload (Frank-Starling mechanism) and from changes in inotropic state in relation to high sympathetic activity or inotropic factors.[77] In chronic anemia, typical for ESRD, long-lasting flow/volume overload and increased cardiac work lead to progressive cardiac enlargement and to the LVH.[78] The alterations in cardiac function are accompanied by simultaneous remodeling of the large conduit arteries.[79] Indeed, in dialysis patients, anemia is associated with LVH, LV dilatation, CHF, increased hospitalization rate, and increased mortality.[69,80–82]

Volume overload between dialyses HD is usually performed 3 times per week and body water accumulates and fluctuates between these dialysis sessions. This fluctuation plays a role in the development of the LVH, which in turn predisposes to CHF.[83–84] Overhydration between dialysis treatments contributes to the pathogenesis of LVH in ESRD by its effects on blood pressure control and also by induction of volume overload.[83–84] The internal dimensions of the LV, stroke volume, and end-diastolic pressure are directly related to circulating blood volume.[85]

Hypertension and arterial wall stiffness CKD can be both the reason and the result of hypertension. This is probably one source for the very high hypertension prevalence in ESRD patients. The ill effects of hypertension are usually attributed to the reduction in the internal diameter of arterioles, resulting in a peripheral resistance increase. Blood pressure is the easiest measurable index of opposition to LV ejection (afterload). In fact, the appropriate term to define the arterial factors opposing LV ejection is the aortic impedance, which depends upon peripheral resistance, the viscoelastic properties of the aorta and central arteries, and the inertial forces represented by the mass of the blood in the aorta and LV.[86] Peripheral resistance, as a determinant of mean blood pressure, sets the general level at which the pressure wave will fluctuate. The amplitude of this fluctuation (pulse pressure) is influenced by the viscoelastic properties of the aorta and large arteries and by the characteristics of the LV ejection (stroke volume and ejection velocity). The viscoelastic properties of the aorta can be described in terms of compliance, distensibility, and stiffness. Stiffening of arterial walls can increase the afterload independently of peripheral resistance. Clinically, high aortic stiffness is suspected in patients with high pulse pressure. The latter can occur in case of diastolic pressure decrease, systolic pressure increase, or both. Arterial stiffening leads to faster pulse wave velocity, which, after the reflections at the level of peripheral arteries, returns earlier to the aorta, amplifies aortic and even ventricular pressures during systole (aortic valve is still open), and reduces aortic pressure during diastole.[87]

VASCULAR ACCESS

A surgically created VA, either "native" (direct connection of patient's artery and vein) or with the use of an artificial graft, serves for repeated entries into the bloodstream during HD. Adequate flow volume (Qa) is needed for the dialysis procedure and also for longer patency of the access. Generally, forearm VAs have Qa 400–800 mL/min, upper arm VAs 800–1500 mL/min.

▶ **The Opening of an Arteriovenous Fistula (AVF)**

Table 22-3 shows the hemodynamic effects determined by the opening of an AVF. Poiseuille law states that the blood flow in any vessel, and therefore also Qa, is determined by the following relationship:[88]

$$Qa = \pi \Delta P r^4 / 8 \eta l$$

ΔP is the pressure difference between the extremities of the vessel, r the radius of the vessel, η the viscosity of the fluid, and l the length of the vessel. From this formula we can imply that an upper arm AVF has a higher Qa than a forearm AVF, since Qa is directly proportional to r (to the fourth power). Since access resistance (AR) is expressed by the following ratio:[89]

$$AR = \text{Mean arterial pressure (MAP)}/Qa$$

TABLE 22–3
Hemodynamic Effects of Arteriovenous Fistulas
Increased cardiac output Decreased systemic peripheral resistances Increased sympathetic activity with increased contractility, heart rate and stroke volume Increased blood volume with increased atrial natriuretic peptide and brain natriuretic peptide, left ventricular end-diastolic volume Increased pulmonary flow and pressure

We can re-write this relationship in the following way.[90]

$$AR = MAP \times 8\eta l / \pi \Delta P r^4$$

It is clearly evident that, among all factors involved, r (raised to the fourth power) of a vessel plays the most important role in determining AR. Since the brachial artery utilized for an upper arm AVF must necessarily have a higher r than the radial artery utilized for a lower arm AVF, the AR of an upper arm AVF will be lower than that of a forearm AVF.[89]

CO increases greatly and immediately on opening an AVF in experimental models.[91] This increase in CO is achieved by means of a reduction in peripheral resistance, an increase in sympathetic nervous system activity (increasing contractility), and an increase in stroke volume and heart rate.[91] Very elegant experiments performed in dogs by Guyton and Sagawa[91] illustrate the adaptive mechanisms underlying the opening of an AVF. They demonstrated that the normal venous return curve crossed the CO curve at a CO of 1.5 L/min and a right atrial pressure of 0 mm Hg. Upon opening an AVF, the venous return curve rises to a much higher level. This new curve crosses the CO curve at a CO of 2.4 L/min and a right atrial pressure of only 0.8 mm Hg. Thus, the right atrial pressure rises only slightly while CO increases greatly upon opening the AVF. Therefore, simply on the basis of Frank-Starling's concept of cardiac adaptation, it is quite easy to explain how the heart compensates for the increased load of blood returning from an AVF.

In ESRD patients, the presence of an AVF lowers systemic vascular resistance, resulting in an increase in stroke volume and CO in order to maintain blood pressure.[92] Circumferential wall stress, calculated with the same value of mean blood pressure (96 ± 14 mm Hg) upon the radial artery feeding the AVF and upon the contralateral radial artery taken as a control, is significantly increased on the AVF side.[93] A 6-fold increase in mean blood flow is observed on the AVF side compared with the contralateral side.[93] In man, there are very little prospective data concerning the impact upon the heart of the opening of an AVF. A prospective short-term echocardiographic study was performed in order to assess the influence that the creation of an AVF exerted on cardiac function.[94] This showed that a significant elevation in LV end-diastolic diameter (+4%), fractional shortening (+8%), and CO (+15%) occurred when comparing data obtained immediately before and 14 days after the creation of an AVF. Furthermore, in a study of 12 pre-dialysis patients, LV mass index increased by 5.1 g/m$^{2.7}$ at 1 month and 8.7 g/m$^{2.7}$ at 3 months post-AVF creation.[95]

Significant elevations in plasma atrial natriuretic peptide (ANP) and brain natriuretic peptide (BNP) levels in patients with CKD are well known.[96] A study showed that both ANP and BNP concentrations increased after the creation of AVF, with peak levels occurring after 10 days. The elevated ANP level was associated with an increase in CO, whereas the elevation of BNP level was associated with an increase in the ratio of the peak velocity of early diastolic to atrial filling.[94]

Pulmonary hypertension (PHT) is an elevation of pulmonary arterial pressure (PAP) that can be the result of heart, lung, or systemic disorders. PHT is defined as a sustained elevation of PAP to >25 mm Hg at rest or to >30 mm Hg with exercise. Recently, a 40–50% incidence of PHT has been detected by Doppler echocardiography in patients starting HD treatment via an arteriovenous access.[97] It is suggested that HD patients have inadequate pulmonary vasodilatation in response to the increased flows caused by the AVF, possibly due to suboptimal production of nitric oxide.[98] Furthermore, the partial restoration of normal PAP and CO that occurs in HD patients undergoing either temporal arteriovenous shunt closure or successful transplantation indicates that excessive pulmonary blood flow is involved in the pathogenesis of the disease.[98] However, the existing evidence does not clearly support the recently proposed policy of not creating an AVF in patients with an increased risk for development of PHT. In fact, PAP did not correlate with either Qa or longevity of AVFs in a prospective study in 20 HD patients.[99]

Maturation of the Arteriovenous Fistula

Maturation of an AVF is a process that involves the entire cardiovascular system through a flow-mediated remodeling of the arterial inflow, the venous outflow, and the cardiac muscle itself. Maturation of a radio-cephalic wrist AVF is an intrinsically dynamic process characterized by an increase in both brachial and radial artery Qa and in both brachial and radial diameter (D).[100] In fact, the acute pressure drop due to the construction of an AVF produces an increase in both brachial and radial artery Qa and, consequently, a flow-mediated increase in both brachial and radial D, which tends to neutralize the increased shear stress.[101] A study showed that acutely (1 day following a radio-cephalic AVF placement), mean shear stress increased by 475% and brachial artery D by 15%.[101] The vascular endothelium responds to the short-term increases in Qa and shear stress by releasing nitric oxide and other endothelium-dependent relaxing factors that dilate the artery and try to reduce shear stress towards normal.[102–103] Vascular remodeling can be seen as the long-term effects of sustained changes in shear stress.

The flow of brachial artery as measured by Duplex Doppler ultrasonography is a reliable expression of Qa of a distal AVF.[100] A study demonstrated that the mean brachial artery flow increases from 56.2 ± 20.0 mL/min before the creation of an AVF to 365.0 ± 129.3 mL/min 1 day after and to 720.4 ± 132.8 mL/min 28 days after the creation of an AVF.[100]

Furthermore, the effects on myocardium, due essentially to the volume overload, translate into a remodeling of the cardiac muscle, which is characterized by 4-chamber enlargement and by the addition of new sarcomeres in series. Thus, an eccentric hypertrophy is realized, which must be distinguished from the concentric hypertrophy in which the addition of the new sarcomeres is parallel and the pathogenetic mechanism is a pressure overload. In both cases, an increase in LV muscle mass occurs with normal relative wall thickness in eccentric hypertrophy.[73]

▶ The AVF in the Long Run

Currently, there is no definition of when a Qa is too high. The concept of using the ratio Qa/CO (cardio-pulmonary recirculation or CPR) has been advanced by Pandeya and Lindsay[104] in their study of stable long-term HD patients. In their study they found that the average Qa was 1.6 L/min and the average CO was 7.2 L/min, thus describing an average CPR of 22%. The Vascular Access Society guidelines define an AVF with a high Qa as one having a Qa of 1.0–1.5 L/min and a CPR > 20%.[105] Basile et al[106] and van den Mark et al[89] showed that a third-order polynomial regression model described the best fit relationship between Qa and CO. In addition, Basile et al[106] showed, in a prospective study involving 96 HD patients, that CO did not vary significantly for Qa values ranging from 0.95 to 2.2 L/min. In other words, the increase in Qa was not accompanied by a parallel increase of CO. The causes of this phenomenon are not known, but one can hypothesize a sort of myocardial functional reserve followed by myocardial adaptation, capable of sustaining increases of Qa in the long term without the precipitation of HF. In that study, the receiver operating characteristic curve analysis showed that Qa values ≥2.0 L/min predicted the occurrence of high-output HF more accurately than 2 other Qa values and 3 CPR values.[106]

In the long run, the AVF of a HD patient can be considered very similar to a "physiological fistula" created in endurance trained older men.[107] Nine highly trained male master athletes (64 ± 2 years old) were compared with 9 sedentary older men (63 ± 1 years old). LV systolic function at peak exercise was higher in master athletes as evidenced by a higher LV functional reserve, a large decrease in end-systolic volume during exercise, a higher LV fractional shortening, and a greater decrease in end-systolic diameter at peak exercise. Thus, cardiac adaptations in older endurance trained men are characterized by volume-overload LVH with enhanced LV function during exercise and excellent prognosis.[107] There are no published prospective studies looking at the changes in LV end-diastolic volume

(LVEDV) or LV mass in patients over extended time periods prior to dialysis or on dialysis. Unfortunately, the only way to determine if AVF creation produces LVH in HD patients is with a prospective randomized study comparing a central venous catheter with an AVF and examining the serial changes in LV dimensions and thickness. Due to the increased morbidity and mortality associated with catheters, this is unlikely to occur.[108]

Recent data[109] of a 1-year prospective cohort study showed that LV mass increased by 12.2% and plasma N-terminal pro-brain natriuretic peptide (NT-proBNP) levels increased by 170% a year after AVF creation. AVF Qa did not correlate with increases in LV mass by echocardiography or plasma levels of NT-proBNP. Another recent study[110] showed that patients with Qa > 1000 mL/min had a lower prevalence of LVH and that relatively higher Qa appears to be associated with a lower level of observed HD-induced cardiac injury. A recent analysis of the US Renal Data System Clinical Performance Measures data comprising 4854 patients showed that AVF use was strongly associated with lower all-cause and CV mortality.[111] After adjustment for covariates, AVF use 90 days after the start of dialysis remained significantly associated with lower CV mortality (hazard ratio 0.69, $P = 0.004$) compared with catheter use. This advantage was persistent even after 4 years and was independent of the effect of other known risk factors.[111] Many possible explanations exist for the association between the use of an AVF and decreased risk of CV-related death. These may include greater delivered dose of dialysis and better blood flow rates among patients with AVF, reduced risk of infection, and lower levels of inflammatory mediators. It may be that central venous catheters, being associated with more infection and inflammation, could contribute to worsening the CVD, or alternatively, that those provided with catheters may not be able to mature an AVF due to poor vascular and cardiac status.[111] Finally, a retrospective study of 820 incident chronic HD patients treated in 3 Canadian cities did not suggest an increased risk of death at higher levels of Qa.[112]

High-flow Rate Vascular Access

It has long been known that a VA with an inappropriately high-flow rate may be the cause of high-output HF.[113–116] The latter is defined as symptoms of cardiac failure (dyspnea either at rest or with varying degrees of exertion, orthopnea, paroxysmal dyspnea, and edema, either pulmonary and/or peripheral) in the presence of an above-normal cardiac index (CI) (>3.0 L/min/m^2).[117] There is a paucity of literature regarding high-output HF in HD patients other than a few case reports.[113–116] The incidence of this complication remains unknown. A study[118] found a 3.7% (17/460) incidence of high-flow rate VAs requiring surgical correction. Some authors[117] have stressed that when the CPR exceeds 30%, the onset of high-output HF is possible independently of the absolute value of Qa. Furthermore, a strong relationship exists between Qa and CO: $Qa = 0.20\,CO + 0.06$ ($r = 0.62$; $P = 0.01$).[104]

When Should an Arteriovenous Access Be Modified Because of a High Blood Flow Rate?

The mechanism(s) that transforms a volume-overload LVH in HF is not known. Specific characteristics of either the patients or the AVFs, or both, may predispose to the development of HF.[119] Some suggest that cardiac decompensation due to the effects of an AVF is likely to only occur in patients with underlying cardiac disease.[73] Patients bearing a high-flow rate AVF and having a greater increase in LVEDV are more likely to develop HF.[119] In fact, preliminary data show that patients with Qa > 2 L/min have a greater tendency to the increase in LVEDV when compared with those with Qa < 1 L/min.[120]

Currently, the evidence linking AVF flow to the development of HF is indirect, but consistent with what is known about high-output HF in other kinds of conditions such as traumatic arteriovenous fistulas. The risk factors for the development of a high-Qa AVF are male gender, an upper arm AVF, and previous access surgery.[106,121–122] The recent study by Basile et al[106] showed that an upper arm AVF is associated with an increased risk of high-output HF. Even though it must be acknowledged that a lower arm AVF is usually positioned in a type of patient with a different phenotype from those who get an upper arm AVF (among them, usually there are less diabetics, younger people with fewer vascular diseases and cardiac dysfunctions), the fact remains that such an association seems to favor the hypothesis of a causative role of the upper arm AVF in the pathogenesis of high-output HF. Even though it is likely that only a small percentage of patients have overt stage D HF, a study[123] reported that only 2.6% of patients with an upper arm AVF underwent banding or ligation due to either steal or high-output syndromes. The message deriving from this study[106] is clear; the upper extremity AVF should be placed as distal as possible, as also underlined by the very recent European Best Practice Guidelines (EBPG) guidelines.[124]

In the presence of HF, the decision to intervene to reduce the Qa of an AVF should include a careful control of the factors leading to HF – anemia, hypertension, overestimated dry weight with subsequent expansion of the extracellular volume. If clinical signs of HF do persist after solving these problems (eg, dyspnea on exertion or at rest, orthopnea, fatigue, and edema), it is reasonable to intervene to correct an AVF with a persistently high Qa (>2.0 L/min) or in the presence of a cardiac index >3.0 L/min/m^2.

How Should an Arteriovenous Access Be Modified Because of a High Blood Flow Rate?

Several surgical techniques have been proposed[125] for the treatment of high-output HF; all are based on an attempt to increase resistance at the level of the anastomosis or of the venous outflow (reduction of the caliber of the AVF anastomosis, interposition of a prosthetic graft, banding)

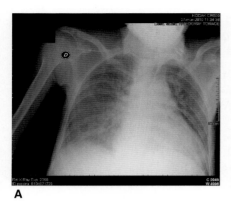
A

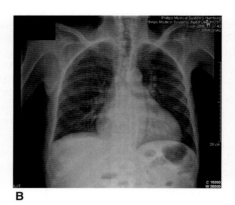
B

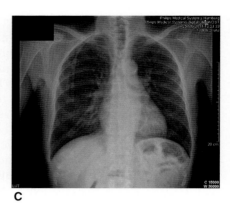
C

Figure 22-2. (**A**) Chest X-rays of a hemodialysis patient affected by high-output HF. His vascular access is a brachial-basilic AVF on the left arm with a blood flow rate of 2.8 L/min. (**B**) Chest X-rays of the patient 10 days after ligation of the AVF and placement of a right internal jugular vein catheter. (**C**) Chest X-rays of the patient 10 months after AVF ligation: cardiomegaly reversed completely.

with the hope of obtaining a reduction of Qa. In such cases an assessment of Qa by means of intra-operative Doppler ultrasound is mandatory.[126] This will avoid failures or aleatory reductions in the caliber, taking into account the fact that a drastic reduction of Qa exposes the AVF to a thrombosis risk. Banding is accomplished by surgical positioning of a circumferential polytetrafluoroethylene (PTFE) band adjacent to the arterial anastomosis, which reduces blood inflow.[127] Alternatively, hemoclips may be applied downstream to the venous supply to further increase resistance. Another technique,[118] described as an inflow reduction procedure, is performed in upper arm AVFs by ligating the brachial artery anastomosis and attaching a synthetic graft from the cephalic vein to the smaller-diameter distal radial artery. In other cases, if the possibility of setting up a VA at the most distal site of the contralateral arm exists, ligation of the AVF may be considered. In severe cases (New York Heart Association class IV) after ligating the AVF, a tunneled central venous catheter, hemodynamically inert, may be the only possible VA (Figures 22-2A–C).[128]

▶ Regression of LVH after AVF Closure

Several studies[129–131] have shown regression of LVH following AVF closure in renal transplant patients. In transplant patients followed for a longer period of time after AVF closure (up to 21 months in a study[129]) there is a regression of eccentric LVH, which implies a reduction in volume overload. However, whether this decrease in volume is caused by either restoration of normal fluid balance or removal of the AVF *per se* is unknown. There is only 1 prospective study of the long-term changes of AVF closure on cardiac functional and structural findings in HD patients.[132] This was a 6-month observational study in 25 HD patients with AVF malfunction undergoing AVF closure and conversion to tunnelled central venous catheter because of exhaustion of alternative vascular sites. This study showed the following echocardiographic modifications—a significant decrease in LV internal diastolic diameter, interventricular septum thickness, and diastolic posterior wall

thickness. These changes were associated with a significant improvement in LV ejection fraction, a significant decrease in LV mass and LV mass index, and a more favorable shift of cardiac geometry toward normality.[132]

CONCLUSION AND FUTURE DIRECTIONS

Is AVF a "lesser evil"[133] or a God's blessing? The right answer is obviously the second one. Actually, the review by Amerling et al[133] denies the life-saving benefit of Brescia-Cimino's basic idea of AVF for millions of human beings. The key word in the case of VA choice is "eligibility."[134] We should aim for a clear "back to the roots" effect. In order to do this, we think that nephrologists must be able to gain the role of coordinator of the VA team. Although important, the problems associated with the management of a VA go beyond the technical details represented by the location (site of arterial inflow), length of anastomosis, blood flow rate, etc.[135] More generally, they are related to the choice of the VA, its planning and timing, and surgical strategies in relation to the characteristics of the patient and to the management of complications. They are also related to the need for careful clinical and instrumental monitoring.[136]

REFERENCES

1. United States Renal Data System: Excerpts from the USRDS 2007 annual data report: atlas of end-stage renal disease in the United States.
2. Coresh J, Astor BC, Greene T, Eknoyan G, Levey AS. Prevalence of chronic kidney disease and decreased kidney function in the adult US population: Third National Health and Nutrition Examination Survey. *Am J Kidney Dis.* 2003;41:1–12.
3. Levin A, Singer J, Thompson CR, Ross H, Lewis M. Prevalent left ventricular hypertrophy in the predialysis population: identifying opportunities for intervention. *Am J Kidney Dis.* 1996;27:347–354.

4. Moran A, Katz R, Jenny NS, et al. Left ventricular hypertrophy in mild and moderate reduction in kidney function determined using cardiac magnetic resonance imaging and cystatin C: the multi-ethnic study of atherosclerosis (MESA). *Am J Kidney Dis.* 2008;52: 839–848.

5. Parfrey PS, Foley RN, Harnett JD, Kent GM, Murray DC, Barre PE. Outcome and risk factors for left ventricular disorders in chronic uraemia. *Nephrol Dial Transplant.* 1996;11:1277–1285.

6. Parfrey PS, Foley RN. The clinical epidemiology of cardiac disease in chronic renal failure. *J Am Soc Nephrol.* 1999;10:1606–1615.

7. Paoletti E, Bellino D, Gallina AM, Amidone M, Cassottana P, Cannella G. Is left ventricular hypertrophy a powerful predictor of progression to dialysis in chronic kidney disease? *Nephrol Dial Transplant.* 2011;26:670–677.

8. Koren MJ, Devereux RB, Casale PN, Savage DD, Laragh JH. Relation of left ventricular mass and geometry to morbidity and mortality in uncomplicated essential hypertension. *Ann Intern Med.* 1991;114:345–352.

9. Verdecchia P, Carini G, Circo A, et al. Left ventricular mass and cardiovascular morbidity in essential hypertension: the MAVI study. *J Am Coll Cardiol.* 2001;38:1829–1835.

10. Haider AW, Larson MG, Benjamin EJ, Levy D. Increased left ventricular mass and hypertrophy are associated with increased risk for sudden death. *J Am Coll Cardiol.* 1998;32:1454–1459.

11. Go AS, Chertow GM, Fan D, McCulloch CE, Hsu C-y. Chronic kidney disease and the risk of death, cardiovascular events, and hospitalization. *N Engl J Med.* 2004;351:1296–1305.

12. Hostetter TH. Chronic kidney disease predicts cardiovascular disease. *N Engl J Med.* 2004;351: 1344–1346.

13. Thorp ML, Eastman L, Smith DH, Johnson ES. Managing the burden of chronic kidney disease. *Dis Manag.* 2006;9:115–121.

14. Shulman NB, Ford CE, Hall WD, et al. Prognostic value of serum creatinine and effect of treatment of hypertension on renal function. Results from the hypertension detection and follow-up program. The Hypertension Detection and Follow-up Program Cooperative Group. *Hypertension.* 1989;13(5 suppl):180–193.

15. Manjunath G, Tighiouart H, Ibrahim H, et al. Level of kidney function as a risk factor for atherosclerotic cardiovascular outcomes in the community. *J Am Coll Cardiol.* 2003;41:47–55.

16. Henry RM, Kostense PJ, Bos G, et al. Mild renal insufficiency is associated with increased cardiovascular mortality: The Hoorn Study. *Kidney Int.* 2002;62: 1402–1407.

17. Fellstrom BC, Jardine AJ, Schmieder RE, et al. Rosuvastatin and cardiovascular events in patients undergoing hemodialysis. *N Engl J Med.* 2009;360:1395–1407.

18. Ganesh SK, Stack AG, Levin NW, Hulbert-Shearon T, Port FK. Association of elevated serum PO(4), Ca × PO(4) product, and parathyroid hormone with cardiac mortality risk in chronic hemodialysis patients. *J Am Soc Nephrol.* 2001;12:2131–2138.

19. Raggi P, Boulay A, Chasan-Taber S, et al. Cardiac calcification in adult hemodialysis patients. A link between end-stage renal disease and cardiovascular disease? *J Am Coll Cardiol.* 2002;39:695–701.

20. Young EW, Albert JM, Satayathum S, et al. Predictors and consequences of altered mineral metabolism: the Dialysis Outcomes and Practice Patterns Study. *Kidney Int.* 2005;67:1179–1187.

21. Sarnak MJ, Levey AS, Schoolwerth AC, et al. Kidney disease as a risk factor for development of cardiovascular disease: a statement from the American Heart Association Councils on Kidney in Cardiovascular Disease, High Blood Pressure Research, Clinical Cardiology, and Epidemiology and Prevention. *Circulation.* 2003;108:2154–2169.

22. United States Renal Data System: Excerpts from the USRDS 2006 annual data report: atlas of end-stage renal disease in the United States.

23. Centers for Disease Control and Prevention (CDC). Prevalence of chronic kidney disease and associated risk factors – United States, 1999–2004. *MMWR Morb Mortal Wkly Rep.* 2007;56:161–165.

24. Coresh J, Byrd-Holt D, Astor BC, et al. Chronic kidney disease awareness, prevalence, and trends among U.S. adults, 1999 to 2000. *J Am Soc Nephrol.* 2005;16:180–188.

25. Cerasola G, Mulè G, Cottone S, Nardi E, Cusimano P. Hypertension, microalbuminuria and renal dysfunction: the Renal Dysfunction in Hypertension (REDHY) study. *J Nephrol.* 2008;21:368–373.

26. Cerasola G, Mulè G, Nardi E, et al. Clinical correlates of renal dysfunction in hypertensive patients without cardiovascular complications: the REDHY study. *J Hum Hypertens.* 2010;24:44–50.

27. Guyton AC, Coleman TG. Quantitative analysis of the pathophysiology of hypertension. 1969. *J Am Soc Nephrol.* 1999;10:2248–2249.

28. Foley RN, Parfrey PS, Harnett JD, et al. Clinical and echocardiographic disease in patients starting end-stage renal disease therapy. *Kidney Int.* 1995;47:186–192.

29. Herzog CA, Ma JZ, Collins AJ. Poor long-term survival after acute myocardial infarction among patients on long-term dialysis. *N Engl J Med.* 1998;339:799–805.

30. Levy D, Garrison RJ, Savage DD, Kannel WB, Castelli WP. Prognostic implication of echocardiographically determined left ventricular mass in the Framingham Heart Study. *N Engl J Med.* 1990;322:1561–1566.

31. Silberberg JS, Barre PE, Prichard SS, Sniderman AD. Impact of left ventricular hypertrophy on survival in end-stage renal disease. *Kidney Int.* 1989;36:286–290.

32. Meeus F, Kourilski O, Guerin AP, Gaudry C, Marchais SJ, London GM. Pathophysiology of cardiovascular disease in hemodialysis patients. *Kidney Int.* 1989;76:S140–S147.

33. Mall G, Huther W, Schneider J, Lundin P, Ritz E. Diffuse intramyocardiocytic fibrosis in uraemic patients. *Nephrol Dial Transplant.* 1990;5:39–44.

34. Amann K, Breitbach M, Ritz E, Mall G. Myocyte/capillary mismatch in the heart of uremic patients. *J Am Soc Nephrol.* 1998;9:1018–1022.

35. London GM, Fabiani F, Marchais SJ, et al. Uremic cardiomyopathy: an inadequate left ventricular hypertrophy. *Kidney Int.* 1987;31:973–980.

36. Locatelli F, Bommer J, London GM, et al. Cardiovascular disease determinants in chronic renal failure: clinical approach and treatment. *Nephrol Dial Transplant.* 2001;16:459–468.

37. Foley RN, Parfrey PS, Harnett JD, Kent GM, Murray DC, Barre PE. The prognostic importance of left ventricular geometry in uremic cardiomyopathy. *J Am Soc Nephrol.* 1995;5:2024–2031.

38. Stack AG, Saran R. Clinical correlates and mortality impact of left ventricular hypertrophy among new ESRD patients in the United States. *Am J Kidney Dis.* 2002;40:1202–1210.

39. Shlipak MG, Fried LF, Cushman M, et al. Cardiovascular mortality risk in chronic kidney disease: comparison of traditional and novel risk factors. *JAMA.* 2005;293:1737–1745.

40. Middleton RJ, Parfrey PS, Foley RN. Left ventricular hypertrophy in the renal patient. *J Am Soc Nephrol.* 2001;12:1079–1084.

41. Harnett JD, Kent GM, Barre PE, Taylor R, Parfrey PS. Risk factors for the development of left ventricular hypertrophy in a prospectively followed cohort of dialysis patients. *J Am Soc Nephrol.* 1994;4:1486–1490.

42. London G. Pathophysiology of cardiovascular damage in the early renal population. *Nephrol Dial Transplant.* 2001;16(suppl 2):S3–S6.

43. Sarnak MJ. Cardiovascular complications in chronic kidney disease. *Am J Kidney Dis.* 2003;41(suppl 5):S11–S17.

44. Cottone S, Mulè G, Nardi E, et al. C-reactive protein and intercellular adhesion molecule-1 are stronger predictors of oxidant stress than blood pressure in established hypertension. *J Hypertens.* 2007;25:423–428.

45. Cottone S, Mulè G, Guarneri M, et al. Endothelin-1 and F2- isoprostane relate to and predict renal dysfunction in hypertensive patients. *Nephrol Dial Transplant.* 2009;24:497–503.

46. Ayerden Ebinç F, Ebinç H, Derici U, et al. The relationship between adiponectin levels and proinflammatory cytokines and left ventricular mass in dialysis patients. *J Nephrol.* 2009;22:216–223.

47. López B, González A, Varo N, Laviades C, Querejeta R, Diez J. Biochemical assessment of myocardial fibrosis in hypertensive heart disease. *Hypertension.* 2001;38:1222–1226.

48. Stella P, Manunta P, Mallamaci F, et al. Endogenous ouabain and cardiomyopathy in dialysis patients. *J Intern Med.* 2008;263:274–280.

49. Gutierrez O, Isakova T, Rhee E, et al. Fibroblast growth factor-23 mitigates hyperphosphatemia but accentuates calcitriol deficiency in chronic kidney disease. *J Am Soc Nephrol.* 2005;16:2205–2215.

50. Gutiérrez OM, Januzzi JL, Isakova T, et al. Fibroblast growth factor-23 and left ventricular hypertrophy in chronic kidney disease. *Circulation.* 2009;119:2545–2552.

51. Aoki J, Ikari Y, Nakajima H, et al. Clinical and pathologic characteristics of dilated cardiomyopathy in hemodialysis patients. *Kidney Int.* 2005;67:333–340.

52. Ahmed A, Rich M, Sanders P, et al. Chronic kidney disease associated mortality in diastolic versus systolic heart failure: a propensity matched study. *Am J Cardiol.* 2007;99:393–398.

53. Bezante GP, Viazzi F, Leoncini G, et al. Coronary flow reserve is impaired in hypertensive patients with subclinical renal damage. *Am J Hypertens.* 2009;22:191–196.

54. Ljungman S, Laragh JH, Cody RJ. Role of the kidney in congestive heart failure. Relationship of cardiac index to kidney function. *Drugs.* 1990;39(suppl 4):S10–S21.

55. Miyazato J, Horio T, Takiuchi S, et al. Left ventricular diastolic dysfunction in patients with chronic renal failure: impact of diabetes mellitus. *Diabet Med.* 2005;22:730–736.

56. Bruch C, Rothenburger M, Gotzmann M, et al. Chronic kidney disease in patients with chronic heart failure - impact on intracardiac conduction, diastolic function and prognosis. *Int J Cardiol.* 2007;118:375–380.

57. Nardi E, Palermo A, Mulè G, Cusimano P, Cottone S, Cerasola G. Left ventricular hypertrophy and geometry in hypertensive patients with chronic kidney disease. *J Hypertens.* 2009;27:633–641.

58. Oh JK, Appleton CP, Hatle LK, Nishimura RA, Seward JB, Tajik AJ. The noninvasive assessment of left ventricular diastolic function with 2-dimensional and Doppler echocardiography. *J Am Soc Echocardiogr.* 1997;10:246–270.

59. Shan K, Bick RJ, Poindexter BJ, et al. Relation of tissue Doppler derived myocardial velocities to myocardial structure and beta-adrenergic receptor density in humans. *J Am Coll Cardiol.* 2000;36:891–896.

60. Sarraf M, Masoumi A, Schrier RW. Cardiorenal syndrome in acute decompensated heart failure. *Clin J Am Soc Nephrol.* 2009;4:2013–2026.

61. Smith GL, Lichtman JH, Bracken MB, et al. Renal impairment and outcomes in heart failure: systematic review and meta-analysis. *J Am Coll Cardiol.* 2006;47:1987–1996.

62. Ezekowitz J, McAlister FA, Humphries KH, et al. The association among renal insufficiency, pharmacotherapy, and outcomes in 6,427 patients with heart failure and coronary artery disease. *J Am Coll Cardiol.* 2004;44:1587–1592.

63. Hillege HL, Girbes AR, de Kam PJ, et al. Renal function, neurohormonal activation, and survival in patients with chronic heart failure. *Circulation.* 2000;102:203–210.

64. Adams KF Jr, Fonarow GC, Emerman CL, et al. Characteristics and outcomes of patients hospitalized for heart failure in the United States: rationale, design, and preliminary observations from the first 100,000 cases in the Acute Decompensated Heart Failure National Registry (ADHERE). *Am Heart J.* 2005;149:209–216.

65. Collins AJ. Cardiovascular mortality in end-stage renal disease. *Am J Med Sci.* 2003;325:163–167.

66. Stack AG, Bloembergen WE. A cross-sectional study of the prevalence and clinical correlates of congestive heart failure among incident US dialysis patients. *Am J Kidney Dis.* 2001;38:992–1000.

67. Trespalacios FC, Taylor AJ, Agodoa LY, Bakris GL, Abbott KC. Heart failure as a cause for hospitalization in chronic dialysis patients. *Am J Kidney Dis.* 2003;41:1267–1277.

68. Harnett JD, Foley RN, Kent GM, Barre PE, Murray D, Parfrey PS. Congestive heart failure in dialysis patients: prevalence, incidence, prognosis and risk factors. *Kidney Int.* 1995;47:884–890.

69. Foley RN, Parfrey PS, Harnett JD, Kent GM, Murray DC, Barre PE. The impact of anemia on cardiomyopathy, morbidity, and mortality in end-stage renal disease. *Am J Kidney Dis.* 1996;28:53–61.

70. Foley RN, Parfrey PS, Kent GM, Harnett JD, Murray DC, Barre E. Long-term evolution of cardiomyopathy in dialysis patients. *Kidney Int.* 1998;54:1720–1725.

71. Levin A, Thompson CR, Ethier J, et al. Left ventricular mass index increase in early renal disease: impact of decline in hemoglobin. *Am J Kidney Dis.* 1999;34:125–134.

72. Rigatto C, Foley R, Jeffery J, Negrijn C, Tribula C, Parfrey P. Electrocardiographic left ventricular hypertrophy in renal transplant recipients: prognostic value and impact of blood pressure and anemia. *J Am Soc Nephrol.* 2003;14:462–468.

73. London GM. Left ventricular alterations and end-stage renal disease. *Nephrol Dial Transplant.* 2002;17(suppl 1): S29–S36.

74. van der Meer P, Voors AA, Lipsic E, van Gilst WH, van Veldhuisen DJ. Erythropoietin in cardiovascular diseases. *Eur Heart J.* 2004;25:285–291.

75. van der Meer P, Lipsic E, Henning RH, et al. Erythropoietin improves left ventricular function and coronary flow in an experimental model of ischemia-reperfusion injury. *Eur J Heart Fail.* 2004;6:853–859.

76. Parsa CJ, Kim J, Riel RU, et al. Cardioprotective effects of erythropoietin in the reperfused ischemic heart: a potential role for cardiac fibroblasts. *J Biol Chem.* 2004;279:20655–20662.

77. Muller R, Steffen HM, Brunner R, et al. Changes in the alpha adrenergic system and increase in blood pressure with recombinant human erythropoietin (rHuEpo) therapy for renal anemia. *Clin Invest Med.* 1991;14: 614–622.

78. Parfrey PS, Harnett JD, Barre PE. The natural history of myocardial disease in dialysis patients. *J Am Soc Nephrol.* 1991;2:2–12.

79. London GM, Guerin AP, Marchais SJ, et al. Cardiac and arterial interactions in end-stage renal disease. *Kidney Int.* 1996;50:600–608.

80. Foley RN, Parfrey PS, Harnett JD, Kent GM, Murray DC, Barre PE. Hypoalbuminemia, cardiac morbidity, and mortality in end-stage renal disease. *J Am Soc Nephrol.* 1996;7:728–736.

81. Ma JZ, Ebben J, Xia H, Collins AJ. Hematocrit level and associated mortality in hemodialysis patients. *J Am Soc Nephrol.* 1999;10:610–619.

82. Madore F, Lowrie EG, Brugnara C, et al. Anemia in hemodialysis patients: Variables affecting this outcome predictor. *J Am Soc Nephrol.* 1997;8:1921–1929.

83. London GM. Cardiovascular disease in chronic renal failure: pathophysiologic aspects. *Semin Dial.* 2003;16: 85–94.

84. London GM. Cardiovascular calcifications in uremic patients: clinical impact on cardiovascular function. *J Am Soc Nephrol.* 2003;14(suppl 4):S305–S309.

85. Chaignon M, Chen WT, Tarazi RC, Nakamoto S, Bravo EL. Effect of hemodialysis on blood volume distribution and cardiac output. *Hypertension.* 1981;3:327–332.

86. Nichols WW, O'Rourke MF. Vascular impedance. In: Nichols RR, O'Rourke MF, eds. *McDonald's blood Flow in Arteries: Theoretical, Experimental and Clinical Principles.* London, Hodder Arnold Publisher; 2005:83–96.

87. Safar ME, Levy BI, Laurent S, London GM. Hypertension and the arterial system: clinical and therapeutic aspects. *J Hypertens.* 1990;8(suppl 7):S113–S119.

88. Pfitzner J. Poiseuille and his law. *Anaesthesia.* 1976;31:273–275.

89. van der Mark WAMA, Boer P, Cramer MJM, Blankestijn PJ. Decreased access resistance in haemodialysis patients with upper arm arteriovenous fistulae. *Nephol Dial Transplant.* 2008;23:2105–2106.

90. Basile C, Vernaglione L, Lomonte C. Reply. *Nephrol Dial Transplant.* 2008;23:2106–2107.

91. Guyton AC, Sagawa K. Compensations of cardiac output and other circulatory functions in areflex dogs with large A-V fistulas. *Am J Physiol.* 1961;200:1157–1163.

92. London GM, Guerin AP, Marchais SJ. Hemodynamic overload in end-stage renal disease patients. *Semin Dial.* 1999;12:77–83.

93. Girerd X, London G, Boutouyrie P, Mourad J-J, Safar M, Laurent S. Remodelling of the radial artery in response to a chronic increase in shear stress. *Hypertension.* 1996;27:799–803.

94. Iwashima Y, Horio T, Takami Y, et al. Effects of the creation of arteriovenous fistula for hemodialysis on cardiac function and natriuretic peptide levels in CRF. *Am J Kidney Dis.* 2002;40:974–982.

95. Ori Y, Korzets A, Katz M, et al. The contribution of an arteriovenous access for hemodialysis to left ventricular hypertrophy. *Am J Kidney Dis.* 2002;40:745–752.

96. Buckley MG, Sethi D, Markandu ND, Sagnella GA, Singer DRJ, MacGregor GA. Plasma concentrations and comparisons of brain natriuretic peptide and atrial natriuretic peptide in normal subjects, cardiac transplant recipients and patients with dialysis-independent or dialysis-dependent chronic renal failure. *Clin Sci.* 1992;83:437–444.

97. Yigla M, Nakhoul F, Sabag A, et al. Pulmonary hypertension in patients with end-stage renal disease. *Chest.* 2003;123:1577–1582.

98. Nakhoul F, Yigla M, Gilman R, Reisner SA, Abassi Z. The pathogenesis of pulmonary hypertension in haemodialysis patients via arterio-venous access. *Nephrol Dial Transplant.* 2005;20:1686–1692.

99. Unal A, Tasdemir K, Oimak S, et al. The long-term effects of arteriovenous fistula creation on the development of pulmonary hypertension in hemodialysis patients. *Hemodial Int.* 2010;14:398–402.

100. Lomonte C, Casucci F, Antonelli M et al. Is there a place for duplex screening of the brachial artery in the maturation of arteriovenous fistulas? *Semin Dial.* 2005;18:243–246.

101. Dammers R, Tordoir JHM, Welten RJTHJ, Kitslaar PJEHM, Hoeks APG. The effect of chronic flow changes on brachial artery diameter and shear stress in arteriovenous fistulas for hemodialysis. *Int J Artif Organs.* 2002;25:124–128.

102. Mitchell GF, Parise H, Vita JA, et al. Local shear stress and brachial artery flow-mediated dilation. The Framingham Heart Study. *Hypertension.* 2004;44:134–139.

103. Vogel RA. Measurement of endothelial function by brachial artery flow-mediated vasodilation. *Am J Cardiol.* 2001;88:31–34.

104. Pandeya S, Lindsay RM. The relationship between cardiac output and access flow during hemodialysis. *ASAIO J.* 1999;45:135–138.

105. Vascular Access Society. Guideline 20.3: Management of high flow in AV fistula and graft. www.vascularaccesssociety.org.

106. Basile C, Lomonte C, Vernaglione L, Casucci F, Antonelli M, Losurdo N. The relationship between flow of arteriovenous fistula and cardiac output in haemodialysis patients. *Nephrol Dial Transplant.* 2008;23:282–287.

107. Seals DR, Hagberg JM, Spina RJ, Rogers MA, Schectman KB, Ehsani AA. Enhanced left ventricular performance in endurance trained older man. *Circulation.* 1994;89:198–205.

108. MacRae JM. Vascular access and cardiac disease: is there a relationship? *Curr Opin Nephrol Hypertens.* 2006;15:577–582.

109. Hiremath S, Doucette SP, Richardson R, Chan K, Burns K, Zimmerman D. Left ventricular growth after 1 year does not correlate with arteriovenous access flow: a prospective cohort study. *Nephrol Dial Transplant.* 2010;25:2656–2661.

110. Korsheed S, Burton JO, McIntyre CW. Higher arteriovenous fistulae blood flows are associated with a lower level of dialysis-induced cardiac injury. *Hemodial Int.* 2009;13:505–511.

111. Wasse H, Speckman RA, McClellan WM. Arteriovenous fistula use is associated with lower cardiovascular mortality compared with catheter use among ESRD patients. *Semin Dial.* 2008;21:483–489.

112. Al.Ghonaim M, Manns BJ, Hirsch DJ, Gao Z, Tonelli M, for the Alberta Kidney Disease Network. Relation between access blood flow and mortality in chronic hemodialysis patients. *Clin J Am Soc Nephrol.* 2008;3:387–391.

113. Ahearn DJ, Maher JF. Heart failure as a complication of hemodialysis arteriovenous fistula. *Ann Intern Med.* 1972;77:201–204.

114. Engelberts I, Tordoir JH, Boons ES, Schreij G. High-output cardiac failure due to excessive shunting in a hemodialysis access fistula: an easily overlooked diagnosis. *Am J Nephrol.* 1995;15:323–326.

115. Kajiwara IS, Kondo J, Matsumoto A. Banding a hemodialysis arteriovenous fistula to decrease blood flow and resolve high output cardiac failure: report of a case. *Surgery Today.* 1994;24:734–736.

116. Young PR Jr, Rohr MS, Marterre WF Jr. High-output cardiac failure secondary to a brachiocephalic arteriovenous hemodialysis fistula: two cases. *Am Surg.* 1998;64:239–241.

117. MacRae JM, Pandeya S, Humen DP, Krivitski N, Lindsay RM. Arteriovenous fistula-associated high-output cardiac failure: a review of mechanisms. *Am J Kidney Dis.* 2004;43:e17–e22.

118. Chemla ES, Morsy M, Anderson L, Whitemore A. Inflow reduction by distalization of anastomosis treats efficiently high-flow high-cardiac output vascular access for hemodialysis. *Semin Dial.* 2007;20:68–72.

119. MacRae JM, Levin A, Belenkie I. The cardiovascular effects of arteriovenous fistulas in chronic kidney disease: a cause for concern? *Semin Dial.* 2006;19:349–352.

120. MacRae JM, Do TH, Rosenbaum D, Levin A, Kiaii M. High flow fistulas and cardiac hemodynamics. *J Am Soc Nephrol.* 2004;15:369A.

121. Begin V, Ethier J, Dumont M, Leblanc M. Prospective evaluation of the intra-access flow of recently created native arteriovenous fistulae. *Am J Kidney Dis.* 2002;40:1277–1282.

122. Wijnen E, Keuter XH, Planken NR et al. The relation between vascular access flow and different types of vascular access with systemic hemodynamics in hemodialysis patients. *Artif Organs.* 2005;29:960–964.

123. Dixon BS, Noval L, Fangman J. Hemodialysis vascular access survival: upper-arm native arteriovenous fistula. *Am J Kidney Dis.* 2002;39:92–101.

124. Tordoir J, Canaud B, Haage P et al. EBPG on vascular access. *Nephrol Dial Transplant.* 2007;22(suppl 2):ii88–ii117.

125. Stern AB, Klemmer PJ. High-output heart failure secondary to arteriovenous fistula. *Hemodial Int.* 2011;15:104–107.

126. Tellioglu G, Berber I, Kilicoglu G, Seymen P, Kara M, Titz I. Doppler ultrasonography-guided surgery for high-flow hemodialysis vascular access: preliminary results. *Transplant Proc.* 2008;40:87–89.

127. Suding PN, Wilson SE. Strategies for management of ischemic steal syndrome. *Semin Vasc Surg.* 2007;20:184–188.

128. Quarello F, Forneris G, Borca M, Pozzato M. Do central venous catheters have advantages over arteriovenous fistulas or grafts? *J Nephrol.* 2006;19:265–279.

129. Unger P, Velz-Roa S, Wissing K, Hoang A, Van de Borne P. Regression of left ventricular hypertrophy after arteriovenous fistula closure in renal transplant recipients: a long-term follow-up. *Am J Transplant.* 2004;4:2038–2044.

130. van Duijnhoven EC, Cheriex EC, Tordoir JH, Kooman JP, van Hooff JP. Effect of closure of the arteriovenous fistula on left ventricular dimensions in renal transplant patients. *Nephrol Dial Transplant.* 2001;16:368–372.

131. Bos WJW, Zietse R, van den Meiracker AH, Schalekamp MADH, Weimar W. Hemodynamic consequences of Cimino fistulas studied with finger pressure measurements during fistula compression. *Kidney Int.* 1995;48:1641–1645.

132. Movilli E, Viola BF, Brunori G, et al. Long-term effects of arteriovenous fistula closure on echocardiographic functional and structural findings in hemodialysis patients: a prospective study. *Am J Kidney Dis.* 2010;55:682–689.

133. Amerling R, Ronco C, Kuhlmann M, Winchester JF. Arteriovenous fistula toxicity. *Blood Purif.* 2011;31:113–120.

134. Dinwiddie L. "Eligibility" is key word in Fistula First Breakthrough Initiative in determining fistula use. *Neph News Issues.* 2006;20:39–40.

135. Konner K, Nonnast-Daniel B, Ritz E. The arteriovenous fistula. *J Am Soc Nephrol.* 2003;14:1669–1680.

136. Lomonte C, Basile C. The role of the nephrologist in the management of vascular access. *Nephrol Dial Transplant.* 2011;26:1461–1463.

HAND ISCHEMIA

STEVEN WU & JENNIFER JOE

INTRODUCTION

There is a wide spectrum of clinical symptoms associated with hand ischemia after dialysis access placement, ranging from mild numbness and tingling to limb-threatening ischemia. Recognition of the developing clinical scenario of arterial "steal" is critical, and can facilitate rapid initiation of treatment in order to avoid potential limb loss.[1–4] The incidence of severe steal ranges from 0.5% to 5%.[5] It is worth mentioning that in the 1998 noteworthy paper by Lazarides et al., the incidence of limb-threatening ischemia was 3.9% (7 of 180 patients).[4]

Physicians and nurses who manage dialysis patients must be able to recognize the clinical situations in which the potential for limb-threatening ischemia can arise. This chapter will focus on pathophysiology, clinical features, diagnosis, and management strategies to combat hand ischemia.

TERMINOLOGY AND PATHOPHYSIOLOGY

The familiar clinical scenario of a dialysis patient who develops a cold and painful hand distal to the site of their dialysis accesses has traditionally been termed "arterial steal syndrome." This focuses attention on the arteriovenous access as the sole cause of the symptoms, which is the traditional view. It has now been recognized that there are other clinical factors contributing to the presentation of hand ischemia.

Recent information has documented that approximately 80% of patients experience decreased digital pressures after arteriovenous access creation.[6] This is considered "physiological steal," or the expected re-routing of blood after the creation of a high flow, low-resistance circuit.[7–10] The blood flow in the artery immediately distal to the anastomosis can be retrograde, antegrade, or "to and fro," depending on the pressure gradients and the timing of the cardiac cycle.[10] In fact, studies show that a great percentage of forearm and proximal arteriovenous accesses have retrograde flow by imaging.[11–13] This "physiological steal" or "steal phenomena" is usually well-tolerated, but can become clinically significant and lead to ischemic symptoms only if the compensatory mechanisms are not adequate (Figure 23-1).

Due to the prevalence of "physiological steal" and the increasing awareness regarding arterial stenosis as an important contribution factor, the term "arterial steal syndrome" is no longer appropriate, and is likely a misnomer. To date, there are several new descriptive phrases that have been proposed to describe hand ischemia related to the dialysis access. These include distal hypoperfusion ischemic syndrome, dialysis-associated steal syndrome, hemodialysis access-induced distal ischemia, and access-related hand ischemia.[8–10,14,15] Out of these the term "distal hypoperfusion ischemic syndrome" (DHIS) most precisely describes the underline pathophysiology of this disorder.[8]

The two other physiological mechanisms felt to play an important role in hand ischemia are the presence of arterial stenosis and distal arteriopathy (Figure 23-2, Figure 23-6 and Figure 23-7).[7–9,16,17]

There is a significant and growing body of current data suggesting that arterial stenosis plays an essential role in

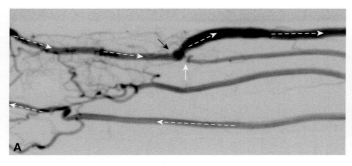
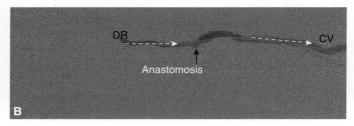

Figure 23-1. Steal phenomena. A severe stenosis (**A**, white solid arrow) in the right radial artery immediately upstream from the AV anastomosis (A, black solid arrow). The direction of blood flow was from right ulnar artery to palmer arch to right distal radial artery to AV anastomosis to cephalic vein (A, white dotted arrow). When a catheter was placed into right distal radial artery (DR) via right cephalic vein (CV), angiogram showed blood flow was from right distal radial artery to AV anastomosis to cephalic vein (**B**, white dotted arrows).

DHIS. Arterial stenotic lesions can occur anywhere within the arterial tree of the hemodialysis vascular access circuit, including central arteries such as a subclavian stenosis and the arteries distal to the arteriovenous access.[9] Arterial stenotic lesions often predate the creation of the vascular access and are particularly common in the diabetic population.[10] The physiological blood flow changes that occur after arteriovenous access creation can induce a previously asymptomatic arterial stenotic lesion to become pathologically symptomatic.

By arteriography, the incidence of arterial stenosis contributing to peripheral ischemia has been reported to range between 62% and 100%, depending upon definition used.[8,16,17] The prospective study by Asif et al found arterial stenotic lesions in 10 of 12 patients (83%). Ten of the 12 were suitable candidates for percutaneous transluminal balloon angioplasty (PTA), and 8 of the 10 successfully underwent PTA. All eight were symptom free at the mean follow-up of 8 months after PTA, without further intervention.[8]

Distal arteriopathy refers to the presence of occlusive disease in the forearm or hand, poor arterial compliance resulting from calcification, and/or decreased vasodilation from endothelial cell dysfunction contributing to symptoms of hand ischemia.[7,8,10] Many hemodialysis patients have significant microvascular and macrovascular disease prior to creation of vascular access. This arteriosclerotic disease may not be clinically significant before access creation. However, in the presence of pre-existing occlusive disease, poor arterial compliance, and decreased vasodilation, normal compensatory mechanisms are not sufficient to overcome the state of "physiological steal" that occurs after access creation, and hand ischemia ensues.

Many pathogenic aspects particular to the dialysis patient likely contribute to the level of high vascular resistance seen in distal arteriopathy. These include disturbances in mineral metabolism in the uremic millieu, calcium-containing phosphate binders, and vitamin D treatment of secondary hyperparathyroidism, increased oxidized LDL cholesterol, increased oxidative stress, and hyperhomocysteinemia.[18]

Yeager et al illustrated the severity of atherosclerotic occlusive disease that can occur in the hand and digits of dialysis patients, and demonstrated that this extreme form of artherosclerotic disease can potentially cause gangrene in both the access and the nonaccess arm.[19] The study retrospectively examined 23 patients with gangrene of the finger, and discovered that only 48% (11 of 23) exhibited this condition in the same arm as the dialysis access. The remaining 52% (12 of 23) had gangrene in the arm opposite that of the dialysis access. Arteriography suggested a diffuse occlusive process involving the distal radial or ulnar arteries, extending into the palmar and digital circulation and consistent with atherosclerotic occlusive disease.[19]

A	B	C
No arterial lesion	Brachial artery stenosis	Distal arteriopathy

Figure 23-2. Arterial stenosis and distal arteriopathy as the causes of DHIS.

EPIDEMIOLOGY

The prevalence of DHIS ranges from 1% to 25%.[5,7,20-23] Ischemia in upper arm (brachial artery based) accesses is more common than forearm (radial artery based) accesses.[7] A review by Tordoir et al in 2004 noted that the brachiocephalic and basilic AVFs have a 10–25% incidence of ischemia, compared with 1–1.8% in radiocephalic AVFs.[7] Ischemia in arteriovenous fistulas is more common than grafts.[24] The location and type of arteriovenous access affects the likelihood of having hand ischemia, but it does not affect the number or intensity of symptoms experienced.[24]

The proposed mechanism for the increased likelihood of ischemia in the setting of proximal AVF is a higher rate of blood flow than seen in distal AVFs.[7,24] In distal AVFs, blood flow rates are usually in the range of 500–800 mL/min, with the systolic finger blood pressure usually above 100 mm Hg.[7] In patients with an elbow AVF, the blood flow can increase to more than 1500–2000 mL/min, with systolic finger blood pressures as low as 50–60 mm Hg, potentially causing ischemic symptoms.[7]

Van Hoek et al were the first to examine the incidence of mild hand ischemia symptoms, which may not be clinically apparent.[24] He distributed a questionnaire to 120 incident chronic hemodialysis patients with stable arteriovenous accesses. The questionnaire included specific hand ischemia questions about cold sensation, pain, diminished sensibility, strength, cramps, and skin quality. The investigators determined that as many as 50% ($n = 14$) of patients with brachiocephalic arteriovenous fistulas, 25% ($n = 26$) of patients with prosthetic forearm loops, and 12% ($n = 12$) of patients with radiocephalic fistulas regularly experience a cold hand. Of patients with brachiocephalic arteriovenous fistulas, 79% reported regularly experiencing one of the symptoms detailed in the questionnaire.[24] Thus, mild hand ischemia symptomatology is likely a very common occurrence.

DIAGNOSIS AND CLINICAL ASSESSMENT

The diagnosis of DHIS is made by clinical assessment. First, one should obtain a full history of the current symptoms and altering factors such as if exercise or dialysis exacerbates the condition. Additionally, when symptoms began in relationship to creation of the access is important to document. Second, one should assess for risk factors for DHIS, such as DM and PVD. Third, one must perform a thorough physical examination, with particular attention paid to comparing the access extremity to the nonaccess extremity. DHIS should be highly suspected if symptoms reverse with temporary blocking of the access outflow tract. Finally, one should evaluate all past radiological studies.

Assessment of the current symptoms should evaluate five different areas—cold sensation, pain, sensibility of the skin, strength, cramps, and quality of the skin.[24] Patients should

be asked about cold sensation, what part of the hand is cold, what fingers are cold, and the severity and frequency of the cold sensation. For pain, patients should be asked a similar set of questions—what part of the hand is painful, what fingers are painful, and the severity and frequency of the pain. Sensibility refers to abnormal sensation, such as numbness and ability to feel light and sharp touch. One should ask the patient if their sensibility is altered or diminished and how frequently so. One should assess if the patient experiences decreased strength, also enquiring about severity and frequency. The presence of cramping should be evaluated with similar questioning. Finally, the patient should be questioned regarding pallor, changes in nail appearance, diminished growth, and ulceration.

Evaluation of the risk factors for DHIS is an important part of the assessment. One should ask if the patient is a diabetic, has peripheral vascular disease, uses tobacco, has high cholesterol, or has coronary artery disease. Female gender is also seems to be a risk factor for DHIS.

On physical examination, it is most important to assess for temperature, skin sensibility, strength, and quality of skin. It is critical to compare the affected with the nonaffected hand. One can subjectively touch the skin of the dorsum and palm of the hand for temperature, or this can be measured with a digital thermometer. Sensibility can be tested using a two-point discrimination test of sharp and soft objects. Grip strength can be assessed subjectively, or measured using hand grip dynamometry.

Evaluating the quality of the skin of the hand is an essential component of the physical examination. One should assess for normal skin color, or whether pallor or cyanosis is visible. Trophic lesions, such as nail bed changes, loss of hair, and muscle atrophy, should be identified. Clearly, any ulceration, necrosis, or area of gangrene should prompt emergent evaluation and intervention.

The health of the vascular bed should be evaluated. Blood pressure should be compared from both arms. A significant discrepancy in blood pressure would suggest a central or large arterial stenosis in the lower blood pressure arm contributing to DHIS. Each extremity should be compared with regard to skin color, presence of lesions, and strength of radial and ulnar pulses. Cold fingers with pale or blue-purple discoloration can be observed. Patients should also be examined while undergoing hemodialysis, as this will often augment the symptoms. In DHIS, often distal radial pulses are only palpable when the AVF has been manually compressed.[7] On the other hand, the radial pulse may be normal on palpation due to reversed blood flow from the ulnar artery to the radial artery (steal phenomenon), masking the presence of DHIS.[9] For this reason, the presence or absence of the radial pulse has limited diagnostic value.

Finally, the pattern of neuropathy is important to differentiate DHIS from the other neuropathies common to dialysis patients. For possible arthropathy or dermatological local lesions, further plain X-ray or skin biopsy may be required.

Prior imaging studies may hold the key to diagnosis of DHIS. As mentioned before, arterial stenosis can be an important contribution to the symptoms of DHIS. Often times, previous imaging prior to surgical construction of AV access may have demonstrated mild to moderate stenosis that was not considered clinically relevant at the time and therefore not explicitly reported as such. In the presence of symptoms of DHIS, these previously documented stenotic lesions may represent the underlying etiology.

SPECTRUM OF SYMPTOMS

DHIS exists on a spectrum, with signs and symptoms ranging from mild to severe. Generally, the natural history of DHIS appears to be similar to the sequence of events that is observed in the progression of peripheral obstructive arterial disease of the lower limbs. Many investigators have proposed a grading system with four tiers.[7,14,15]

Conventionally, the occurrence of DHIS has been divided into two categories, early and late. Early has traditionally been referred to as less than 30 days after access creation, with late being greater than 30 days after access creation.[2,25]

Traditionally, the diagnosis is still made clinically by physical examination. It is important to stage the condition during the clinical assessment, because this will determine the urgency of the situation.

Stage 1
- Pale/blue/cool hand without pain
- No or slight cyanosis of nail beds, mild coldness of skin or hand, reduced arterial pulsations at the wrist (not a reliable sign for forearm AVF), reduced systolic finger pressures

Stage 2
- Pain during hand exercise and/or with dialysis
- Pain, cramps, numbness, or disturbing coldness in fingers or hand

Stage 3
- Pain at rest or motor dysfunction of fingers or hand

Stage 4
- Tissue loss, including ulcers, necrosis, or gangrene

DIFFERENTIAL DIAGNOSIS FOR DISTAL HYPOPERFUSION ISCHEMIA SYNDROME

Rheumatic disorders with joint complications are frequent in the dialysis population.[26] There is a significant differential diagnosis in the evaluation of hand pain in the extremity with a dialysis access, which often requires a detailed history and a thorough physical examination (Tables 23-1 and 23-2). This differential diagnosis includes carpal tunnel syndrome, tendopathies, arthropathies, and neuropathies.[9] A study by Valji et al focused on the potential distribution of these varying diagnoses. They presented 14 cases

of hemodialysis grafts which underwent arteriography for possible hand ischemia, 7 of which proved to be due to obstructive arterial disease (3 with superimposed steal), 3 of which were due to graft steal alone, 2 due to ischemic monomelic neuropathy, and 2 due to carpal tunnel syndrome.[16]

Ischemic monomelic neuropathy (IMN) is a complication almost exclusive to diabetics on dialysis, particularly those with preexisting neuropathy.[9,27,28] It was first reported by Bolton in 1979.[29] It is characterized by the acute development of pain, weakness, and paralysis of the forearm and hand muscles, often associated with sensory changes, and occurs immediately (minutes to hours) after the creation of an arteriovenous access.[9,28] Typically, the hand is warm and the radial pulse present.[9] IMN is felt to be caused by the sudden diversion or transient occlusion of blood supply to the nerves of the forearm and hand, with the acute ischemic insult being severe enough to damage nerve fibers, but not severe enough to cause necrosis of other tissues.[28] It can be thought of as steal affecting only the nerves.[28] This selective neural injury is thought to be due to the greater metabolic requirement and the more tenuous blood supply of the peripheral nerves compared with other tissues.[30]

First described in 1975, carpal tunnel syndrome occurs frequently in the dialysis population.[31] The carpal tunnel syndrome associated with dialysis has a different clinical picture and natural progression than idiopathic carpal tunnel syndrome.[32] Males and females are equally affected. It is often bilateral, and will readily recur after surgical decompression. It is frequently associated with tenosynovitis of the flexor tendons.[26] Wasting of the lateral thenar muscle is often present and will denote advanced nerve compression.[33–35] An electromyelogram illustrating reduction in motor conduction can help to establish the diagnosis.[34]

Destructive arthropathy of the hands is common to chronic dialysis patients, and has been previously called "dialysis-associated arthropathy." It is felt to be a later onset complication of hemodialysis, usually occurring after 5–7 years of treatment.[26] Arthralgia is a frequent complaint, often noted in the wrist, knee, hip, and spine.[26,36] It can be accompanied by stiffness and limitation of function, or by joint effusion or deformation. It is generally associated with radiographic destructive changes.[26]

EVALUATION OF DISTAL HYPOPERFUSION ISCHEMIA SYNDROME

▶ Arteriogram

Complete arteriography is the most important tool in confirming the diagnosis of DHIS and also in developing a strategy for treating DHIS (Figure 23-3 and Table 23-3). This is best achieved by digital subtraction angiography. As steal from the distal vessels can be expected, images with and without compression of the AVF are usually required.[7,9] It is important to study the entire arterial tree, from the aortic to the palmar arch and the digits so that

TABLE 23–1

Common Causes of Hand Pain in Dialysis Patients and Their Differentiating Features

	Distal Hypoperfusion Ischemic Syndrome (DHIS)	Ischemic Monomelic Neuropathy (IMN)	Carpal Tunnel Syndrome (CTS)	Destructive Arthropathy (DA)	Peripheral Neuropathy	Local skin lesions (Dermatological)	Hypertensive venous compression syndrome
Predominant feature	Cold and painful hand, worse on dialysis	Muscle weakness and paralysis with prominent sensory loss, warm hand with good pulse	Hand weakness and pain, finger numbness	Pain localized mainly to phalangeal joints	Finger numbness, tingling, pain	Skin lesion, gangrene-like, warm hand with good pulse	Central venous stenosis, arm edema
Time to presentation	Acute and chronic	Acute	Chronic	Chronic	Chronic	Acute or chronic	Acute or chronic
Access type	More common with upper arm accesses	Only with upper arm accesses	—	—	—	—	—
Tissue involved	Skin > muscle > nerve	Nerve	Nerves	Joints and phalangeal bones	Nerves	Skin, subcutaneous tissue	Subcutaneous tissue
Cause	Vascular insufficiency leading to distal hypoperfusion	Vascular insufficiency causing nerve damage	Accumulation of B2-microglobulin amyloidosis	Poorly understood	DM, poorly understood increase in dialysis patients	Local trauma or irritation	Central venous stenosis with increased tissue pressure and compressive arterial flow
Radial pulse	Usually diminished (but not a reliable sign for forearm AVF)	Usually present	Present	Present	Present	Present	Usually diminished
Diagnostic evaluation	History, physical, arteriography	History and clinical features	History, physical, nerve conduction velocity study	History, physical, hand X-rays	History, physical	History, physical, skin biopsy	History, fistulagram and/or arteriogram
Groups commonly found in	DM, PVD, smokers	DM, PVD	Long-term HD patients	Long-term HD patients	DM	—	—
Management strategies	Percutaneous and surgical interventions	Immediate access ligation	Supportive, surgery	Supportive	Medical management	Local skin lesion care and treat underlying cause	Correct central venous stenosis

Data from Asif.[9]

TABLE 23–2

Clinical Assessment

1. Chief complaints and associated symptoms/signs
   a. Detailed questions about sensation changes (such as coldness, pain, numbness, muscle weakness or cramping), skin discoloration, tissue loss (such as dry or wet gangrene), hand or joint deformation, arm swelling.
   b. Acute versus chronic onset
   c. Persistent versus intermittent
   d. Triggering or aggregation factors: post- surgical creation or post-declot procedure (may suggest arterial embolism), during dialysis or exercise, or at rest
2. Risk factors for DHIS
   a. Diabetic
   b. Peripheral vascular disease
   c. Female gender
   d. Previous multiple failed access
3. Physical exam
   a. Compare access arm to non-access arm.
   b. Evaluate skin color, skin temperature, the degree of tissue loss, muscle strength, and test other sensations.
   c. Palpate both radial and ulnar pulses of both hand.
   d. Evaluate microcirculation
   e. Observe reversal of ischemic symptoms and/or signs seconds to few minutes after blocking the venous outflow
   f. Measure blood pressure in both upper arms to determine any discrepancy.
4. Review of past radiologic studies
   Look for previous clinically significant or insignificant arterial stenotic lesions

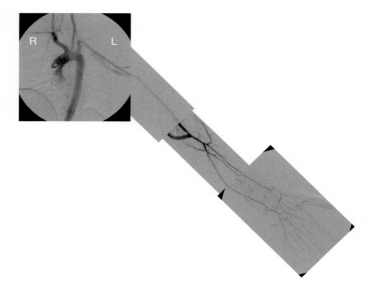

Figure 23-3. Complete arteriogram.

course depend upon the configuration of the access, with catheterization possible if the acute angle at the AV anastomosis can be traversed.

▶ CT Angiogram

Computed tomographic angiogram (CTA) is emerging as a promising technique because it is a less invasive means of imaging the lower extremity arteries.[37–40] It would be most useful in detecting stenotic lesions contributing to DHIS

lesions in the more proximal as well as in the more distal arteries are not missed. This is even more critical when no local arterial stenosis is identified. Recorded images should be carefully evaluated for occlusive arterial disease.[8,9]

Two approaches have been used for arteriography in DHIS. The traditional approach uses the femoral artery antegrade approach, which is ideal because it allows one to evaluate the entire arterial tree. This has been the customary approach and may still be performed for DHIS.

An alternative approach is performance of the arteriogram via the dialysis access, which is retrograde, technically easier, and probably more appropriate in the dialysis setting. We recommend this approach because it is easy, safe, less invasive, and has reasonably good results as long as the catheter is deep in the ascending aorta. Of note, the literature supporting this approach is less than optimum because most studies do not evaluate the entire arterial tree, with the catheter placed only distal to the level of the vertebral artery instead of deep in the aorta because of a theoretical concern for stroke. However, the risk for stroke with the retrograde approach is theoretically comparable to the risk involved with the antegrade approach. Given the ease of using the dialysis access and its relative safety, we feel that this approach with cannulation of the ascending aorta should be the standard of care. This will of

TABLE 23–3

Algorithm of DHIS Management

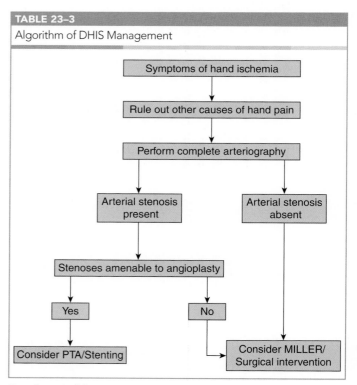

Data from Asif .[9]

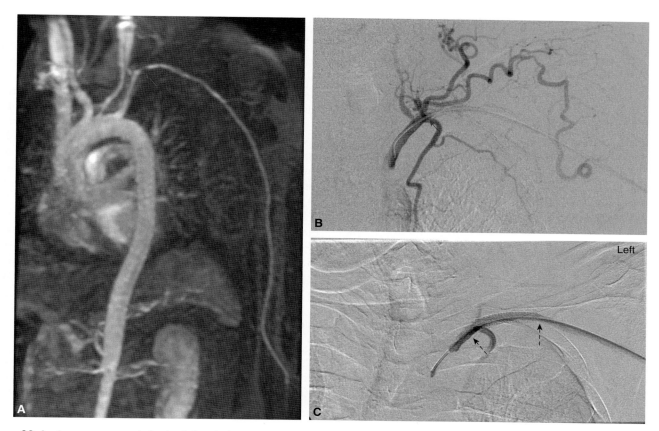

Figure 23-4. A severe stenosis in the left subclavian artery. The stenosis was present at a MR angiogram (A, red arrow) years prior, but neglected at the time of surgical creation of a left upper arm AV graft. The stenosis (B, red arrow) was identified by arteriogram via access approach, and then successfully stented (C, dotted arrows).

as it has been widely used in the investigation of arterial stenosis and general fistula/graft dysfunction.

Multidetector-row CT (MDCT) technology is making rapid advances.[37] The advantages include fast scan times, high spatial resolution, detailed anatomic reformations, and three-dimensional renderings from raw data that can quickly be reprocessed.[38] Fraioli et al compared radiation exposure and image quality during MDCT angiography and digital subtraction angiography (DSA), and found that MDCT angiography provided a substantial reduction in the radiation dosage delivered to the patient while maintaining optimal diagnostic accuracy.[40] Of course, compared to DSA, the drawback to using CT angiography is that intervention cannot be performed simultaneously as it is in DSA.

► Magnetic Resonance Angiogram

Magnetic resonance angiography (MRA) has also been useful in quantifying the severity of peripheral vascular disease and in detecting stenosis in dysfunctional hemodialysis accesses (Figure 23-4).[41–44] Duijm et al prospectively compared MRA with DSA in evaluating inflow stenosis in 6 dysfunctional AVFs and 35 AVGs in 56 men and 45 women. MRA discovered 19 arterial stenotic lesions, and DSA confirmed 18 of those lesions.[41] Although the

sensitivity of MRA is comparable to that of DSA, we no longer recommend using MRA because of the high rates of nephrogenic systemic fibrosis (NSF) associated with gadolinium use.

► Other Diagnostic Studies

Noninvasive investigation is helpful in the diagnosis. Digital blood pressure measurement, duplex ultrasonography, and transcutaneous PO_2 measurement are all useful.[7,45] Digital pressures of less than 50 mm Hg, a digit/brachial index of less than 0.6, and a $TcPO_2$ of less than 20–30 mm Hg are suggestive of ischemia.[7]

Duplex ultrasonography

Duplex ultrasonography can measure the amount of blood flow through the AVF. In addition, it can be used to evaluate stenotic and obstructive lesions in the peripheral and collateral vessels, though we would normally recommend the arteriogram as the gold standard.[7]

Digital/brachial index

A digit/brachial index (DBI) of less than 0.6 has generally been accepted to suggest risk for DHIS, but this demarcation is controversial.[7,9] In the study by Valentine et al with

109 patients, the DBI had a specificity of only 59% and a positive predictive value of 18%.[46] On the other hand, a study with 35 cases concluded that the DBI less than 0.6 on the day of surgery was a reasonable predictive risk for the symptoms of DHIS.[6]

Oxygen saturation

Oxygen saturation can be a valuable tool. Generally, a $TcPO_2$ of less than 20–30 mm Hg is suggestive of ischemia.[7] Halevy et al looked at five patients with symptoms of DHIS, and it was determined that the oxygen saturation ranged from 42% to 63% before intervention. The oxygen saturation increased to 80–100% following intervention.[47] Despite this, a digital oxygen level below which ischemic symptoms are inevitable has not been established, and oxygen saturation testing can be suggestive, but is not definitive of DHIS.[9]

Digital pressure monitoring

In most asymptomatic patients with healthy fistulas, digital pulse volume recordings show a phasic waveform that is augmented by occluding the venous limb of the fistula.[48] In the patient with DHIS, the digital systolic pressures in the fistula are usually less than 50 mm Hg, and the resting digital pulse volume recordings are flat but return to a pulsatile waveform after occlusion of the venous limb.[48] In a study by Goff et al, this group found that a digital/brachial artery pressure less than 0.6 had the best test characteristics for DHIS.[49]

However, most studies report considerable overlap in physiological test results of symptomatic and asymptomatic patients, and thus these tests should be interpreted in the context of the clinical situation.[2,49,50]

It is necessary to decide if there is true DHIS because, if present, this requires surgical intervention. Depending on the site of the AVF, various publications have suggested AVF flow and digital pressure demarcations may be helpful in identifying the presence of true DHIS.[7]

Intravascular ultrasound

Intravascular ultrasound (IVUS) is a new catheter-based imaging modality that is becoming widely accepted in cardiology to provide high-resolution cross-sectional images of the coronary arteries.[51] It requires the insertion of a catheter with a transducer embedded in its tip into a vessel and provides tomographic 2D cross-sectional images. The lumen, outer vessel wall, and stent (if implanted) can be identified and accurate measurements can be obtained. In the field of cardiology, IVUS is useful in estimating the severity of a lesion, helping in clinical decision making such as identification of a pseudoaneurysm, and helping to guide treatment such as the selection of angioplasty balloon dimensions and inflation pressures and selection of optimal stent sizes.[51] However, intravascular ultrasound techniques have not been applied to the evaluation of dialysis accesses because of the poor image quality with larger vessels.

TREATMENT

Treatment of DHIS depends on the level of symptoms and the clinical situation as well as hemodialysis adequacy. With mild symptoms, watchful waiting is all that is necessary. With more severe symptoms, percutaneous and/or surgical interventions are often necessary. The goal of the treatment is to save both limb and hemodialysis vascular access. If hemodialysis adequacy secondary to poor blood flow is in question, even in mild forms of hand ischemia, further investigation of possible etiologies is mandatory to assure the correction of underlying lesions and resolution of symptoms.

When severe DHIS with tissue loss occurs or IMN is diagnosed, immediate ligation or physiological restoration of blood flow is crucial.[52] If intervention is delayed greater than a week in patients with severe symptoms, then results are poor and intervention is likely to produce little change or improvement.[52–54]

For hand ischemia itself, the following staging system and suggested treatment are offered:

Stage 1: Conservative treatment. Watchful waiting.
Stage 2: Conservative or invasive treatment (endovascular or surgical) depending on the timing and the clinical situation.
Stage 3: Urgent invasive treatment supported by conservative measures.
Stage 4: Urgent invasive treatment supported by conservative measures. Amputation may be required.

▶ Endovascular Intervention

Once it has been decided that invasive treatment is necessary, one must decide on percutaneous versus surgical interventions (Table 23-3). As mentioned previously, arterial stenosis can be a major contributor to the symptoms of DHIS. The correction of arterial stenosis with percutaneous balloon angioplasty has been repeatedly shown to be safe and effective.[8,9] In a study by Asif et al, 12 patients were prospectively evaluated with comprehensive arteriography and percutaneous transluminal balloon angioplasty (PTA) for symptoms of DHIS. Eight of the 12 (67%) were treated with PTA alone and were symptom-free at the mean followup of 8.3 months. There were no procedure-related complications.[8] Because a good percentage of DHIS may be treated safely and effectively with PTA alone, we suggest the first step in treatment is the evaluation and treatment of arterial stenotic lesions.

Treatment of arterial stenotic lesions before consideration of surgical intervention such as banding may help to prevent dialysis access compromise.[8,55] For example, a banding procedure applied to correct DHIS in the setting of significant arterial stenosis proximal to the anastomosis can cause a critical decrease in access blood flow, culminating in access thrombosis, as has been described by DeCaprio et al.[55]

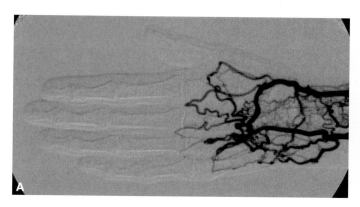
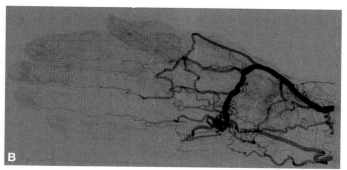

Figure 23-5. Hand blood perfusion without and with blocking the venous outflow. (**A**) While the venous outflow was not blocked, there was virtually no blood perfusion to patient's digits. (**B**) On the other hand, while the venous outflow was blocked, blood perfusion to patient's digits occurred.

▶ Surgical Options

Ligation or deconstruction of the access

The simplest and most reliable method for treating DHIS is ligation of the conduit. Clearly, the downside of this is immediate and absolute loss of the arteriovenous access. This should be avoided given that the access is the lifeline of the dialysis patient and a limited number of access options. Loss of the AV access would also mean that the patient would require an alternative, often an indwelling catheter, which has much higher risk of infection and complications.

Fistula banding

Fistula banding is a well-established surgical technique that has commonly been used to correct DHIS.[56] Banding increases resistance in the vascular access, slowing flow through the access, and thus diverting flow down the native artery[50] (Figure 23-5). Banding was first described shortly after the introduction of AV shunts for hemodialysis.[57] The biggest challenge to this technique is the increased risk of thrombosis due to reduced flow.

Estimating the correct size band to achieve the appropriate results has been problematic.[56] Because of this, surgeons have used different clinical measurements intraoperatively in attempts to predict the necessary degree of decrease in blood flow through the vascular access that will reverse symptoms of ischemia. These include measurement of distal perfusion and access blood flow.

In the Odland series, distal artery flow was monitored by digital plethysmography to achieve a digital pressure of greater than 50 mm Hg and a digital/brachial pressure index greater than 0.6.[16] In all 16 patients studied, DHIS symptoms were relieved, but only 63% (10 of 16) had satisfactory graft function for more than 6 months.[58]

Zanow et al had relatively better success in his series of 78 patients with DHIS and high fistula flow when his group tailored their banding to reduce fistula flow to 400 mL/min in autogenous grafts, and 600 mL/min in prosthetic grafts. Eighty-six percent of patients had relief of symptoms, and 91% of autogenous fistulae were patent at 12 months.[59]

Using intraoperative measures of distal perfusion and access blood flow is severely limited by the false physiological situation that general anesthesia creates.[56,58,60] Under general anesthesia, a patient's blood pressure is generally lower and heart rate usually much slower than in the normal clinical settings.

Altogether, banding with estimating the correct size band is technically difficult and requires an experienced surgeon. Many different banding techniques have been described, but the complexities in sizing the band and poor long-term outcomes have led to near abandonment of this approach.[56,61,62] Instead, procedures that reroute arterial inflow, such as distal revascularization with interval ligation (DRIL) and proximalization of the arterial inflow (PAI), are now favored.

DRIL procedure

DRIL involves ligation of the artery distal to the fistula to prevent reversal of flow in the distal artery, and a bypass graft is placed from the brachial artery well above the fistula to the antecubital or forearm artery distal to the ligation.[60] Because the DRIL procedure creates a low-resistance collateral artery to the distal arm, it improves symptoms in over 90% of patients, while also preserving fistula function in 73–100% of cases.[5,48,62–64] Drawbacks to the DRIL procedure include the fact that the entire distal arm will be dependent on a graft for blood supply and that distal anastomoses are technically difficult in patients with diffuse arterial disease (Figure 23-6 and Figure 23-7).[50]

Alternatives to the DRIL: RUDI and PAI

The revision using distal inflow (RUDI) and PAI are surgical variations on the DRIL procedure. The RUDI, or revision using distal inflow, is designed to treat DHIS in a brachial artery fistula. In contrast to ligating the native artery as in the DRIL procedure, RUDI ligates the fistula at its origin and creates a bypass to the fistula from one of the more distal forearm arteries.[65]

The proximal arterial inflow (PAI) converts the arterial supply of the arteriovenous access to a more proximal

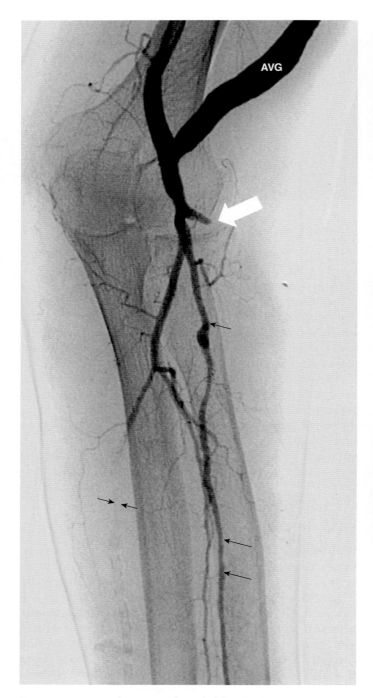

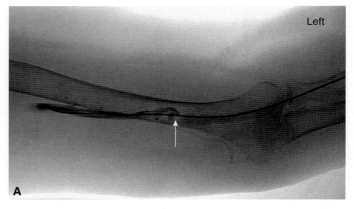

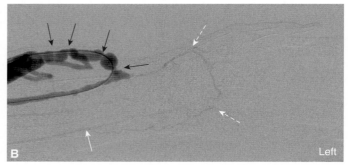

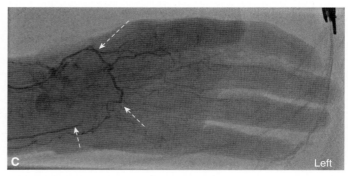

Figure 23-7. Co-existing of brachial artery stenosis with distal arteriopathy. 65-year-old with left radio-cephalic AVF, presented with left-hand DHIS. Arteriogram showed a severe stenosis in the left brachial artery (**A**, arrow), which co-exited with distal arteriopathy (**B** and **C**, white arrows) and diseased palmer arch (B and C, white dotted arrows). Juxta-anastomatic cephalic vein stenosis (B, blue arrows) was also noticed.

Figure 23-6. Distal arteriopathy. A left brachial artery to cephalic vein AV graft (AVG) with previous failed AV access (white arrow). Left ulnar artery was calcified and totally occluded (thin arrows), and left radial artery had multiple stenoses (thick arrows).

artery with higher capacity by using a small-caliber polytetraflueoroethylene graft as a feeder. It was developed as an alternative to the DRIL procedure for surgeons who are reluctant to ligate an axial artery. Concern over ligation of the axial artery lies in the fact that distal perfusion is then maintained only by the construction of an arterial bypass. Thus, the advantage to the PAI is that the natural arterial pathway is preserved (Figure 23-7).[66]

MILLER technique

First making its appearance in a cohort of 16 patients in 2006, the MILLER technique is a new, exciting procedure for the treatment of DHIS.[56,67] MILLER stands for minimally invasive limited ligation endoluminal-assisted revision, and is considered a precision modified banding procedure.[50,56,67]

The authors report four major benefits of the MILLER technique over those previously discussed. First, it is the least invasive of all current treatments. Second, the authors report that the use of an intraluminal balloon as a sizing dowel allows for band sizing with great precision, eliminating the need for complex flow and perfusion measurements.

Third, the procedure is more cost-effective than those previously discussed. And finally, the MILLER technique is easily reversed if necessary. In cases of slow blood flow or access thrombosis, the bands can be safely stretched or even broken with a larger diameter angioplasty balloon.[56]

For this procedure, an angioplasty balloon is introduced into the fistula and inflated. This balloon acts as the sizing dowel for the band creation. In the initial report by Goel et al, the site for banding required a transverse skin incision with full exposure of the access. With the even less invasive modification proposed by Miller et al, two small parallel lateral incisions are made, and a tunnel where the band will be placed is dissected subcutaneously.[56] A nonresorbable suture is then tied around the inflated balloon and vein to achieve a defined reduction in balloon diameter.[56]

In the original report by Goel et al in 2006, all 16 patients reported symptom improvement, 2 required further revision, and all were patent at the mean 3 month followup.[67]

Miller et al retrospectively analyzed 183 patients undergoing the MILLER procedure, of which 114 were being treated for steal symptoms and 69 for pathological high access flow such as congestive heart failure. The report showed complete symptomatic relief in 96% ($n = 109$ of 114) of those being treated for steal syndrome, and 100% ($n = 69$ of 69) in those being treated for pathological high access flow. The average primary patency at 6 months was 75% in those with steal syndrome. The average secondary patency at 24 months was 90% in all patients.[56]

Choice of rerouting arterial inflow (DRIL, PAI, RUDI) versus the MILLER technique

Given the limited use of the MILLER technique in clinical practice thus far, it is not established what intervention is best for treatment of DHIS. The decision will likely relate to the qualities of the vascular access causing the hand ischemia symptoms and to the overall vasculature of the patient.

Fistula banding is generally considered most appropriate for accesses with normal to high flow.[4,61,66] In fact, Miller et al reported 100% clinical success in the accesses that were treated for clinically defined pathological high access flow.[56] Both fistula banding and the MILLER technique selectively slow blood flow through the vascular access. Thus physiologically, it is practical to assume that use of these techniques would be appropriate in settings in which the original vascular access had normal to high blood flow.

On the other hand, rerouting arterial inflow with techniques such as the DRIL, PAI, or RUDI all extend the existing vascular circuit. These techniques tend to enhance total extremity flow and therefore may be better for hand ischemia caused by accesses with low flow[56] (Figure 23-8).

These techniques can be performed singly or in combination. Miller et al reported the success of three patients who underwent the MILLER technique after a DRIL procedure.[56]

PREVENTION OF DHIS WITH APPROPRIATE PRESURGICAL EVALUATION

We suggest performing the modified Allen test in both hands in order to assess the radial arterial blood supply. In this test, the patient is first asked to make a fist for about 30 seconds. Then pressure is applied over the ulnar and radial arteries to occlude them both. With the hand still elevated, then the patient's fist is opened. It should appear blanched so that pallor can be observed at the fingernails.

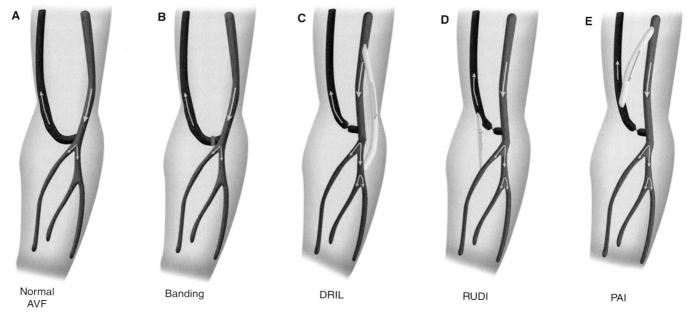

A	B	C	D	E
Normal AVF	Banding	DRIL	RUDI	PAI

Figure 23-8. Certain surgical options for treatment of DHIS.

Finally, ulnar pressure is released, and the color should return to the hand within 7 seconds. If it does not, then this is considered a negative test, and the ulnar arterial supply to the hand may be compromised. The presence of a high bifurcation of brachial artery is also an important element.[68] Preoperative assessment performed by simple ultrasound test can detect this variation and provide more information to the surgeon before the creation of an access.

SUMMARY

Distal hypoperfusion ischemic syndrome can have a wide spectrum of clinical symptoms from mild to severe. It is important for healthcare workers to immediately recognize the severe presentation of distal hypoperfusion ischemic syndrome. This can range from simply hand pain at rest and/or hand motor dysfunction to tissue loss with ulceration, necrosis, and gangrene. These presentations need immediate referral to interventionalists or surgeons. Timely referral can prevent catastrophic consequences such as amputation.

The pathophysiology of DHIS is more complex than the traditional steal syndrome. A significant proportion of cases are caused by arterial stenotic lesions. Distal arteriopathy also likely plays an important role. Because of this, we prefer the term "distal hypoperfusion ischemic syndrome" over the traditional term "arterial steal syndrome."

The clinical diagnosis of DHIS is made on history and physical examination. DHIS should be highly suspected if symptoms reverse with blocking of the access outflow tract.

Once the clinical diagnosis of DHIS is made, imaging needs to be performed to pinpoint the underlying lesion causing the symptoms. The gold standard is digital subtraction angiography where the entire arterial tree, from deep in the aortic arch to the palmar arch, is evaluated. The benefit of this approach is that the lesion can be treated during the same session as the diagnostic imaging. There are also a variety of less invasive imaging modalities available for evaluation.

Both endovascular and surgical approaches are very effective. Because percutaneous balloon angioplasty of arterial stenotic lesions has been shown to successfully treat DHIS without surgical intervention, we prefer this as the first method of intervention.

REFERENCES

1. Unek IT, Birklik M, Cavdar C, et al. Reflex sympathetic dystrophy syndrome due to arteriovenous fistula. *Hemodial Int.* 2005;9:344–348.
2. Lazarides MK, Staramos DN, Kopadis G, et al. Onset of arterial "steal" following proximal angioaccess: immediate and delayed types. *Nephrol Dial Transplant.* 2003;18: 2387–2390.
3. Miles AM. Vascular steal syndrome and ischaemic monomelic neuropathy: two variants of upper limb ischaemia after haemodialysis vascular access surgery. *Nephrol Dial Transplant.* 1999;14:297–300.
4. Lazarides MK, Staamos DN, Panagopoulos GN, et al. Indications for surgical treatment of angioaccess-induced arterial "steal." *J Am Coll Surg.* 1998;187:422–426.
5. Berman SS, Gentile AT, Glickman MH, et al. Distal revascularization-interval ligation for limb salvage and maintenance of dialysis access in ischemic steal syndrome. *J Vasc Surg.* 1997;26:393–402.
6. Papasavas PK, Reifsnyder R, Birdas TJ, et al. Prediction of arteriovenous access steal syndrome utilizing digital pressure measurements. *Vasc Endovascular Surg.* 2003;37:179–184.
7. Tordoir JHM, Dammers R, van der Sande FM. Upper extremity ischemia and hemodialysis vascular access. *Eur J Vasc Endovasc Surg.* 2004;27:1–5.
8. Asif A, Leon C, Merrill D, Bhimani B, et al. Arterial steal syndrome: a modest proposal for an old paradigm. *Am J Kidney Dis.* 2006;48:88–97.
9. Leon C, Asif A. Arteriovenous access and hand pain: the distal hypoperfusion ischemic syndrome. *Clin J Am Soc Nephrol.* 2007;2:175–183.
10. Scali ST, Huber TS. Treatment strategies for access-related hand ischemia. *Semin Vasc Surg.* 2011;24:128–136.
11. Duncan H, Ferguson L, Faris I. Incidence of the radial steal syndrome in patients with Brescia fistula for hemodialysis: its clinical significance. *J Vasc Surg.* 1986;4:144–147.
12. Kwun KB, Schanzer H, Finkler N. Hemodynamic evaluation of angioaccess procedures for hemodialysis. *Vasc Surg.* 1979;13:170–177.
13. DeMasi RJ, Gregory RT, Sorrell KA, et al. Intraoperative non-invasive evaluation of arteriovenous fistulae and grafts. The steal study [abstract]. *J Vasc Tech.* 1994;18:192.
14. Scheltinga MR, van Hoek F, and Bruinjinckx CMA. Time of onset in haemodialysis access-induced distal ischaemia (HAIDI) is related to the access type. *Nephrol Dial Transplant.* 2009;24:3198–3204.
15. Thermann F, Wollert U, Dralle H, Brauckhoff M. Dialysis shunt-associated steal syndrome with autogenous hemodialysis accesses: proposal for a new classification based on clinical results. *World J Surg.* 2008;32: 2309–2315.
16. Valji, K, Hye RJ, Roberts AC, et al. Hand ischemia in patients with hemodialysis access grafts: aniographic diagnosis and treatment. *Radiology.* 1995;196:697–701.
17. Guerra A, Raynaud A, Beyssen B, et al. Arterial percutaneous angioplasty in upper limbs with vascular access devices for haemodialysis. *Nephrol Dial Transplant.* 2002;17:843–851.
18. Derici U, El Nahas AM. Vascular calcifications in uremia: old concepts and new insights. *Semin Dial.* 2006;19: 60–68.
19. Yeager RA, Moneta GL, Edwards JM, et al. Relationship of hemodialysis access to finger gangrene in patients with end-stage renal disease. *J Vasc Surg.* 2002;36:245–249.
20. Morsy A, Kulbaski M, Chen C, Isiklar H, Lumsden AB. Incidence and characteristics of patients with hand ischemia after a hemodialysis access procedure. *J Surg Res.* 1998;74:8–10.
21. Haimov M, Baez A, Neff M, Sliftin R. Complications of arteriovenous fistulae for hemodialysis. *Arch Surg.* 1975;110:708–712.
22. Rinnaert P, Struyvan J, Mathieu J. Intermittent claudication of the hand after creation of an arteriovenous fistula in the forearm. *Am J Surg.* 1980;139:838–843.

23. Miles AM. Upper limb ischemia after vascular access surgery: differential diagnosis and management. *Semin Dial.* 2000;13:312–315.

24. Van Hoek F, Scheltinga MR, Kouwenberg I, et al. Steal in hemodialysis patients depends on type of vascular access. *Eur J Vasc Endovasc Surg.* 2006;32:710–717.

25. Yu SH, Cook PR, Canty TG, et al. Hemodialysis-related steal syndrome: predictive factors and response to treatment with the distal revascularization-interval ligation procedure. *Ann Vasc Surg.* 2008;22:210–214.

26. Kessler M, Netter P, Azoulay E, et al. Dialysis-associated arthropathy: a multicentre survey of 171 patients receiving haemodialysis for over 10 years. *Brit J Rheumatol.* 1992; 31:157–162.

27. Riggs JE, Moss AH, Labosky DA, et al. Upper extremity ischemic monomelic neuropathy: a complication of vascular access procedures in uremic diabetic patients. *Neurology.* 1989;39:997–998.

28. Miles AM. Vascular steal syndrome and ischaemic monomelic neuropathy: two variants of upper limb ischaemia after haemodialysis vascular access surgery. *Nephrol Dial Transplant.* 1997;14: 297–300.

29. Bolton CF, Driedger AA, Lindsay RM. Ischemic neuropathy in uremic patients cause by bovine arteriovenous shunt. *J Neurol Neurosurg Psychiatry.* 1979;42:810–814.

30. Milnor W. Regional circulations. In: Mountcastle VB, ed. *Medical Physiology.* St Louis: CV Mosby, 1974;993–1007.

31. Warren DJ, Otieno LS. Carbal tunnel syndrome in patients on intermittent haemodialysis. *Postgrad Med J.* 1975;51: 450–452.

32. Kessler M, Netter P, Delons S, et al. Complications articulaires chez insuffisant srenauxchroniques hemodialysis despuis plus de 10 ans (40cs). *Presse Med.* 1988;17: 679–682.

33. Vellani G, Dallari D, Fatone F, et al. Carpal tunnel syndrome in hemodialyzed patients. *Chir Organi Mov.* 1993;78: 15–18.

34. Bartova V, Zima T. Diagnosis and treatment of carpal tunnel syndrome. *Ren Fail.* 1993;15:533–537.

35. Asencio G, Rigout C, Ramperez P, et al. Hemodialysis-related lesions of the hand. *Rev Rhum Engl Ed.* 1995;62:233–240.

36. Brown EA, Arnold IR, Gower PE. Dialysis arthropathy: complication of long term treatment with hemodialysis. *Br Med J.* 1986;292:163–166.

37. Willman JK, Wildermuth S. Multidetector-row CT angiography of upper- and lower-extremity peripheral arteries. *Eur Radiol.* 2005;15:D3–D9.

38. Hiatt MD, Fleischmann D, Hellinger JC, et al. Aniographic imaging of the lower extremities with multidetector CT. *Radiol Clin North Am.* 2005;43:1119–1127.

39. Ouwendijk R, de Vries M, Pattynama PM, et al. Imaging peripheral arterial disease: a randomized controlled trial comparing contrast-enhanced MR angiography and multi-detector row CT angiography. *Radiology.* 2005;1094–1103.

40. Fraioli, F, Catalano C, Napoli A, et al. Low-dose multidetector-row CT angiography of the infra-renal aorta and lower extremity vessels: image quality and diagnostic accuracy in comparison with standard DSA. *Eur Radiol.* 2006;16:137–146.

41. Duijm LEM, Liem YS, van der Rijt RHH, et al. Inflow stenosis in dysfunctional hemodialysis access fistulae and grafts. *Am J Kidney Dis.* 2006;48:98–105.

42. Pavlovic C, Futamatsu H, Angiolillo DJ, et al. Quantitative contrast enhanced magnetic resonance imaging for the evaluation of peripheral arterial disease: a comparative study versus standard digital angiography. *Int J Cardiovasc Imaging.* 2007;23:225–232.

43. Planken RN, Torcoir JH, Dammers R, et al. Stenosis detection in forearm hemodialysis arteriovenous fistulae by multiphase contrast-enhanced magnetic resonance angiography: preliminary experience. *J Magn Reson Imaging.* 2003;17:54–64.

44. Smits JH, Bos C, Elgersma OE, et al. Hemodialysis access imaging: comparison of flow-interrupted contrast-enhanced MR angiography and digital subtraction angiography. *Radiology.* 2002;225:829–834.

45. Rutherford RB. The value of noninvasive testing before and after hemodialysis access in the prevention and management of complications. *Semin Vasc Surg.* 1997;10:157–161.

46. Valentine RJ, Bouch CW, Scott DJ, et al. Do preoperative finger pressures predict early arterial steal in hemodialysis access patients? A prospective analysis. *J Vasc Surg.* 2002;36:351–356.

47. Halevy A, Halpern Z, Negri M, et al. Pulse oximetry in the evaluation of the painful hand after arteriovenous fistula creation. *J Vasc Surg.* 1991;14:537–539.

48. Wixon CL, Hughes JD, Mills JL. Understanding strategies for the treatment of ischemic steal syndrome after hemodialysis access. *J Am Coll Surg.* 2000;191:301–310.

49. Goff CD, Sato DT, Bloch PH, DeMasi RJ, Gregory RT, Gayle RG, Parent FN, Meier GH, Wheeler JR. Steal syndrome complicating hemodialysis access procedures: can it be predicted? *Ann Vasc Surg.* 2000;14(2):138–144.

50. Zamani, P, Kaufman J, Kinlay S. Ischemic steal syndrome following arm arteriovenous fistula for hemodialysis. *Vasc Med.* 2009;14:371–376.

51. Bourantas CV, Naka KK, Garg S, et al. Clinical indications for intravascular ultrasound imaging: review article. *Echocardiography.* 2010;27:1282–1290.

52. Padberg FT, Calligaro KD, Sidaway AN. Complications of arteriovenous hemodialysis access: recognition and management. *J Vasc Surg.* 2008;48:55S–80S.

53. Redfern AB, Zimmerman ND. Neurologic and ischemic complications of upper extremity vascular access for dialysis. *J Hand Surg (AM).* 1995;20:199–204.

54. Riggs JE, Moss AH, Labosky DA, et al. Upper extremity ischemic monomelic neuropathy: a complication of vascular access procedures in uremic diabetic patients. *Neurology.* 1989;39:997–998.

55. DeCaprio JD, Valentine RJ, Kakish HB, et al. Steal syndrome complicating hemodialysis access. *Cardiovasc Surg.* 1997;5:648–653.

56. Miller GA, Goel N, Friedman A, et al. The MILLER banding procedure is an effective method for treating dialysis-associated steal syndrome. *Kidney Int.* 2010;77:359–366.

57. Quinton W, Dillard D, Scribner BH. Cannulation of blood vessels for prolonged hemodialysis. *Trans Am Soc Artif Intern Organs.* 1960;6:104–113.

58. Odland MD, Kelly PH, Ney AL, et al. Management of dialysis-associated steal syndrome complicating upper extremity arteriovenous fistulas: use of intraoperative digital photoplethysmography. *Surgery.* 1991;110:664–669.

59. Zanow J, Petzold K, Petzold M, et al. Flow reduction in high-flow arteriovenous access using intraoperative flow monitoring. *J Vasc Surg.* 2006;44:1273–1278.

60. Schanzer H, Schwartz M, Harrington E, et al. Treatment of ischemia due to "steal" by arteriovenous fistula with distal artery ligation and revascularization. *J Vasc Surg.* 1988;7:770–773.

61. Lebow MH, Cassada DC, Freeman MB, et al. Preemptive distal revascularization-interval ligation to prevent ischemic steal after hemodialysis access surgery. *J Surg Educ.* 2007;64: 171–173.

62. Mickley V. Steal syndrome—strategies to preserve vascular access and extremity. *Nephrol Dial Transplant.* 2008;23: 19–24.

63. Knox RC, Berman SS, Hughes JD, et al. Distal revascularization-interval ligation: a durable and effective treatment for ischemic steal syndrome after hemodialysis access. *J Vasc Surg.* 2002;36:250–255.

64. Schanzer H, Skladany M, Haimov M. Treatment of angioaccess-induced ischemia by revascularization. *J Vasc Surg.* 1992;16:861–864.

65. Minion DJ, Moore E, Endean E. Revision using distal inflow: a novel approach to dialysis-associated steal syndrome. *Ann Vasc Surg.* 2005;19:625–628.

66. Zanow J, Kruger U, Scholz H. Proximalization of the arterial inflow: a new technique to treat access-related ischemia. *J Vasc Surg.* 2006;43:1216–1221.

67. Goel N, Miller GA, Jotwani MC, et al. Minimally invasive limited ligation endolluminal-assisted revision (MILLER) for treatment of dialysis access-associated steal syndrome. *Kidney Int.* 2006;70:765–770.

68. Kian K, Shapiro JA, Salman L, Khan RA, Merrill D, Garcia L, Eid N, Asif A, Aldahan A, Beathard G. High brachial artery bifurcation: clinical considerations and practical implications for an arteriovenous access. *Semin Dial.* 2011 Sep 19. (the online version can be accessed at http://onlinelibrary.wiley.com/doi/10.1111/j.1525-139X.2011.00964.x/abstract)

24

PERIPHERAL ARTERIAL DISEASE

STEVEN WU & DIEGO COVARRUBIAS

1. To review the prevalence, risk factors, prevention, diagnosis, and management of peripheral arterial disease (PAD) in the chronic kidney disease (CKD) population.
2. To explore the role of PAD in hemodialysis (HD) arteriovenous (AV) access (fistula or graft) presurgical planning and dysfunction.
3. To understand the epidemiology, physiology, clinical features, assessment, imaging diagnosis, and intervention of PAD in dysfunctional HD AV access.

INTRODUCTION

Peripheral arterial disease (PAD) affects nearly 8 million Americans, and its prevalence is rapidly rising worldwide.[1] A large percentage of patients with chronic kidney disease (CKD) are commonly affected by PAD, with vasculopathy complicating the management of their underlying renal disease. For late-stage CKD patients requiring hemodialysis (HD), the establishment of a functional arteriovenous (AV) access (fistula or graft) is critical to survival, with many measurable clinical outcomes dependent on the reliability and consistency of access. Creation and maintenance of AV access is fraught with inherent challenges for HD access specialists, including interventional nephrologists, interventional radiologists, and surgeons. The presence of PAD and its risk factors in the HD population clearly further amplify these challenges, playing a key role in management decisions related to AV access.

PAD is traditionally defined as obstructive atherosclerosis of the lower extremities with an ankle-brachial index (ABI) of <0.9.[2] Given the common use of an upper extremity site for surgically created HD AV access, for this chapter, particularly for the discussion of HD AV access with concurrent PAD, we expand this definition to further include the upper extremities with symptomatic arterial luminal stenosis leading to dysfunctional AV access due to inadequate arterial inflow, and, potentially, distal ischemia. The chapter focuses on PAD in patients with AV access on HD, with a general overview of PAD in CKD patients.

PERIPHERAL ARTERIAL DISEASE IN CHRONIC KIDNEY DISEASE

▶ Prevalence of Peripheral Arterial Disease in Chronic Kidney Disease

PAD and CKD often coexist and share many cardiovascular risk factors. Diabetic nephropathy is the leading cause of CKD, and diabetes is a major risk factor for the development of PAD. Studies have shown the prevalence of PAD in CKD patients to range from 24 to 32% overall, with a 15% prevalence in patients on dialysis.[3] Conversely, patients with PAD have a high prevalence of CKD, present in up to 61% of patients with an ABI <0.89.[4] The prevalence of moderate to severe CKD increases with the severity of PAD.[5] Clinical PAD has an associated high mortality rate, up to 29% after 5 years, as well as a two- to threefold increased risk of lethal cardiovascular events.[6] Patients who suffer from PAD also demonstrate increased functional impairment and an accelerated rate of functional decline compared to nonaffected individuals.

The specific causative factors underlying the increased incidence of PAD in the CKD patient population remain unclear. It is thought that manifestations of CKD such as hyperparathyroidism, hyperphosphatemia, and chronic inflammation from prolonged uremic state contribute to the development and progression of PAD, especially in the dialysis population.[7,8]

▶ Risk Factors Associated with Peripheral Arterial Disease in Chronic Kidney Disease

Traditional risk factors for the development of PAD include smoking, diabetes, hypertension, dyslipidemia, male gender, black race, and age. CKD and end-stage renal disease (ESRD) are also considered major independent risk factors, likely representing an underestimated causative etiology.[9] The most important modifiable risk factor is tobacco use. Indeed, recent long-term studies have shown that stopping smoking reduced risk proportionately to the length of abstinence, but still not to the level of risk in never-smokers.[10,11] Strict control of diabetes, hypertension, and other associated conditions is essential for slowing progression of PAD. Obviously, nonmodifiable risk factors include gender, age, and race.

The presence of PAD clearly increases morbidity and mortality in patients with CKD. CKD patients with associated PAD are more likely to undergo limb amputation compared with the general population. Patients with concomitant PAD and CKD also have a lower event-free survival time relative to those with CKD alone.[12] Patients with PAD have a six times higher risk of death, with even asymptomatic PAD conveying an increased risk of adverse cardiovascular event.[13]

▶ Challenges in the Diagnosis and Intervention

Despite the widespread coexistence of PAD in CKD, screening for its presence is controversial, as many patients with CKD may not be candidates for intervention, such as revascularization. Even diagnosis in this population presents challenges. The diagnosis of PAD is commonly made with performance of the ABI, a noninvasive study. The abnormal ABI in PAD is due to decreased blood pressure in the lower extremity relative to the upper extremity because of arterial narrowing. In the setting of CKD, ABI may be inaccurate due to the higher likelihood of the presence of calcified vessels specific to this population. Alternative diagnostic strategies include magnetic resonance (MR) angiography and computed tomographic (CT) angiography. While both of these modalities have been shown to be reliably accurate in providing information regarding the presence and extent of vascular disease, they are not without problematic characteristics and limitations. CT uses ionizing radiation and requires the use of iodinated contrast, which is nephrotoxic and could potentially exacerbate CKD due to contrast-induced nephropathy. MR can be performed without contrast using certain parameters, but unfortunately the acquired datasets with these techniques are not as accurate as their contrast-enhanced counterparts and are rife with artifactual pitfalls. Contrast MR

angiography of the lower extremities is a highly accurate modality, which does not utilize ionizing radiation. The emergence of nephrogenic systemic fibrosis (NSF) as a complication of gadolinium use in patients with compromised renal failure has limited the continued use of MRA in the CKD population.[14,15] Patients with vascular stents pose a significant problem for evaluation with MRA as the stents will create artifacts limiting evaluation of patency and adjacent vascular segments.

Conventional angiography is the gold standard, highly accurate method for evaluation of PAD. Although invasive, it offers the distinct advantage of allowing for treatment with percutaneous transluminal angioplasty (PTA) or stenting of significant lesions discovered at the time of assessment. Disadvantages include the use of iodinated contrast and ionizing radiation, relative cost, need for patient sedation and monitoring, and the potential occurrence of associated complications. Complications of conventional angiography include bleeding, infection, and vascular injury. Major complications, though rare, do occur, and patients may require emergent surgery. Patients with CKD not yet on dialysis may not be able to safely undergo conventional angiography due to the use of iodinated contrast. In these cases, carbon dioxide can be used as a substitute contrast agent as necessary.[16]

▶ Prevention and Medical Management

The clinical manifestations of PAD lead to progressive debilitation in many patients, and morbidity and mortality is greatly increased in affected individuals. Furthermore, PAD is considered a coronary artery disease (CAD) equivalent, conveying added risks.[17] Medical management is often difficult, and current strategies focus on prevention.[18] Prevention of PAD depends on modification of risk factors. Similar to CAD, prevention of PAD entails blood pressure control, use of statins or other equivalent for control of lipids, and cessation of smoking. In diabetics, strict glucose control is imperative. A focused exercise program including up to 60 minutes of lower limb aerobic activity three times per week has been shown to improve symptoms of claudication.[19] Finally, there is evidence that antiplatelet therapy with aspirin or clopidogrel can have a positive impact on symptom reduction.[20]

Treatment of PAD in the CKD population has not specifically been studied, and the above-mentioned strategies, while applicable, have only been validated in the general population. The underlying chronic inflammatory state of CKD is postulated to accelerate the development and severity of PAD in these patients. Given this additional mechanism at play, reduction of inflammatory metabolites should be considered a primary goal in management of PAD in CKD patients.[21] In CKD patients not on dialysis, effective therapies for inflammation control are limited. In HD patients, this is achieved through adequate dialysis, with reduction of proteinuria, control of phosphorus, and optimization of PTH hormone.

PERIPHERAL ARTERIAL DISEASE IN HEMODIALYSIS ARTERIOVENOUS ACCESS

▶ Arterial Inflow and Hemodialysis Vascular Access Circuit

A brief review of AV access principles is warranted prior to discussion of the relevance of PAD in patients on HD. The HD AV access can be conceptualized as a circuit, with arterial inflow starting from the heart and flowing into the ascending aorta, to the peripheral arteries, and to the AV anastomosis. Flow continues through the fistula body (arterialized venous portion used for HD needling) or graft, and then courses through the outflow to the draining veins, progressing centrally back to the heart.[22,23] This model is helpful as it reminds the clinician that problems can arise at any point along the course of the circuit and provides a framework for systematic evaluation. Application of this concept should begin prior to AV access creation, during the process of planning for surgery. The importance of certain characteristics of the venous outflow is well known, and the veins of the extremities are duly evaluated with venography prior to surgery. Less emphasis has been placed on pre-placement arterial evaluation. The high prevalence of PAD in the CKD and HD population warrants a thorough investigation of the status of limb arteries prior to surgical construction of AV access. Although PAD is more common in the lower extremities, surgical placement of a low vascular resistance HD AV access in an upper extremity could potentially unmask subclinical arterial stenosis due to increasing demand. Compromised arterial inflow can impair AV access maturation and function and lead to hand ischemia. In the case of AV access dysfunction, the circuit model is also useful. Systematic examination of the venous outflow, the AV access itself (fistula body or graft), and the arterial inflow is critical to ensure the best possible outcomes. For example, outflow stenoses are commonly encountered and easily treated, therefore rarely neglected. However, successful treatment of an outflow stenosis without addressing the less obvious and more often neglected presence of a compromised inflow will not completely resolve the underlying clinical issues.

▶ Presurgical Evaluation of Artery for AV Fistula or Graft Creation

Evaluation prior to surgical creation of AV access begins with a detailed history. Patients should be questioned regarding ischemic symptoms, such as claudication, the presence of cold hands or feet, and rest pain. History of previous surgery or trauma to the extremities should be recorded, as well as a history of prior failed AV access. Physical exam should include measurement of blood pressure bilaterally, with careful attention to the presence of discrepancies. A significantly lower blood pressure in one limb relative to the other may reflect the presence of PAD. The Allen's test should be performed to verify adequate radial and ulnar arterial supply to the hand.

Following thorough history and physical, any prior imaging studies should be reviewed, as these could potentially demonstrate vascular lesions or abnormalities that would predispose to AV access failure. The widespread acceptance of PACS and the longitudinal storage of historical studies have facilitated this process. Studies performed for other reasons in the past may not address lesions that could be important in the consideration of AV access planning. Recognizing the presence of such abnormalities is a cost-effective and time-saving method of avoiding unnecessary surgery and preserving limited resources (see Figure 24-1).

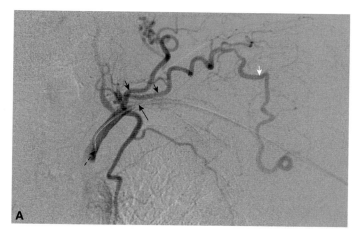

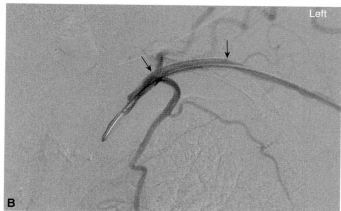

Figure 24-1. A 68-year-old male with CKD Stage 5 on hemodialysis, presented with thrombosis of left brachio-antecubital looped AV graft, which was created 6 month prior. Despite of successful declot with adequate angioplasty of a stenosis at venous-graft anastomosis, the graft kept thrombosis. Patient's previous imaging studies were retrieved and reviewed via the PACS system; interestingly, a severe left subclavian artery stenosis was diagnosed through a MR angiography 4 years prior and the stenosis was left untreated due to lacking of hand ischemia. Apparently, surgical creation of AVG was performed without complete reviewing of history and imaging studies. (**A**) Left subclavian arteriogram with a Kumpe catheter (long dot arrow) placed in the proximal left subclavian artery. The arteriogram showed a near-occlusion stenosis in the left subclavian artery (long solid arrow) with large collaterals (short arrows). (**B**) The stenosis was successfully treated with angioplasty and stenting (arrow). The graft became thrombosis-free since.

If prior imaging studies are not available or unhelpful, dedicated imaging for the purpose of surgical planning can be obtained. Similar to the evaluation of PAD, available diagnostic modalities include sonography, CTA, MRA, and digital subtraction angiography (DSA). These will be further addressed in a later section of this chapter.

Documentation of suitable vessels is essential prior to AV access creation. The minimal diameter of the artery that can successfully be utilized for AV access should be greater than or equal to 2 mm.[24] Consensus on minimal venous size is less certain, but most authors advocate a minimum diameter of 2.5 mm for AV fistulas and 4 mm for grafts.[25,26] Imaging studies can provide information regarding lesions such as arterial calcification burden or central venous stenosis. A seemingly insignificant lesion may become hemodynamically significant after AV access creation when exposed to the demanding flow rates of dialysis, leading to access failure or even limb ischemia. Treatment of pre-existing lesions with PTA and/or stenting can allow for successful creation of AV access.

▶ Postsurgical Complications

Surgical creation of AV access is not without potential complications. These include typical complications relevant to vascular surgeries in general, such as infection and bleeding or hematoma formation. Additionally, there can be resultant nerve damage or hand ischemia. If a pre-existing arterial lesion existed and was either unknown or unaddressed, thrombosis of the newly created access is a recognized possibility. This can also occur due to problems with the venous outflow, again tying in to the model of AV access as a functional circuit. Complications specific to the AV access are detailed below.

Early failure of AV access due to inadequate arterial inflow

As mentioned previously, compromise of arterial inflow can have a host of negative results on the AV access. These range from thrombosis, to failure of maturation, to complete failure, to hand ischemia. Adequate inflow is imperative for the AV access circuit to function properly. The causes of poor inflow are multifactorial, including the existence of pre-existing lesions and surgical complications. The tenuous status of the distal limb arteries may drive some surgeons to pursue a conservative approach in the creation of the access. While factors such as arterial diameter, degree of calcification/atherosclerosis, and the general health of the feeding arteries are usually not directly in the surgeon's control, difficulties in these areas can usually be avoided with a complete pre-procedure evaluation. The experience and skill of the surgeon is a key factor in the success of viable AV access creation.[27] An experienced surgeon will possess familiarity with the characteristics of a suitable AV access and will be more successful in facilitating their creation. Also, the experienced surgeon is less likely to create problematic juxta-anastomotic lesions by careful handling of the artery, thus avoiding possible contributors to AV access failure or dysfunction.

Steal phenomena

A commonly encountered situation following surgical AV access creation is the steal phenomenon. This is characterized by the presence of retrograde flow (ie, flow into the AV access and away from the distal limb) in the arterial segments distal to the anastomosis. The steal phenomenon occurs in a majority of patients with surgical AV access, but is rarely symptomatic or associated with ischemia. It can be seen in the immediate post-surgical period and can persist indefinitely. There is no proven significant association with steal phenomenon and early AV access failure or dysfunction.[28] Although steal phenomena is common in functional AV access, it usually associated with steal syndrome as well (see Figure 24-2).

Steal syndrome

The so-called steal syndrome in the setting of AV access is actually a misnomer. While some cases are indeed caused

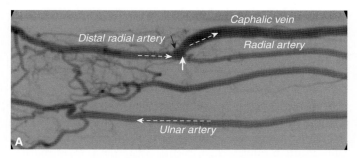

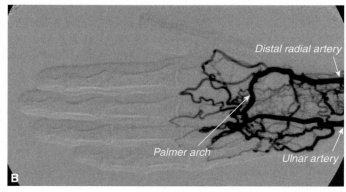

Figure 24-2. A 60-year-old hemodialysis patient with a right radio-cephalic AV fistulae, presented with cold and painful right hand. DHHIS was suspected. The aortogram, the right subclavian arteriogram, and run-offs were performed. (**A**) Steal phenomena was confirmed by observing blood flow (dotted arrows) from ulnar artery to palmar arch to distal radial artery to the AV anastomosis (blue arrow) and then to the cephalic vein. There was an occlusive stenosis (short solid arrow) in the radial artery immediately proximal to the AV anastomosis. (**B**) Although palmar arch (long arrow) was intact, digits of the right hand are virtually lacking of blood perfusion due to the stenosis in the radial artery as mentioned above (A, short solid arrow).

by high-flow AV fistulas essentially sucking blood away from the more distal extremity leading to clinically significant ischemia, the overwhelming majority is due to underlying arterial disease.[29] The more descriptive and perhaps better-suited nomenclature of distal hypoperfusion hand ischemia syndrome (DHHIS) is synonymous with steal syndrome.[30] The condition has also been referred to as dialysis-associated steal syndrome.[31] DHHIS may present with extremity pallor, decreased temperature, parasthesia, pain, and diminished pulses distal to the fistula. Urgent evaluation and immediate attention is required when the condition is suspected, as failure to recognize this entity can lead to potential tissue or limb loss. The diagnosis is clinically straightforward, with immediate relief or reversal of symptoms when the AV access is manually blocked. The goal of treatment is to save both the distal limb and the access, and begins with determination of the underlying cause, necessitating angiography. In cases due to high flow, the flow to the AV access can be restricted, whether by surgical restriction or banding or recently by the MILLER procedure. In cases due to arterial disease, one should focus on finding and treating underlying arterial stenoses to preserve both the affected limb and the HD AV access. This again emphasizes the importance of PAD in this specific population as well as the need for a complete evaluation of the arteries prior to surgery (see Figure 24-2).

PERIPHERAL ARTERIAL DISEASE IN DYSFUNCTIONAL HEMODILAYSIS ARTERIOVENOUS ACCESS

▶ Epidemiology

Despite the known association of PAD with the CKD/HD patient population, traditionally arterial inflow stenoses were considered to be a rare cause of dysfunctional AV access, estimated to occur in 0–4% of patients.[32] A vascular stenosis is defined as a greater than or equal to 50% reduction in luminal diameter relative to adjacent normal vessel. Analysis of the recent literature provides evidence that arterial stenosis is actually relatively common, with an incidence ranging from 14 to 42% depending on definitions.[33] While a large percentage of these were anastomotic lesions, up to one-third were due to PAD, involving the more proximal feeding arteries, from the subclavian artery to just before the level of the anastomosis. A higher incidence of inflow stenoses is seen in forearm AV access compared to the upper arm location.[34] Also, a higher incidence of these lesions is seen in fistulas than grafts.[35] Most commonly, nonanastomotic stenoses are seen in the subclavian artery, followed by the radial artery.[36] The likelihood of arterial lesions increases with increasing age.[37] Arterial stenoses are likely a significantly under-recognized and therefore undertreated source of AV access dysfunction.

Perhaps the major challenge in diagnosing and treating nonanastomotic arterial stenoses lies in the lack of a standardized algorithmic approach to evaluation. Physical examination often fails to detect clinically significant lesions. Common interventional practice is to use the fistula or graft itself as the point of access for diagnosis or treatment, facilitating assessment of the venous outflow and anastomosis. This approach allows for relatively simple and straightforward treatment of lesions on the venous side of the AV access circuit, while discouraging analysis of the complete arterial inflow due to the added procedural complexity. Furthermore, a complete evaluation of the arterial inflow should include the ipsilateral subclavian artery, a time-consuming endeavor that carries unique complications, such as acute neurovascular event and spinal cord injury. Interventions performed on arterial lesions typically have excellent results, with an up to 20% increase of flow in 90% of cases.

Due to the nature of current practice patterns, many interventionalists may deem depiction of the entire arterial tree in every patient unfeasible. However, given the excellent clinical results of endovascular PTA or stenting of arterial stenoses, the presence of arterial disease should be sought in certain high-risk patients. Venous stenoses coexist with arterial lesions up to 54% of the time in patients with fistulas and up to as high as 100% of the time in patients with grafts.[38] If poor blood flow persists after adequate treatment of the venous stenoses, this is a sensitive and specific sign that should prompt thorough investigation of the entire arterial inflow.[38] Noninvasive imaging methods such as Duplex ultrasound and CTA also play a role in evaluation of the arterial inflow, and may further help select patients that require complete angiographic assessment.

▶ Pathophysiology

The pathogenesis of arterial inflow stenosis in dysfunctional AV access remains unclear and is likely multifactorial. An exact causal relationship can be difficult to elucidate, with some degree of disease likely present prior to surgical creation of the access in a proportion of cases and others likely due to the high-flow state the vessels endure under regular hemodialysis.[39] A combination of these mechanisms is also a possibility. Studies have clearly documented the presence of pre-existing stenoses in the HD population with surgically created AV access.[40] Unfortunately, no studies have followed these lesions through initiation of dialysis nor are there studies that have demonstrated how or when the high-flow state of HD causes its effects on healthy native arteries.

The underlying lesions leading to arterial stenoses include neointimal hyperplasia and atherosclerotic plaques, both calcified and noncalcified.[41] The altered physiologic state during hemodialysis contributes to both initiation and accelerated progression of these lesions, likely due to its inflammatory nature.[42] As these lesions develop and advance in severity, they lead to luminal narrowing and eventually stenosis. Stenosis leads to decreased blood flow to the extremity and AV access, resulting in dysfunction, and, potentially, distal ischemia.

▶ Clinical Features and Assessment

Clinical features of dysfunctional AV access secondary to arterial inflow stenosis include infiltration of the access, poor clearance, poor blood flow, increasing negative arterial pressure, thrombosis, and distal ischemia. Physical examination, as previously mentioned, is somewhat limited. The AV access will usually have a weak thrill with decreased tension. Manual blockage of the venous outflow can cause significant augmentation of tension in this setting, and in the setting of distal ischemia, cause reversal of symptoms. A discrepancy in blood pressures of the limbs may be seen if the lesion in question involves the more central arterial tree. In some cases presenting without clinical hand ischemia, the signs and symptoms that suggest arterial inflow stenosis can be nonspecific, and the fact that venous disease frequently coexists with arterial disease renders them less likely to be appreciated as well. A high index of suspicion and attention to subtle changes are the key to the diagnosis of arterial inflow stenosis. After successful and complete treatment of the venous stenoses, persistence of clinical features of inadequate arterial inflow as mentioned above, or observation of sluggish flow on postangioplasty angiogram warrants further investigation of the inflow/arterial tree. While clinical assessment can raise the index of suspicion for the presence of a problem on the arterial side of the AV access circuit, the mainstay of diagnosis is via imaging.

▶ Imaging

As with diagnostic imaging evaluation of PAD in general, the assessment of the vascular system in patients with problematic AV access can be performed using various modalities. Each has its own advantages and disadvantages, and while noninvasive studies may provide a diagnosis, treatment will typically require either endovascular intervention or surgery. Conventional angiography in the form of a fistulogram or graftogram is an acceptable first option for evaluation of dysfunctional AV access as it provides both a diagnosis and the potential to render treatment simultaneously.

Noninvasive modalities include Duplex sonography, CT angiography, and MR angiography. Duplex sonography has the advantage of low cost and nearly universal availability, as well as the ability to quantify flow velocity and direction in real time.[43] Limitations include inability to evaluate the central vasculature and heavy operator dependence. Sonography is particularly useful for direct visualization of the anastomosis as this is often superficial. CT angiography provides excellent spatial resolution and allows for visualization of the entire arterial tree as well as the venous outflow (see Figure 24-3 and Figure 24-4). Three-dimensional reconstruction of the acquired data is also possible, increasing diagnostic accuracy (see Figure 24-4). CT is also widely available and technically does not depend on the operator for

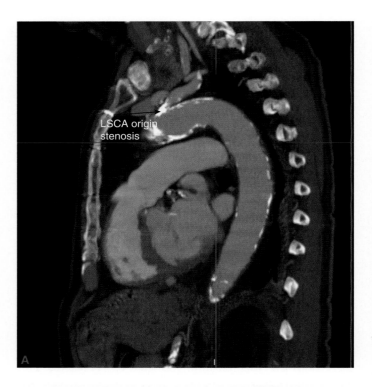

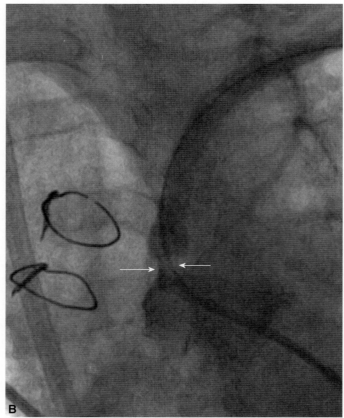

Figure 24-3. (**A**) CT angiogram identified a possible stenosis at the origin of the left subclavian artery (arrow). (**B**) The stenosis (arrows) was confirmed by an arteriogram via the right femoral artery approach.

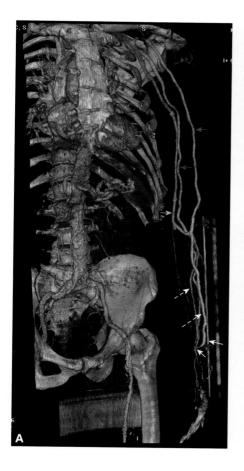
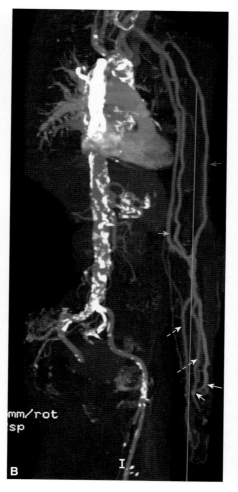
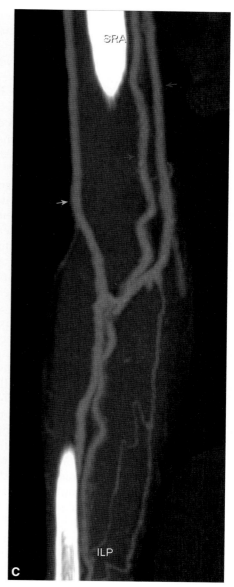

Figure 24-4. CT angiography with 3D reconstruction (**A**, **B**, **C**) demonstrating detailed arterial and venous structures of the left arm. Red arrow: the left brachial artery; blue arrow: the cephalic vein of the left upper arm; yellow arrow: the basilica vein of the left upper arm; long solid white arrow: the cephalic vein of the left forearm; short solid white arrow: the AV anastomosis; long dotted white arrow: the left radial artery; and short dotted white arrow: the left ulnar artery.

high-quality images. Image acquisition is rapid, allowing for better patient tolerance. The major disadvantage of CT is the use of ionizing radiation, although this has been somewhat mitigated in the present era by the recent acceptance of low-dose protocols.[44] CT angiography requires the use of intravenous contrast, which in the HD AV access population does not pose a problem as renal function is not a concern. MR angiography is similar to CT in respect of its ability to depict the entire AV access circuit, including the central vasculature. For diagnostic purposes, use of intravenous contrast is required. Unfortunately, the recognition of the association of NSF with poor clearance of gadolinium has limited the use of MR in the HD population.[45] MR also demands longer imaging times relative to CT, which may be difficult for elderly patients. Additionally, many HD patients have co-morbid conditions that may preclude exposure to a magnetic field, such as an indwelling pacemaker.

▶ Locations and Types of Lesions

Lesions can be classified according to location and/or type. Locations include central and feeding artery, juxta-anastomotic, and distal arterial stenoses. Types include lesions due to intrinsic factors such as underlying atherosclerosis, PAD, etc, versus those due to external factors, such as compression by adjacent anatomic structures. The degree of stenosis is usually described as mild, moderate, or severe. A severe stenosis is usually obviously hemodynamically significant, but the lower grades are not so easily qualifiable. In other words, radiological mild to moderate arterial stenoses may not convey a hemodynamic abnormality. In the nondialysis population especially, clinically insignificant mild to moderate stenoses may be the norm.[46] In HD patients, even a mild arterial stenosis can be problematic if it limits the inflow to the AV access or causes limb ischemia. Further adding to the difficulty in clarifying the actual clinical effects of a stenosis is the fact that there are no reliable signs or symptoms to assist in differentiation. Typically, the only recourse is to treat the lesion and observe whether the problem with the AV access resolves; if so, then it can be concluded that the treated lesion was the cause.

Anastomotic and juxta-anastomotic locations are by far the most common regions for the development of arterial stenoses in the setting of HD AV access. Together these represent approximately 50% of lesions.[47] Stenoses of the central and feeding arteries are not uncommon, accounting for up to roughly 30–40% of lesions.[48] Diagnosis of these lesions during fistulogram or graftogram can be problematic, as a retrograde injection has a limited coverage, useful for evaluating only the arteries adjacent to the AV access itself. If the index of suspicion for a central lesion is high, diagnosis may require retrograde cannulation of the aorta through the AV access to perform aortagraphy and runoff. An alternative is to use an antegrade approach via femoral artery puncture (see Figure 24-5). These maneuvers incur greater risk, including complications such as stroke and spinal cord injury due to the potential for showering of clot or debris into the carotid or vertebral arteries.

Distal arterial stenoses are less frequently encountered but are not uncommon. The association of PAD and general vasculopathy with the CKD/HD patient population predisposes these patients to diffuse arterial disease. While the distal lesion may not affect the AV access function, the potential for clinically significant events such as hand ischemia or tissue loss in the limb make recognition of such lesions important. Distal arterial stenoses often coexist with abnormalities of the venous outflow. If these are treated without awareness of distal arterial disease, the interventionalist can inadvertently trigger a steal phenomenon in which the newly treated AV access shunts blood away from the more distal territories supplied by the diseased arterial segments because of markedly lower resistance to flow. A thorough retrograde angiogram of the anastomosis and adjacent arteries and post-procedure examination of hand should be included in the evaluation of a dysfunctional AV access to ensure avoidance of this scenario (see Figure 24-6).

External compression of the venous outflow or arterial inflow by anatomic structures such as an enlarged aorta or a cervical rib is rare causes of AV access dysfunction. Treatment of these lesions via an endovascular approach will inevitably fail, as the underlying compressing structure cannot be addressed in this way. Surgical decompression is required. Occasionally, an arterial stenosis at the AV anastomosis and/or the juxta-anastomotic region of a previous failed AV access in the same limb acts as the direct cause of failure of a functional downstream HD AV access and/or hand ischemia.

▶ Treatment

Endovascular intervention is the norm for treatment of arterial inflow stenoses. In some cases, an endovascular approach is not possible, such as in the severe or occlu-

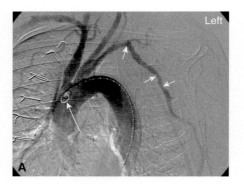

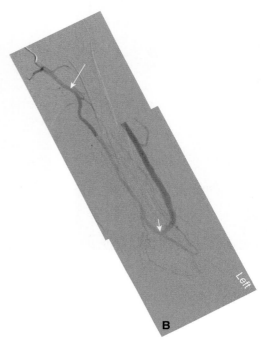

Figure 24-5. (A) Aortogram via a femoral approach. A pigtail catheter (long white arrow) was placed into the ascending aorta, and aortogram was performed. Multiple stenoses (short white arrows) were identified. **(B)** Selective left axillary arteriogram and run-offs. Long arrow: the left axillary artery; short arrow: the AV anastomosis.

sive stenosis that cannot be recanalized with a guide wire (Figure 24-7). In these cases, surgical bypass graft is a satisfactory option with a reasonable patency rate. Endovascular treatments have excellent long-term results and safety profile compared to surgery.[49] Recurrence of an arterial inflow stenosis appear to occur at very low rates, with many studies documenting no need for additional interventions within their specified follow-up periods after successful angioplasty or stenting.[50] An additional advantage is that treatment can be delivered in the same session as diagnosis.

Percutaneous transluminal angioplasty (PTA)

PTA is the main weapon in the endovascular arsenal. It is used on both arterial and venous stenoses. On the venous side, angioplasty usually requires an oversized

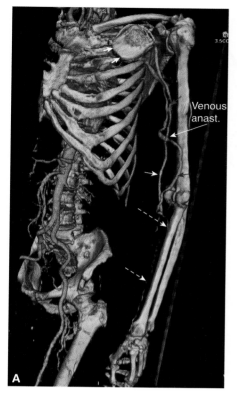
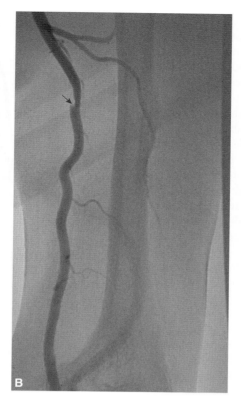
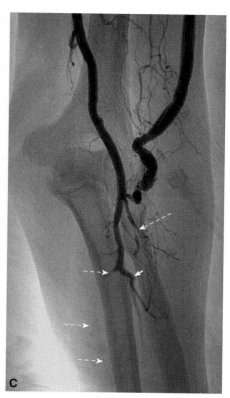

Figure 24-6. A 75-year-old male with a left brachial artery to left basilic vein AV graft (blue arrow), presented with ischemic left hand with fingertips necrosis after angioplasty of venous stenosis at the venous anastomosis (**A**, solid long white arrow) and the left subclavian vein (the stenosis in the left subclavian vein was induced by a pacer). The hand ischemia was induced by increasing flow to the graft after angioplasties on the basis of severe distal arterial disease, such as radial artery stenosis (long dot arrows) and ulnar artery stenosis (short dot arrow), as well as the proximal feeding artery stenosis (A and B, red arrows). The hand was only perfused by the left interosseous artery (**C**, short solid arrow).

balloon under high pressure with longer durations of inflation to achieve acceptable results. On the arterial side, the balloon should be sized according to the vessel diameter, lower pressures are required, and less inflation time is necessary.[51] These differences in approach to PTA are due to natural factors, such as the compliance of the vessels and potential for complications among others. PTA of arterial lesions carries a higher risk profile, with associated complications including dissection, occlusion, thrombosis, distal embolization, and arterial rupture.[52]

Pseudo-aneurysm formation at the procedure puncture site (ie, common femoral artery, etc) may also occur.

Stent placement

Stents are an adjunct to PTA, providing a treatment option when significant residual stenosis or a resistant lesion is seen after or during angioplasty. Additionally, should complications such as dissection or rupture of the artery arise due to PTA attempts, stents can be used to quickly and safely

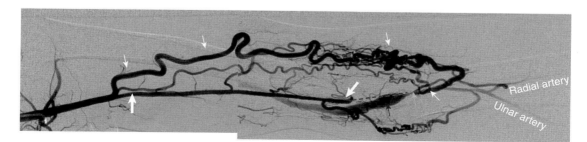

Figure 24-7. A 43-year-old female with a left brachio-cephalic AV fistula, which was not maturing. Left-arm arteriogram showed a total occlusion (short fat arrow) of the left brachial artery (long fat arrow) with enlarged and torturous profunda brachii (thin white arrow) and many collaterals. Red dot line: occluded brachial artery; blue arrow: the cephalic vein; yellow arrow: arteriovenous anastomosis.

treat these lesions while preserving the native vascular channels and the AV access. The most common stent varieties are bare metal and covered systems. Other options include self-expanding and balloon mounted. Each variety or combination thereof offers its own advantages and disadvantages, such as differences in patency rates, precision of delivery, delivery systems, etc. Although a complete review of the characteristics of stents is beyond the scope of this chapter, a few significant principles are worth mentioning. For peripheral arterial lesions, balloon-mounted stents should generally be avoided due to the concern of stent fracture/malfunction from the high degree of external force encountered. Self-expandable stents are preferred in this setting because of their generally greater tensile and radial strength. In addition, the placement of stents across joints or points of flexion should as rule be avoided whenever possible. Repeated motion in these locations can theoretically cause stent occlusion or fracture. Obviously, if complications occur during angioplasty, a self-expanding covered stent is a reasonable option regardless of anatomic location. Bare metal stent appear to be less problematic in the arterial system relative to the venous system and are commonly used for resistant or recoiling stenosis.[53]

Endovascular approaches

The interventionalist can choose to access the arterial tree via a number of approaches. Commonly, the AV access itself is cannulated, and the upstream arteries are accessed in a retrograde fashion. This has been proven to be a safe and effective approach, with the advantages addressed earlier in the chapter. Utilizing the AV access as the site of cannulation site also avoids complications associated with arterial puncture, such as pseudoaneurysm formation. Other possible routes include common femoral, upstream arterial, and downstream arterial approaches (see Figure 24-8). Studies have shown that the antegrade approach is associated with detecting a higher degree of luminal stenosis, with retrograde angiography underestimating the presence of inflow lesions by up to 20% in comparison.[54] Regardless of the chosen approach, the principles of angiography are the same: access is gained, and a guide wire and catheter system are used to cannulate the vessel of interest under fluoroscopic guidance, allowing for injection of contrast material.

Anticoagulation therapy

Standard use of anticoagulation during angiographic intervention varies by institution. Although anticoagulation therapy with heparin is usually not required, the interventionalist may choose to administer a dose prior to angioplasty. If stents are placed, antiplatelet therapy with aspirin and clopidrogel will be initiated after the procedure.

SUMMARY

Arterial disease plays a significant role in AV access dysfunction. The high association of PAD with the CKD/HD population underscores the prevalence of arterial

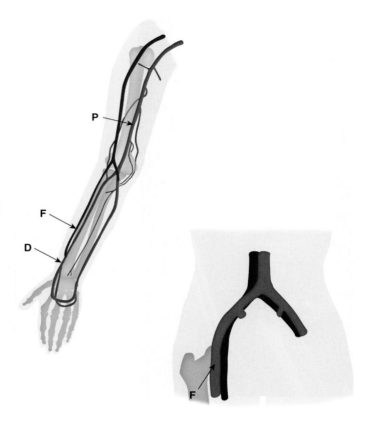

Figure 24-8. Investigation of arterial tree via different cannulation approaches. F: via femoral artery, antegrade approach; F: via fistula or graft retrograde approach; P: via proximal artery approach; D: via distal artery approach.

lesions in this setting. While treatment of arterial stenoses with an endovascular approach such as PTA or stenting usually has excellent results, diagnosis can pose a significant challenge. Noninvasive imaging may help to clarify the situation in certain cases, but the gold standard of diagnosis remains angiography. Complete evaluation of the arterial tree, including the central arteries and feeding arteries as well as the juxta-anastomotic region is important but may be time consuming and not without risk. A combination of clinical and noninvasive imaging findings can help stratify patients that require thorough arterial evaluation. The interventionalist should be familiar with the multitude of available approaches to arterial diagnosis, as well as the potential complications. Also, a thorough understanding of the characteristics of arterial stenoses will allow the interventionalist to deliver the best possible solution while minimizing adverse outcomes.

REFERENCES

1. Mukherjee D, Cho L. Peripheral arterial disease: considerations in risks, diagnosis, and treatment. *J Natl Med Assoc*. 2009;101(10):999–1008.
2. Stephanie S. DeLoach, Emile R. Mohler, III. Peripheral arterial disease: a guide for nephrologists. *Clin J Am Soc Nephrol*. 2007;2:839–846.

3. Selvin E, Erlinger TP. Prevalence of and risk factors for peripheral arterial disease in the United States: results from the National Health and Nutrition Examination Survey, 1999–2000. *Circulation.* 2000;110:738–743.

4. O'Hare AM. High prevalence of peripheral arterial disease in persons with renal insufficiency: results from the National Health and Nutrition Examination Survey. *Circulation.* 2004;109:320–323.

5. Wattanakit K, Folsom AR, Selvin E, Coresh J, Hirsch AT, Weatherley BD. Kidney function and risk of peripheral arterial disease: results from the Atherosclerosis Risk in Communities (ARIC) Study. *J Am Soc Nephrol.* 2000;18:629–636.

6. Hirsch AT, Criqui MH, Treat-Jacobson D. Peripheral arterial disease detection, awareness, and treatment in primary care. *JAMA.* 2000;286:1317–1324.

7. Boaz M, Weinstein T, Matas Z, Green MS, Smetana S. Peripheral vascular disease and serum phosphorus in hemodialysis: a nested case-control study. *Clin Nephrol.* 2005;63:98–105.

8. Cooper BA, Penne EL, Bartlett LH, Pollack CA. Protein malnutrition and hypoalbuminemia as predictors of vascular events and mortality in ESRD. *Am J Kidney Dis.* 2004;43:61–66.

9. Schiffrin EL, Lipman ML, Mann JF. Chronic kidney disease: effects on the cardiovascular system. *Circulation.* 2007;116(1):85–97.

10. Conen D, Everett BM, Kurth T, Creager MA, Buring JE, Ridker PM, Pradhan AD. Smoking, smoking status, and risk for symptomatic peripheral artery disease in women: a cohort study. *Ann Intern Med.* 2011;154(11):719–726.

11. Suriñach JM, Alvarez LR, Coll R, Carmona JA, Sanclemente C, Aguilar E, Monreal M. FRENA Investigators. Differences in cardiovascular mortality in smokers, past-smokers and non-smokers: findings from the FRENA registry. *Eur J Intern Med.* 2009;20(5):522–526. Epub 2009 Jun 12.

12. Ungprasert P, Pornratanarangsi S. Correlation between peripheral arterial disease and stage of chronic kidney disease. *J Med Assoc Thai.* 2011;94(suppl 1):S46–S50.

13. Suominen V, Uurto I, Saarinen J, Venermo M, Salenius J. PAD as a risk factor for mortality among patients with elevated ABI—a clinical study. *Eur J Vasc Endovasc Surg.* 2010;39(3):316–322. Epub 2010 Jan 20.

14. Abu-Alfa AK. Nephrogenic systemic fibrosis and gadolinium-based contrast agents. *Adv Chronic Kidney Dis.* 2011;18(3):188–198.

15. Wang Y, Alkasab TK, Narin O, Nazarian RM, Kaewlai R, Kay J, Abujudeh HH. Incidence of nephrogenic systemic fibrosis after adoption of restrictive gadolinium-based contrast agent guidelines. *Radiology.* 2011;260(1):105–111. Epub 2011 May 17.

16. Hawkins IF, Cho KJ, Caridi JG. Carbon dioxide in angiography to reduce the risk of contrast-induced nephropathy. *Radiol Clin North Am.* 2009;47(5):813–825, v–vi.

17. Parikh SV, Saya S, Divanji P, Banerjee S, Selzer F, Abbott JD, Naidu SS, Wilensky RL, Faxon DP, Jacobs AK, Holper EM. Risk of death and myocardial infarction in patients with peripheral arterial disease undergoing percutaneous coronary intervention (from the National Heart, Lung and Blood Institute Dynamic Registry). *Am J Cardiol.* 2011;107(7):959–964. Epub 2011 Jan 20.

18. Weinberg MD, Lau JF, Rosenfield K, Olin JW. Peripheral artery disease. Part 2: medical and endovascular treatment. *Nat Rev Cardiol.* 2011;8(8):429–441.

19. Parmenter BJ, Raymond J, Dinnen P, Singh MA. A systematic review of randomized controlled trials: walking versus alternative exercise prescription as treatment for intermittent claudication. *Atherosclerosis.* 2011;218(1):1–12.

20. Poredos P, Jezovnik MK. Antiplatelet and antithrombotic treatment of patients with peripheral arterial disease. *Int Angiol.* 2010;29(1):20–26.

21. Luo Y, Li X, Li J, Wang X, Xu Y, Qiao Y, Hu D, Ma Y. Peripheral arterial disease, chronic kidney disease, and mortality: the Chinese Ankle Brachial Index Cohort Study. *Vasc Med.* 2010;15(2):107–112. Epub 2010 Feb 4.

22. Beathard GA. Percutaneous transvenous angioplasty in the treatment of vascular access stenosis. *Kidney Int.* 1992;42:1390.

23. Beathard, GA. Physical examination of AV grafts. *Semin Dial.* 1992;5:74.

24. Ives CL, Akoh JA, George J, et al. Pre-operative vessel mapping and early post-operative surveillance duplex scanning of arteriovenous fistulae. *J Vasc Access.* 2009;10:37.

25. Lauvao LS, Ihnat DM, Goshima KR, Chavez L, Gruessner AC, Mills JL Sr. Vein diameter is the major predictor of fistula maturation. *J Vasc Surg.* 2009;49(6):1499–1504.

26. Beathard GA. Interventionalist's role in identifying candidates for secondary fistulas. *Semin Dial.* 2004;17(3):233–236.

27. Fassiadis N, Morsy M, Siva M, Marsh JE, Makanjuola AD, Chemla ES. Does the surgeon's experience impact on radiocephalic fistula patency rates? *Semin Dial.* 2007;20(5):455–457.

28. Duncan H, Ferguson L, Faris I. Incidence of the radial steal syndrome in patients with Brescia fistula for hemodialysis: its clinical significance. *J Vasc Surg.* 1986;4(2):144–147.

29. Salman L, Maya ID, Asif A. Current concepts in the pathophysiology and management of arteriovenous access-induced hand ischemia. *Adv Chronic Kidney Dis.* 2009;16(5):371–377. Review.

30. Leon C, Asif A. Arteriovenous access and hand pain: the distal hypoperfusion ischemic syndrome. *Clin J Am Soc Nephrol.* 2007;2(1):175–183.

31. Malik J, Tuka V, Kasalova Z, Chytilova E, Slavikova M, Clagett P, Davidson I, Dolmatch B, Nichols D, Gallieni M. Understanding the dialysis access steal syndrome. A review of the etiologies, diagnosis, prevention and treatment strategies. *J Vasc Access.* 2008;9(3):155–166. Review.

32. Long B, Brichart N, Lermusiaux P, Turmel-Rodrigues L, Artru B, Boutin JM, Pengloan J, Bertrand P, Bruyère F. Management of perianastomotic stenosis of direct wrist autogenous radial-cephalic arteriovenous accesses for dialysis. *J Vasc Surg.* 2011;53(1):108–114. Epub 2010 Sep 22.

33. Kumakura H, Kanai H, Aizaki M, Mitsui K, Araki Y, Kasama S, Iwasaki T, Ichikawa S. The influence of the obesity paradox and chronic kidney disease on long-term survival in a Japanese cohort with peripheral arterial disease. *J Vasc Surg.* 2010;52(1):110–117. Epub 2010 May 15.

34. Bonforte G, Rossi E, Auricchio S, Pogliani D, Mangano S, Mandolfo S, Galli F, Genovesi S. The middle-arm fistula as a valuable surgical approach in patients with end-stage renal disease. *J Vasc Surg.* 2010;52(6):1551–1556. Epub 2010 Aug 25.

35. Schild AF, Perez E, Gillaspie E, Seaver C, Livingstone J, Thibonnier A. Arteriovenous fistulae vs. arteriovenous grafts: a retrospective review of 1,700 consecutive vascular access cases. *J Vasc Access*. 2008;9(4):231–235.

36. Hong HP, Kim SK. Usefulness of percutaneous intervention with transarterial approach in the salvage of nonmaturing native fistulas status-post transvenous approach failure: transarterial approach in the salvage of nonmaturing native fistulas. *Cardiovasc Intervent Radiol*. 2009;32(6): 1252–1256. Epub 2009 Jul 31.

37. Escobar C, Blanes I, Ruiz A, Vinuesa D, Montero M, Rodríguez M, Barbera G, Manzano L. Prevalence and clinical profile and management of peripheral arterial disease in elderly patients with diabetes. *Eur J Intern Med*. 2011;22(3):275–281. Epub 2011 Mar 15.

38. Asif A, Gadalean FN, Merrill D, et al. Inflow stenosis in arteriovenous fistulas and grafts: a multicenter, prospective study. *Kidney Int*. 2005; 67:1986–1992.

39. Rattanasompattikul M, Chanchairujira K, On-Ajyooth L, Chanchairujira T. Evaluation of atherosclerosis, arterial stiffness and related risk factors in chronic hemodialysis patients in Siriraj Hospital. *J Med Assoc Thai*. 2011;94(suppl 1):S117–S124.

40. Jourde-Chiche N, Dou L, Cerini C, Dignat-George F, Brunet P. Vascular incompetence in dialysis patients-protein-bound uremic toxins and endothelial dysfunction. *Semin Dial*. 2011;24(3):327–337.

41. Puntmann VO, Bigalke B, Nagel E. Characterization of the inflammatory phenotype in atherosclerosis may contribute to the development of new therapeutic and preventative interventions. *Trends Cardiovasc Med*. 2010;20(5):176–181.

42. Swaminathan S, Shah SV. Novel inflammatory mechanisms of accelerated atherosclerosis in kidney disease. *Kidney Int*. 2011;80(5):453–463.

43. Grogan J, Castilla M, Lozanski L, Griffin A, Loth F, Bassiouny H. Frequency of critical stenosis in primary arteriovenous fistulae before hemodialysis access: Should duplex ultrasound surveillance be the standard of care? *J Vasc Surg*. 2005;41:1000–1006.

44. Marin D, Nelson RC, Schindera ST, Richard S, Youngblood RS, Yoshizumi TT, Samei E. Low-tube-voltage, high-tube-current multidetector abdominal CT: improved image quality and decreased radiation dose with adaptive statistical iterative reconstruction algorithm–initial clinical experience. *Radiology*. 2010;254(1):145–153.

45. Coelman C, Duijm LEM, Liem YS, et al. Stenosis detection in failing hemodialysis access fistulas and grafts: comparison of color Doppler ultrasonography, contrast-enhance magnetic resonance angiography and digital subtraction angiography. *J Vasc Surg*. 2005;42:739–746.

46. Khan FA, Vesely TM. Arterial problems associated with dysfunctional hemodialysis grafts: evaluation of patients at high risk for arterial disease. *J Vasc Interv Radiol*. 2002;13:1109–1114.

47. Kanterman RY, Vesely TM, Pilgram TK, et al. Dialysis access grafts: anatomic location of venous stenosis and results of angioplasty. *Radiology*. 1995;195:135–139.

48. Duijm LE, Liem YS, van der Rijt RH, Nobrega FJ, van den Bosch HC, Douwes-Draaijer P, Cuypers PW, Tielbeek AV. Inflow stenosis in dysfunctional hemodialysis access fistulae and grafts. *Am J Kidney Dis*. 2006;48(1):98–105.

49. Duijm LEM, van der Rijt RHH, Cuypers PWM, et al. Outpatient treatment of arterial inflow stenoses of dysfunctional hemodialysis access fistulas by retrograde venous access puncture and catheterization. *J Vasc Surg*. 2008;47:591–598.

50. Guerra A, Raynaud A, Beyssen B, et al. Arterial percutaneous angioplasty in upper limbs with vascular access device for haemodialysis. *Nephrol Dial Transplant*. 2002;17:843–851.

51. Yevzlin AS, Asif A. Arterial stenosis in patients with arteriovenous dialysis access. *US Nephrol*. 2009;4(2): 72–74.

52. Duijm LE, Overbosch EH, Liem YS, et al. Retrograde catheterization of haemodialysis fistulae and grafts: angiographic depiction of the entire vascular access tree and stenosis treatment. *Nephrol Dial Transplant*. 2009;24: 539–547.

53. Beathard GA. Angioplasty for arteriovenous grafts and fistulae. *Semin Nephrol*. 2002;22:202–210.

54. Chan MR, Chhokar VS, Young HN, et al. Retrograde occlusive arteriography of hemododialysis access: failure to detect inflow lesions? *Semin Dial*. 2010;24(4):452–455.

25

TEMPORARY HEMODIALYSIS CATHETERS

JAMIE ROSS

LEARNING OBJECTIVES

1. Understand the training issues for placement of central venous catheters.
2. Know the preferred technique for catheter placement.
3. Understand the indications for temporary dialysis catheters.
4. Know the complications of catheter placement and how to manage them.

INTRODUCTION

Late referral for symptomatic renal failure requiring acute dialysis using a temporary catheter has been shown to adversely alter the first year outcome of the patient.[1] While the use of temporary venous access for a hospitalized patient is less than ideal, it is unavoidable when there is an urgent need for treatment and no prior opportunity to intervene. It is incumbent upon those physicians providing venous access services to become proficient in the intellectual as well as has technical aspects of placing and managing temporary central venous catheters. This chapter will summarize the current information and thinking with regard to this small but important aspect of care. Whether these procedures are performed by hospitalists, critical care physicians, or nephrologists will become a matter of training, timing, equipment, interest, and economics. Nephrologists have and will continue to have a vested interest in making sure that these procedures are done with the optimum safety and expedience for the dialysis patient population. Interventional nephrology is able to provide both the immediate care of the patients and future physician training in this area.

WHAT CONSTITUTES ADEQUATE TRAINING IN CENTRAL LINE PLACEMENT?

Who performs these procedures may become more of an issue in the near future, since as of 2010 it is no longer required that internal medicine residents become proficient in the basic procedures once thought to be essential to the practice of an internist.[2] This does include central venous access. The present system of training internal medicine residents to place central lines is likely to be deferred to fellowship. Then, the specialties likely to be interested in training their fellows in this skill will be hospital-based internists, critical care medicine, cardiology and nephrology. Oncology physicians may be interested in learning this in the future but at the present time it has not been a part of oncology practice. The predominant teaching method of hands on training during the course of patient care is still practiced as the sole method of learning in most training programs. Some programs have begun using computer simulations and anatomic models to assist in this process.[3,4] This might make the access of such skills more readily available in the future.

At present several surveys suggest not all nephrologists have adequate training during fellowship in placing central lines.[5-8] It has been demonstrated that training is essential and repeated performance of procedural skills improves the outcome for the patients.[5,6] For instance, the placement of subclavian lines while not the first or second choice of a dialysis access location is a skill which is needed for those physicians placing temporary catheters for patients who have normal renal function. The subclavian temporary line is the preferred choice in most medicine and surgical patients.[9,10] This particular approach is highly operator dependent and the incidence of pneumothorax can range from 1 to 5% depending on operator experience.[11,12] It is reasonable to assume a similar pattern would emerge from all central line procedures.

The American Society of Diagnostic and Interventional Nephrology (ASDIN) has stated in their certification guidelines that at least 25 temporary dialysis and 25 tunneled dialysis central venous lines be placed in order to be considered for certification in this skill.[13] The placement of tunneled lines involves some additional skills but at least involves the same skills needed to place temporary central venous access. If we assumed the majority of these lines were internal jugular and some were femoral, then we may have arrived at the number of lines it takes to attain enough experience to be certified in central venous access. This would be somewhere between 25 and 50 placements.

Regardless of the location of placement, it is essential that the procedural physician maintain use of their skills after initial training so that they become proficient. This is the same principle supported by most surgical specialties. Evidence suggests that creating a service that repeatedly performs such procedures increases the success and decreases the complications of these procedures.[14-16] It remains to be established what constitutes adequate continued experience. If we use the example of moderate sedation skills that have to be renewed at most hospitals, then it would be about 25 procedures a year at a minimum.[17]

INDICATIONS FOR USE OF TEMPORARY CENTRAL VENOUS ACCESS

There are multiple medical indications for placement of central venous access but they can be divided by the intent use. There are only three major classifications for use: infusion, apheresis, and dialysis. The last two procedures require at least two larger lumens, which can tolerate movement of blood to at least 200 cc/min. The expectations for a temporary dialysis catheter would be at least 250 cc/min flow.[18] Temporary catheters are used predominately in the hospital and are no longer considered standard of care for outpatient treatment. The physician must weigh the clinical and prognostic data available to determine if a temporary or tunneled catheter is to be chosen. The choice of a temporary versus a tunneled catheter would be influenced by both the patient's immediate medical condition as well as the expectation of duration of treatment. If a patient is hemodynamically unstable, has an uncorrected coagulopathy, or actively infected, then placement of a tunneled catheter is not warranted. If the patient cannot tolerate a prolonged procedure due to hyperkalemia, acidosis, or volume overload, then a tunneled catheter procedure would be somewhat contraindicated. In these situations, the use of a temporary catheter is the only reasonable alternative.

There is some evidence, which indicates that the length of infection free survival and functionality of a temporary dialysis catheter is less than 2–3 weeks.[19,20] It should be noted that the rate of recovery of acute kidney injury is usually longer than that and the time for healing of the subcutaneous tunnel for a tunneled catheter is at least 2 weeks. This makes the length of expected use an important clinical assessment tool in choosing a temporary catheter.[21]

At present, the length of treatment recommended for choosing a temporary over a tunneled catheter is recommended by the kidney/dialysis outcomes quality initiative (K/DOQI) is 1 week.[18] Each case would require a balanced view of expected length of recovery with the risk of infection in either the temporary catheter or the unhealed tunnel of the new tunneled catheter to arrive at an appropriate choice of catheter.

HOW TO PLACE CENTRAL VENOUS ACCESS

The techniques involved in placing temporary or tunneled access involve selecting a site, selecting a catheter type and size, use of sterile procedure, ultrasound guidance, use of the traditional catheter over a wire (Seldinger) method, reading a chest X-ray or fluoroscopy if needed and suturing. Each of these areas involves both a knowledge and procedural component.

▶ Site Selection

When considering site selection for patients with acute or chronic kidney disease, the decision has been narrowed to the one best site by multiple studies and experience. The internal jugular (IJ) vein is the best location by far for dialysis access whether it is temporary or tunneled. The rate of stenosis of the right IJ is about 10% compared to about 50% stenosis in the subclavian vein.[22,23] Stenosis of the subclavian vein would limit or eliminate the ability to use the ipsilateral arm for arteriovenous fistulae or grafts in the future. The recommendations for catheter placement by the K/DOQI of 2006 recommend the choice of sites in this order right IJ/then right external jugular (EJ)/then left IJ.[18] Studies have shown that the right-sided central lines outperform the left-sided ones.[24] The location on the neck in relation to the clavicle is not vital for temporary line placement. However, if these lines are used as a conversion site for tunneled catheter, it is worth noting the closer to the clavicle the less likely the tunnel will "kink" the intravascular portion of the catheter. While many people create a new venotomy site to place a tunneled catheter, there is some evidence that use of a temporary catheter as a conversion to a tunneled catheter can be safe and effective.[25,26] Therefore when placing temporary catheters, it is prudent to think of the tunneled catheter that may follow.

A clearly inferior choice after the IJs is the femoral veins. The rate of infection makes this an unacceptable choice for more than 3–5 days. The infection rate increases rapidly as the femoral catheters are left in place over time.[27-29] Another problem with extended use of femoral lines is the immobility, which can result in delayed recovery and contribute to the formation of deep venous thrombosis. However, it is still a safe and reasonable location for an emergent catheter placement especially in a patient with a bleeding diathesis. The ideal location along the femoral vein for placing a catheter is one, which will allow obtuse angle of the catheter as it enters under the inguinal ligament. This is likely to be below the inguinal ligament and can be safely performed with ultrasound.[30,31]

A distant third location would be the subclavian vein. However, a temporary subclavian infusion catheter is the standard of care for medicine patients according to the Center for Disease Control and the Infectious Disease Society. This is because the rate of infection is about one-third of that seen with internal jugular placement.[9,10] The issue of prevention of catheter related blood stream infection (CRBSI) is far more important for patients without significant renal disease rather than overall venous preservation.

As our dialysis patients receive more and more catheters for central venous access, it is becoming more common that some of their central circulation is damaged or destroyed. The damaged circulation results in fewer locations for future access both arteriovenous and central venous. This fact emphasizes the need for planned venous preservation in the CKD patients.[32] When traditional sites are no longer available, there are some other "exotic" locations for central placement such as the supraclavicular approach, the transhepatic, translumbar, or even the femoral artery.[33–36] These are all meant to be the choices of last resort and therefore should be reserved primarily for tunneled or semipermanent access.

▶ Catheter Choice

The options for types of temporary catheters for dialysis are limited in regard to tip type. Discussion of types of infusion catheters is beyond the scope of this chapter. The majority of temporary dialysis catheters are a staggered tip or Mahurkar type of catheter (Figure 25-1). This allows blood to be pulled from the more proximal "arterial" lumen treated and then returned to the distal or "venous" lumen. There have been many studies to evaluate if recirculation is present. These studies show consistently less than 10% recirculation in these types of catheters.[37,38] This number can double if the lines are reversed.[38] The length of the catheter should be so that the tip is at the appropriate location as approved by the FDA, which is the governing body for medical devices. The approved location for temporary catheters is about 3 cm above the right atrium.[39,40] While some tunneled catheters have been approved by the FDA to be placed in the more optimal location of the atrial–caval junction, there has not be an approval of a temporary catheter to be placed in this location at this time. The original literature reviewed by the

FDA to make their decision about tip location reflected a concern for cardiac and vascular erosion which occurred approximately less than 0.2% of the time but was fatal in up to two-thirds of the cases.[41,42] The material of the catheters at that time may be an issue since most of the original studies were done showing vascular damage, stenosis, and/or thrombosis using catheters that were made of "stiffer" materials compared to those available in some of the temporary catheters at present.[43,44] Since the FDA has not changed its stance, the length of the catheter needs to be adjusted to the point of access. It is usually 13–16 cm from the right IJ and about 15–20 cm on the left.[38,45] The length needed to ensure effective dialysis in femoral catheters has been demonstrated to be at least 16 cm and preferably greater than 19 cm.[37]

Some note should be made about the number of lumens. There is data that support that the frequency of "break-ins" is related to the frequency of infections. In the past, this issue has been managed by limiting the number of lumens.[9,10] Recent evidence shows that this is not significant, and the infection rate of temporary catheters is not significantly different whether they are double or triple lumen.[46] Therefore, the choice of a triple lumen catheter with an extra infusion port or a double lumen catheter solely for dialysis or apheresis is a clinical decision. Limiting the number of lumens to that needed is still prudent. There are triple lumen dialysis catheters available made by several companies so no specific type of catheter is identified as a single option.

The rate of infections based on tip cultures show that antibiotic or antiseptic coating can decrease the rate of catheter colonization for approximately 2 weeks.[47–49] This makes complete sense in the choice of temporary infusion catheters. Unfortunately, there is not a lot of choice in this regard in temporary dialysis catheters. This may result in the patient receiving a catheter that is softer or functions more efficiently but does not have antibiotic coating.

▶ Use of Sterile Technique

It is essential for the procedural physician to adhere strictly to sterile technique. By definition this involves the use of an appropriate antiseptic technique over the area selected, total draping, mask, hat, gown, and gloves. Use of the sterile technique is just as important in temporary catheters as it is in a procedure for permanent device placement. Evidence clearly shows that strict use of the sterile technique reduces the rate of CRBSIs to less than expected national standards.[50–52] With the Federal and some state governments interested in tracking the rate of CRBSI to ensure patient safety, the knowledge about and use of sterile procedures has taken on a matter of urgency.[53,54]

Infectious disease literature and the CDC have clearly outlined the choice of antiseptic agent, 2% chlorhexidine, used to prepare the skin for most procedures. The comparison of this agent to povidone–iodine and 70% alcohol clearly shows that chlorhexidine is superior. Both the number of organisms on the skin as well as the number of

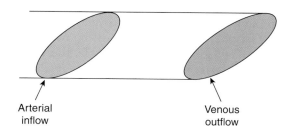

Figure 25-1. Mahurkur staggered catheter tip.

Arterial inflow

Venous outflow

catheter infections are reduced. It is essential for all anti-septic agents to be allowed to dry completely for them to be effective. This drying period is at least 30 seconds for chlorhexidine and longer for povidone–iodine.[9,10,55,56]

Ultrasound Guidance and Anatomic Location

It has become standard of care to use simultaneous ultrasound to place central venous access per K/DOQI, ASDIN.[18,30,32] Multiple studies have demonstrated the improved success and safety of these procedures even with the most inexperienced operators.[57,58,59] While use of ultrasound is an essential part of the procedure, it is still necessary to know the anatomy well to avoid complications and assist in appropriately placing the ultrasound for optimal visualization. Some proceduralists have used EKG guidance as well but this has not become either popular or standard of care as a sole "imaging" technique.[60]

Understanding how ultrasound imaging works improves the ability to place access successfully. The range of vascular access ultrasound probes usually allows a visual depth of between 2.2 and 7.1 cm. The deeper the object imaged, the lower the hertz needed to visualize the object. Some probes have a fixed hertz, and some can vary allowing the operator to adjust the depth of field to the needs of the procedure. The patient vein will appear dark and flatten with compression (see Figure 25-2). The partially or completely thrombosed vein will have some material in the lumen that may appear "white" on ultrasound and will not be easily compressible. Arteries will not compress without a great deal of force and will be visibly pulsatile.[61]

The beam of sound will make the vessel visible but will not allow optimal visualization of the tip of the needle unless it is as close to 90° from the direction of the beam at the point of intersection in the vessel. The extent of the entire needle can be more easily seen longitudinally, and some operators prefer this.[61,62,63] Adjusting the probe and the angle of the needle to the depth of the patient's vessel can take some practice but will allow the operator to directly observe the tip of the needle not just the path of the needle as the procedure is performed. There are etched needles that allow the tips to be imaged more clearly with the ultrasound probe as well.

Technique of Catheter Placement

Prior to the use of ultrasound, a number of internal jugular vein approaches were described. However since the advent of ultrasound use, the principal approach for an IJ access is the anterior one. The usual location of the vessel is superior lateral to the artery. Using ultrasound, this relationship is seen only 66% of the time. The remaining 33% of the time, the vessels can be in any other direction in relation to the artery.[51] This points out the utility of preprocedure assessment of the vessels to ensure the correct approach and that the vessel is patent.[64]

There have been no clear-cut recommendations with regard to the use of the traditional 18-gauge hollow needle or Seldinger needle versus a micropuncture needle. Each operator is free to choose the method with which they are most comfortable. However, the majority of physicians, who regularly perform these procedures, use the micropuncture needle and kit. These materials are not provided in the standard catheter placement trays but must be ordered separately. There is no clear study showing evidence that use of the 21-gauge micropuncture needle with a 0.018-in. wire, and use of a 4–5 French dilator and sheath have fewer complications associated with it.[65] The number of punctures and presence of a hematoma have been demonstrated to be an increased risk for the development of stenosis or thrombosis. Given the essential need for venous preservation for CKD patients, it is imperative to use the optimum technique for all catheter placements.[32]

Once access has been obtained with the needle, then the initial wire is placed through the needle into the superior vena cava (SVC) and possibly even further into the inferior vena cava (IVC). This is not easy to do without the proper equipment. The ease of the passage of the wire has in the past been the primary means of confirming the proper location. If no resistance is met, then evidence suggests that the wire can be safely inserted "blindly" to approximately 16 cm on the right IJ approach and 20 cm on the left IJ approach.[39,45] This can be deceptive. For instance, the path of the right Azygous vein can mimic the path of the SVC until the atrial–caval junction.[66] Only placement of the wire in the IVC assures that the catheter will not ultimately reside in the Azygous vein. To truly confirm the wire placement, fluoroscopy must be used. However, since fluoroscopy is not always available, the importance of knowing the anatomy and appropriately reading a chest x-ray become a greater priority.

The location of the wire entering the skin can be enlarged slightly with a scalpel, thus becoming the venotomy site. Most wires used for central venous catheters are placed either directly into the 18-gauge hollow

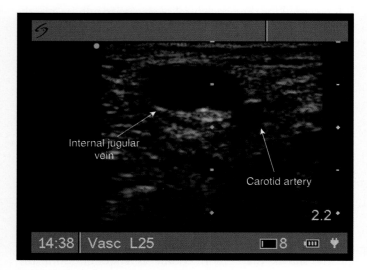

Figure 25-2. Ultrasound image of neck vessels.

needle or the sheath of the micropuncture kit. They are typically 0.032–0.035 in nonhydrophilic and stiff enough to support the use of the dilators and catheters passing over them. The tip can be a J-type or a soft floppy end. The dilators are meant to enlarge the venotomy site and allow passage of the larger catheter. While each kit provides dilators appropriately sized to increase the venotomy site to that of the catheter, there are a few things worth knowing about the use of the dilator. The dilator does not have to feed all the way into the vessel just to dilate the entrance of the catheter as it goes over the wire. It should be noted that the dilator is capable of causing severe damage and even perforation of the vessel even with the wire in place. Ideally if fluoroscopy is available, one should watch as the dilator goes over the wire especially when negotiating any curves or direction changes in the vessel. This means that the safest procedures to perform "blind" are accessing either the right IJ or the femoral vessels. Do not force the dilator. This will only lead to increased risk of complications. Once the venotomy site is dilated, the catheter can be fed directly over the wire. The catheter tip is adjusted to be in the appropriate position. This initially is done by estimation in a "blind" procedure and by direct visualization when using fluoroscopic guidance. The catheter is then sutured in place after the flow and draw are confirmed to be adequate for dialysis.

▶ Location of the Catheter Tip

For a catheter placed in the chest vessels, the tip location is confirmed by an x-ray or fluoroscopy. As stated above, the FDA approved position for temporary catheters is at least 3 cm above the right atrium. The right atrium is below the right main stem bronchus on x-ray. Several publications have delineated the appropriate location for the tip of the catheter on x-ray.[67] Since the atrial–caval junction provided the best and most consistent flow for dialysis, it is now standard of care for tunneled soft tip catheters to be placed in this location. There are several brands of catheters that have approval from the FDA to be placed in this proximal position.[62] Some the newer soft tip temporary catheters may be able to be safely placed in this location but no FDA approval has been granted for this at this time (see Figure 25-3).

Regardless of the location at the time of placement, it must be remembered that the catheter will likely change position with the posture of the patient. When the patient is flat, it will be at the most proximal point, and when the patient is upright, the tip will be at its most distal point in the chest. On and off dialysis, the patient should be without discomfort or ectopy in all positions with the catheter in place. For femoral catheters, ideally the tip should be in the IVC or at least a few centimeters away from a junction of two vessels. Femoral catheters are more likely to malfunction based on location compared to internal jugular catheters.[68–70] If the tip of any catheter is at the junction of two vessels, it is likely to malfunction due to abutting against a vessel wall.

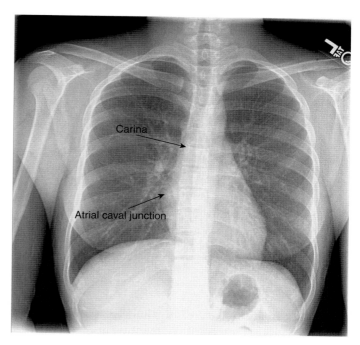

Figure 25-3. Normal chest x-ray.

COMPLICATIONS

In performing any procedure, it is important for the operator to know the possible complications and how to manage them. The rate of complications as a measure of performance has been a standard measure in most continuous quality improvement programs. These complications are listed in Table 25-1.[71] Knowledge of the management of these complications can be lifesaving and needs to be learned prior to performing the procedure. Some of the most frequent and/or important complications are discussed below. Some of the other complications listed occur less frequently but can be reduced as the operator increases their knowledge of the anatomy involved. For instance, awareness of the location of the thoracic duct is the only way to avoid it.

▶ Short-Term Complications

Arterial puncture is probably the most common acute complication in placement of central lines. Recognizing this has occurred is the first step in management. Then if the size of the puncture or laceration is small enough, external pressure can be the primary mode of management in the carotid and femoral locations. However for obvious reasons it will not be effective in the chest. Pressure treatment for an arterial puncture should be proximal from the entrance of the needle and be held for 6–10 minutes depending on the coagulation status of the patient.[72,73] In the case of the carotid vessel, the timing might be limited by causing decreased flow to the cerebral cortex in some patients. If the procedure has progressed to placement of the catheter or the use of dilators over 8 French in size, it would be wise to consult with a vascular surgeon prior to

TABLE 25–1

Complications of Central Venous Catheter Placement

Short Term	Long Term
• Arterial puncture	• Infection
• Bleeding/hematoma	○ Exit site
• Pneumo or hemothorax	○ Bacteremia
• Vascular injury or perforation	○ Metatstatic/endocarditis
• Arrhythmia	• Stenosis
• Neurological injuries	• Thrombosis
○ Brachial plexus	• Fibrin sheath development
○ Horner's syndrome	• Vascular erosion and perforation
• Thoracic duct injuries (left side only)	• Catheter fracture or embolism
• Air embolus	• Superior vena cava syndrome

removing catheter or decrease manual pressure from the vessel as a surgical intervention might be needed.

Bleeding not related to arterial puncture can be managed with both pressure and optimization of the patient's coagulation factors and platelets. If a patient has significant bleeding from a procedure on one side of their neck, then a second procedure should not be performed on the contralateral side until bleeding has ceased and observation occurs for at least 24 hours to ensure that there is no tracheal compression. This same precaution, delaying a contralateral procedure, should be taken for lines thought to enter the thoracic cavity. If a patient has bleeding from a subclavian vessel or a vessel in the chest cavity, then a hemothorax can result and the treatment can range from observation, a chest tube or even an open thoracotomy. If the bleeding is from an intra-thoracic vessel or the pericardium has been damaged during placement, then an open heart/thoracic surgery is usually needed immediately.[71,74–76] The patient's survival will depend on the speed with which the physician recognizes the problem and the patient is given definitive treatment. If the bleeding is not brisk, then the patient can be monitored with serial x-rays and blood counts and may need a chest tube.

A special case is associated with femoral line placement. Bleeding into the retroperitoneal space can occur with both arterial and venous bleeding. The most important management of this complication is diagnosis prior to significant blood loss. Unfortunately the diagnosis is usually made after there is an alteration in vital signs and/or a decrease in blood counts. The most common method of diagnosis is with computerized tomography.[77,78] Management of this complication can run from removing the catheter to endovascular repair or surgery. There are some important anatomical issues to be aware of when placing femoral catheters that might improve the results. The inguinal ligament is the traditional location of femoral line placement. There is a peritoneal reflection around this ligament at this point that allows passage of blood into the retroperitoneal

space. Using ultrasound the operator can access the vessel several centimeters below this ligament and reduce the risk of bleeding in the retroperitoneal space. While bleeding can still occur, it would be contained in the thigh compartment. In addition the more distal approach has the advantage of not resulting in such an acute angle of entrance and is less likely to cause difficulty passing under the inguinal ligament with the dilator or catheters. This approach will likely reduce catheter malfunction due to kinking. This improved outcome must be balanced with the fact that the more distal in the thigh the vessel goes, the more likely the operator is to encounter arterial branches and risk injury to those vessels.

Air embolus is one of the most frightening complications of central line placement in the chest. The highest risk is with a hypovolemic patient, who is not flat or in Trendelenburg, has a good size opening in their vein with a direct connection to the atmosphere and then inhales. If the amount of air is a large enough volume, it will behave like a pulmonary embolus and cause tachycardia, hypoxia, hypotension, chest pain, and even death. The management of this complication is by immediately placing the patient left side down and the right side elevated so the air remains in the right side of the heart and does not move forward. Then aspirate the air out of the venous access if the catheter is still in place at this point.[79]

Pneumothorax is less likely to occur with an internal jugular approach than the subclavian approach. It is important to realize the potential for this problem. The cupola of the left lung is higher than the right making the left-sided approach a higher risk for this complication. The usual incidence of pneumothorax with an IJ catheter placement is 0.1%. This is likely to increase if the tip of the needle itself went below the clavicle during placement. The acute symptoms would be similar to an air embolus but the exam would reveal decreased breath sounds over the involved lung. While a large pneumothorax would be immediately symptomatic, it may take 4 hours or more for a small pneumothorax to be symptomatic or even radiographically visible. It is important to image the patient with an upright x-ray so that the air is superior in location and not anterior. While anything greater than a 10% pneumothorax will need a chest tube, it is possible to manage the smaller ones more expectantly depending on the clinical situation.[71,80,81]

Arrhythmia can be a complication of using wires near the heart. A few ectopic beats resolving immediately as the wire is withdrawn is not a true complication of the procedure. However, a prolonged arrhythmia is a serious complication of these procedures requiring monitoring and sometimes prolonged hospitalization. This is not a frequent complication of the procedure and an arrhythmia that is associated with a brief exposure to a wire as it nears the right atrium or ventricle should not be confused with a prolonged and sustained cardiac abnormality.[71] If a prolonged cardiac arrhythmia results from the manipulation of the catheter or wire, then this is a direct complication of the procedure. The risk of this even transient alteration in cardiac rhythm should encourage the proceduralists to have a cardiac monitor on the patient to ensure safety. In addition it would be prudent for all operators in this area to be Advanced Cardiac Life Support certified.

▶ Long-Term Complications

Infection is the most common longer-term complication of this procedure and is extensively reviewed in other articles and texts. The full discussion of diagnosis and management of CRBSIs is beyond the scope of this chapter. However, the treatment of infections in temporary catheters is initially managed by removing the catheter. This is different from the current recommendations for treatment of tunneled catheters.[9,10] The incidence, morbidity, mortality, and cost of catheter-related infections have become a national patient safety initiative.[53,54] The prevention of infection by an appropriate sterile technique is the most important part rather than managing the infection after it occurs.

Antibiotic choice and length of treatment is dependent on the organism cultured. The most common organisms are *Staphylococcus epidermidis* and *Staphylococcus aureus* followed by gram negatives and increasingly Enterococcus in hospital-based patients.[82,83] If the organisms are gram positive and likely to have a high risk for metastatic infections, then a prolonged course of antibiotics will be needed.[84-86] The duration of treatment is dependent on many variables such as patient symptoms, underlying medical comorbidities, clearance of bacteremia, and type of organism.[9,10,87] Of note the frequency of metastatic infections in patients using catheters for dialysis can be as high as 25% when associated with *S. aureus* bacteremia.[9,10,87] The mortality associated with this type of infection, especially endocarditis, is between 19 and 65%. The location of the metastatic infection may not be obvious and can vary[71,88] (Table 25-2).

Stenosis and thrombosis are the next two most frequent problems associated with both temporary and tunneled catheters. The frequency of right atrial thrombi is not trivial.[89,90] It is often associated with a concomitant infection. Suspicion of this diagnosis and awareness of the issue is needed in order to diagnosis the problem. The treatment for thrombosis can be up to 6 months of anticoagulation.[90] Evidence suggests that the catheter-associated femoral thrombus may be related to immobility with the use of these catheters as well as obstruction of the vessel. This is demonstrated by the frequency of ipsilateral as well as

contralateral popliteal thrombi associated with use of these femoral catheters.[91] The patients at highest risk are oncology patients and those with underlying abnormalities in their vessels with or without procoagulants.

The issue of frequency of stenosis associated with either temporary or tunneled central venous access is not defined. It is clear that the presence of these catheters cause damage to these vessels.[92-96] Even a 5–7 French peripherally inserted central catheters (PICC lines) can have a 7% incidence of central venous stenosis.[32] The frequency of total central stenosis or superior vena cava (SVC) syndrome in patients with previous multiple dialysis lines may be higher than reported. The case reports in the literature of symptomatic central venous stenosis and/or SVC syndrome resulting from central venous catheters are likely just the tip of the iceberg. The number of patients on dialysis with evidence of central stenosis may be higher than 25%.[71,92-96] These patients require repeated treatments for symptoms or failed accesses if the arteriovenous access is ipsilateral to the central venous lesion.

▶ Maintenance and Troubleshooting

The locking of catheters has become more of a research area of interest in the last several years. There is some data to suggest that antibiotic locks in tunneled catheters may be useful as infective prophylaxis and treatment. However since the definitive treatment for infected temporary catheter is to remove them, the use of lock solutions with temporary catheters is limited to prophylaxis.[97,98,99] The use of an anticoagulant to prevent thrombosis is essential to catheter function. In the past this has been heparin. Some studies show the risk for bleeding is increased as heparin is slowly released from the catheter.[100,101] The result has been to reduce the amount of heparin or use sodium citrate to "pack" the catheter. Citrate has the risk of binding intravascular calcium in larger quantities or concentrations but using the volume of the catheter and the solutions now commercially available (2–4%), this is unlikely. The advantage of citrate is that it is both an antiseptic and anticoagulant. There is also some interest in using 70% alcohol as well for these reasons. Alcohol is not widely accepted as a catheter lock due to the lack of experience in adult medicine and the known use as a sclerotic agent. In the past, many of the materials used to manufacture catheters were intolerant to alcohol.[102]

If there is a malfunction, it is likely to be a malposition, thrombosis, or even kinking of the catheter.[103-105] The diagnosis of a malposition would be by x-ray, and the catheter could be rewired if it had been dislodged. Another length can be chosen if needed to avoid an area where two vessels adjoin. If the exit site is clean and there is no evidence of infection, the operator may choose to rewire the catheter. The only reason to rewire a catheter is for malfunction not for infection. The risk of infection is increased with rewiring, and the strict sterile technique must be maintained. The treatment of intracatheter thrombus is acceptable if

TABLE 25–2
Metastatic Infections

- Endocarditis
- Osteomyelitis
- Epidural abscess
- Septic arthritis
- Infections of remotely implanted devices such as old dialysis grafts

the catheter is not infected or malpositioned. This is done usually with 1–2 mg of Alteplase™, and the dwell time should be between 30 minutes and 2 hours. The longer dwell times are thought more likely to allow full effective use of this agent; however, no difference has been noted in the actual success related to time.[106] The success rate can be over 60–70% in the catheters, which have clot as the reason for malfunction. Kinking rarely occurs in IJ catheters but is a frequent problem in the femoral catheters as people move their hip joints. This is especially true with the stiffer temporary catheters and may be avoided by selecting a softer more flexible catheter for initial placement. If the catheter is kinked, then it can be rewired with the same caveats described above. Lastly, if no other problems are found, then the catheter might have developed a fibrin sheath. In tunneled catheters, this may be worthwhile to treat. Treatment involves angiography and possible angioplasty of the fibrin sheath.[107] Fibrin sheaths in temporary catheters may be reasonably treated with removal and subsequent replacement.

CONCLUSION

The information presented crosses multiple specialties. It is important to understand this issue from the point of view of not only nephrology but also infectious disease, oncology, critical care, and multiple other specialties. Each literature contributes to the physician's ability to care for these patients in the most appropriate fashion. The essentials for a procedural physician transcend the specialty and the particular procedure performed. The physician needs to know the risks and benefits involved in the procedure, the anatomy involved, mechanics of performing the procedure, and the frequency and management of the complications. In the case of central venous access, it has long been under appreciated by the medical community at large and thought of as a minor procedure. For the patients whose life depends on venous access, it is a very important and significant procedure in the scope of their medical care and should be treated as such.

REFERENCES

1. Goncalves EA, Andreoli MC, Watanabe R, Freitas MC, Pedrosa AC, Manfredi SR, et al. Effect of temporary catheter and late referral on hospitalization and mortality during the first year of hemodialysis treatment. *Artif Organs*. 2004;28:1043–1049.
2. American Board of Internal Medicine Policies and Procedures Required procedural knowledge. Revised August 2009 pg 4 www.abim.org.
3. Britt RC, Reed SF, Britt LD. Central line simulation: a new training algorithm. *Am Surg*. 2007;73(7):682–683.
4. Karakitsos D, Labropoulos N, De Groot E, Patrianakos AP, Kouraklis G, Poularas J, et al. Real-time ultrasound-guided catheterization of the internal jugular vein: a prospective comparison with the landmark technique in critical care patients. *Crit Care*. 2006;10(6):R162.
5. Feller-Kopman D. Ultrasound guided internal jugular access: a proposed standardized approach and implications for training and practice. *Chest*. 2007;132:302–307.
6. Barsuk JH, Ahya SN, Cohen ER, McGaghie WC, Wayne DB. Mastery learning of temporary hemodialysis catheter insertion by nephrology fellows using simulation technology and deliberate practice. *Am J Kid Dis*. 2009;54(1):70–76.
7. Berns, JS. A survey-based evaluation of self-perceived competency after nephrology fellowship training. *Clin J Am Soc Nephrol*. 2010;5:490–496.
8. Berns, JS, O'Neill WC. Performance of procedures by nephrologists and nephrology fellows at U.S. nephrology training programs. *Clin J Am Soc Nephrol*. 2008;3:941–947.
9. O, Grady NP, Alexander M, Dellionger EP, et al. Guidelines for the prevention of intravascular catheter-related infection. Centers for Disease Control and Prevention. *MMWR Recomm Rep*. 2002;51:1–29.
10. Mermel LA, Allon M, Bouza E, Craven DE, Flynn P, O'Grady NP, et al. Clinical practice guidelines for the diagnosis and management of intravascular catheter-related infection: 2009. Update by the Infectious Disease Society of America. *Clin Infect Dis*. 2009;49(1):1–45.
11. Mullins, R. Shock, electrolytes and fluid. In: Townsend CM Jr, Beauchamp RD, et al, eds. *Sabiston Textbook of Surgery*. 18th ed. Philadelphia, PA: Sunders Elsevier; 2008:96–98.
12. Kilbourne MJ, Bochicchio GV, Scalea T, Xiao Y. Avoiding common technical errors in subclavian central venous catheter placement. *J Am Coll Surg*. 2009;208(1):104–109.
13. American Society of Diagnostic and Interventional Nephrology. Application for Certification of Hemodialysis Vascular Access Procedures. Revised June 2010;5 www.abim.org
14. Walters G, Kahn A, Jescovitch A Jr, Astor R Jr, Jones CE. Efficacy of a central venous access service. *South Med J*. 1997;90(1):37–39.
15. Lee MK, Mossop PJ, Vrazas JI. Central venous catheter placement by an Interventional Radiology Unit: an Australian experience. *Australas Radiol*. 2007;51(1):35–41.
16. Ross JL. An innovative approach to temporary hemodialysis vascular access. *Am J Kid Dis*. 1999;33:718–721.
17. Krauss B, Greene S. Training and credentialing in procedural sedation and analgesia in children: lessons from the United States Model. *Pediatr Anesthesia*. 2008;18:30–35.
18. Besarab A, Work J, chairs. Kidney Dialysis Outcomes Quality Initiative Vascular Access Workgroup 2006. *Am J Kid Dis*. 2006;48(suppl 1):S192–S200.
19. Weijmer MC, Vervloet MG, ter Wee PM. Compared to tunneled cuffed haemodialysis catheters, temporary untunneled catheters are associated with more complications already within 2 weeks of use. *Nephrol Dial Transplant*. 2004;19(3):670–677.
20. Kairaitis LK, Gottlieb T. Outcome and complication of temporary hemodialysis catheters. *Nephrol Dial Transplant*. 1999;14:1710–1714.
21. Canaud B, Desmeules S, Klouche K, Leray-Moragués H, Béraud JJ. Vascular access for dialysis in the intensive care unit. *Best Pract Res Clin Anaesthesiol*. 2004;18(1):159–174.

22. Beenen L, van Leusen R, van Leusen R, Deenik B, Bosch FH. The incidence of subclavian vein stenosis using silicone catheters for hemodialysis. *Artif Organs.* 1994;18:289–292.

23. Cimochowski GE, Worley E, Rutherford WE, Sartain J, Blondin J, Harter H. Superiority of the internal jugular over the subclavian access for temporary dialysis. *Nephron.* 1990;54(2):154–161.

24. Oliver MJ, Edwards LJ, Treleaven DJ, Lambert K, Margetts PJ. Randomized study of temporary hemodialysis catheters. *Int J Artif Organs.* 2002;25(1):40–44.

25. Falk A, Prabhuram N, Parthasarathy S. Conversion of temporary hemodialysis catheters to permanent hemodialysis catheters: a retrospective study of catheter exchange versus classic de novo placement. *Semin Dial.* 2005;18(5):425–430.

26. Van Ha TG, Fimmen D, Han L, Funaki BS, Santeler S, Lorenz J. Conversion of non-tunneled to tunneled hemodialysis catheters. *Cardiovasc Intervent Radiol.* 2007;30(2):222–225.

27. Deshpande KS, Hatem C, Ulrich HL, Currie BP, Aldrich TK, Bryan-Brown CW, Kvetan V. The incidence of infectious complications of central venous catheters at the subclavian, internal jugular, and femoral sites in an intensive care unit population. *Crit Care Med.* 2005;33(1):13–20.

28. Oliver MJ, Callery SM, Thorpe KE, Schwab SJ, Churchill DN. Risk of bactermia from temporary hemodialysis catheters by site of insertion and duration of use: a prospective study. *Kidney Int.* 2000;58(6):2543–2545.

29. Naumovic RT, Jovanovic DB, Djukanovic LJ. Temporary vascular catheters for hemodialysis: a 3 year prospective study. *Int J Artif Organs.* 2004;27(10):848–854.

30. Pervez A, Abreo K. Central vein cannulation for hemodialysis: techniques and tips for quick and safe temporary catheter placement. *Semin Dial.* 2007;20:621–625.

31. Prabhu MV, Juneja D, Gopal PB, Sathyanarayanan M, Subhramanyam S, Gandhe S, Nayak KS. Ultrasound-guided femoral dialysis access placement: a single-center randomized trial. *Clin J Am Soc Nephrol.* 2010;5(2):235–239.

32. Hoggard J, Saad T, Schon D, Vesely TM, Royer T. Guidelines for venous access in patients with chronic kidney disease: a position statement from the American Society of Diagnositic and Interventional Nephrology Clinical Practice Committee and the Association for Vascular Access. *Semin Dial.* 2008;21(2):186–191.

33. Gupta A, Karak PK, Saddekni S. Translumbar inferior vena cava catheter for long-term hemodialysis. *J Am Soc Neprol.* 1995;5(12):2094–2097.

34. Moimi M, Rasoulo MR, Kenari MM, Mahmoodi HR. Non-cuffed dual lumen catheters in the external jugular veins versus other central veins for hemodialysis. *Saudi J Kidney Dis Transpl.* 2009;20:44–48.

35. Ross, J. An alternative approach to the central circulation from about the diaphragm. *Semin Dial.* 2004;17:307–309.

36. Frampton AE, Kessaris N, Hossain M, Morsy M, Chemla ES. Use of the femoral artery rout for the placement of temporary catheters for emergency dialysis when all usual central venous access sites are exhausted. *Nephrol Dial Transplant.* 2009;24(3):913–918.

37. Little MA, Conlon PJ, Walshe JJ. Access recirculation in temporary dialysis catheters as measured by saline dilution technique. *Am J Kid Dis.* 2000;36(6):1135–1139.

38. Atapour A, Mosakazemi M, Mortazavi M, Beigi A, Shahidi S. Access recirculation in jugular venous catheter in regular and reversed lines. *Iran J Kid Dis.* 2008;2(2):91–94.

39. McGee WT, Ackerman BL, Rouben LR, Prasad VM, Bandi V, Mallory DL. Accurate placement of central venous catheters: a prospective, randomized multicenter trial. *Critical Care Med.* 1993;21(8):1118–1123.

40. Vesely TM. Central venous catheter tip position: a continuing controversy. *J Vasc Interv Radiol.* 2003;14:527–534.

41. Collier PE, Goodman GB. Cardiac Tamponade caused by central venous catheter perforation of the heart: a preventable complication. *J Am Coll Surg.* 1996;181:459–463.

42. Duntley P, Siever J, Korwes ML, Harpel K, Heffner JE. Vascular erosion by central venous catheters: clinical features and outcome. *Chest.* 1992;101(6):1633–1638.

43. Canaud B, Leray-Moraques H. Temporary vascular access for extracorporeal renal replacement in acute renal failure patients. *Kidney Int Suppl.* 1998;66:S142–S1450.

44. Bersten AD, Williams DR, Phillips GD. Central venous catheter stiffness and its relation to vascular perforation. *Anaesth Intensive Care.* 1988;16(3):342–351.

45. Andrews RT, Bova DA, Venbrux AC. How much guidewire is too much? Direct measurement of the distance from the subclavian and internal jugular vein access sites to the superior vena cava–atrial junction during central venous catheter placement. *Crit Care Med.* 2000;28(1):138–142.

46. Contreras G, Lui PY, Elzinga L, Anger MS, Lee J, Robert N, et al. A multicenter, prospective, randomized comparative evaluation of the dual-versus triple-lumen catheters for hemodialysis and apheresis. *Am J Kid Dis.* 2003;42(2):315–324.

47. Rupp ME, Lisco SJ, Lipsett PA, Perl TM, Keating K, Civetta JM, et al. Effect of a second-generation venous catheter impregnated with chlorhexidine and silver sulfadiazine on central catheter-related infections. *Ann Intern Med.* 2005;143(8):570–580.

48. Civetta JM, Hudson-Civetta J, Ball S. Decreasing catheter-related infection and hospital costs by continuous quality improvement. *Crit Care Med.* 1996;24(10):1660–1665.

49. Maki DG, Stolz SM, Wheeler S, Mermel LA. Prevention of central venous catheter-related blood stream infection by use of an antiseptic-impregnated catheter. A randomized, controlled trial. *Ann Intern Med.* 1997;127(4):257–266.

50. Hu KK, Veenstra DL, Lipsky BA, Saint S. Use of maximal sterile barriers during central venous catheter insertion: clinical and economic outcomes. *Clin Infect Dis.* 2004;39(10):1441–1445.

51. Young EM, Commiskey ML, Wilson SJ. Translating evidence into practice to prevent central venous catheter-associated bloodstream infections: a systems-based intervention. *Am J Infect Control.* 2006;34(8):503–506.

52. Safdar N, Maki DG. The pathogenesis of catheter-related bloodstream infection with noncuffed short-term central venous catheters. *Intensive Care Med.* 2004;30:62–67.

53. Ranji SR, Shojania KG. Implementing patient safety interventions in your hospital: what to try and what to avoid. *Med Clin N Am*. 2008;92:275–293.

54. Catalano K, Fickensher K. Complying with the 2008 National Patient Safety Goals. *AORN J*. 2008;87: 547–556.

55. Maki DG, Ringer M, Alvarado CJ. Prospective randomized trial of povidone–iodine and chlorhexidine for prevention of infection associated with central venous and arterial catheters. *Lancet*. 1991;338(8763):339–343.

56. Langgartenr J, Linde HJ. Combined skin disinfection with chlorhexidine/propanol and aqueous povidone–iodine reduces bacterial colonization of central venous catheters. *Intensive Care Med*. 2004;30:1081–1088.

57. Lin BS, Kong CW, Tarng DC, Huang TP, Tang GJ. Anatomical variation of the internal jugular vein and its impact on temporary haemodialysis vascular access: an ultrasonographic survey in uraemic patients. *Nephrol Dial Transplant*. 1998;13(1):134–138.

58. Hind D, Calvert N, McWilliams R, Davidson A, Paisley S, Beverley C, Thomas S. Ultrasonic locating devices for central venous cannulation: meta-analysis. *BMJ* 2003;327(7411):361.

59. Geddes CC, Walbaum D, Fox JG, Mactier RA. Insertion of internal jugular temporary hemodialysis cannulae by direct ultrasound guidance—a prospective comparison of experienced and inexperienced operators. *Clin Nephrol*. 1998;50(5):320–325.

60. Dionisio P, Cavatorta F, Zollo A, Valenti M, Chiappini N, Bajardi P. The placement of central venous catheters in hemodialysis: role of the endocavitary electrocardiographic trace. Case reports and literature review. *J Vasc Access*. 2001;2(2):80–88.

61. Adams BD, Lyon ML, DeFlorio PT. Central venous catheterization and central venous pressure monitoring. In: Roberts JR, Hodges JR, eds. *Clinical Procedures in Emergency Medicine*. 5th ed. Philadelphia, PA: Saunders Elsevier; 2009:1263–1267.

62. Chapman GA, Johnson D, Bodenham AR. Visualisation of needle position using ultrasonography. *Anaesthesia*. 2006;61(2):148–158.

63. Stone MB, Moon C, Sutijono D, Blaivas M. Needle tip visualization during ultrasound-guided vascular access: short-axis vs long-axis approach. *Am J Emerg Med*. 2010;28(3):343–347.

64. Forauer AR, Glockner JF. Importance of US findings in access planning during jugular vein hemodialysis catheter placements. *J Vasc Interv Radiol*. 2000;11:233–238.

65. Niyyar VD, Work J. Interventional nephrology: core curriculum 2009. *Am J Kidney Dis*. 2009;54:160–182.

66. Granata A, Figuera M. Azygos arch cannulation by central venous catheters for hemodialysis. *J Vasc Access*. 2006;7:43–45.

67. Stonelake PA, Bodenham AR. The Carina as a landmark for central venous catheter tip position. *Br J Anaesth*. 2006;96: 335–340.

68. Abidi SM, Khan A, Fried LF, Chelluri L, Bowles S, Greenberg A. Factors influencing the function of temporary dialysis catheters. *Clin Nephrol*. 2000;53(3):199–205.

69. Hryszko T, Brzosko S, Mazerska M, Malyszko J, Mysliwiec M. Risk factors of nontunneled noncuffed hemodialysis catheter malfunction. A prospective study. *Nephron Clin Pract*. 2004;96(2):c43–c47.

70. Leblanc M, Fedak S, Mokris G, Paganini EP. Blood recirculation in temporary central catheters for acute hemodialysis. *Clin Nephrol*. 1996;45(5):315–319.

71. Kusminsky RE. Complications of central venous catheterization. *J Am Coll Surg*. 2007;204:681–696.

72. Filis K. Management of early and late detected vascular complications following femoral arterial puncture for cardiac catheterization. *Hellenic J Cardiol*. 2007;48: 134–142.

73. Guibert MC. Arterial trauma during central venous catheter insertion: case series, review and proposed algorithm. *J Vasc Surg*. 2008;48:918–925.

74. Schmiege LM. A fatal cardiac tamponade during hemodialysis. *Semin Dial*. 2006;19:434–437.

75. Tong MK, Siu YP, Ng YY, Kwan TH, Au TC. Misplacement of a right internal jugular vein haemodialysis catheter into the mediastinum. *Hong Kong Med J*. 2004;10(2):135–138.

76. Kaupke CJ, Ahdout J, Vaziri ND, Deutsch LS. Perforation of the superior vena cava by a subclavian hemodialysis catheter: early detection by angiography. *Int J Artif Organs*. 1992;15(11):666–668.

77. Akata T, Nakayama T, Kandabashi T, Kodama K, Takahashi S. Massive retroperitoneal hemorrhage associated with femoral vein cannulation. *J Clin Anesth*. 1998;10(4): 321–326.

78. Sreeram S, Lumsden AB, Miller JS, Salam AA, Dodson TF, Smith RB. Retroperitoneal hematoma following femoral arterial catheterization: a serious and often fatal complication. *Am Surg*. 1993;59(2):94–98.

79. Mirski MA, Lele AV, Fitzsimmons L, Toung TJ. Diagnosis and treatment of vascular air embolism. *Anesthesiology*. 2007;106(1):164–177.

80. Plewa MC, Ledrick D. Delayed tension pneumothorax complicating central venous catheterization and positive pressure ventilation. *Am J Emerg Med*. 1995;13:532–535.

81. Giacomini M, Iapichino G, Armani S, Cozzolino M, Brancaccio D, Gallieni M. How to avoid and manage a pneumothorax. *J Vasc Access*. 2006;7(1):7–14.

82. Alexandraki I, Sullivan R, Zaiden R, Bailey C, McCarter Y, Khan A, et al. Blood culture isolates in hemodialysis vascular catheter-related bacteremia. *Am J Med Sci*. 2008;336(4):297–302.

83. Hung KY, Tsai TJ, Yen CJ, Yen TS. Infection associated with double lumen catheterization for temporary haemodialysis: experience of 168 cases. *Nephrol Dial Transplant*. 1995;10(2):247–251.

84. Unver S, Atasoyu EM, Evrenkaya TR, Ardic N, Ozyurt M. Risk factors for the infections caused by temporary double-lumen hemodialysis catheters. *Arch Med Res*. 2006;37(3):348–352.

85. Roberts TL, Obrador GT, St Peter WL, Pereira BJ, Collins AJ. Relationship among catheter insertions, vascular access infections and anemia management in hemodialysis patients. *Kidney Int*. 2004;66(6):2429–2436.

86. Mokrzycki MH, Zhang M, Cohen H, Golestaneh L, Laut JM, Rosenberg SO. Tunneled haemodialysis catheter bacteraemia: risk factors for bacteraemia recurrence, infectious complications and mortality. *Nephrol Dial Transplant*. 2006;21(4):1024–1031.

87. Bouza E, Burillo A, Munoz P. Empiric therapy for intravenous central line infections and nosocomially acquired acute bacterial endocarditis. *Crit Care Clin*. 2008;24(2):293–312, viii–ix.

88. Schubert C, Moosa MR. Infective endocarditis in a hemodialysis patient: a dreaded complication. *Hemodial Int.* 2007;11:379–384.

89. Shah A, Murray M, Nzerue C. Right atrial thrombi complicating use of central venous catheters in hemodialysis. *J Vasc Access.* 2005;6(1):18–24.

90. Kingdon EJ, Holt SG, Davar J, Pennell D, Baillod RA, Burns A, et al. Atrial thrombus and central venous dialysis catheters. *Am J Kidney Dis.* 2001;38(3):631–639.

91. Durbec O, Viviand X, Potie F, Vialet R, Albanese J, Martin C. A prospective evaluation of the use of femoral venous catheters in critically ill adults. *Crit Care Med.* 1997;25(12):1986–1989.

92. Gonsalves CF, Eschelman DJ, Sullivan KL, DuBois N, Bonn J. Incidence of central vein stenosis and occlusion following upper extremity PICC and port placement. *Cardiovasc Intervent Radiol.* 2003;26(2):123–127.

93. Oguzkurt L, Tercan F, Torun D, Yildirim T, Zümrütdal A, Kizilkilic O. Impact of short-term hemodialysis catheters on the central veins: a catheter venographic study. *Eur J Radiol.* 2004;52(3):293–299.

94. Madan AK, Allmon JC, Harding M, Cheng SS, Slakey DP. Dialysis access induced superior vena cava syndrome. *Am Surg.* 2002;68(10):904–906.

95. Ansari MJ, Syed A, Wongba W, Shaikh Y, Hug S, Karamally Z, Salem M. Superior vena cava obstruction presenting as a complication of repeated central venous cannulations. *Compr Ther.* 2006;32(3):189–191.

96. Weyde W, Badowski R, Krajewska M, Penar J, Moron K, Klinger M. Femoral and iliac vein stenosis after prolonged femoral vein catheter insertion. *Nephrol Dial Transplant.* 2004;19(6):1618–1621.

97. Manierski C, Besarb A. Antimicrobial locks: putting the lock on catheter infections. *Adv Chronic Kidney Dis.* 2006;13:245–258.

98. Chiou PF, Chang CC. Antibiotic lock technique reduces the incidence of temporary catheter-related infections. *Clin Nephrol.* 2006;65:419–422.

99. Mandolfo S, Borlandelli S, Elli A. Catheter lock solutions: it's time for a change. *J Vasc Access.* 2006;7(3):99–102.

100. Moran JE, Ash SR, Beathard GA, Hoggard J, Lewis J, Lichfield T, et al. Locking solutions for hemodialysis catheters; heparin and citrate—a position paper by ASDIN. *Semin Dial.* 2008;21(5):490–492.

101. Yevzlin AS, Sanchez RJ, Hiatt JG, Washington MH, Wakeen M, Hofmann RM, Becker YT. Concentrated heparin lock is associated with major bleeding complications after tunneled dialysis catheter placement. *Semin Dial.* 2007;20(4):351–354.

102. Vercaigne LM, Takla TA. Long-term effect of an ethanol/sodium citrate locking solution on the mechanical properties of hemodialysis catheters. *J Vasc Access.* 2010;11:12–16.

103. Parienti JJ, Mégarbane B, Fischer MO, Lautrette A, Gazui N, Marin N, et al. Catheter dysfunction and dialysis performance according to vascular access among 736 critically ill adults requiring renal replacement therapy: a randomized controlled study. *Crit Care Med.* 2010;38(4):1118–1125.

104. Wong JK, Sadler DJ, McCarthy M, Saliken JC, So CB, Gray RR. Analysis of early failure of tunneled hemodialysis catheters. *AJR Am J Roentgenol.* 2002;179(2):357–363.

105. Suhocki PV, Conlon PJ Jr, Knelson MH, Harland R, Schwab SJ. Silastic cuffed catheters for hemodialysis vascular access: thrombolytic and mechanical correction of malfunction. *Am J Kidney Dis.* 1996;28(3):379–386.

106. Macrae JM, Loh G, Djurdjev O, Shalansky S, Werb R, Levin A, Kiaii M. Short and long alteplase dwells in dysfunctional hemodialysis. *Hemodial Int.* 2005;9(2):189–195.

107. Faintuch S, Salazar GM. Malfunction of dialysis catheters: management of fibrin sheath and related problems. *Tech Vasc Interv Radiol.* 2008;11:195–200.

26

TUNNELED CATHETER DESIGNS AND THE PLACEMENT CONUNDRUM

STEPHEN R. ASH

1. Understand the many requirements for a properly functioning of central venous catheters (CVC) for dialysis.

2. Understand the importance of position of catheter tip placement on function of CVC for dialysis.

3. Understand the difference between acute and chronic CVC for dialysis.

4. Understand the effects of various tip designs and side holes on function and complications of CVC for dialysis.

5. Understand why it is difficult to follow the K-DOQI recommendation to have both lumen tips of CVC placed in the right atrium for proper hydraulic function.

6. Understand the remaining challenges of CVC for dialysis and future directions to resolve the remaining problems.

INTRODUCTION

Over 70% of patients initiating chronic hemodialysis in the United States have a tunneled central venous catheter (CVC) for dialysis as their first blood access device. Tunneled CVC for dialysis have requirements for blood flow that are unparalleled by other chronic access devices. There have been numerous designs of the tip of tunneled CVC for dialysis, each designed to maximize flow through the catheter. Also there have been conflicting recommendations regarding whether the tips of

the catheter should be placed within the SVC or within the right atrium. This chapter reviews the numerous tip designs of tunneled CVC and evaluates the advantages and disadvantages of each design, reviewing supporting evidence for differences in outcomes. This chapter also reviews data and recommendations indicating that the tips of standard single-body and split-tip dialysis catheters should reside within the right atrium, while the Centros catheter arterial tip functions properly in the lower part of the SVC.

PREVALENCE AND PROBLEMS OF CENTRAL VENOUS CATHETERS FOR HEMODIALYSIS

Over 70% of patients initiating chronic hemodialysis in the United States have a tunneled CVC as their first blood access device.[1] As shown by CMS and in Figure 26-1, at 90 days of dialysis, the catheter is still the access of use in over 50% of patients, often in patients in whom the fistula or graft has not matured, was not workable, or was not indicated.[2] Over the period from 2002 to 2005, the number of grafts being used at 90 days decreased and the number of fistulas increased, but the percentage of catheters being used remained about the same.

Many patients would be better served if an AV fistula had been placed some months earlier, and if it were fully developed and functional when dialysis was implemented. Although this is the desired situation, it is not often the actual course. One reason that fistulas can be created after the start of dialysis is that tunneled CVC are fairly effective in providing dialysis therapy, at least for a period of some months. As summarized by Beathard,[3,4] tunneled CVC for dialysis have numerous advantages (noted in Table 26-1) as well as some significant disadvantages.

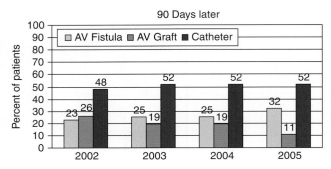

Figure 26-1. Distribution of access types 90 days after initiation of chronic outpatient dialysis (CMS[2]).

The requirements for a tunneled CVC for dialysis are actually multiple and stringent, unlike requirements for any other access device[5]:

- High blood flow rates at moderate pressure drops, with few instances of outflow failure and pressure alarms regardless of patient fluid status and catheter position relative to the vein wall.
- Minimal trauma to the vein intima to avoid thrombosis and venous stenosis.
- Resistance to occlusion by fibrous sheathing.
- Prevention of bacterial migration around the catheter after placement.
- Avoidance of contamination of the catheter lumen.
- Avoidance of seeding of the outside of the catheter during bacteremia.

TABLE 26–1
Advantages and Disadvantages of Tunneled Central Venous Catheters for Dialysis

Advantages	Disadvantages
• Universally applicable (functional in nearly 100% of patients) • Ability to insert into multiple sites • Maturation time not required • Venipuncture not required • No hemodynamic consequences (no CP recirculation) • Ease and low cost of placement and replacement • Ability to provide access over a period of months • Ease of correcting thrombotic complications	• High morbidity due to thrombosis and infection • Ricks of permanent central venous stenosis or occlusion • Discomfort and cosmetic disadvantage of external appliance • Lower blood flow rates, requiring longer dialysis times

From Beathard et al.[3,4]

- Avoidance of clotting at the tip or within the catheter.
- Biocompatibility of the catheter surfaces, avoiding removal of white cells or platelets.
- Avoidance of lumen collapse under negative pressure.
- Avoidance of kinking of catheter segments at points of bending.
- Physical strength and integrity to avoid breaks or disconnections of any component (ability to replace broken connectors is desirable).
- Resistance to antiseptic agents that might be applied at the skin exit site.
- Placement procedures with minimal trauma, difficulty, and risk.
- Radiopaque appearance on x-ray, for evaluation of location during placement and after use.

Each tunneled CVC has a risk of failing one or more of these requirements, and each failure results in significant medical problems.

The use of dual lumen CVC for removing and returning blood during dialysis is commonplace now but in the late 1970s, this concept revolutionized dialysis.[6] Before the development of CVC for dialysis, dialysis was possible only with an arterial access, through an internal/external arterio–venous silicone shunt or through separate catheters placed into an artery and a vein and removed after each treatment.

The development of CVC for dialysis was not simple, especially for single-body catheters. Drawing blood from a central vein at 200–400 mL/min is a delicate and somewhat unpredictable process. The pressure in central veins is much lower than in arteries, and vein walls are thinner and more distensible, even though the flow of blood though central veins is the same as through central arteries. Removal of blood through the ports of a CVC in a vein creates a negative pressure around these ports due to direct suction and due to the Bernoulli effect. This negative pressure can cause the vein wall to collapse around the ports and obstruct flow into the ports, even if the flow through the vein is much higher than the flow of blood through the catheter. If a fibrous tissue sheath forms around the catheter and reaches the tip or if clots form around the tip, the entry port to the catheter becomes smaller and the velocity of blood flow is increased. The increased blood velocity creates a greater negative pressure around the ports, and increases the tendency to pull the vein wall over the tip.

There are four classic approaches to the problem of providing sufficient blood outflow through dual-lumen CVC for dialysis:

- Place the removal and return lumens into the left atrium, pointing downward from the left side of the SVC. At this location, the tips cannot rest against a venous or atrial wall (this position works well for IJ catheters placed on the right side).

- Position the catheter with the removal lumen on the inside of the catheter curve, directing this lumen away from the vein or atrial wall and towards the flowing blood stream (this position is the only choice for IJ catheters placed on the left side).

- Use a large catheter so that the removal lumen cannot be blocked by a small clot or a small amount of fibrous tissue at the point of contact with a vein or atrial wall.

- Provide multiple blood entry ports in all directions around the circumference of each catheter tip, so that some of the ports are always facing away from the vein wall.

There are problems and limitations of each of these approaches. Positioning the tips of the removal and return lumens at the middle of the atrium is somewhat difficult, especially since the relative positions of the catheter and the heart change when the patient stands up after lying on the procedure table and since the removal lumen is shorter than the return lumen (see further discussion below). Catheters placed from the right IJ lay against the left border of the SVC due to the tendency of the catheter to straighten. From this position, the tips can enter the mid portion of the right atrium. For catheters placed from the left IJ will lie against the right border of the SVC and the right wall of the atrium. These catheters are much more prone to outflow failure due to wall apposition, clotting, and sheathing. Positioning the catheter so that the removal lumen is on the inside of the catheter curve is not always easy, as the catheter course through the subcutaneous tissue and central veins are rather complex and tortuous. Placing a larger catheter is always more difficult and somewhat more traumatic than placing a smaller catheter, especially if the larger catheter is not round in shape. Providing multiple side holes in all directions around the catheter tips requires that two catheters be placed or that one catheter must separate into two separate tips. Side holes in a catheter also have disadvantages. If they are too large or too many, blood will quickly flow through the tip of the catheter after placement and between uses, removing catheter lock solutions and promoting clotting at the tip. If the side holes are too small or too few, then blood will flow in and out only through the tip of the catheter; thus diminishing any advantage of the side holes. Further, any single-body catheter that becomes covered by a sheath will lose function, whether there are side holes or not. Sheathing of catheters occurs wherever the catheter contacts a vein or atrial wall.[7] When sheathing develops, it is difficult to correct by tPA infusion, stripping, or catheter replacement.[8]

TYPES OF CVC FOR DIALYSIS AND A SHORT HISTORY

CVC for dialysis are classified into either "acute" or "chronic" catheters, depending on whether the catheters are expected to be used for only several days or months to years. Acute CVC are designed to be placed with a minimum amount of effort. Historically, acute catheters for dialysis were relatively rigid, pointed catheters with a conically shaped tip, which could be advanced into the vein directly over a guidewire. The catheter body dilates the entry site as it is advanced into the vein. Acute CVC for dialysis have no subcutaneous cuff or locking device and a short linear tunnel. More recently, some acute catheters have become available with soft tips similar to chronic tunneled catheters. The tract around the guidewire is dilated, and the catheter is stiffened using a stylet and then advanced over a guidewire in a manner similar to over-the-wire placement of a tunneled catheter (described below).

Tunneled CVC for dialysis are soft, blunt-tipped catheters with a subcutaneous Dacron® "cuff" for tissue in-growth or a plastic "grommet" to immobilize the catheters below the skin surface. Tunneled CVC are generally placed through internal jugular veins into the SVC with the goal of placing the tips of the catheter at the junction of the SVC and the right atrium. Alternative venous access points are external jugular veins, subclavian veins, and femoral veins. Due to their blunt shape tunneled CVC have traditionally been placed through a "splitsheath," which is a cylindrical thin-walled plastic device advanced into the vein over a dilator. The dilator has a central lumen that follows the guidewire. The guidewire and dilator are then removed, and the splitsheath opening is closed with a finger or valve to prevent excessive bleeding. The catheter is then inserted through the splitsheath into the central vein. The splitsheath is split along two preformed grooves, and the halves are retracted around the catheter, leaving the catheter in position within the central vein. More recently, techniques have been developed to allow placement of tunneled CVC to be performed over a guidewire placed through a previously dilated tract, in a manner similar to acute central venous catheters for dialysis. A plastic catheter or stylet within the catheter stiffens the catheter to allow it to follow the guidewire more easily.

Tunneled CVC for dialysis have a curved subcutaneous tunnel leading from the vein insertion site to a distant exit site. The cuff or plastic grommet fixes the catheter in position and prevents bacteria at the exit site from migrating around the catheter. The cuff also serves as the outer limit for a fibrous tunnel that leads to the entrance point of the central vein. This tunnel is similar to a vein wall and is contiguous with the internal jugular vein (or other vein of insertion), creating a passageway for blood or air when the catheter is removed. The tunnel stops at the Dacron cuff where it melds into the fibrous tissue surrounding the cuff. Without the cuff, as in acute catheters, this tunnel continues all of the way to the skin exit site over time, creating potential for back-and-forth movement of the catheter and potential peri-catheter bacterial migration around the catheter.

A pictorial history of tunneled dialysis catheters is included in Figure 26-2, and this history is discussed more fully in a recent review.[5] Canaud devised a catheter system comprised of two 10 French catheters, each placed into the vena cava and with tips leading to the right atrium. Flow

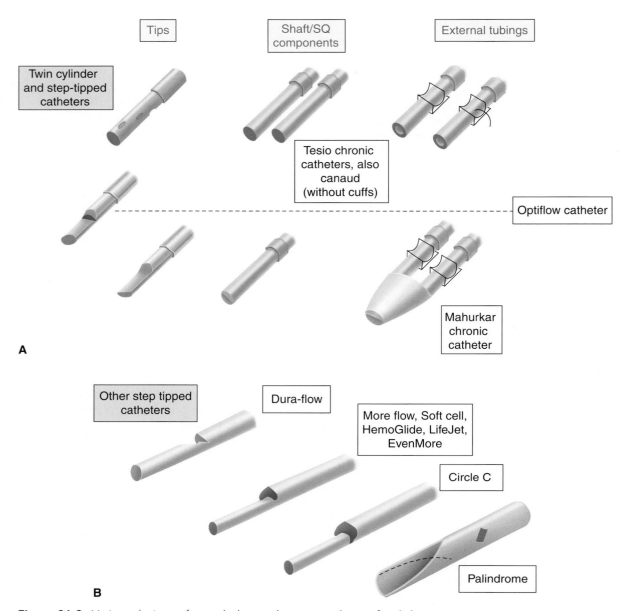

Figure 26-2. Various designs of tunneled central venous catheters for dialysis.

rate was excellent over many months of use.[9,10] Tesio added subcutaneous cuffs, and the catheter became more popular. More recent versions of the Canaud catheters have included a subcutaneous plastic grommet to fix the catheter limbs in place; the Schon catheter has a similar device. Quinton designed the PermCath dual lumen chronic catheter, an oval-shaped chronic catheter of about 20 French circumference and including two cylindrical 8 French lumens.[11,12] Mahurkar designed a chronic CVC of soft materials and blunt tips and double-d blood flow lumens.[13] The Ash Split Cath chronic catheter has a double-d configuration in the mid-body, but separates into two separate distal tips, each with side holes in all directions. The Palindrome catheter is a double-d catheter with both lumens having the same length, but with oppositely angled and symmetrical side

ports.[14] The Centros™ catheter has outward bends of the tips that contact the inferior vena cava in two places and inward bends to place the arterial and venous ports in the middle of the vena cava.[15]

ADVANTAGES AND DISADVANTAGES OF VARIOUS TUNNELED CVC DESIGNS

▶ Hydraulic Performance of Tunneled CVC Versus Grafts and Fistulas with Needles

In spite of the wide variety of designs of tunneled CVC for dialysis, there are few comparative studies to define advantages of one design over another. The best way to characterize the effectiveness of flow in a dialysis access

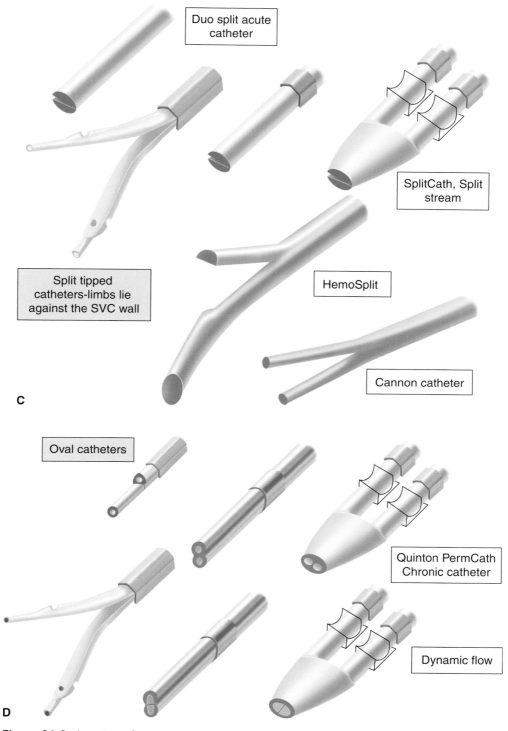

Duo split acute catheter

Split tipped catheters-limbs lie against the SVC wall

SplitCath, Split stream

HemoSplit

Cannon catheter

C

Oval catheters

Quinton PermCath Chronic catheter

Dynamic flow

D

Figure 26-2. (continued)

is to determine the "conductance" of the access, which is the flow rate divided by the pressure drop on the arterial (blood removal) limb.[4,5] Merely describing the achieved blood flow rate during an entire dialysis is not very descriptive, since the blood flow rate depends upon many factors such as number of pressure alarms, volume status of the patient, physician's prescription, pressure gradients, etc. General experience in a dialysis unit indicates that the hydraulic conductance of tunneled catheters and fistula or graft needles is about the same, until one or the other develops flow problems. Twardowski in 1999 showed that although there is considerable scatter, the hydraulic conductance of most catheters is similar to a 15- or 16-gauge needle in a graft or fistula during dialysis.[16]

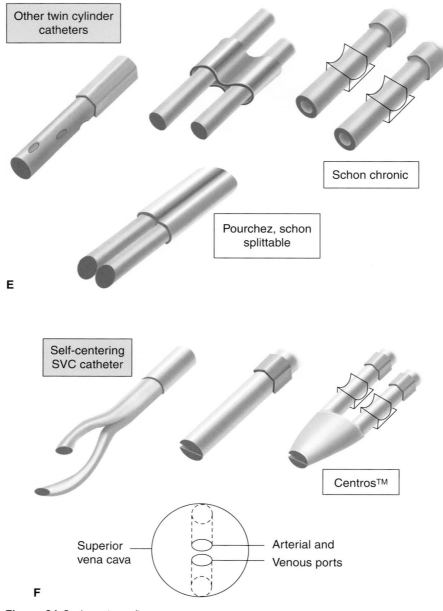

Figure 26-2. (continued)

Split-Tip Catheters Versus Single-Body Step Tips

The basic concept of a split-tipped catheter is to provide side holes around each limb of the catheter, similar to a Canaud or Tesio catheter. This assures that even if each limb lies against the surface of the vena cava or atrium that some side holes will be facing the lumen, and away from the wall. In vitro studies demonstrate the hydraulic advantage of this design, using models as shown in Figure 26-3. Mareels et al performed studies using computational flow dynamics and particle imaging and demonstrated that the Split Cath design had a considerably lower shear rate than any other catheter design, with only 32% of the tip portion having a shear stress over 10 Pa as shown in Figure 26-4. However, the downside of the Split Cath design was that it also creates areas of stagnation in the tip, with blood residence time at this location over 0.03 seconds.[17]

Clinically which is better, catheters with a split tip or a single body? Several studies have shown a slight advantage to the Split Cath versus step-tip catheters. Trerotola et al performed a randomized study of 12 ESRD patients receiving 14 F Split Cath catheters placed versus 12 patients receiving 13.5 F Hickman catheters.[18] Weekly for 6 weeks the blood flow rate was measured using Transonic flow monitors, while the blood pump was

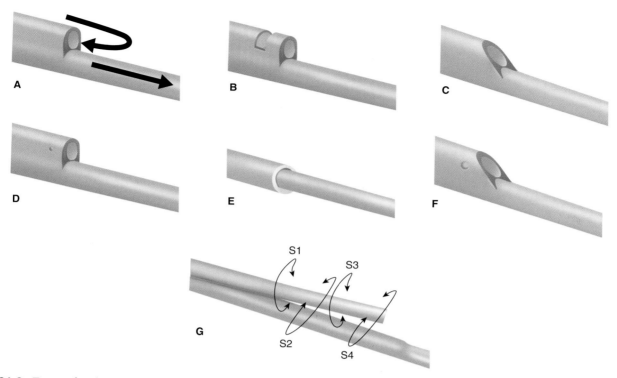

Figure 26-3. Types of catheters evaluated in CFD and PIV studies. (From Mareels et al.[17])

Parameters calculated in the tip zone of the arterial lumen of each catheter

	Cut straight (Reference)	Cut angle	Cut straight hole	Cut angle hole	Cut straight sleeve	Concentric	Ash split–based
Flow division							
End-opening	100%	100%	48.8%	46.6%	18.0%	100%	6.6%
Side entrance	N/A	N/A	51.2%	53.4%	82.0%	N/A	S4: 4.2% S3: 8.6%
							S2: 15.6% S1: 65.0%
Avg. SS	12.6 Pa	16.3 Pa +29%	14.2 Pa +13%	14.6 Pa +17%	12.8 Pa +2%	44.8 Pa +255%	11.6 Pa −8%
% Vol. SS > 10 Pa	41.8%	54.7% +31%	45.8% +10%	47.9% +15%	41.0% −2%	87.9% +110%	32.2% −23%
% Vol. RT > 0.015 s	16.8%	13.9% −17%	9.8% −42%	10.2% −39%	19.7% +17%	18.9% +13%	60.8% +262%
% Vol. RT > 0.030 s	0.1%	2.6% ×26	0.1% ×1	0.1% ×1	2.7% ×27	8.3% ×83	31.4% ×314
Avg. SS where RT ≤ 0.015 s	10.7 Pa	15.3 Pa +43%	13.4 Pa +25%	13.7 Pa +28%	10.6 Pa −1%	37.1 Pa +247%	11.0 Pa +3%
Avg. SS where RT ≥ 0.015 s	21.3 Pa	22.7 Pa +6%	21.3 Pa 0%	22.6 Pa +6%	22.0 Pa +3%	77.6 Pa +264%	12.0 Pa −44%
Platelet lysis index	0.0071	0.0448 ×6.3	0.0154 ×2.2	0.0249 ×3.5	0.0497 ×7.0	0.1260 ×17.7	0.0357 ×5.0

SS, Shear stress; RT, blood residence time.
The following parameters were calculated in the tip zone of the arterial lumen of each catheter: (1) tip volume average SS, (2) percentage of tip volume with SS > 10 Pa, (3) percentage of tip volume with RT > 0.015 second, (4) percentage of tip volume with RT > 0.030 second, (5) average SS in zones with RT ≤ 0.015 second, (6) average SS in zones with RT > 0.015 second, and (7) Platelet Lysis Index. Percentages show relative difference compared with reference case.

Figure 26-4. Measured shear rate and residence time for various parts of various catheter designs.[17]

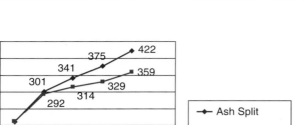

Figure 26-5. Relationship between roller pump setting of dialysis machine and actual flow rate by Transonic™ device, for Split Catheter and Bard Hickman. (From Trerotola et al.[18])

set at speeds of 200, 300, 350, 400, and as high as possible with sustained flow. The measured blood flow rate at the highest pump setting was 422 ± 12 mL/min for the Split Cath and 359 ± 13 for the Hickman ($P < 0.005$) as shown in Figure 26-5. Recirculation was significantly less at all pump settings for the Split Cath patients ($P = 0.01-0.06$), though for both catheters it remained below 6% as shown in Figure 26-6.

Long-term functional survival of CVC is probably the most significant measure of the success of their use. One problem with such studies is a lack of firm definitions for patency failure or catheter-related blood stream infection (CRBSI), to serve as endpoints. Many catheters are removed in these studies for presumed failure to flow or sepsis. In the Trerotola study above, the Split Cath had slightly better 6-week survival than the Hickman catheter. Richard et al performed a randomized study comparing the Split Cath, Opti-Flow, and Tesio catheters in 113 placements in ESRD patients.[19] Maximum (effective) blood flow rates were compared between the catheters immediately after placement, and 30 and 90 days after placement. Blood flow rate tended to be higher with the Split Cath but results were not significantly different. Failure-

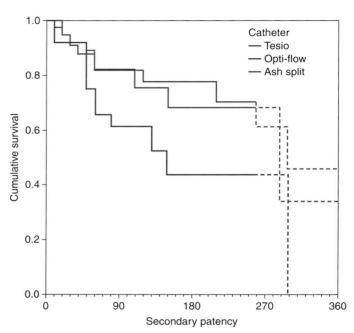

Figure 26-7. Survival of catheters to primary failure, for Split Cath, Optiflow, and Tesio Catheters. (From Richard.[19])

free survival of the catheters was analyzed with an average follow-up of 120 days. Though statistically not significant, predicted lifespan appeared higher for the Split Cath and Tesio catheters than the Opti-Flow. Placement complications occurred only with Tesio and Opti-Flow catheters. These results are shown in Figure 26-7.

Trerotola and Kraus also performed a randomized study comparing the Split Cath and Opti-Flow catheters in 132 placements in ESRD patients.[20] Complications during placement were no different for the two catheters and ranged 15–17% (mostly, kinking). Opti-Flow delivered significantly higher flow rates when tested at 1 month, but there was no significant difference in flow at 6 months. Recirculation was always lower with the Split Cath catheter but not always significantly different. The Split Cath had significantly longer half life, partly due to lower infection rate but also due to some mechanical failures of the Opti-Flow. Postulating on reasons that the Split Cath might have lower infection rates, the authors suggested that the "self-cleaning" function of the Split Cath, with high velocity flow through the side holes created by the "step down" tip, may diminish fibrin sheath and therefore decrease opportunity for bacterial colonization. The results of seven nonrandomized studies of the Split Cath confirming catheter survival rates of about 9 months on average are summarized in our review in Seminars in Dialysis.[5] However, overall longevity of Split Caths is not any better than that of Tesio/Canaud catheters, which have been shown to have up to 2 years average assisted function.[21]

One problem with both single-body and split-tip catheters is that both lay against the vena cava or atrial wall,

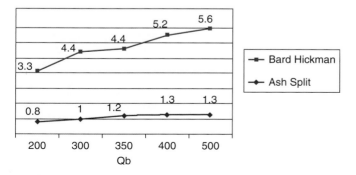

Figure 26-6. Recirculation in forward flow measured by Transonic, for recently placed Split Caths versus Bard Hickman. (Data from Trerotola et al.[18])

rather than in the center of the vena cava. This means that both types of catheters function much better if placed from the right IJ with tips extending into the atrium from the left border of the SVC.

▶ Side Holes Versus No Side Holes in Tunneled CVC

As discussed above regarding the Split Cath design, catheter side holes have advantages and disadvantages. They can decrease overall resistance and provide lower shear rate and better flow in the short run especially on the arterial side. However, they can also create relative dead space at the end of the tip promoting clotting. They allow flow of blood through the tip to wash out locking solution almost as soon as the catheter is filled with it.[5,22,23] Side holes also allow clots to adhere to the catheter tip, a process facilitated by lumens with rough edges. Tesio/Canaud catheters have six side holes in a spiral shape. It is not uncommon for these catheters to clot completely within several hours after placement. Removing the clot with forceful irrigation, using the catheter for dialysis, and then relocking the catheter with heparin usually results in a catheter that functions for a long time. Presumably this is because the catheter becomes "biolized" or protein-coated and is therefore more resistant to clotting.

Side holes can also increase overall catheter resistance. To understand this, it is important to understand more about how blood flows within a catheter. A curious phenomenon is that the relationship between flow and pressure is not the same on both lumens of the catheter. As shown in Figure 26-8, the higher the blood flow rate, the higher the hydraulic resistance on the arterial side. The relationship

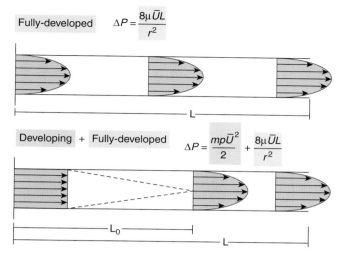

Figure 26-9. Depiction of the difference between fully developed and developing flow within dialysis catheters. At the arterial inlet port, blood enters as developing flow rather than parabolic flow, and this flow has high resistance. The higher the flow rate, the greater the proportion of developing flow in the catheter lumen. (From Fricker et al.[25])

between flow and pressure is not a straightline as it is on the venous lumen.[24] The best explanation for this phenomenon is given by Fricker et al, who demonstrated that at the arterial inlet port, blood enters the catheter as "developing" flow pattern, not a parabolic or developed flow pattern, as shown in Figure 26-9. This "plug" flow results in higher shear at the catheter inner surface. The higher the flow rate, the greater the distance it takes the blood to develop parabolic flow within the catheter lumen, and the greater the hydraulic resistance of the catheter.[25] Also, the more complicated the tip shape, the greater the distortion of flow and the greater the distance of developing flow, as shown in Figure 26-10. If the tip is blocked and all of the flow is through the side holes, then hydraulic resistance can increase markedly with blood flow rate, regardless of the size of the side holes.[25]

Do side holes provide any advantage clinically? Tal et al performed a prospective study of Mahurkar-type single-body tunneled catheters, comparing catheters with side holes to catheters without side holes.[26] On removal, many of the catheters with side holes had adherent clots, while those without side holes had fewer adherent clots, as shown in Figure 26-11. In follow-up over 12 weeks, there was a slightly higher flow rate for catheters with side holes, though not a significant difference. Surprisingly there was a significantly higher rate incidence of CRBSI in the catheters with side holes versus those without (2.54/1000 catheter days versus 0.254/1000 catheter days). The authors surmised that clots adherent to the catheter tip served as a nidus for infection, after seeding from systemic bacteremia or lumen contamination.

Thus, side holes have advantages and disadvantages. If a catheter limb rests against a vein or atrial wall and

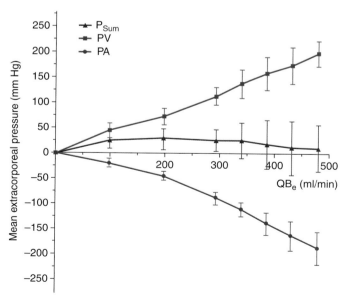

Figure 26-8. Relationship between flow and pressure during in vitro experiments with DD catheters. The hydraulic resistance of the venous lumen is fairly constant, but that of the arterial lumen increases with increasing flow. (From Kindgen-Milles.[24])

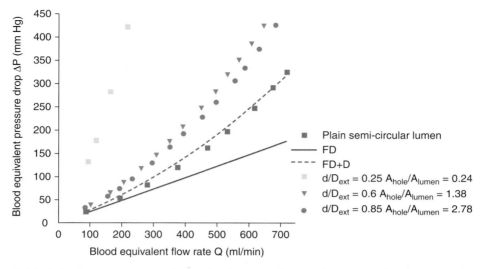

Figure 26-10. Effect of side-hole tip geometry on relationship between flow and pressure. The more complicated the tip design, the less developed is the flow pattern and the greater the catheter resistance. (From Fricker et al.[25])

the tip is blocked by sheath or thrombus, side holes allow continued flow though at a higher hydraulic resistance. However, if a catheter tip can be positioned away from a wall, as in the atrium or within the SVC blood stream, then side holes would not be necessary and in fact may be disadvantageous.

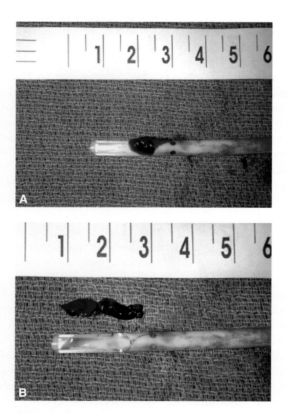

Figure 26-11. Clots adherent to the side holes of Mahurkar-type step tipped catheters, in the study by Tal et al.[26]

▶ Symmetric Tipped Tunneled CVC, the Palindrome™

In 2005, Tal reported on a new catheter design with symmetric tips and biased ports, as shown in Figure 26-12.[27] In an animal study, the percentage recirculation was compared to that of step-tip and split-tip catheters, immediately after placement. All of the catheters were run in reverse flow and tips placed in the SVC or the right atrium. As shown in Figure 26-13, the Palindrome had less recirculation than any of the other catheters. Surprisingly, all catheters had slightly more recirculation when placed in the atrium than when in the SVC. The stepped tip catheters had no flow when placed in the SVC of the pig though the split tip and Palindrome allowed flow.

In the patient and over time, any catheter lying on the vein or atrial wall will be affected by sheaths, clots, and the relation of the catheter tip to the vascular surfaces, and these factors affect recirculation. In a recent survey study of recirculation in a dialysis unit, Moossavi et al measured recirculation in patients with step-tip, split-tip, and

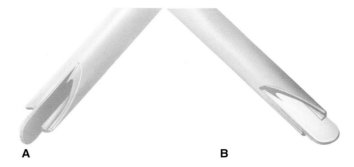

Figure 26-12. The symmetrical Palindrome catheter of Dr. Tal, with bias-cut ports. Kinetic energy carries returning blood downstream, and pressure gradient brings blood through the closest part of the removal blood lumen. (From Tal et al.[27])

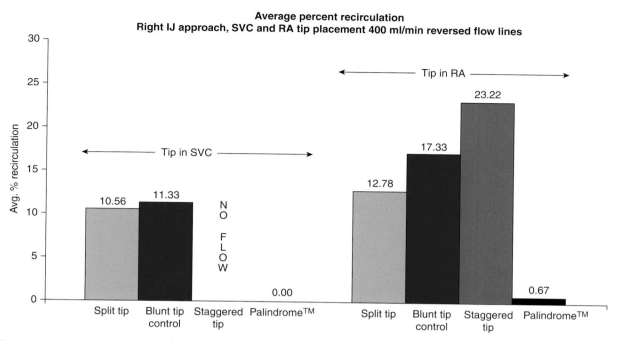

Figure 26-13. Recirculation rates with reversed flow for step tip, split tip, and Palindrome catheters, in an animal model. (From Tal et al.[27])

symmetrical (Palindrome) catheters, while the catheters were run in the usual flow direction. All tunneled catheters delivered the same recirculation, between 6% and 8%. Acute dialysis catheters however delivered blood flow with 23% recirculation. Though the Palindrome catheter appears successful, there are no clinical data yet showing that it diminishes recirculation or has higher flow rates over time than other catheters.[28]

▶ Self-Centering SVC Catheter, the Centros™

The idea of the Centros™ catheter is fairly simple. The best way to avoid complete sheathing of the catheter is to hold a portion of the catheter in the middle of the vena cava, since sheaths develop only at points of contact with the vein. As shown in Figure 26-12, the Centros™ catheter has a distal end that is planar with two outward bends of the distal tips that create two points of contact with the SVC. The ports bend inward from the two contact points toward the center of blood flow in the vena cava and away from the wall of the vein wall. Side holes are not necessary since the ports should not be in contact with the vena cava wall, and therefore the ports should not become occluded. If fibrous sheathing near the ports is avoided, the blood flow rate of the Centros™ should be maintained over many months of use, and recirculation should be minimal (in vitro tests demonstrate zero recirculation). The catheter is designed to be placed in the lower third of the SVC rather than within the atrium, so positioning is made easier and if the catheter rides up or down a few centimeters, then this will not change the relationship of the ports to the vein wall and flowing blood and therefore will not affect blood flow.

Total area of contact of the catheter at two points with the vena cava is much less than for single-body or split-tip catheters, which lie in a line along the SVC, and there is no more separation of the "jet" of blood entering and leaving the tips than with standard catheters.

Animal trials have demonstrated that a catheter supported within the SVC will remain free of sheathing and thrombosis and diminish evidence of trauma in the SVC. In 1998, Kohler and Kirkman reported an animal trial in which single lumen 3.2 mm diameter catheters were placed in the SVC of pigs and left for 1–8 weeks.[29] No anticoagulant was administered, and the catheters were not used for infusion or blood removal. Some of the catheters had a 2 cm diameter loop attached to them, to center the tip in the distal SVC. During placement of the catheters without a loop, fluoroscopy demonstrated a continued relative motion of the catheter and vena cava wall with each heartbeat; however, catheters with the loop remained stationary at the point of contact with the vena cava wall. As shown in Figure 26-14 when the loop catheters were examined at the end of the 8 weeks period, the SVC and catheter were completely free of fibrous sheathing and thrombosis. In pigs with nonlooped catheters, the catheter was completely covered by sheath and thrombus, and the SVC had a greater number and size of intimal lesions and was nearly occluded by fibrosis and clot. From this study, it is apparent that a catheter, which is supported in the vena cava by two points of contact, should have considerably less sheathing and fibrosis, and therefore more constant flow over time, versus straight, single-body or split-tip catheters. Catheters of this design should also cause less damage to the vena cava and might have a lower incidence of eventual SVC stenosis.

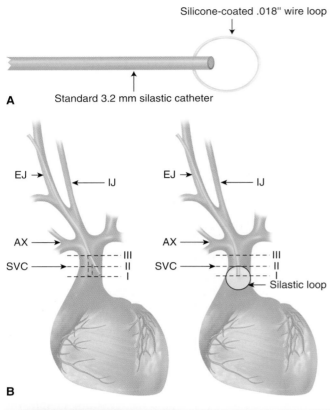

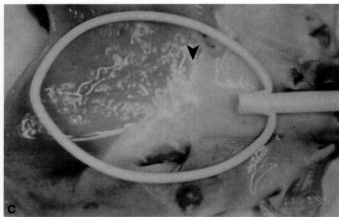

Figure 26-14. (**A**) Catheter design of Dr. Kohler with loop to support the distal tip in the middle of the vena cava; (**B**) position of loop in SVC; (**C**) appearance of SVC in area of tip of catheter, 8 weeks after placement. (From Kohler et al.[29])

In June of 2007, the FDA approved the Centros™ catheter for use in dialysis access. A small number of these catheters were created of 28 and 24 cm length (hub to tip) and a gentle bend at the apex. All catheters had a self-sealing opening on the venous limb to allow threading over a single guidewire, though this feature is not needed for placement through a split sheath. After IRB approval, we initiated a clinical trial at four independent centers to determine the hydraulic properties of the catheter and permanence of flow. Inclusion criteria were quite broad:

- adult patients initiating or continuing in-center HD who were scheduled to receive a tunneled dialysis catheter in the right IJ vein;
- patients who may have had a prior tunneled catheter for dialysis in the right IJ site were eligible for inclusion in the study; and
- patients were expected to require use of the catheter for more than 45 days.

Exclusion criteria were few:

- patients with a prior history of right IJ vein thrombosis, or
- with documented stenosis of the right IJ, innominate, or SVC;
- patients in whom the catheter would be placed into the same site as an existing catheter; and
- patients who were unable to sign a consent form.

Nine catheters were placed into patients, in all cases through the right IJ, under local anesthesia using fluoroscopy, ultrasound, and a 16 French split sheath. Tips of the catheters were placed in the lower third of the SVC rather than in the atrium. An example of a postplacement x-ray is in Figure 26-15. The catheters were used three times per week for outpatient hemodialysis treatments. Once per week at the start of dialysis, the blood pump was set to deliver a negative arterial pressure of -200 mm Hg on the arterial line. The blood flow rate associated with this modestly negative pressure was recorded (Qb_{-200}). The same measurement was also performed on 120 prevalent DD tunneled CVC for dialysis in 20 dialysis centers, as part of a study of catheter locks. In the current study, reasons for catheter removal were recorded as were any significant problems with the catheters.

Figure 26-16 demonstrates the average Qb_{-200} flow rate for all nine catheters, over the 7 week study. The mean Qb_{-200} was 390 mL/min (SD $\pm$ 49) at catheter insertion and was 401 mL/min (SD $\pm$ 80) at 7 weeks of use (NS). By comparison, 120 standard tunneled dialysis IJ catheters being used in several dialysis units had a lower Qb_{-200}, 348 mL/min (SD $\pm$ 64, $P < 0.05$). During 7 weeks of follow up, one of the nine self-centering catheters was removed due to presumed exit infection, and one was removed when no longer needed. No catheter failed to provide adequate flow for dialysis during the study.

At the end of the study catheters continued to be used for dialysis, in some patients up to 18 months. All catheters continued to function without any loss of flow for duration of catheter use. Two patients volunteered for a CT scan of the chest after 4 months of catheter use. Figure 26-17 demonstrates that the catheters were in the expected position, limbs in a plane across the vena cava with at least one distal limb separated from the wall of the vena cava. No sheath was seen but, of course, a standard CT could not detect sheaths of less than 1 mm thickness. For comparison, Figure 26-18 includes two CT scans performed on patients with Split Cath catheters, demonstrating that both limbs of these catheters are adjacent to the vena cava wall,

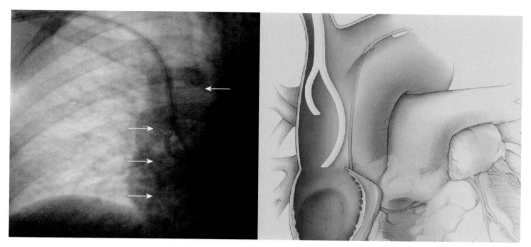

Figure 26-15. X-ray of chest showing placement of the Centros™ tips in the lower third of the SVC and drawing of same position (left side). Arrows indicate (from top) right tracheo-broncheal angle, split point of Centros, arterial port, and venous port. All arrows are approximately 3 cm apart. For comparison, a drawing of the usual placement position of the Centros™ (right).

as is always the case. One of these Split Cath catheters has a clot and/or sheath covering the catheter. At removal, none of the Centros™ catheters exhibited any resistance to retraction, and none came out with remnants of any thickened sheath. In fact, most catheters were remarkably free of any clots or evidence of sheath.

This preliminary study indicated that the self-centering Centros™ catheter provides highly acceptable flow rate at modest negative pressure, without deterioration in flow rate over 7 weeks of use. This high flow rate occurred despite positioning of the tips of the catheter in the SVC (rather than within the atrium). The Centros™ catheter was marketed briefly in 2008 but a production problem led to some process redesign, and the catheter was reintroduced in 2010. An observational multicenter study of catheter function has indicated high flow at modest negative pressure in almost all catheters, for periods of up to 18 months. It has been observed that in

patients with pacemaker wires and a history of previous IJ dialysis catheters, there is sometimes a limitation in arterial or venous port flow noted during placement of a Centros from the right IJ.

THE CATHETER TIP CONUNDRUM

Further, if the Centros catheter is inserted too far into the right atrium, the venous limb may rest against the right wall of the atrium, and outflow through the venous limb can be impeded. For this reason, current recommendation is that the arterial lumen should be placed toward the left, in all patients (as in K/DOQI recommendations). As described above and confirmed in a review by Vesely in 2003, standard tunneled IJ single-body or split-tip catheters work best if the arterial port (or tip) is placed well within the right atrium.[30] NKF K/DOQI recommendations in 2000 stated "The catheter tip should be adjusted to the level of the caval atrial junction or into the right

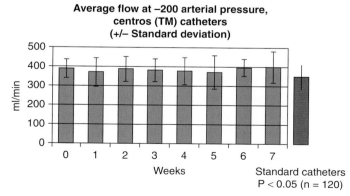

Figure 26-16. Flow rate of the Centros catheters at modestly negative arterial side pressure (QB_{-200}), over 7 weeks of dialysis use. For comparison, same measurement done on 120 prevalent DD tunneled dialysis catheters.

Average flow at −200 arterial pressure, centros (TM) catheters (+/− Standard deviation)

Standard catheters
$P < 0.05$ (n = 120)

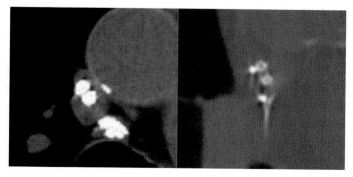

Figure 26-17. CT scans of the chest done 4 months after Centros placement in two patients, demonstrating that the catheter limbs form a plane within the vena cava and at least one port is separated from the vena cava wall. The SVC on the right includes two pacemaker wires.

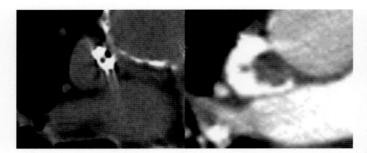

Figure 26-18. CT scans of two patients with Split Cath catheters in place for several months. Note that both limbs of the catheter lie against the vena cava wall. Clot surrounds the catheter in the CT angiogram on the right.

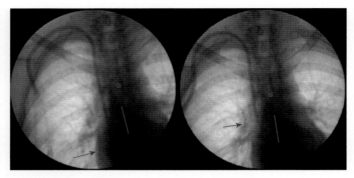

Figure 26-19. Two successive x-rays of a patient and a newly placed single-body tunneled CVC for dialysis, when supine (left) and on standing immediately after placement (right). The red arrows indicate the tip of the catheter, the red dots indicate the level of the right tracheo-bronchial angle, and the red line the approximate extent of the superior vena cava (3–7 cm below the right tracheo-bronchial angle). (Courtesy of Dr. Beathard.[3])

atrium to ensure optimal blood flow. (Atrial positioning is only recommended for catheters composed of soft compliant material, such as silicone.)" However, due to the recommendations of many on the committee in 2006, the language was updated to "At the time of placement, the tip(s) of the catheter should be in the midatrium, with the arterial lumen facing the mediastinum."[31] However, the FDA stated in 1989 that for all central venous catheters "the catheter tip should not be placed in or allowed to migrate into the heart" and this position is unchanged at present.[32] Most instructions for use included with tunneled IJ dialysis catheters still say that the tips should be placed "at the junction of SVC and right atrium." In 2000, the SCVIR Technology Assessment Committee published "Reporting Standards for Central Venous Access" which states that the "ideal tip location for central venous access catheters has yet to be determined."[33]

Aside from the general confusion and conflict in the opinions expressed by these influential organizations, there are physical impossibilities regarding recommendations for keeping the tip position either "at the junction" or "in the right atrium":

- It is not possible to have both tips reside at any one point since the tips are separated, usually by 3 cm.
- The SVC/atrial junction is not a single point, but rather a slanted oval.
- The location of this junction is not clear from commonly used landmarks such as the intersection of the right border of the mediastinum and the heart shadow.[30] Aslamy et al have demonstrated by MRI that in 38% of patients the right border of the heart is formed by the left atrial appendage.[34] The best landmark for determining the SVA/atrial junction is the right tracheobronchial angle, but this landmark is rarely used during catheter placement.[30] The median distance from the origin of the SVC to the right tracheobronchial angle is 1.5 cm (range, 0.1–3.8 cm), and the median distance from the right tracheobronchial angle to the SVC/atrial junction is 4.9 cm (range, 2.9–6.8 cm). A catheter tip positioned 3 cm below the right tracheobronchial angle would always be within the SVC, not the atrium.[34]

- The tip of a catheter often is not clearly visible on x-ray due to the rapid movement of the tip with heartbeat and inspiration.[30]
- When a patient rises from supine position to sitting the abdominal contents descend, the central veins lengthen, the right atrium expands, and the anterior chest wall shifts inferiorly because of gravity. All of these changes result in a tip movement up into the SVC of 2–3 cm in all patients (not just obese patients).[30] An example of the range of tip motion between supine and standing positions is shown in Figure 26-19.
- If the arterial port is placed 2–3 cm into the right atrium, then the venous tip will be 5–6 cm into the right atrium, bringing the venous port into apposition with the lower atrium or even through the tricuspid valve when the patient is supine.
- If the arterial port is placed less than 2 cm into the right atrium, then retraction of the catheter on standing will cause the tips to enter the lower portion of the SVC, and heart and respiratory motion will cause the tips to "piston" in and out of the SVC-atrial junction, as shown in Figure 26-19.
- Due to the material memory of tunneled dialysis catheters, it is not possible to place the tips of a catheter placed in the left IJ anywhere except on the right atrial wall or right wall of the SVC.
- The recommendation of tip placement is not relevant to catheters that are designed to function in the SVC, such as the Centros, although the usual placement of the Centros does place the venous port at or below the SVC/atrial junction.
- The NKF K/DOQI recommendations for catheters placed through femoral veins are only that they be longer than 20 cm in length. "This length dependency may result from the ultimate tip position of longer catheters in the IVC as opposed to the common iliac vein with

shorter catheters. The greater blood flow available to the catheter at the IVC site reduces recirculation." Thus, it would appear that catheters placed in the SVC should reach the SVC/atrial junction or be within the atrium, but catheters in the IVC can work OK.

In spite of all of these inconsistencies, there is general agreement that the best location for single-body or split-tip catheters is to have them placed through the right IJ route and with the tips as far as possible into the right atrium.

CURRENT CHALLENGES AND FUTURE DIRECTIONS FOR TUNNELED CVC FOR DIALYSIS

The advent of successful tunneled CVC for dialysis has been a great advance for patients with ESRD, both for beginning hemodialysis and for continuing dialysis. Tunneled CVC now allow dialytic support of patients for many months if needed, allowing patients to be supported long enough for fistulas and grafts to be created, corrected, and become the best long-term access choices.

In spite of advances, tunneled CVC still have significant problems and limitations. For each of these problems, there will someday exist a solution that will advance the technology and benefits of tunneled CVC for dialysis:

- *Catheter-related infections*: Catheter materials, chemical impregnation methods, or catheter locks are now being investigated to kill bacteria in the biofilm layers both on the outside and inside of tunneled CVC, in order to decrease this most common complication of the catheters. The antibacterial effect of impregnated chemicals and new catheter materials in a tunneled CVC must remain for many months rather than a week or so (as with acute catheters), and this implies the need for some method of regeneration of the active component over time, or use of covalently bound enzymatic or catalytic materials. Two recent reviews have confirmed that every antibacterial catheter lock that has been studied in randomized, prospectively controlled trials has demonstrated a 50–80% decrease in incidence of CRBSI.[35,36] Recently, a new antiseptic catheter lock comprised of 7% sodium citrate, and parabens and methylene blue has been studied in a large randomized trial and found to have a diminished incidence of CRBSI and improved catheter patency.[37]

- *Catheter tip position*: As discussed above, for when IJ catheters are placed from the left side, the natural elasticity of the catheter places the tips against the right side of the vena cava or right atrial wall. If catheters were specifically created for left IJ placement and had a curved shape to fit the innominate vein and vena cava, then the memory of the material might position tips against the left side of the lower vena cava and direct them into the middle of the right atrium.

- *Catheter tip clotting*: As mentioned above, catheters without side holes have some advantage in avoiding clotting.

Catheters that open and close at the tip would allow the catheter to retain anticoagulant and completely avoid blood clotting within the ports. Heparin-coated catheters have not been shown to prolong patency of the catheter.

- *Catheter fibrous sheathing*: As described above, one solution for catheter sheathing may be a catheter that centers itself in the vena cava (the Centros™). Other approaches include chemical impregnation of the catheter to prevent the growth of macrophages and fibroblasts around the catheter bodies, though this is likely to be difficult since the irritation of the vein wall by the catheter is such a strong stimulus for sheath formation.

- *Central venous stenosis*: Methods to distribute or diminish "wear" on the vena cava must be evolved to avoid this serious and still frequent complication. Avoiding use of acute dialysis catheters diminishes the frequency of central venous stenosis. Catheters that are supported at only two points in the SVC diminish the contact area of the catheter to the vein but might increase wear at two points. Whether these catheters diminish the risk of SVC stenosis in the long run is unproven.

- *External component bulk*: Patients bandage and keep dry the hubs, extension tubings, clamps, and connectors, but many also complain about the general bulk of the catheters components on their bodies. Also, the preclusion of showering is a real bother to many patients. Subcutaneous ports were proposed as one solution (LifeSite and BioLink) but clearly are not the answer for most long-term patients. Eventually more radical skin-level "connectology" will be necessary.

- *External component breakage*: More durable yet still lightweight components are possible. Simplifying the entire catheter design to limit the size and number of glued connections is a partial solution.

With a few significant improvements, tunneled CVC for dialysis could become a painless, effective, and safe long-term access for the majority of dialysis patients and perfectly acceptable as an alternative to AV grafts. For those patients in whom they are possible, the fistula will likely remain the optimal access for some years. However, when looked at objectively, none of our dialysis access devices are completely maintenance-free, safe, or reliable and vascular access remains the "Achilles Heel" of dialysis therapy. What is needed is a fourth option, which has been slow in coming. What we need to do is to mimic nature's design of vascular connections and model our dialysis access to the end-to-side anastomoses of the natural body.

REFERENCES

1. Beathard GA. Strategy for maximizing the use of arteriovenous fistulae. *Semin Dial.* 2000;13(5):291–296.
2. 2006 Annual Report ESRD Clinical Performance Measures Project, CMS.
3. Beathard GA. ASDIN Curriculum. Published 2008 by ASDIN through Lippincott.

4. K/DOQI Guideline updates and clinical practice guidelines from 2006. CPG 2.4 (Basic Principles for Catheter Insertions).

5. Ash SR. Fluid mechanics and clinical success of central venous catheters for dialysis— answers to simple but persisting problems. *Semin Dial.* 2007;20:237–256.

6. Schwab SJ, Beathard G. The hemodialysis conundrum: hate living with them, but can't live without them. *Kidney Int.* 1999;56:1–17.

7. Foraner AR, Theohasis C. Histologic changes in the human vein wall adjacent to indwelling central venous catheters. *J Vasc Interv Radiol.* 2003;14:1163–1168.

8. D'Othee BJ, Than JC, Sheiman RG. Restoration of patency in failing hemodialysis catheters. *J Vasc Interv Radiol.* 2006; 17:1011–1015.

9. Canaud B, Leray-Moragues H, Garrigues V, Mion C. Permanent twin catheter: a vascular access option of choice for haemodialysis in elderly patients. *Nephrol Dial Transplant.* 1998;7:82–88.

10. Canaud B, Leray-Moragues H, Kamoun K, Garrigue V. Temporary vascular access for extracorporeal therapies. *Ther Apher.* 2000;4:249–255.

11. Blake PG, Huraib S, Wu G, Uldall PR. The use of dual lumen jugular venous catheters as definitive long term access for haemodialysis. *Int J Artif Organs.* 1990;13: 26–31.

12. Schwab SJ, Buller GL, McCann RL, Bollinger RR, Stickel DL. Prospective evaluation of a Dacron cuffed hemodialysis catheter for prolonged use. *Am J Kidney Dis.* 1988;1: 166–169.

13. Tapson JS, Hoenich NA, Wilkinson R, Ward MK. Dual lumen subclavian catheters for haemodialysis. *Int J Artif Organs.* 1985;8(4):195–200.

14. Tal MG. Comparison of recirculation percentage of the palindrome catheter and standard hemodialysis catheters in a swine model. *J Vasc Interv Radiol.* 2005; 16:1237–1240.

15. Ash SR, Brown K, Asif A, Yevzlin S, Samaha AL. Preliminary clinical study of a self-centering central venous catheter for dialysis (Centros™). American Society of Diagnostic and Interventional Nephrology (ASDIN) Accepted Abstracts—Fourth Annual ASDIN Scientific Meeting February 9–10, 2008. *Semin Dial.* 2008;21(1): 105–111.

16. Twardowski Z. Blood flow, negative pressure and hemolysis during hemodialysis. *Home Hemodial Int.* 1999;3:45–50.

17. Mareels G, Kaminsky R., Verdonck PR. Particle image velocimetry-validated, computational fluid dynamics-based design to reduce shear stress and residence time in central venous hemodialysis catheters. *ASAIO J.* 2007;53(4): 438–446.

18. Trerotola SO, Shah H, Johnson M, Namyslowski J, Moresco K, Patel N, Kraus M, Gassensmith C, Ambrosius WT. Randomized comparison of high-flow versus conventional hemodialysis catheters. *JVIR.* 1999;10:1032–1038.

19. Richard HM, Hastings GS, Boyd-Kranis RL, Murthy R, Radack DM, Santilli JG, Ostergaard C, Coldwell DM. A randomized, prospective evaluation of the Tesio, Ash Split, and Opti-flow hemodialysis catheters. *J Vasc Interv Radiol.* 2001;12(4):431–435.

20. Trerotola SO, Kraus M, Shah H, Namyslowski J, Johnson MS, Stecker MS, Ahmad I, McLennan G, Patel NH, O'Brien E, Lane KA, Ambrosius WT. Randomized comparison of split tip versus step tip high flow hemodialysis catheters. *Kidney Int.* 2002;62:282–289.

21. Wang J, LaBerge JM, Chertow GM, Kerlan RK. Tesio catheter access for long-term maintenance hemodialysis. *Radiology.* 2006;241(1):284–290.

22. Polaschegg HD, Shah C. Overspill of catheter locking solution: safety and efficacy aspects. *ASAIO J.* 2003;49(6): 713–715.

23. Polaschegg HD. Loss of catheter locking solution caused by fluid density. *ASAIO J.* 2005;51(3):230–235.

24. Kindgen-Milles D, Kram R, Kleinekofort W. Assessment of Temporary Dialysis Catheter Performance on the basis of flow and pressure measurements in vivo and in vitro. *ASAIO J.* 2007;53(3):351–356.

25. Fricker ZP, Rockwell DO. Pressure drop through generic lumens of hemodialysis catheters. *ASAIO J.* 2007;53(4): 428–433.

26. Tal MG, Peixoto AJ, Crowley ST, Denbow N, Eliseo D, Pollak J. Comparison of side hole versus nonside hole high flow hemodialysis catheters. *Hemodial Int.* 2006;10(1): 63–67.

27. Tal MG. Comparison of recirculation percentage of the palindrome catheter and standard hemodialysis catheters in a swine model. *J Vasc Interv Radiol.* 2005;16:1237–1240.

28. Moossavi S, Kaufman T, Jordan J, Moossavi S, Vachharajani T. Retrospective evaluation of factors influencing the catheter recirculation in prevalent dialysis patients. *Semin Dial.* 2008;21(2):197–199.

29. Kohler TR, Kirkman, TR. Central venous catheter failure is induced by injury and can be prevented by stabilizing the catheter tip. *J Vasc Surg.* 1998;28(1):59–65.

30. Vesely T. Central venous catheter tip position: a continuing controversy. *J Vasc Interv Radiol.* 2003;14:527–534.

31. National Kidney Foundation. K/DOQI Clinical Practice Guidelines for Vascular Access. *Am J Kidney Dis.* 2001;37(suppl 1):S137–S181; Clinical Practice Guidelines and Clinical Practice Recommendations 2006 Updates, www.kidney.org/professionals/kdoqi.

32. Food and Drug Administration Task Force. Precautions necessary with central venous catheters. *FDA Drug Bull.* 1989;15–16.

33. Silberzweig JE, Sacks D, Khorsandi AS, Bakal CW. Reporting standards for central venous access. *J Vasc Interv Radiol.* 2000;11:391–400.

34. Aslamy Z, Dewald CL, Heffner JE. MRI of central venous anatomy. Implications *for central venous c*atheter insertion. *Chest.* 1998;114:820–826.

35. Jaffer Y, Selby NM, Taal MW, et al. A meta-analys*is of hemodialysis c*atheter locking sol*utions* in the prevention of catheter-related infection. *Am J Kidney Dis.* 2008;51: 233–241.

36. Labriola L, Ralph Crott R, Jadoul M. Preventing haemodialysis catheter-related bacteraemia with an antimicrobial lock solution: a meta-analysis of prospective randomized trials. *Nephrol Dial Transplant.* 2008;23(5): 1666–1672.

37. Maki DG, Ash SR, Winger RK, Lavin P. A novel antimicrobial and antithrombotic lock solution for hemodialysis catheters, a Multi-center Controlled Randomized Trial. *Crit Care Med.* 2011;39(4):613–620.

CATHETER DYSFUNCTION—RECIRCULATION, THROMBOSIS, AND FIBROEPITHELIAL SHEATH

TUSHAR J. VACHHARAJANI

LEARNING OBJECTIVES

1. To understand the various mechanical causes leading to tunneled catheter dysfunction.
2. To understand the strategies to treat noninfectious causes of catheter dysfunction.

Mechanical dysfunction of the central venous catheter (CVC) is the second most common problem (after infection) encountered in clinical practice. The NKF/DOQI guidelines define CVC malfunction as "failure to attain and maintain an extracorporeal blood flow sufficient to perform hemodialysis (HD) without significantly lengthening the HD treatment." The Work Group considered sufficient extracorporeal blood flow to be 300 mL/min.[1] The current definition is opinion-based and has been disputed recently in a study comparing adequacy of dialysis with blood flows ranging from 250 to 300 mL/min.[2] Recirculation of blood during hemodialysis is considered to be a marker of CVC dysfunction. Early dysfunction of CVC is often related to poor placement techniques and malpositioned catheter tips.[3] Appropriate use of fluoroscopy and postprocedure radiographic evaluation can help avoid such a complication in most cases. Late catheter dysfunction is generally related to either a thrombus[4] or fibroepithelial sheath formation.[5]

RECIRCULATION

Recirculation occurs when blood returning from the venous limb of the catheter re-enters the arterial limb of the catheter without passage through the circulation (Figure 27-1).

Catheter recirculation rate is generally considered to be significant when it exceeds 10% of the blood flow. Typically, the arterial and venous ports of the CVC are connected to the arterial and venous lines of the dialyzer, respectively, to achieve maximum solute clearance during dialysis. The ports of a poorly functioning CVC can be reversed for one dialysis treatment before being definitively evaluated. Often this practice is unavoidable due to the lack of an immediate alternative solution, resulting in the patient receiving inadequate dialysis therapy. Frequent monitoring and implementing the guidelines by Kidney/Dialysis Outcomes and Quality Initiatives for immediate referral for catheter evaluation with an appropriate intervention may prevent inadequate dialysis.[6]

The incidence of blood recirculation is common with nontunneled CVC,[7] especially when the connections are reversed.[8] Laurin et al reported that 42% of their study population, who were being dialyzed using temporary catheters with reversed connections, had a three- to sixfold increase in recirculation rate compared to patients with standard connections.[8] Leblanc et al reported that temporary CVC for acute hemodialysis had lower recirculation rates when placed in the subclavian vein than when placed in the femoral vein.[9] A shorter length (13.5 vs 19.5 cm) of the temporary CVC, especially when placed in the femoral vein, was also associated with an increase (22% vs 12%) in the recirculation rate.[9]

The recirculation rates, both with standard and reversed connections, have been investigated in animal models. Tal evaluated a symmetric tip catheter (Palindrome™), staggered tip catheter without side holes, a split-tip catheter, and a "blunt tip" catheter (created by cutting the tip of the staggered tip catheter) in three animals.[10] Twelve catheters were used, and recirculation rates were measured at 300, 400, and 500 mL/min with standard connections. The recirculation was measured at 400 mL/min with each

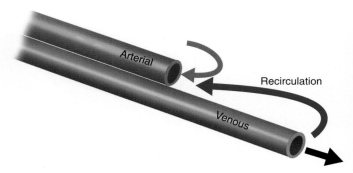

Figure 27-1. Schematic representation of recirculation in a double lumen catheter.

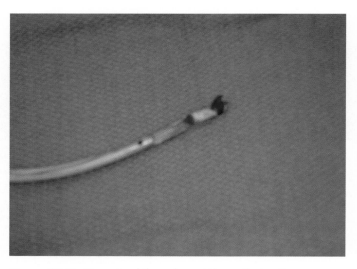

Figure 27-2. Organized thrombus at the catheter tip occluding the lumen.

catheter after reversal of lines. The measurements were obtained with tips positioned in the superior vena cava and in the right atrium. The study concluded that the symmetric tip catheter had minimal recirculation with reversal of dialysis lines compared to currently marketed split tip and staggered tip catheters.

Similar data on various catheter designs and recirculation rates with reversed connections in human subjects in a single study are not available. However, there are published data from observational studies. Senecal et al reported 18–24% recirculation rate in 37 step tip CVC with line reversal.[11] The recirculation rate with standard connections in tunneled CVC in humans is controversial. Trerotola et al reported a higher recirculation rate in step tip catheters compared to split tip catheter design[12] at blood flows of 300–400 mL/min in 123 patients. Moossavi et al reported CVC recirculation rate to be independent of the catheter design, site, or time on dialysis in 165 catheters.[13]

Dysfunctional CVC are routinely connected with line reversal to achieve adequate blood flow during dialysis. A higher rate of recirculation when lines are reversed is not without consequences, as it often leads to inadequate dialysis.[14] To circumvent the possible reduction in dialysis adequacy with CVC reversal, the alternatives are to increase the duration of therapy or maximize blood flow.[11,15] Moist et al reported a 41.7% incidence of recirculation in their prevalent dialysis population. Nearly 30% (28.7%) of these CVC were in standard connections whereas 71.3% were in reversed connections. Moreover, the authors reported that when blood flow was maintained at >250 mL/min, 80% of the dialysis population maintained adequate clearance, defined as urea removal rate >65%.[2] Recirculation rate in CVC can be a marker for catheter dysfunction and should not be considered as the only indicator for intervention.

THROMBOSIS

Thrombosis is a common cause of catheter dysfunction. Catheter-associated thrombus can be intraluminal or extraluminal. The physiological process of thrombosis begins with damage to the vascular endothelium during

catheter insertion, resulting in propagation of the coagulation and inflammatory cascades.[16] The process may be further enhanced by inadequate flushing of catheters after dialysis or inadequate filling of the catheter lumen with anticoagulants.

▶ Intraluminal Thrombus

Thrombus formation within the lumen or at the catheter tip can result in catheter dysfunction as shown in Figure 27-2.

Proper maintenance and care of the catheter by the dialysis staff can generally reduce the incidence of intraluminal thrombus formation. Adequate flushing of the catheter after dialysis treatment is completed is the key to preventing thrombus formation. The incidence of thrombosis is higher in CVC placed in femoral veins as compared to internal jugular veins.[17] The effect of gravity and difference in viscosity between heparin and blood leads to leakage of the anticoagulant.[18] The anticoagulant leakage is prominent with catheters with multiple side holes at the tip, which will not retain the heparin. A thrombus at the tip can be occlusive or act like a one-way valve preventing free blood flow through the catheter.

▶ Extraluminal Thrombus

Extraluminal thrombus formation can be categorized as either central vein thrombosis or right atrial thrombosis. The mere presence of a catheter in the central vein can lead to thrombus formation in the central vein (Figure 27-3).

The true incidence of central vein thrombus formation is unknown, as many patients remain asymptomatic. The incidence has been reported as ranging from 2% to 64% depending on the study design.[19,20]

Asymptomatic formation of a thrombus in the internal jugular vein has been reported in 29.5% of 143 patients with a history of having a tunneled catheter and 62% of

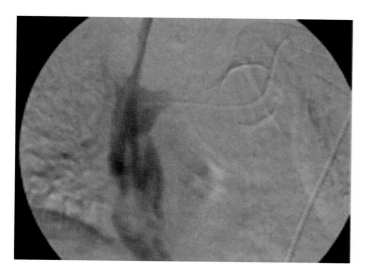

Figure 27-3. Thrombus in the central vein. (Courtesy Aslam Pervez.)

these with occluded internal jugular veins.[21] The common risk factors associated with catheter-related thrombosis are infection and a longer duration of having the catheter in the central vein.

Thrombosis of the axillary and subclavian veins has been reported but rarely. Superior vena caval thrombosis manifests commonly when there is a significant associated stenosis or when the thrombosis occurs in the presence of multiple hardware, as seen with patients with transvenous cardiac rhythm devices.[22] The incidence of central vein stenosis is higher if the CVC is placed in the left-sided central veins.[23] The common presenting symptoms of acute central vein thrombosis include facial, neck, upper extremity, and/or breast swelling. The symptoms are pronounced in the presence of a maturing or functioning ipsilateral permanent dialysis vascular access. Less frequently noticed symptoms such as cyanosis, dysphagia, chest pains, hoarseness of the voice, and headaches have been reported with thrombosis of the superior vena cava. Physical examination will reveal edema of the face, head, neck, and upper extremities with congested conjunctiva along with multiple collateral vein development in the chest and shoulder area.

▶ Right Atrial Thrombus

Large intra-atrial thrombus is an uncommon complication of CVC. More commonly a thrombus that is attached to the atrium at its point of contact is often detected on angiographic studies.[24] The differentiation from a large atrial thrombus (defined as >2 cm in diameter) may be difficult on initial angiographic study and requires further investigations with transesophageal echocardiography. The CVC may malfunction because of its tip being embedded in the thrombus.[25] The presence of an atrial thrombus can have serious consequences resulting in hemoptysis or dyspnea, as reported by Kingdon et al.[26] Negulescu et al reported 27% mortality in patients with CVC who developed atrial thrombosis.[27]

MANAGEMENT OF CATHETER THROMBOSIS

The medical care of catheter thrombosis can be divided into prevention and treatment.

▶ Prevention of CVC Thrombosis

Preventing thrombosis in CVC can be attempted by using a catheter lock solution with anticoagulant properties. The most commonly used locking solution is heparin. Various concentrations of heparin ranging from 1000 to 10,000 units/lumen have been used as CVC lock solutions. Although heparin has been used for several decades for preventing catheter thrombosis, the incidence reported in the literature remains between 4.0 and 5.5 episodes/1000 catheter days.[28,29]

Trisodium citrate lock is used as an alternative to heparin. Several studies have found trisodium citrate to be equivalent or superior to heparin as a catheter lock solution.[28,29] The risk of systemic bleeding events has been reported to be lower with trisodium citrate than with heparin.[30,31] Proper flushing of the catheter lumen with saline followed by instillation of the appropriate volume (not to exceed the internal catheter volume) of 1000 units/mL heparin or 4% citrate was recommended by the working group of American Society of Diagnostic and Interventional Nephrology in 2008.[32] The use of fibrinolytic agents like tissue plasminogen activator (tPA) as a locking solution is currently being studied and, until the results are available, routine use of tPA is not recommended.

Prophylaxis for CVC thrombosis using oral agents has been evaluated in randomized studies. Mokrzycki et al studied mini dose warfarin (1 mg/day) to prevent CVC thrombosis and did not find any improvement in CVC patency.[33] Another study, using warfarin (target INR 1.8–2.5) and ticlopidine (250 mg/day), reported significant improvement in CVC thrombosis when used as primary prevention compared with secondary prevention. However, fewer patients in the secondary prevention group had achieved adequate anticoagulation.[34] In the absence of controlled safety and efficacy studies using antiplatelet agents alone for the prevention of CVC thrombosis and with the additional risk of bleeding, such therapy should be reserved for high-risk patients with recurrent CVC malfunction.

▶ Primary Treatment of CVC Thrombosis

Once recognized, CVC malfunction must be addressed immediately. The initial approach is to administer a forceful saline flush and reposition the patient. The catheter can be flushed forcefully with a 10 mL syringe filled with saline, and an attempt to aspirate blood should be made. This technique is simple and can be repeated several times. If this technique fails, intraluminal lytic enzyme should be used. Urokinase and stretokinase were used in the past but have been replaced by recombinant tissue plasminogen activators (tPA). tPA activates the fibrinolytic system by cleaving the plasminogen, resulting in active plasmin formation, which eventually lyses fibrin. Several tPAs (alteplase, reteplase, and tenecteplase) have been used to treat CVC thrombosis but none have yet been approved for this indication. The reported short-term success rate for these tPAs is between 40% and 92% with no clear recommendation of dwell duration or dose.[35–38] In general, the effect of tPA should be expected to be temporary, and repeated instillations may be required for recurrent CVC thrombosis.

tPA infusion has been used to treat CVC thrombosis. 2.5 mg tPA in 50 mL of normal saline at 17 mL/h per port has been used, but the 90-day survival of catheter patency is reported to be 25%.[39] The value of tPA infusion is questionable, primarily due to the logistic difficulty in administering an infusion, and it has limited advantages over standard luminal instillation.

▶ Catheter Exchange Over a Guide Wire

Failure to achieve CVC patency with pharmacotherapy is an indication to perform catheter exchange over a guide wire. It is imperative to exclude fibrin sheath formation before inserting a new catheter as advocated by NKF-DOQI Clinical Practice Guideline 7.[1] Catheter exchange over a guide wire preserves the exit and venotomy site. The technical success rate has been reported to be 93%, with infection rates comparable to de novo CVC insertions.[40] The primary and secondary patency rates of catheters exchanged over a wire were no different from de novo CVC insertions.[40] In patients with limited life expectancy and limited central vascular sites, this strategy prolongs the patency of CVC. Complications during this procedure are rare.[40] No bleeding from the exit site was observed with this technique in a report of 51 consecutive catheter exchanges.[41]

▶ Treatment of Right Atrial Thrombus

The presence of a large atrial thrombus necessitates removal of the CVC along with systemic anticoagulation. Systemic anticoagulation is recommended for a minimum period of 6 months.[27] Low surgical risk patients should be considered for surgical thrombectomy, especially if there is any evidence of infection.[25,27,42] Appropriate management strategies have not been established for high surgical risk patients. The mortality reported in these patients is high, and long-term anticoagulation with weekly echocardiographic monitoring for resolution has been suggested.[43]

FIBROEPITHELIAL SHEATH

Fibrin sheath formation needs to be considered in every dysfunctional CVC that fails to respond to pharmacotherapy. The development of a fibrin sheath occurs within 24 hours of CVC placement. It develops at the point of CVC contact with the endothelium and eventually extends to cover the entire length of the catheter. A full-length fibrin sheath can develop as early as 5–7 days after placement, as a result of an inflammatory reaction in response to vessel injury and the biocompatibility of the catheter material.[5]

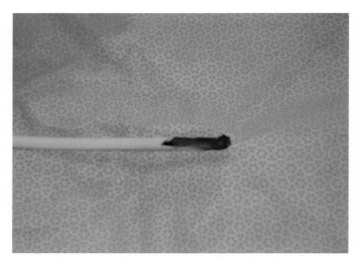

Figure 27-4. Fibrin sheath with thrombus encasing the entire tip of the catheter.

In an autopsy study, 100% of 55 cases were found to have a fibrin sheath around the CVC.[5] The fibrin sheath is not actually fibrin but connective tissue.[44,45] The endothelial injury from vessel puncture is covered with a collagenous layer produced by smooth muscle cells creating a one-way valve mechanism limiting the flow in a CVC. Further, formation of a thrombus at the tip of this sleeve eventually occludes the catheter lumen (Figure 27-4).

The presence of a fibrin sheath can be demonstrated in about 40% of cases with angiographic study[46] (Figure 27-5).

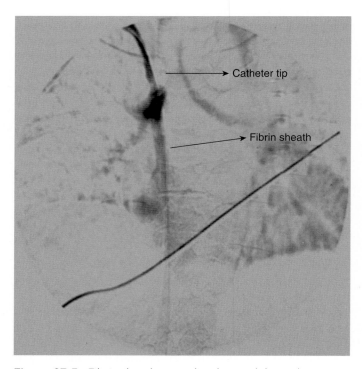

Catheter tip

Fibrin sheath

Figure 27-5. Fibrin sheath extending beyond the catheter tip.

Currently, there is no clear intervention available to prevent fibrin sheath formation.

▶ Treatment of Fibrin Sheath

Fibrin sheath can be treated with stripping or disruption. Stripping of the fibrin sheath is performed using a snare catheter. The snare is introduced through a femoral puncture, and the CVC is stripped along its entire length. The reported immediate success for this procedure is 78–98%.[47–49] Three-month and 6-month primary CVC patency has been reported as 45–60% and 28–45%, respectively.[47,48,50,51] The studies reported in the literature have used different techniques and study populations, making it difficult to draw any definitive conclusions. No major complications have been reported while performing this procedure. The major disadvantages are increasing the cost and duration of the procedure and added discomfort to the patient from femoral puncture. A newer internal snare device has been in limited use, with a reported 6-week primary success rate of 100%.[52]

Catheter exchange over a wire with simultaneous fibrin sheath disruption with a balloon has been used as an alternative to fibrin sheath stripping (Figure 27-6). The fibrin sheath is confirmed with angiography and, through the use of a noncompliant balloon, is disrupted from the confluence of brachiocephalic veins to the mid-right atrium. In a randomized, controlled pilot trial, 33/47 (70%) patients with dysfunctional CVC despite pharmacotherapy had a fibrin sheath. The median time to repeat dysfunction in the group assigned to sheath disruption was 373 days compared with 97.5 days in patients who

did not undergo disruption, and the median time to repeat catheter exchange was 411 days and 198 days, respectively. The dialysis blood flow (340 vs 329 mL/min) and adequacy (URR 73% vs 66%) were significantly better in the group assigned to sheath disruption.[53] The study was not adequately powered to evaluate the patency rate. A retrospective, nonrandomized small study compared catheter exchange over a guide wire, catheter exchange after fibrin sheath disruption and fibrin sheath stripping technique in 66 consecutive procedures on dysfunctional CVC. The authors reported the technical success rate, complication rate, and cumulative catheter patency rate at 1, 3, and 6 months to be identical.[54] A larger randomized study is needed to definitively determine the correct strategy to treat CVC with fibrin sheath.

SUMMARY

Catheter dysfunction due to mechanical problems remains a major clinical hurdle in patients receiving hemodialysis via tunneled central venous catheters. Early recognition and management can prevent or minimize the incidence of underdialysis. The management of mechanical dysfunction of a catheter as currently practiced in the United States is summarized in Table 27-1.

TABLE 27–1

Management of Catheter Dysfunction

Catheter Dysfunction	Treatment Options
Recirculation	• Appropriate catheter length • Avoid reversal of ports during dialysis • Early diagnosis and intervention
Catheter thrombus	• Prevention with proper locking solution • Use of thrombolytic agents • Catheter exchange over a wire
Fibroepithelial sheath formation	• Fibrin sheath disruption with a balloon • Stripping of fibrin sheath

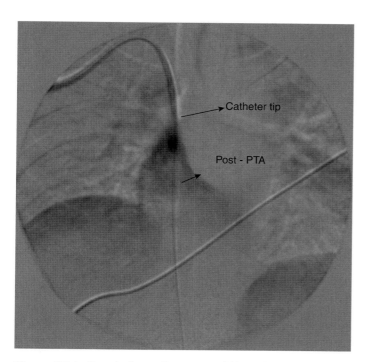

Figure 27-6. Post balloon disruption of fibrin sheath, radiocontrast filling the right atrium.

REFERENCES

1. Clinical practice guidelines for vascular access. *Am J Kidney Dis.* 2006;48(suppl 1):S176–S247.
2. Moist LM, Hemmelgarn BR, Lok CE. Relationship between blood flow in central venous catheters and hemodialysis adequacy. *Clin J Am Soc Nephrol.* 2006;1(5):965–971.
3. Wong JK, Sadler DJ, McCarthy M, Saliken JC, So CB, Gray RR. Analysis of early failure of tunneled hemodialysis catheters. *AJR Am J Roentgenol.* 2002;179(2):357–363.
4. Schwab SJ, Beathard G. The hemodialysis catheter conundrum: hate living with them, but can't live without them. *Kidney Int.* 1999;56(1):1–17.

5. Hoshal VL, Jr., Ause RG, Hoskins PA. Fibrin sleeve formation on indwelling subclavian central venous catheters. *Arch Surg.* 1971;102(4):353–358.

6. Clinical practice guidelines for vascular access. *Am J Kidney Dis.* 2006;48(suppl 1):S248–S273.

7. Leblanc M, Bosc JY, Paganini EP, Canaud B. Central venous dialysis catheter dysfunction. *Adv Ren Replace Ther.* 1997;4(4):377–389.

8. Laurin L, Twolan C. Study of access recirculation in reversed temporary indwelling catheters. *J Cannt.* 1994;4(2):11–12.

9. Leblanc M, Fedak S, Mokris G, Paganini EP. Blood recirculation in temporary central catheters for acute hemodialysis. *Clin Nephrol.* 1996;45(5):315–319.

10. Tal MG. Comparison of recirculation percentage of the palindrome catheter and standard hemodialysis catheters in a swine model. *J Vasc Interv Radiol.* 2005; 16(9):1237–1240.

11. Senecal L, Saint-Sauveur E, Leblanc M. Blood flow and recirculation rates in tunneled hemodialysis catheters. *ASAIO J.* 2004;50(1):94–97.

12. Trerotola SO, Kraus M, Shah H, et al. Randomized comparison of split tip versus step tip high-flow hemodialysis catheters. *Kidney Int.* 2002;62(1):282–289.

13. Moossavi S, Vachharajani TJ, Jordan J, Russell GB, Kaufman T, Moossavi S. Retrospective analysis of catheter recirculation in prevalent dialysis patients. *Semin Dial.* 2008;21(3):289–292.

14. Hassan HA, Frenchie DL, Bastani B. Effect of reversal of catheter ports on recirculation: comparison of the PermCath with Tesio Twin Catheter. *ASAIO J.* 2002;48(3): 316–319.

15. Pannu N, Jhangri GS, Tonelli M. Optimizing dialysis delivery in tunneled dialysis catheters. *ASAIO J.* 2006; 52(2):157–162.

16. Weiss MF, Scivittaro V, Anderson JM. Oxidative stress and increased expression of growth factors in lesions of failed hemodialysis access. *Am J Kidney Dis.* 2001;37(5):970–980.

17. Brzosko S, Hryszko T, Malyszko J, Malyszko JS, Mazerska M, Mysliwiec M. Femoral localization and higher ultrafiltration rate but not concentration of heparin used for canal locking of hemodialysis catheter are negative predictors for its malfunction. *Am J Nephrol.* 2008;28(2):298–303.

18. Markota I, Markota D, Tomic M. Measuring of the heparin leakage into the circulation from central venous catheters—an in vivo study. *Nephrol Dial Transplant.* 2009; 24(5):1550–1553.

19. Agraharkar M, Isaacson S, Mendelssohn D, et al. Percutaneously inserted silastic jugular hemodialysis catheters seldom cause jugular vein thrombosis. *ASAIO J.* 1995;41(2):169–172.

20. Karnik R, Valentin A, Winkler WB, Donath P, Slany J. Duplex sonographic detection of internal jugular venous thrombosis after removal of central venous catheters. *Clin Cardiol.* 1993;16(1):26–29.

21. Wilkin TD, Kraus MA, Lane KA, Trerotola SO. Internal jugular vein thrombosis associated with hemodialysis catheters. *Radiology.* 2003;228(3):697–700.

22. Vachharajani TJ, Moossavi S, Kaufman T, Rocco M. Central vein hardware: cannot live with it, cannot live without it. *Semin Dial.* 2009;22(5):588–589.

23. Salgado OJ, Urdaneta B, Colmenares B, Garcia R, Flores C. Right versus left internal jugular vein catheterization for hemodialysis: complications and impact on ipsilateral access creation. *Artif Organs.* 2004;28(8):728–733.

24. Fuchs S, Pollak A, Gilon D. Central venous catheter mechanical irritation of the right atrial free wall: a cause for thrombus formation. *Cardiology.* 1999;91(3):169–172.

25. Ghani MK, Boccalandro F, Denktas AE, Barasch E. Right atrial thrombus formation associated with central venous catheters utilization in hemodialysis patients. *Intensive Care Med.* 2003;29(10):1829–1832.

26. Kingdon EJ, Holt SG, Davar J, et al. Atrial thrombus and central venous dialysis catheters. *Am J Kidney Dis.* 2001;38(3):631–639.

27. Negulescu O, Coco M, Croll J, Mokrzycki MH. Large atrial thrombus formation associated with tunneled cuffed hemodialysis catheters. *Clin Nephrol.* 2003;59(1):40–46.

28. Lok CE, Appleton D, Bhola C, Khoo B, Richardson RM. Trisodium citrate 4%—an alternative to heparin capping of haemodialysis catheters. *Nephrol Dial Transplant.* 2007;22(2):477–483.

29. Buturovic J, Ponikvar R, Kandus A, Boh M, Klinkmann J, Ivanovich P. Filling hemodialysis catheters in the interdialytic period: heparin versus citrate versus polygeline: a prospective randomized study. *Artif Organs.* 1998;22(11):945–947.

30. Macrae JM, Dojcinovic I, Djurdjev O, et al. Citrate 4% versus heparin and the reduction of thrombosis study (CHARTS). *Clin J Am Soc Nephrol.* 2008;3(2):369–374.

31. Weijmer MC, van den Dorpel MA, Van de Ven PJ, et al. Randomized, clinical trial comparison of trisodium citrate 30% and heparin as catheter-locking solution in hemodialysis patients. *J Am Soc Nephrol.* 2005;16(9): 2769–2777.

32. Moran JE, Ash SR. Locking solutions for hemodialysis catheters; heparin and citrate—a position paper by ASDIN. *Semin Dial.* 2008;21(5):490–492.

33. Mokrzycki MH, Jean-Jerome K, Rush H, Zdunek MP, Rosenberg SO. A randomized trial of minidose warfarin for the prevention of late malfunction in tunneled, cuffed hemodialysis catheters. *Kidney Int.* 2001;59(5): 1935–1942.

34. Coli L, Donati G, Cianciolo G, et al. Anticoagulation therapy for the prevention of hemodialysis tunneled cuffed catheters (TCC) thrombosis. *J Vasc Access.* 2006;7(3): 118–122.

35. Zacharias JM, Weatherston CP, Spewak CR, Vercaigne LM. Alteplase versus urokinase for occluded hemodialysis catheters. *Ann Pharmacother.* 2003;37(1):27–33.

36. O'Mara NB, Ali S, Bivens K, Sherman RA, Kapoian T. Efficacy of tissue plasminogen activator for thrombolysis in central venous dialysis catheters. *Hemodial Int.* 2003;7(2):130–134.

37. Little MA, Walshe JJ. A longitudinal study of the repeated use of alteplase as therapy for tunneled hemodialysis catheter dysfunction. *Am J Kidney Dis.* 2002;39(1):86–91.

38. Tumlin J, Goldman J, Spiegel DM, et al. A phase III, randomized, double-blind, placebo-controlled study of tenecteplase for improvement of hemodialysis catheter function: TROPICS 3. *Clin J Am Soc Nephrol.* 2010;5(4):631–636

39. Savader SJ, Ehrman KO, Porter DJ, Haikal LC, Oteham AC. Treatment of hemodialysis catheter-associated fibrin sheaths by rt-PA infusion: critical analysis of 124 procedures. *J Vasc Interv Radiol.* 2001;12(6):711–715.

40. Duszak R, Jr., Haskal ZJ, Thomas-Hawkins C, et al. Replacement of failing tunneled hemodialysis catheters through pre-existing subcutaneous tunnels: a comparison of catheter function and infection rates for de novo placements and over-the-wire exchanges. *J Vasc Interv Radiol.* 1998;9(2):321–327.

41. Garofalo RS, Zaleski GX, Lorenz JM, Funaki B, Rosenblum JD, Leef JA. Exchange of poorly functioning tunneled permanent hemodialysis catheters. *AJR Am J Roentgenol.* 1999;173(1):155–158.

42. Sontineni SP, White M, Singh S, et al. Thrombectomy reduces the systemic complications in device-related right atrial septic thrombosis. *Can J Cardiol.* 2009;25(2): e36–e41.

43. Shah A, Murray M, Nzerue C. Right atrial thrombi complicating use of central venous catheters in hemodialysis. *Int J Artif Organs.* 2004;27(9):772–778.

44. Xiang DZ, Verbeken EK, Van Lommel AT, Stas M, De Wever I. Composition and formation of the sleeve enveloping a central venous catheter. *J Vasc Surg.* 1998; 28(2):260–271.

45. O'Farrell L, Griffith JW, Lang CM. Histologic development of the sheath that forms around long-term implanted central venous catheters. *JPEN J Parenter Enteral Nutr.* 1996;20(2):156–158.

46. Haskal ZJ, Leen VH, Thomas-Hawkins C, Shlansky-Goldberg RD, Baum RA, Soulen MC. Transvenous removal of fibrin sheaths from tunneled hemodialysis catheters. *J Vasc Interv Radiol.* 1996;7(4):513–517.

47. Crain MR, Mewissen MW, Ostrowski GJ, Paz-Fumagalli R, Beres RA, Wertz RA. Fibrin sleeve stripping for salvage of failing hemodialysis catheters: technique and initial results. *Radiology.* 1996;198(1):41–44.

48. Brady PS, Spence LD, Levitin A, Mickolich CT, Dolmatch BL. Efficacy of percutaneous fibrin sheath stripping in restoring patency of tunneled hemodialysis catheters. *AJR Am J Roentgenol.* 1999;173(4):1023–1027.

49. Gray RJ, Levitin A, Buck D, et al. Percutaneous fibrin sheath stripping versus transcatheter urokinase infusion for malfunctioning well-positioned tunneled central venous dialysis catheters: a prospective, randomized trial. *J Vasc Interv Radiol.* 2000;11(9):1121–1129.

50. Suhocki PV, Conlon PJ, Jr., Knelson MH, Harland R, Schwab SJ. Silastic cuffed catheters for hemodialysis vascular access: thrombolytic and mechanical correction of malfunction. *Am J Kidney Dis.* 1996;28(3):379–386.

51. Johnstone RD, Stewart GA, Akoh JA, Fleet M, Akyol M, Moss JG. Percutaneous fibrin sleeve stripping of failing haemodialysis catheters. *Nephrol Dial Transplant.* 1999; 14(3):688–691.

52. Reddy AS, Lang EV, Cutts J, Loh S, Rosen MP. Fibrin sheath removal from central venous catheters: an internal snare manoeuvre. *Nephrol Dial Transplant.* 2007;22(6): 1762–1765.

53. Oliver MJ, Mendelssohn DC, Quinn RR, et al. Catheter patency and function after catheter sheath disruption: a pilot study. *Clin J Am Soc Nephrol.* 2007;2(6):1201–1206.

54. Janne d'Othee B, Tham JC, Sheiman RG. Restoration of patency in failing tunneled hemodialysis catheters: a comparison of catheter exchange, exchange and balloon disruption of the fibrin sheath, and femoral stripping. *J Vasc Interv Radiol.* 2006;17(6):1011–1015.

EXIT-SITE, TUNNEL INFECTION, AND CATHETER-RELATED BACTEREMIA

SHAHRIAR MOOSSAVI

LEARNING OBJECTIVES

1. Understand the definition of exit-site and tunnel infection.
2. Understand the definitions of catheter-related bacteremia.
3. Describe the pathogenesis of biofilm and catheter-related bacteremia.
4. Discuss the risk factors for developing catheter-related bacteremia.
5. Describe the most common pathogens involved in catheter-related bacteremia.
6. Discuss the treatment of catheter-related bacteremia.

INTRODUCTION

Despite rigorous educational efforts and national initiatives, the majority of dialysis patients start their treatment with a central venous catheter (CVC). The CVC use among incident end-stage renal disease patients ranges from 56.8% to 71%.[1] At any given time about 22–25% of dialysis patients use a CVC as their primary dialysis access.[2] The catheter use is a major cause of morbidity and mortality in dialysis patients and infection is the major contributor to the high morbidity and mortality associated with catheter use. The risk of developing an infection is fivefold higher for patients with a CVC as compared to patients with an arteriovenous fistula.[3] Patients who undergo dialysis via a CVC have a 30% higher relative risk of death as compared to patients using an arteriovenous fistula or graft as their dialysis access.[4] Unfortunately, septicemia has a higher cumulative mortality rate in dialysis patients than in the general population.[5] Prevention and successful treatment of catheter-related bacteremia (CRB) could save about 5500 lives annually.[6]

There have been major advances in the understanding of catheter-related bacteremia and its pathogenesis. The knowledge about biofilm matrix and its formation has opened new avenues in prevention and treatment of CRB. This has led to development of new therapeutic and preventive tools that may not be readily available or may be costly to use. With the move in decreasing the healthcare cost, there is a strong momentum to avoid catheter use. However, central venous catheters will likely not be eliminated and the catheter-related infection and its complications will remain a challenge in treating dialysis patients.

Infection is the most common reason for catheter loss. The infection can involve the exit-site, the tunnel, or the blood stream (Figure 28-1). The anatomic location of the infection has an impact on the treatment, possible consequences, and the prevention strategy.

EXIT-SITE INFECTION

Exit-site infection is a soft tissue infection that is localized to the area extending from the catheter cuff to the catheter exit site (Figure 28-1). It is a localized cellulitis. The exit site may be red, tender, with purulent drainage. By definition the tunnel is not involved and there is no sign of inflammation over the tunnel. However, an exit-site infection can spread to the tunnel tract if not treated in a timely fashion. It may be difficult to distinguish between an exit-site infection and tunnel infection especially if the catheter cuff is deep in the soft tissue or further away from the exit-site. A swab culture from the exit-site should be obtained to guide the therapy. Of all exit-site infections, 75% are due to Gram-positive species, with coagulase-negative *Staphylococcus* leading the list. The incidence of exit-site infection is reported to be 0.6 infections per 1000 catheter days.[7]

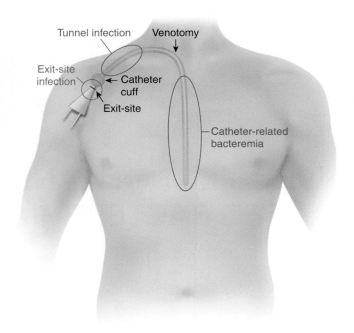

Figure 28-1. Localization of infection.

The treatment consists of oral or systemic antibiotics in addition to local skin care with judicious use of topical antibiotics. If the infection does not respond to these measures or if the infection spreads to the tunnel tract, the catheter may need to be removed. In some cases it is technically possible to perform a cut down at the venotomy and exchange the catheter with creation of a new tunnel away from the infected tunnel and surrounding soft tissue.

To prevent an exit-site infection, the exit site should be cleaned and redressed at each dialysis session only by trained dialysis staff. The patient and the staff need to wear surgical mask during catheter manipulation. No specific patient characteristics have been found to be associated with an exit-site infection. However, the type of dressing and the cleansing solution used have been shown to influence the incidence of exit-site infection.[8] The preferred cleansing solution is a chlorhexidine-based solution if this is compatible with the catheter material. A nonocclusive dressing is preferable.

A chlorhexidine-impregnated dressing is now available commercially and is being commonly used in the hospital setting. A recent retrospective study in pediatric hemodialysis patients showed a significant reduction in the incidence of exit-site infections ($P < 0.05$) with the use of this dressing. However, there was no difference in the incidence of CRBs.[7]

TUNNEL INFECTION

Tunnel infection is defined as an infection that involves part or the entire subcutaneous tissue from the venotomy to the cuff (Figure 28-1). The tunnel tract is red, swollen, and tender. There is frequently drainage from the exit site. If a purulent drainage is not visible, pus can be expressed from the exit site by milking the tunnel. The drainage should be cultured to confirm the diagnosis and guide the treatment. The infection can spread centrally leading to CRB. The treatment includes administration of intravenous antibiotics and removal of the CVC catheter. In very few and selective cases if the infection does not involve the venotomy site and there is enough healthy subcutaneous tissue, the catheter might be replaced with creation of a new tunnel. This requires a cut down at the venotomy to dissect the catheter and free up the catheter at a site that is not infected. The catheter can be then clamped and severed. A wire is then placed down the catheter into the inferior vena cava and the proximal portion of the catheter is removed. A new catheter is now placed while creating a new tunnel away from the infected tunnel. Once the new catheter is placed and dressing is applied, the remainder distal portion of the catheter is removed. The catheter cuff is usually loose and can be dissected with minimal effort.

CATHETER-RELATED BACTEREMIA

A precise definition of CRB is important, both in clinical setting and research. However, in clinical practice and in many papers related to this subject the term catheter-related bacteremia may reflect physicians' or investigators' interpretation and not a standard definition. The Centers for Disease Control and Prevention (CDC) has established a detailed definition for central line-associated bloodstream infection (CLABSI). Based on the CDC definitions, the 2006 update of the National Kidney Foundation's Kidney Disease Quality Initiative (KDOQI) guidelines for vascular access has formulated the following definitions for definite, probable, and possible CLABSI.

If the same organism is obtained from a semiquantitative culture of the catheter tip (>15 colony-forming units per catheter segment) and from a peripheral or catheter blood sample in a symptomatic patient with no other apparent source of infection, it is a definite CLABSI.

Probable CLABSI in a symptomatic patient with no other apparent source of infections is defined as defervescence of symptoms after antibiotic therapy with or without removal of catheter, in the setting in which blood cultures confirm infection, but catheter tip does not (or catheter tip does, but blood cultures do not) in a symptomatic patient with no other apparent source of infection.

However, defervescence of symptoms after antibiotic treatment or after removal of catheter in the absence of laboratory confirmation of bloodstream infection in a symptomatic patient with no other apparent source of infection is classified as a possible CLABSI.[9]

There are many limitations to the application of these definitions in the clinical practice. The work up to exclude other sources of infection is not well defined and is limited to the available resources. In most cases a physician is not present at the outpatient dialysis center. The patient may not get a chest x-ray or may not be able to produce urine for culture. In many instances the CVC is not removed prior to administration of antibiotics. If the CVC is removed after the initiation of the intravenous antibiotics, the catheter tip culture may not grow significant number of colonies.

It is not always possible to obtain peripheral blood cultures from a hemodialysis patient as there may not be any suitable veins for venipuncture. In fact in one study in almost 40% of patients a peripheral blood culture could not be obtained.[10] In cases that the patient does have a suitable vein for venipuncture, it may need to be preserved for a future vascular access. If the patient becomes symptomatic while receiving dialysis treatment, a blood culture cannot practically be obtained from the catheter lumen. Given the high blood flows through the catheter, any blood culture obtained from the catheter or the dialysis tubing as the patient is receiving dialysis will likely be similar to obtaining blood from a peripheral site.

Semiquantitative cultures are costly and not readily available at all laboratories. Outpatient dialysis centers are often not close to the laboratory. Time to positivity is not being reported at all labs and it may not have a meaning if the samples are being shipped.[11]

The Infectious Diseases Society of America (IDSA) has acknowledged some of these limitations in their 2009 updated "Clinical Practice Guidelines for the Diagnosis and Management of Intravascular Catheter-Related Infection." The criteria for definitive diagnosis of CRBSI are very similar to the KDOQI guidelines. It requires that the same organism grows from at least one percutaneous blood culture and from a culture of the catheter tip. The definite diagnosis can also be made if instead of a catheter tip culture, one of the blood samples is obtained from a catheter hub and the colony count of organisms grown from blood obtained through the catheter hub is at least threefold greater than the colony count from blood obtained from a peripheral vein. Or if the laboratory is reporting differential time to positivity (DTP), a catheter hub culture should become positive at least 2 hours before microbial growth is detected in a blood sample obtained from a peripheral vein.

Possible CRBSI can be diagnosed as per ISDA guidelines if two quantitative blood cultures are obtained through two catheter lumens and the colony count for the sample drawn through one lumen is at least threefold greater than the colony count for the blood culture obtained from the second lumen.

Alternatively, when a peripheral blood sample cannot be obtained, blood samples may be drawn during hemodialysis from bloodlines connected to the CVC as recommended in the special section of IDSA guidelines addressing the hemodialysis CVC.[12]

This practical approach has been also recommended by the European Renal Best Practice (ERBP). The therapeutic relevance of culturing catheter tips in symptomatic patients is low when blood cultures are collected appropriately and the patient is started on appropriate antibiotic treatment. It is more practical and realistic to obtain blood cultures

TABLE 28–1

Source of Infection

Migration along the exterior surface of catheter
Contamination of catheter hub and luminal colonization
Hematogenous seeding
Contaminated infusate

during dialysis through the dialysis circuit linked to the catheter to isolate an organism related to catheter-associated infection.[13,14]

▶ Pathogenesis

The first step in the pathogenesis of CRB is the attachment of the microorganism to the catheter. The skin microorganism can colonize the tunnel tract and migrate along the exterior surface of the catheter. A possible contributing factor here is improper manipulation of the catheter by the patient or staff. Contamination of the catheter hub can lead to luminal colonization. Hematogenous seeding of the catheter surface from another source of infection or from temporary bacteremia may play a role in some patients. A less frequent source of bacterial colonization is a contaminated infusate as a result of inadequate water treatment or improper dialyzer reuse practices (Table 28-1).

Once the microorganism is attached to the catheter, it produces a biofilm also called "slime." The biofilm is composed of extracellular polymers mainly polysaccharides. The polysaccharides form the matrix that connects the microorganisms to each other and to the catheter surface. Host factors such as fibrinogen and fibronectin have been shown to be involved in biofilm formation as well. Some cells are completely embedded in the polymer and receive nutrients via convective flow trough small channels. It is important to make the distinction between the sessile bacteria in the biofilm and the free-floating (planktonic) bacteria as they are biologically different. The bacteria in biofilm are much more active and show a distinct gene expression pattern that is different from their planktonic counterparts. In addition to producing adhesion molecules and matrix materials, they interact in the biofilm community by secreting regulatory and signaling molecules (Figure 28-2).

The biofilm formation and its growth is influenced by the type of microorganism, the type of catheter material, the flow rate, and the type of fluid flowing through the catheter.

Catheters made of polytetrafluoroethylene (PTFE), silicone elastomer, or polyurethane are more resistant to bacterial adherence than catheters made of polyvinyl chloride or polyethylene. Currently, most available tunneled central venous catheters are made of polyurethane that is more resistant to bacterial adherence.

Biofilm will form on all central venous catheters if they are left in place long enough. The type of microorganism involved may be influenced by host factors. It is very

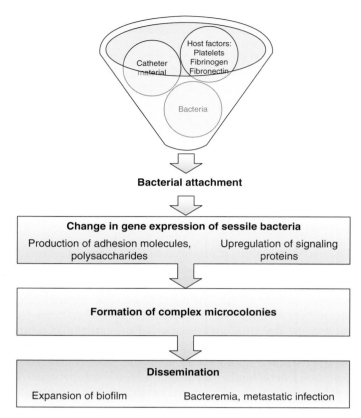

Figure 28-2. Pathogenesis of catheter-related bacteremia.

difficult for antibiotics or host defense mechanisms to penetrate the biofilm.

The biofilm is capable of causing an infection. If few bacteria are shed into the blood, the host-immune mechanisms may overcome them. However, if the host becomes immunocompromised or large number of bacteria is disseminated, overt infection is the result.

Unfortunately, the host defense mechanism specifically the neutrophils might be dysfunctional in dialysis population. Uremic toxins, such as *p*-cresol, polyamines or aminoguanidine, trace element deficiencies, malnutrition, hyperparathyroidism, and impaired glucose metabolism have been shown to contribute to neutrophil dysfunction in dialysis population.[15–18]

▶ Epidemiology

Bloodstream infections are the second most common cause of death among end-stage renal disease patients counting for about 11% of all deaths. The incidence of catheter-related bacteremia is reported per 1000 catheter days in the literature. It ranges from 1.6 to 5.5 episodes per 1000 catheter days, which translates to 0.6–2.0 episodes of bacteremia per catheter year. This is significantly higher than the infection rate for arteriovenous fistula or graft, which has been reported to range from 0.04 to 0.55 per 1000 patient-days or 0.01–0.2 per year.[9,16] The cumulative likelihood of having an episode of catheter-related bacteremia at 3 and 6 months

has been reported to be 35% and 48%, respectively.[19] In the United States, between 67,500 and 150,000 dialysis patients acquire CRB each year.[20] Clinical studies have shown that it is possible to decrease the infection rate with good clinical practices.[9,21] Any center with rates greater than 2/1000 should initiate a CQI project to reduce the infection rate.[17] Adherence to a protocol, patient re-education, and staff re-training is a major part of such an initiative. However, the primary objective should be to convert the access from CVC to an arteriovenous fistula or if a fistula cannot be created then to an arteriovenous graft. Multiple analyses have shown a significant decrease in death risk after the conversion from a catheter to a permanent access.

The incidence of exit-site infection for tunneled central venous catheters ranges from 0.35 to 8.3 per 1000 catheter days.[22]

▶ Risk Factors

Previous episode of bacteremia has been shown in multiple studies as a major risk factor for bacteremia. During a 6-month follow-up, the probability of bacteremia was more than sixfold in patients who had experienced a previous infection in a multicenter Canadian study. The increased risk for the recurrence of an infection could be related to impaired host-defense mechanisms or poor hygiene. In this study, poor patient hygiene, as perceived by the clinical staff caring for the patient, was associated with a 2.4 times increased risk of infection. This factor may be modifiable with patient education regarding the care of the CVC.[23] Placement of a tunneled CVC in femoral position is generally believed to have a higher incidence of CRB than catheters placed in the internal jugular or subclavian position. The risk of CRB is lowest for temporary catheters placed in the subclavian vein; however placing a catheter in the subclavian vein position is associated with greater risk of central vein stenosis, which will limit the patient's options for future access creation. Hence the preferable site for placement of a dialysis catheter is the internal jugular vein.[16] Diabetes, peripheral vascular disease, hypoalbuminemia, *Staphylococcus aureus* nasal carriage, and local infection have been identified as risk factors for catheter-related bacteremia. Interestingly, use of aspirin has been shown to be associated with a decreased risk of *S. aureus* CRB in a retrospective study. This effect was mostly seen with the 325 mg aspirin dose. Use of aspirin resulted in a 54% reduction in the risk of developing a first episode of *S. aureus* bacteremia. This effect is not surprising. Salicylic acid has been shown to reduce the virulence of *S. aureus* by downregulating the transcription of proteins necessary for bacterial replication in host tissues.[9,16,21]

▶ Microbiology

Gram-positive bacteria are the most common cause of CRB. Up to 68% of isolates in patients with CRB are *Staphylococcus* species. Coagulase-negative staphylococci are part of normal skin flora and are the most common contaminant as well. This leads to a diagnosis dilemma when interpreting blood cultures that are positive for coagulase-negative staphylococci. If blood cultures drawn from multiple sites are positive for coagulase-negative *Staphylococcus*, it indicates a CRB rather than contamination. Most patients with coagulase-negative *Staphylococcus* infection have a benign clinical course, except for *Staphylococcus* lugdunensis that can cause metastatic infections and endocarditis similar to *S. aureus*. Hematogenous complications have been reported in 25–30% of infections related to *S. aureus*. Identifying patients at high risk for developing a hematogenous complication is clinically valuable. A positive blood culture 72 hours after the start of the appropriate antibiotics and catheter removal is one of the best predictors of hematogenous complications in patients with *Staphylococcus* bacteremia.[12] Endocarditis is one such complication. The rates of valvular vegetations have been found to be between 25% and 32% in studies using transesophageal echocardiogram (TEE) in patients with *S. aureus* bacteremia.[12] To minimize the possibility of false-negative results, a TEE should be done 5–7 days after the onset of bacteremia as per IDSA recommendations. Unfortunately, the *S. aureus* infections are also associated with more treatment failures and hospitalizations.[16] Methicillin-resistant *S. aureus* (MRSA) is especially common in the dialysis population. The risk of invasive MRSA in about 100 times greater in dialysis population as compared to general population. The reported incidence of invasive MRSA infections was 45.2 cases per 1000 in dialysis population as compared to 0.4 infections per 1000 in general population.[24] In a retrospective study of 11,572 admissions of hemodialysis patients related to *S. aureus* bacteremia 21% of patients had one or more complications; 11.8% were readmitted within 12 weeks of the hospital discharge for recurrence of the infection or treatment of a complication related to *S. aureus*. CVC was the most common known access type in these patients.[25]

Differences in the mortality risk among organisms that cause septicemia were evaluated in a retrospective study of over 22,000 hospitalizations. *S. aureus* was identified in 27% of hospitalizations. No other organism had an incidence >10%. The adjusted death rate was 20% higher for *S. aureus* septicemia compared to all other specified organisms for both the in-hospital period and the 3 months following the hospital discharge.[26] Overall Gram-negative CRB is less common. Enterobacter and Pseudomonas are the leading cause of Gram-negative CRB. Fungal infections and polymicrobial infections are rare. They may be more common in immunocompromised patients.

▶ Prevention

The presence of catheter-related bacteremia within 72 hours of placement is likely related to the procedure itself. To reduce the risk of infection associated with the interventional procedures, all tunneled CVC should be placed in an operating room under conditions of maximum sterile barrier.[17,27] Using 2% chlorhexidine as skin antisepsis

TABLE 28–2
Prevention of Catheter-Related Bacteremia
Placement of CVC in operating room Use of 2% chlorhexidine as skin prep Use of aseptic technique to access the catheter by trained staff only Use of antibiotic lock solution Use of t-PA as catheter lock Use of topical antibiotics to the exit-site after placement of a nontunneled catheter

prior to CVC insertion has been shown to be superior to 10% povidone-iodine or 70% alcohol. CDC recommends 2% chlorhexidine (Table 28-2).[28-30]

Administration of prophylactic antibiotic prior to CVC insertion is common in some centers. A recent retrospective study of 283 catheter insertion or exchange procedures without administration of prophylactic antibiotics showed only one infection within 72 hours of the procedure.[31] Other studies have shown no reduction in the incidence of catheter-related bacteremia with administration of oral or parenteral antibiotics preprocedure.[32-34]

Protection of the catheter hub from contamination is essential. KDOQI Clinical Practice Guidelines for Vascular Access emphasizes the need for using aseptic technique including correct hand-washing, masks for patient and staff (not a face shield), "no-touch" technique, and disposable clean gloves. A chlorhexidine solution is preferred for cleansing. In a study of 700 dialysis patients, the incidence of catheter-related bacteremia was decreased from 6.97 per 1000 to 1.68 per thousand by adherence to a catheter hub care protocol.[21]

Multiple studies have shown the benefit of topical antibiotic application to the exit site. Topical mupirocin and povidone-iodine have been shown to reduce the rate of bacteremia. A recent meta-analysis was able to demonstrate a reduction in bacteremia from 4.5 to 1.0 cases per 1000 catheter-days, a reduction in exit-site infection from 4.1 to 0.6 cases per 1000 catheter-day, and a reduction in the need for catheter removal, and hospitalization for infection.[35] However, routine use of topical antibiotics may lead to emergence of resistant microorganisms. It may also promote colonization of the catheter with fungi. Many of these studies were in temporary catheters that are not tunneled. The topical antibiotic was used until the insertion site was healed.[17]

S. aureus nasal colonization among hemodialysis patients has been shown to be associated with more frequent infections. Rifampin can be used to eradicate the *S. aureus* nasal carriage. The colonization recurs within 3 months of rifampin administration. Readministration of rifampin at 3 months intervals has been shown to reduce the infection rate. However, this may lead to emergence of resistant strains.[36]

Lock solutions have emerged as a promising strategy to prevent catheter-related bacteremia (Table 28-3). The

TABLE 28–3

Possible Antibiotic Lock Solutions

Gentamicin/citrate
Vancomycin
Ceftazidime
Cefazolin
Minocycline
Ethanol 70%

antibiotic lock solution has been also studied as an adjuvant to systemic antibiotics in treatment of catheter-related bacteremia. The lock solution may contain more than one ingredient. It is usually a mixture of an antibiotic with an anticoagulant. The perfect lock solution would inhibit the formation of biofilm in the catheter and would not promote the development of resistant organisms. It would be inexpensive, easy to store and administer. The perfect lock solution would be without systemic side effects.

The lock solution can be citrate- or antibiotic based. A well-designed European study comparing 30% trisodium citrate with 5000 U/mL heparin lock solution was stopped prematurely because of a significant lower rate of bacteremia in citrate group. In the heparin group, 46% of catheters had to be removed because of any complication compared with 28% in the citrate group ($P = 0.005$). Catheter-related bacteremia rates were 1.1 per 1000 catheter-days for citrate versus 4.1 in the heparin group ($P < 0.001$). There were no deaths related to bacteremia in the citrate group. However, five deaths related to bacteremia were reported in the heparin group ($P = 0.028$). There were no differences in catheter thrombosis or flow problems ($P = 0.75$). Major bleeding episodes were significantly lower in the citrate group ($P = 0.010$).[37]

A recent meta-analysis of eight prospective randomized trials, involving 829 patients, 882 catheters, and 90,191 catheter-days, showed a threefold reduction in catheter-related bacteremia with the use of lock solutions.[38] Recombinant tissue plasminogen activator (rt-PA) has been used as catheter lock solution. In a recently published prospective randomized study comparing rt-PA to heparin, the risk of CRB was threefold higher in heparin group as compared to rt-PA group.[39]

A systematic review of antimicrobials in prevention of catheter-related infections showed a significant reduction in catheter-related bacteremia and exit-site infection with the use of lock solutions. However, use of antimicrobial-impregnated catheters and perioperative systemic antimicrobial administration was not found to be beneficial in the reduction of catheter-related bacteremia.[40]

A drawback of using lock solution is the spillage into the circulation. The listed catheter volume as labeled by the manufacturer is frequently 0.1 or 0.2 mL higher than the actual volume. In addition, the laminar flow down the center of the lumen results in the spillage of the injected lock solution into the circulation.[6]

To decrease the adherence of bacteria to the catheter and prevent CRB, antibiotic-coated CVC have been developed and studied. Minocycline/rifampin, chlorhexidine/silver sulfadiazine, silver sulfadiazine, silver platinum, and more recently 5-fluorouracil have been investigated in nontunneled catheters in the critical care setting. In dialysis patients, silver sulfadiazine has been used with limited data and inconsistent results.[4]

More recently, heparin-coated catheters have been developed to combat thrombus formation. Heparin is bonded covalently to the catheter surface to achieve the antithrombotic coating. There are currently two different heparin coatings available on the market: the Carmeda BioActive Surface and the Trillium Biosurface.

The Carmeda treatment consists of covalently bonding of the heparin molecules to the catheter surface. The active heparin sequence is exposed to the circulation.[4] The CRB was significantly lower in a retrospective analysis of 175 tunneled dialysis catheters including 89 heparin-coated catheters and 86 noncoated catheters (34% vs 60%, $P < 0.001$). The cumulative catheter survival and the frequency of thrombolytic instillation were similar in both groups.[41]

The Trillium treatment is structurally different. It consists of a copolymer containing heparin, polyethylene glycol, sulfate, and sulfonate groups. The polyethylene glycol groups in the coating material have been shown to minimize both protein adsorption and platelet adhesion. The coating also contains sulfate and sulfonate groups that are negatively charged and have been shown to repel cells and reduce cellular attachment of erythrocytes and platelets.[42]

Heparin-coated catheters should not be used in patients with history of heparin-induced thrombocytopenia (HIT). In addition, HIT should be suspected in patients dialyzing with heparin-coated catheters who develop thrombocytopenia, venous or arterial thrombosis, or acute extremity ischemia. The durability of the Carmeda BioActive surface has been reported to be 90 days. Trillium Biosurface reduces platelet adhesion to the catheter for up to 720 hours of dialysis treatment.[43]

► Treatment

Most catheters are lost secondary to an infection or the complications of an infection. The initial treatment consists of broad-spectrum antibiotic coverage (Figure 28-3). However, intravenous antibiotics alone are usually not successful in treating the catheter-related bacteremia. Studies have shown recurrence of infection in 75% of patients after the discontinuation of antibiotics if the catheter is left in place. The combination of intravenous antibiotics and catheter exchange over a guidewire has proven to be more effective. The catheter is often exchanged after 48–72 hours of antibiotic treatment. This approach is also known as "salvage of site rather than salvage of catheter." The success rate of "salvage of site" approach has been shown to be 80–88% without any apparent ill effects. The expected 3-month patient survival for CVC exchange over the wire was similar to the immediate CVC removal approach (93%). Exchanging the CVC

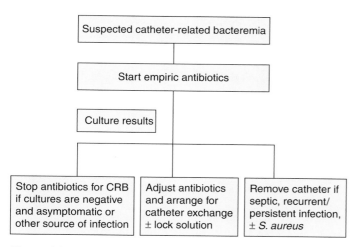

Figure 28-3. Approach to catheter-related bacteremia.

over the guidewire has been shown to be cost effective. The hypothetical cost savings were estimated at $5200 as compared to catheter salvage approach and at around $700 as compared to immediate catheter removal approach.[9] If the CRB can be treated in an outpatient setting, the estimated expenditures would be between $7000 and $15,000 per episode. However, if the treatment requires hospital admission the health-care cost increases by at least 66%.[2]

The antibiotic coverage needs to be modified once the result of the initial blood culture and the sensitivity is available. The dose of antibiotic may need to be adjusted for residual renal function or for use of a high-flux dialyzer. In a recent position paper, the ERBP recommended 3 weeks of antibiotic therapy for uncomplicated catheter-related bacteremia, 6 weeks of antibiotics for endocarditis or if the bacteremia/fungemia persists 72 hours after initiating the antibiotic therapy. Eight weeks of antibiotics was recommended for osteomyelitis due to catheter-related bacteremia. A followup culture 1 week after the completion of the antibiotic therapy is recommended if the CVC was exchanged over the guidewire or catheter salvage was attempted.[13]

Not every CRB can be treated by exchanging the catheter over the guidewire after initiating the antibiotic therapy. The catheter may need to be removed if there is septicemia, metastatic infection, fungemia, or recurrence of CRB after a catheter exchange. A temporary catheter is used for dialysis until a new tunneled CVC can be placed.

An innovative approach is the combination of the intravenous antibiotic with a lock solution, especially if catheter removal is deemed undesirable or impossible. This may be the situation if the patient is on his "last access" or placing a new tunneled CVC after removing the current catheter will be technically challenging if not impossible. The success rate of the combination therapy (intravenous antibiotics and catheter lock solution) depends largely on the type of microorganism and the type of lock solution used. This approach is very effective in treating CRB related to Gram-negative organisms. The cure rate is 87–100% for

Gram-negative infections, 75–84% for *S. epidermidis* infections, 61% for *Enterococcus* infections, and only 40–55% for *S. aureus* infections.[11]

The initial antibiotic coverage needs to be effective against both Gram-positive and Gram-negative microorganisms. Vancomycin is the first choice for Gram-positive coverage, given the high prevalence of methicillin-resistant *Staphylococcus* species in dialysis population. Vancomycin is given as a loading dose (20 mg/kg) followed by a maintenance dose (500–1000 mg) after each dialysis session. It can be administered in the last 30 minutes of dialysis treatment. If vancomycin levels can be obtained in timely fashion the dose can be adjusted based on the level.

Most Gram-negative organisms that cause CRB in dialysis patients are sensitive to aminoglycosides or third-generation cephalosporins. Both medications could be administered after the dialysis. However, the toxicity profile of aminoglycosides makes it a less preferable choice. Ceftazidime dose is 1 g after each dialysis session. Gentamicin may be given after each dialysis session at a dose of 1 mg/kg, not to exceed 100 mg per dose. A gentamicin trough level can be obtained before the start of the dialysis session to help adjust the dose and decrease the risk of toxicity.

The antibiotic choice needs to be adjusted accordingly once the sensitivity result becomes available. As an example, treating methicillin-sensitive *Staphylococcus* infection with vancomycin instead of switching to cefazolin has a threefold higher failure rate. The dose for cefazolin is 20 mg/kg after each dialysis treatment. When minimum inhibitory concentration for vancomycin exceeds 2 µg/mL, vancomycin should be discontinued and daptomycin therapy should be initiated. Daptomycin is also effective against VRE; 6 mg/kg of daptomycin can be given after each dialysis session. Amphotericin B and fluconazole have been successfully used to treat candidemia in dialysis patients.[11]

▶ **Complications**

Untreated or poorly treated CRB can result is sepsis, infective endocarditis, osteomyelitis, septic thrombophlebitis, or metastatic infection. Persistent symptoms or continued positive blood cultures despite appropriate antibiotic coverage are suggestive of such a complication and warrant removal of the CVC. Patient's symptoms and the organism are important in choosing the diagnostic tests that can localize the focus of infection. *S. aureus* is the most common offending organism. Complicated CRB requires prolonged antibiotic therapy. The duration of the antibiotic therapy may be 6–8 weeks depending on the type of organism and the location of the infection.[2,12]

CONCLUSION

Use of CVC for dialysis is associated with multiple adverse events including CRB. Despite major advances in understanding the pathogenesis of the infection, CRB remains the leading cause of dialysis access loss in patients using CVC for dialysis. All efforts need to be concentrated in avoiding CVC as dialysis access. If their use cannot be avoided, then the goal should be minimizing the duration of CVC use as well as limiting the number of blood vessels that are used to place a CVC. There is evidence that lock solutions could be used for prevention or for treatment of CRB in conjunction with intravenous antibiotics. However, avoiding a CVC will remain the best strategy to prevent CRB.

REFERENCES

1. Wasse H. Catheter-related mortality among ESRD patients. *Semin Dial*. 2008;21:547–549.

2. Lok CE, Mokrzycki MH. Prevention and management of catheter-related infection in hemodialysis patients. *Kidney Int*. 2011;79:587–598.

3. Rayner HC, Besarab A, Brown WW, Disney A, Saito A, Pisoni RL. Vascular access results from the Dialysis Outcomes and Practice Patterns Study (DOPPS): performance against Kidney Disease Outcomes Quality Initiative (K/DOQI) Clinical Practice Guidelines. *Am J Kidney Dis*. 2004;44:22–26.

4. Dwyer A. Surface-treated catheters—a review. *Semin Dial*. 2008;21:542–546.

5. U.S. Renal Data System, USRDS 2007 Annual Data Report: Atlas of Chronic Kidney Disease and End-Stage Renal Disease in the United States, National Institutes of Health, National Institute of Diabetes and Digestive and Kidney Diseases, Bethesda, MD. 2007. (Ref Type: Report.)

6. Bleyer AJ. Use of antimicrobial catheter lock solutions to prevent catheter-related bacteremia. *Clin J Am Soc Nephrol*. 2007;2:1073–1078.

7. Onder AM, Chandar J, Coakley S, Francoeur D, Abitbol C, Zilleruelo G. Controlling exit site infections: does it decrease the incidence of catheter-related bacteremia in children on chronic hemodialysis? *Hemodial Int*. 2009;13:11–18.

8. Harwood L, Wilson B, Thompson B, Brown E, Young D. Predictors of hemodialysis central venous catheter exit-site infections. *CANNT J*. 2008;18:26–35.

9. National Kidney Foundation: K/DOQI Clinical Practice guidelines for vascular access. *Am J Kidney Dis*. 2006;48:S248–S257.

10. Poole CV, Carlton D, Bimbo L, Allon M. Treatment of catheter-related bacteraemia with an antibiotic lock protocol: effect of bacterial pathogen. *Nephrol Dial Transplant*. 2004;19:1237–1244.

11. Allon M. Treatment guidelines for dialysis catheter-related bacteremia: an update. *Am J Kidney Dis*. 2009;54:13–17.

12. Mermel LA, Allon M, Bouza E, Craven DE, Flynn P, O'Grady NP, Raad II, Rijnders BJ, Sherertz RJ, Warren DK. Clinical practice guidelines for the diagnosis and management of intravascular catheter-related infection: 2009 update by the Infectious Diseases Society of America. *Clin Infect Dis*. 2009;49:1–45.

13. Vanholder R, Canaud B, Fluck R, Jadoul M, Labriola L, Marti-Monros A, Tordoir J, Van BW. Catheter-related blood stream infections (CRBSI): a European view. *Nephrol Dial Transplant*. 2010;25:1753–1756.

14. Vanholder R, Canaud B, Fluck R, Jadoul M, Labriola L, Marti-Monros A, Tordoir J, Van Biesen W. Diagnosis, prevention and treatment of haemodialysis catheter-related bloodstream infections (CRBSI): a position statement of European Renal Best Practice (ERBP). *NDT Plus*. 2010;3:234–246.

15. Costerton W, Veeh R, Shirtliff M, Pasmore M, Post C, Ehrlich G. The application of biofilm science to the study and control of chronic bacterial infections. *J Clin Invest*. 2003;112:1466–1477.

16. Lafrance JP, Rahme E, Lelorier J, Iqbal S. Vascular access-related infections: definitions, incidence rates, and risk factors. *Am J Kidney Dis*. 2008;52:982–993.

17. Beathard GA, Urbanes A. Infection associated with tunneled hemodialysis catheters. *Semin Dial*. 2008;21:528–538.

18. Jaber BL. Bacterial infections in hemodialysis patients: pathogenesis and prevention. *Kidney Int*. 2005;67:2508–2519.

19. Lee T, Barker J, Allon M. Tunneled catheters in hemodialysis patients: reasons and subsequent outcomes. *Am J Kidney Dis*. 2005;46:501–508.

20. Allon M. Dialysis catheter-related bacteremia: treatment and prophylaxis. *Am J Kidney Dis*. 2004;44(5):779–791.

21. Beathard GA. Catheter management protocol for catheter-related bacteremia prophylaxis. *Semin Dial*. 2003;16:403–405.

22. McCann M, Moore ZE. Interventions for preventing infectious complications in haemodialysis patients with central venous catheters. *Cochrane Database Syst Rev*. 2010;(1):CD006894.

23. Taylor G, Gravel D, Johnston L, Embil J, Holton D, Paton S. Incidence of bloodstream infection in multicenter inception cohorts of hemodialysis patients. *Am J Infect Control*. 2004;32:155–160.

24. Invasive methicillin-resistant Staphylococcus aureus infections among dialysis patients—United States, 2005. *MMWR Morb Mortal Wkly Rep*. 2007;56:197–199.

25. Nissenson AR, Dylan ML, Griffiths RI, Yu HT, Dean BB, Danese MD, Dubois RW. Clinical and economic outcomes of *Staphylococcus aureus* septicemia in ESRD patients receiving hemodialysis. *Am J Kidney Dis*. 2005;46:301–308.

26. Danese MD, Griffiths RI, Dylan M, Yu HT, Dubois R, Nissenson AR. Mortality differences among organisms causing septicemia in hemodialysis patients. *Hemodial Int*. 2006;10:56–62.

27. Raad II, Hohn DC, Gilbreath BJ, Suleiman N, Hill LA, Bruso PA, Marts K, Mansfield PF, Bodey GP. Prevention of central venous catheter-related infections by using maximal sterile barrier precautions during insertion. *Infect Control Hosp Epidemiol*. 1994;15:231–238.

28. Maki DG, Ringer M, Alvarado CJ. Prospective randomised trial of povidone-iodine, alcohol, and chlorhexidine for prevention of infection associated with central venous and arterial catheters. *Lancet*. 1991;338:339–343.

29. Chaiyakunapruk N, Veenstra DL, Lipsky BA, Saint S. Chlorhexidine compared with povidone-iodine solution for vascular catheter-site care: a meta-analysis. *Ann Intern Med*. 2002;136:792–801.

30. O'Grady NP, Alexander M, Dellinger EP, Gerberding JL, Heard SO, Maki DG, Masur H, McCormick RD, Mermel LA, Pearson ML, Raad II, Randolph A, Weinstein RA. Guidelines for the prevention of intravascular catheter-related infections. *Infect Control Hosp Epidemiol*. 2002;23:759–769.

31. Salman L, Asif A. Antibiotic prophylaxis: is it needed for dialysis access procedures? *Semin Dial*. 2009;22:297–299.

32. McKee R, Dunsmuir R, Whitby M, Garden OJ. Does antibiotic prophylaxis at the time of catheter insertion reduce the incidence of catheter-related sepsis in intravenous nutrition? *J Hosp Infect*. 1985;6:419–425.

33. Ranson MR, Oppenheim BA, Jackson A, Kamthan AG, Scarffe JH. Double-blind placebo controlled study of vancomycin prophylaxis for central venous catheter insertion in cancer patients. *J Hosp Infect*. 1990; 15:95–102.

34. Ljungman P, Hagglund H, Bjorkstrand B, Lonnqvist B, Ringden O. Peroperative teicoplanin for prevention of Gram-positive infections in neutropenic patients with indwelling central venous catheters: a randomized, controlled study. *Support Care Cancer*. 1997;5:485–488.

35. James MT, Conley J, Tonelli M, Manns BJ, Macrae J, Hemmelgarn BR. Meta-analysis: antibiotics for prophylaxis against hemodialysis catheter-related infections. *Ann Intern Med*. 2008;148:596–605.

36. Yu VL, Goetz A, Wagener M, Smith PB, Rihs JD, Hanchett J, Zuravleff JJ. *Staphylococcus aureus* nasal carriage and infection in patients on hemodialysis. Efficacy of antibiotic prophylaxis. *N Engl J Med*. 1986;315:91–96.

37. Weijmer MC, van den Dorpel MA, Van d, V, ter Wee PM, van Geelen JA, Groeneveld JO, van Jaarsveld BC, Koopmans MG, le Poole CY, Schrander-Van der Meer AM, Siegert CE, Stas KJ. Randomized, clinical trial comparison of trisodium citrate 30% and heparin as catheter-locking solution in hemodialysis patients. *J Am Soc Nephrol*. 2005;16:2769–2777.

38. Labriola L, Crott R, Jadoul M. Preventing haemodialysis catheter-related bacteraemia with an antimicrobial lock solution: a meta-analysis of prospective randomized trials. *Nephrol Dial Transplant*. 2008;23:1666–1672.

39. Hemmelgarn BR, Moist LM, Lok CE, Tonelli M, Manns BJ, Holden RM, LeBlanc M, Faris P, Barre P, Zhang J, Scott-Douglas N. Prevention of dialysis catheter malfunction with recombinant tissue plasminogen activator. *N Engl J Med*. 2011;364:303–312.

40. Rabindranath KS, Bansal T, Adams J, Das R, Shail R, MacLeod AM, Moore C, Besarab A. Systematic review of antimicrobials for the prevention of haemodialysis catheter-related infections. *Nephrol Dial Transplant*. 2009;24: 3763–3774.

41. Jain G, Allon M, Saddekni S, Barker JF, Maya ID. Does heparin coating improve patency or reduce infection of tunneled dialysis catheters? *Clin J Am Soc Nephrol*. 2009;4:1787–1790.

42. Mojibian H, Spector M, Ni N, Eliseo D, Pollak J, Tal M. Initial clinical experience with a new heparin-coated chronic hemodialysis catheter. *Hemodial Int*. 2009;13: 329–334.

43. Falk A. The role of surface coatings on central venous and hemodialysis catheters. Endovascular Today, Buyer's Guide. 2009. (Ref Type: Report.)

CATHETER LOCK SOLUTIONS

VANDANA DUA NIYYAR

1. Identify the rationale behind the use of catheter lock solutions.
2. Familiarity with different types of catheter lock solutions available.
3. Differentiate between the use of catheter lock solutions for prophylaxis and management of thrombosis and infection.
4. Differentiate between the use of catheter lock solutions for prophylaxis and management of infection.
5. Understand the limitations of currently available catheter lock solutions.
6. Discuss potential future directions for development of "ideal" catheter lock solutions.

INTRODUCTION

At present, hemodialysis (HD) is the predominant modality for renal replacement therapy for patients with end-stage renal disease (ESRD) in the United States.[1] Although the incidence of patients with ESRD is relatively stable, the prevalent dialysis population continues to increase rapidly. Additionally, as the HD population ages,[2] multiple comorbidities affecting the vasculature have led to a dearth of suitable options for vascular accesses. Vascular access dysfunction is thus a major cause of morbidity in HD patients and the need to provide a suitable vascular access is an ongoing challenge.

An upper extremity autogenous arteriovenous fistula (AVF) that preferentially involves the cephalic vein is the access of choice for hemodialysis patients, followed by autogenous AVF utilizing the basilic vein and then the use of prosthetic arteriovenous grafts (AVG).[3,4] Despite these recommendations, central venous catheter (CVC) use is widespread among both incident and prevalent HD patients[1] and their use has remained fairly constant over the years, even with the continued and successful efforts of the fistula first initiative. Although CVCs have the distinct advantage of providing immediate access for use,[5] they are primarily intended as bridge therapy. Their long-term use is fraught by complications including a high rate of infection,[6] thrombus-related dysfunction,[7,8] and the potential for central venous stenosis.[9]

Catheter-locking solutions have been used both prophylactically and therapeutically for catheter thrombosis as well as catheter-related infections, with varying degrees of success. This chapter aims to address the different catheter-locking solutions, their advantages and disadvantages, and new directions in this field.

CATHETER THROMBOSIS

▶ Pathogenesis of Thrombus Formation

Central venous catheters were first introduced for dialysis access in the 1980s.[10,11] Since then, catheter design has evolved over the years,[12] with constant modifications in an attempt to provide maximal blood flow while at the same time minimizing infections and intimal trauma leading to thrombosis.[5] The phenomenon of thrombus formation was first described in an in vivo study from Belgium, where the investigators placed silicone catheters in rats and studied histological changes in their veins at scheduled intervals.[13] A pericatheter thrombus formed as early as 24 hours within insertion as a result of endothelial damage to the cell wall. As the injury was sustained (with the continued presence of the central venous catheter), they noted smooth muscle migration and the addition of collagenous matrix, transforming the thrombus into an organized sheath. There is thus a continuum from clot formation to an organized sheath that disrupts flow through the catheter.

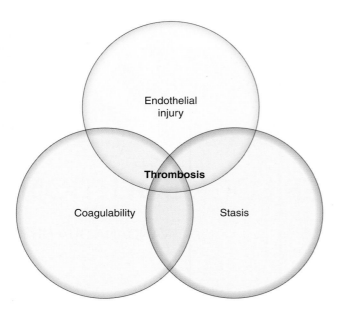

Figure 29-1. Pathophysiology of thrombus formation. The pathophysiology of thrombus formation in CVCs used for HD can be elucidated by application of Virchow's triad—*disruption in vessel walls* (initial insertion of catheter leading to endothelial damage of the vessel wall), *coagulability* (initiation of the coagulation and inflammatory cascade), and *stasis/ changes in blood flow* (intraluminal stasis of blood in the interdialytic period), which leads to the continuum of thrombus and fibrin sheath formation.

The pathophysiology of thrombus formation in CVCs used for HD can be further elucidated by application of Virchow's triad—*disruption in vessel walls* (initial insertion of catheter leading to endothelial damage of the vessel wall), *coagulability* (initiation of the coagulation and inflammatory cascade), and *changes in blood flow* (intraluminal stasis of blood in the interdialytic period), which leads to the continuum of thrombus and fibrin sheath formation (Figure 29-1). Attempts have been made to address each one of these factors in order to minimize catheter dysfunction including changes in catheter design, individual catheters, placed side by side; dual-lumen catheters; step-tip versus spilt-tip catheter which showed no significant differences in flow and recirculation, though the split-tip catheters had a significantly longer half-life (78% vs 64% at 120 days)[14]; addition of side holes, which lead to higher flow rates, but increased adherent clots and CRBI (2.54 vs 0.254/1000 catheter days); symmetric tipped tunneled catheters,[15] and the self-centering superior vena cava catheter.[5] Surface-coated catheters, with heparin covalently bonded to the surface of catheter, have the theoretical advantage of reduction in thrombin-activated factors, reduced proliferation of smooth muscle cells, and reduction in biofilm, fibrin sheath, and thrombus formation. Both thrombus weight and fibrin sheath formation were reduced in unpublished animal studies, though the results are yet to be validated in the HD population. At present, it is difficult to justify the increased cost of surface-treated catheters for chronic hemodialysis in the absence of robust clinical data demonstrating that they reduce catheter-related complications in this patient population.

▶ **Catheter Lock Solutions: Prophylaxis Against Thrombus Formation**

Historically, the standard prophylaxis for intraluminal thrombus formation has been to "lock" the catheter in between hemodialysis treatments with varying concentrations of an anticoagulant such as heparin or citrate. However, neither of these has been shown to be optimal and the ideal catheter lock solution is yet to be identified.

Heparin as prophylaxis against thrombus formation

Heparin is a sulfated polysaccharide that produces its major anticoagulant effect by inactivating thrombin and activated factor X (factor Xa) through an antithrombin (AT)-dependent mechanism.[16] The amount of heparin is based on the luminal volume of the catheter and is specific to each catheter. However, heparin is associated with significant risks, including inadvertent systemic anticoagulation,[17] heparin-induced thrombocytopenia, and an increased potential for bleeding,[18] particularly in uremic patients already predisposed to it. In in vitro studies, even when the fill volume is calculated precisely, there is a 20% leakage of the lock solution due to parabolic flow within the catheter.[19] In vivo studies have confirmed elevation in aPTT (activated partial thromboplastin time) greater than two times normal in patients receiving high-dose heparin locks,[17] and the increase is proportional to the concentration of heparin used (5000–10,000 units/mL > 1000 units/mL).

To minimize these unintended side effects of high-dose heparin in catheter-locking solutions, investigators have evaluated the efficacy of low-dose heparin (1000 units/mL) in maintaining catheter patency. Although there was no change in the incidence of catheter malfunction, there was a significant increase in the use of tissue plasminogen activator (tPA) to maintain patency.[20–22] A decrease in the heparin concentration is also associated with a lower risk of bleeding. A retrospective study evaluating the change in heparin lock concentration from 5000 units/mL to 1000 units/mL found the risk of postinsertion bleeding to be 11.9 times higher in the high-dose heparin group.[18]

Based on the above evidence, ASDIN recommends the use of heparin 1000 units/mL or 4% sodium citrate as suitable choices for catheter lock solutions,[23] as the risk associated with higher concentrations is decreased. However, with the potential for an increased requirement of tPA to maintain catheter patency, higher concentrations of heparin should be reserved for patients with evidence of catheter thrombosis. In addition, recent issues with contamination[24] of the manufacturing process have led to a renewed effort to identify alternatives to heparin for locking solutions.

TABLE 29–1

Catheter-Locking Solutions in Prophylaxis of Thrombosis

Year	Drugs Used	Results
2000 (Schenk et al)[32]	rTPA vs heparin	Flow significantly better in the rTPA group; small n = 12, limited 4-month crossover
2005 (Weijmer et al)[29]	30% Trisodium citrate vs heparin	Comparable patency, citrate with lower costs and decreased CRB
2006 (Lok et al)[27]	4% Trisodium citrate vs heparin	Comparable patency
2007 (Grudzinski et al)[26]	4% Trisodium citrate vs heparin	Comparable patency
2008 (Macrae et al)[25]	4% Trisodium citrate vs heparin	Comparable patency

Citrate as prophylaxis against thrombus formation

Sodium citrate is an effective anticoagulant that acts by chelating ionized calcium, which prevents activation of calcium-dependent coagulation pathways. It was first used medically as an anticoagulant to preserve blood during transfusions and has been used in continuous renal replacement therapy as an anticoagulant for many years. Investigators have shown that trisodium citrate 4% is at least as effective in maintaining catheter patency as heparin.[25–28] A higher concentration of trisodium citrate (30%) was compared with heparin in a randomized, clinical trial and found no difference in catheter thrombosis.[29] The results of these trials are summarized in Table 29-1. Although interdialytic catheter locking has been reported with higher concentrations of citrate, there are potential complications.[30] Some patients report a perioral or peripheral paresthesia or a metallic taste immediately after locking with a high (30%) concentration of trisodium citrate.[29] A case report of a fatal cardiac arrest following the use of trisodium citrate 46.7% led to the withdrawal of TriCitrasol, a commercially available product, by the FDA in 2000.[31]

Alternative locking solutions as prophylaxis against thrombus formation

A myriad of other locking solutions as well as oral anticoagulants have been investigated as possible replacement for heparin, albeit in small, uncontrolled studies. Recombinant tissue plasminogen activator (rtPA)[32] has been compared to heparin, and even though the flow was better in the (rtPA) group, the sample size was small

and there was a limited followup time. A randomized, prospective study comparing 5000 units/mL heparin, 4% citrate, and 3.5% polygeline found comparable patency rates in temporary catheters used for dialysis.[28] Low-dose warfarin and aspirin have also been studied, but the authors found no improvement in thrombosis-free survival.[33,34] The Pre-CLOT study investigated the substitution of rtPA (1 mg in each lumen) in the mid-week session instead of heparin.[35] This group was compared to a group receiving conventional heparin therapy as a lock solution (5000 units/mL). The primary outcome was catheter patency and the secondary outcome was catheter-related bacteremia. The authors reported a statistically significant decrease in the incidence of both catheter dysfunction (40/115 in the heparin group vs 22/110 in the treatment group) and catheter-related bacteremia (15/115 vs 5/110). The risk of adverse events, including bleeding, was similar within the two groups. The authors concluded that the use of once-weekly rtPA significantly reduced the incidence of catheter malfunction and catheter-related bacteremia.

▶ Catheter Lock Solutions: Treatment of Thrombus

A number of studies using thrombolytic agents, either as catheter-locking solutions[36–38] or as infusions[39,40] have been reported in the management of catheter dysfunction. Thrombolytics offer certain advantages in that they restore catheter patency noninvasively and allow for catheter salvage while still preserving the primary access site. Early K-DOQI guidelines recommended the use of urokinase and streptokinase as thrombolytics. These are however no longer widely used due to the potential risks for anaphylaxis with repeated streptokinase and contamination concerns with urokinase.[36] Reteplase has also shown to be effective in restoring flow through occluded and poorly functioning catheters safely and effectively. Instillation of reteplase in each port with dwell times in one study from 30 to 60 minutes or until the next HD session resulted in restoration of flow in >85% cases.[37,41] In another prospective study, a low-dose, 3-hour infusion of recombinant tissue plasminogen activator (rTPA) resulted in a 91% technical success rate. Although primary patency rates were relatively short, dysfunctional catheters were retreated, resulting in significantly improved secondary patency rates.[40] The use of alteplase (tPA, tissue plasminogen activator) in short (1 hour) or long (>48 hours) dwells demonstrated that though restoration of patency is achievable with either regimen, it is quite short-lived.[38] The authors concluded that tPA is ineffective in the long-term management of catheter dysfunction and provided a median gain of catheter function of only 14 days after tPA use. Their results were similar to another group of investigators who found that after repeated tPA use, the median time until the next intervention was five to seven HD treatments.[42] The results of these studies are summarized in Table 29-2.

TABLE 29–2

Catheter-Locking Solutions in Management of Thrombosis

Year	Drugs Used	Results
1994 (Haire et al)[73]	Urokinase (10,000 IU/mL) vs tPA (2 mg)	tPA significantly better in restoring catheter function
2001 (Savader et al)[40]	rTPA infusion (2.5 mg over 3 h)	91% technical success rate, primary patency low, but improved secondary patency
2002 (Little et al)[43]	tPA (1 mg/mL)—dwell time 2–8 h	Patency declined with successive use, median patency only 5–7 treatments
2004 (Haire et al)[74]	Urokinase (5000 IU/mL) vs placebo	UK significantly better in restoring catheter function
2004 (Falk et al)[37]	Reteplase (0.4 units), dwell time 30 min to 1 h	Initial patency 88%, no adverse events
2005 (Macrae et al)[38]	tPA (1mg/mL)—dwell time 1 h vs 48–96 h	Initial patency 78%, but short-lived, median patency only 6 treatments

CATHETER RELATED BACTEREMIA

► Pathogenesis of Catheter-related Bacteremia

Catheter-related bacteremia (CRB) is a serious complication limiting the use of central venous catheters.[43] Contamination of the catheter hub, subsequent colonization of the catheters by intraluminal spread, and the formation of a biofilm by bacteria are major risk factors for catheter-related infections. Bacteria are introduced to the lumen through the flora of the surrounding skin or the hands of health-care workers during catheter-hub manipulation for dialysis. The bacteria then attach to the HD catheter and proliferate to transform into bacterial colonies. Subsequently, they generate a coating of exopolysaccharide and a sticky glycocalyx matrix called the biofilm (Figure 29-2). As the bacterial colonies mature, the biofilm stabilizes and attracts other microorganisms to adhere to each other. Biofilm formation shields the bacteria and prevents diffusion of antibiotics to them and is thus an adaptive strategy that allows the bacteria to survive in an adverse environment.[44] In addition, though a clear link between biofilms and fibrin sheaths has not been established, it has been shown that once a pericatheter thrombus or fibrin sheath is formed, the patient is predisposed to infections[45] and vice versa—infectious complications increase the risk of catheter-related thrombosis.[46] As a result, successful treatment of catheter-related bacteremia usually requires catheter exchange in addition to systemic antibiotics,[47] though the use of concentrated antibiotic locks in conjunction with systemic antibiotics has also been advocated.[48] The uses of antimicrobial locks for prophylaxis as well as for management of catheter-related bacteremia are discussed below.

Prophylaxis against catheter-related bacteremia with lock solutions

The use of an interdialytic catheter lock solution with antimicrobial effects may potentially reduce colonization and biofilm formation, and minimize the risk of catheter-related bacteremia. It is important to differentiate antiseptic solutions (that inhibits the growth and development of microorganisms without necessarily killing them) from antibiotic solutions (that inhibit the growth of or kill other microorganisms), as subtherapeutic levels of antibiotic solutions may induce resistant strains, though this is not the case with antiseptic solutions.

The hitherto standard catheter lock solution, heparin, has been shown to induce biofilm formation in the presence of

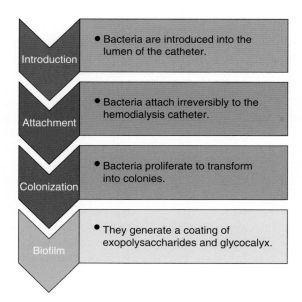

Figure 29-2. Pathophysiology of biofilm formation. Bacteria are introduced to the lumen through the flora of the surrounding skin or the hands of health-care workers during catheter-hub manipulation for dialysis. The bacteria then attach to the HD catheter and proliferate to transform into bacterial colonies. Subsequently, they generate a coating of exopolysaccharide and a sticky glycocalyx matrix called the biofilm. As the bacterial colonies mature, the biofilm stabilizes and attracts other microorganisms to adhere to each other.

Staphylococcus aureus, with higher concentrations increasing biofilm formation faster than lower concentrations.[49,50] On the other hand, in vitro testing of the antimicrobial efficacy of four concentrations of trisodium citrate (TSC 2.2%, 7.5%, 15%, 30%), heparin (5000 units/mL) and gentamicin 1mg/mL in 7.5% trisodium citrate showed superior antimicrobial activity of TSC, especially in higher concentrations.[51] A recent prospective observational study evaluated the characteristics of biofilm formation in tunneled HD catheters in patients with and without catheter-related bacteremia, accounting for catheter lock solutions.[52] The authors found that though the biofilm was present in all catheters, the extent and thickness of the biofilm was significantly higher in patients with bacteremia than those without bacteremia. Further, all biofilm parameters were lower in catheters in which 4% citrate was used as a locking solution as compared to 1000 units/mL heparin.

A catheter lock solution containing 1.35% taurolidine and 4% sodium citrate was evaluated in 20 patients and though it showed a lower frequency of catheter-related bacteremia, the unassisted catheter patency was significantly lower as compared to a control group using heparin (5000 units/mL).[53] Additionally, though antibiotic-lock solutions containing gentamicin are potent and have been shown to decrease the incidence of catheter-related bacteremia, they are not recommended due to the concern for development of resistant organisms.[54]

A meta-analysis of seven trials[55] with a total of 624 patients and 819 catheters showed a 7.72 times less risk of CRB with antibiotic and/or antimicrobial lock solution as compared to heparin alone. Five of the studies used an antibiotic lock,[56–60] one used taurolidine,[61] and one used 30% citrate.[29] An accompanying editorial noted barriers to the widespread use of antimicrobial locks including the potential for systemic toxicity and resistance, short duration of follow-up of the original studies, and the economic ramifications.[62] Another meta-analysis, evaluating eight randomized, controlled trials (seven listed above and the eighth using a catheter lock solution containing minocycline and EDTA; disodium *e*thylene *d*iamine *t*etra *a*cetate[63] concluded that the use of antimicrobial locking solutions decreased the risk of catheter-related bacteremia by a factor of 3. However, they concluded that the achieved incidence of CRB in the groups with antimicrobial catheter locks was similar to published reports from HD units with low CRB incidence, and presumably stricter hygienic measures. They, along with others,[64] advocated intensifying the education of all dialysis staff on adequate catheter care and reserving antibiotic-lock solutions for patients at high risk of infection or those in whom a catheter-related bacteremia would have devastating consequences.

A solution containing 7% sodium citrate, 0.05% methylene blue, and 0.165% parbens has been tested in vitro and has shown strong antimicrobial properties against both planktonic and sessile microorganisms.[65] The solution also has a rapid bactericidal effect on the preformed, mature biofilm of *S. aureus* and significantly reduced biofilm mass

and thickness.[66] This solution (Zuragen™) has recently been evaluated in a multicenter prospective randomized open-label clinical trial (AZEPTIC) to determine its safety and efficacy in maintaining catheter patency and decreasing the incidence of catheter-related bacteremia. A total of 407 patients participated in the trial—201 in the treatment group and 206 in the control group (5000 units of heparin). Catheters locked with the citrate/methylene blue/parabens solution were significantly less likely to cause catheter-related bloodstream infections. They were also less likely to be lost secondary to patency failure but the difference was not statistically significant. This solution is currently awaiting FDA approval and a detailed cost-benefit analysis.

Treatment of catheter-related bacteremia with lock solutions

An alternative approach to the now standard management of catheter-related bacteremia (catheter exchange over guidewire vs removal of the catheter with replacement after eradication of infection) in use by some authors is installation of antibiotic lock into the lumen of the catheter to eradicate the bacteria in the biofilm in addition to systemic antibiotics. The antibiotic regimens for both the systemic and antibiotic-lock solutions are the same—initially broadspectrum and later modified once the identity and sensitivity of the organism are available.[48] In a study over 6 months, use of an antibiotic-lock protocol resulted in a clinical and bacteriological cure of catheter-related bacteremia in 64.5% patients.[67] However, 14% of the patients developed subsequent fungemia on surveillance cultures and required catheter exchange with antifungal therapy. In a small case series of 32 episodes of catheter-related bacteremia, the authors were able to successfully treat 62% patients with the protocol outlined above.[68] However, the salvage rate is highly dependent on the infecting organism—in one report, an antibiotic-lock solution was successful in treating 70% of the cases with catheter-related bacteremia, but a subanalysis revealed that the likelihood of a clinical cure was 87% for Gram-negative infections, 75% for *S. epidermidis* infections, and only 40% for *S. aureus* infections.[69] Another quality improvement report found a 59% failure rate and a 25% incidence of serious complications in patients with *S. aureus* catheter-related bacteremia.[70] Another study from the same center found a 61% catheter salvage rate with a 6% incidence of serious complications in patients with enterococcal catheter-related bacteremia.[71] Thus, an antibiotic-lock solution as an adjunct to systemic antibiotics may not be the solution for every catheter-related bacteremia and should only be used in carefully selected patients.

FUTURE DIRECTIONS

The varying uses of catheter lock solutions—in both prophylaxis and treatment of catheter thrombosis and catheter-related bacteremia—have led to the development of an assortment of solutions, none of which is "just right." The use of heparin (previously the gold standard) has been called into question secondary to the risks of inadvertent systemic anticoagulation, adverse events, and its propensity to induce biofilm formation. Citrate 4% has been shown to be equivalent to heparin in maintaining catheter patency, but shows no advantage over heparin in preventing catheter-related bacteremias. On the other hand, though in vitro studies demonstrate that higher concentrations of citrate inhibit biofilm formation, infusions of higher concentrations are associated with significant toxicity if injected rapidly. EDTA has been shown to decrease biofilm formation but all reported data is in conjunction with antibiotic solutions and it was recently (2008) withdrawn from the market. Taurolidine is an antiseptic agent that inhibits and kills a broad range of microorganisms, but is ineffective in preventing thrombosis and needs to be combined with citrate or heparin as an anticoagulant. tPA is an effective thrombolytic but is too expensive for routine prophylactic use.

So, where do we go from here? What would be an ideal catheter-locking solution? Preferably, it should be one that *prevents* both thrombosis and infection, as the adage "prevention is better than cure" is applicable in this situation too. It is preferable to prevent these complications rather than manage them after they occur. Dr Stephen Ash identified the desired characteristics in a recent review[72]:

- a solution with anticoagulant properties comparable to heparin;
- safe for prophylactic use with infusion of both lumen values;
- lack of caustic effects and protein denaturation;
- ability to kill planktonic bacteria and fungi;
- ability to kill sessile bacteria in biofilm;
- no known bacterial resistance to components;
- not an antibiotic;
- relative density equivalent to that of blood;
- preferably have a color so that it is apparent when catheters are locked.

Although central venous catheters are the least preferred mode of vascular access, a catheter lock solution that improves patency while decreasing catheter-related infections may decrease the morbidity and mortality associated with them. The search is on for the perfect solution and though there have been tremendous improvements in the development of catheter-locking solutions; the field is still wide open for future innovation.

REFERENCES

1. U.S. Renal Data System, USRDS 2010 Annual Data Report: Atlas of Chronic Kidney Disease and End-Stage Renal Disease in the United States, National Institutes of Health, National Institute of Diabetes and Digestive and Kidney Diseases, Bethesda, MD, 2010.
2. Chan MR, Sanchez RJ, Young HN, Yevzlin AS. Vascular access outcomes in the elderly hemodialysis population: a USRDS study. *Semin Dial*. 2007;20(6):606–610.
3. Clinical practice guidelines for vascular access. *Am J Kidney Dis*. 2006;48(suppl 1):S176–S247.
4. Fistula First National Vascular Access Improvement Initiative; www.fistulafirst.org; accessed 2011.
5. Ash SR. Advances in tunneled central venous catheters for dialysis: design and performance. *Semin Dial*. 2008;21(6):504–515.
6. Saad TF. Bacteremia associated with tunneled, cuffed hemodialysis catheters. *Am J Kidney Dis*. 1999;34(6):1114–1124.
7. Beathard GA. Dysfunction of new catheters by old fibrin sheaths. *Semin Dial*. 2004;17(3):243–244.
8. Oliver MJ, Mendelssohn DC, Quinn RR, Richardson EP, Rajan DK, Pugash RA, et al. Catheter patency and function after catheter sheath disruption: a pilot study. *Clin J Am Soc Nephrol*. 2007;2(6):1201–1206.
9. MacRae JM, Ahmed A, Johnson N, Levin A, Kiaii M. Central vein stenosis: a common problem in patients on hemodialysis. *ASAIO J*. 2005;51(1):77–81.
10. Bregman H. Double lumen subclavian hemodialysis cannulas. *Int J Artif Organs*. 1985;8(1):17–18.
11. Snider HC, Ingalls CE, Schloeder FX, Sivanna P. Use of subclavian catheters for hemodialysis. *South Med J*. 1982;75(9):1093–1094, 1098.
12. Ash SR. Fluid mechanics and clinical success of central venous catheters for dialysis—answers to simple but persisting problems. *Semin Dial*. 2007;20(3):237–256.
13. Xiang DZ, Verbeken EK, Van Lommel AT, Stas M, De Wever I. Composition and formation of the sleeve enveloping a central venous catheter. *J Vasc Surg*. 1998;28(2):260–271.
14. Trerotola SO, Kraus M, Shah H, Namyslowski J, Johnson MS, Stecker MS, et al. Randomized comparison of split tip versus step tip high-flow hemodialysis catheters. *Kidney Int*. 2002;62(1):282–289.
15. Tal MG. Comparison of recirculation percentage of the palindrome catheter and standard hemodialysis catheters in a swine model. *J Vasc Interv Radiol*. 2005;16(9):1237–1240.
16. Hirsh J, Anand SS, Halperin JL, Fuster V. AHA scientific statement: guide to anticoagulant therapy: heparin: a statement for healthcare professionals from the American Heart Association. *Arterioscler Thromb Vasc Biol*. 2001;21(7):E9–E33.
17. Karaaslan H, Peyronnet P, Benevent D, Lagarde C, Rince M, Leroux-Robert C. Risk of heparin lock-related bleeding when using indwelling venous catheter in haemodialysis. *Nephrol Dial Transplant*. 2001;16(10):2072–2074.
18. Yevzlin AS, Sanchez RJ, Hiatt JG, Washington MH, Wakeen M, Hofmann RM, et al. Concentrated heparin lock is associated with major bleeding complications after tunneled hemodialysis catheter placement. *Semin Dial*. 2007;20(4):351–354.
19. Sungur M, Eryuksel E, Yavas S, Bihorac A, Layon AJ, Caruso L. Exit of catheter lock solutions from double lumen acute haemodialysis catheters—an in vitro study. *Nephrol Dial Transplant*. 2007;22(12):3533–3537.
20. Thomas CM, Zhang J, Lim TH, Scott-Douglas N, Hons RB, Hemmelgarn BR. Concentration of heparin-locking solution and risk of central venous hemodialysis catheter malfunction. *ASAIO J*. 2007;53(4):485–488.

21. Holley JL, Bailey S. Catheter lock heparin concentration: effects on tissue plasminogen activator use in tunneled cuffed catheters. *Hemodial Int*. 2007;11(1):96–98.

22. Ivan DM, Smith T, Allon M. Does the heparin lock concentration affect hemodialysis catheter patency? *Clin J Am Soc Nephrol*. 2010;5(8):1458–1462.

23. Moran JE, Ash SR. Locking solutions for hemodialysis catheters; heparin and citrate—a position paper by ASDIN. *Semin Dial*. 2008;21(5):490–492.

24. Blossom DB, Kallen AJ, Patel PR, Elward A, Robinson L, Gao G, et al. Outbreak of adverse reactions associated with contaminated heparin. *N Engl J Med*. 2008;359(25):2674–2684.

25. Macrae JM, Dojcinovic I, Djurdjev O, Jung B, Shalansky S, Levin A, et al. Citrate 4% versus heparin and the reduction of thrombosis study (CHARTS). *Clin J Am Soc Nephrol*. 2008;3(2):369–374.

26. Grudzinski L, Quinan P, Kwok S, Pierratos A. Sodium citrate 4% locking solution for central venous dialysis catheters—an effective, more cost-efficient alternative to heparin. *Nephrol Dial Transplant*. 2007;22(2):471–476.

27. Lok CE, Appleton D, Bhola C, Khoo B, Richardson RM. Trisodium citrate 4%—an alternative to heparin capping of haemodialysis catheters. *Nephrol Dial Transplant*. 2007;22(2):477–483.

28. Buturovic J, Ponikvar R, Kandus A, Boh M, Klinkmann J, Ivanovich P. Filling hemodialysis catheters in the interdialytic period: heparin versus citrate versus polygeline: a prospective randomized study. *Artif Organs*. 1998;22(11):945–947.

29. Weijmer MC, van den Dorpel MA, Van de Ven PJ, ter Wee PM, van Geelen JA, Groeneveld JO, et al. Randomized, clinical trial comparison of trisodium citrate 30% and heparin as catheter-locking solution in hemodialysis patients. *J Am Soc Nephrol*. 2005;16(9):2769–2777.

30. Polaschegg HD, Sodemann K. Risks related to catheter locking solutions containing concentrated citrate. *Nephrol Dial Transplant*. 2003;18(12):2688–2690.

31. FDA. 2000 [cited 2010 9/30/2010]. Available at http://www.fda.gov/Safety/MedWatch/SafetyInformation/SafetyAlertsforHumanMedicalProducts/ucm173095.htm. Accessed 2011.

32. Schenk P, Rosenkranz AR, Wolfl G, Horl WH, Traindl O. Recombinant tissue plasminogen activator is a useful alternative to heparin in priming quinton permcath. *Am J Kidney Dis*. 2000;35(1):130–136.

33. Mokrzycki MH, Jean-Jerome K, Rush H, Zdunek MP, Rosenberg SO. A randomized trial of minidose warfarin for the prevention of late malfunction in tunneled, cuffed hemodialysis catheters. *Kidney Int*. 2001;59(5):1935–1942.

34. Traynor JP, Walbaum D, Woo YM, Teenan P, Fox JG, Mactier RA. Low-dose warfarin fails to prolong survival of dual lumen venous dialysis catheters. *Nephrol Dial Transplant*. 2001;16(3):645.

35. Hemmelgarn BR, Moist LM, Lok CE, Tonelli M, Manns BJ, Holden RM, et al. Prevention of dialysis catheter malfunction with recombinant tissue plasminogen activator. *N Engl J Med*. 2011;364(4):303–312.

36. Paulsen D, Reisoether A, Aasen M, Fauchald P. Use of tissue plasminogen activator for reopening of clotted dialysis catheters. *Nephron*. 1993;64(3):468–470.

37. Falk A, Samson W, Uribarri J, Vassalotti JA. Efficacy of reteplase in poorly functioning hemodialysis catheters. *Clin Nephrol*. 2004;61(1):47–53.

38. Macrae JM, Loh G, Djurdjev O, Shalansky S, Werb R, Levin A, et al. Short and long alteplase dwells in dysfunctional hemodialysis catheters. *Hemodial Int*. 2005;9(2):189–195.

39. Webb A, Abdalla M, Russell GI. A protocol of urokinase infusion and warfarin for the management of the thrombosed haemodialysis catheter. *Nephrol Dial Transplant*. 2001;16(10):2075–2078.

40. Savader SJ, Ehrman KO, Porter DJ, Haikal LC, Oteham AC. Treatment of hemodialysis catheter-associated fibrin sheaths by rt-PA infusion: critical analysis of 124 procedures. *J Vasc Interv Radiol*. 2001;12(6):711–715.

41. Hilleman DE, Dunlay RW, Packard KA. Reteplase for dysfunctional hemodialysis catheter clearance. *Pharmacotherapy*. 2003;23(2):137–141.

42. Little MA, Walshe JJ. A longitudinal study of the repeated use of alteplase as therapy for tunneled hemodialysis catheter dysfunction. *Am J Kidney Dis*. 2002;39(1):86–91.

43. Little MA, O'Riordan A, Lucey B, Farrell M, Lee M, Conlon PJ, et al. A prospective study of complications associated with cuffed, tunnelled haemodialysis catheters. *Nephrol Dial Transplant*. 2001;16(11):2194–2200.

44. Dasgupta MK. Biofilms and infection in dialysis patients. *Semin Dial*. 2002;15(5):338–346.

45. Mehall JR, Saltzman DA, Jackson RJ, Smith SD. Fibrin sheath enhances central venous catheter infection. *Crit Care Med*. 2002;30(4):908–912.

46. van Rooden CJ, Schippers EF, Barge RM, Rosendaal FR, Guiot HF, van der Meer FJ, et al. Infectious complications of central venous catheters increase the risk of catheter-related thrombosis in hematology patients: a prospective study. *J Clin Oncol*. 2005;23(12):2655–2660.

47. Beathard GA. Management of bacteremia associated with tunneled-cuffed hemodialysis catheters. *J Am Soc Nephrol*. 1999;10(5):1045–1049.

48. Maya ID. Antibiotic lock for treatment of tunneled hemodialysis catheter bacteremia. *Semin Dial*. 2008;21(6):539–541.

49. Shanks RM, Sargent JL, Martinez RM, Graber ML, O'Toole GA. Catheter lock solutions influence staphylococcal biofilm formation on abiotic surfaces. *Nephrol Dial Transplant*. 2006;21(8):2247–2255.

50. Shanks RM, Donegan NP, Graber ML, Buckingham SE, Zegans ME, Cheung AL, et al. Heparin stimulates *Staphylococcus aureus* biofilm formation. *Infect Immun*. 2005;73(8):4596–4606.

51. Weijmer MC, Debets-Ossenkopp YJ, Van De Vondervoort FJ, ter Wee PM. Superior antimicrobial activity of trisodium citrate over heparin for catheter locking. *Nephrol Dial Transplant*. 2002;17(12):2189–2195.

52. Jones SM, Ravani P, Hemmelgarn BR, Muruve D, Macrae JM. Morphometric and biological characterization of biofilm in tunneled hemodialysis catheters. *Am J Kidney Dis*. 2011;57(3):449–455.

53. Allon M. Prophylaxis against dialysis catheter-related bacteremia with a novel antimicrobial lock solution. *Clin Infect Dis*. 2003;36(12):1539–1544.

54. Landry DL, Braden GL, Gobeille SL, Haessler SD, Vaidya CK, Sweet SJ. Emergence of gentamicin-resistant bacteremia in hemodialysis patients receiving gentamicin lock catheter prophylaxis. *Clin J Am Soc Nephrol*. 2010;5:1799–1804.

55. Jaffer Y, Selby NM, Taal MW, Fluck RJ, McIntyre CW. A meta-analysis of hemodialysis catheter locking solutions in the prevention of catheter-related infection. *Am J Kidney Dis*. 2008;51(2):233–241.

56. Dogra GK, Herson H, Hutchison B, Irish AB, Heath CH, Golledge C, et al. Prevention of tunneled hemodialysis catheter-related infections using catheter-restricted filling with gentamicin and citrate: a randomized controlled study. *J Am Soc Nephrol*. 2002;13(8):2133–2139.

57. Kim SH, Song KI, Chang JW, Kim SB, Sung SA, Jo SK, et al. Prevention of uncuffed hemodialysis catheter-related bacteremia using an antibiotic lock technique: a prospective, randomized clinical trial. *Kidney Int*. 2006;69(1):161–164.

58. McIntyre CW, Hulme LJ, Taal M, Fluck RJ. Locking of tunneled hemodialysis catheters with gentamicin and heparin. *Kidney Int*. 2004;66(2):801–805.

59. Nori US, Manoharan A, Yee J, Besarab A. Comparison of low-dose gentamicin with minocycline as catheter lock solutions in the prevention of catheter-related bacteremia. *Am J Kidney Dis*. 2006;48(4):596–605.

60. Saxena AK, Panhotra BR, Sundaram DS, Morsy MN, Al-Ghamdi AM. Enhancing the survival of tunneled haemodialysis catheters using an antibiotic lock in the elderly: a randomised, double-blind clinical trial. *Nephrology (Carlton)*. 2006;11(4):299–305.

61. Betjes MG, van Agteren M. Prevention of dialysis catheter-related sepsis with a citrate-taurolidine-containing lock solution. *Nephrol Dial Transplant*. 2004;19(6):1546–1551.

62. Allon M. Prophylaxis against dialysis catheter-related bacteremia: a glimmer of hope. *Am J Kidney Dis*. 2008;51(2):165–168.

63. Bleyer AJ, Mason L, Russell G, Raad, II, Sherertz RJ. A randomized, controlled trial of a new vascular catheter flush solution (minocycline-EDTA) in temporary hemodialysis access. *Infect Control Hosp Epidemiol*. 2005;26(6):520–524.

64. Bleyer AJ. Use of antimicrobial catheter lock solutions to prevent catheter-related bacteremia. *Clin J Am Soc Nephrol*. 2007;2(5):1073–1078.

65. Steczko J, Ash SR, Nivens DE, Brewer L, Winger RK. Microbial inactivation properties of a new antimicrobial/antithrombotic catheter lock solution (citrate/methylene blue/parabens). *Nephrol Dial Transplant*. 2009;24(6):1937–1945.

66. Sauer K, Steczko J, Ash SR. Effect of a solution containing citrate/methylene blue/parabens on *Staphylococcus aureus* bacteria and biofilm, and comparison with various heparin solutions. *J Antimicrob Chemother*. 2009;63(5):937–945.

67. Krishnasami Z, Carlton D, Bimbo L, Taylor ME, Balkovetz DF, Barker J, et al. Management of hemodialysis catheter-related bacteremia with an adjunctive antibiotic lock solution. *Kidney Int*. 2002;61(3):1136–1142.

68. Vardhan A, Davies J, Daryanani I, Crowe A, McClelland P. Treatment of haemodialysis catheter-related infections. *Nephrol Dial Transplant*. 2002;17(6):1149–1150.

69. Poole CV, Carlton D, Bimbo L, Allon M. Treatment of catheter-related bacteraemia with an antibiotic lock protocol: effect of bacterial pathogen. *Nephrol Dial Transplant*. 2004;19(5):1237–1244.

70. Maya ID, Carlton D, Estrada E, Allon M. Treatment of dialysis catheter-related *Staphylococcus aureus* bacteremia with an antibiotic lock: a quality improvement report. *Am J Kidney Dis*. 2007;50(2):289–295.

71. Peterson WJ, Maya ID, Carlton D, Estrada E, Allon M. Treatment of dialysis catheter-related *Enterococcus bacteremia* with an antibiotic lock: a quality improvement report. *Am J Kidney Dis*. 2009;53(1):107–111.

72. Ash S. Catheter locks for central vein catheters for dialysis. *Davita Quest*. 2008;(14):18–24.

73. Haire WD, Atkinson JB, Stephens LC, Kotulak GD. Urokinase versus recombinant tissue plasminogen activator in thrombosed central venous catheters: a double-blinded, randomized trial. *Thromb and Haemost*. 1994;72(4):543–547.

74. Haire WD, Deitcher SR. Mullane KM, Jaff MR, Firszt CM, Schulz GA, Schuerr DM, Schwartz LB, Mouginis TL, Barton RP. Recombinant urokinase for restoration of patency in occluded central venous access devices. A double-blind, placebo-controlled trial. *Thromb and Haemost*. 2004;92(3):575–582.

30

SURFACE COATINGS FOR TUNNELED CATHETERS

AMY DWYER

1. Understand the scope of catheter complications.
2. Define the three most common types of catheter complications.
3. Understand the pathophysiology of biofilm formation.
4. Define the typical organisms involved in hemodialysis catheter infections.
5. Understand how catheters can become infected.
6. Understand the pathophysiology of catheter failure due to thrombosis.
7. Define an intrinsic and extrinsic thrombus.
8. List the different types of catheter surface treatments.
9. Discuss the use of surface-treated, central venous catheters.
10. Discuss the use of nontunneled, antimicrobial-treated hemodialysis catheters.
11. Discuss the use of tunneled, surface-treated hemodialysis catheters.

INTRODUCTION

An arteriovenous fistula (AVF) is the preferred hemodialysis vascular access because it is associated with the lowest rate of complications from thrombosis and infection and the highest patient survival rate compared to grafts and catheters. In 1997, the Kidney Disease Outcomes Quality Initiative (K/DOQI) developed guidelines to improve patient care and reduce costs by recommending that 50% of dialysis patients have an AVF. In 2003, the Centers for Medicare and Medicaid Services (CMS) in a joint effort with the End Stage Renal Disease Networks and dialysis health-care providers implemented the National Vascular Access Improvement initiative later called the "Fistula First Initiative," with the primary goal to exceed the K/DOQI guidelines by recommending an increase in the AVF rate to 66% nationwide.[1-3]

Despite the Fistula First campaign, more than 60% of incident and almost 30% of prevalent patients on chronic hemodialysis use a tunneled catheter as their vascular access[4-6] and catheter complications are a major cause of morbidity and mortality in hemodialysis patients. According to the Dialysis Outcomes and Practice Patterns Study, dialysis patients with a tunneled catheter have a five-fold increased risk of developing infection compared to patients with an AVF.[7] The relative risk of death for patients starting dialysis with a tunneled catheter is 1.31 compared to patients with an AVF or synthetic graft. It has been estimated that costs of access-related complications are approaching $1 billion annually, with catheters accounting for a large portion of this expenditure.[8] Thus, catheter complications have a negative impact on patient outcomes while increasing the burden to the health-care budget.

▶ Catheter-Related Complications

The three most common causes of catheter dysfunction and failure are as follows:

1. Biofilm formation
2. Infection
3. Thrombus formation

Many approaches to prevention and treatment of catheter-related complications have been studied. This chapter will focus on the use of surface-treated catheters and their role in combating catheter-related complications.

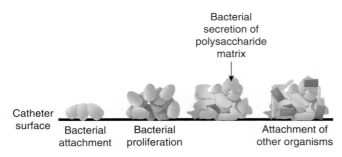

Figure 30-1. Formation of catheter biofilm.

Approaches to determining the best type of catheter, insertion site, skin preparation, and use of adjunctive medications are beyond the scope of this chapter.

Biofilm formation

A biofilm is a complex structure formed by bacteria that have attached to an artificial surface or dead tissue. Biofilm formation is an important factor in both early and late catheter failure and in catheter failure associated with infection. There is evidence that soon after catheter placement, bacteria attach to the catheter surface and begin to produce biofilm. Electron microscopy studies demonstrate bacterial attachment to the surfaces of indwelling vascular catheters as early as 24 hours after insertion.[9] After bacterial attachment, the bacteria proliferate and secrete a polysaccharide matrix that provides a medium for the attachment of additional organisms (Figure 30-1). This bacterial colonization intensifies with increasing endovascular dwelling time. Published studies support that most organisms involved in biofilm formation are indigenous to the host and that these organisms form biofilm on all artificial surfaces inserted in the body. The mere formation of a biofilm does not necessarily produce clinical manifestations of infection. In many instances, the biofilm grows too slowly to produce clinical symptoms such as fever, chills, and bacteremia. In a study comparing bacterial isolates from catheter biofilm and catheter-related bacteremia (CRB) with central venous catheters, no clear association between biofilm formation and pathogenic virulence was seen.[10]

The pathogenesis of biofilm development to fibrin sheath formation is not well understood. There is considerable debate as to whether fibrin sheath formation can occur without the initial development of a biofilm. The best evidence supports the theory that a biofilm evolves over weeks to months into a more complex structure, a fibrin sheath. In addition to fibrin, these sheaths contain multiple other molecular and cellular components, including laminin, fibronectin, collagen, and even smooth muscle cells.[8] A fibrin sheath surrounds the catheter surface beginning at the venipuncture site and progressively extends down the length of the catheter until it eventually covers the catheter tip, thereby occluding the catheter lumen.[11] The rate of catheter malfunction due to fibrin sheath formation has been reported to be as high as 50%.[12]

TABLE 30-1

Microbiologic Isolates from 123 Episodes of Catheter-Related Bacteremia[13]

Organism	Isolates (%)
Gram-positive cocci	104 (64.5%)
Staphylococcus epidermidis	46
Staphylococcus aureus	37
Enterococcus faecalis	15
Other group D enterococci	6
Gram-positive rods	2 (1.6%)
Corynebacterium species	4
Gram-negative rods	41 (33.3%)
Enterobacter cloacae	11
Other Enterobacter species	2
Pseudomonas species	8
Acinetobacter baumannii	5
Citrobacter species	5
Serratia species	2
Klebsiella pneumoniae	4
Proteus mirabilis	1
Escherichia coli	1
Agrobacterium radiobacter	1
Alcaligenes species	1
Acid-fast organism	2 (1.6%)

Catheter infection

The typical organisms involved in hemodialysis catheter infections include coagulase-negative staphylococci, *Staphylococcus aureus*, *Pseudomonas*, enterococci, and *Candida* (Table 30-1).[13]

Catheters become infected by different routes depending on the time from catheter insertion[6]:

- ≤30 days catheters become infected by external routes:
  - from the patient's skin microflora
  - from the hands of the medical personnel during insertion
- >30 days catheters become infected by internal routes: contamination of the catheter hub that leads to hematogenous spread and bacteremia.

Catheter infection is typically resistant to antimicrobial treatment alone due to failure of the antibiotics to penetrate all layers of the biofilm, and the slow growing nature of the organisms involved. Although bacteria in a biofilm release antigens that stimulate antibody production by the host, organisms imbedded in a biofilm are resistant to these antibodies.[14,15] The resistance to both endogenous and exogenous antibacterial agents has led to the recommendation that treatment of infected catheters includes removal or exchange, in addition to antimicrobial agents, as part of the treatment of an infected biofilm.[16–19]

Catheter thrombosis

Catheter failure due to thrombosis is a common problem in hemodialysis patients. There are unique physiologic factors that make hemodialysis patients more susceptible to thrombosis formation. These factors include both platelet and plasma abnormalities. As reviewed by Smits et al,[16] there may also be an abnormal expression of platelet membrane proteins that leads to thrombosis in dialysis patients. In addition, platelets become activated upon attachment to the dialyzer membrane, to the catheter surface, or with shear stress during catheter use.[16] Finally, plasma factors such as hyperfibrinogenemia, reduced levels of antithrombin III and protein C anticoagulant activity, and increased levels of homocysteine are also postulated to make hemodialysis patients more susceptible to thrombus formation.[20]

In addition to platelet and plasma factors as a cause, catheter failure due to thrombus can develop from both intrinsic and extrinsic sources,[21] occluding the catheter and causing it to fail:

- *Intrinsic thrombus*: a thrombus that forms within the catheter lumen or on the catheter tip
- *Extrinsic thrombus*: a thrombus that forms around the catheter *in the vein* that leads to catheter attachment to the vessel wall, or form in the atria

The relationship between catheter infection, fibrin sheath, and thrombus formation is unclear. A recent prospective study, examining the risk of catheter thrombosis with infection, concluded that there was indeed an association between infection and thrombosis, and that the risk of developing thrombosis increased with the severity of infection.[22] Catheters in patients with bacteremia demonstrated a higher risk of developing thrombosis, compared to those catheters in patients with a local infection. In addition, Timsit et al reported also that the incidence of vein thrombosis was 18.8% in patients with catheter-related bacteremia, compared to 7.2% in patients without catheter-related bacteremia.[23] Suojanen et al performed a histologic evaluation of fibrin sheaths associated with 10 indwelling central venous catheters removed from 8 patients. They found that 70% of the fibrin sheaths contained organizing thrombus.[24,25]

▶ Catheter Surface Treatments

To combat all three causes of catheter failure, the ideal catheter coating or surface treatment should be biocompatible, prevent both thrombus and fibrin sheath formation, be effective long-term, and have broad-spectrum antimicrobial activity without inducing resistance. Two types of catheter coatings have been developed: those with antimicrobial coatings and those with antithrombotic coatings. Although numerous catheters with different types of surface treatments have been developed, only a few surface-treated catheters are available for use in the United States (Table 30-2).

For more than 10 years, the Critical Care community has studied the effectiveness if catheters impregnated with rifampin compounds, chlorhexidine and silver sulfadiazine, or silver platinum compounds. The primary and secondary endpoints for most studies were the rate

TABLE 30–2

Surface-Treated Catheters Available in the United States

Nontunneled Catheters	Coating Type	Surface Coated	Catheter Length (cm)	Catheter Diameter (French)
ARROWgard Blue® (Arrow International)	Chlorhexidine/silver sulfadiazine	External (hub to tip)	13, 16, 20, 25	12, 14
ARROWgard Blue PLUS® (Arrow International)	Chlorhexidine/silver sulfadiazine	Internal/external (hub to tip)	16, 20	7, 8
Glide Spectrum® (Cook Critical Care)	Minocycline/rifampin	Internal/external (hub to tip)	15, 20, 25	8, 9.5
Vantex® (Edwards Lifesciences)	Silver-platinum-carbon (SPC)	Internal/external (hub to tip)	16, 20	7, 8.5
BioBloc® Coating (CR Bard)	Silver sulfadiazine	External (hub to cuff and tip)	20, 24, 28, 32, 36, 40, 47	14.5
Vitacuff® (CR Bard) available on HemoGlide® and Hohn® catheters	Silver sulfadiazine	Dacron fiber cuff only	24, 28, 32, 36	14
Palindrome Ruby® (Tyco-Kendall)	Silver sulfadiazine	External (hub to cuff only)	36, 40, 45, 50	14.5
Palindrome Emerald® (Tyco-Kendall)	Trillium Biosurface®	Internal/external (hub to tip)	36, 40, 45, 50	14.5
Palindrome Sapphire® (Tyco-Kendall)	Silver sulfadiazine/ Trillium Biosurface®	Silver (external hub to cuff), heparin (internal/external from hub to tip)	36, 40, 45, 50	14.5

of catheter colonization and occurrence of CRB. None of the published studies evaluated the effect of coated catheter use on fibrin sheath or thrombus formation, or determined the influence of these complications on the rate of infection.

Data with surface-treated, central venous catheters (CVC)

- A meta-analysis of randomized controlled trials using rifampin-impregnated central venous catheters concluded that surface-treated catheters were safe and effective for reducing catheter colonization and CRB compared to a standard catheter.[26] In the groups with coated catheters, the odds ratio for developing infection was 0.23 and the odds ratio for bacterial colonization was 0.46 compared to an uncoated catheter.

- In a meta-analysis of central venous catheters impregnated with chlorhexidine and silver sulfadiazine (CH-SS), the risk of CRB was reduced from 4.1% to 1.9% compared to the standard catheter.[27]

- A prospective, randomized study compared minocycline and rifampin coated catheters (Cook Spectrum, Cook Critical Care, Bloomington, IN) to chlorhexidine and silver sulfadiazine-coated catheters (ARROWgard® Blue Plus, Arrow International, Reading, PA). This study concluded that catheter colonization was 1/3 as likely and CRB was 1/12 as likely with minocycline and rifampin coated catheters.[28]

- In 2008, Gilbert and Harden performed a systematic review of 37 randomized, controlled trials involving 11,568 patients with various types of central venous catheters.[29] The catheter types in the studies included in the review were uncoated, heparin-coated, antibiotic-coated, and antiseptic-coated central venous catheters. The review compared differential efficacy of the various coatings as well as comparing coated versus uncoated catheters in critically ill patients. The primary endpoints were episodes of CRB and bacterial colonization.

A Forest-plot analysis showed the following:

1. Reduction in CRB with heparin-coated catheters and antibiotic-coated catheters compared to the standard (uncoated) catheter.

2. Reduction in CRB with antibiotic-coated catheters compared to CH-SS catheters.

3. No effect on CRB with silver-coated catheters compared to a standard catheter.

4. No effect on CRB with antibiotic coating compared to a silver-coated catheter.

5. No difference in CRB in studies comparing heparin-coated catheters with CH-SS coated catheters.

The authors concluded that the best options for reducing CRB in critically ill patients were to use either a heparin-coated or antibiotic-coated catheter.

Summary and recommendations for CVC The Centers for Disease Control (CDC) published guidelines for the prevention of catheter-related infections.[30] They recommended the use of antimicrobial-coated catheters in populations in which the rate of infection exceeded 3.3 per 1000 catheter days. This recommendation would apply to the hemodialysis population as CRB has been reported at rates ranging from 2.2 to 5.5 per 1000 catheter days using a tunneled catheter,[31] and this rate can be as high as 6.3 per 1000 catheter days in dialysis patients using a non-tunneled catheter.[32] In addition, a recent comprehensive review of all published studies on catheter-related blood stream infections between 1990 and 2005 recommended that "antibiotic-coated catheters are clinically effective and cost saving compared with either aseptic-coated or standard catheters."[33]

Surface-treated catheters for hemodialysis

Although the critical care data and CDC recommendations support the use of antimicrobial-coated catheters in the acute setting, to date there are few published studies examining the use of antimicrobial-coated catheters in the hemodialysis patient population.

Nontunneled, antimicrobial-treated hemodialysis catheters

- A prospective, randomized study by Chatzinikolaou et al examined the frequency of CRB in patients with acute kidney injury (AKI).[34] One-hundred and three patients were randomized to receive either a femoral vein nontunneled catheter coated with minocycline and rifampin on both internal and external surfaces (Cook Spectrum, Cook Critical Care, Bloomington, IN) or a femoral vein nontunneled, uncoated catheter. Catheter dwell times were the same for both groups (8 ± 6 days) (Figure 30-2). All seven episodes of CRB occurred in the patients with uncoated catheters ($P = 0.006$).

- A randomized trial showed that use of a nontunneled, antimicrobial-coated dialysis catheter (ARROWgard® Blue Plus, Arrow International, Reading, PA), with both internal and external surface coatings, chlorhexidine and chloracetate on the internal surface and chlorhexidine

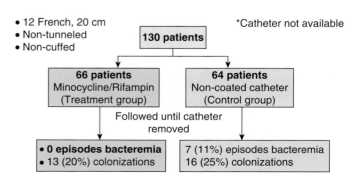

Figure 30-2. Study design. (Data from Chatzinikolaou et al.[34])

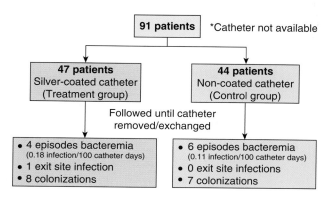

Figure 30-3. Study design. (Data from Trerotola et al.[36])

and silver sulfadiazine on the external surfaces, reduced bacterial colonization in central venous catheters.[35]

Tunneled, surface-treated hemodialysis catheters *Silver-coatings*: Data with the use of tunneled, silver-coated hemodialysis catheters are limited and the results are inconsistent.

- In 91 patients randomly assigned to receive either a silver-coated tunneled hemodialysis catheter (Silvergard, MedComp, Harleysville, PA) or an uncoated tunneled catheter (Figure 30-3), Trerotola et al found no reduction in colonization or CRB with the coated catheter.[36]

- Bambauer et al found an 8% colonization rate using a silver-coated catheter (Spi-Argent, Spire Biomedical, Bedford, MA) compared to 46.4% with uncoated catheters.[37] In addition, the silver-coated catheters had a reduced rate of thrombus formation.

- A prospective trial comparing the silver-impregnated cuff (Hohn catheter, Bard Access Systems, Inc., Salt Lake City, UT) to a standard cuff showed that the incidence of CRB was actually increased with the silver cuff (17.2% vs 3.2%).[38] In addition, patients with silver cuffs experienced an increase in pulmonary embolism.

Two antithrombotic coatings have been developed on tunneled, hemodialysis catheters: the Carmeda® BioActive Surface (CBAS) developed by Carmeda (Upplands Väsby, Sweden) and the Trillium® Biosurface developed by Bio-Interactions Ltd. (Reading, Berks, UK). However, only the Trillium® Biosurface treated catheters are available for use today in the United States. Both surfaces use heparin bonded to the catheter as an anticoagulant. Heparin is not only a strong anticoagulant, but has been shown in many studies to both reduce thrombin-activated factors and reduce the proliferation of smooth muscle cells.[39] As a result, surface heparinization on medical devices has the potential not only to reduce biofilm and fibrin sheath formation, but also to reduce infection and thrombus formation.

The CBAS treatment consists of heparin molecules covalently bonded in an endpoint fashion to the catheter surface, exposing its active heparin sequence to the blood stream. CBAS has been used in clinical trials on numerous implanted medical devices including coronary stents, ventricular assist devices, central venous catheters, vascular

grafts, and intraocular lenses. Central venous catheters coated with CBAS are associated with reduced rates of catheter-related bacteremia.[34,40] In unpublished animal studies using a CBAS-coated Decathlon® hemodialysis catheter (Spire Biomedical®, Bedford, MA), both thrombus weight and fibrin sheath formation were reduced.[41] However, the CBAS-coated Decathlon® hemodialysis catheter is no longer available.

The Trillium® Biosurface treatment also uses heparin as its anticoagulant, but it is structured differently. It has a hydrophilic polyethylene oxide layer with negatively charged sulfate polymers to hold water at the catheter surface and to repel blood cells. In addition, it has heparin covalently bonded to the polyethylene oxide layer for anticoagulation. In clinical trials with various implanted devices, this surface treatment has been shown to reduce platelet, complement, and granulocyte activation, and to reduce the requirement for blood product transfusions.[42,43]

Data with the use of heparin-coated catheters in hemodialysis patients

There are only two studies evaluating the effect of tunneled, heparin-treated catheters in the chronic hemodialysis population.

- In 2008, Kakkos et al[44] published a case-control study of 200 newly placed or exchanged tunneled catheters in 163 chronic hemodialysis patients. They consecutively placed or exchanged 100 tunneled catheters using an uncoated, tunneled dialysis catheter (control group, HemoSplit, Angiotech) until October 2006 at which time they changed their practice to place or exchange only heparin-coated tunneled catheters (treatment group, Palindrome Ruby, Kendall/Tyco Healthcare). One hundred catheters in the control group were followed for 9765 catheter days and 100 catheters in the treatment group were followed for 11,173 catheter days (Figures 30-4 and 30-5). The primary endpoints were (1) thrombosis rate, (2) catheter infection rate, (3) reintervention rate, (4) rate of exit-site infection, and (5) rate of tunnel infection.

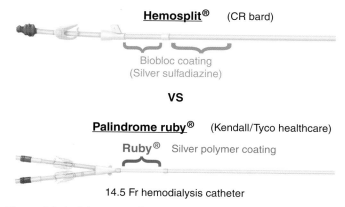

Figure 30-4. Schematic of catheter characteristics in Kakkos et al.[44]

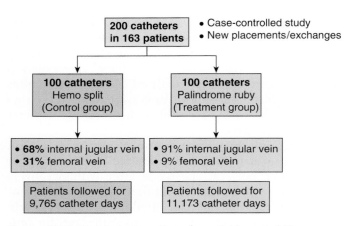

Figure 30-5. Study design. (Data from Kakkos et al.[44])

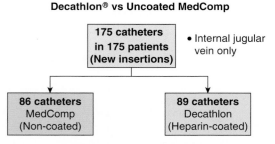

Figure 30-6. Study design. (Data from Jain et al.[45])

The results are shown in Table 30-3. The control group had a higher rate of exit-site infection, catheter thrombosis, and reintervention rate compared to the treatment group. The authors attributed the significantly lower rate of thrombosis and catheter reintervention in the treatment group to the unique tip design of the Palindrome Ruby catheter. There was a surprising, statistically significant reduction in the rate of CRB (18%) in the control group compared to the treatment group (24%) even though 31% of the control catheters were inserted into the femoral vein, a location with a known higher incidence of CRB.

- Jain et al[45] published a retrospective study in 2009 that compared the CRB rates of newly inserted internal jugular vein uncoated, tunneled catheters (control group, MedComp, Harleysville, PA) with heparin-coated, tunneled catheters (treatment group, Spire Biomedical®, Bedford, MA) in hemodialysis patients. Eighty-six patients were included in the control and 89 patients were in the treatment group (Figure 30-6). Retrospective data collected included time to catheter removal, catheter failure, exchange, catheter infection rates, tPA installations, and catheter blood flow rates (Table 30-4). The authors concluded that catheters coated with heparin had a decreased frequency of CRB compared to the standard catheter but no difference was seen in catheter malfunction rates in the two groups.

Summary and conclusions on the use of surface-treated catheters Substantial clinical data support the use of antimicrobial- and antithrombotic-coated catheters to decrease both bacterial colonization and CRB in the critical care setting. In addition, cost analysis studies favor the use of surface-treated catheters in high-risk patient populations.

The only prospective studies with nontunneled, surface-treated catheters performed in hemodialysis patients are in the setting of acute kidney injury; therefore, there is no evidence on which to base application of the CDC guidelines recommending the use of nontunneled, surface-treated catheters in the chronic hemodialysis patient population.

Few, randomized clinical trials have evaluated the use of tunneled, surface-treated catheters in hemodialysis patients. Surface-treated tunneled dialysis catheters cost about $100 more than standard catheters. In the absence of adequate clinical data to support the use of surface-treated tunneled catheters, the increased expense cannot be justified. More randomized, controlled clinical trials are necessary to determine the effectiveness of this new technology in the hemodialysis patient population.

TABLE 30–3		
Outcomes of HemoSplit Compared to Palindrome Ruby		
Endpoint	**HemoSplit®**	**Palindrome Ruby®**
Thrombosis	32%	5%
Infection	18%	24%
Reintervention (thrombosis/infection)	50%	29%
Exit-site infection	1%	0
Tunnel infection	0	1%

Source: Adapted from Kakkos et al.[44]

TABLE 30–4		
Study Outcomes		
Study Outcome	**Heparin Coated (Decathlon®)**	**Noncoated (MedComp)**
Number of patients	89	86
Catheter malfunction	17 (19%)	13 (15%)
Catheter-related bacteremia	30 (34%)	52 (60%)
Elective removal	31 (35%)	17 (20%)
Remained patent	11 (12%)	4 (5%)
tPA installations (per 1000 catheter days)	1.8	1.8

Source: Adapted from Jain et al.[45]

REFERENCES

1. Lok C. Fistula first initiative: advantages and pitfalls. *Clin J Am Soc Nephrol.* 2007;2:1043–1053.
2. Bazan H. Why "fistula first" matters: increased durability, less interventions, and decreased costs. *Catheter Cardiovasc Interv.* 2009;75:22.
3. "National Vascular Access Improvement Initiative." The Institute for Healthcare Improvement. www.fistulafirst.org, Web. September 22, 2010.
4. Allon M. Dialysis catheter-related bacteremia: treatment and prophylaxis. *Am J Kidney Dis.* 2004;44(5): 779–791.
5. Lee T, Barker J, Allon M. Tunneled catheters in hemodialysis patients: reasons and subsequent outcomes. *Am J Kidney Dis.* 2005;46(3):501–508.
6. Nori U, Manoharan A, Yee J, Besarab A. Comparison of low dose gentamicin with minocycline as catheter lock solutions in the prevention of catheter-related bacteremia. *Am J Kidney Dis.* 2006;48(4):596–605.
7. Rayner HC, Besarab A, Brown WW, Disney A, Saito A, Pisoni RL. Vascular access results from the Dialysis Outcomes and Practice Patterns Study (DOPPS): performance against kidney disease outcomes quality initiative (K/DOQI) clinical practice guidelines. *Am J Kidney Dis.* 2004;44(5):S22–S26.
8. Manerski C, Besarab A. Antimicrobial locks: putting the lock on catheter infections. *Adv Chronic Kidney Dis.* 2006;13(3):245–258.
9. Trautner B, Darouiche R. Catheter-associated infections. *Arch Intern Med.* 2004;164:842–850.
10. Vogel L, Sloos JH, Spaargaren J, Suiker I, Dijkshoorn L. Biofilm production by *Staphylococcus epidermis* isolates associated with catheter-related bacteremia. *Diagn Microbiol Infect Dis.* 2000;26:139–141.
11. Beathard G. Catheter thrombosis. *Semin Dial.* 2001;14(6):441–445.
12. Liangos O, Gul A, Madias NE, Jaber BL. Long-term management of the tunneled venous catheter. *Semin Dial.* 2006;19(2):158–164.
13. Beathard G. Management of bacteremia associated with tunneled-cuffed hemodialysis catheters. *J Am Soc Nephrol.* 1999;10:1045–1049.
14. Costerton JW, Stewart PS, Greenberg EP. Bacterial biofilms: a common cause of persistent infections. *Science.* 1999;284:1318–1322.
15. Mehall JR, Saltzman DA, Jackson RJ, Smith SD. Fibrin sheath enhances central venous catheter infection. *Crit Care Med.* 2002;30(4):908–912.
16. Robinson D, Suhocki P, Schwab SJ. Treatment of infected tunneled venous access hemodialysis catheters with guidewire exchange. *Kidney Int.* 1998;53:1792–1794.
17. Sullivan R, Samuel V, Le C, Khan M, Alexandraki I, Cuhaci B, et al. Hemodialysis vascular catheter-related bacteremia. *Am J Med Sci.* 2007;334(6):458–465.
18. Kovalik E, Schwab S. Treatment approaches for infected hemodialysis vascular catheters. *Curr Opin Nephrol Hypertens.* 2002;11:593–596.
19. Saad T. Central venous dialysis catheters: catheter-associated infection. *Semin Dial.* 2001;14(6):446–451.
20. Smits JH, van der Linden J, Blankestijn PJ, Rabelink TJ. Coagulation and haemodialysis access thrombosis. *Nephrol Dial Transplant.* 2000;15:1755–1760.
21. Beathard G. Catheter thrombosis. *Semin Dial.* 2001;14(6): 441–445.
22. van Rooden CJ, Schippers EF, Barge RM, Rosendaal FR, Guiot HF, van der Meer FJ, et al. Infectious complications of central venous catheters increase the risk of catheter-related thrombosis in hematology patients: a prospective study. *J Clin Oncol.* 2005;23(15):2655–2660.
23. Timsit JF, Farkas JC, Boyer JM, Martin JB, Misset B, Renaud B, et al. Central vein catheter-related thrombosis in intensive care patients: incidence, risk factors, and relationship with catheter-related sepsis. *Chest.* 1998;114(1):207–213.
24. Suojanen JN, Brophy DP, Nasser I. Thrombus on indwelling central venous catheters: the histopathology of "fibrin sheaths." *Cardiovasc Intervent Radiol.* 2000;23:194–197.
25. Forauer A, Theoharis C. Histologic changes in the human vein wall adjacent to indwelling central venous catheters. *J Vasc Intervent Radiol.* 2003;14:1163–1168.
26. Falgas ME, Fragoulis K, Bliziotis IA, Chatzinikolaou I. Rifampin-impregnated central venous catheters: a meta-analysis of randomized controlled trials. *J Antimicrob Chemother.* 2007;59:359–369.
27. Walder B, Pittet D, Tramer MR. Prevention of bloodstream infections with central venous catheters treated with anti-infective agents depends on catheter type and insertion time: evidence from a meta-analysis. *Infect Control Hospital Epidemiol.* 2002;23(12):748–756.
28. Darouiche RO, Raad II, Heard SO, Thronby JI, Wenker OC, Gabrielli A, et al. A comparison of two antimicrobial impregnated central venous catheters. *N Engl J Med.* 1999;341(1):1–8.
29. Gilbert RE, Harden M. Effectiveness of impregnated central venous catheters for catheter related blood stream infection: a systematic review. *Curr Opin Infect Dis.* 2008;21(3):235–245.
30. Centers for Disease Control and Prevention. Guidelines for the Prevention of Intravascular Catheter-Related Infections. *MMWR* 2002;51(RR-10):1–26.
31. Beathard G. Catheter management protocol for catheter-related bacteremia prophylaxis. *Semin Dial.* 2003;16(5):403–405.
32. Sullivan R, Samuel V, Le C, Khan M, Alexandraki I, Cuhaci B, et al. Hemodialysis vascular catheter-related bacteremia. *Am J Med Sci.* 2007;334(6):458–465.
33. Halton K, Graves N. Economics of preventing catheter-related bloodstream infections. *Emerg Infect Dis.* 2007; 13(6):815–823.
34. Chatzinikolaou I, Finkel K, Hanna H, Boktour M, Foringer J, Ho T, et al. Antibiotic-coated hemodialysis catheters for the prevention of vascular catheter-related infections: a prospective, randomized study. *Am J Med.* 2003;115:352–357.
35. Rupp ME, Lisco SJ, Lipsett PA, Perl TM, Keating K, Civetta JM, et al. Effect of a second-generation venous catheter impregnated with chlorhexidine and silver sulfadiazine on central catheter-related infections. *Ann Intern Med.* 2005;143(8):570–581.
36. Trerotola SO, Johnson MS, Shah H, Kraus MA, McKusky MA, Ambrosius WT, et al. Tunneled hemodialysis catheters: use of a silver-coated catheter for prevention of infection—a randomized study. *Radiology.* 1998;207:491–496.

37. Bambauer R, Mestres P, Schiel R, Bambauer S, Sioshansi P, Latza R. Long-term catheters for apheresis and dialysis with surface treatment with infection resistance and low thrombogenicity. *Ther Apher Dial.* 2003;7(2):225–231.

38. Alderman R, Sugarbaker P. Prospective nonrandomized trial of silver impregnated cuff central lines. *Int Surg.* 2005;90(4):219–222.

39. Lumsden A. A unique combination technology of ePTFE and proprietary end-point covalent bonding of heparin for lower extremity revascularization: the GORE PROPATEN vascular graft. *Vasc Dis Manag.* 2007;4(suppl B):11B–14B.

40. CBAS: *CBAS® Compendium. Carmeda®*, Reading, UK: Biointeractions Ltd., 2000.

41. Spire Biomedical: *In vitro and Animal Data on File, Sheep Study Duration: 25–30 days*, Medical Device Evaluation Center, Salt Lake City, UT, USA. Spire Biomedical, 2005.

42. Sandhu S, Luthra A. Developments in biointeracting materials for medical application. *Med Device Manufac Tech.* 2004;13(8):1–4.

43. *Trillium® Biosurface*. Retrieved April 29, 2008, from http://www.medtronic.com/cardsurgery/arrested_heart/biopassive.html

44. Kakkos SK, Haddad GK, Haddad RK, Scully MM. Effectiveness of a new tunneled catheter in preventing catheter malfunction: a comparative study. *J Vasc Interv Radiol.* 2008;19:1018–1026.

45. Jain G, Allon M, Saddekni S, Barker JF, Maya ID. Does heparin coating improve patency or reduce infection of tunneled dialysis catheters? *Clin J Am Soc Nephrol.* 2009;4:1787–1790.

31

CARDIAC RHYTHM DEVICES IN RENAL PATIENTS

ARIF ASIF, LOAY SALMAN, & GERALD A. BEATHARD

INTRODUCTION

Patients with chronic kidney disease (CKD) have a high incidence of cardiovascular disease. In fact, this is the leading cause of death in patients with end-stage renal disease (ESRD).[1] In the United States Renal Data System database, more than one-fourth of cardiac deaths are attributable to arrhythmic mechanisms.[1,2] As a result of these problems, there is a frequent need for the placement of cardiac rhythm devices (CRDs) such as pacemaker, implantable cardioverter defibrillator, and cardiac resynchronization therapy. Traditionally, the transvenous route has been the most frequently used pathway for the insertion of the electrical leads used by these devices. However, the use of this route of placement can cause major problems for chronic hemodialysis patients.

In the dialysis patient, central venous flow and pressure is markedly increased due to the diversion of arterial flow into the venous circuit. Central venous obstruction or even nonobstructive stenosis makes the patient particularly vulnerable to the development of severe progressive edema of the ipsilateral arm, shoulder, breast, neck, and face.[3-6] These symptoms cause considerable patient discomfort and place the patient at risk for serious complications. Dialysis therapy becomes increasingly difficult due to problems with cannulation. The patient's vascular access is frequently lost if this problem is allowed to progress.[7] Additionally, the development of central vein obstruction obviates the possibility of vascular access creation on the affected side. Many dialysis patients have a life expectancy of several decades. With the loss of central venous patency, the potential for realizing this longevity is materially diminished.

Transvenous CRD wires can also have an adverse effect by inducing or aggravating tricuspid insufficiency which is already common in these patients.[8-10] Dialysis patients are prone to recurrent episodes of bacteremia; the presence of any intravascular device represents a significant risk factor for serious complications especially in cases with catheter-related bacteremia.[11,12]

This chapter focuses on transvenous CRD-associated central venous stenosis, CRD infection, and tricuspid regurgitation in chronic hemodialysis patients and highlights epicardial leads as an alternative approach that carries great potential of minimizing the above-cited complications in renal patients. Because the effectiveness of the epicardial leads is often brought into question, this report also provides information regarding the functionality of epicardial and transvenous leads.[13-20]

CENTRAL VENOUS STENOSIS

Central venous stenosis is a recurrent problem that is observed with the use of transvenous leads (Figure 31-1).[3–6,21,22] This complication is not infrequent, it has been reported to occur in up to 64% of the nonhemodialysis-dependent patients.[6,21,22] Because of the absence of a dialysis access in their extremity, only a minority of these patients ever develop symptoms. The situation is vastly different, however, in end-stage renal disease patients receiving dialysis therapy with an arteriovenous access in the upper extremity ipsilateral to the CRD device. These cases are particularly vulnerable to the development of edema of the face, neck, breast, shoulder, and the arm due to the development of progressive central venous stenosis.[3–6]

Elevated venous pressure and high recirculation rates for arteriovenous accesses in patients with transvenous cardiac devices have been reported.[5,23] Teruya et al[4] found that 71% (10/14) of chronic hemodialysis patients with a pacemaker ipsilateral to an arteriovenous dialysis access developed symptoms of central venous stenosis and demonstrated subclavian vein stenosis and thrombosis on angiography. The average time for the onset of symptoms was 12.6 months. None of their patients had a prior history of a catheter; dialysis was initiated through an arteriovenous dialysis access. The patients that did not develop central venous stenosis had expired within 6 months of AV access/PM placement of unrelated causes. The high incidence of symptoms in this report is attributable to the high blood flow of an arteriovenous access in the affected extremity compared to patients with no access in the upper extremity. In addition to the underlying stenosis, the fibrous tissue covering the leads and the development of binding sites or pedicles between the vein wall and the fibrous tissue covering the leads can compound the occlusive problem and restrict blood flow to the atrium.[5,24–26] Avoiding this process with the use of epicardial leads in hemodialysis patients would represent a major advantage.

In some instances, it has become necessary to ligate the dialysis access in order to control the patient's symptoms.[4] This leaves the patient with the need to create a new access. This has generally been accomplished by moving it to the opposite arm in the belief that the symptoms of central stenosis are less common when the arteriovenous access is located contralateral to the cardiac device.[7] While this approach is generally successful in alleviating the immediate symptoms, it does not obviate the fact that the patient has lost the entire venous capital of one extremity. Also, since the superior vena cava (SVC) is the final pathway for the leads, stenosis can develop in this vessel as well. SVC stenosis has been documented in multiple reports[27–31] and confirmed by a multicenter study that documented that lead-induced stenosis of the superior vena cava occurred in nearly 18% of the cases.[5] In fact, it is possible for a patient to develop SVC stenosis subsequent to a lesion that was initially localized to the brachiocephalic vein.[23] If this occurs, recurrence of symptoms would be expected. Epicardial leads bypass the central veins altogether and provide a meaningful solution to this difficult problem.

In view of the general success obtained with the treatment of venous lesions with percutaneous balloon angioplasty (PTA) with primary patency rates ranging from 41% to 76% at 6 months and 31% to 45% at 1 year,[32–40] this modality might be considered a reasonable approach to the problem of lead-induced central vein stenosis (Figure 31-2). However, a large multicenter study evaluating the role of PTA in the treatment of this problem found primary patency rates of only 18% and 9% at 6 and 12 months, respectively.[5] Secondary patency rates were 95%, 86%, and 73% at 6, 12, and 24 months, respectively, with an average of 2.1 procedures per year required to maintain secondary patency. Unfortunately, PTA is not always successful and in some cases the results are short-lived. In one study, two patients with transvenous lead-associated central stenosis were treated with simple PTA. Both patients experienced a recurrence of stenosis in less than 3 months. The transvenous leads were replaced by epicardial leads and the PTA treatment was repeated for the central stenotic lesions. The duration of angioplasty was greater than 8 months in both.[23]

Over the past decade, the use of endovascular stents for the management of dialysis access dysfunction has increased dramatically.[41] Several investigators have considered using stents as an adjunct to PTA in the treatment of lead-induced central

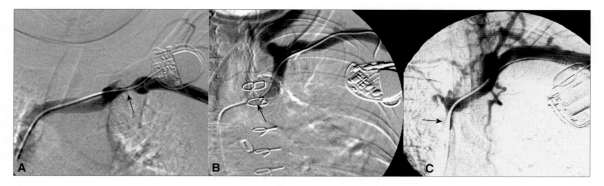

Figure 31-1. Central venous stenosis secondary to transvenous wires (arrows). (**A**) Subclavian vein, (**B**) brachiocephalic vein, and (**C**) superior vena cava.

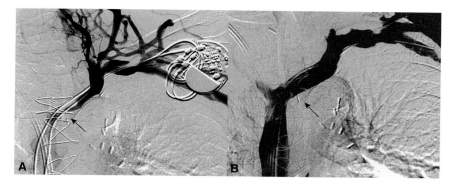

Figure 31-2. Angioplasty of lesion associated with transvenous wires. (**A**) Lesion (arrow) and (**B**) postangioplasty.

vein stenosis.[42–44] In this regard, there are three possible approaches to stent placement: (1) ignore the transvenous leads and place the stent over them, (2) remove the leads and replace them after the stent is inserted, and (3) convert the transvenous leads to epicardial.

For a number of years many interventionalists have ignored the presence of the leads and approached the problem as though they did not exist. This was the approach analyzed in a retrospective study which employed 17 bare metal stents/stent grafts in 15 patients placed over transvenous CRD leads.[42] A primary patency at 6 and 12 months of 41.7% and 8.3%, respectively, was recorded. A total of 45 total repeat interventions were required, 33 were performed on the target lesion. During repeat interventions, five additional bare metal stents/stent grafts were placed. The incidence of sepsis (*Staphylococcus aureus*) in this small series was 6.6%. The authors successfully treated sepsis with antibiotic therapy without the removal of the intravascular devices that were present and reported success. This approach is potentially problematic, however. Transvenous leads are exposed in many areas within the vessel lumen. When sepsis occurs, it can result in a biofilm infection upon the leads (see below). Microbes within a biofilm are more resistant to antibiotics and host defenses. For this reason, it is recommended by the American Heart Association that an essential part of the treatment of all infected CRDs include a complete removal of all hardware.[45] Unfortunately, when a stent is inserted over transvenous leads, they become entrapped (Figure 31-3). This can present a major impediment to their removal with simple percutaneous techniques and often necessitate open thoracotomy.

The second approach, the one recommended by the Hearth Rhythm Society expert consensus,[46] is to remove the leads prior to stent placement and then reinsert new ones afterward. This was recommended because of the serious nature of lead infections and the inherent risk involved in removing them after they have been covered with a stent. However, because these new leads still traverse through the central veins and serve as a source of constant endothelial irritation, the potential for future development of stenosis elsewhere within the central veins and within the stent

itself remains. Nevertheless, this should be regarded as the minimal approach when stent placement is felt to be mandatory in a patient with transvenous CRD leads.

The third approach is to convert the case to epicardial leads. This has a dual benefit. It gets them out of the central circulation and offers the benefit of avoiding the risk of lead infection secondary to the frequent bacteremias that plague hemodialysis patients. It also avoids further exposure of the central veins to the irritation of the devices and its contribution to venous pathology.

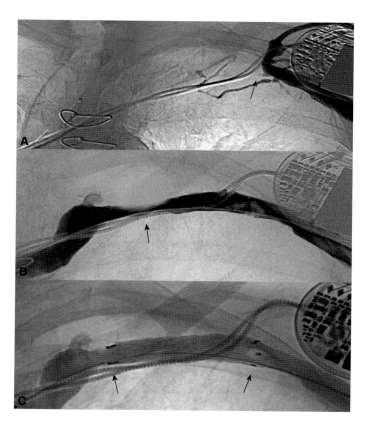

Figure 31-3. Ill-advised stent placed over transvenous wires. (**A**) Obstruction of subclavian secondary to transvenous wires (arrow), (**B**) postangioplasty shown significant residual (arrow), (**C**) poststent placement (between arrows).

CARDIAC DEVICE INFECTION

The incidence of pacemaker infection in the general population ranges from 0.8% to 5.7%.[45,46] However, CKD is a risk factor for the development of this problem.[47,48] In a case-control study ($n = 152$), it was found that moderate to severe renal disease (glomerular filtration rate of ≤ 60 mL/min/1.73 m^2) was the most potent risk factor among all those identified for infection of a pacemaker with a prevalence of 42% in infected patients as compared to 13% in the control group (odds ratio 4.8).[47]

Staphylococcal species cause the bulk of CRD infections and account for 60%–80% of cases in most reported series.[45] In one study examining ESRD patients with CRDs, all patients (7 cases) with an infected CRD had *S. aureus* bacteremia and in more than half, the organism was methicillin resistant.[23] A variety of coagulase-negative *Staphylococcus* species have also been described to cause CRD infections.[49] Gram-negative bacilli[50,51] including *Pseudomonas aeruginosa*[52] and *Candida* species account for a minority of cases.

A major concern in the hemodialysis patient with a CRD is the high frequency of infection in this patient group and the potential for infection spreading to the transvenous leads. Infection has been reported to account for 20% of all dialysis access complications[53] and to be the second leading cause of graft loss. Additionally, it is the second most common cause of death in this patient group.[54–57] In one report, infection was reported to occur at a frequency of 1.3 episodes per 100 dialysis months and be associated with bacteremia at a rate of 0.7 cases per 100-dialysis months.[58] In a prospective Canadian study in which surveillance for hemodialysis-related bloodstream infections was performed in 11 centers during a 6-month period, it was found that the relative risk for bloodstream infection was 15.5 with cuffed and tunneled central venous catheter access, and 22.5 with uncuffed CVC access per 1000 dialysis procedures.[59]

Since transvenous CRD leads do not become completely covered over, even after a long period in place, an episode of bacteremia can lead to hematogenous spread of the infection to the device. This is more likely to occur with Staphylococcus than with a Gram-negative bacteremia. By means of surface adhesins, bacteria can adhere to host matrix proteins such fibrinogen, fibronectin, and collagen that are deposited on newly implanted biomaterials.[60,61] Staphylococci have a variety of surface adhesins, some known collectively by the acronym MSCRAMM (microbial surface components reacting with adherence matrix molecules), that allow this pathogen to be especially adept at establishing a focus of infection.[62] When a bacterial cell switches modes from planktonic (free-floating) organisms to sessile (attached), two things happen—they become encased in a layer of slime[63] referred to as a biofilm and they undergo phenotypic changes.[64] Staphylococcus, being a "slime former," creates a more exuberant biofilm that does most other organisms. The hallmark of biofilm-related infections is a marked resistance to antimicrobials and to host defenses. Biofilm microorganisms have been shown to be 100 to 1000 times less susceptible to antibiotics than their planktonic counterparts.[65,66]

The treatment of a biofilm infection requires a dual approach; antibiotics are required to treat the planktonic (free-floating) organisms and, because it is resistant to antibiotics, the biofilm must be removed. This removal generally involves extraction of the surface to which the biofilm is attached. For this reason, it has been recommended by the American Heart Association (class I indication) that an essential part of the treatment of all infected CRDs include a complete removal of all hardware to get rid of the biofilm.[45] Lead entrapment by a bare metal or a stent graft can complicate this process considerably. Percutaneous lead extraction may no longer be feasible leaving complex open-heart surgery as the only option. It is for this reason that the Heart Rhythm Society expert consensus on transvenous lead extraction recommends (class I indication) lead removal in patients with planned stent deployment in a vein already containing a transvenous lead.[51]

When CRD infection occurs it can be life threatening.[67–70] Although lead infection can occur alone, it may also be associated with cardiac valve involvement.[2,71,72] Lead-associated endocarditis (LAE) is a major contributor to the high mortality observed with this problem.[69] Unfortunately, LAE is not an uncommon condition and has been shown to occur in approximately 50% of the patients presenting with device-related infection.[69] Transesophageal echocardiography (TEE) is especially useful in evaluating these cases for both lead infection and cardiac valvular involvement.[45] Because of its poor sensitivity, transthoracic echocardiography is frequently not helpful in ruling out a diagnosis of LAE. Moreover, patients can develop both right-sided (lead associated) and left-sided (hematogenous) endocarditis; the sensitivity of TEE for left-sided involvement and for perivalvular extension of infection is superior to that of transthoracic echocardiography. Additionally, visualization of the leads in the proximal superior vena cava from TEE views may identify tissue along that region that is difficult to visualize by other methods. Lead vegetation has been reported to be present in 90%–96% of the cases.[67,71,72] TEE examination is critical among patients with *S. aureus* bacteremia, because the rate of endocarditis is so significant.[73] Staphylococcus continues to be a major culprit (60%) causing of the LEA cases many of which are methicillin-resistant *S. aureus*.[70]

TRICUSPID REGURGITATION

In the hemodialysis patient, TR can be a serious problem. This problem is characterized by the backflow of blood into the right atrium during systole. Both the right atrial and ventricular pressures are increased. The elevated right ventricular pressures can eventually lead to right ventricular systolic dysfunction and low forward cardiac output.[74] The right ventricle can eventually fail and become hypokinetic. In this setting, right ventricular systolic function may not accurately reflect the severity of TR on echocardiography.[74] Additionally, when the regurgitation is severe, right ventricular volume overload causes diastolic interventricular septal flattening displacing the septum toward the left complicating left ventricular output.

Tricuspid regurgitation is associated with decreased survival.[74-76] In a Veterans Affairs study of 5223 patients, the 1-year survival for moderate and severe TR was only 79% and 64%, respectively.[75] Similar findings have been documented in other studies ($n = 1421$).[76] Decreased survival in these cases was significant even in the absence of pulmonary hypertension and left ventricular dysfunction.[74-76] TR can be especially problematic in the hemodialysis patient because of increased cardiac output related to the arteriovenous access. This is compounded by the fact that these patients have a tendency to become fluid overloaded and there is a high incidence of cardiac disease in this patient population.

Transvenous CRD leads, either single or multiple, cause tricuspid valve regurgitation (TR) ranging from mild to severe in a significant number of cases.[9,77-84] There are several mechanisms to explain the development of CRD lead-induced TR. It has been shown that CRD leads can cause fibrosis and valve adhesions.[9,25,26,85,86] This makes the valve stiff and interferes with its function. Lead-induced adhesions can tether these devices at multiple sites to the walls of central veins including the superior vena cava causing problems.[25,26,85,86] Impingement and entanglement of the valve due to the leads can result valvular dysfunction.[9] Finally, perforation of the valve can also be caused by transvenous CRD leads and result in TR.[9,77-81]

In a large retrospective study,[9] the role of pacemaker and ICD leads on the development of TR was evaluated. The investigators examined 156 patients who had PM or ICD and severe symptomatic TR (New York Heart Association functional class III or IV). All underwent surgical repair to correct severe TR. At the time of surgery, 26.2% (41) of the patients were found to have direct evidence of tricuspid value damage with severe symptomatic regurgitation due to the leads. Operative findings included lead adherence to the valve ($n = 14$), lead-induced perforation of the valve ($n = 7$), lead-induced impingement of the valve ($n = 16$), and lead entanglement ($n = 4$). The strength of the study was the fact that the direct surgical evidence of valvular involvement was documented compared to indirect measures. In this study, both transthoracic ($n = 41$) and transesophageal echocardiogram ($n = 38$) were available for analysis. Of note, valvular malfunction due to PM/ICD leads was diagnosed by transthoracic echocardiography in only 5/41 (12%) of cases that demonstrated lead-induced valvular damage during surgery. In contrast, transesophageal echocardiogram was able to visualize the lead as a cause of TR in 17/38 (45%) of the patients.

EPICARDIAL LEADS

In the past, epicardial leads for pacing have been used primarily in children. This approach to pacing is often required because of the patient's small size and concern about vascular obstruction, AV valve integrity, and the limitations of lead accommodation with somatic growth.[19,87-89] Even though they were being used, early reports suggested that they did not work as well as the transvenous devices. In one study,[90] conventional epicardial leads showed an inferior 2-year lead survival (71% ± 10%) compared to endocardial leads (93% ± 7%). Because of this type of data, concerns have continued to be raised among healthcare providers regarding the effectiveness of this approach to cardiac pacing. However, epicardial lead technology has changed dramatically. Advances in lead technology and in surgical approach, such as steroid epicardial leads and left atrial leads, have resulted in major improvements.[14,91-93] Today, this concern is ill founded.

Dodge-Khatami et al[18] conducted a study to compare the function of steroid-eluting epicardial ($n = 38$) versus steroid-eluting transvenous leads ($n = 47$). Atrial and ventricular sensing and capture thresholds (acute and chronic) as well as impedance were evaluated. The study demonstrated practically identical results for these parameters for the two groups. It was concluded that steroid-eluting epicardial and transvenous leads were functionally equivalent. The differences between the survival of the epicardial and transvenous devices has also been evaluated. In one report,[20] the 2-year survival for epicardial leads (91% ± 5%) was similar to that obtained for the endocardial leads (86% ± 7%) ($p = 0.97$). Lead failure occurred in four leads in both epicardial and endocardial devices ($p = 0.85$). In both of these reports,[18,20] the pacing and sensing thresholds were similar for both the epicardial and endocardial systems.

Cohen et al[19] reported their 17-year experience (over 1200 outpatient visits) with over 200 epicardial leads. The 1-, 2-, and 5-year lead survival was 96%, 90%, and 74%, respectively, for this long-term study. The authors concluded that steroid-eluting epicardial leads provided stable acute chronic sensing and pacing thresholds and demonstrated lead survival that was similar to endocardial leads. Other studies evaluating the epicardial versus endocardial leads have also found no difference in lead recalls or fracture between the endocardial or epicardial leads.[15,16]

Although these data represent studies done in pediatric patients, excellent results have also been reported in adult cases. Approximately 30% of patients with heart failure have intraventricular conduction delay, defined by left bundle-branch block with QRS duration greater than 120 ms.[94] Studies have shown that dyssynchronous ventricular contraction is inefficient, leading to as much as 20% loss of myocardial stroke work. The importance of a highly synchronized ventricular contraction has been recognized, but not all modes of synchronization are efficient, dual-chamber right-sided pacing worsens heart failure.[95,96] Cardiac resynchronization therapy (CRT, biventricular pacing) has been proposed for the treatment for heart failure patients.[97–101] A meta-analysis of this therapeutic strategy revealed a significant reduction in mortality from heart failure.[102]

Usually, left ventricular lead implant for CRT is accomplished by passing the lead through the coronary sinus,[103] advancing it into a major cardiac vein. Unfortunately, this technique is associated with long fluoroscopic times and is not applicable to all patients because of coronary sinus and coronary venous anatomy limitations. Early and late failure occurs in approximately 12% and 10% of procedures, respectively.[104] Additionally, attempts to pass the lead through the coronary sinus can result in complications such as coronary sinus dissection (up to 4%), cardiac perforation (<1%), and diaphragmatic pacing from phrenic nerve stimulation.[105]

Epicardial lead placement has been shown to be successful and offers advantages related to its safety and shorter implant time. Moreover, it allows visual selection of the best pacing site and multiplicity of pacing sites. Minimally invasive surgical procedures facilitate left ventricular lead placement and can be accomplished with low risk and similar or superior results to full thoracotomy.[106–110]

Ailawadi et al[13] investigated whether an epicardial lead inserted into the left ventricle offered the same benefit as a transvenous lead passed through the coronary sinus. In this study, 452 patients undergoing transvenous left ventricular lead placement for cardiac resynchronization therapy were included. Forty-five patients had failed transvenous leads and underwent epicardial insertion. These 45 patients were matched with 135 patients in whom transvenous placement was successful. The follow-up period was 32.4 ± 17.5 months and 39.4 ± 14.8 months for the epicardial and transvenous leads, respectively. During the follow-up, there was no difference between the two approaches for readmissions due to congestive heart failure (epicardial = 26.2%, transvenous = 31.5%; $p = 0.53$), improvement in New York Heart functional class (epicardial = 60.1%, transvenous = 49.6%, $p = 0.17$) or all-cause mortality (epicardial = 30.6%, transvenous = 23.8%; $p = 0.22$).

In a randomized prospective study,[111] 80 consecutive patients with an indication for CRT were randomized to receive either a transvenous ($n = 40$) or an epicardial ($n = 40$) lead placement. The mean age of the two groups was 61.7 and 64 years, respectively. There were no significant differences in any of their clinical parameters prior to the procedure. At 6 months, there were no major differences in lead parameters (threshold, sensing, and impedance).

In view of the results from studies such as these and the ability to place epicardial leads using minimally invasive techniques, it has been proposed that this approach be considered a primary option for these problems. Because they bypass major complicating issues, epicardial leads are particularly relevant in renal failure patients receiving hemodialysis therapy.

PERCUTANEOUS EPICARDIAL AND SUBCUTANEOUS CRD

To eliminate the need for venous access, percutaneous and subcutaneous approaches have been tried for the placement of an ICD.[112–115] The percutaneous technique is accomplished by introducing a needle into the pericardial space from the subxiphoid region with fluoroscopic guidance. Then a defibrillation coil is inserted through a sheath.[112] An entirely subcutaneous ICD has also been used.[114] In nonrandomized studies, system was shown to successfully and consistently detect and convert episodes of ventricular fibrillation that were induced during electrophysiological testing. The device also successfully detected and treated episodes of spontaneous, sustained ventricular tachyarrhythmia. While preliminary results are encouraging, there is a great need for the optimal configuration of these devices.[115] Future development of efficient electrode configurations that would maximize shock vector alignment and lower defibrillation threshold would be beneficial. Because of the problems associated with transvenous leads, the development of such device is critically important and holds promise particularly for hemodialysis patients.

CONCLUSIONS

There are multiple advantages of epicardial leads (Table 31-1). These leads do not traverse through the central veins or cause central venous stenosis. Epicardial leads are not directly exposed to blood flow and hence are not readily available for bacterial seeding. These leads do not cross the tricuspid valve and consequently avoid the risk of valve injury and associated TR. Data have indicated that epicardial leads are equivalent endocardial leads regarding performance and can be placed using minimally invasive techniques.

The approach to CRD lead placement in all patients with ESRD should be guided by a set of principles designed

TABLE 31–1

Advantages and Disadvantages of Subcutaneous Epicardial and Transvenous Endocardial Cardiac Devices are Presented

	Subcutaneous Epicardial Cardiac Devices	Transvenous Endocardial Cardiac Devices
Central venous stenosis	Not observed	Common
Infection	Uncommon	Not uncommon
Preservation of central venous real estate	Available	Compromised
Tricuspid valve problems	Not observed	Observed

to protect the patient's potential for an optimum vascular access. The following seem appropriate:

- The indications for use of CRDs are well defined in the practice guidelines published by cardiology professional societies. In patients with CKD, these guidelines should be interpreted very conservatively.

- Wherever possible, epicardial leads should be used in CKD patients who need a CRD.

- Wherever possible, epicardial CRD leads should be considered in patients receiving hemodialysis therapy with an arteriovenous access or tunneled dialysis catheter.

- CKD patients with existing CRDs with transvenous leads who are in need for an arteriovenous access should undergo detailed vessel mapping. Specifically, the superior vena cava (SVC) should be imaged to evaluate the presence or absence of stenosis. If SVC stenosis is absent, an arteriovenous access might be created contralateral to the CRD. This approach would effectively avoid the subclavian vein (the most common site of stenosis) that harbors the leads. However, if SVC stenosis is present, lead removal, treatment of stenosis, and insertion of an epicardial system should be considered before access placement.

- CKD/ESRD patients with an existing transvenous CRD who meet requirements for lead removal should be considered for subsequent epicardial lead placement if continued CRD use is required.

REFERENCES

1. *US Renal Data System, USRDS 2006 Annual Data Report.* National Institutes of Health, National Institute of Diabetes and Digestive and Kidney Diseases, Bethesda, MD, 2006.
2. Herzog CA, Mangrum JM, Passman, R. Sudden cardiac death and dialysis patients. *Semin Dial.* 2008;21:300.
3. Korzets A, Chagnac A, Ori Y, et al. Subclavian vein stenosis, permanent cardiac pacemakers and the haemodialysed patient. *Nephron.* 1991;58:103.
4. Teruya TH, Abou-Zamzam AM, Jr., Limm W, Wong L. Symptomatic subclavian vein stenosis and occlusion in hemodialysis patients with transvenous pacemakers. *Ann Vasc Surg.* 2003;17:526.
5. Asif A, Salman L, Carrillo RG, et al. Patency rates for angioplasty in the treatment of pacemaker-induced central venous stenosis in hemodialysis patients: results of a multi-center study. *Semin Dial.* 2009;22:671.
6. Sticherling C, Chough SP, Baker RL, et al. Prevalence of central venous occlusion in patients with chronic defibrillator leads. *Am Heart J.* 2001;141:813.
7. Tourret J, Cluzel P, Tostivint I, et al. Central venous stenosis as a complication of ipsilateral haemodialysis fistula and pacemaker. *Nephrol Dial Transplant.* 2005; 20:997.
8. Paniagua D, Aldrich HR, Lieberman EH, et al. Increased prevalence of significant tricuspid regurgitation in patients with transvenous pacemakers leads. *Am J Cardiol.* 1998; 82:1130.
9. Lin G, Nishimura RA, Connolly HM, et al. Severe symptomatic tricuspid valve regurgitation due to permanent pacemaker or implantable cardioverter-defibrillator leads. *J Am Coll Cardiol.* 2005;45:1672.
10. Iskandar SB, Ann Jackson S, Fahrig S, et al. Tricuspid valve malfunction and ventricular pacemaker lead: case report and review of the literature. *Echocardiography.* 2006; 23:692.
11. Carrillo RG, Garisto JD, Salman L, Asif A. Arteriovenous dialysis access-associated transvenous pacemaker infection. *Clin Nephrol.* 2011;75:174.
12. Carrillo RG, Garisto JD, Salman L, et al. Contamination of transvenous pacemaker leads due to tunneled hemodialysis catheter infection: a report of 2 cases. *Am J Kidney Dis.* 2010;55:1097.
13. Ailawadi G, Lapar DJ, Swenson BR, et al. Surgically placed left ventricular leads provide similar outcomes to percutaneous leads in patients with failed coronary sinus lead placement. *Heart Rhythm.* 2010;7:619.
14. Bauersfeld U, Nowak B, Molinari L, et al. Low-energy epicardial pacing in children: the benefit of autocapture. *Ann Thorac Surg.* 1999;68:1380.
15. Walker F, Siu SC, Woods S, et al. Long-term outcomes of cardiac pacing in adults with congenital heart disease. *J Am Coll Cardiol.* 2004;43:1894.
16. Cecchin F, Frangini PA, Brown DW, et al. Cardiac resynchronization therapy (and multisite pacing) in pediatrics and congenital heart disease: five years experience in a single institution. *J Cardiovasc Electrophysiol.* 2009;20:58.
17. Odim J, Suckow B, Saedi B, et al. Equivalent performance of epicardial versus endocardial permanent pacing in children: a single institution and manufacturer experience. *Ann Thorac Surg.* 2008; 85:1412.
18. Dodge-Khatami A, Johnsrude CL, Backer CL, et al. A comparison of steroid-eluting epicardial versus transvenous pacing leads in children. *J Card Surg.* 2000;15:323.
19. Cohen MI, Bush DM, Vetter VL, et al. Permanent epicardial pacing in pediatric patients: seventeen years of experience and 1200 outpatient visits. *Circulation.* 2001; 103:2585.
20. Beaufort-Krol GC, Mulder H, Nagelkerke D, et al. Comparison of longevity, pacing, and sensing characteristics of steroid-eluting epicardial versus conventional endocardial pacing leads in children. *J Thorac Cardiovasc Surg.* 1999;117:523.
21. Da Costa SS, Scalabrini Neto A, Costa R, et al. Incidence and risk factors of upper extremity deep vein lesions after permanent transvenous pacemaker implant: a 6-month follow-up prospective study. *Pacing Clin Electrophysiol.* 2002;25:1301.
22. Riezebos RK, Schroeder-Tanka J, de Voogt WG. Occlusion of the proximal subclavian vein complicating pacemaker lead implantation. *Europace.* 2006;8:42.
23. Asif A, Carrillo R, Garisto JD, Lopera G, Ladino M, Barakat U, Eid E, Salman L. Epicardial cardiac rhythm devices for dialysis patients: minimizing the risk of infection and preserving central veins. *Semin Dial.* 2012; 25:88–94.
24. Lagergren H, Dahlgren S, Nordenstam H. Cardiovascular tissue response to intracardiac pacemaking. *Acta Chir Scand.* 1966;132:696.

25. Friedberg HD, D'Cunha GF. Adhesions of pacing catheter to tricuspid valve: adhesive endocarditis. *Thorax.* 1969;24:498.

26. Becker AE, Becker MJ, Claudon DG, Edwards JE. Surface thrombosis and fibrous encapsulation of intravenous pacemaker catheter electrode. *Circulation.* 1972;46:409.

27. Pipili C, Cholongitas E, Tzanatos H. Two cases of silent superior vena cava syndrome associated with vascular access and end-stage renal disease. *Int J Artif Organs.* 2009; 32:883.

28. Lenard L, Szabados S, Imre J, et al. Vena cava superior syndrome: surgical treatment of the thrombosis of the superior vena cava after implantation of a hemodialysis catheter—a case report and review of the literature. *Orv Hetil.* 2008;149:29.

29. Madan AK, Allmon JC, Harding M, et al. Dialysis access-induced superior vena cava syndrome. *Am Surg.* 2002;68:904.

30. Stockx L, Raat H, Donck J, et al. Repositioning and leaving in situ the central venous catheter during percutaneous treatment of associated superior vena cava syndrome: a report of eight cases. *Cardiovasc Intervent Radiol.* 1999;22:224.

31. Saval N, Pou M, Lopez Pedret J, et al. Superior vena cava thrombosis in a patient on hemodialysis. *Nefrologia.* 2004;24(suppl 3):35.

32. Beathard GA. Percutaneous transvenous angioplasty in the treatment of vascular access stenosis. *Kidney Int.* 1992;42:1390.

33. Beathard GA. Angioplasty for arteriovenous grafts and fistulae. *Semin Nephrol.* 2002;22:202.

34. Glanz S, Gordon DH, Butt KM, et al. The role of percutaneous angioplasty in the management of chronic hemodialysis fistulas. *Ann Surg.* 1987;206:777.

35. Hunter DW, So SK. Dialysis access: radiographic evaluation and management. *Radiol Clin North Am.* 1987;25:249.

36. Kanterman RY, Vesely TM, Pilgram TK, et al. Dialysis access grafts: anatomic location of venous stenosis and results of angioplasty. *Radiology.* 1995;195:135.

37. Turmel-Rodrigues L, Pengloan J, Baudin S, et al. Treatment of stenosis and thrombosis in haemodialysis fistulas and grafts by interventional radiology. *Nephrol Dial Transplant.* 2000;15:2029.

38. Lilly RZ, Carlton D, Barker J, et al. Predictors of arteriovenous graft patency after radiologic intervention in hemodialysis patients. *Am J Kidney Dis.* 2001;37:945.

39. Beathard G. Percutaneous angioplasty for the treatment of venous stenosis: a nephrologist's view. *Semin Dial.* 1995; 8:166.

40. Katz SG, Kohl RD. The percutaneous treatment of angioaccess graft complications. *Am J Surg.* 1995; 170:238.

41. Yevzlin A, Asif A. Stent placement in hemodialysis access: historical lessons, the state of the art and future directions. *Clin J Am Soc Nephrol.* 2009;4:996.

42. Saad TF, Myers GR, Cicone J. Central vein stenosis or occlusion associated with cardiac rhythm management device leads in hemodialysis patients with ipsilateral arteriovenous access: a retrospective study of treatment using stents or stent-grafts. *J Vasc Access.* 2010;11:293.

43. Slonim SM, Semba CP, Sze DY, Dake MD. Placement of SVC stents over pacemaker wires for the treatment of SVC syndrome. *J Vasc Interv Radiol.* 2000;11:215.

44. Bolad I, Karanam S, Mathew D, et al. Percutaneous treatment of superior vena cava obstruction following transvenous device implantation. *Catheter Cardiovasc Interv.* 2005;65:54.

45. Baddour LM, Epstein AE, Erickson CC, et al. Update on cardiovascular implantable electronic device infections and their management: a scientific statement from the American Heart Association. *Circulation.* 2010;121:458.

46. Wilkoff BL, Love CJ, Byrd CL, et al. Transvenous lead extraction: Heart Rhythm Society expert consensus on facilities, training, indications, and patient management: this document was endorsed by the American Heart Association (AHA). *Heart Rhythm.* 2009;6:1085.

47. Bloom H, Heeke B, Leon A, et al. Renal insufficiency and the risk of infection from pacemaker or defibrillator surgery. *Pacing Clin Electrophysiol.* 2006;29:142.

48. Lekkerkerker JC, van Nieuwkoop C, Trines SA, et al. Risk factors and time delay associated with cardiac device infections: Leiden device registry. *Heart.* 2009;95:715.

49. Kloos WE, Bannerman TL. Update on clinical significance of coagulase-negative staphylococci. *Clin Microbiol Rev.* 1994;7:117.

50. Chua JD, Wilkoff BL, Lee I, et al. Diagnosis and management of infections involving implantable electrophysiologic cardiac devices. *Ann Intern Med.* 2000;133:604.

51. Sohail MR, Uslan DZ, Khan AH, et al. Management and outcome of permanent pacemaker and implantable cardioverter-defibrillator infections. *J Am Coll Cardiol.* 2007;49:1851.

52. Chacko ST, Chandy ST, Abraham OC, et al. Pacemaker endocarditis caused by *Pseudomonas aeruginosa* treated successfully. *J Assoc Physicians India.* 2003;51:1021.

53. Butterly DW. A quality improvement program for hemodialysis vascular access. *Adv Ren Replace Ther.* 1994; 1:163.

54. Sarnak MJ, Jaber BL. Mortality caused by sepsis in patients with end-stage renal disease compared with the general population. *Kidney Int.* 2000;58:1758.

55. Butterly DW, Schwab SJ. Dialysis access infections. *Curr Opin Nephrol Hypertens.* 2000;9:631.

56. Lafrance JP, Rahme E, Lelorier J, Iqbal S. Vascular access-related infections: definitions, incidence rates, and risk factors. *Am J Kidney Dis.* 2008;52:982.

57. Sexton DJ. Vascular access infections in patients undergoing dialysis with special emphasis on the role and treatment of *Staphylococcus aureus. Infect Dis Clin North Am.* 2001;15:731.

58. Kaplowitz LG, Comstock JA, Landwehr DM, et al. A prospective study of infections in hemodialysis patients: patient hygiene and other risk factors for infection. *Infect Control Hosp Epidemiol.* 1988;9:534.

59. Taylor G, Gravel D, Johnston L, et al. Prospective surveillance for primary bloodstream infections occurring in Canadian hemodialysis units. *Infect Control Hosp Epidemiol.* 2002;23:716.

60. Vaudaux PE, Francois P, Proctor RA, et al. Use of adhesion-defective mutants of *Staphylococcus aureus* to define the role of specific plasma proteins in promoting bacterial adhesion to canine arteriovenous shunts. *Infect Immun.* 1995;63:585.

61. Francois P, Vaudaux P, Lew PD. Role of plasma and extracellular matrix proteins in the physiopathology of foreign body infections. *Ann Vasc Surg.* 1998;12:34.

62. Heilmann C, Schweitzer O, Gerke, C, et al. Molecular basis of intercellular adhesion in the biofilm-forming Staphylococcus epidermidis. *Mol Microbiol.* 1996;20:1083.

63. Bayston R, Penny SR. Excessive production of mucoid substance in staphylococcus SIIA: a possible factor in colonisation of Holter shunts. *Dev Med Child Neurol Suppl.* 1972;27:25.

64. Vuong C, Otto M. Staphylococcus epidermidis infections. *Microb Infect.* 2002;4:481.

65. Mah TF, Pitts B, Pellock B, et al. A genetic basis for *Pseudomonas aeruginosa* biofilm antibiotic resistance. *Nature.* 2003;426:306.

66. Gilbert P, Maira-Litran T, McBain AJ, et al. The physiology and collective recalcitrance of microbial biofilm communities. *Adv Microb Physiol.* 2002;46:202.

67. Karchmer A. Infection of cardiac pacemaker and implantable cardioverter defibrillator. UpToDate 2009.

68. Uslan D. Infections of electrophysiologic cardiac devices. *Exp Rev Med Devices.* 2008;5:183.

69. Greenspon AJ, Rhim ES, Mark G, et al. Lead-associated endocarditis: the important role of methicillin-resistant *Staphylococcus aureus.* *Pacing Clin Electrophysiol.* 2008; 31:548.

70. Anselmino M, Vinci M, Comoglio C, et al. Bacteriology of infected extracted pacemaker and ICD leads. *J Cardiovasc Med (Hagerstown).* 2009;10:693.

71. Chamis AL, Peterson GE, Cabell CH, et al. *Staphylococcus aureus* bacteremia in patients with permanent pacemakers or implantable cardioverter-defibrillators. *Circulation.* 2001;104:1029.

72. Durack DT, Lukes AS, Bright DK. New criteria for diagnosis of infective endocarditis: utilization of specific echocardiographic findings. Duke Endocarditis Service. *Am J Med.* 1994;96:200.

73. Fowler VG, Jr., Li J, Corey GR, et al. Role of echocardiography in evaluation of patients with *Staphylococcus aureus* bacteremia: experience in 103 patients. *J Am Coll Cardiol.* 1997;30:1072.

74. Otto C. Pathophysiology, clinical features and management of tricuspid regurgitation. UpToDate 2010.

75. Nath J, Foster E, Heidenreich PA. Impact of tricuspid regurgitation on long-term survival. *J Am Coll Cardiol.* 2004;43:405.

76. Koelling TM, Aaronson KD, Cody RJ, et al. Prognostic significance of mitral regurgitation and tricuspid regurgitation in patients with left ventricular systolic dysfunction. *Am Heart J.* 2002;144:524.

77. Fishenfeld J, Lamy Y. Laceration of the tricuspid valve by a pacemaker wire. *Chest.* 1972;61:697.

78. Petterson SR, Singh JB, Reeves G, Kocot SL. Tricuspid valve perforation by endocardial pacing electrode. *Chest.* 1973;63:125.

79. Gould L, Reddy CV, Yacob U, et al. Perforation of the tricuspid valve by a transvenous pacemaker. *J Am Med Assoc.* 1974;230:86.

80. Vecht RJ, Fontaine CJ, Bradfield JW. Fatal outcome arising from use of a sutureless "corkscrew" epicardial pacing electrode inserted into apex of left ventricle. *Br Heart J.* 1976;38:1359.

81. Christie JL, Keelan MH, Jr. Tricuspid valve perforation by a permanent pacing lead in a patient with cardiac amyloidosis: case report and brief literature review. *Pacing Clin Electrophysiol.* 1986;9:124.

82. Rubio PA, al-Bassam MS. Pacemaker-lead puncture of the tricuspid valve. Successful diagnosis and treatment. *Chest.* 1991;99:1519.

83. Postaci N, Eksi K, Bayata S, Yesil M. Effect of the number of ventricular leads on right ventricular hemodynamics in patients with permanent pacemaker. *Angiology.* 1995;46:421.

84. Champagne J, Poirier P, Dumesnil JG, et al. Permanent pacemaker lead entrapment: role of the transesophageal echocardiography. *Pacing Clin Electrophysiol.* 2002;25:1131.

85. Lagergren H, Dahlgren S, Nordenstam H. Cardiovascular tissue response to intracardiac pacemaking. *Acta Chir Scand.* 1966;132:696.

86. Robboy SJ, Harthorne JW, Leinbach RC, et al. Autopsy findings with permanent pervenous pacemakers. *Circulation.* 1969;39:495.

87. Figa FH, McCrindle BW, Bigras JL, et al. Risk factors for venous obstruction in children with transvenous pacing leads. *Pacing Clin Electrophysiol.* 1997;20:1902.

88. Angeli SJ. Superior vena cava syndrome following pacemaker insertion post atrial septal defect repair. *Am Heart J.* 1990;120:433.

89. Old WD, Paulsen W, Lewis SA, Nixon JV. Pacemaker lead-induced tricuspid stenosis: diagnosis by Doppler echocardiography. *Am Heart J.* 1989;117:1165.

90. Kerstjens-Frederikse MW, Bink-Boelkens MT, de Jongste MJ, Homan van der Heide JN. Permanent cardiac pacing in children: morbidity and efficacy of follow-up. *Int J Cardiol.* 1991;33:207.

91. Johns JA, Fish FA, Burger JD, Hammon JW, Jr. Steroid-eluting epicardial pacing leads in pediatric patients: encouraging early results. *J Am Coll Cardiol.* 1992;20:395.

92. Ramesh V, Gaynor JW, Shah MJ, et al. Comparison of left and right atrial epicardial pacing in patients with congenital heart disease. *Ann Thorac Surg.* 1999;68:2314.

93. Schmid FX, Nowak B, Kampmann C, et al. Cardiac pacing in premature infants and neonates: steroid eluting leads and automatic output adaptation. *Ann Thorac Surg.* 1999;67:1400.

94. Stevenson WG, Stevenson LW, Middlekauff HR, et al. Improving survival for patients with advanced heart failure: a study of 737 consecutive patients. *J Am Coll Cardiol.* 1995;26:1417.

95. Blanc JJ, Etienne Y, Gilard M, et al. Evaluation of different ventricular pacing sites in patients with severe heart failure: results of an acute hemodynamic study. *Circulation.* 1997;96:3273.

96. Yu CM, Lin H, Fung WH, et al. Comparison of acute changes in left ventricular volume, systolic and diastolic functions, and intraventricular synchronicity after biventricular and right ventricular pacing for heart failure. *Am Heart J.* 2003;145:E18.

97. Young JB, Abraham WT, Smith AL, et al. Combined cardiac resynchronization and implantable cardioversion defibrillation in advanced chronic heart failure: the MIRACLE ICD Trial. *J Am Med Assoc.* 2003;289:2685.

98. Auricchio A, Stellbrink C, Sack S, et al. Long-term clinical effect of hemodynamically optimized cardiac resynchronization therapy in patients with heart failure and ventricular conduction delay. *J Am Coll Cardiol.* 2002;39:2026.

99. Linde C, Braunschweig F, Gadler F, et al. Long-term improvements in quality of life by biventricular pacing

in patients with chronic heart failure: results from the Multisite Stimulation in Cardiomyopathy study (MUSTIC). *Am J Cardiol.* 2003;91:1090.

100. Abraham WT. Rationale and design of a randomized clinical trial to assess the safety and efficacy of cardiac resynchronization therapy in patients with advanced heart failure: the Multicenter InSync Randomized Clinical Evaluation (MIRACLE). *J Card Fail.* 2000; 6:369.

101. Bristow MR, Saxon LA, Boehmer J, et al. Cardiac-resynchronization therapy with or without an implantable defibrillator in advanced chronic heart failure. *N Engl J Med.* 2004;350:2140.

102. Bradley DJ, Bradley EA, Baughman KL, et al. Cardiac resynchronization and death from progressive heart failure: a meta-analysis of randomized controlled trials. *J Am Med Assoc.* 2003;289:730.

103. Daubert JC, Ritter P, Le Breton H, et al. Permanent left ventricular pacing with transvenous leads inserted into the coronary veins. *Pacing Clin Electrophysiol.* 1998;21:239.

104. Alonso C, Leclercq C, d'Allonnes FR, et al. Six year experience of transvenous left ventricular lead implantation for permanent biventricular pacing in patients with advanced heart failure: technical aspects. *Heart.* 2001;86:405.

105. Philippon F. Cardiac resynchronization therapy: device-based medicine for heart failure. *J Card Surg.* 2004;19:270.

106. DeRose JJ, Ashton RC, Belsley S, et al. Robotically assisted left ventricular epicardial lead implantation for biventricular pacing. *J Am Coll Cardiol.* 2003; 41:1414.

107. Navia JL, Atik FA. Minimally invasive surgical alternatives for left ventricle epicardial lead implantation in heart failure patients. *Ann Thorac Surg.* 2005;80:751.

108. Navia JL, Atik FA, Grimm RA, et al. Minimally invasive left ventricular epicardial lead placement: surgical techniques for heart failure resynchronization therapy. *Ann Thorac Surg.* 2005;79:1536.

109. Mair H, Jansens JL, Lattouf OM, et al. Epicardial lead implantation techniques for biventricular pacing via left lateral mini-thoracotomy, video-assisted thoracoscopy, and robotic approach. *Heart Surg Forum.* 2003;6:412.

110. Maessen JG, Phelps B, Dekker AL, Dijkman B. Minimal invasive epicardial lead implantation: optimizing cardiac resynchronization with a new mapping device for epicardial lead placement. *Eur J Cardiothorac Surg.* 2004;25:894.

111. Doll N, Piorkowski C, Czesla M, et al. Epicardial versus transvenous left ventricular lead placement in patients receiving cardiac resynchronization therapy: results from a randomized prospective study. *Thorac Cardiovasc Surg.* 2008;56:256.

112. Jacob S, Lieberman RA. Percutaneous epicardial defibrillation coil implantation: a viable technique to manage refractory defibrillation threshold. *Circ Arrhythm Electrophysiol.* 2010;3:214.

113. Bove T, Francois K, De Caluwe W, et al. Effective cardioverter defibrillator implantation in children without thoracotomy: a valid alternative. *Ann Thorac Surg.* 2010; 89:1307.

114. Bardy GH, Smith WM, Hood MA, et al. An entirely subcutaneous implantable cardioverter-defibrillator. *N Engl J Med.* 2010;363:36.

115. Lobodzinski, SS. Subcutaneous implantable cardioverter-defibrillator (S-ICD). *Cardiol J.* 2011;18:326.

32

CENTRAL VEIN STENOSIS

ANIL K. AGARWAL

1. Describe epidemiology of central vein stenosis.
2. Consider etiopathology and pathogenesis of central vein stenosis.
3. Describe clinical features and diagnosis of central vein stenosis.
4. Discuss current methods of management of central vein stenosis.
5. Consider possible future directions in management of central vein stenosis.

INTRODUCTION

Hemodialysis (HD) vascular access circuit originates with cardiac output from the left side of heart, requires patent arterial tree to provide adequate inflow to the arteriovenous (AV) anastomosis, continues as outflow via patent venous drainage, and eventually returns venous blood into the right side of heart. An optimally functioning vascular access (arteriovenous fistula—AVF or arteriovenous graft—AVG) mandates patent inflow and outflow to allow adequate dialysis without complications or discomfort. Outflow of the access is often the most crucial component due to its vulnerability to the fallacies of the physiologic processes that mature it to be able to sustain adequate outflow. Anatomic demands of a mature AVF to remain easily accessible for cannulation on a frequent basis over long periods of time are yet another challenge affecting the fistula outflow.

The venous outflow of an AV access can further be subdivided into peripheral veins and central veins. The "peripheral" venous outflow starts at the arterial anastomosis and ends at its confluence into the intracavitary veins, that is, subclavian vein in upper extremity and iliac veins in lower extremity, the anatomical site that also marks the beginning of "central" veins. Thus, the major intrathoracic veins including subclavian vein, innominate vein, and superior vena cava are considered the central veins in the upper extremity, whereas the iliac veins and inferior vena cava are the central veins draining the lower extremity (Figure 32-1). These central veins have characteristics distinct from the peripheral veins being significantly larger and thicker, having higher blood flow and being more elastic than the peripheral veins. Central veins are also less accessible to surgical intervention due to the overlying bony cage. Presence of central vein stenosis (CVS) or occlusion jeopardizes the venous outflow from the whole extremity and can result in symptoms and signs related to venous pooling and hypertension. Severe CVS or occlusion often precludes successful use of vascular access (Figure 32-2 to 32-4). Moreover, the presence of CVS has other clinical consequences associated with increased morbidity, hospitalization, and mortality.

Although CVS can occur in conditions unrelated to dialysis therapy, it is far more commonly encountered in patients on dialysis (Table 32-1). This occurs primarily due to previous or concomitant use of central venous devices including central venous catheters (CVC) and cardiac rhythm devices (CRD). The diagnosis and treatment of CVS are essential for continuation of adequate dialysis. Due to lack of a definitive treatment of CVS, it is even more important to implement effective strategies to prevent its development. This chapter will focus on CVS in primary context of vascular access and intravascular device use in patients on hemodialysis.

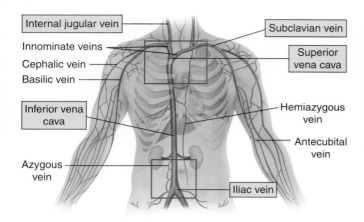

Figure 32-1. Anatomy of venous system showing central veins in upper and lower extremities.

PREVALENCE AND INCIDENCE

The clinical syndrome of CVS has been well recognized and acknowledged for over a century. In patients with end-stage renal disease (ESRD), it is not uncommon to encounter clinical symptoms and signs of CVS only after AVF or AVG has been placed. Because the occurrence of CVS has not been studied systematically in asymptomatic patients, it is not possible to accurately determine the true incidence or prevalence of CVS in ESRD. Such estimation becomes even more difficult due to the frequent absence of clinical findings suggestive of CVS in many patients with CVS.[1] Nevertheless, the awareness of CVS has increased with growing interest in interventional nephrology procedures

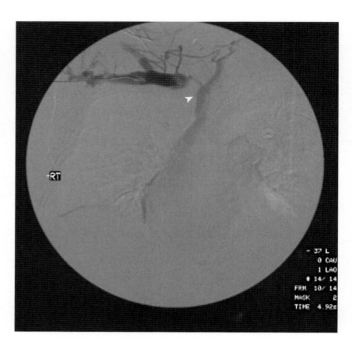

Figure 32-3. Near occlusion of right subclavian vein with collateralization in neck.

during the last decade and more frequent diagnosis and reporting of CVS. It is also important to note that recent emphasis on increasing placement of AVF has significantly improved prevalent AVF rate, although AVF failure rate has remained high due to frequent utilization of suboptimal veins in a complex population of patients with extensive co-morbidities. AVG utilization has declined and CVC

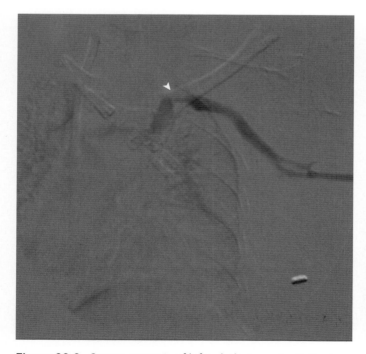

Figure 32-2. Severe stenosis of left subclavian vein. Patient has a left IJ dialysis catheter in place.

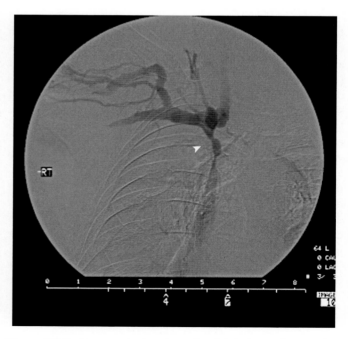

Figure 32-4. Near occlusive stenosis of right innominate vein with retrograde flow to IJ vein and presence of collaterals.

TABLE 32–1

Causes of CVS

Unrelated to intravascular device
  Idiopathic
  Extrinsic compression of vein
  Fibrosing mediastinitis
  Retroperitoneal fibrosis
  Post radiation therapy
Related to intravascular device
  Central vein catheters-
    Tunneled dialysis catheters
    Nontunneled dialysis catheters
    Peripherally inserted central catheters
    Other central venous catheters and ports
  Cardiac rhythm devices
    Pacemakers
    Defibrillators

prevalence has remained static and CVC remains the initial VA in nearly 80% of incident dialysis patients which has the potential to distort venous anatomy and cause CVS.[2] Due to the paucity of data, it is not possible to assess the impact of this recent surge in AVF placement on incidence or prevalence of CVS.

Most reports of CVS come from the studies of symptomatic patients with dysfunctional vascular access. A high prevalence of CVS has been noted in patients with subclavian CVC. Nearly a fourth of all patients having subclavian CVC were found to develop subclavian vein stenosis in an early report of 47 hemodialysis patients.[3] In another study of the symptomatic dialysis patients, half of the patients were found to have subclavian vein stenosis.[4] An angiographic study of CVS in 36 patients referred for evaluation prior to AVF placement and history of subclavian vein catheterization showed 34% prevalence of subclavian vein stenosis while other 4 patients already on hemodialysis but with fistula dysfunction showed stenosis of subclavian vein in 3 and occlusion in 1.[5] Significantly, 30 extremities with no history of subclavian vein cannulation had no stenosis.

Although the internal jugular (IJ) CVC have been felt to be rather innocuous, a retrospective investigation of symptomatic HD patients undergoing angiography found 19% of all patients and 27% of those with previous history of CVC placement to have CVS, similar to the finding of 16% in another duplex and angiographic study.[6,7] Most of these patients had IJ catheters. Another study of 133 hemodialysis patients with vascular access dysfunction and minimal use of subclavian vein catheters found 41% of patients to have CVS.[8] As the long-term femoral vein catheters are being used more frequently for dialysis due to the loss of other suitable veins, it is not uncommon to find iliac vein stenosis but the literature is lacking a systematic description of this complication.

Temporary (nontunneled) dialysis catheters are not immune to CVS development that can occur after only a short dwell (Figure 32-5). A recent study of color Doppler sonography of 100 consecutive patients undergoing temporary double lumen dialysis catheters showed CVS in 18%.[9]

▶ Risk Factors for CVS

CVS can be idiopathic or can occur in association with placement of AV access, CVC for HD, or other intravascular device. Occurrence of CVS in HD patients has been reported on the ipsilateral side of AV access without history of previous CVC placement.[10,11] Preoperative venography of patients prior to right IJ vein tunneled catheter placement also showed presence of CVS or angulation in 30% of patients without previous history of CVC placement.[12] There are many risk factors for occurrence of CVS:

Number and duration of CVC

Higher number and longer duration of CVC placement increase the risk of developing CVS.[4] This risk seems to apply to both subclavian and IJ catheters. The mean number of ipsilateral subclavian catheters was 1.6 and mean duration of line placement was 5.5 weeks in another study of subclavian vein stenosis.[3] One prospective study of 42 consecutive subclavian vein catheterizations showed persistent stenosis at 6 months in those with greater number of inserted catheters (2 vs 1.58), longer dwell time (49 vs 29 days), more dialysis sessions (21 vs 12) and more catheter-related infections (66.6% vs 33.3%) than in those recanalizing spontaneously.[13] Similar results were found with IJ vein catheters in another study.[14]

Location of CVC

Subclavian location of CVC is particularly prone to lead to development of CVS. One study showed a significantly higher prevalence of CVS with subclavian dialysis catheters as compared to IJ dialysis catheters (42% vs 10%).[15] The subclavian group had placement on the right side in 58% of patients, as compared to 78% in IJ group. Similarly, a higher incidence of CVS was noted in a study of short-term temporary dialysis catheters in 32 subclavian and 20 IJ placements, with 50% incidence of CVS in subclavian group and none in IJ group.[16] Another study of temporary hemodialysis catheters in 57 HD patients found thrombus formation in 28%, subclavian stenosis in 14% and SVC stenosis in 2%, with no difference between subclavian and IJ catheterization.[17] The lack of difference in the incidence of CVS may have been due to a small number of subclavian catheters in these studies.

IJ CVC were initially considered much less risky for development of CVS, but recent research has found that even this location is prone to venous thrombosis and CVS in much higher proportion of patients than recognized earlier.[18-20] It is possible that such an increase is related to more frequent use of IJ catheters and longer duration of use. An ultrasonographic evaluation of 143 patients with right IJ dialysis catheter placement showed 25.9% of patients to have thrombosis; 62% of these patients had venous occlusion.[21] A study of 133 patients utilizing

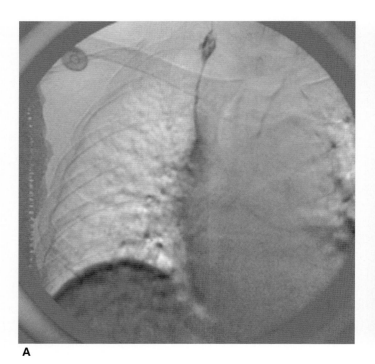

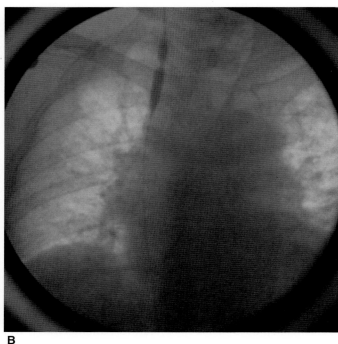

A

B

Figure 32-5. (**A**) Right IJ vein stenosis occurring only 1 week after placement of temporary hemodialysis catheter. (**B**) During balloon angioplasty, the waist on the balloon defines severe stenosis of the vein. (Picture courtesy Tony Samaha MD.)

venograms to diagnose CVS found CVS in 41% of patients, with only 18 patients with history of subclavian vein catheterization.[8] Routine venography of 69 patients undergoing placement of tunneled right IJ catheters showed CVS or angulation of central veins in 42%, with 65% of those with previous IJ catheters and in 30% of those without such history.[12] Thus, it seems that the frequency and duration of CVC placement are more important determinant of CVS than simply the location of CVC, although there may be a lower incidence of CVS with IJ CVC as compared to subclavian CVC.

As noted above, CVCs on the left side are significantly more likely to be associated with CVS than the ones on the right. An analysis of 403 right IJ CVC and 77 left IJ CVC in 294 HD patients revealed a higher number of complications related to infections in left IJ group.[22] There were four patients with central venous occlusion in the left IJ group as compared to none in the right IJ group. Another retrospective study of 127 patients with IJ CVC showed that 50% (7/14) of the patients with left IJ CVC developed CVS compared with 0.9% (1/117) with right IJ CVC ($p < 0.05$). Seven of 13 patients with left CVC and left AVF developed signs and symptoms of CVS in comparison to 1 of 24 patients with right CVC and right AVF.[14]

Higher propensity to the development of CVS on the left side may be related to multiple peculiar anatomic features on the left as compared to on the right side. There are at least three sites of sharp angle in the course of an IJ catheter placed on the left side—between left IJ vein and left innominate vein, mid innominate vein as it drapes around mediastinal vessels, and between innominate vein and superior

vena cava (Figure 32-6).[23] The extended length of vein traversed from the left side necessitates increased contact of catheter with the vein wall and increased pressure at points of angulation with movements during respiration, cardiac cycle, and with external movements, which may contribute to increased endothelial trauma and fibrotic response.

There is a significant difference in the size of right and left IJ veins. An ultrasound study showed a significantly smaller cross-sectional area of left internal jugular vein than the right IJ in a majority of healthy adults.[24] Additionally, the left innominate vein may be compressed by external mediastinal structures (Figure 32-7).[25]

CVS has been reported in association with femoral catheters and the incidence might increase as the utilization of this access site increases.[26]

PICC lines

Although the size (diameter) of the CVC is thought to impact the occurrence of CVS and venous thrombosis, CVC with smaller caliber (such as PICC lines and triple lumen CVC) can also be associated with thrombus formation and CVS over a short term.[27-30] A 7% incidence of CVS or occlusion was found in 150 patients undergoing PICC line placement during the course of venography before and after insertion, especially in those with longer catheter dwell time.[31] The true clinical incidence and prevalence of CVS is uncertain in patients with PICC lines as not all patients with history of PICC lines are studied with angiography or challenged by high blood flow from an AV access. Increasing use of PICC lines in patients with

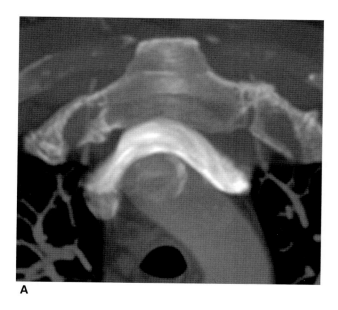

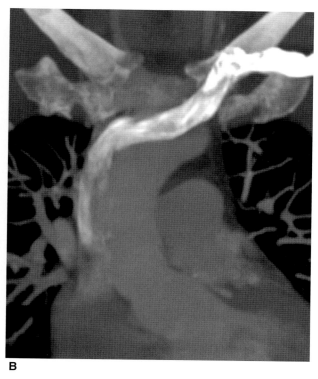

Figure 32-6. (**A**) Thick slab MIP image demonstrating a sharp angulation of the brachiocephalic vein as it crosses the aorta and great vessels. (**B**) Coronal MIP image in the same patient. The angulation of the brachiocephalic vein cannot be appreciated in this projection.[23]

or at risk of chronic kidney disease (CKD) is concerning, as CVS can endanger future hemodialysis vascular access. Preferential use of single lumen central infusion catheters can preserve arm veins for future AVF placement but it is unknown if this would also reduce occurrence of CVS.

▶ Cardiac Rhythm Device Associated CVS

Cardiovascular disease and CKD co-exist frequently and intravascular devices such as pacemakers or defibrillators are commonly placed in these patients.[32,33] Left upper extremity is commonly preferred for vascular access placement and cardiac rhythm devices are preferentially placed on the left side as well. Pacemaker leads can cause persistent friction and inflammation of the vein over long period of dwell (Figure 32-8). In a venography study of 30 patients with chronic transvenous defibrillators in place for 45 ± 21 months, 50% had subclavian vein stenosis.[34] A shorter duration of placement of these devices is also not necessarily harmless. Abnormality of central veins was found in 64% of patients on routine angiography after 6 months in a study.[35] Other studies of such devices have

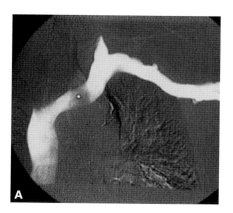

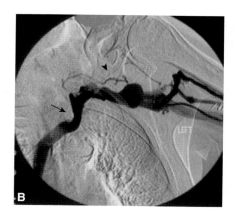

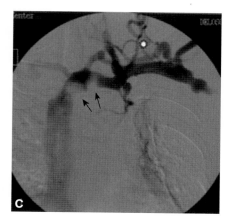

Figure 32-7. Left upper extremity fistulography demonstrates different degrees of LIV compression. (**A**) Splaying of the LIV (star) of a patient with mild (grade 1) compression. (**B**) Indentation of the LIV (arrow) and collaterals (arrowhead) in a patient with moderate (grade 2) compression. (**C**) Marked indentation of the LIV (arrows) and prominent collaterals (star) in a patient with severe (grade 3) compression by what appear to be the innominate and left common carotid arteries. (From Maxim I Kraus MJ, Trerotola SO. Extrinsic compression of the left innominate vein in hemodialysis patients. *J Vasc Interv Radiol.* 2004;Jan:15(1 Part 1):51–56.)

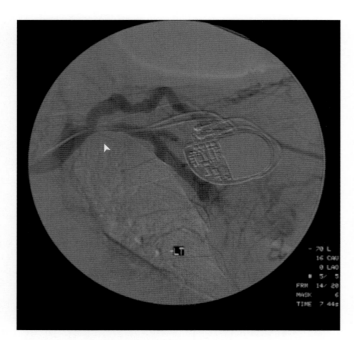

Figure 32-8. Stenosis of left subclavian vein due to the presence of pacemaker wires. Note the presence of collateralization in upper arm and retrograde filling of cephalic vein.

also shown high prevalence of central vein abnormality.[36–38] While many such stenoses remain asymptomatic, it is not uncommon for CVS to become clinically manifest when challenged by increased blood flow after creation of a dialysis access.[32,39,40] Appearance of clinical manifestations after placement of ipsilateral access for hemodialysis leads to detection of CVS in patients on HD with ultimate loss of vascular access.

In the presence of cardiac rhythm devices, CVS should be seriously considered and investigated prior to the placement of AV access on ipsilateral side. If it is necessary to place ipsilateral AV access, it may be important to preemptively treat if stenosis seems to be significant. Similarly, if a device is to be placed in a dialysis patient, it should not be placed on the side of the AV access if possible. While it is technically feasible to do angioplasty and stenting of the CVS associated with device wires, this should be avoided due to the risk of lead erosion over months to years. Stent placement over the leads makes it difficult to extract the wires trapped between the stent and the vein wall in the event of an infection.

PATHOGENESIS

The pathogenesis of CVS due to CVC is not well defined, although there is evidence of inflammation with activation of leukocytes, release of myeloperoxidase, and activation of coagulation cascade after CVC placement.[41] The inflammatory response of the endothelium may result from a number of factors, individually or in combination. These include initial trauma of CVC cannulation, persistently indwelling foreign body with variable degree of bio-incompatibility, movement of catheter with respiration, movements of head and changes in posture, and increased flow and turbulence from AV access. Turbulence can also cause platelet deposition and venous wall thickening.[42] Trauma to the vessel wall results in thrombin generation, platelet activation, and expression of P-selectin with inflammatory response.[43] Activation of leukocytes results in release of myeloperoxidase and formation of platelet aggregates results in intravascular thrombosis.[44] Venous thrombosis is often found in conjunction with stenosis, which may be causally interrelated.[45] This may also lead to formation of platelet thrombi and thrombus at the tip of the catheter which can cause early catheter dysfunction. Additionally, a fibrin sleeve starts forming on the outer surface of the catheter, as a result of mechanical as well as chemical factors related to inflammation from a constantly mobile and bio-incompatible catheter. This process starts early and has potential to form a full-length sleeve within a week.[46,47] It is unclear if the presence of fibrin sheath is causally related to development of CVS.

There is only minimal direct evidence available for histopathological changes related to CVS in the patients on HD. Experimental models using animal veins show that the structural changes in the vein wall result within 24 hours after endothelial denudation, with the development of platelet microthrombi.[48] Over the next 7 to 8 days, several layers of smooth muscle cells develop in the injured areas. However, such a response is felt to require a "critical area" of injury, without which the proliferative response would not occur. Human evidence comes from subclavian vein specimens from directional atherectomy in patients with symptomatic stenosis or occlusion that show intimal hyperplasia and presence of fibrous tissue.[49] Autopsy finding of adherent clot with intimal injury in patients with <14 days of catheter use and presence of smooth muscle proliferation and thickened venous wall in those with >90 days of catheter use support this hypothesis.[50] These catheters were also found to be focally attached to the vein wall by organizing thrombus, endothelial cells, and collagen. It is plausible that these initial adhesions were the precursor of fibrin sheath or CVS.

Biocompatibility of intravascular device is likely to be an issue in causation of venous injury and inflammation. Catheter material may have varying degrees of biocompatibility resulting in different levels of antigenicity, potential for tissue growth, and fibrogenesis. Silastic IJ catheters were initially felt to produce little thrombosis.[51] Use of silicone catheters in 22 patients with subclavian cannulation showed stenosis in only 2 and thrombosis in only 3 and lower incidence of subclavian vein stenosis than with polytetrafluoroethylene and polyurethane catheters.[52] In a rabbit model, polyethylene and Teflon catheters caused more inflammation than silicone and polyurethane.[53] Both silicone (eg, Tesio® Medcomp, Harleysville, PA and Schon®

Angiodynamics, Queensbury, NY) and polyurethane (eg, Opti-Flow® Bard Access Systems, Salt Lake City, Utah and Ash Split® Medcomp, Harleysville, PA) are commonly used to manufacture long-term dialysis catheters. This issue deserves further study.

As inflammation is considered an important risk factor for the development of CVS, disease states with high degree of inflammation, such as systemic lupus erythematosus (SLE), may also predispose to CVS. In a study of 77 patients with SLE and ESRD, 17 patients (15 females) had documented CVS, leading to 22% prevalence of CVS.[54] However, this was similar to the non-SLE group. Number of CVC, but not the degree of inflammation was found to be associated with CVS in this retrospective cohort study. Lack of a difference in the prevalence could possibly be due to a basal state of high inflammation in patients with ESRD from any cause.

Infections associated with CVC may also predispose to the development of CVS. In one study of 54 chronic HD patients, venograms after 6 months of removal showed 75% prevalence of CVS in those with previous catheter infections as compared to 28% in those with no infection.[55] This study supports the hypothesis that the inflammation plays a role in the causation of CVS. It is also plausible that CVS was the predisposing factor for infection, pointing to a possible vicious cycle.

Anatomical factors may also contribute to the development of CVS. Relatively high incidence of CVS on the left side of neck, as previously mentioned, can be attributed to a closer apposition of catheters and wires to the wall of the vein due to the angulations of the left-sided veins, smaller cross-sectional area of the left IJ vein in a third of the patients and longer and tortuous course traversed by the left-sided catheters.[23–25,56] Three-dimensional model of the left-sided veins suggests an additional angulation of the innominate vein over the brachiocephalic artery and the aortic arch.[23] Continuous movement of the catheter in this tight space may be causally related to occurrence of stenosis. In a swine model, stabilizing the tip of the catheter during the cardiac cycle with a thin wire loop resulted in less injury, thrombosis, and thickening in the vessel wall.[57] This supports the mechanical theory of the development of CVS. Whether gender-specific differences exist in occurrence of CVS is not well substantiated.

In patients without history of intravascular device placement, occurrence of CVS remains unexplained. It is plausible that the changes in blood flow pattern and speed after placement of access alter shear stress, produce oxidative radicals, and lead to venous wall hyperplasia and eventual stenosis.

CLINICAL FEATURES

CVS is often asymptomatic in HD patients and is undetected unless dysfunction of the vascular access develops. In symptomatic patients, the clinical features vary according to the site of obstruction of blood flow that result in

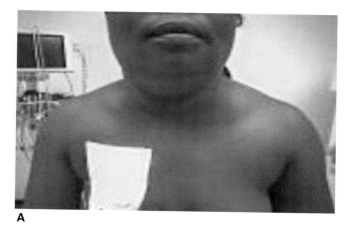

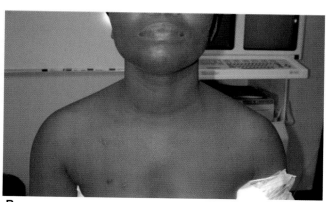

Figure 32-9. (**A**) Severe stenosis of SVC with edema of face, lips and thorax at presentation. A. At presentation. B. After successful angioplasty of SVC stenosis. (**B**) Dramatic resolution of edema after successful angioplasty of SVC stenosis. (Picture courtesy Arif Asif, MD.)

development of venous hypertension and collaterals behind the obstruction.

There are two main varieties of clinical symptoms and signs:

1. *Related to venous hypertension behind the obstruction*: CVS can lead to edema, swelling, pain, tenderness, and erythema of the ipsilateral extremity. Ipsilateral breast swelling is not uncommon. Bilateral stenosis of the innominate veins or the superior vena cava (SVC) can lead to the features of SVC syndrome, which can be relieved by angioplasty (Figure 32-9). Pleural effusion may develop in severe cases. In chronic SVC obstruction, alternative venous drainage into the azygos system can develop (Figure 32-10). Clinical features of CVS are almost invariably present in these cases. CVS is not always obvious or may be minimally apparent if the augmentation in the blood flow by creation of an AV shunt is not sufficient to precipitate the symptoms. In such cases, the presence of CVS is recognized only by venography done for other reasons. Only about half of the patients with subclavian vein obstruction develop edema of the arm.[3]

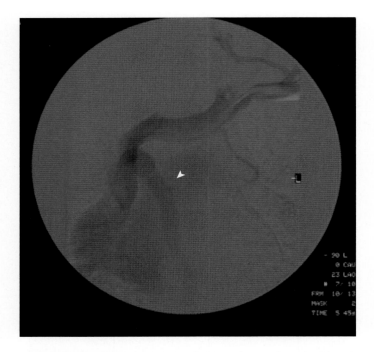

Figure 32-10. Severe stenosis of SVC with significantly dilated azygos vein (arrowhead).

2. *Related to vascular access dysfunction on dialysis*: Poor adequacy of dialysis and its consequences can develop if CVS remains untreated. It is not uncommon to see recurrent hyperkalemia in such patients. Back-pressure due to the stenosis can cause aneurysmal dilatation of veins, development of collaterals, prolonged bleeding after dialysis, or thrombosis of the access.

DIAGNOSIS

Angiography remains the gold standard for diagnosis of CVS. It is superior to duplex ultrasound and is recommended as a screening test prior to the placement of permanent access for those with history of previous CVC placement, especially in subclavian location.[58,59] Duplex ultrasound is useful but limited by bony thorax and in obese. Clues to the presence of CVS by color flow duplex ultrasound include the absence of respiratory variations in vessel diameter, lack of polyphasic atrial waves, and presence of collateral channels.[60] A study comparing Duplex ultrasound and phlebography in symptomatic patients with liver transplant, dialysis, or with tumors showed significant yield with duplex with 90% agreement with phlebography.[61] The study also suggested that the best criterion by duplex ultrasonography to detect a >50% stenosis was a poststenotic to prestenotic peak vein velocity ratio of 2.5.

Magnetic resonance angiography to evaluate central veins has been used previously, but has to be avoided due to the possibility of nephrogenic systemic fibrosis after gadolinium use in patients with advanced kidney dysfunction.[62]

Asymptomatic CVS is incidentally detected by angiography done either in preparation of access placement or after placement of AV access due to its dysfunction. A high index of suspicion, especially in those with a history of multiple CVC placement or longstanding CVC use, can lead to clinical diagnosis of CVS. Particular attention should be paid to the number and duration of previous CVC or intravascular device placement. Careful physical examination reveals limb or breast swelling and development of collaterals, particularly around neck and upper part of chest. Retrograde flow in collateral veins, detected on physical examination, is another clue to the upstream outflow obstruction. Extrinsic causes of CVS should be considered and investigated.

TREATMENT OF CVS

Not all CVS need immediate treatment. Those with chronic obstruction and adequately developed collaterals may be able to maintain AV access function without much compromise in adequacy of dialysis. A heightened state of vigilance and close follow-up is indicated for these accesses. As the performance of dialysis deteriorates (inadequate dialysis) or when symptoms appear, treatment of CVS is indicated.

▶ Conservative Approach

For only mildly symptomatic accesses with CVS, often the first choice is limited conservative treatment. Simple measures such as elevation of the extremity may help. If there is associated thrombus in the vein, anticoagulation is indicated. Occasionally, watchful observation may allow collateralization as symptoms improve. However, there is no evidence-based strategy for mild CVS. These measures may bridge dysfunctional accesses while more definitive therapy is planned.

▶ Endovascular Intervention

Endovascular intervention should be considered with caution keeping in mind that the endovascular approaches to correction of CVS remain suboptimal at this time, and can possibly be even detrimental. More aggressive neointimal hyperplasia and proliferative lesion was found in restenotic area after angioplasty than in the original stenosis, probably in response to the endovascular trauma.[63] Indeed, in one study of >50% CVS in 35 asymptomatic HD patients with 38 AVG, 86 venograms were reviewed.[64] No intervention was done in 28%, and none of these patients progressed to symptoms, stent placement, or additional CVS. In contrast, 72% of the patients who underwent percutaneous angioplasty (PTA) had escalation of CVS after PTA in 8%, which required further interventions. These findings corroborate the theory that endothelial damage from an angioplasty can aggravate the venous response and accelerate the stenotic process. It is also possible that a rather high residual stenosis (40%) in the intervention group was an indication of its already refractory nature and that a more aggressive approach with stent placement might have been beneficial.[65] Thus, endovascular intervention for CVS should be individualized and planned very carefully.

PTA with or without stent placement has been recommended as the preferred approach to CVS, depending upon the rapidity of recurrence (Guideline 20 of K/DOQI).[66] The initial success of angioplasty is good, although poor patency rates after PTA alone were seen in two earlier studies of patients with CVS (28.9% at 180 days, and 25% at 1 year, respectively).[67,68] Intravascular ultrasound study after angioplasty of central veins has shown that central veins are much more likely to recoil than the peripheral veins.[69] However, a more recent study showed better results with PTA alone with primary patency of 60% at 6 months and 30% at 12 months.[70] Better results in this study may suggest either a difference in patient population or advances in the technique. Since high-pressure balloons were used, this study argues for the use of primary PTA alone with high-pressure balloon for the treatment of asymptomatic CVS. Similarly, better results were also noted in another study.[71] Significantly, secondary patency can be achieved with repeated angioplasty without use of stent.

Unimpressive results with PTA have led to the use of stents for CVS. Guidelines recommend placement of stent for elastic recoil of the vein leading to significant residual stenosis after PTA or for lesions recurring within 3 months after angioplasty.[66] Use of Wallstents for elastic lesions has shown better outcomes, as compared to the angioplasty alone. Stent placement in the treatment of CVS typically achieves a high degree of technical success. However, the primary patency and secondary patency of stents is modest at best (Table 32-2).[72] It is difficult to make inter study comparisons because earlier studies used stainless steel stents. In one study of 52 HD patients with 56 lesions, 51 Wallstents were placed.[73] The primary and secondary patency rates were 46% and 76% at 6 months and 20% and 33% at 12 months, respectively. However, another study of 57 Wallstents in 50 patients with CVS showed primary patency rates of 92%, 84%, 56%, and 28% at 3, 6, 12, and 24 months, respectively.[74] The secondary patency was also significantly better—97% after 6 and 12 months, 89% after 24 months, and 81% after 36 and 48 months. Another study of central vein angioplasty ($n = 101$) and stent placement ($n = 46$) showed that while angioplasty alone was superior to stent placement in terms of primary patency, assisted (secondary) patency of both angioplasty and stent placement was similar, pointing to the benefit of stenting in angioplasty resistant group.[75] Similar patency with angioplasty and stent placement was seen in another recent study.[76]

Although the primary patency after stent placement is poor, repeated interventions can maintain patency for a much longer period of time. As these patients are already nearing exhaustion of their accesses, allowing the use of access at the cost of multiple interventions may be appropriate for some patients. In a retrospective study, 23 patients with symptomatic, refractory CVS were treated with various types of stent placement.[77] In this study, the median primary patency was 138 days with 1-year patency of only 19%. Median secondary patency was 1036 days with 64% patency at 1 year. A recent retrospective analysis of the Nitinol shape memory alloy stents in 64 patients (with 15 central and 54 peripheral vein stents) showed primary patency of 14.9 months in central veins and 8.9 months in peripheral veins.[78] Significantly, better results in this study can be attributed to the more advanced nature of the stent material, although the retrospective nature of the study does not allow such a conclusion to be made.

Use of covered stents is also becoming common place and these "stent grafts" have also been found to be effective. One study of PTFE covered stent placement showed 360-day primary patency of 32% and secondary patency of 39%.[79] Results of Dacron-covered stents showed patency rates of 29% and 64% at 1 year in a similar study.[80]

Venous stents may be associated with complications such as migration, fracture, intrastent neointimal hyperplasia, and appearance of unrelated stenoses. Stents placed in the low-pressure venous system are inherently less likely to remain patent than in the high-pressure arterial system. Despite these shortcomings, stent placement offers an immediate, lifesaving intervention for those with difficult access with refractory lesions, who require a bridge to more definitive treatment later.

▶ Special Considerations

A novel approach to CVS has recently become available in the form of hybrid graft- catheter. When CVS is refractory, but placement of a CVC is possible, this approach allows use of an internal arteriovenous access with reduced risk of infection.[81] Long-term results from this device are awaited.

▶ Cardiac Rhythm Device-Related CVS

Management of CRD-related CVS is more complex due to the presence of wires and leads. The management of CVS in these situations may require angioplasty, stent placement or ligation of access.[82] Ligation of access should be the treatment of last resort because angioplasty has been shown to be safe and provides poor primary but acceptable secondary patency rates at 1 year. Placement of stent over the lead wire is generally not recommended, primarily due to a higher risk of infection in dialysis patient.[83] If a stent is placed over the wire, it makes transvenous removal of wire difficult in case of infection. Perhaps, if stenting is needed, the device can first be removed, vein stented, and device replaced through the patent vein to avoid such a dilemma in future.[84] It may be preferable to place epicardial leads to preserve central veins and avoid lead infection.[85]

TABLE 32–2

Noted Studies of Stent Placement in Central Venous Stenosis[74]

Authors	Study Design	Year of Publication	Number of Central Lesions	Primary Patency	Secondary Patency	Notes
Rajan, DK	Observational	2007	6	83.3% (95% CI 0.5–1.2) at 3 months, and 66.7% at 6 and 12 months (0.2–1.1, 0.1–1.2)	Secondary patency was 100% at 12 months with 3 patients censored over that time period	
Rajan, DK	Observational	2007	89	In the fistula group the rates were 88.5 ± 4.8%, 59.4 ± 7.6%, and 46 ± 7.9% at 3, 6, and 9 months, respectively. In the graft group, the rates were 78.1 ± 7.3%, 40.7 ± 9%, and 16 ± 7.3%, respectively	n/a	
Maya, ID	Observational	2007	23	19% at 1 year	64% at 1 year	All stent had restenosis on follow-up venogram
Sprouse, LR	Observational	2004	32	n/a	Symptoms related to central stenosis were controlled for 6.5 months on average	
Aytekin, C	Observational	2004	14	1-, 3-, 6- and 12-month primary stent patency rates were 92.8%, 85.7%, 50%, and 14.3%	3-, 6-, and 12-month, and 2-year secondary patency rates were 100%, 88.8%, 55.5%, and 33.3%	
Chen, CY	Observational	2003	18	3, 6, 12 and 18 months were 100% and 89%, 73% and 68% 49% and 42%, and 16% and 0%, respectively	100% after 3 months, 93% and 100% after 6 months, 85% and 91% after 12 months, and 68% and 72% after 24 months	
Hatzimpaloglou, A	Observational	2002	15	70% at 12 and 24 months	n/a	
Smayra, T	Observational	2001	9	56% at 1 year	75% 1 year	
Haage, P	Observational	1999	50	3-, 6-, 12-, and 24-months were 92%, 84%, 56%, and 28%	97% after 6 and 12 months, 89% after 24 months, and 81% after 36 and 48 months	
Vesely, TM	Observational	1997	20	1 month, 3 months, 6 months, and 1 year: 90%, 67%, 42%, and 25%	at 3 months, 6 months, 1 year, and 2 years: 89%, 64%, 56%, and 22%	
Mickley, V	Observational	1997	15	1year was 100%, 2 year was 85%	1 year was 70%, 2 year was 50%	
Lumsden, AB	Observational	1997	25	84% at 1 month, 42% at 6 months, and 17% at 1 year		
Vesely, TM	Observational	1997	20	1 month, 3 months, 6 months, and 1 year: 90%, 67%, 42%, and 25%	at 3 months, 6 months, 1 year, and 2 years: 89%, 64%, 56%, and 22%	
Mickley, V	Observational	1997	15	100% at 1 year, 85% at 2 years	70% at 1 year, 50% at 2 years	
Gray, RJ	Observational	1995	32	46% at 6 months, 20% at 12 months	76% at 6 months, 33% at 12 months	Peripheral and central outcomes were mixed in the data reporting. Two central stents migrated after catheter placement
Beathard, GA	Observational	1992	24	n/a	70.4% at 1 month, 62.1% at 2 months, 48.6% at 3 months, and 28.9% at 4 months	
Matthews, R	Case report	1992	2	n/a	n/a	

Surgery

Surgery for correction of CVS is invasive and difficult, often requiring claviculectomy. It remains a procedure of last resort and can be used in those situations where choices for percutaneous treatment have been tried and exhausted. Direct repair using saphenous vein grafts or ringed PTFE graft can be done. Jugular vein turndown has been used to bypass a stenosed subclavian vein. Creative surgical techniques have been described to create vein-to-vein or even vein to right atrium anastomosis to bypass the area of stenosis. A common approach is axillary to jugular vein bypass.[86] Bypasses connecting subclavian vein to SVC, cephalic vein to external jugular vein, and axillary vein (or artery) to SVC or auricular appendage have been described. In lower extremity, common femoral vein to iliac vein or IVC and external iliac vein to IVC bypass have also been used. A detailed description of these techniques is beyond the scope of this article but has been discussed elsewhere.[87] Systematic studies of the surgical treatment of CVS are also lacking. When another access site is available, new access should be created and symptomatic CVS can be treated with ligation of access. Preemptive creation of another access may avoid interim use of catheters.

Access occlusion, if all other measures fail, can be achieved by surgical ligation. It is sometimes also possible to occlude the access manually or by inflating a balloon inside the access for prolonged period of time.

Considering Alternative Approaches to the Renal Replacement Therapy in CVS

HD is the most commonly used treatment for ESRD. It is important to consider access for HD in a different location if CVS develops. However, in case of CVS and poor vascular access options, other options must be considered including change of modality to peritoneal dialysis. If possible, expedited renal transplantation should also be considered.

PREVENTION

Over 80% of the patients initiating HD in United States do so with a CVC.[2,88] Ultimately, development of CVS, in most cases, represents insufficient planning for vascular access during late CKD care, either due to late referral of the patient to nephrologist or late referral to access surgeon. As placement of a CVC is the single most important risk factor for later development of CVS, it is highly desirable to avoid CVC placement to preserve central veins. Although the fistula first approach has improved the fistula rate, the new focus on "catheter last" approach is likely to influence the outcomes of the prevalent dialysis access in future. Early referral to the nephrologist and early placement of AVF are likely to be the most effective approaches to achieve low catheter rates at the initiation of HD.

In patients with earlier stages of CKD, it would be important to continue and strengthen current strategies of preserving veins and raising the awareness of the risk of using CVC, including the risks of infusion catheters and PICC lines. PICC lines need special attention due to their prevalent use. In patients with CKD use of alternative intravenous access such as single lumen central venous infusion catheters should be seriously considered to avoid the loss of arm veins for the future creation of AVF. More liberal use of PD as initial modality of renal replacement is also likely to provide ample time to place and mature an AVF when transition to HD is imminent. It is important to note that in more recent times dialysis is being initiated at a higher level of renal function as compared to previous decade, although there is little evidence for benefits of such a practice.[89] This practice can be substituted to utilize the early start time for better CKD care to prepare patients for renal replacement, including placement of AVF prior to initiation of HD.

There are other strategies to avoid catheter use and development of CVS. Effective early salvage of immature AVF and improving use of relatively difficult AVF using special techniques, such as creation of a buttonhole are often critical. Subclavian catheters are recommended only as an access of last resort, only after IJ (and external jugular) approaches have been explored and exhausted.[90] If a future access in the ipsilateral extremity is to be planned in future, it is preferable to place a femoral access rather than using a subclavian catheter.

FUTURE DIRECTIONS IN MANAGEMENT OF CVS

Vascular access management requires a proactive approach and prevention of CVC placement. Despite significant advances in technology, optimal treatment of CVS remains elusive and ill-defined at this time. Benefits and harms of angioplasty and stent placement need to be better defined. A prudent approach would emphasize preventive strategies promoting early referral to surgeon and early placement of AV access.

As CVC are unlikely to completely disappear in foreseeable future, research to investigate catheter-like approaches to vascular access would be necessary. Search should continue for the least antigenic catheter material and for the most hemodynamically advanced design to avoid trauma to the endothelium. Animal and in vitro studies of the newer heparin-coated catheters have shown lower thrombosis and fibrin-sheath formation, although human data is still limited. Impact on development of CVS should become a routine endpoint in such studies. Whether treatment with more effective balloons or better stents will improve treatment of resistant stenoses and cause less intimal hyperplasia also remains to be investigated. Use of drug eluting stents for the venous system has not been attempted at this time. Newer therapies to prevent intimal hyperplasia should also be considered. Brachytherapy of CVS after PTA or stent placement has not shown prolongation of patency of the vein because despite suppression of the original stenosis by irradiation, recurrent stenosis develops in new locations in the peripheral portions of the stent or in the adjacent area even with inclusion in the field of irradiation.[91] Pharmacologic approaches to reduce inflammation, development of fibrotic response and infection should be investigated.

REFERENCES

1. Clark DD, Albina JE, Chazan JA. Subclavian vein stenosis and thrombosis: a potential serious complication in chronic hemodialysis patients. *Am J Kidney Dis.* 1990;15:265–268.
2. *U.S. Renal Data System 2010 Annual Data Report. Atlas of Chronic Kidney Disease and End-Stage Renal Disease in the United States* National Institutes of Health, National Institute of Diabetes and Digestive and Kidney Diseases, Bethesda MD, 2010.
3. Schwab SJ, Quarles LD, Middleton JP, Cohan RH, Saeed M, Dennis VW. Hemodialysis-associated subclavian vein stenosis. *Kidney Int.* 1988;33:1156–1159.
4. Barrett N, Spencer S, McIvor J, Brown EA. Subclavian stenosis: a major complication of subclavian dialysis catheters. *Nephrol Dial Transplant.* 1988;3:423–425.
5. Al-Salman MM, Rabee H, Abu-Aisha H, Trengganu N, Al-Damegh S, Al-Smeyer S, Freigoun T. Central vein stenosis in patients with prior subclavian vein catheterization for maintenance dialysis. *Saudi J Kidney Dis Transpl.* 1997;8:119–122.
6. Agarwal AK, Patel BM, Farhan NJ. Central venous stenosis in hemodialysis patients is a common complication of ipsilateral central vein catheterization. *J Am Soc Nephrol.* 2004;15:368A–369A.
7. MacDonald MJ, Martin LG, Hughes JD, Kikeri D, Scout DC, Harker LA. Distribution and severity of stenoses in functioning arteriovenous grafts: a duplex and angiographic study. *J Vasc Tech.* 1996;20:131–136.
8. MacRae JM, Ahmed A, Johnson N, Levin A, Kiaii M. Central vein stenosis: a common problem in patients on hemodialysis. *ASAIO J.* 2005;51:77–81.
9. Naroienejad M, Saedi D, Rezvani A. Prevalence of central vein stenosis following catheterization in patients with end-stage renal disease. *Saudi J Kidney Dis Transplant.* 2010;21:975–978.
10. Morosetti M, Meloni C, Gandini R, Galderisi C, Pampana E, Nicoletti M, Gallucci MT, Simonetti G, Casciani U. Late symptomatic venous stenosis in three hemodialysis patients without previous central venous catheters. *Artificial Organs.* 2000;24:929–931.
11. Oguzkurt L, Tercan F,m Yildirim S, Torun D. Central venous stenosis in haemodialysis patients without a previous history of catheter placement. *Eur J Radiol.* 2005;55:237.
12. Taal MW, Chesterton IJ, McIntyre CW. Venography at insertion of tunneled internal jugular vein dialysis catheters reveals significant occult stenosis. *Nephrol Dial Transplant.* 2004;19:1542–1545.
13. Hernandez D, Diaz F, Rufino M, Lorenzo V, Perez T, Rodriguez A, DeBonis E, Losada M, Gonzalez-Posada JM, Torres A. Subclavian vascular access stenosis in dialysis

patients: natural history and risk factors. *J Am Soc Nephrol.* 1998;9:1507–1510.
14. Koh KH, Tan C. Central vein stenosis in end stage renal failure patients. *J R Coll Physicians Edinb.* 2005;35:116–122.
15. Schillinger F, Schillinger D, Montagnac R, Milcent T. Post catheterisation vein stenosis in haemodialysis: comparative angiographic study of 50 subclavian and 50 internal jugular accesses. *Nephrol Dial Transplant.* 1991;6:722–724.
16. Cimochowski GE, Worley E, Rutherford WE, Sartain J, Blondin J, Harter H. Superiority of the internal jugular over the subclavian access for temporary dialysis. *Nephron.* 1990;54:154–161.
17. Oguzkurt L, Tercan F, Torun D, Yildirim T, Zümrütdal A, Kizilkilic O. Eur Impact of short-term hemodialysis catheters on the central veins: a catheter venographic study. *J Radiol.* 2004;52:293–299.
18. Jean G, Vanel T, Chazot C, Charra B, Terrat JC, Hurot JM. Prevalence of stenosis and thrombosis of central veins in hemodialysis after a tunneled jugular catheter. *Nephrologie.* 2001;22:501–504.
19. Jassal SV, Pierratos A, Roscoe JM. Venous stenosis and thrombosis associated with the use of internal jugular vein catheters for hemodialysis. *ASAIO J.* 1999;45:356–359.
20. Forauer AR, Glockner JF. Importance of US findings in access planning during jugular vein hemodialysis catheter placements. *J Vasc Interv Radiol.* 2000;11:233–238.
21. Wilkin TD, Krause MA, Lane KA, Trerotola SA. Internal Jugular vein thrombosis associated with hemodialysis catheters. *Radiology.* 2003;228:697–700.
22. Salgado OJ, Urdaneta B, Colmenares B, Garcia R, Flores C. Right versus left internal jugular vein catheterization for hemodialysis: complications and impact on ipsilateral access creation. *Artif Organs.* 2004;28:728–733.
23. Salik E, Daftary A, Tal MG. Three-dimensional anatomy of the left central veins: implications for dialysis catheter placement. *J Vasc Interv Radiol.* 2007;18:361–364.
24. Lobato EB, Sulek CA, Moody RL, Morey TE. Cross sectional area of the right and left internal jugular veins. *J Cardiothorac Vasc Anesth.* 1999;13:136–138.
25. Maxim I Kraus MJ, Trerotola SO. Extrinsic compression of the left innominate vein in hemodialysis patients. *J Vasc Interv Radiol.* 2004;15:51–56.
26. Hegarty J, Picton M, Chalmers N, Kalra PA. Iliac vein stenosis secondary to femoral catheter placement. *Nephrol Dial Transplant.* 2001;16:1520–1521.
27. Wu X, Studer W, Skarvan K, Seeberger MD. High incidence of intravenous thrombi after short-term central venous catheterization of the internal jugular vein. *J Clin Anesth.* 1999;11:482–485.
28. Grove JR, Pevec WC. Venous thrombosis related to peripherally inserted venous catheters. *J Vasc Interv Radiol.* 2000;11:837–840.
29. Ryder MA. Peripherally inserted central venous catheters. *Nurs Clin North Am.* 1993;28:937–971.
30. Allen AW, Megargell JL, Brown DB, Lynch FC, Singh H, Singh Y, Waybill PN. Venous thrombosis associated with placement of peripherally inserted central catheters. *J Vasc Interv Radiol.* 2000;11:1309.
31. Gonsalves CF, Eschelman DJ, Sullivan KL, DuBois N, Bonn J. Incidence of central vein stenosis and occlusion following upper extremity PICC and port placement. *Cardiovasc Intervent Radiol.* 2003;26:123–127.

32. Korzets A, Chagnac A, Ori Y, Katz M, Zevin D. Subclavian vein stenosis, permanent cardiac pacemakers and the haemodialysed patient. *Nephron.* 1991;58:103–105.

33. Chuang C, Tarng D, Yang W, Huang T. An occult cause of arteriovenous access failure: central vein stenosis from permanent pacemaker wire. *Am J Nephrol.* 2001;21:406–409.

34. Sticherling C, Chough SP, Baker RL, Wasmer K, Oral H, Tada H, Horwood L, Kim MH, Pelosi F, Michaud GF, Strickberger SA, Morady F, Knight BP. Prevalence of central venous occlusion in patients with chronic defibrillator leads. *Am Heart J.* 2001;141:813–816.

35. Da Costa SS, Scalabrini Neto A, Costa R, Caldas JG, Martinelli Filho M. Incidence and risk factors of upper extremity deep vein lesions after permanent transvenous pacemaker implant: a 6-month follow-up prospective study. *Pacing Clin Electrophysiol.* 2002;25:1301.

36. Lickfett L, Bitzen A, Arepally A, Nasir K, Wolpert C, Jeong KM, Krause U, Schimpf R, Lewalter T, Calkins H, Jung W, Lüderitz B. Incidence of venous obstruction following insertion of an implantable cardioverter defibrillator. A study of systematic contrast venography on patients presenting for their first elective ICD generator replacement. *Europace.* 2004;6:25–31.

37. Rozmus G, Daubert JP, Huang DT, Rosero S, Hall B, Francis. Venous thrombosis and stenosis after implantation of pacemakers and defibrillators. *J Interv Cardiac Electrophys.* 2005;13:9–19.

38. Oginosawa Y, Abe H, Nakashima Y. The incidence and risk factors for venous obstruction after implantation of transvenous pacing leads. *PACE.* 2002;25:1605–1611.

39. Deighan CJ, McLaughlin KJ, Simipson K, Boulton JM. Unsuspected subclavian stenosis esulting from a permanent pacing wire. *Nephrol Dial Transplant.* 1996;11:2333–2334.

40. Teruya TH, Abou-Zamzam AM, Limm W, Wong L, Wong L. Symptomatic subclavian vein stenosis and occlusion in hemodialysis patients with transvenous pacemakers. *Ann Vasc Surg.* 2003;17:526–529.

41. Weiss MF, Scivittaro V, Anderson JM. Oxidative stress and increased expression of growth factors in lesions of failed hemodialysis access. *Am J Kidney Dis.* 2001;37:970–980.

42. Glanz S, Gordon DH, Lipkowitz GS, Butt KM, Hong J, Sclafani SJ. Axillary and subclavian vein stenosis: percutaneous angioplasty. *Radiology.* 1988;168:371–373.

43. Palabrica T, Lobb R, Furie BC, Aronovitz M, Benjamin C, Hsu YM, Sajer SA. Leukocyte accumulation promoting fibrin deposition is mediated by P-selectin on adherent platelets. *Nature.* 1992;359:848–851.

44. Weiss MF, Scivittaro V, Anderson JM. Oxidative stress and increased expression of growth factors in lesions of failed hemodialysis access. *Am J Kidney Dis.* 2001;37:970–980.

45. Vanherweghem JL, Yassine T, Goldman M, Vandenbosch G, Delcour C, Struwen J, Kinnaert P. Subclavian vein thrombosis: a frequent complication of subclavian vein cannulation for hemodialysis. *Clin Nephrol.* 1986;26: 235–238.

46. Hoshal Jr VL, Ause RG, Hoskins PA. Fibrin sleeve formation on indwelling subclavian central venous catheters. *Arch Surg.* 1971;102:253–258.

47. Forauer AR, Theoharis CGA, Dasika NL. Jugular vein catheter placement: histologic features and development of catheter-related (fibrin) sheaths in a Swine model. *Radiology.* 2006;240:427–434.

48. Manderson J, Campbell GR. Venous response to endothelial denudation. *Pathology.* 1986;18:77–87.

49. Gray RJ, Dolmatch BL, Buick MK. Directional atherectomy treatment for hemodialysis access: early results. *J Vasc Interv Radiol.* 1992;3:497–503.

50. Forauer AR, Theoharis C. Histologic changes in the human vein wall adjacent to central venous catheters. *J Vasc Interv Radiol.* 2003;14:1163–1168.

51. Agraharkar M, Isaacson S, Mendelssohn D, Muralidharan J, Mustata S, Zevallos, Besley M, Uldall R. Percutaneously inserted Silastic jugular hemodialysis catheters seldom cause jugular vein thrombosis. *ASAIO J.* 1995;41:169–172.

52. Beenen L, van Leusen R, Deenik B, Bosch FH. The incidence of subclavian vein stenosis using silicone catheters for hemodialysis. *Artif Organs.* 1994;18:289–292.

53. Di Costanzo J, Sastre B, Choux R, Kasparian M. Mechanism of thrombogenesis during total parenteral nutrition: role of catheter composition. *Parenter Enteral Nutr.* 1988;12:190–194.

54. Waheed U, Brown C, Haddad N, Van Cleef S, Agarwal A, Bhatt U. Central venous stenosis in systemic lupus erythematosus associated ESRD. *Semin Dial.* 2008;106–107.

55. Hernandez D, Dıaz F, Suria S, Machado M, Lorenzo V, Losada M, Gonzalez-Posada JM, De Bonis E, Domı́nguez ML, Rodrı́guez AP. Subclavian catheter-related infection is a major risk factor for the late development of subclavian vein stenosis. *Nephrol Dial Transplant.* 1993;8:227–230.

56. Nazarian G, Bjarnason H, Dietz CA, Bernadas CA, Hunter DW. Changes in catheter tip position when a patient is upright. *J Vasc Interv Radiol.* 1997;8:437–441.

57. Kohler TR, Kirkman TR. Central venous catheter failure is induced by injury and can be prevented by stabilizing the catheter tip. *J Vasc Surg.* 1998;28:59–66.

58. Lumsden AB, MacDonald MJ, Isiklar H, Martin LG, Kikeri D, Harker LA, Allen RC. Central venous stenosis in the hemodialysis patient: incidence and efficacy of endovascular treatment. *Cardiovasc Surg.* 1997;5:504–509.

59. National Kidney Foundation – Dialysis Outcomes Quality Initiative: Clinical Practice Guidelines for Vascular Access. New York: National Kidney Foundation, 20–21, 1997.

60. Rose SC, Kinney TB, Bundens WP, Valji K, Roberts AC. Importance of Doppler analysis of transmitted atrial waveforms prior to placement of central venous access catheters. *J Vasc Interv Radiol.* 1998;9:927–934.

61. Labropoulos N, Borge M, Pierce K, Pappas PJ. Criteria for defining significant central vein stenosis with duplex ultrasound. *J Vasc Surg.* 2007;46:101–107.

62. Paksoy Y, Gormus N, Tercan MA. Three-dimensional contrast enhanced magnetic resonance angiography (3-D CE-MRA) in the evaluation of hemodialysis access complications, and the condition of central veins in patients who are candidates for hemodialysis access. *J Nephrol.* 2004;7:57.

63. Chang CJ, Ko PJ, Hsu LA, Ko YS, Ko YL, Chen CF, Huang CC, Hsu TS, Lee YS, Pang JH. Highly increased cell proliferation activity in the restenotic hemodialysis vascular access after percutaneous transluminal angioplasty: implication in prevention of restenosis. *Am J Kidney Dis.* 2004;43:74–84.

64. Levit RD, Cohen RM, Kwak A, Shlansky-Goldberg RD, Clark TW, Patel AA, Stavropoulos SW, Mondschein JI, Solomon JA, Tuite CM, Trerotola SO. Asymptomatic central venous stenosis in hemodialysis patients. *Radiology*. 2006;238:1051–1056.

65. Aruny JE, Lewis CA, Cardella JF, Cole PE, Davis A, Drooz AT, Grassi CJ, Gray RJ, Husted JW, Jones MT, McCowan TC, Meranze SG, Van Moore A, Neithamer CD, Oglevie SB, Omary RA, Patel NH, RhollKS, Roberts AC, Sacks D, Sanchez O, Silverstein MI, Singh H, Swan TL, Towbin RB, Trerotola SO, Bakal CW, Society of Interventional Radiology Standards of Practice Committee: Quality improvement guidelines for percutaneous management of the thrombosed or dysfunctional dialysis access. *J Vasc Interv Radiol*. 2003;14:S247–S253.

66. Guideline 20. NKF-K/DOQI clinical practice guidelines for vascular access, 2000. *Am J Kidney Dis*. 2001;37:s137–s181.

67. Beathard GA. Percutaneous transvenous angioplasty in the treatment of vascular access stenosis. *Kidney Int*. 1992;42:1390–1397.

68. Beathard GA. The treatment of vascular access graft dysfunction: a nephrologist's view and experience. *Adv Ren Replace Ther*. 1994;1:131.

69. Davidson CJ, Newman GE, Sheikh KH, Kisslo K, Stack RS, Schwab SJ. Mechanisms of angioplasty in hemodialysis fistula stenoses evaluated by intravascular ultrasound. *Kidney Int*. 1991;40(1):91–95.

70. Burtankova E, Kocher M, Bachleda P, Utikal P, Kojecky Z, Cerna M, Herman M. Endovascular treatment of central venous stenoses in patients with dialysis shunts. *Biomed Papers*. 2003;147:203–206.

71. Surowiec SM, Fegley AJ, Tanski WJ, Sivamurthy N, Illig KA, Lee DE, Waldman DL, Green RM, Davies MG. Endovascular management of central venous stenoses in the hemodialysis patient: results of percutaneous therapy. *Vasc Endovascular Surg*. 2004,38:349.

72. Yevzlin AS. Hemodialysis catheter-Associated central venous stenosis. *Semin Dial*. 2008;21:522–527.

73. Gray RJ, Horton KM, Dolmatch BL, Rundback JH, Anaise D, Aquino AO, Currier CB, Light JA, Sasaki TM. Use of Wallstents for hemodialysis access-related venous stenoses and occlusions untreatable with balloon angioplasty. *Radiology*. 1995;195:479–484.

74. Haage P, Vorwerk D, Piroth W, Schuermann K, Guenther RW. Treatment of hemodialysis-related central venous stenosis or occlusion: results of primary Wallstent placement and follow-up in 50 patients. *Radiology*. 1999;212:175–180.

75. Ozyer U, Harman A, Yildirim E, Aytekin C, Karakayali F, Boyvat F. Long-term results of angioplasty and stent placement for treatment of central venous obstruction in 126 hemodialysis patients: a 10-year single-center experience. *Am J Roentegenol*. 2009;193:1672–1679.

76. Kim YC, Won JY, Choi SY, Ko H-K, Lee K-H, Lee DY, Kang B-C, Kim S-J. Percutaneous treatment of central venous stenosis in hemodialysis patients: long-term outcomes. *Cardiovasc Intervent Radiol*. 2009;32:271–278.

77. Maya ID, Saddekhi S and Allon M. Treatment of refractory central vein stenosis in hemodialysis patients with stents. *Semin Dial*. 2006;20:78–82.

78. Vogel PM, Parise C. SMART Stent for salvage of hemodialysis access grafts. *J Vasc Interv Radiol*. 2004;15:1051–1060.

79. Quinn SF, Kim J, Sheley RC. Transluminally placed endovascular grafts for venous lesions in patients on hemodialysis. *Cardiovasc Intervent Radiol*. 2003;6:365–369.

80. Farber A, Barbey MM, Grunert JH, Gmelin E. Access-related venous stenoses and occlusions: treatment with percutaneous transluminal angioplasty and Dacron-covered stents. *Cardiovasc Intervent Radiol*. 1999;22:214–218.

81. Katzman HE, McLafferty RB, Ross JR, Glickman MH, Peden EK, Lawson JH. Initial experience and outcome of a new hemodialysis access device for catheter-dependent patients. *J Vasc Surg*. 2009;50:600–607.

82. Asif A, Salman L, Carrillo RG, Garisto JD, Lopera G, Barakat U, Lenz O, Yevzlin A, Agarwal A, Gadalean F, Sachdeva B, Vachharajani TJ, Wu S, Maya ID, Abreo K. Patency rates for angioplasty in the treatment of pacemaker-induced central venous stenosis in hemodialysis patients: results of a multicenter study. *Semin Dial*. 2009;22:671.

83. Baddour LM, Epstein AE, Erickson CC, Knight BP, Levison ME, Lockhart PB, Masoudi FA, Okum EJ, Wilson WR, Beerman LB, Bolger AF, Estes NA 3rd, Gewitz M, Newburger JW, Schron EB, Taubert KA. Update on cardiovascular implantable electronic device infections and their management: a scientific statement from the American Heart Association. *Circulation*. 2010;121:458.

84. Wilkoff BL, Love CJ, Byrd CL, Bongiorni MG, Carrillo RG, Crossley GH 3rd, Epstein LM, Friedman RA, Kennergren CE, Mitkowski P, Schaerf RH, Wazni OM. Transvenous lead extraction: Heart Rhythm Society expert consensus on facilities, training, indications, and patient management: this document was endorsed by American Heart Association. *Heart Rhythm*. 2009;6:1085–1104.

85. Asif A, Carrillo R, Juan-Domingo G, Lopera G, Ladino M, Barakat U, Eid N, Salman L. Epicardial cardiac rhythm devices for dialysis patients: minimizing the risk of infection and preserving central veins. *Semin Dial*. 2012;25:88–94.

86. Currier CB Jr, Widder S, Ali A, Kuusisto E, Sidawy A. Surgical management of subclavian and axillary vein thrombosis in patients with a functioning arteriovenous fistula. *Surgery*. 1986;100:25.

87. Anaya-Ayala JE, Bellows PH, Ismail N, Cheema ZF, Naoum JJ, Bismuth J, Lumsden AB, Reardon MJ, Davies MG, Peden EK. Surgical management of hemodialysis-related central venous occlusive disease: a treatment algorithm. *Ann Vasc Surg*. 2011;25:108–119.

88. Pisoni RL, Young EW, Dykstra DM, Greenwood RN, Hecking E, Gillespie B, Wolfe RA, Goodkin DA, Held PJ. Vascular access use in Europe and the United States: results from the DOPPS. *Kidney Int*. 2002;16:305–316.

89. Cooper BA, Branley P, Bulfone L, Collins JF, Craig JC, Fraenkel MB, Harris A, Johnson DW, Kesselhut J, Li JJ, Luxton G, Pilmore A, Tiller DJ, Harris DC, Pollock CA. A randomized, controlled trial of early versus late initiation of dialysis. *N Engl J Med*. 2010;363:609–619.

90. Falk A. Use of the brachiocephalic vein for placement of tunneled hemodialysis catheters. *Am J Roentegenol*. 2006;187:773–777.

91. Kwok PC, Wong KM, Ngan RK, Chan SC, Wong WK, Wong KY, Wong AK, Chau KF, Li CS. Prevention of recurrent central venous stenosis using endovascular irradiation following stent placement in hemodialysis patients. *Cardiovasc Intervent Radiol*. 2001;4:400–406.

33

VASCULAR ACCESS IN SPECIAL POPULATIONS

MICAH R. CHAN

LEARNING OBJECTIVES

1. Discuss the vascular access hierarchy in relation to the Fistula First Breakthrough Initiative.
2. Understand the importance of population-specific risk factors in vascular access outcomes.
3. Describe the landmark clinical studies describing the association of risk factors and vascular access outcomes.
4. Understand the pathophysiology of vascular access failure and their association with population-specific factors.

INTRODUCTION

Vascular access procedures and their complications represent a major cause of morbidity for the U.S. hemodialysis population.[1-4] The annual cost of access-related morbidity is estimated to be nearly \$1 billion.[5] Despite these facts, there has never been a large, multicenter, randomized, controlled trial (RCT) comparing arteriovenous fistulae (AVF), arteriovenous grafts (AVG), and central venous catheters (CVC) vis-à-vis patency rates, morbidity, and mortality. However, the ethical dilemma of placing patients' autonomy and choice in jeopardy, and the fact that one or another form of access leads to better outcomes suggests such a trial would never occur. Therefore, based on population cohort studies, it remains a widely held belief that AVF are superior to AVGs, and that both are superior to CVCs. Based on this vascular access hierarchy, the National Kidney Foundation Kidney Disease Outcome Quality Initiative (NKF K/DOQI) guidelines have recommended the use of AVF, AVGs, and CVCs, in 50%, 40%, and 10%, respectively, in the U.S. prevalent hemodialysis population.[6]

Despite the increase in arteriovenous fistulae placement as a result of the Fistula First Breakthrough Initiative (FFBI), consisting of the Centers for Medicare & Medicaid Services (CMS) and ESRD Networks, there still appears to be a substantial number of patients who have early and late fistula failure. Many in the ESRD community began to question whether one of the unforeseen consequences of increasing fistulae use was an increase in catheter prevalence.[7-9] Indeed, the Fistula First campaign has stipulated that patients be referred to surgery for "fistula only" evaluations.[10] The question arises whether certain subsets of patients should be scrutinized differently for the placement of AVF. While AVF have been shown to be superior to AVGs and CVCs in terms of thrombosis, morbidity, and mortality in certain hemodialysis populations,[4,5,11,12] they continue to have a higher primary failure rate. In this chapter, we will review the literature on dialysis-dependent special populations and their associations with vascular access outcomes.

BACKGROUND

The first large population study examining the predictors of vascular access use in the United States was accomplished by Hirth et al.[13] They showed in a United States Renal Data System (USRDS) Special Studies cross-sectional analysis of 4150 incident dialysis patients in 1986, 1987, and 1990 that 56% of patients had an AVG and 44% had an AVF 30 days into chronic dialysis. In multivariate logistic regression analysis, they found that female gender adjusted odds ratio (aOR) 1.93; 95% CI: 1.66–2.24, $P < 0.001$), age per 10 years (aOR 1.17; 95% CI: 1.12–1.22, $P < 0.001$), diabetes (aOR 1.27; 95% CI: 1.08–1.49, $P < 0.01$), and peripheral vascular disease (aOR 1.31; 95% CI: 1.08–1.59, $P < 0.01$) were all significant factors favoring grafts as opposed to fistulae placement. Due to these findings, these variables or risk factors are now commonly used as historical covariates in vascular access outcome studies. Other notable findings were that insurance status, living in poverty, and census region in the U.S. were associated with more AVG placement. This large, nationally representative sample confirmed for the first time that perhaps factors such as technically challenging vasculature favors grafts over fistulae placement. Other factors including wide regional practice pattern variations may be due to differences in predialysis nephrology care or referral patterns as suggested by the authors. They comment that perhaps more focus should be placed on referring patients early, teaching surgeons how to place fistulae, and nurses how to access these AVF.

This landmark study generated more questions on population-specific risk factors in vascular access outcomes. Soon, a plethora of studies explored different hypotheses on why this occurs, including a few major clinical studies.

CLINICAL STUDIES

▶ USRDS DMMS Wave I and II

The first large national prospective trial looking at vascular access associations with all-cause mortality was the USRDS [Dialysis Morbidity and Mortality Study (DMMS) Wave I study by Dhingra et al].[12] This landmark study was a representative sample from 550 hemodialysis facilities with 5507 incident patients that initiated dialysis between October 2, 1993 and December 31, 1993. Follow-up mortality data over 2 years showed that in diabetics the relative risk of mortality was significantly higher in patients with AVG (RR 1.41, 95% CI: 1.13–1.77, $P < 0.003$) and CVC (RR 1.54, 95% CI: 1.17–2.02, $P < 0.002$) as compared to AVF. In nondiabetic patients, those with CVC had a higher associated mortality (RR = 1.70, 95% CI: 1.41–2.05, $P < 0.001$), as did to a lesser degree those with AVG (RR = 1.08, 95% CI: 0.92–1.26, $P = 0.35$) when compared with AVF.

Next, DMMS Wave II was a prospective longitudinal study of adult patients sampled from 25% of the dialysis units in the United States. All incident (new) end-stage renal disease (ESRD) patients as of January 1, 1996, over the age of 18, receiving either hemodialysis (HD) or peritoneal dialysis (PD) were eligible for inclusion. Among other variables, data collected for the DMMS Wave 2 included: type and location of vascular access, date of first vascular access creation, AVF maturity (fistula adequate for use), revision (open or endovascular procedure), and failure (primary unassisted/assisted or secondary). Data were collected for the DMMS Wave II by dialysis unit personnel through chart review or were recorded at time of initiation of HD and follow-up. Stehman-Breen et al showed in a cohort of 1449 patients that 33% initiated

with an AVF and 67% with an AVG as permanent access (CVCs were not considered permanent).[14] Using multivariate logistic regression, age (per decade; aOR = 0.84, $P < 0.001$), female gender (aOR = 0.52, $P < 0.001$), and sharing in decision making (aOR = 1.50, $P = 0.02$) were all significant predictors of what type of permanent access was initially placed (AVF vs AVG). Also, patients who had one visit to a nephrologist prior to initiation of dialysis were 79% less likely not to have a permanent access in place (aOR 0.21, 95% CI: 0.10–0.43, $P < 0.001$) as compared to those with great than five visits.

The same group then demonstrated in another compelling analysis on vascular access patency that AVGs had a significantly higher rate of primary failure (RR 1.41; 95% CI: 1.22–1.64, $P < 0.001$) and revision (RR 1.91; 95% CI: 1.60–2.28, $P < 0.001$).[15] At 1 and 2 years, primary patency rates for simple AVFs were 56.1% and 39.8% ($P < 0.001$) respectively, compared with 38.2% and 24.6% for AVG ($P < 0.001$). When compared with simple fistulas, vein transpositions demonstrated equivalent secondary patency at 2 years (61.5% vs 64.3%, $P = 0.43$) but poorer primary patency (27.7% vs 39.8%, $P = 0.008$) and had a 32% increased incidence of revision ($P = 0.04$).

Overall, the data from the USRDS DMMS datasets suggest that predialysis care have an integral role in vascular access type at initiation of dialysis and that more studies are needed to investigate how certain patient subgroups confer a higher risk of vascular access failure.

HEMO

The hemodialysis (HEMO) study was a randomized multicenter clinical trial that recruited patients from over 65 dialysis facilities and 15 clinical centers over a time period from 1995 to 1999. The study was originally designed to test two interventions: the dialysis dose (or K_t/V) intervention and the membrane flux intervention and determine if there is an association with mortality.[16] There have been many secondary analyses of the HEMO study, one of them by Allon et al who aimed to look at risk factors associated with prevalence of AVF.[17] Over a 4-year period, they were able to analyze 1824 patients that were dialyzing with an AVG or AVF. On multivariable regression analysis, six factors that were independently associated with a lower prevalence of AV fistulas were dialysis unit ($P < 0.001$), female gender (aOR 0.37, 95% CI: 0.28–0.48, $P < 0.001$), BMI per 5 kg/m^2 (aOR 0.76, 95% CI: 0.65–0.87, $P < 0.001$), peripheral vascular disease (aOR 0.55, 95% CI: 0.38–0.79, $P < 0.001$) age per 10 years (aOR 0.85, 95% CI: 0.78–0.94, $P < 0.001$), and black race (aOR 0.64, 95% CI: 0.46–0.89, $P = 0.008$). Interestingly, a significantly lower prevalence of fistulas in black subjects was observed in both hemodialysis units with a high or low proportion of black subjects. This was one of the first national cohort studies to demonstrate an independent association of certain subsets of patients to fistula prevalence. The authors suggest three ways to improve these numbers that would be to a concerted effort to place AVF in females, to use preoperative venous mapping, and to construct AVF in the upper arm first rather than distally in certain populations.

CHOICE

The Choices for Healthy Outcomes in Caring for End-Stage Renal Disease (CHOICE) study was a national prospective cohort study of 1041 incident dialysis patients initiated in 1995 and followed to 1998, from 80 dialysis facilities to study treatment choices of dialysis, dose and outcomes of dialysis. A secondary analysis by Astor et al demonstrated that out of 356 patients that had type of vascular access and referral times to nephrologists recorded, that an overwhelmingly higher odds of initiation with a catheter was seen in patients referred late prior to initiation of dialysis.[18] After 6 months on hemodialysis, 70% of patients with data available had used an AV access for at least one dialysis session. Of these accesses, 87 (39%) were AVF and 137 (61%) were AVGs. Of those patients referred to a nephrologist late (<1 month prior to initiation of dialysis), only 56% had an AV access, 65% of those patients referred 1–4 months had an AV access, 63% for those referred 4–12 months, and 82% for those referred >12 months prior to initiation of dialysis (P_{trend} < 0.001). This association remained after adjustment for other variables such as race, age, gender, education, and primary cause of ESRD (aOR for ≥4 months vs <4 months, 2.05; 95% CI: 1.20–3.50). The authors followed up this study looking at type of vascular access and survival in the same cohort followed up 3 years after initiation of dialysis.[19] A total of 616 incident dialysis patients with 1084 vascular accesses were recorded over 1382 person years. At initiation of hemodialysis, 410 (66.6%) patients were using a catheter, 121 (19.6%) were using an AVG, and 85 (13.8%) were using an AVF. The adjusted relative hazards (RH) of death of CVC use as compared with AVF (RH 1.5 (95% CI: 1.0–2.2) was significantly higher, however, AVG as compared with AVF was higher but not significant [RH 1.2 (0.8–1.8) for AVG]. In addition, this increased risk associated with catheter use after adjustment for multiple confounders was higher among men (RH 1.98; 95% CI: 1.16–3.38) than among women (RH 0.96; 95% CI: 0.50–1.87; P < 0.05 for interaction). The authors suggest that more emphasis should be placed on earlier referral and better care for these patients prior to dialysis and catheter avoidance strategies to minimize mortality and attendant complications of vascular access.

DOPPS

The Dialysis Outcomes and Practice Patterns Study (DOPPS) is an international prospective longitudinal study that compared vascular access use between the United States and five European countries (France, Germany, Italy, Spain,

and United Kingdom). Data between the countries were gathered between 1996 and 2000 consisting of 145 dialysis facilities in the United States and over 20 centers in each European country to include over 6000 patients. Pisoni et al reported that 80% of European patients and only 24% of U.S. prevalent dialysis patients were using arteriovenous fistulae as vascular access of choice during study period.[20] After adjusting for multiple covariates (age, gender, diabetes, peripheral vascular disease, angina, BMI, and years on HD), AVF use as compared to AVG was significantly higher in Europe than in the United States (aOR 21, P < 0.0001). In incident dialysis patients only 15% of U.S. patients used an AVF as compared to 66% in Europe (aOR 39, P < 0.0001). CVCs were used in 60% of the U.S. patients as compared to 31% in Europe. Interestingly, pre-ESRD care was associated with a significant odds for having an AVF as compared to an AVG (aOR 1.9, P = 0.01) and only 68% of patients in the United States see a nephrologist 4 months prior to initiating dialysis as compared to 80% in Europe (P < 0.0001). Since this original landmark study demonstrating the differences in practice patterns between the United States and Europe, there have been many secondary analyses and opinions on why this occurs. Some think that perhaps there is a better multidisciplinary cohesiveness in Europe, especially with nephrologists placing vascular access and cannulating themselves. Others believe it is how the health care system in Europe is set up with the ability to provide more staffing, training, and education in early cannulation, surveillance, and monitoring. However, a recurring theme seems to be pre-ESRD nephrology care. A recent study by Bradbury et al which analyzed data from DOPPS I and II (1996–2004) demonstrated that among incident patients the risk of death was increased during the first 120 days as compared to 121–365 days (27.5 deaths per 100 person-years vs 21.9 deaths per 100 person-years; P = 0.002, respectively).[21] Pre-ESRD care >1 month prior to initiation of dialysis was associated with a lower risk of death during these first 120 days (HR 0.65; 95% CI: 0.51–0.83).

PATHOPHYSIOLOGY

▶ Neointimal Hyperplasia

These population studies generated much speculation on why certain sectors of the population were more prone to AVG placement and perhaps the pathophysiology of development of stenosis or primary failure contributes to this phenomenon. Parameters such as changes in blood volume, inflammation, and aberrant electrolyte states could all incite stimuli that trigger aspects of neointimal hyperplasia (NH), the pathologic *sine quo non* of access dysfunction. Added to those chronic physiological stimuli are the serial changes of hydrostatic pressure, shear stress, and repeated vessel injury that accompany a dialysis procedure. An elegant study by Rehkter et al[22] demonstrated, in seven stenosed vein segments of AVG anastomoses, that neointimal hyperplasia was predominantly made of smooth muscle cells, macrophages (CD68+), and lymphocytes (CD45RB+). The authors postulate that perhaps multiple growth factors such as transforming growth factor beta (TGF-β) or platelet-derived growth factor (PDGF) on the graft surface may be intimally involved in the proliferation of hyperplastic cells. More recently, this has been corroborated with studies in polymorphisms of TGF-β, heme oxygenase 1 (HO-1), and the methylene tetrahydrofolate reductase gene and their link to AVF patency.[23–26] Other studies of inflammation in surgically harvested thrombosed fistulae have found elevated levels of inflammatory biomarkers including IGF-1, TGF-β, IL-6, and vascular cellular adhesion molecule 1 (VCAM-1).[27] The question remains, as to how these stimuli accelerate the process of neointimal hyperplasia in certain patient populations and not others.

▶ Race

Since neointimal hyperplasia as a purely pathological entity induces thrombosis in hemodialysis vascular access, Goldwasser and colleagues studied a number of variables including serum lipoprotein (a) [Lp(a)], systolic BP, and race, among others.[28] They showed in a cohort of 124 dialysis patients studied over 14 months that access occlusion was associated with age, diabetes, AVG, serum fibronectin, reduced systolic BP, and lipoprotein (a) > or = 57 mg/dL. Since black patients have significantly elevated levels of Lp (a), on Cox proportional hazards model including race and Lp(a) as interaction terms, they showed that having an AVG and low systolic BP correlated independently to access thrombosis. In a small study by Obialo et al they demonstrated in an analysis of three subsets of black patients; HIV, hypertensives, and focal segmental glomerulosclerosis (FSGS) that 1-year primary patency was 85%, 65%, and 0%, respectively.[29] The significantly increased thrombosis rate in the FSGS subgroup correlated to their weight ($R = 0.8$, $P = 0.003$) and predialysis protein excretion ($R = 0.9$, $P = 0.001$). This was a novel study because for the first time, risk factors within a race that is predisposed to vascular access failure was examined. The authors suggest that shear stress, accelerated atherosclerosis, and vessel diameter may all contribute to these findings and more studies need to be done.

▶ Intra-access Blood Flow

Tonelli et al subsequently examined access blood flow (Qa) in a retrospective study of 294 patients to determine which factors were independently associated with a feasibility of utilizing it as a screening method for subclinical stenoses.[30] Qa was significantly lower in diabetics as compared to nondiabetics (788 ± 580 vs 1054 ± 681 mL/min, $P = 0.002$, respectively), and Qa was lower in patients >65 years old compared with younger patients (883 ± 620 vs 1118 ± 706 mL/min, $P = 0.004$, respectively). On multivariate analysis, for both forearm and upper arm AVF, blood pressure, overweight status (BMI > 25), and diabetic status were independently associated with Qa. This study showed that perhaps hemodynamic status and serial changes of shear stress and endothelial injury may be a pathogenic mechanism for differences in vascular access outcomes in population subsets. A recent article by Monroy-Cuadros et al showed in a 3.5-year retrospective Canadian study that initial intra-access blood flow less than 500 mL/min was most predictive of 6-month primary functional patency odds ratio (OR) 29, $P < 0.001$), along with known variables of diabetes, age, and distal AVF.[31]

Access blood flow has long been an argument why certain people have higher primary failure rates than others. Plumb and colleagues recently published a report showing two women with increased BMI and adequate vessels by vein mapping who had early failures of their brachiocephalic fistulas. They demonstrated with venogram how excess axillary tissue compresses venous outflow when the arm is in the adducted position and offer this as a possible explanation to early fistula failure in patients with high BMI.[32] In a single-center, retrospective cohort, Kats et al demonstrated that obesity was the only significant factor in predicting secondary fistula failure (HR 2.93; 95% CI: 1.44–5.93; $P = 0.004$) on multivariable survival analysis.[33] However, obesity did not predict a lower likelihood of fistula placement and primary failure was not significantly different between the obese and nonobese groups. The authors conclude that perhaps obese patients with AVF should be scrutinized more for evidence of fistula failure but tempered by the fact this was a single-center study that diminishes the generalizability of results. Studies have suggested pathogenetic mechanisms for fistula failure in the obese subpopulation. One of the earliest studies in 1996 by DeMarchi et al attempted to explain biochemical parameters that predict AVF failure. They elegantly demonstrated that compared to patients without fistula dysfunction, higher levels of monocyte chemoattractant protein-1 (MCP-1), IL-6, hyperinsulinemia, hyperlipidemia, and plasminogen activator inhibitor type-1 (PAI-1) and factor VII were associated with stenosis and thrombosis of AVF.[34] Increased levels of these cytokines, hyperinsulinemia, and dyslipidemia, as well as PAI-1 is upregulated in obese patients.[34,35] Furthermore, Irish et al showed that PAI-1 was independently correlated with BMI, triglycerides, and lipoprotein(a) in CKD and hemodialysis patients.[36] However, one could argue that there may be other mediators which compensate the effects of the latter and provide a beneficial effect on fistula survival. Chan et al showed in a retrospective analysis using the DMMS Wave 2 dataset that obesity did not emerge as a factor in predicting vascular access revisions or failures.[37] Of 1486 patients, 1146 (77.1%) subjects were classified as nonobese and 340 obese based on BMI <30 or ≥30 kg/m². Results from logistic regression models using the National Heart, Lung and Blood Institute (NHLBI) BMI criteria, showed that obesity failed to predict AVF failure to mature. However, results from the regression model using BMI quartiles to define obesity indicated an increased risk of AVF failure

TABLE 33–1

Odds Ratio of Factors Associated with Arteriovenous Fistula (AVF) Failure to Mature (BMI Quartiles)

Covariates	*P* value	aOR[†]	95% CI
Mean BMI (kg/m²)			
Quartile			
1 (<25 kg/m²)	Reference		
2 (25–29.9)	0.18	1.76	0.77–4.04
3 (30–34.9)	0.69	0.73	0.15–3.51
4 (≥35)	0.017*	3.66	1.27–10.56
Age (per year)	0.72	1.00	0.98–1.03
Gender (female)	0.67	0.84	0.36–1.93
Black ethnicity (compared to Caucasian and other)	0.17	1.73	0.79–3.75
Comorbidities			
Peripheral vascular disease	0.78	1.15	0.44–3.03
Diabetes	0.44	1.34	0.64–2.82

*Significance based on multivariable logistic regression.
[†]Adjusted odds ratio based on multivariable analysis.
Reprinted with permission from Chan.[37]

to mature for the highest BMI quartile (≥35 kg/m²) only (aOR 3.66 [95% CI: 1.27–10.56], *P* = 0.017). All other patient characteristics such as age, gender, black ethnicity, diabetes, and peripheral vascular disease were not associated with AVF failure to mature (Table 33-1). Findings also indicated that neither obesity nor any other variable was associated with AVF or AVG access revision. The authors concluded that obesity was not associated with increased vascular access revision rates or failure and was only associated with poorer AVF maturity at highest BMI quartile.

Therefore, obesity should not preclude placement of AVF as vascular access of choice, except in the very obese where assessment should be individually based. Also, a recent prospective study by Weyde et al demonstrated, in 71 obese patients with a mean BMI 34.6 kg/m², results of acceptable dialysis adequacy based on set parameters and primary patency rates of 65% and 59% at 6 and 12 months and secondary patency of 83% at both 6 and 12 months, respectively (Figures 33-1 and 33-2). These patency rates are comparable to normal weight individuals with the authors concluding that obesity should not preclude placement of AVF and may even protect venous vessels from iatrogenic insult.[38]

▶ **Vascular Anatomy**

Other population subgroups of concern for higher primary and secondary failure rates include women with smaller vessel diameters and the growing majority of elderly diabetics. Perhaps vessel caliber, vascular calcification and endothelial dysfunction all contribute to higher failure rates in these patients (Figure 33-3). A meta-analysis conducted by Lazarides et al showed that in 10 studies consisting of 1171 nonelderly patients and 670 elderly patients, that pooled 12-month (OR 1.525, 95% CI: 1.189–1.957, *P* = 0.001) and 24-month patency rates (OR 1.357, 95% CI: 1.062–1.751, *P* = 0.019) favored the nonelderly cohort.[39] Primary radial-cephalic AVF failure was also in favor of nonelderly adults (OR, 1.79; *P* = 0.012) and secondary analysis revealed a pooled effect in favor of brachiocephalic AVF (*P* = 0.004) compared with distal AVF in elderly patients. Multiple studies have suggested that these individuals have decreased AVF patency rates and higher failure to mature due to their vascular anatomy given the higher incidence of atherosclerosis, systolic hypertension, and arterial stiffness.[40–43] Given

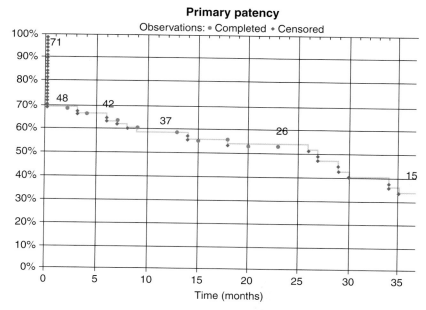

Figure 33-1. Primary patency rates were 65%, 59%, 53%, and 33% at 6, 12, 24, and 36 months, respectively. (Reprinted with permission from Weyde W, et al. Obesity is not an obstacle for successful autogenous arteriovenous fistula creation in haemodialysis. *Nephrol Dial Transplant.* 2008:Apr;23(4):1318–1322.)

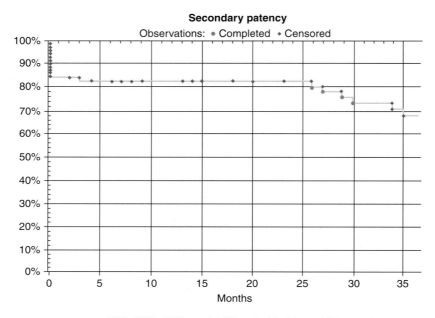

Figure 33-2. Secondary patency rates were 83%, 83%, 80%, and 68% at 6, 12, 24, and 36 months respectively. (Reprinted with permission from Weyde W, et al. Obesity is not an obstacle for successful autogenous arteriovenous fistula creation in haemodialysis. *Nephrol Dial Transplant.* 2008:Apr;23(4):1318–1322.)

these findings, Konner recommends strategies that place more focus on the feeding artery rather than vein, phlebography in certain patients, and Doppler/duplex evaluation of both artery and vein just to name a few.[44] Over a 2-year period in his series of 347 patients, no AVGs were needed to be placed; also there was no significant difference in primary patency or need for revisions between diabetics and nondiabetics. Recently, Chan et al explored whether there are significant predictors of access patency and survival in elderly hemodialysis patients using the DMMS Wave 2 dataset.[45] Of 1471 hemodialysis patients with AVF or AVGs,

764 patients were greater than age 65. Elderly diabetics had no significant mortality benefit from the use of AVF compared to AVG (OR 1.34 [95% CI: 0.92–1.95], $P = 0.123$) (Figure 33-4). Likewise, elderly nondiabetics had no significant mortality benefit from the use of AVF compared to AVG (OR 1.05 [95% CI: 0.81–1.36], $P = 0.735$). Elderly diabetics had no difference in access patency for AVF compared to AVG (OR 1.49 [95% CI: 0.76–2.9], $P = 0.24$) (Figure 33-5). Elderly nondiabetics had no difference in access patency for AVF compared to AVG (OR 1.48 [95% CI: 0.95–2.3], $P = 0.08$). Given the data, the authors argue

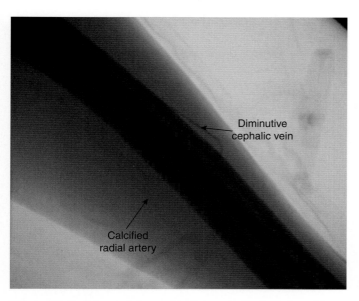

Figure 33-3. Primary failure of radial cephalic AVF placed in a 72-year-old male diabetic.

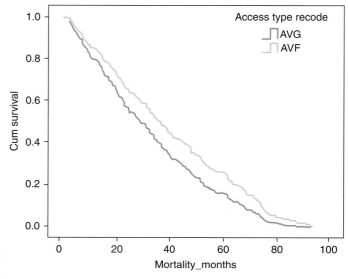

Figure 33-4. Kaplan–Meier curve of patient survival versus time for diabetic elderly patients. (From Chan,[45] reprinted with permission.)

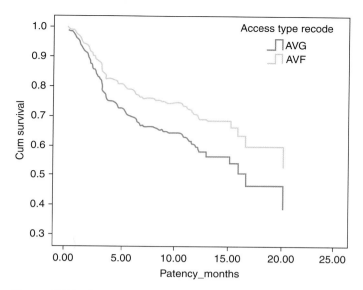

Figure 33-5. Cox regression curve of vascular access patency versus time for diabetic elderly patients. (From Chan,[45] reprinted with permission.)

persuasively that differences in patient populations should be taken into account for the purposes of vascular access planning. Most compelling is the assertion that the primary selection of PTFE graft placement in the elderly population may be beneficial due to their high death rates on dialysis with 2-year mortality of greater than 50%.[46–48]

SUMMARY

Arteriovenous fistulae and grafts have mortality benefits over catheters, however, their patency rates are much to be desired. The Fistula First Initiative and efforts of the Kidney Disease Outcome Quality Initiative (KDOQI) have shifted the paradigm of vascular access use in the United States, however, primary failure rates are still high and catheter usage is still at more than 20%. Pharmacologic, endovascular, and surgical methods to improve these patency rates have been disappointing and the number of robust clinical trials few. Given the current changes in Medicare reimbursement and quality improvement performance measures, nephrologists are under more pressure than ever to develop prudent strategies to improve vascular access outcomes.

Predialysis nephrologist care will be one of the key steps in integrating these strategies. Patients and providers will need to be engaged in novel educational and access planning programs in order to accomplish this. With the implementation of the Medicare Improvements for Patients and Providers Act (MIPPA), more emphasis will be geared toward chronic kidney disease (CKD) education, patient autonomy, and shared decision making.

While it is clear that certain subgroups of the dialysis population are less likely to have an AVF placed or result in poorer patency rates, the issue of whether or not this practice is justified by poorer outcomes in these populations

remains controversial. Therefore, until more compelling data is published, the guidelines established by NKF K/DOQI and the Fistula First Breakthrough Initiative should be followed according to the hierarchy of vascular access of choice as stipulated for the general population alike.

REFERENCES

1. Fan PY, Schwab SJ. Vascular access: concepts for the 1990s. *J Am Soc Nephrol.* 1992;3:1–11.
2. Windus DW. Permanent vascular access: a nephrologist's view. *Am J Kidney Dis.* 1993;21:457–471.
3. Porile JL, Richter M. Preservation of vascular access. *J Am Soc Nephrol.* 1993;4:997–1003.
4. Allon M, Robbin ML. Increasing arteriovenous fistulas in hemodialysis patients: problems and solutions. *Kidney Int.* 2002;62:1109–1124.
5. Feldman HI, Kobrin S, Wasserstein A. Hemodialysis vascular access morbidity. *J Am Soc Nephrol.* 1996;7:523–535.
6. National Kidney Foundation. NKF-K/DOQI Clinical Practice Guidelines for Vascular Access: Update 2000. *Am J Kidney Dis.* 2001;37: S137–S181.
7. U.S. Renal Data System: *USRDS 2006 Annual Data Report: Atlas of End-Stage Renal Disease in the United States,* National Institutes of Health, National Institute of Diabetes and Digestive and Kidney Diseases, Bethesda, MD, 2006.
8. Lacson E, Jr., Lazarus JM, Himmelfarb J, Ikizler TA, Hakim RM. Balancing fistula first with catheters last. *Am J Kidney Dis.* 2007;50:379–395.
9. Rehman R, Schmidt RJ, Moss AH. Ethical and legal obligation to avoid long-term tunneled catheter access. *Clin J Am Soc Nephrol.* 2009;4:456–460.
10. National Vascular Access Improvement Initiative. Change of Concept #3. Available at: http://www.fistulafirst.org/. Accessed August, 2010.
11. Schwab SJ, Harrington JT, Singh A, et al. Vascular access for hemodialysis. *Kidney Int.* 1999;55:2078–2090.
12. Dhingra RK, Young EW, Hulbert-Shearon TE, Leavey SF, Port FK. Type of vascular access and mortality in U.S. hemodialysis patients. *Kidney Int.* 2001;60:1443–1451.
13. Hirth RA, Turenne MN, Woods JD, et al. Predictors of type of vascular access in hemodialysis patients. *J Am Med Assoc.* 1996; 276:1303–1308.
14. Stehman-Breen CO, Sherrard DJ, Gillen D, Caps M. Determinants of type and timing of initial permanent hemodialysis vascular access. *Kidney Int.* 2000;57:639–645.
15. Gibson KD, Gillen DL, Caps MT, Kohler TR, Sherrard DJ, Stehman-Breen CO. Vascular access survival and incidence of revisions: a comparison of prosthetic grafts, simple autogenous fistulas, and venous transposition fistulas from the United States Renal Data System Dialysis Morbidity and Mortality Study. *J Vasc Surg.* 2001;34:694–700.
16. Greene T, Beck GJ, Gassman JJ, et al. Design and statistical issues of the hemodialysis (HEMO) study. *Control Clin Trials.* 2000;21:502–525.
17. Allon M, Ornt DB, Schwab SJ, et al. Factors associated with the prevalence of arteriovenous fistulas in hemodialysis patients in the HEMO study. Hemodialysis (HEMO) Study Group. *Kidney Int.* 2000;58:2178–2185.
18. Astor BC, Eustace JA, Powe NR, et al. Timing of nephrologist referral and arteriovenous access use: the CHOICE Study. *Am J Kidney Dis.* 2001;38:494–501.

19. Astor BC, Eustace JA, Powe NR, Klag MJ, Fink NE, Coresh J; CHOICE Study. Type of vascular access and survival among incident hemodialysis patients: the Choices for Healthy Outcomes in Caring for ESRD (CHOICE) Study. *J Am Soc Nephrol.* 2005;16:1449–1455.

20. Pisoni RL, Young EW, Dykstra DM, et al. Vascular access use in Europe and the United States: results from the DOPPS. *Kidney Int.* 2002; 61:305–316.

21. Bradbury BD, Fissell RB, Albert JM, et al. Predictors of early mortality among incident US hemodialysis patients in the Dialysis Outcomes and Practice Patterns Study (DOPPS). *Clin J Am Soc Nephrol.* 2007;2:89–99.

22. Rekhter M, Nicholls S, Ferguson M, Gordon D. Cell proliferation in human arteriovenous fistulas used for hemodialysis. *Arterioscler Thromb.* 1993;13:609–617.

23. Fukasawa M, Matsushita K, Kamiyama M, et al. The methylentetrahydrofolate reductase C677T point mutation is a risk factor for vascular access thrombosis in hemodialysis patients. *Am J Kidney Dis.* 2003;41:637–642.

24. Heine GH, Ulrich C, Sester U, Sester M, Kohler H, Girndt M. Transforming growth factor beta1 genotype polymorphisms determine AV fistula patency in hemodialysis patients. *Kidney Int.* 2003;64:1101–1107.

25. Lazo-Langner A, Knoll GA, Wells PS, Carson N, Rodger MA. The risk of dialysis access thrombosis is related to the transforming growth factor-beta1 production haplotype and is modified by polymorphisms in the plasminogen activator inhibitor-type 1 gene. *Blood.* 2006;108:4052–4058.

26. Lin CC, Yang WC, Lin SJ, et al. Length polymorphism in heme oxygenase-1 is associated with arteriovenous fistula patency in hemodialysis patients. *Kidney Int.* 2006;69: 165–172.

27. Goldwasser P, Avram MM, Collier JT, Michel MA, Gusik SA, Mittman N. Correlates of vascular access occlusion in hemodialysis. *Am J Kidney Dis.* 1994;24:785–794.

28. Goldwasser P, Michel MA, Collier J, et al. Prealbumin and lipoprotein(a) in hemodialysis: relationships with patient and vascular access survival. *Am J Kidney Dis.* 1993;22: 215–225.

29. Obialo CI, Robinson T, Brathwaite M. Hemodialysis vascular access: variable thrombus-free survival in three subpopulations of black patients. *Am J Kidney Dis.* 1998;31:250–256

30. Tonelli M, Hirsch DJ, Chan CT, et al. Factors associated with access blood flow in native vessel arteriovenous fistulae. *Nephrol Dial Transplant.* 2004;19:2559–2563.

31. Monroy-Cuadros M, Yilmaz S, Salazar-Bañuelos A, Doig C. Risk factors associated with patency loss of hemodialysis vascular access within 6 months. *Clin J Am Soc Nephrol.* 2010;5:1787–1792.

32. Plumb TJ, Adelson AB, Groggel GC, Johanning JM, Lynch TG, Lund B. Obesity and hemodialysis vascular access failure. *Am J Kidney Dis.* 2007;50:450–454.

33. Kats M, Hawxby AM, Barker J, Allon M. Impact of obesity on arteriovenous fistula outcomes in dialysis patients. *Kidney Int.* 2007;71:39–43.

34. De Marchi S, Falleti E, Giacomello R, et al. Risk factors for vascular disease and arteriovenous fistula dysfunction in hemodialysis patients. *J Am Soc Nephrol.* 1996;7: 1169–1177.

35. Dixon BS. Weighing in on fistula failure. *Kidney Int.* 2007;71:12–14.

36. Irish AB. Plasminogen activator inhibitor-1 activity in chronic renal disease and dialysis. *Metabolism.* 1997;46: 36–40.

37. Chan MR, Young HN, Becker YT, Yevzlin AS. Obesity as a predictor of vascular access outcomes: analysis of the USRDS DMMS Wave II study. *Semin Dial.* 2008;21: 274–279.

38. Weyde W, Krajewska M, Letachowicz W, et al. Obesity is not an obstacle for successful autogenous arteriovenous fistula creation in haemodialysis. *Nephrol Dial Transplant.* 2008;23:1318–1322.

39. Lazarides MK, Georgiadis GS, Antoniou GA, Staramos DN. A meta-analysis of dialysis access outcome in elderly patients. *J Vasc Surg.* 2007;45:420–426.

40. Staramos DN, Lazarides MK, Tzilalis VD, Ekonomou CS, Simopoulos CE, Dayantas JN. Patency of autologous and prosthetic arteriovenous fistulas in elderly patients. *Eur J Surg.* 2000;166:777–781.

41. Latos D. Hemodialysis in the elderly: vascular access and initiation of renal replacement therapy. *Semin Dial.* 2002;15:91–93.

42. Hayakawa K, Miyakawa S, Hoshinaga K, Hata K, Marumo K, Hata M. The effect of patient age and other factors on the maintenance of permanent hemodialysis vascular access. *Ther Apher Dial.* 2007;11:36–41.

43. Leapman SB, Boyle M, Precovitz MD, Milgrom ML, Jindal RM, Filo RS. The arteriovenous fistula for hemodialysis access: gold standard or archaic relic? *Am Surg.* 1996;62:652–656.

44. Konner K. Primary vascular access in diabetic patients: an audit. *Nephrol Dial Transplant.* 2000;15:1317–1325.

45. Chan MR, Sanchez RJ, Young HN, Yevzlin AS. Vascular access outcomes in the elderly hemodialysis population: A USRDS study. *Semin Dial.* 2007;20:606–610.

46. Letourneau I, Ouimet D, Dumont M, Pichette V, Leblanc M. Renal replacement in end-stage renal disease patients over 75 years old. *Am J Nephrol.* 2003;23:71–77.

47. Joly D, Anglicheau D, Alberti C, et al. Octogenarians reaching end-stage renal disease: cohort study of decision-making and clinical outcomes. *J Am Soc Nephrol.* 2003;14:1012–1021.

48. Culp K, Taylor L, Hulme PA. Geriatric hemodialysis patients: a comparative study of vascular access. *J Am Nephrol Nurses Assoc.* 1996;23:583–590.

34

THE ROLE OF PHARMACOLOGIC AGENTS IN PRESERVING VASCULAR ACCESS

MICAH R. CHAN

LEARNING OBJECTIVES

1. Discuss the vascular access hierarchy in relation to the fistula first breakthrough initiative.
2. Understand the epidemiology and pathophysiology behind vascular access patency in tunneled catheters, arteriovenous grafts, and arteriovenous fistula.
3. Describe the landmark clinical studies that describe the role pharmacologic agents have in preserving vascular access

INTRODUCTION

Sustaining hemodialysis vascular access is and has remained one of the most challenging aspects of nephrology care. Dating back to the 1960s when Scribner and Quinton established their arteriovenous shunt via silastic tubes inserted into the radial artery and cephalic vein, maintaining permanent vascular access continues to mystify experts in the field.[1] Scribner shunts are no longer used due to the invasiveness of the technique, high bleeding and thrombosis rates. However, even though the complications have changed, long-term accesses used today, arteriovenous fistulae (AVF), arteriovenous grafts (AVG), and tunneled dialysis catheters (TDCs) are still plagued by poor patency rates.

It goes without saying that the efforts of the National Kidney Foundation's Kidney Dialysis Outcome and Quality Initiative (NKF/KDOQI) along with the Fistula First Breakthrough Initiative (FFBI), have increased AVF rates and decreased AVGs in the United States. However, central venous catheters (CVCs) still represent a large modality of vascular access in existing and newly diagnosed dialysis patients. According to the Forum of End-Stage Renal Disease Networks, 21% of prevalent hemodialysis patients were dialyzing with a CVC for 90 days or longer.[2] This is far greater than the NKF/KDOQI published recommendations of less than 10% CVC prevalence.[3] According to the CMS Clinical Performance Measures (CPM) data, at 90 days the dialysis catheter is still the access of choice (Figure 34-1).[4] The reasons for this sobering data are multifactorial, however, one cannot overlook the poor primary and secondary patency rates of arteriovenous access as a contributor to this phenomenon. TDCs also have their attendant complications and dysfunction all contributing to their tremendous morbidity, mortality, and cost to the health care system.

In this chapter, one should not forget the fact that early referral to nephrologists prior to the initiation of renal replacement therapy may be the single most important step in establishing and preserving a permanent access for patients. It has been shown that those who have been under nephrologists' care, 22% have a functioning fistula compared to 14% of patients who have not been under a nephrologists' care.[5] Furthermore, patients with predialysis nephrologist care and functioning fistulae have significantly better survival and decreased hospitalization rates than those without nephrologist care and initiation with catheter.[6-8] We will review the important role of pharmacologic agents in preserving vascular access in the dialysis patient.

ENDOVASCULAR AND SURGICAL TECHNIQUES

It would be remiss not to mention the role of endovascular and surgical techniques in preserving arteriovenous access first before reviewing pharmacologic agents. Although it is out of the scope of this chapter and discussed in detail

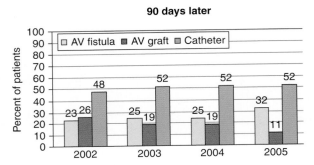

Figure 34-1. Graph from 2006 ESRD CPM Project[4] (Figure 30, p 36) shows percent of incident* adult in-center hemodialysis patients with different types of vascular access 90 days after initiation of dialysis (Reprinted with permission). *Incident patient defined as patient initiating in-center HD on or between January 1, 2005 and August 31, 2005.

elsewhere, we will give a brief overview. The KDOQI Work Group recommends prospective surveillance of arteriovenous access in order to permit the early detection of hemodynamic significant stenoses that may in turn lead to decreased access patency and/or thrombosis.[9] The Work Group recommends treatment of hemodynamically significant stenosis of arteriovenous fistulae and grafts with either endovascular or surgical techniques depending on the expertise of each dialysis center.[3] Although there is a paucity of robust clinical trials in this field, the comparison of surgical versus endovascular repair of thrombosed AVG have been reviewed in the literature. Historically, thrombosed and stenosed AVG were treated with mechanical thrombectomy and revision of the access, however, given the technological improvement and advantages of endovascular treatment, these surgical procedures have decreased dramatically. These advantages may include decreased morbidity, healthcare costs, and hospitalization rates.[10–12] Green et al performed the first meta-analysis comparing surgical versus endovascular treatment of thrombosed AVGs.[10] They showed that at 30, 60, and 90 days as well as at 1 year, the primary patency and technical success rate of surgery was significantly better than endovascular thrombectomy. The study, however, suffered from limitations of a lack of standard reporting methodology and an assessment of quality of analyzed studies. Furthermore, the poor technical success rate of 76% of endovascular thrombectomy does not mirror current rates and is likely responsible for the lower patency. More recently, Tordoir et al showed in their review, with current endovascular methods, technical success rates of 79% to 95%.[13] In their analysis of eight randomized trials and one meta-analysis, on AVG thrombosis, studies conducted before 2002 showed better technical success rates and primary patency of surgical versus endovascular treatment. However, after 2002, there has been a marked improvement of initial success rates (mean 92%), which has translated to comparable patency rates to surgery. One randomized trial reported AVG patency

at 30 and 90 days of 79% and 75%, respectively, for the endovascular group and 73% and 68% for the surgical group, respectively.[14] The authors attribute these recent findings to better thrombolytic devices and the use of potent thrombolytic agents such as tPA. Their review of thrombosed AVF revealed only population-based studies that showed comparable initial success rates for surgical versus endovascular intervention but a clear advantage of surgical over endovascular technique on 1-year primary and secondary patency. This advantage, however, is limited, by the anatomic location of the arteriovenous access, the surgical procedure performed, and experience in technique of each independent center. It goes without saying that the hemodialysis access circuit starts with the heart and ends with the heart, specifically the entire circuit including the artery and inflow, the access and outflow veins, and finally the central vasculature.[15] The prevalence of central venous stenosis whether from previous access or de novo has been recognized as a contraindication for ipsilateral placement of an arteriovenous access.[16] Endovascular techniques have largely replaced surgical management of these often inaccessible lesions and avoided complicated mediastinal surgeries. Whether endovascular interventions on the central veins definitively improve the patency of involved arteriovenous access remains to be seen.

TUNNELED DIALYSIS CATHETERS

▶ Epidemiology

Tunneled dialysis catheters for renal replacement therapy represent a major modality of vascular access in the United States. CVCs were first described as a form of hemodialysis (HD) access in 1959 by Teschan, which required venous cutdown into the saphenous vein to the inferior vena cava. Later, percutaneous methods of cannulation gained wide acceptance and reports surfaced in the early 1960s of the more "convenient" double-lumen cannula that was inserted in the femoral vein.[17,18] TDCs were later developed in the 1980s as an alternative to these temporary catheters. The newer catheters were more soft and pliable than the temporary catheters and provided greater blood flows as well as prevented higher rates of infection given the use of the tunnel and Dacron cuff.[19] Despite significant innovations along the way, after 50 years of hemodialysis access with catheters, this modality is still universally regarded as inadequate. Their associated complications are attended by tremendous morbidity, mortality, and cost to the health care system.[20] These complications include catheter-related bacteremia (CRB), thrombosis-related occlusion, venous stenosis, and dialysis inadequacy. Catheter dysfunction has a variety of definitions, ranging from decreased blood flow rates, frequent arterial and venous pressure alarms, poor conductance, and poor dialysis efficiency based on URR or K_t/V calculations.[9] Ultimately, the consequences of these parameters translate into diminished quality of dialysis that may affect mortality and morbidity as previously discussed.

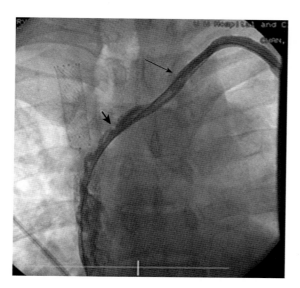

Figure 34-2. Central venogram via left internal jugular vein. Note extensive fibrin sheath from catheter tip (arrow) to superior vena cava (arrowhead).

► Pathophysiology

There are a myriad of causes of catheter dysfunction including patient positioning, mechanical kinking, malpositioning of catheter tip, leakage, drug precipitation, thrombus accumulation, and the growth of fibrin sheath.[21,22] Thrombus-related occlusion, which typically occurs as delayed, or late dysfunction, may occur with or without the presence of a fibrin sheath (Figure 34-2). Early dysfunction typically occurs with the mechanical problems previously mentioned but also may occur with early fibrin formation which can present within 24 hours of placement and occlude the lumen of the catheter or cause a vacuum effect preventing blood aspiration.[23,24] However, both are inexorably related to blood flow, mechanical and intimal vessel injury, and changes in patient-related coagulability.[25] Primary patency of TDCs has been reported to be 65–75% at 1 year.[26,27] Intraluminal or periluminal thrombosis has been reported as the primary reason for CVC dysfunction with 17–33% requiring untimely removal.[28] One large study showed that a majority of patients (51%) with tunneled CVCs develop thrombosis >30 days from time of implantation to catheter dysfunction.[29] Therefore, the pharmacologic inhibition of the coagulation cascade has been targeted as a distinct mode of prophylactic intervention. There have been a number of randomized prospective clinical trials that compare antiplatelet or anticoagulant therapy to control groups or placebo.[30–42]

► Clinical Studies

The first such study in 1998 by Buturović et al compared the efficacy of heparin, citrate, or polygeline in preventing catheter dysfunction in 30 patients.[30] Polygeline is a gelatin-based colloid previously used as a plasma expander. Patients were randomized into three groups and followed

for catheter failure and clot burden. There was no difference in catheter usage time or clot volume and the authors concluded that citrate or polygeline could be used as a filling solution in place of heparin without the risk of systemic anticoagulation. Schenk et al then compared recombinant tissue plasminogen activator (rTPA) with heparin for priming the Quinton Permcath in a prospective, randomized, crossover study.[31] He showed that flow was significantly improved in the rTPA group ($P = 0.0001$) and there was no clot formation or need for fibrinolysis compared to a 20–40% rate in the heparin group, respectively. However, the study was very small ($n = 12$) and suffered from a limited 4-month crossover design. Approximately a year later, Mokrzycki et al intended to show that low dose anticoagulation with warfarin could prevent fibrin sheath or thrombosis formation on tunneled hemodialysis catheters.[31] Their randomized, placebo-controlled trial of 105 patients showed with multivariate analysis that warfarin use (1 mg) and aspirin did not confer an improved thrombosis-free tunneled catheter survival as compared to placebo. This study did demonstrate a significant risk of late malfunction and incipient thrombosis when mean INR was less than 1.0 ($P = 0.04$, RR 4.0, 95% CI: 1.1–14.5; $P = 0.009$, RR 2.8, 95% CI: 1.3–6.1, respectively). Unfortunately, these results have never been reproduced and higher target INRs have never been shown to prevent catheter dysfunction without significant complications.[41]

Recently, Hemmelgarn et al reported on a pivotal randomized controlled trial on 225 patients across Canada comparing low dose (1 mg/lumen) rTPA once per week versus heparin (5000 U/mL) three times per week in catheter malfunction.[42] They showed that the rTPA group decreased catheter malfunction by 50% and surprisingly also CRB by two-thirds. This was the largest study to date showing such a significant benefit of a fibrinolytic agent on catheter patency and infection rates. However, the results are tempered by the fact that this was a study of early catheter dysfunction which most likely is caused by thrombotic occlusion and less likely a result of fibrin sheath which is much more difficult to prevent. Also, the incremental cost of using rTPA even once a week was almost $13,000 more than that of heparin per episode of catheter-related bacteremia prevented. Nevertheless, it was a very well-conducted study and sets the stage for more trials comparing rTPA with low-dose heparin, citrate, and other anticoagulants.

A number of studies have examined the use of citrate as an intraluminal catheter lock to prevent thrombosis-related catheter failure. Trisodium citrate has anticoagulant properties by chelating free ionized calcium making it unavailable to the coagulation cascade.[43] Weijmer et al compared trisodium citrate 30% with heparin 5000 U/mL in a multicenter, double-blind, randomized trial.[34] Their study showed no difference in catheter flow problems or premature removal for the heparin as compared to the citrate group (3.6 per 1000 catheter-days vs 3.2 per 1000 catheter-days; RR 0.92; 95% CI: 0.54–1.55; $P = 0.75$). Citrate also decreased the risk of CRB by 75%, which stopped the study prematurely. The authors conclude that citrate should be considered as an alternative agent to heparin as a catheter lock given its comparable patency, lower costs, and catheter-related bacteremia. More recently, Macrae et al demonstrated that even citrate 4% was as effective as heparin 5000 U/mL in episodes of catheter dysfunction as measured by access flow and use of fibrinolytics.[35] Given the potential for severe systemic complications associated with heparin use in the latter study, as well as by Yevzlin et al perhaps the time has come to abandon the use of concentrated heparin lock for thrombosis prevention.[44] All in all, however, the results of prophylactic therapies in inhibiting the accumulation of fibrin and thrombus in TDCs have generally been disappointing. Therefore, tremendous efforts have been placed on catheter avoidance strategies and preservation of vascular access for autogenous AVF placement.

ARTERIOVENOUS GRAFTS

▶ Epidemiology and Pathophysiology

Recent clinical studies have confirmed that arteriovenous fistulae prevalence has steadily risen and that arteriovenous graft prevalence has declined since 1998 as a result of KDOQI guideline recommendations and the Centers for Medicare and Medicaid (CMS) breakthrough initiative, "Fistula First."[5,45,46] However, in the United States, the poor early and long-term patency of both AVF and AVG remain a major challenge in the post-KDOQI era.[5,47–49] The primary cause of arteriovenous access dysfunction is turbulent flow primarily within stenotic lesions at the artery-to-vein or graft-to-vein anastomoses.[50–52]

It is this natural course of neointimal hyperplasia (NH) that induces AVGs to thrombose more readily; therefore, poorer patency rates as compared to autogenous AVF. Patency rates of (polytetrafluoroethylene) PTFE grafts range from 62% to 83% at 1 year and 50% to 77% at 2 years.[53] In AVGs, histological and immunohistochemical analysis of NH have revealed smooth muscle cell (SMC) and myofibroblast proliferation at the venous anastomosis and downstream vein.[54] Angiogenesis was prominent in the adventitia and neointima at these sites. In addition, there is increased growth factor expression by SMC, myofibroblasts, microvessels, and macrophages in these areas. In other models, cytokines related to oxidative stress have also been shown to be expressed in conjunction with growth factors.[55] A number of other inflammatory cytokines are also likely to play a role in this process of venous NH.[56]

Given this pathogenic mechanism for NH, local pharmacologic interventions are being tested such as a perivascular paclitaxel wrap, implantation of sirolimus-eluting collagen matrix, and administration of edifoligide, an E2F transcription factor decoy.[57–59] Other vasoactive drugs with the potential to regulate NH in AVGs such as calcium channel blockers, angiotensin-converting enzyme inhibitors, and recombinant human erythropoietin have been tried

with mixed results.[60–62] Perhaps all of these therapies may be successful in the short term in altering NH. However, long-term patency remains elusive and the ability to regulate NH, not just eradicate or prevent it for any potential benefit is unknown. Moreover, the lack of randomized clinical trials in NH makes it difficult to make conclusive arguments for or against these pharmacologic agents.

Antiplatelet and anticoagulant therapy, on the other hand, has been studied extensively in the prevention of AVG thrombosis in randomized clinical trials.[63–72] Not only do many of these agents block thromboxane synthesis and the coagulation cascade, but some even have antiproliferative effects locally.

▶ Clinical Studies

Wing et al first described utilizing warfarin to reduce clotting events in Scribner shunts, by targeting prothrombin times at 1.5 times control.[63] They showed a decrease in clotting episodes from one in every 2.6 patient months to one in every 8.6 patient months. However, the study design was a retrospective cohort and complications of hemorrhage were significant. This study likely set the stage for multiple historical landmark trials. Kaegi et al demonstrated in two randomized controlled trials, one in 1974 and the other in 1975, that sulfinpyrazone could decrease the incidence of thrombosis in straight siliconized rubber shunts.[64,65] Sulfinpyrazone is a uricosuric agent typically used for gout but previously used in cardiovascular and cerebral vascular events as an antiplatelet agent which inhibits cyclooxygenase. Its use in a 12-month randomized crossover study by Kaegi showed that there was an overall mean reduction of 0.43 thrombi per patient month ($P < 0.001$). This latter study was an interim analysis of their previous 6-month study that also demonstrated a decrease in thrombosis events and venous shunt revisions. Then, Harter et al studied the effects of 160 mg of aspirin in a double blind randomized controlled trial.[66] In this landmark study, 44 patients were randomized to aspirin or placebo, 25 patients were given placebo, and 19 patients were given aspirin. Over a period of 20-months, 32% patients on aspirin developed one or more thrombi and 72% in the placebo group ($P < 0.01$). Also, the total number of thrombi in the aspirin group was only 14 as compared to 53 in the placebo group. However, this study lacked sufficient sample size, follow-up time, and has never been reproduced in a long-term robust clinical trial. Not until 15 years later, did Sreedhara et al study the potential benefits of dipyridamole and aspirin in improving risk of thrombosis in PTFE grafts.[67] The mechanism of action of dipyridamole is thought to be inhibitory on vascular smooth muscle proliferation as well as a potent inhibitor of platelet aggregation via inhibition of cAMP-phosphodiesterase. In combination with aspirin, there appears to be a synergistic effect on decreasing vascular stenosis.[68] This study for the first time looked at two separate groups, that is, those patients with virgin PTFE grafts and those that already had grafts in place that had previously been thrombosed and revised or thrombectomized. They showed in 96 patients that completed the study protocol that aspirin alone conferred a higher risk of thrombosis than dipyridamole. Newly placed AVGs had cumulative thrombosis rates of 21% on dipyridamole alone, compared with 25% on dipyridamole and aspirin combination, 42% on placebo, and 80% on aspirin alone. Those patients that had previously thrombosed grafts had an overall 78% thrombosis rate and no difference in treatment groups. The authors concluded that in newly placed AVGs, there is a role to use dipyridamole with or without aspirin. However, even as the authors suggest, this was a single center study, and therefore results need to be replicated in larger, multicenter trials. It was not until another 15 years later, that Dixon et al accomplished this feat in their Dialysis Access Consortium (DAC) study.[68] This trial was originally designed to randomize 1056 subjects over 4 years with 6-months follow-up. Patients with newly placed AVG would receive a capsule (Aggrenox) of combination dipyridamole (200 mg) and aspirin (25 mg) to take twice daily or placebo. For the first time, primary unassisted patency was measured as the primary outcome and cumulative access patency as a secondary outcome. The study ultimately only enrolled 649 patients even with extending the enrollment period by one-half year. The duration of primary unassisted patency was increased with treatment of dipyridamole and aspirin (HR 0.82; 95% CI: 0.68–0.98; $P = 0.03$) as compared to placebo. Cumulative access patency, however, did not differ significantly between study groups. The main limitation of this study was the substantial 400 patient fewer enrollment target, which affects the generalizability of the study. The benefits of a modest 6 weeks in improved duration of primary patency have many questioning whether it is worth the cost and side effects to use these medications at all. Other studies including clopidogrel, clopidogrel and aspirin, fish oil, and warfarin have generated these same questions with varying results that still leave us to ponder if pharmacologic agents can truly offset the complex interactions of the coagulation cascade, inflammation, and hemodynamic mechanisms at play in NH.[69–73]

ARTERIOVENOUS FISTULAE

▶ Epidemiology and Pathophysiology

It remains a widely held belief that AVFs are superior to AVGs, and that both are superior to CVCs. Based on this vascular access hierarchy, the NKF K/DOQI guidelines have recommended the use of AVF, AVGs, and CVCs, in 50%, 40%, and 10%, respectively, in the U.S. prevalent hemodialysis population.[3] Indeed, the Fistula First campaign has stipulated that patients be referred to surgery for "fistula only" evaluations.[44] Primary patency rates of AVF after 5 years of placement are greater than 50%, whereas only 10% of AVGs are still patent.[74] While AVFs have been shown to be superior to AVGs and CVCs in terms of thrombosis, morbidity, and mortality in certain

hemodialysis populations, they continue to have a higher primary failure rate.[75–78] Because of this, many believe that the increased use of AVF may have contributed to the dramatic increase in the placement of CVCs since 1996.[79]

Again, NH has been characterized as the primary pathologic lesion in hemodialysis access fistulae that develop stenosis.[80] There is also evidence, though limited, that implicates NH in fistula nonmaturation.[81] In this study, human venous tissue obtained from three patents and one thrombosed AVF was examined. NH was present together with medial hypertrophy resulting in greater than 80% stenosis. The predominant cell type was myofibroblasts by immunohistochemistry. There are also studies that have described increased expression of TGF-β1, latent TGF-β1 binding protein-1 and TGF-β1 mRNA in stenotic AVF.[82,83] Interestingly, TGF-β1 increases plasminogen activator inhibitor-1 (PAI-1) expression and has in turn been shown to be higher in stenotic AVF and increase risk of access thrombosis.[84,85] Other studies have confirmed that higher levels of plasma fibrinogen and circulating activated platelets are associated with AVF failure.[86,87]

▶ Clinical Studies

Given these pathogenic mechanisms of NH and thrombosis, and their effect on the patency of AVF, a number of medications have been investigated. Unfortunately, there are only a handful of randomized clinical trials that have been accomplished.[88–95] At least in the United States, this was likely in part due to the waning interest of nephrologists in vascular access management in the 1960s and 1970s and the growth of AVG placement after Wilbert Gore patented the GoreTex/ePTFE in 1976.[96] Nevertheless, a number of population cohort studies such as the Dialysis Outcomes and Practice Patterns Study (DOPPS) examined primary and secondary AVF patency and its association with medication use, adjusted for multiple covariates.[97] In this study, 900 AVF in 802 patients showed that ACE inhibitors are associated with a 44% risk reduction ($P = 0.010$) in secondary patency rates. Other antiplatelet agents, such as clopidogrel, dipyridamole, and ticlopidine, failed to show statistically significant associations. Yevzlin et al later showed in an analysis of the USRDS Dialysis Morbidity and Mortality Study (DMMS) Wave 2 that the use of antiplatelet agents, ticlopidine, and dipyridamole (HR 3.54; $P = 0.04$) and aspirin (HR 2.49; $P = 0.005$) conferred a higher risk of AVF failure (Figure 34-3).[98] In another secondary analysis of the DOPPS, Hasegawa et al showed in 2815 incident hemodialysis patients that consistent aspirin use which was defined as using aspirin at baseline and 1 year later, was associated with decreased final AVF failure (aHR 0.63; 95% CI: 0.42–0.95, $P = 0.03$).[99] These mixed results confirm the limitations in database studies including selection and confounding biases which affect the generalizability of the results. The only large multicenter randomized clinical trial to date was published by Dember et al when they investigated the effects of clopidogrel on AVF failure.[91] This was named the DAC

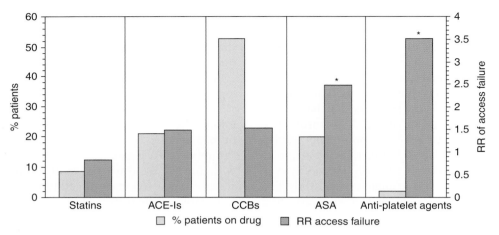

Figure 34-3. Risk of AVF failure and medication use. (Data from Saran,[97] reprinted with permission.)

Early Thrombosis AVF trial that was originally designed to randomize 1284 patients over a 4-year enrollment period. Patients were to receive either clopidogrel or placebo for 6 weeks after AVF creation and then followed for primary patency (thrombosis) at 6 weeks and for AVF suitability for dialysis. AVF suitability was defined as the ability to obtain adequate blood flows and cannulation during a 30-day suitability ascertainment period. Ultimately, 877 patients were randomized to receive placebo or a loading dose of 300 mg of clopidogrel 1-day after fistula placement and then 75 mg each day for 41 days. AVF thrombosis occurred in 53 (12.2%) patients assigned to clopidogrel compared with 84 (19.5%) patients assigned to placebo (RR, 0.63; 95% CI: 0.46–0.97; $P = 0.018$). Failure to attain suitability for dialysis did not differ between the clopidogrel and placebo groups. Although the data is fairly compelling in the significantly less early thrombosis of AVF, there are several limitations in the study. First, there was a very high primary failure rate of 61.8% and 59.6% in the clopidogrel and placebo groups, respectively. This is much higher than that reported in the literature and points to the fact that practice patterns and surgical expertise was not examined carefully. Second, even the authors point out that the statistical power was compromised given the 32% smaller sample size from target. Third, the primary outcome of primary failure or thrombosis by physical exam that the authors equate, may not in fact be apropos. Beathard showed that under angiographic examination, most AVF that do not mature are due to stenotic lesions rather than clot.[100] It is unlikely therefore, that antiplatelet medications such as clopidogrel would have real practical benefits in early AVF failure. Rather, surgical or endovascular therapies that correct these stenoses may have more efficacy than pharmacologic means in primary failure. The multifactorial cellular and signaling mechanisms and series of biological interactions that characterize NH are being studied extensively *in vitro* and *in vivo*. The biology of this "venopathy," whether it relates solely to the venous arm of the dialysis access or to more fundamental mechanisms of venous endothelial biology per se, has the potential to help us develop new pharmacologic and nonpharmacologic technologies to test out targeted therapies.

SUMMARY

Catheter-dependent (incident or prevalent) dialysis patients have steadily increased in numbers for a variety of reasons. Although it is an inferior form of access for dialysis, many patients rely on its use as their "lifeline." Catheter thrombosis and dysfunction diminish the quality of dialysis and is a major cause of access removal, which perpetuates a cycle of poor dialysis, morbidity, and mortality. Prophylactic medications have fallen short in improving catheter patency and therefore arteriovenous access is preferred.

Arteriovenous fistulae and grafts have mortality benefits over catheters; however, their patency rates are much to be desired. The Fistula First Initiative and efforts of the KDOQI have shifted the paradigm of vascular access use in the United States, however, primary failure rates are still high and catheter usage is still at more than 20%. Pharmacologic mechanisms to improve these patency rates have been disappointing and the number of robust clinical trials is few.

Early pre-ESRD nephrologist referral will be one of the key steps in integrating strategies to improve vascular access outcomes. Patients and providers will need to be engaged in novel educational and access planning programs with a multidisciplinary approach in order to accomplish this.

REFERENCES

1. Quinton W, Dillard D, Scribner BH. Cannulation of blood vessels for prolonged hemodialysis. *Trans Am Soc Artif Intern Organs.* 1960;6:104–113.
2. Forum of End Stage Renal Disease Networks, Available at: http://www.esrdnetworks.org/. Accessed July, 2010.
3. National Kidney Foundation: K/DOQI clinical practice guidelines for vascular access, 2000. *Am J Kidney Dis.* 2001;37:S137–S181.

4. 2006 Annual Report: ESRD Clinical Performance Measures Project. Department of Health and Human Services, Centers for Medicare & Medicaid Services, Office of Clinical Standards & Quality, Baltimore, MD: CMS, 2006.

5. US Renal Data System: USRDS 2009 Annual Data Report: Atlas of Chronic Kidney Disease and End-Stage Renal Disease in the United States. Bethesda, MD, National Institutes of Health, National Institute of Diabetes and Digestive and Kidney Diseases 2009.

6. Lorenzo V, Martn M, Rufino M, Hernandez D, Torres A, Ayus JC. Predialysis nephrologic care and a functioning arteriovenous fistula at entry are associated with better survival in incident hemodialysis patients: an observational cohort study. *Am J Kidney Dis.* 2004;43:999–1007.

7. Chan MR, Dall AT, Fletcher KE, Lu N, Trivedi H. Outcomes in patients with chronic kidney disease referred late to nephrologists: a meta-analysis. *Am J Med.* 2007;120:1063–1070.

8. Navaneethan SD, Nigwekar SU. Lack of permanent access in late referrals and its implications: not to be forgotten. *Am J Med.* 2008;121:e17; author reply e19.

9. National Kidney Foundation: K/DOQI clinical practice guidelines for vascular access, 2006. *Am J Kidney Dis.* 2006;48:S248–S257.

10. Green LD, Lee DS, Kucey DS. A metaanalysis comparing surgical thrombectomy, mechanical thrombectomy, and pharmacomechanical thrombolysis for thrombosed dialysis grafts. *J Vasc Surg.* 2002;36:939–945.

11. Sands JJ, Patel S, Plaviak DJ, Miranda CL. Pharmacomechanical thrombolysis with urokinase for treatment of thrombosed hemodialysis access grafts. A comparison with surgical thrombectomy. *ASAIO J.* 1994;40:M886–M888.

12. Tessitore N, Mansueto G, Lipari G, et al. Endovascular versus surgical preemptive repair of forearm arteriovenous fistula juxta-anastomotic stenosis: analysis of data collected prospectively from 1999 to 2004. *Clin J Am Soc Nephrol.* 2006;1:448–454.

13. Tordoir JH, Bode AS, Peppelenbosch N, van der Sande FM, de Haan MW. Surgical or endovascular repair of thrombosed dialysis vascular access: is there any evidence? *J Vasc Surg.* 2009;50:953–956.

14. Uflacker R, Rajagopalan PR, Selby JB, Hannegan C. Thrombosed dialysis access grafts: randomized comparison of the Amplatz thrombectomy device and surgical thromboembolectomy. *Eur Radiol.* 2004;14:2009–2014.

15. Asif A, Gadalean FN, Merrill D, et al. Inflow stenosis in arteriovenous fistulas and grafts: a multicenter, prospective study. *Kidney Int.* 2005;67:1986–1992.

16. Agarwal AK, Patel BM, Haddad NJ. Central vein stenosis: a nephrologist's perspective. *Semin Dial.* 2007;20:53–62.

17. Piazza A, Chanamé W, Cauti D. Double lumen percutaneous cannula for dialysis with the artificial kidney. *Trans Am Soc Artif Intern Organs.* 1964;10:136–139

18. Cimino JE. Historical perspective on more than 60 years of hemodialysis access. *Semin Vasc Surg.* 2007;20:136–140.

19. Schwab SJ, Beathard G. The hemodialysis catheter conundrum: hate living with them but can't live without them. *Kidney Int.* 1999;56:1–17.

20. Little MA, O'Riordan A, Lucey B, et al. A prospective study of complications associated with cuffed, tunneled haemodialysis catheters. *Nephrol Dial Transplant.* 2001;16:2194–2200.

21. Janne d'Othée B, Tham JC, Sheiman RG. Restoration of patency in failing tunneled hemodialysis catheters: a comparison of catheter exchange, exchange and balloon disruption of the fibrin sheath, and femoral stripping. *J Vasc Interv Radiol.* 2006;17:1011–1015.

22. Dinwiddie LC. Managing catheter dysfunction for better patient outcomes: a team approach. *Nephrol Nurs J.* 2004;31:653–660.

23. Leblanc M, Bosc JY, Paganini EP, Canaud B. Central venous dialysis catheter dysfunction. *Adv Ren Replace Ther.* 1997;4:377–389.

24. Schwab SJ, Beathard G. The hemodialysis catheter conundrum: hate living with them but can't live without them. *Kidney Int.* 1999;56:1–17.

25. Mandolfo S, Piazza W, Galli F. Central venous catheter and the hemodialysis patient: a difficult symbiosis. *J Vasc Access.* 2002;3:64–73.

26. Moss AH, Vasilakis C, Holley JL, Foulks CJ, Pillai K, McDowell DE. Use of a silicone dual-lumen catheter with a Dacron cuff as a long-term vascular access for hemodialysis patients. *Am J Kidney Dis.* 1990;16:211–215.

27. Gibson SP, Mosquera D. Five years experience with the Quinton Permcath for vascular access. *Nephrol Dial Transplant.* 1991;6:269–274.

28. Blankestijn P. Cuffed tunneled catheters for long-term vascular access. In: Conlon PJ, Nicholson M, Schwab S, eds. *Hemodialysis Vascular Access: Practice and Problems.* New York: Oxford University Press, 2001:67–84.

29. Moureau N, Poole S, Murdock MA, Gray SM, Semba CP. Central venous catheters in home infusion care: outcomes analysis in 50,470 patients. *J Vasc Interv Radiol.* 2002;13:1009–1916.

30. Buturović J, Ponikvar R, Kandus A, Boh M, Klinkmann J, Ivanovich P. Filling hemodialysis catheters in the interdialytic period: heparin versus citrate versus polygeline: a prospective randomized study. *Artif Organs.* 1998;22:945–947.

31. Schenk P, Rosenkranz AR, Wölfl G, Hörl WH, Traindl O. Recombinant tissue plasminogen activator is a useful alternative to heparin in priming quinton permcath. *Am J Kidney Dis.* 2000;35:130–136.

32. Mokrzycki MH, Jean-Jerome K, Rush H, Zdunek MP, Rosenberg SO. A randomized trial of minidose warfarin for the prevention of late malfunction in tunneled, cuffed hemodialysis catheters. *Kidney Int.* 2001;59:1935–1942.

33. Meeus G, Kuypers DR, Claes K, Evenepoel P, Maes B, Vanrenterghem Y. A prospective, randomized, double-blind crossover study on the use of 5% citrate lock versus 10% citrate lock in permanent hemodialysis catheters. *Blood Purif.* 2005;23:101–105.

34. Weijmer MC van den Dorpel MA, Van de Ven PJ, et al. CITRATE Study Group: Randomized, clinical trial comparison of trisodium citrate 30% and heparin as catheter-locking solution in hemodialysis patients. *J Am Soc Nephrol.* 2005;16:2769–2777.

35. Macrae JM, Dojcinovic I, Djurdjev O, et al. Citrate 4% versus heparin and the reduction of thrombosis study (CHARTS). *Clin J Am Soc Nephrol.* 2008;3:369–374.

36. Tumlin J, Goldman J, Spiegel DM, et al. A phase III, randomized, double-blind, placebo-controlled study of tenecteplase for improvement of hemodialysis

catheter function: TROPICS 3. *Clin J Am Soc Nephrol.* 2010;5:631–636.

37. Malo J, Jolicoeur C, Theriault F, Lachaine J, Senecal L. Comparison between standard heparin and tinzaparin for haemodialysis catheter lock. *ASAIO J.* 2010;56:42–47.

38. Power A, Duncan N, Singh SK, et al. Sodium citrate versus heparin catheter locks for cuffed central venous catheters: a single-center randomized controlled trial. *Am J Kidney Dis.* 2009;53:1034–1041.

39. Macrae JM, Loh G, Djurdjev O, et al. Short and long alteplase dwells in dysfunctional hemodialysis catheters. *Hemodial Int.* 2005;9:189–195.

40. Hendrickx L, Kuypers D, Evenepoel P, Maes B, Messiaen T, Vanrenterghem Y. A comparative prospective study on the use of low concentrate citrate lock versus heparin lock in permanent dialysis catheters. *Int J Artif Organs.* 2001;24:208–211.

41. Traynor JP, Walbaum D, Woo YM, Teenan P, Fox JG, Mactier RA. Low-dose warfarin fails to prolong survival of dual lumen venous dialysis catheters. *Nephrol Dial Transplant.* 2001;16:645.

42. Hemmelgarn BR, Moist LM, Lok CE, et al. Prevention of dialysis catheter malfunction with recombinant tissue plasminogen activator. *N Engl J Med.* 2011;364:303–12.

43. Ash SR, Mankus RA, Sutton JM, et al. Concentrated Sodium Citrate (23%) for Catheter Lock. *Hemodialysis Int.* 2000;4:22–31.

44. Yevzlin AS, Sanchez RJ, Hiatt JG, et al. Concentrated heparin lock is associated with major bleeding complications after tunneled hemodialysis catheter placement. *Semin Dial.* 2007;20:351–354.

45. National Vascular Access Improvement Initiative. Available at: http://www.fistulafirst.org/. Accessed August, 2010.

46. Pisoni RL, Young EW, Dykstra DM, et al. Vascular access use in Europe and the United States: results from the DOPPS. *Kidney Int.* 2002;61:305–316.

47. Biuckians A, Scott EC, Meier GH, Panneton JM, Glickman MH. The natural history of autologous fistulas as first-time dialysis access in the KDOQI era. *J Vasc Surg.* 2008;47:415–421.

48. Maya ID, Allon M. Outcomes of thrombosed arteriovenous grafts: Comparison of stents vs. angioplasty. *Kidney Int.* 2006;69:934–937.

49. Lilly RZ, Carlton D, Barker J, et al. Predictors of arteriovenous graft patency after radiologic intervention in hemodialysis patients. *Am J Kidney Dis.* 2001;37:945–953.

50. Saeed M, Newman GE, McCann RL, Sussman SK, Braun SD, Dunnick NR. Stenoses in dialysis fistulas: treatment with percutaneous angioplasty. *Radiology.* 1987;164:693–697.

51. Kanterman RY, Vesely TM, Pilgram TK, Guy BW, Windus DW, Picus D. Dialysis access grafts: anatomic location of venous stenosis and results of angioplasty. *Radiology.* 1995;195:135–139.

52. Beathard GA, Arnold P, Jackson J, Litchfield T. Physician Operators Forum of RMS Lifeline. Aggressive treatment of early fistula failure. *Kidney Int.* 2003;64:1487–1494.

53. Henrich WL, ed. *Principles and Practice of Dialysis.* Philadelphia, PA: Lippincott Williams & Wilkins; 2004

54. Roy-Chaudhury P, Kelly BS, Miller MA, et al. Venous neointimal hyperplasia in polytetrafluoroethylene dialysis grafts. *Kidney Int.* 2001; 59:2325–2334.

55. Weiss MF, Scivittaro V and Anderson JM. Oxidative stress and increased expression of growth factors in lesions of failed hemodialysis access. *Am J Kidney Dis.* 2001;37:970–980.

56. Rectenwald JE, Moldawer LL, Huber TS, Seeger JM, Ozaki CK. Direct evidence for cytokine involvement in neointimal hyperplasia. *Circulation.* 2000;102: 1697–1702.

57. Kelly B, Melhem M, Zhang J, et al. Perivascular paclitaxel wraps block arteriovenous graft stenosis in a pig model. *Nephrol Dial Transplant.* 2006;21:2425–2431.

58. Paulson WD, Kipshidze N, Kipiani K, et al. Safety and efficacy of locally eluted sirolimus for prolonging AV graft patency (PTFE graft plus Coll-R)-First in man experience. *J Am Soc Nephrol.* 2008; 19:252A.

59. Hoel AW, Conte MS. Edifoligide: a transcription factor decoy to modulate smooth muscle cell proliferation in vein bypass. *Cardiovasc Drug Rev.* 2007;25:221–234.

60. Martino MA, Vogel KM, O'Brien SP, Kerstein MD. Erythropoietin therapy improves graft patency with no increased incidence of thrombosis or thrombophlebitis. *J Am Coll Surg.* 1998;187:616–619.

61. Gradzki R, Dhingra RK, Port FK, Roys E, Weitzel WF, Messana JM. Use of ACE inhibitors is associated with prolonged survival of arteriovenous grafts. *Am J Kidney Dis.* 2001;38:1240–1244.

62. Pisoni R, Barker-Finkel J, Allon M. Statin therapy is not associated with improved vascular access outcomes. *Clin J Am Soc Nephrol.* 2010;5:1447–1450.

63. Wing AJ, Curtis JR, De Wardener HE. Reduction of clotting in Scribner shunts by long-term anticoagulation. *Br Med J.* 1967;3:143–145.

64. Kaegi A, Pineo GF, Shimizu A, Trivedi H, Hirsh J, Gent M. The role of sulfinpyrazone in the prevention of arterio-venous shunt thrombosis. *Circulation.* 1975;52:497–499.

65. Kaegi A, Pineo GF, Shimizu A, Trivedi H, Hirsh J, Gent M. Arteriovenous-shunt thrombosis. Prevention by sulfinpyrazone. *N Engl J Med.* 1974;290:304–306.

66. Harter HR, Burch JW, Majerus PW, et al. Prevention of thrombosis in patients on hemodialysis by low-dose aspirin. *N Engl J Med.* 1979;301:577–579.

67. Sreedhara R, Himmelfarb J, Lazarus JM, Hakim RM. Anti-platelet therapy in graft thrombosis: results of a prospective, randomized, double-blind study. *Kidney In.* 1994;45:1477–1483.

68. Dixon BS, Beck GJ, Vazquez MA, et al. Effect of dipyridamole plus aspirin on hemodialysis graft patency. *N Engl J Med.* 2009;360:2191–2201.

69. Schmitz PG, McCloud LK, Reikes ST, Leonard CL, Gellens ME. Prophylaxis of hemodialysis graft thrombosis with fish oil: double-blind, randomized, prospective trial. *J Am Soc Nephrol.* 2002;13:184–190.

70. Bowden RG, Wilson RL, Gentile M, Ounpraseuth S, Moore P, Leutholtz BC. Effects of omega-3 fatty acid supplementation on vascular access thrombosis in polytetrafluorethylene grafts. *J Ren Nutr.* 2007; 17:126–131.

71. Kaufman JS, O'Connor TZ, Zhang JH, et al. Randomized controlled trial of clopidogrel plus aspirin to prevent hemodialysis access graft thrombosis. *J Am Soc Nephrol.* 2003;14:2313–2321.

72. Trimarchi H, Young P, Forrester M, Schropp J, Pereyra H, Freixas E. Clopidogrel diminishes hemodialysis access graft thrombosis. *Nephron Clin Pract.* 2006;102:c128–c132.

73. Crowther MA, Clase CM, Margetts PJ, et al. Low-intensity warfarin is ineffective for the prevention of PTFE graft failure in patients on hemodialysis: a randomized controlled trial. *J Am Soc Nephrol.* 2002;13:2331–2337.

74. Mehta S. Statistical summary of clinical results of vascular access procedures for haemodialysis, in Vascular Access fro Hemodilaysis-II, edited by Summer B, Henry M, W.L. Gore & Associates, 1991;145–157.

75. Allon M, Robbin ML. Increasing arteriovenous fistulas in hemodialysis patients: problems and solutions. *Kidney Int.* 2002;62:1109–1124.

76. Feldman HI, Kobrin S, Wasserstein A. Hemodialysis vascular access morbidity. *J Am Soc Nephrol.* 1996;7:523–535.

77. Schwab SJ, Harrington JT, Singh A, et al. Vascular access for hemodialysis. *Kidney Int.* 1999;55:2078–2090.

78. Dhingra RK, Young EW, Hulbert-Shearon TE, Leavey SF, Port FK. Type of vascular access and mortality in U.S. hemodialysis patients. *Kidney Int.* 2001;60:1443–1451.

79. Levey A, Coresh J, Balk E, et al. National Kidney Foundation practice guidelines for chronic kidney disease: evaluation, classification, and stratification. *Ann Intern Med.* 2003;139:137–147.

80. Chang CJ, Ko PJ, Hsu LA, et al. Highly increased cell proliferation activity in the restenotic hemodialysis vascular access after percutaneous transluminal angioplasty: implication in prevention of restenosis. *Am J Kidney Dis.* 2004;43:74–84.

81. Roy-Chaudhury P, Arend L, Zhang J, et al. Neointimal hyperplasia in early arteriovenous fistula failure. *Am J Kidney Dis.* 2007;50:782–790.

82. Stracke S, Konner K, Köstlin I, et al. Increased expression of TGF-beta1 and IGF-I in inflammatory stenotic lesions of hemodialysis fistulas. *Kidney Int.* 2002;61:1011–1019.

83. Ikegaya N, Yamamoto T, Takeshita A, et al. Elevated erythropoietin receptor and transforming growth factor-{beta}1 expression in stenotic arteriovenous fistulae used for hemodialysis. *J Am Soc Nephrol.* 2000;11:928–935.

84. De Marchi S, Falleti E, Giacomello R, et al. Risk factors for vascular disease and arteriovenous fistula dysfunction in hemodialysis patients. *J Am Soc Nephrol.* 1996;7: 1169–1177.

85. Lazo-Langner A, Knoll GA, Wells PS, Carson N, Rodger MA. The risk of dialysis access thrombosis is related to the transforming growth factor-beta1 production haplotype and is modified by polymorphisms in the plasminogen activator inhibitor-type 1 gene. *Blood.* 2006;108:4052–4058.

86. Chuang YC, Chen JB, Yang LC, Kuo CY. Significance of platelet activation in vascular access survival of haemodialysis patients. *Nephrol Dial Transplant.* 2003;18:947–954.

87. Song IS, Yang WS, Kim SB, Lee JH, Kwon TW, Park JS. Association of plasma fibrinogen concentration with vascular access failure in hemodialysis patients. *Nephrol Dial Transplant.* 1999;14:137–141.

88. Fiskerstrand CE, Thompson IW, Burnet ME, Williams P, Anderton JL. Double-blind randomized trial of the effect of ticlopidine in arteriovenous fistulas for hemodialysis. *Artif Organs.* 1985;9:61–63.

89. Gröntoft KC, Larsson R, Mulec H, Weiss LG, Dickinson JP. Effects of ticlopidine in AV-fistula surgery in uremia. Fistula Study Group. *Scand J Urol Nephrol.* 1998;32:276–283.

90. Gröntoft KC, Mulec H, Gutierrez A, Olander R. Thromboprophylactic effect of ticlopidine in arteriovenous fistulas for haemodialysis. *Scand J Urol Nephrol.* 1985;19:55–57.

91. Dember LM, Beck GJ, Allon M, et al. Effect of clopidogrel on early failure of arteriovenous fistulas for hemodialysis: a randomized controlled trial. *JAMA.* 2008;299: 2164–2171.

92. Andrassy K, Malluche H, Bornefeld H, Comberg M, Ritz E, Jesdinsky H, Möhring K. Prevention of p.o. clotting of av. cimino fistulae with acetylsalicyl acid: Results of a prospective double blind study. *Klin Wochenschr.* 1974;52(7):348–349.

93. Michie DD, Wombolt DG. Use of sulfinpyrazone to prevent thrombus formation in arteriovenous fistulas and bovine grafts of patients on chronic hemodialysis. *Curr Ther Res Clin Exp.* 1977;22:196–204.

94. Albert FW, Schmidt U, Harzer R. Postoperative thromboprophylaxis for Cimino-fistulae with sulfinpyrazone in comparison to acetylsalicylic acid. *Krankenhausarzt.* 1978;51:712–718.

95. Janicki K, Bojarska SA, Pietura R, Janicka L. Preventive effects of ticlopidine on the incidence of late A-V fistula thrombosis complications in haemodialyses patients. *Annales Universitatis Mariae Curie Sklodowska Sectio D: Medicina.* 2003;58:215–218.

96. Sachdeva B, Abreo K. The history of interventional nephrology. *Adv Chronic Kidney Dis.* 2009; 16:302–308.

97. Saran R, Dykstra DM, Wolfe RA, Gillespie B, Held PJ, Young EW. Dialysis Outcomes and Practice Patterns Study. Association between vascular access failure and the use of specific drugs: the Dialysis Outcomes and Practice Patterns Study (DOPPS). *Am J Kidney Dis.* 2002;40:1255–1263.

98. Yevzlin AS, Conley EL, Sanchez RJ, Young HN, Becker BN. Vascular access outcomes and medication use: a USRDS study. *Semin Dial.* 2006;19:535–539.

99. Hasegawa T, Elder SJ, Bragg-Gresham JL, et al. Consistent aspirin use associated with improved arteriovenous fistula survival among incident hemodialysis patients in the dialysis outcomes and practice patterns study. *Clin J Am Soc Nephrol.* 2008;3:1373–1378.

100. Beathard GA, Arnold P, Jackson J, Litchfield T. Aggressive treatment of early fistula failure. *Kidney Int.* 2003;64:1487–1494.

35

SEDATION AND ANALGESIA FOR ENDOVASCULAR PROCEDURES

GERALD A. BEATHARD

LEARNING OBJECTIVES

1. Describe the features of the various levels of the depth of sedation.
2. Describe the components of a proper patient safety protocol as it relates to the performance of endovascular procedures.
3. Understand the importance of a close adherence to the patient safety protocol.
4. Describe the patient preevaluation as it is related to airway assessment.
5. Describe the General Clinical Status (GCS) scoring system and its use.
6. Define the American Society of Anesthesiology Physical Status system and its relevance.
7. Discuss intraprocedure patient monitoring, its components, and methods of accomplishment.
8. Define contemporaneous recording of monitored parameters and its importance.
9. Discuss criteria for the discharge of a patient from recovery following an endovascular procedure.
10. Discuss the actions and side-effects of the medications commonly used for sedation/analgesia in interventional nephrology practice.
11. Understand the importance of titrating sedation/analgesia medications.
12. Discuss the action and uses of reversal agents for the sedation/analgesia medication commonly used.

SEDATION

All hemodialysis patients, but especially those whose treatments are provided via a catheter or synthetic graft are subject to recurrent problems, necessitating repeated trips to an interventional facility. Pain management through effective sedation/analgesia becomes an important aspect of the conduct of these procedures; however, this aspect of management carries with it a degree of risk. This risk may be enhanced in this population of patients because the nature of their basic disease and the associated comorbidities. Additionally, an unpleasant episode or one associated with pain and discomfort adds greatly to the anxiety and stress associated with subsequent episodes of access dysfunction.

▶ Sedation and Analgesia

"Sedation and analgesia" describes a specific sedated state that allows a patient to tolerate unpleasant procedures while maintaining adequate cardiorespiratory functions and the ability to respond purposely to verbal command and/or tactile stimulation.[1] With appropriate sedation/analgesia, the patient retains the ability to maintain their airway independently and continuously and to respond appropriately to physical stimulation and verbal command. Although this is quite different from anesthesia, it definitively creates an increased level of risk to the patient.

▶ Definitions

In order to administer and manage sedation/analgesia, it is important that certain definitions be understood (Table 35-1).

TABLE 35–1

Depth of Sedation Continuum[1]

	Minimal Sedation (Anxiolysis)	Moderate Sedation/ Analgesia (Conscious Sedation)	Deep Sedation/Analgesia	General Anesthesia
Responsiveness	Normal response to Verbal stimulation	Purposeful* response to verbal or tactile stimulation	Purposeful* response after repeated or painful stimulation	Unarousable, even with painful stimulus
Airway	Unaffected	No intervention required	Intervention may be required	Intervention often required
Spontaneous Ventilation	Unaffected	Adequate	May be adequate	Frequently inadequate
Cardiovascular Function	Unaffected	Usually maintained	Usually maintained	May be impaired

*Reflex withdrawal from a painful stimulus is not considered a purposeful response.

Minimal sedation (anxiolysis)

Minimal sedation is a drug-induced state during which patients respond normally to verbal commands. Although cognitive function and coordination may be somewhat impaired, ventilatory and cardiovascular functions are unaffected. This is basically a state of decreased anxiety.

Moderate sedation/analgesia (conscious sedation)

Moderate sedation/analgesia is a drug-induced depression of consciousness during which patients respond purposefully to verbal commands, either alone or accompanied by light tactile stimulation. No interventions are required to maintain a patent airway, and spontaneous ventilation is adequate. Cardiovascular function is usually maintained. This state is often referred to as conscious sedation.

Deep sedation/analgesia

Deep sedation/analgesia is a drug-induced depression of consciousness during which patients cannot be easily aroused but respond purposefully following repeated or painful stimulation. The ability to independently maintain ventilatory function may be somewhat impaired. There is a potential for patients to require assistance in maintaining a patent airway, and spontaneous ventilation may be inadequate. Cardiovascular function is usually maintained.

General anesthesia

General anesthesia is a drug-induced loss of consciousness during which patients are not arousable, even by painful stimulation. The ability to independently maintain ventilatory function is often impaired. Patients require assistance in maintaining a patent airway, and positive pressure ventilation may be required because of depressed spontaneous ventilation or drug-induced depression of neuromuscular function. Cardiovascular function may also be impaired.

Even though four distinct states of sedation can be defined, it is important to realize that sedation is actually a continuum. Each patient is an individual and it is not always possible to predict how an individual will respond. Therefore, it is critical that practitioners intending to produce a given level of sedation be able to rescue patients whose level of sedation becomes deeper than initially intended. The goal for the interventionalist performing dialysis access procedures is patient comfort. What is required to accomplish this goal will vary according to the procedure and the tolerance of the patient upon whom the procedure is being performed. It is important that individual variations be taken into consideration. In actuality, in the vascular access interventional facility, the first three of these categories will be used to some varying degree. It is unlikely that general anesthesia will ever be applied. To do this would require special equipment, supplies, and personnel (anesthesiologist) that are not typically included in such a facility.

▶ Patient Safety Protocol

The complications associated with dialysis vascular access interventional procedures done with sedation/analgesia fall into two categories, those associated with the performance of the procedure and those that might result from the use of the drugs that are administered. The nephrologist working in a free-standing outpatient facility dealing with hemodialysis patients, administering sedation/analgesia presents several issues of potential concern. First, the patient is being cared for away from a hospital setting; second, sedation/analgesia is being administered by a nonanesthesia trained physician; and third, hemodialysis patients have a high incidence of comorbidities that could make them at high risk for these types of procedures.

The physician who administers sedation/analgesia must be experienced in the use of the necessary drugs and the ability to recognize and deal with the complications that might ensue. Expertise in airway management is essential. The use of a carefully designed patient safety protocol is important.[1]

▶ **Patient Presedation/Analgesia Evaluation**

A careful evaluation of the patient should be conducted prior to any procedure that might require sedation/analgesia. This is necessary to assure that the patient has no unforeseen risks and to minimize the chances of a complication.

Medical history and physical examination

Positive pressure ventilation, with or without tracheal intubation, may be necessary if respiratory compromise develops during sedation–analgesia. This may be more difficult in patients with atypical airway anatomy. In addition, some airway or breathing abnormalities may increase the likelihood of airway problems during spontaneous ventilation. Appropriate preprocedure evaluation (history and physical examination) increases the likelihood of satisfactory sedation and decreases the likelihood of adverse outcomes for both moderate and deep sedation.

Physicians administering sedation/analgesia should be familiar with sedation-oriented aspects of the patient's medical history (Table 35-2) and how these might alter the patient's response to sedation/analgesia.[1] These include: (1) abnormalities of the major organ systems; (2) previous adverse experience with sedation/analgesia as well as regional and general anesthesia; (3) drug allergies, current medications, and potential drug interactions; (4) time and nature of last oral intake; and (5) history of tobacco, alcohol, or substance use or abuse.

Patients presenting for sedation/analgesia should undergo a focused physical examination (Table 35-2), including vital signs, auscultation of the heart and lungs, and evaluation of the airway. These evaluations should be confirmed immediately before sedation is initiated. In this evaluation, one is looking for evidence of issues that adversely affect respiratory function and issues that make airway management more difficult should an adverse event occur. Positive pressure ventilation, with or without tracheal intubation, may be necessary if respiratory compromise develops during sedation/analgesia. This may be more difficult in patients with atypical airway anatomy. In addition, some airway abnormalities may increase the likelihood of airway obstruction during spontaneous ventilation. If the patient cannot be easily intubated, one might elect to have the case done at the hospital, if significant sedation is going to be required.

The question is—what can be reasonably done that would suffice for this evaluation and still not be difficult or time consuming to accomplish. The following quick examination has been recommended:[2]

- Check to see if the patient can open their mouth widely. One should be able to insert two large fingers (three small ones) between the incisors (Figure 35-1). This indicates the mobility of the TM joint.

- Have the patient protrude their tongue. They should be able to do this maximally; the posterior pharynx should be clearly visible. This will indicate how easily the laryngoscope can be inserted. Some anesthesiologists use the

TABLE 35–2
History and Physical for Airway Assessment

History
  Previous problems with anesthesia or sedation
  Stridor, snoring or sleep apnea
  Advanced rheumatoid arthritis
Physical examination
  Habitus
    Significant obesity (especially involving the neck and facial structures)
  Head and neck
    Short neck
      Decreased hyoid-mental* distance, or (should be at least 4 cm or 3 finger breadths)
      Decreased thyroid-mental† distance (should be at least 6.5 cm or 4 finger breadths)
  Limited neck extension
  Cervical spine disease
Mouth
  Small opening (should be 2 large finger breadths or 3 cm‡ between upper and lower incisors)
  High Mallampati score
  Edentulous
  Protruding incisors
  Loose or capped teeth
  Dental appliance
  High, arched palate
Jaw
  Temporomandibular joint disease
  Micrognathia
  Significant malocclusion

*Measurement of midline distance from hyoid to chin (mental).
†Measurement of midline distance from thyroid cartilage to chin (mental).
‡Opened maximally.

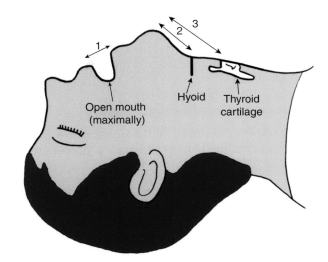

Figure 35-1. (1) Size of mouth should be two large finger breaths or 3 cm when opened maximally. (2) Hyoid-mental distance should be at least three finger breaths or 4 cm. (3) Thyroid-mental distance should be 4 finger breaths or 6.5 cm.

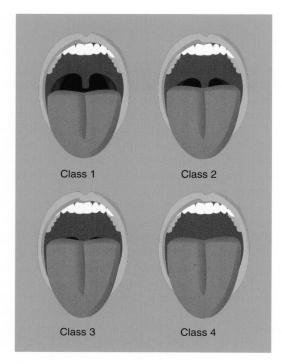

Figure 35-2. Mallampati classification.

Mallampati score to predict the ease of oropharyngeal intubation.[3] This classification is determined by looking at the anatomy of the oral cavity. Based upon the visibility of the base of uvula, faucial pillars (the arches in front of and behind the tonsils), and soft palate, one of four classes is assigned (Figure 35-2 and Table 35-3). A high Mallampati score (class 4) is associated with more difficult intubation.

- Check to see if the patient can move their jaw forward and from side to side. This will indicate how easily the laryngoscope can be manipulated once inserted.
- Check to determine if the patient can flex their neck fully (touch chin to chest) and extend fully. This degree of mobility is important to the process of intubation. Some anesthesiologists recommend measuring either the hyoid-mental[4] or thyroid-mental distance[5] (Figure 35-1 and Table 35-2).

General clinical status (GCS) score

It is important to evaluate and document the patient's general clinical status before, and after a procedure. The risk of the procedure and more importantly the risk of sedation/analgesia relate directly to the patient's overall clinical status. It is suggested that two systems be used—a General Clinical Status system and the American Society of Anesthesiologists Physical Status (ASA-PS) Classification system.

General clinical status (GCS) score A clinical scale assigning numeric values to parameters indicating a patient's status prior to treatment, changes during the procedure, and progress during recovery is of much greater value than merely charting vital signs with accompanying nurse's notes. A numerical scale is more easily understood and transmitted to others. It allows for more accurate communicate using a common defined language. The Aldrete Scoring System has been used in anesthesiology for more than 30 years,[6] but is outdated and includes factors that may have very little relationship to recovery from anesthesia in general and to the hemodialysis patient specifically. A three-level numerical clinical scoring system that included five parameters—consciousness, airway status, oxygen saturation, movement, and ambulation—has been developed specifically for use with dialysis patients undergoing sedation/analgesia.[7] This is referred to as the General Clinical Status (GCS). This classification system (Table 35-4) includes several factors listed as individual complications, but in this system they are utilized in a composite fashion to convey the patient's overall physical status. This classification

TABLE 35–3	
Mallampati Score	
Class 1: Full visibility of tonsils, uvula, and soft palate	
Class 2: Visibility of hard and soft palate, upper portion of tonsils, and uvula	
Class 3: Soft and hard palate and base of the uvula are visible	
Class 4: Only hard palate visible	

TABLE 35–4	
General Clinical Status (GCS)	
Criterion	**Score**
Consciousness	
Awake or at baseline	2
Responding to stimuli	1
Not responding	0
Airway	
Coughing on command or at baseline	2
Maintaining good airway	1
Airway requires maintenance	0
Oxygen saturation	
92% or greater, or at baseline or better	2
90% or greater on supplemental O_2	1
Less than 90% on supplemental O_2	0
Movement	
Movement purposeful or at baseline	2
Nonpurposeful movement	1
Not moving	0
Ambulation	
Ambulate unassisted or at baseline	2
Ambulate only with assistance	1
Unable to ambulate	0
Total	Score

TABLE 35–5

American Society of Anesthesiologists Physical Status Classification

Class I: Patient has no systemic disturbance (eg, healthy and no medical problems)
Class II: Patient has mild to moderate systemic disturbance (eg, hypertension and diabetes).
Class III: Patient has severe systemic disturbance (eg, heart disease that limits activity).
Class IV: Patient has severe systemic disturbance that is life threatening (eg, unstable angina and active congestive heart failure).
Class V: Patient is moribund and has little chance of survival (eg, ruptured abdominal aortic aneurysm).
Class VI: Patient who has been declared brain dead and having procedure for organ donation.

should be performed before and after a procedure at a minimum in order to quantitate changes that might have occurred.

American society of anesthesiologists physical status (ASA-PS) classification The ASA-PS Classification (Table 35-5) was developed and is routinely used to facilitate risk assessment for perioperative morbidity and mortality. It consists of six classes that are based upon the patient's physical and medical status. The sixth category relates only to procedures involving organ donation, therefore it is useful to think in terms of five categories for our purposes. This system is also useful in documenting the overall status of patients having interventional procedures. It has been shown in a number of studies to have a high level of correlate with the risk of surgical procedures in individual patients.

Preprocedure fasting

Sedatives and analgesics tend to impair airway reflexes in proportion to the degree of sedation–analgesia achieved. There is a lack of good evidence to show that preprocedure fasting results in a decreased incidence of adverse outcomes in patients undergoing either moderate or deep sedation.[1] However, it is generally felt that fasting probably does decreases risks during moderate sedation and definitively decreases risks during deep sedation. In situations, when preprocedure fasting is not practical or one is dealing with an urgent situation, the target level of sedation should be modified (ie, less sedation should be administered). If preprocedure fasting is felt to be necessary it should consist of 2 hours for clear liquids and 6 hours for a light meal.[1] Although these times do not totally guarantee that the stomach will be empty, they are felt to be adequate for most cases. It is to be noted that fasting can often cause a slight increase in the serum potassium level due to the lack of normal insulin response to food.

▶ **Intraprocedure Evaluation and Monitoring**

Issues that are important are:

Supplemental oxygen

Equipment to administer supplemental oxygen should be present when sedation/analgesia is administered. Supplemental oxygen should be administered for all cases in which sedation/analgesia is used. In general, nasal oxygen at 2 L/min is appropriate.

Intravenous access

In patients receiving sedation/analgesia, vascular access is mandatory and should be maintained throughout the procedure and until the patient is no longer at risk for cardiorespiratory depression.[1] This generally means a dedicated intravenous line, peripheral or central. However, dialysis access procedures are somewhat unique in that as a general rule, they cannot be done unless vascular access is established for the purposes of the treatment. This access can then be used for the purposes of administering medications, both for sedation/analgesia or to manage adverse events. Since there is no pressing need for vascular access until the medications are given and medications are not needed until the procedure begins, a dedicated intravenous line is not necessary in these cases.

Monitoring

The use of sedation/analgesia creates a mandatory requirement for careful patient monitoring (Table 35-6). This is true for all patient categories; however, it is especially critical for the types of patients who are being treated in a dialysis vascular access interventional facility. It may not be possible for the individual performing a procedure to be fully cognizant of the patient's condition during sedation/analgesia. However, the physician is responsible for the patient's welfare and must be kept constantly aware of their status.

Availability of monitoring nurse The availability of a nurse to monitor the patient's status improves patient comfort

TABLE 35–6

Monitored Variables During Sedation/Analgesia

From the patient
    Level of consciousness
    Sensation of pain
    Quality of respirations
    Respiratory rate
From the monitor
    Pulse oximeter
    Cardiac rhythm
    Heart rate
    Blood pressure

and satisfaction and reduces the risk of adverse events and should be considered mandatory. It is recommended that during the procedure, the nurse be constantly present with the primary duty of carrying out this responsibility. During deep sedation, this individual should have no other responsibilities. However, during moderate sedation, this individual may assist with minor, interruptible tasks once the patient's level of sedation–analgesia and vital signs have stabilized, provided that adequate monitoring for the patient's level of sedation is maintained.[1]

In addition to watching the patient monitor screen, this nurse should be positioned so that the patient's face can be observed. Pain is an important variable and often this is expressed only by facial grimacing that can go undetected unless this is being monitored. Additionally, changes in pulmonary ventilation can frequently be detected early if the patient's ventilatory function is being monitored by observation.

The monitoring nurse should understand the pharmacology of the agents that are administered, as well as the role of pharmacologic antagonists for opioids and benzodiazepines. Additionally, they should be able to recognize the complications associated with sedation/analgesia.

Level of consciousness The response of patients to commands during procedures performed with sedation/analgesia serves as a guide to their level of consciousness. Spoken responses also provide an indication that the patients are breathing. Patients whose only response is reflex withdrawal from painful stimuli are deeply sedated, approaching a state of general anesthesia, and should be treated accordingly.[1] Patients can experience cardiovascular decompensation or cerebral hypoxia as a result of over sedation or as a consequence of an idiosyncratic reaction to drugs (eg, radio-contrast) that are administered during the procedure. The timely detection and treatment of these complications is dependent upon careful patient monitoring.

Pulmonary ventilation The primary causes of morbidity associated with sedation/analgesia are drug-induced respiratory depression and airway obstruction.[1] This must be monitored carefully. Monitoring of ventilatory function by observation will reduce the risk of adverse outcomes associated with sedation/analgesia.

Oxygenation Oximetry monitoring effectively detects oxygen desaturation and hypoxemia in patients who are administered sedatives/analgesics. Early detection of hypoxemia through the use of oximetry during sedation/analgesia decreases the likelihood of adverse outcomes such as cardiac arrest and death. Hypoxemia during sedation/analgesia is more likely to be detected by oximetry than by clinical assessment alone.[1]

Hemodynamics Sedative/analgesia drugs can blunt the appropriate autonomic compensation for hypovolemia and procedure-related stresses. Additionally, if sedation/analgesia is inadequate, patients may develop potentially harmful autonomic stress responses (eg, hypertension and

tachycardia). Early detection of changes in patients' heart rate and blood pressure is important. The physician needs to be able to detect problems and intervene in a timely fashion, reducing the risk of these complications. Regular monitoring of vital signs reduces the likelihood of adverse outcomes during both moderate and deep sedation. Vital signs should be monitored at 5-minute intervals once a stable level of sedation is established.[1] Continuous electrocardiography is also important to reducing the risks of sedation/analgesia.

Pain Pain monitoring during the procedure is important.[1] As stated above, pain can lead to potentially harmful autonomic stress responses. It is also important for humane reasons. Patients need to be as comfortable as possible during the procedure. Repeat procedures are to be expected for the dialysis patient as part of vascular access management. An unpleasant experience will serve to increase the level of anxiety that the patient will experience on return visits. If the initial dose of sedation/analgesia agent is inadequate, detection of pain will indicate the need for additional medication. If the procedure time is prolonged, a painful response on the part of the patient will indicate the need for a repeat dose. This will be recognized only if pain is being monitored.

Recording of monitored parameters

Contemporaneous recording (either automatic or manual) of monitored parameters is important.[1] One should not rely on memory to record values after the procedure. Scribbled notes on a piece of scrap paper are not much better. Unless technically impossible to accomplish, vital signs and respiratory variables should be recorded before initiating sedation/analgesia, after administration of sedative/analgesic medications, at regular intervals during the procedure, on initiation of recovery, and immediately before discharge. The frequency for assessed and recorded monitored parameters should be based upon the type and amount of medication administered, the length of the procedure, and the general condition of the patient.

Pharmacologic antagonists

No sedation/analgesia should ever be administered unless the pharmacological antagonist for the drug(s) used is readily and immediately available.[1] This should be taken to mean that the drug is setting out and available for immediate access, not in a locked cabinet. When there is a need for reversal of sedation/analgesia, it is because there is an emergent problem. Delay can lead to anoxia and the risk on neurological injury.

Availability of crash cart

The immediate availability of a "crash cart" with equipment for establishing a patent airway, including intubation, and providing positive pressure ventilation with supplemental oxygen is required whenever sedation/analgesia is administered.[1] Suction and a defibrillator in good working order should be on the cart. A full battery of resuscitation medications should also be considered essential supplies for this piece of emergency equipment.

It is not enough to simply have a full supplied and equipped "crash cart" available, it must be totally functional with current medications. This will mean that a protocol for checking, inventorying, and updating supplies and equipment should be in place. In general, the "crash cart" should be checked at the beginning of each day.

▶ Postprocedure Patient Management

After a procedure requiring sedation/analgesia is completed, the patient should be sent to a recovery area where continuous monitoring and resuscitative equipment are available. Patients need to recover fully to their presedation level of consciousness and exhibit stable vital signs and intact protective reflexes prior to discharge. The patient's GCS score should be compared to that obtained prior to the procedure to assure that they have returned to their baseline status. If they have not, a careful evaluation should be made to determine the reason. The patient should not be discharged until they are fully and completely recovered.

A responsible adult should be available to drive the patient home. If the patient is to go directly to the dialysis facility for treatment, a responsible adult should accompany them. It is also important that the dialysis nurse be knowledgeable in the effects of the medications that were used and be experienced in monitoring patients following sedation/analgesia. A protocol should be developed for patient discharge that specifies the discharge criteria (Table 35-7) that must be met prior to the patient leaving the recovery area.[1]

MEDICATIONS FOR SEDATION/ANALGESIA

It is imperative that every physician who administers sedation/analgesia have a good working knowledge of the medications that they plan to administer—their appropriate dosages, side effects, and how to reverse inadvertent over sedation should that occur.[1] There are important caveats that should be followed when using sedation/

TABLE 35–7
Discharge Criteria
Stable vital signs and oxygen saturation level
Swallow, cough, gag reflexes present, or appropriate to baseline
Alert or appropriate to baseline
Able to sit unaided or appropriate to baseline
Walk with assistance or appropriate to baseline
Minimal nausea and dizziness
Dressing/procedure site checked
Standard time set in protocol has elapsed

TABLE 35–8
General Caveats of Sedation/Analgesia
Avoid using a "recipe"—no two patients will react the same, individualize
Use reduced doses in patients that are:
Elderly
Small
Debilitated
Hypovolemic
Have COPD
Have sleep apnea
Be aware of the synergistic effects between narcotics and other sedatives
Give only the medication that is needed when it is needed
Titrate all drugs according to desired clinical response

analgesia (Table 35-8). Patients differ considerably in their responses to similar doses of these medications. Additionally, many patients especially dialysis patients have a variety of comorbidities that must be taken into account when administering drugs of this type. For this reason, sedative/analgesic drugs should be given in small, incremental doses that are titrated to the desired end points of analgesia and sedation. Sufficient time must elapse between doses to allow the effect of each dose to be assessed before subsequent drug administration.

For use in performing procedures for dialysis access maintenance, characteristics that are important are—rapid onset of action, short duration of action, predictable response, and availability of rapidly acting reversal agents with few side-effects. The intravenous medications commonly used for sedation/analgesia include benzodiazepines and opioids, alone or in combination.

▶ Benzodiazepine Agents

Benzodiazepines enhance the effect of the neurotransmitter gamma-aminobutyric acid, which results in sedative, hypnotic (sleep-inducing), anxiolytic (anti-anxiety), anticonvulsant, muscle relaxant, and amnesic action.[8] These properties make benzodiazepines particularly useful for dialysis access maintenance procedures, although they are not analgesic. These agents exert their pharmacologic action by binding to benzodiazepine-γ-aminobutyric acid (GABA)-type A-chloride receptors in the central nervous system. This action results in increased inhibitory action of GABA, producing a state of relaxation and inducing anterograde amnesia. It is believed that benzodiazepine receptors in the brain stem control the sedative effects while receptors in the forebrain control the anamnestic effects of these drugs. In general, benzodiazepines are safe and effective in the short term. Unfortunately, some patients experience paradoxical reactions to these agents.[9] These reactions are characterized by increased talkativeness, emotional release, excitement, excessive movement, and even hostility and rage. In some instances, the paradoxical activity can become so disruptive as to prevent the performance of the procedure.[10]

▶ Midazolam (Versed)

Although it is not an analgesic, midazolam is ideal as a single agent to provide the degree of sedation required for in performing short minor surgical procedures.[11] When it is used appropriately, patients generally have no significant indications of pain or discomfort during the procedure or memory of pain afterwards. The onset of action with midazolam is rapid, 1–2 minutes, and the duration of action is short, in the range of 30 minutes. With procedures of long duration, multiple doses can be given successfully.

Action and metabolism

Midazolam has the classic pharmacologic actions of the benzodiazepines including sedative, hypnotic, anticonvulsant, anterograde amnestic, and muscle relaxant properties (Table 35-9). It is 1½–2 times as potent as diazepam. It has a relatively short distribution half-life and elimination half-life, a relatively large volume of distribution, and high plasma clearance. Midazolam has a very rapid onset of action after intravenous administration.[12] It also has a very high metabolic clearance rate and a rapid rate of elimination. This causes it to have a short duration of activity. The drug has a half-life ranging from 1 to 4 hours in healthy individuals.[13,14] There is evidence that the total metabolic clearance of benzodiazepines is impaired in the elderly.[15] Additionally, it appears that this effect is more evident in elderly men than in women. Similar results have been reported for midazolam.[13]

The drug is biotransformed in the liver to hydroxylated metabolites that have considerably less pharmacologic activity than the parent drug. There is minimal renal excretion of the active drug. Studies comparing the pharmacodynamic profile of midazolam in normal subjects and those with chronic renal failure have shown no differences in the distribution, elimination, or clearance of unbound midazolam when tested at a dose of 0.2 mg/kg.[11] This indicates that there is no need for dosage adjustments in patients with renal failure.

Dosage

There are a variety of uses for midazolam in the perioperative period. It can be used for premedication, anesthesia induction, and maintenance and sedation for diagnostic and therapeutic procedures. The application determines the dose range used. It has been referred to as an ideal agent for producing the degree of sedation needed for short minor surgical procedures.[11] When used for this purpose, it is important that the dose administered be titrated to the effect obtained because of individual patient differences. Titrated doses in the range of 0.05–0.15 mg/kg fall into the sedation range, doses in the range of 0.1–0.4 mg/kg generally induce sleep (anesthesia).[16] For a 70 kg person, this would be 3.5–10.5 mg for sedation.

Dosage adjustments are needed if combined with opioids,[17] elderly patients,[16] and American Society of Anesthesiology physical status class (ASA) III and IV patients.[18] There is a combined effect of age over 55 and ASA status of III or IV.[16] Patients in this category require about 20% less of a desired clinical effect than do younger healthy individuals.

In reviewing the sedation/analgesia records of 12,896 hemodialysis patients undergoing dialysis access maintenance procedures, it was found that when midazolam was administered for sedation as the sole agent, the mean dosage used was 3.4 ± 1.5 mg. This dosage is in line with that reported for other procedures of a like nature.[19,20]

Adverse effects

The major adverse effects associated with midazolam administration are related to pulmonary and cardiovascular events and are dose dependent.[16,21] Hypnotic doses of midazolam are without effect on respiration in normal subjects, but special care must be taken in the treatment of children[6] and individuals with impaired hepatic function, such as alcoholics.[7] However, doses at this level may worsen sleep-related breathing disorders by adversely affecting control of the upper airway muscles or by decreasing the ventilatory response to CO_2. The latter effect may cause hypoventilation and hypoxemia in some patients with severe chronic obstructive pulmonary disease (COPD).[8] In patients with obstructive sleep apnea, hypnotic doses may decrease muscle tone in the upper airway and exaggerate the impact of apneic episodes on alveolar hypoxia, pulmonary hypertension, and cardiac ventricular load.

At higher doses, such as those used for interventional procedures, midazolam can depress alveolar ventilation slightly and cause respiratory acidosis as the result of a decrease in hypoxic rather than hypercapnic drive. These effects are exaggerated in patients with COPD, and alveolar hypoxia and/or CO_2 narcosis may result.[8]

TABLE 35–9

Characteristics of Midazolam (Versed)

Exerts effect by binding to the GABA receptor complex in CNS
Onset of action is rapid: 1 to 2 minutes
Duration of action is short: 30 minutes
Produces anxiolysis, amnesia, sedation, and skeletal muscle relaxation
Adverse effects
  Hiccups
  Nausea, vomiting
  Coughing
  Hyperactive and agitated
  Hypoventilation (decrease in tidal volume)
  Decreased respiratory rate
  Apnea
  Hypotension
  Variations in pulse rate

Midazolam can cause apnea during anesthesia or when given with opioids.

Respiratory effects of three different intravenous doses of midazolam (0.05 mg/kg, 0.1 mg/kg, and 0.2 mg/kg) and placebo were measured in a double-blind and randomized fashion in healthy volunteers.[22] After injection of the medication, tidal volume decreased by 40% with all the three doses and respiratory frequency increased to the same extent, minute ventilation remained constant. Only the largest dose of the drug (0.2 mg/kg) produced a significant decrease in oxygen saturation. In two other studies of normal healthy volunteers who received a sedation dose of midazolam (0.05 or 0.075 mg/kg), no decrease in oxygen saturation was observed and there was no decrease in spontaneous ventilation or ventilatory response to CO_2.[21,23] These studies suggest that some effect on respiration is seen even at low doses, but that at lower dose levels, clinically important respiratory depression does not occur.[16,21]

It is probable that midazolam will produce additive respiratory depression when used in conjunction with other CNS depressants such as opioids.[17] It is generally agreed that the risks of adverse respiratory function is greater at any dosage level for the older patient as well as the patient with COPD.[21,23,24]

In normal volunteers,[25] midazolam at a dose of 0.15 mg/kg (10.5 mg in a 70 kg individual) produces a reduction in systolic (5%) and diastolic blood pressure (10%). It also causes an increase in heart rate (18%). The cardiac index and left- and right-heart filling pressures usually are maintained after midazolam, but the systemic vascular resistance is decreased.[26–28] If the individual has cardiac disease, it does not appear to significantly influence the hemodynamic response to induction with midazolam. In patients who have elevated pulmonary artery pressure and reduced cardiac index, midazolam in doses of 0.2 mg/kg have been found to cause a reduction in pulmonary artery pressure and a return of the cardiac index to normal.[29]

When midazolam has been given to American Society of Anesthesiology physical status class III and IV patients,[18,30] the mean arterial pressure was reduced similar to changes that were observed in healthy patients and patients with cardiac disease.

In total, the cardiovascular effects of midazolam involve direct and indirect (reflex) action (Figure 35-3). A decrease in systemic vascular resistance,[28] vasodilation,[28] and a transient change in portal blood flow[31] combine to reduce cardiac filling. Midazolam also decreases myocardial contractility by direct action.[32] A reduction in blood pressure presumably activates the baroreflexes, simultaneously increasing heart rate and contractility with mobilization of splanchnic and other blood volumes into the central circulation. The net effect of these responses makes midazolam relatively safe as far as hemodynamic variables are concerned,[33] indicating a wide safety margin.[16] However, in large doses, midazolam decreases cerebral blood flow and oxygen assimilation considerably.[9]

Other adverse effects include hiccups, nausea, vomiting, and coughing. Occasionally, a patient will become hyperactive and even agitated.[34] Reactions such as agitation, involuntary movements (including tonic/clonic movements and muscle tremor), hyperactivity and combativeness have been reported. This paradoxical reaction may necessitate the avoidance of midazolam in such cases.

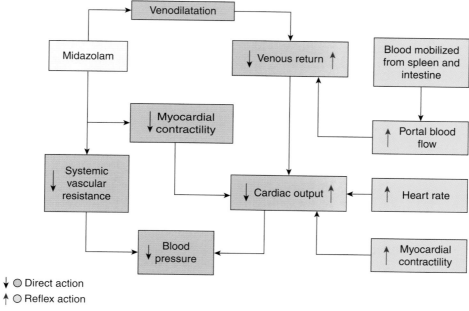

Hemodynamic effects of midazolam

Figure 35-3. Hemodynamic effects of midazolam showing direct and reflex actions.

TABLE 35–10

Characteristics of Fentanyl (Sublimaze)

Exerts effect by binding to mu receptors in the central
   nervous system
Onset of action is rapid: 30 seconds
Duration of action for a single intravenous dose of 100 μg is
   30–60 minutes
Produces analgesia and sedation
   Adverse effects
   Muscle rigidity
   Bradycardia
   Hypotension
   Nausea, vomiting
   Depresses brain stem ventilation, reduction in
     respiratory rate
   Decreased sensitivity to CO_2 stimulation
   Apnea can occur

▶ Opioid Agents

Opioids may be given during sedation/analgesia to provide analgesia as well as sedation (Table 35-10). Opioids produce effects on neurons by acting on receptors located on neuronal cell membranes.[35] There are three major types of opioid receptor, mu, delta, and kappa. Each of these receptors has a unique anatomical distribution in the brain, spinal cord, and periphery. Most of the clinically used opioids are relatively selective for mu receptors. The opioid antagonist, naloxone, inhibits all opioid receptors.[36]

▶ Fentanyl (Sublimaze)

Fentanyl is the opioid most commonly used for sedation/analgesia because of its short duration of action.[37] It is selective for the mu receptors.[35]

Action and metabolism

Fentanyl is approximately 600 times more lipid soluble and 100 times more potent than morphine, with 100 μg of fentanyl being approximately equivalent to 10 mg of morphine and 75 mg of meperidine in analgesic activity.[38] Because of its lipid solubility, fentanyl is able to quickly cross from the blood into the brain. As a result, the onset of action of fentanyl is almost immediate when the medicine is given intravenously. However, the maximal analgesic and respiratory depressant effect may not be noted for several minutes. The usual duration of action of analgesic effect is 30–60 minutes after a single I.V. dose of up to 100 μg.[39] In elderly patients and patients with liver disease, the half-life of fentanyl is prolonged, therefore these patients should have a reduced dosage.[38]

After intravenous administration, fentanyl is rapidly cleared primarily by hepatic microsomal biotransformation.[40] Less than 8% administered to healthy volunteers was excreted unchanged. In these individuals, more than 80% of the dose was recovered as metabolites, mostly from the urine.[41] The major metabolite (99%) is norfentanyl.[40]

Dosage

Dosage should be individualized. Some of the factors to be considered in determining the dose are: age, body weight, physical status, underlying pathological condition, use of other medicines, type of anesthesia to be used, and the surgical procedure involved. The initial dose should be reduced in the elderly and in debilitated patients. The effect of the initial dose should be taken into account in determining supplemental doses.

When used to induce sedation/analgesia for dialysis vascular access interventional procedures, 50–100 μg should be administered initially intravenously and may be repeated at 2–3-minute intervals until the desired effect is achieved. A reduced dose as low as 25–50 μg is recommended in elderly and poor-risk patients. The dose may need to be adjusted if given with a benzodiazepine.[17]

Adverse effects

The clinical utility of many analgesic drugs is altered in the presence of patients with impaired renal or hepatic function not simply because of altered clearance of the parent drug, but also through production and accumulation of toxic or therapeutically active metabolites. Some analgesic agents may also aggravate preexisting renal and hepatic disease. In the presence of renal impairment, fentanyl is considered to be one of the safest drugs available because it does not deliver a high active metabolite load, or have a significantly prolonged clearance.[42] Nevertheless, it can have adverse effects. All adverse effects of fentanyl are dose related.

Like any of the opioids, nausea, vomiting, and itching can be observed with fentanyl.[35] Fentanyl can cause muscle rigidity, particularly involving the muscles of respiration.[43,44] This effect is related to the speed of injection (bolus injection) and its incidence can be reduced by a slow intravenous injection.[35] Nonepileptic (myoclonic) movements can occur.[35] Use with benzodiazepines may be beneficial.

The major adverse reaction is altered respiration. Like all opioids, analgesia is accompanied by marked respiratory depression, but with fentanyl its onset is more rapid.[35] This can persist or recur in the postoperative period. There is a direct depression of brain stem ventilation and a dose-dependent reduction in respiratory rate.[45] Sensitivity to CO_2 stimulation is also decreased and may persist longer than depression of respiratory rate. This diminished sensitivity frequently slows the respiratory rate. Minute ventilation is decreased chiefly by the decreasing respiratory rate that can progress to the point of apnea. There is very little effect on tidal volume. The duration of the respiratory depressant effect of fentanyl may be longer than the analgesic effect.[46,47] The peak respiratory depressant effect of a single intravenous dose of fentanyl is noted 5–15 minutes following injection. Duration and degree of respiratory depression is dose related. However, even with smaller doses (in the range used for interventional dialysis access procedures), a respiratory depressant effect may be evident for 2–4 hours after drug administration.[48,49]

Because of these respiratory effects, fentanyl should be used with caution in patients with severe impairment of pulmonary function because of the possibility of respiratory depression, for example, patients with chronic obstructive pulmonary disease, patients with decreased respiratory reserve, or any patient with potentially compromised respiration. In such patients, narcotics may additionally decrease respiratory drive and increase airway resistance.

Other opioids such as morphine which can cause tachycardia in high dose, thought to be related at least in part by histamine release.[50] Fentanyl does not cause histamine release and in higher doses, its administration may produce bradycardia.[51–54] The mechanism of this bradycardic effect is thought to be due to vagal stimulation.[55] Although this may be treated effectively with atropine,[56] care should be used in patients with cardiac bradyarrhythmias.

Morphine and other opioids can cause hypotension, which can be severe. The etiology of this effect is thought to be secondary to the effects of histamine release.[57] Hypotension rarely occurs with fentanyl even at high doses, possibly because it does not result in histamine release. In fact, fentanyl provides a marked degree of cardiovascular stability.[35] This makes this drug particularly good for patients with poor cardiac function.

▶ Combinations of Drugs

While midazolam is frequently used alone for sedation with dialysis access interventional procedures, fentanyl is generally used in combination with this benzodiazepine when it is given in this setting. The advantage to this approach is that smaller doses of both agents may be used. However, there are also risks. The interaction of midazolam and fentanyl on healthy volunteers breathing room air was investigated.[21] This study revealed that when doses of 0.05 mg/kg (70 kg subject—3.5 mg) of midazolam were given alone, there were no episodes of hypoxemia or apnea. When given 2.0 μg/kg (70 kg subject 140 μg) of fentanyl alone, 50% of the volunteers became hypoxemic with an oxygen saturation less than 90% for more than 10 seconds, but none experienced apnea (defined as a period of more than 10 seconds without spontaneous respiration). When the two drugs were used in combination at these same doses, 91% of the volunteers experienced hypoxemia and 50% became apneic.

▶ Antagonists

The availability of antagonists that can rapidly and safely reverse the depressant effects of the drugs commonly used for sedation/analgesia further improves the overall safety of this procedure. The inclusion of a pharmacologic antagonist in the physician's armamentarium permits rapid reversal of excessive sedation or respiratory depression that might result from inadvertent drug overdosage in unexpectedly sensitive individuals. It may also be useful in the treatment of paradoxical excitatory reactions that occasionally occur following the administration of benzodiazepines.

▶ Flumazenil

Flumazenil (Romazicon) is a benzodiazepine antagonist. Used intravenously, it has been shown to antagonize sedation, impairment of recall, psychomotor impairment, and ventilatory depression produced by benzodiazepines in healthy human volunteers.[58] It is particularly useful in patients who become excessively drowsy after benzodiazepines are used for either diagnostic or therapeutic procedures.[59] Flumazenil (Romazicon) is a specific benzodiazepine antagonist structurally related to midazolam, flumazenil is only 50% bound to plasma proteins, thereby providing significant unbound drug for rapid distribution to the CNS following intravenous administration.[60]

The initial signs of reversal are generally seen within 1 minute, depending on the dose of flumazenil administered as well as the degree of benzodiazepine-induced sedation. Flumazenil competitively inhibits the activity at the benzodiazepine recognition site on the GABA/benzodiazepine receptor complex. By competing for benzodiazepine receptor sites, flumazenil reduces the number of receptors available to interact with midazolam, or other benzodiazepine agonists.[61,62] Flumazenil does not antagonize the central nervous system effects of drugs affecting GABAergic neurons by means other than the benzodiazepine receptor (including ethanol, barbiturates, or general anesthetics) and does not reverse the effects of opioids.

The onset of action is rapid and usually effects are seen within 1–2 minutes (faster if given centrally). The peak effect is seen at 6–10 minutes. Since benzodiazepine effects are dose dependent and appear to correspond to the proportion of receptors that bind agonist drug, a titrated dose of flumazenil may initially reverse hypnosis, and, upon continued titration, reverse sedation as well.[63,64] Significantly, larger doses of flumazenil are required to occupy enough receptors to reverse anxiolysis. In many instances, the patient who is experiencing an adverse event related to sedation/analgesia has been given both a benzodiazepine and an opioid. It has been shown that in cases such as this where the problem is respiratory depression, the reversal of only the benzodiazepine by the administration of flumazenil alone is effective.[65]

High plasma clearance, coupled with rapid hepatic metabolism, results in a rapid elimination of flumazenil (elimination half-life of 0.7–1.3 hours).[66] Therefore, resedation is possible, especially when flumazenil is used to reverse a long-acting benzodiazepine (ie, diazepam or lorazepam) or to reverse large cumulative doses of a short-acting benzodiazepine (ie, >10 mg of midazolam).

Flumazenil is available as a clear, colorless solution for intravenous injection, containing 500 μg in 5 mL. For the reversal of the sedative effects of benzodiazepines administered for sedation/analgesia, the recommended initial dose of flumazenil is 200 μg (2 mL) administered intravenously over 15 seconds. If the desired level of consciousness is not obtained after waiting an additional 45 seconds, a second dose of 200 μg (2 mL) can be injected and repeated at 60-second intervals where necessary to a maximum total dose of 1 mg (10 mL). The dosage should be individualized based on the patient's response in achieving the desired clinical effect. It is well tolerated at the recommended doses in individuals who have no tolerance to (or dependence on) benzodiazepines. Although not recommended, single intravenous doses of flumazenil up to 100 mg have been well tolerated by healthy volunteers.[67]

Elimination of radiolabeled drug is essentially complete within 72 hours, with 90–95% of the radioactivity appearing in urine and 5–10% in the feces. Clearance of flumazenil occurs primarily by hepatic metabolism and is dependent on hepatic blood flow.[68] Caution should be exercised with initial and/or repeated dosing to patients with liver disease. For patients with moderate liver dysfunction, their mean total clearance is decreased to 40–60%. In patients with severe liver dysfunction; it is decreased to 25% of normal value, compared with age-matched healthy subjects. This results in a prolongation of the half-life to 1.3 hours in patients with moderate hepatic impairment and 2.4 hours in severely impaired patients.[69]

The pharmacokinetics of flumazenil is not significantly affected in patients with renal failure or those on dialysis.

▶ Naloxone

Naloxone (Narcan) is a synthetic congener of oxymorphone. It is a pure opioid antagonist preventing or reversing the effects of opioids, including respiratory depression, sedation, and hypotension, by direct competition at mu, kappa, and sigma opioid receptor binding sites. In patients with respiratory depression, an increase in respiratory rate is generally seen within 1 or 2 minutes. Sedative effects are reversed and blood pressure, if depressed, returns to normal.[35] Naloxone will reduce the systemic side effects of opioids in a dose-dependent manner. Higher doses will reverse analgesia; lower doses will reverse opioid-related side effects without antagonizing analgesia.[70] Naloxone has no agonist properties; and, in the absence of opioids, it exhibits little or no significant pharmacologic activity so there are few adverse effects associated with its use.[71–73] However, the abrupt reversal of an opioid by naloxone in patients with physiologic dependence may produce symptoms of acute withdrawal such as agitation, nausea and vomiting, diarrhea, diaphoresis, tachycardia, hypertension, shivering, yawning, tremors, or seizures. In postoperative patients, particularly those with underlying cardiac disease, the administration of naloxone has been associated with changes in blood pressure, ventricular tachycardia or fibrillation, asystole, and pulmonary edema. The mechanism for these reactions may be an increase in sympathetic tone induced directly by naloxone or mediated indirectly through hypercapnia.[10–26]

The drug is administered parenterally. After intravenous administration, naloxone is rapidly distributed throughout the body. It is highly lipophilic and readily crosses into the brain. Onset of action after IV dosing is within 2 minutes. Duration of action following intravenous dosing is 20–60 minutes. Naloxone is hepatically metabolized, primarily through conjugation to naloxone-3-glucuronide. The elimination half-life in adults is approximately 60 minutes.[2,3]

All patients considered to have opioid intoxication should have a stable airway and adequate ventilation established before the administration of naloxone. When treating a patient demonstrating the adverse effects of fentanyl, an initial dose of 0.4–2.0 mg of naloxone may be administered intravenously. If the desired degree of reversal of respiratory function is not obtained, the dose may be repeated at 2–3-minute intervals. If no response is observed after 10 mg has been administered, the diagnosis of narcotic overdose should be questioned.[2,3,6–13]

The duration of action for naloxone depends upon the dose, but is usually 1–4 hours.[35] This may be shorter that some opioids, so patients must be closely monitored for recurrence of opioid toxicity when the antagonist effects of naloxone wane. Additional doses, given at intervals of 20 minutes to 2 hours, may be necessary to maintain reversal. It has been recommended that patients who receive naloxone be continuously observed for a minimum of 2 hours after the last dose.[9] Antagonism of opioid effects by naloxone may be accompanied by an "overshoot" phenomenon. If this occurs, the respiratory rate depressed by opioids transiently becomes higher than that before the period of depression. Rebound release of catecholamines may cause hypertension, tachycardia, and ventricular arrhythmias. Pulmonary edema has been reported.[35]

Naloxone is available as Narcan® (Endo Pharmaceuticals) and as a generic product. The 0.4 mg/mL strength is produced in 1 mL amps and 1 mL syringes, as well as 1, 2, and 10 mL vials. The 1 mg/mL concentration is available in 2 mL amps and 10 mL vials.

REFERENCES

1. American Society of Anesthesiologists Task Force on Sedation and Analgesia by Non-Anesthesiologists. Practice guidelines for sedation and analgesia by non-anesthesiologists. *Anesthesiology.* 2002;96:1004.
2. Gupta S, Sharma R, Jain D. Airway assessment: predictors of difficult airway. *Indian J Anaesth.* 2005;49:257.
3. Mallampati SR, Gatt SP, Gugino LD, et al. A clinical sign to predict difficult tracheal intubation: a prospective study. *Can Anaesth Soc J.* 1985;32:429.
4. Chou HC, Wu TL. Mandibulohyoid distance in difficult laryngoscopy. *Br J Anaesth.* 1993;71:335.
5. Patil V, Stehling L, Zauder H. Predicting the difficulty of intubation utilizing an intubation guide. *Anaesthesiology.* 1983;10:32.
6. Aldrete JA, Kroulik D. A postanesthetic recovery score. *Anesth Analg.* 1970;49:924.

7. Beathard GA, Urbanes A, Litchfield T. The classification of procedure-related complications—a fresh approach. *Semin Dial.* 2006;19:527.

8. Page C, Michael C, Sutter M, et al. *Integrated Pharmacology*, 2nd edition, St. Louis, MO: C.V. Mosby, 2002.

9. Hall RC, Zisook S. Paradoxical reactions to benzodiazepines. *Br J Clin Pharmacol.* 1981;11(suppl 1):99S.

10. Fiset L, Milgrom P, Beirne OR, Roy-Byrne P. Disinhibition of behaviors with midazolam: report of a case. *J Oral Maxillofac Surg.* 1992;50:645.

11. Vinik HR, Reves JG, Greenblatt DJ, et al. The pharmacokinetics of midazolam in chronic renal failure patients. *Anesthesiology.* 1983;59:390.

12. Arendt RM, Greenblatt DJ, deJong RH, et al. In vitro correlates of benzodiazepine cerebrospinal fluid uptake, pharmacodynamic action and peripheral distribution. *J Pharmacol Exp Ther.* 1983;227:98.

13. Greenblatt DJ, Abernethy DR, Locniskar A, et al. Effect of age, gender, and obesity on midazolam kinetics. *Anesthesiology.* 1984;61:27.

14. Heizmann P, Eckert M, Ziegler WH. Pharmacokinetics and bioavailability of midazolam in man. *Br J Clin Pharmacol.* 1983;16(suppl 1):43S.

15. Greenblatt DJ, Sellers EM, Shader RI. Drug therapy: drug disposition in old age. *N Engl J Med.* 1982;306:1081.

16. Reves J, Fragen R, Vinik R, Greenblatt D. Midazolam: pharmacology and uses. *Anesthesiology.* 1985;62:310.

17. Kanto J, Sjovall S, Vuori A. Effect of different kinds of premedication on the induction properties of midazolam. *Br J Anaesth.* 1982;54:507.

18. Lebowitz PW, Cote ME, Daniels AL, et al. Cardiovascular effects of midazolam and thiopentone for induction of anaesthesia in ill surgical patients. *Can Anaesth Soc J.* 1983;30:19.

19. Bergese SD, Patrick Bender S, McSweeney TD, et al. A comparative study of dexmedetomidine with midazolam and midazolam alone for sedation during elective awake fiberoptic intubation. *J Clin Anesth.* 2010;22:35.

20. Koshy G, Nair S, Norkus EP, et al. Propofol versus midazolam and meperidine for conscious sedation in GI endoscopy. *Am J Gastroenterol.* 2000;95:1476.

21. Bailey PL, Pace NL, Ashburn MA, et al. Frequent hypoxemia and apnea after sedation with midazolam and fentanyl. *Anesthesiology.* 1990;73:826.

22. Forster A, Morel D, Bachmann M, Gemperle M. Respiratory depressant effects of different doses of midazolam and lack of reversal with naloxone—a double-blind randomized study. *Anesth Analg.* 1983;62:920.

23. Power SJ, Morgan M, Chakrabarti MK. Carbon dioxide response curves following midazolam and diazepam. *Br J Anaesth.* 1983;55:837.

24. Gross JB, Zebrowski ME, Carel WD, et al. Time course of ventilatory depression after thiopental and midazolam in normal subjects and in patients with chronic obstructive pulmonary disease. *Anesthesiology.* 1983;58:540.

25. Forster A, Gardaz JP, Suter PM, Gemperle M. I.V. midazolam as an induction agent for anaesthesia: a study in volunteers. *Br J Anaesth.* 1980;52:907.

26. Reves JG, Samuelson PN, Lewis S. Midazolam maleate induction in patients with ischaemic heart disease: haemodynamic observations. *Can Anaesth Soc J.* 1979; 26:402.

27. Al-Khudhairi D, Whitwam JG, Chakrabarti MK, et al. Haemodynamic effects of midazolam and thiopentone during induction of anaesthesia for coronary artery surgery. *Br J Anaesth.* 1982;54:831.

28. Samuelson PN, Reves JG, Kouchoukos NT, et al. Hemodynamic responses to anesthetic induction with midazolam or diazepam in patients with ischemic heart disease. *Anesth Analg.* 1981;60:802.

29. Revel J, Samuelson P, Linnan M (Eds). Effects of midazolam maleate in patients with elevated pulmonary artery occluded pressure, *Trends in Intravenous Anesthesia*, Chicago: Year Book Medical Publishers, 1980.

30. Reitan, JA, Soliman, IE. A comparison of midazolam and diazepam for induction of anaesthesia in high-risk patients. *Anaesth Intensive Care.* 1987;15:175.

31. Gelman S, Reves JG, Harris D. Circulatory responses to midazolam anesthesia: emphasis on canine splanchnic circulation. *Anesth Analg.* 1983;62:135.

32. Reves JG, Kissin I, Fournier S. Negative inotropic effects of midazolam. *Anesthesiology.* 1984;60:517.

33. Reves JG, Mardis M, Strong S. Cardiopulmonary effects of midazolam. *Ala J Med Sci.* 1978;15:347.

34. Catterall W, Mackie K. *Goodman and Gilman's The Pharmacological Basis of Therapeutics*, 11th edition, New York: McGraw-Hill, 2006.

35. Gutstein H, Akil H. Opiod analgesics. In: Brunton L, Lazo J, Parker K, eds. *Goodman and Gilman's The Pharmacological Basis of Therapeutics*, 11th ed. New York: McGraw-Hill, 2006:547.

36. Reisine T, Bell GI. Molecular biology of opioid receptors. *Trends Neurosci.* 1993;16:506.

37. Akil H, Simon E (Eds). *Opioids I and II. Handbook of Experimental Pharmacology*, Berlin: Springer-Verlag, 1993.

38. Haberer JP, Schoeffler P, Couderc E, Duvaldestin P. Fentanyl pharmacokinetics in anaesthetized patients with cirrhosis. *Br J Anaesth.* 1982;54:1267.

39. Fassoulaki A, Theodoraki K, Melemeni A. Pharmacology of sedation agents and reversal agents. *Digestion.* 2010; 82:80.

40. Labroo RB, Paine MF, Thummel KE, Kharasch ED. Fentanyl metabolism by human hepatic and intestinal cytochrome P450 3A4: implications for interindividual variability in disposition, efficacy, and drug interactions. *Drug Metab Dispos.* 1997;25:1072.

41. McClain DA, Hug CC, Jr. Intravenous fentanyl kinetics. *Clin Pharmacol Ther.* 1980;28:106.

42. Murphy EJ. Acute pain management pharmacology for the patient with concurrent renal or hepatic disease. *Anaesth Intensive Care.* 2005;33:311.

43. Turski L, Havemann U, Schwarz M, Kuschinsky K. Disinhibition of nigral GABA output neurons mediates muscular rigidity elicited by striatal opioid receptor stimulation. *Life Sci.* 1982;31:2327.

44. Havemann U, Turski L, Kuschinsky K. Role of opioid receptors in the substantia nigra in morphine-induced muscular rigidity. *Life Sci.* 1982;31:2319.

45. Arunasalam K, Davenport HT, Painter S, Jones JG. Ventilatory response to morphine in young and old subjects. *Anaesthesia.* 1983;38:529.

46. Holmes CM. Supplementation of general anaesthesia with narcotic analgesics. *Br J Anaesth.* 1976;48:907.

47. Becker LD, Paulson BA, Miller RD, et al. Biphasic respiratory depression after fentanyldroperidol or fentanyl alone used to supplement nitrous oxide anesthesia. *Anesthesiology.* 1976;44:291.

48. Harper MH, Hickey RF, Cromwell TH, Linwood S. The magnitude and duration of respiratory depression produced by fentanyl and fentanyl plus droperidol in man. *J Pharmacol Exp Ther.* 1976;199:464.

49. Hug CC, Jr., Murphy MR. Fentanyl disposition in cerebrospinal fluid and plasma and its relationship to ventilatory depression in the dog. *Anesthesiology.* 1979;50:342.

50. Rosow CE, Moss J, Philbin DM, Savarese JJ. Histamine release during morphine and fentanyl anesthesia. *Anesthesiology.* 1982;56:93.

51. Stanley TH, Webster LR. Anesthetic requirements and cardiovascular effects of fentanyl-oxygen and fentanyl-diazepam-oxygen anesthesia in man. *Anesth Analg.* 1978;57:411.

52. Lunn JK, Stanley TH, Eisele J, et al. High dose fentanyl anesthesia for coronary artery surgery: plasma fentanyl concentrations and influence of nitrous oxide on cardiovascular responses. *Anesth Analg.* 1979;58:390.

53. Graves CL, Downs NH, Browne AB. Cardiovascular effects of minimal analgesic quantities of Innovar, fentanyl, and droperidol in man. *Anesth Analg.* 1975;54:15.

54. Bovill JG, Sebel PS, Stanley TH. Opioid analgesics in anesthesia: with special reference to their use in cardiovascular anesthesia. *Anesthesiology.* 1984;61:731.

55. Reitan JA, Stengert KB, Wymore ML, Martucci RW. Central vagal control of fentanyl-induced bradycardia during halothane anesthesia. *Anesth Analg.* 1978;57:31.

56. Liu W, Bidwai AV, Stanley TH, Isern-Amaral J. Cardiovascular dynamics after large doses of fentanyl and fentanyl plus N_2O in the dog. *Anesth Analg.* 1976;55:168.

57. Philbin DM, Moss J, Akins CW, et al. The use of H1 and H2 histamine antagonists with morphine anesthesia: a double-blind study. *Anesthesiology.* 1981;55:292.

58. Jensen S, Kirkegaard L, Anderson BN. Randomized clinical investigation of Ro 15-1788, a benzodiazepine antagonist, in reversing the central effects of flunitrazepam. *Eur J Anaesthesiol.* 1987;4:113.

59. Reversal of central benzodiazepine effects by flumazenil after conscious sedation produced by intravenous diazepam. The Flumazenil in Intravenous Conscious Sedation with Diazepam Multicenter Study Group I. *Clin Ther.* 1992;14:895.

60. Hunkeler W, Mohler H, Pieri L, et al. Selective antagonists of benzodiazepines. *Nature.* 1981;290:514.

61. Darragh A, Lambe R, Kenny M, et al. RO 15-1788 antagonises the central effects of diazepam in man without altering diazepam bioavailability. *Br J Clin Pharmacol.* 1982;14:677.

62. Mohler H, Burkard WP, Keller HH, et al. Benzodiazepine antagonist Ro 15-1788: binding characteristics and interaction with drug-induced changes in dopamine turnover and cerebellar cGMP levels. *J Neurochem.* 1981;37:714.

63. Klotz U, Ziegler G, Ludwig L, Reimann IW. Pharmacodynamic interaction between midazolam and a specific benzodiazepine antagonist in humans. *J Clin Pharmacol.* 1985;25:400.

64. Amrein R, Leishman B, Bentzinger C, Roncari G. Flumazenil in benzodiazepine antagonism. Actions and clinical use in intoxications and anaesthesiology. *Med Toxicol Adverse Drug Exp.* 1987;2:411.

65. Gross J, Blouin R, Zandsberg S, et al. Effect of flumazenil on ventilatory drive during sedation with midazolam and alfentanil. *Anesthesiology.* 1996;85:713.

66. Klotz U, Kanto J. Pharmacokinetics and clinical use of flumazenil (Ro 15-1788). *Clin Pharmacokinet.* 1988;14:1.

67. Darragh A, Lambe R, Kenny M, Brick I. Tolerance of healthy volunteers to intravenous administration of the benzodiazepine antagonist Ro 15-1788. *Eur J Clin Pharmacol.* 1983;24:569.

68. Roncari G, Ziegler WH, Guentert TW. Pharmacokinetics of the new benzodiazepine antagonist Ro 15-1788 in man following intravenous and oral administration. *Br J Clin Pharmacol.* 1986;22:421.

69. Klotz U, Ziegler G, Reimann IW. Pharmacokinetics of the selective benzodiazepine antagonist Ro 15-1788 in man. *Eur J Clin Pharmacol.* 1984;27:115.

70. Gan TJ, Ginsberg B, Glass PS, et al. Opioid-sparing effects of a low-dose infusion of naloxone in patient-administered morphine sulfate. *Anesthesiology.* 1997;87:1075.

71. Chamberlain JM, Klein BL. A comprehensive review of naloxone for the emergency physician. *Am J Emerg Med.* 1994;12:650.

72. Burnham T (Ed). *Drug Facts and Comparisons*, St. Louis, MO: C.V. Mosby, 2002.

73. Kallos T, Hudson HE, Rouge JC, Smith TC. Interaction of the effects of naloxone and oxymorphone on human respiration. *Anesthesiology.* 1972;36:278.

36

ADVERSE REACTIONS TO RADIOCONTRAST AGENTS IN VASCULAR ACCESS CENTERS

ADRIAN SEQUEIRA, ZULQARNAIN ABRO, & KENNETH ABREO

LEARNING OBJECTIVES

1. Discuss the classification of contrast agents.
2. Discuss the types of adverse reactions.
3. Discuss the misconception between seafood allergy and contrast reactions.
4. Understand the prophylaxis and treatment of contrast reactions.
5. Describe radiocontrast-induced nephropathy and its prophylaxis.

INTRODUCTION

Radiocontrast use is absolutely necessary for the diagnosis and treatment of dysfunctional or clotted vascular accesses. The potential toxicity of these agents has decreased as newer agents have been developed. The use of contrast agents is generally safe but at times may place patients at risk. There are two unique types of risk: allergic reactions to radiocontrast agents and direct renal toxicity especially in patients with chronic kidney disease. Therefore, it behooves the interventionalist to have a thorough understanding of contrast agents and their adverse effects so that these reactions can be prevented and in the event that they do occur, a specific treatment plan can be immediately embarked upon. The first part of this chapter will be devoted to allergic reactions to contrast agents and the second to radiocontrast-induced renal injury.

ALLERGIC REACTIONS TO RADIOCONTRAST AGENTS

▶ Classification

Radiocontrast media (RCM) are iodinated benzoic acid derivatives whose iodine content is responsible for the property of radiographic visualization. A monomer is a contrast molecule that contains one benzene ring with three iodine atoms, whereas a dimer contains two benzene rings with six iodine atoms.

As shown in Table 36-1, these agents are classified based on their osmolality as follows:

1. High osmolar contrast media (HOCM): These have osmolality ranging from 1200 to 2400 mOsm/kg and are ionic monomers.
2. Low osmolar contrast media (LOCM): These have osmolality between 600 and 860 mOsm/kg and are either ionic (dimers) or nonionic (monomers).
3. Isoosmolar contrast media (IOCM): These have osmolality close to the plasma osmolality of 290 mOsm/kg and are nonionic dimers.

▶ Classification of Reactions

Clinically, based on severity, adverse reactions can be classified as (Table 36-2):

1. mild (self-limiting and no treatment required)
2. moderate (can become life threatening and requires treatment).
3. severe (life threatening and needs hospitalization)
4. fatal

TABLE 36–1

Classification of Contrast Agents

Classification	Contrast Agent
High osmolar agents (Ionic monomers)	Meglumine iothalamate (Conray)
Low osmolar agents • Ionic dimer • Nonionic monomer	• Ioxaglate (Hexabrix) • Iohexol (Omnipaque)
Isoosmolar agents (Nonionic dimer)	Iodixanol (Visipaque)

TABLE 36–2

Classification Based on Severity

Mild	Moderate	Severe
Dizziness	Bronchospasm (mild)	Convulsions
Headache	Head/chest/abdominal pain	Cyanosis
Nausea/vomiting	Hypo/hypertension	Paralysis
Pain at injection site	Severe vomiting	Profound hypotension
Rash/pruritus	Tachy/bradycardia	Unresponsiveness
Urticaria (limited)	Thrombophlebitis	Cardiopulmonary arrest
Warmth	Cutaneous reactions/extensive urticaria	Pulmonary edema
Diaphoresis	Facial and laryngeal edema	Arrhythmias

An alternative classification is the Ring and Messmer's classification (Table 36-3) that provides a grade to specific signs and symptoms that involve the skin, abdomen, respiratory, or cardiovascular system.[1]

Based on timing, reactions to contrast media may be classified as either immediate or delayed reactions. Immediate reactions occur within 60 minutes of contrast administration and comprise two-thirds of all reactions. They are classified as anaphylactoid or nonanaphylactoid based on their pathogenic mechanisms.[2] Another way to classify these reactions is based on the organ system involved (Table 36-4).

▶ **Immediate Reactions**

Anaphylactoid Reactions

These are independent of the dose administered. They are idiosyncratic and unpredictable. Unlike anaphylactic reactions that require prior exposure to the agent, these reactions can occur with first exposure to the agent. Clinically, both (anaphylactic and anaphylactoid) may present identically. Vasovagal reactions, panic attacks, and vocal cord dysfunction are important differentials that must be considered.[1] Anaphylactoid reactions are believed to be non-IgE mediated. The pathogenesis of these reactions remains controversial. Ninety percent of these reactions are believed to be secondary to the release of preformed mediators such as

histamine from basophils and eosinophils, and tryptase from mast cells.[3] This release may occur by direct interaction with cell membrane receptors of mast cells and basophils, by the generation of anaphylatoxins (C3a, C5a), activation of cascade pathways—kinin, coagulation, and fibrinolytic systems, and complement activation by enzyme induction.[4] There is also a theoretical possibility of contrast media behaving as pseudo antigens that bind to IgE and cause histamine release.[5] However, there are reports that suggest that in a small subset (less than 4%) the reactions are IgE mediated,[6,7] and in such cases the reactions are severe. Such patients have demonstrated the presence of anti-RCM IgE antibodies and positive intradermal and basophil degranulation tests.[4,8]

Nonanaphylactoid Reactions

These are predictable and dose dependent and are related to the physiochemical properties of the contrast media

TABLE 36–3

Ring and Messmer Classification

Grade	Skin	Abdomen	Respiratory	Cardiovascular
1	Erythema, urticaria, angioedema			
2	Erythema, urticaria, angioedema	Nausea, cramping	Dyspnea	Tachycardia, hypotension, arrhythmia
3	Erythema, urticaria, angioedema	Vomiting, diarrhea	Bronchospasm, cyanosis, laryngeal edema	Shock
4	Erythema, urticaria, angioedema	Vomiting, diarrhea	Respiratory arrest	Cardiac arrest

TABLE 36–4

Symptoms Based on Organs Involved

Organ System	Signs and Symptoms
Cardiovascular	Hypotension, hypertension, tachy- or bradycardia, cardiac arrest, arrhythmia, and chest pain
Respiratory	Laryngeal edema, pulmonary edema, dyspnea, and wheezing
Gastrointestinal	Vomiting, diarrhea, nausea, and abdominal pain
Neurological	Convulsions, headache, and confusion
Skin	Erythema, urticaria, angioedema, pruritus, and maculopapular rash
Salivary gland	Parotitis
Kidney	Contrast-induced nephropathy

such as the ionicity, osmolality, viscosity, and iodine concentration (Table 36-5). Debilitated and medically unstable patients are more prone to these reactions.[9]

1. *Osmolality*: HOCM when given intravascularly produce rapid fluid shifts into the vascular space causing volume expansion. This may cause pain, flushing, or cardiac decompensation in those with impaired cardiac function.[10,11] HOCM can also deform RBCs in sickle cell patients, potentially precipitating a sickle cell crisis.[10–12] Osmolality of contrast media may also cause degranulation of mast cells and basophils.[1,10] RCM (HOCM and LOCM) can increase serum potassium by causing a shift from RBCs and vascular endothelium into plasma due to solvent drag.[13]

2. *Ionicity*: Ionicity is the property of a compound to ionize in solution, which increases its osmolality. Ionic monomers dissociate into two components (an anion and cation) in solution. This increases osmolality. They provide three iodine atoms and hence a ratio of 2:3 osmolar particles to iodine in solution. Nonionic agents do not ionize, and therefore their osmolality is half of ionic agents. Nonionic monomers have a ratio of 1:3, while nonionic dimers

TABLE 36–5

Nonanaphylactoid Reactions

Physiochemical Properties	Manifestations
Ionicity	Arrhythmias, neurotoxicity
Osmolality	Renal injury, hypotension, tachycardia, sickling, flushing, nausea, vomiting, and hyperkalemia
Viscosity	Pain during injection
Iodine concentration	Hyperthyroidism, thyroid storm, and suppression of I-131 uptake

have a ratio of 1:6 osmolar particles to iodine. Therefore, nonionic dimers provide more iodine without affecting osmolality, thereby improving contrast visualization. The older ionic agents dissociate to produce charged particles, which may interfere with cardiac and cerebral electrical activity.[10,11] In addition, ionic contrast media can bind calcium and magnesium, thereby affecting cardiac rhythm and function.[10,11]

3. *Viscosity*: Viscosity affects the rate of IV injection. High viscosity agents may not mix well with blood and therefore affect optimal visualization. It also contributes to the patient discomfort during injection.[10] By warming to body temperature, the viscosity decreases enabling faster rates of injection and thereby decreasing discomfort. While this may improve radio-opacification, it may also increase the risk of adverse reactions.[11] Isoosmolar agents are more viscous compared to LOCM or HOCM.[10]

4. *Other effects*: Histamine release is also influenced by the chemical structure, size, and iodine content of the molecule.[14] These agents can also stimulate release of serotonin from platelets causing vasodilatation.[4] The protein-binding effect (older agents) may cause inhibition of cholinesterase, which causes flushing, bronchospasm, and cardiovascular arrest.[4,14] Iodinated contrast agents may precipitate iodine-induced hyperthyroidism or a thyroid storm in poorly controlled hyperthyroid states.[10] In addition, iodinated contrast media can suppress I-131 uptake by the thyroid (by 50%). This takes a few weeks to normalize.[15] This should be kept in mind in individuals requiring I-131 therapy. HOCM may also induce the release of catecholamines and precipitate a hypertensive crisis. This does not appear to happen with LOCM.[16] RCMs (HOCM and LOCM) can induce granulocytosis with neutrophilia.[17,18] In the lung, RCMs can cause bronchospasm and noncardiogenic pulmonary edema.[19,20]

INCIDENCE

The incidence of mild adverse reactions to HOCM varies from 5% to 15%,[21,22] whereas with LOCM it is believed to be 1–3%.[21,22] Moderate reactions to HOCM have an incidence of 1–2% and 0.2–0.4% with LOCM.[9,21] The incidence of severe reactions with HOCM is 0.2–0.06%,[21] while with LOCM it is 0.04%.[9] Fatal reactions are rare and occur at the rate of 1/100,000 with both types of agents.[23] Thus, there is a fivefold decrease in the incidence of adverse reactions with the use of LOCM with majority of the reactions being mild.

RISK FACTORS

Table 36-6 provides a general idea of risk factors. Generally, these reactions occur commonly in women[5] and in individuals between 20 and 50 years of age.[5,9] The elderly tend to have more severe reactions, as they are unable to

TABLE 36–6

Risk Factors for Contrast Media Reactions

- History of allergies: 2–3× increased risk[4,5,9,10]
- Pulmonary conditions: asthma (2–6× increased risk)[9,10,30,58]
- Heart disease[10,27,28]
- Hematological conditions: myeloma, sickle cell anemia[9,58]
- Drugs : Nonsteroidal anti-inflammatory drugs (NSAIDS), β-blockers, IL-2[9,58]
- History of previous contrast reactions: 3–5× increased risk[4,10,25,26]
- Endocrine conditions: Thyroid disease, pheochromocytoma[10]
- Renal insufficiency[9,10]
- Anxiety[4, 10,58]

tolerate reactions secondary to coexisting comorbid conditions.[9] Ansell reports that in the United Kingdom, people of Mediterranean origin and those from the Indian subcontinent have a higher risk of having reactions.[24] A history of a previous reaction also increases the risk for a recurrent reaction by a factor of five for both ionic and nonionic media.[25,26] There is a fourfold reduction in the incidence of repeat reactions when a nonionic contrast media is used in patients with a history of a previous reaction to an ionic contrast media.[25] β-Blockers increase the risk of anaphylactoid reactions (bronchospasm) because they impair the response to epinephrine.[10,21,27–29] However, these drugs are not routinely held prior to contrast study.[30] Anxiety may contribute to vasovagal reactions. Risk factors for death include the four W's: White, Women, Wrinkled (elderly), and Weakened (debilitating medical conditions).[9]

DELAYED REACTIONS

These occur 1 hour to 7 days after contrast injection and are T-cell mediated. The incidence of delayed reactions is 2–3% when followed for a week after contrast administration.[31] There is no significant difference in the incidence between ionic and nonionic agents or between the various nonionic monomers,[32] though reactions are more frequent with isoosmolar agents.[32,33] Iotrolan (isoosmolar nonionic dimer) was withdrawn from the market because of a high incidence of skin reactions.[32] Patients may present with flu-like symptoms, GI symptoms, or skin reactions. Hypotension and wheezing occur rarely. Skin reactions are more common. Sutton et al noted two specific forms of skin reaction: diffuse, itchy macular rash and a peeling reaction confined to the face, hands, and feet.[33] Angioedema is another common dermatologic presentation.[34] Serious reactions include erythema multiforme, fixed drug eruptions, Stevens–Johnson syndrome, toxic epidermal necrosis, and cutaneous vasculitis.[31] Since these reactions may occur a week later, other drugs that patients are on or have been initiated later on are usually blamed.

Risk factors include patients with a history of a previous reaction, adults in the third to fifth decades, women and

history of IL-2 therapy (Interleukin-2).[10,35] The recurrence rate in those with a previous reaction varies between 13% and 27%.[35,36] Japanese seem to have a higher incidence.[21] Women and those with a history of allergy have a twofold risk of such reactions.[34] Reactions tend to be more common during the pollen season.[34] Comorbid conditions like diabetes, cardiac, renal, and liver disease also predispose to delayed reactions. Systemic lupus erythematosus, patients on hydralazine, and bone marrow transplant recipients have been reported to have severe skin reactions.[37]

IODIDE MUMPS

Iodide mumps, first described by Sussman and Miller in 1956, is a peculiar reaction that can occur with all classes of iodinated RCM.[38] Painful bilateral swelling of the salivary glands occurs within a few minutes to 5 days after contrast administration (Figure 36-1). It may be associated with thyroiditis, facial nerve paralysis, and enlargement of the lacrimal glands.[39] The mechanism is not entirely clear. It might be an idiosyncratic reaction or result from the accumulation of iodide within the ducts of the salivary glands. Renal failure is a risk factor because 98% of the contrast media is excreted unchanged in the urine, while 2% is excreted from the liver, salivary, lacrimal, and sweat glands.[11,40] With renal failure, the elimination half life increases from 30 to 60 minutes to 20 to 140 hours.[11] Contrast media contain a small amount of inorganic iodide and a large amount of organically bound iodine. In renal failure, the retained iodine undergoes deiodination to nonorganic iodide, which accumulates in the salivary glands and induces inflammation. Treatment consists of

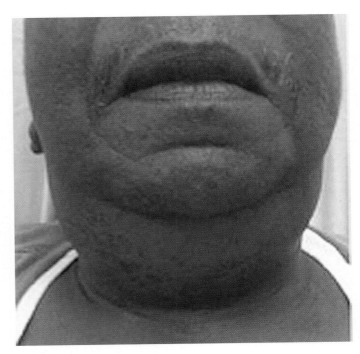

Figure 36-1. Iodide mumps.

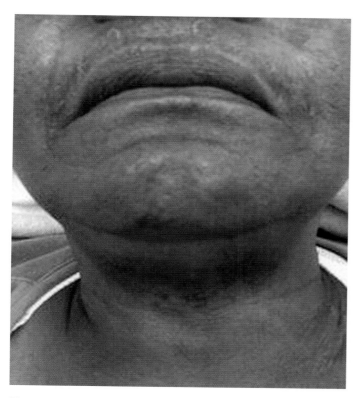

Figure 36-2. Resolution of iodide mumps postdialysis.

analgesics for pain relief and 2–3 sessions of hemodialysis to remove these agents completely (Figure 36-2).[11] Switching contrast media does not help, and premedication with steroids and antihistaminics does not prevent a recurrence.[39] In patients without renal failure, the reaction may spontaneously subside within a few days. This condition is not a contraindication for recurrent contrast administration, as no serious reactions have been described.[39]

SEAFOOD ALLERGY AND CONTRAST MEDIA

There is a common misconception that seafood (fish and shellfish) allergy predisposes to a disproportionately higher risk for contrast media reactions. This view is prevalent among physicians as well.[41] The earliest record in literature may have been from Witten et al (1973)[42] and Shehadi (1975). Shehadi reported that 15% of patients with an allergy to seafood had an adverse reaction to RCM. However, in the same study, a similar percentage of patients with allergies to egg, chocolate, and milk were also predisposed to an adverse reaction to RCM.[43] Iodine is an essential trace mineral, and therefore it is unlikely that people are allergic to iodine itself. The iodine atom is too small to initiate an antigen–antibody reaction, though it might act as a hapten.[44] In vitro animal studies have shown that iodine can induce the formation of iodinated protein antigens under certain conditions and this can generate an immune response.[45] While it is true

that a history of allergy or atopy increases the risk of a reaction to RCM (2–3 times that of general population), seafood allergy does not disproportionately increase the risk. In fact, 85% of those with seafood allergy will not have an adverse reaction to RCM.[43,44] True IgE-mediated reactions to seafood are directed specifically toward fish protein (parvalbumin) and in shellfish to tropomysin and not iodine.[42] Hence, people who are allergic to shellfish (crustaceans and mollusks) can eat scaled fish. True seafood allergy that usually occurs within 2 hours of exposure should be differentiated from seafood intolerance. The latter occurs after the ingestion of food rich in histamine together with drugs or alcohol that inhibit histaminases. This produces a pruritic skin rash, diarrhea, and bronchospasm.[46] Hence, patients with seafood allergy should always be questioned about the nature of the reaction. There is also no relationship between contact dermatitis to iodine containing antiseptics and anaphylactoid reactions to contrast media.[44]

PREVENTION OF ADVERSE REACTIONS IN HIGH-RISK PATIENTS

There are a number of steps that one can take to minimize an adverse reaction. All patients at high risk should be identified by history and such patients must have a clear reason for an intervention. If possible, other modalities should be considered for evaluation of an access, for example, CO_2 venography, ultrasound, or direct surgical intervention (surgical thrombolysis) instead of the contrast study. In individuals with a past history of a reaction, a detailed history into the nature of the reaction and the type of agent used should be obtained. There may be reasons other than a contrast allergy causing the reaction such as latex allergy, antibiotic allergy, or a reaction to opioids.[47] The use of premedication with steroids and antihistaminics has been advocated for patients with a history of moderate-to-severe reactions by the American College of Radiology.[3] The initial study in 1987 by Lasser et al showed that premedication decreases the risk of adverse reactions when used with HOCM.[48] Methyl prednisone was given in two doses, 32 mg PO at 12 hours and at 2 hours prior to the procedure. This study reported that steroids given as a single dose 2 hours before a procedure did not offer any protection. In 1994, Lasser et al reported that using the two-dose protocol of steroids also decreased the incidence of adverse reactions when LOCM was used.[49] The study also demonstrated that this protocol should be given at least 6 hours prior to a procedure for any benefit. Golberger et al used a three-dose protocol, prednisone 50 mg given 13 hours, 7 hours, and 1 hour prior to a procedure along with 50 mg diphenhydramine (1 hour before a procedure) and use of a LOCM in patients with a previous reaction to HOCM.[50] This protocol also decreased the number of total adverse reactions. However, the use of premedication has associated risks. Diphenhydramine can cause hypotension, tachycardia, and chest tightness, while steroids can exacerbate manic symptoms. Steroids should also be used cautiously in patients with peptic ulcer disease and diverticulitis.[3] The mechanism by which premedication works is not well understood. Steroids have been shown to decrease the number of circulating basophils and eosinophils and decrease levels of histamine. These effects are of maximal benefit between 4 and 8 hours after administration.[51] Steroids inhibit the production of prostaglandins and leukotrienes. In addition, steroids increase the functional C1 esterase inhibitor level that inhibits activated factor XII (Hageman factor), which is involved in the activation of the kinin system with the subsequent production of bradykinin.[52] Antihistaminics block histamine receptors. The use of H-2 blockers is optional, but H-2 blockers should not be used in the absence of H-1 blockers especially in patients with coronary artery disease. When used alone, there is unopposed stimulation of H-1 receptors causing coronary vasoconstriction.[22] Switching from one form of LOCM to another may help.[3] LOCM including IOCM induce less histamine release than HOCM. In addition, nonionic monomers induce less histamine release compared to ionic dimers and isoosmolar dimers.[53]

Despite premedication and the use of LOCM, breakthrough reactions can still occur in 10% of patients.[54] These reactions tend to be similar to the original reaction in a majority of patients, but in 10% of cases the reaction may increase in severity.[54,55] If the previous reaction is mild, then in 70–90% the breakthrough reaction is also mild.[54,55] If the initial reaction is moderate or severe, then in 40–60% the breakthrough reaction will be of similar severity.[55] Table 36-7 provides a list of the different premedication protocols. Table 36-8 provides a brief protocol that can be followed in high-risk individuals. Steroids are of no benefit in chemotoxic reactions. Drug rechallenges and test doses are not recommended, as they can be fatal. In those patients with a previous reaction, it may be prudent to keep a record of the reaction including the type of RCM that was used. It is best to avoid RCM in patients with a severe reaction and in those who develop noncardiogenic pulmonary edema.[8,20] It has also been suggested that patients with a history of a reaction should be referred to an allergologist for testing. These tests may determine if the reaction in severe cases is IgE mediated as well as determine cross-reacting RCMs that can be avoided.[6]

TABLE 36–7

Premedication Protocols

Premedication Protocols[3]

1. Prednisone 50 mg PO at 13, 7, and 1 h prior to study + diphenhydramine 50 mg IV/PO/IM 1 h prior to study
2. Methyl prednisone 32 mg PO at 12 and 2 h prior to study with or without diphenhydramine 50 mg 1 h prior to study

---

TABLE 36–8

Steps to Prevent an Adverse Reaction

1. Identify high-risk individuals
2. Enquire as to the nature of the previous reaction keeping in mind the differentials. Make sure the previous reaction is not noncardiogenic pulmonary edema
3. Evaluate other noncontrast modalities that can be used instead of RCM
4. Stop β-blockers if possible prior to study
5. Premedicate with steroids and antihistaminics
6. Use a different LOCM agent or switch from LOCM to IOCM
7. Use small amounts of RCM and fewest doses when possible
8. Minimize anxiety
9. Be prepared for breakthrough reactions that maybe severe
10. Refer to an allergologist

TREATMENT OF REACTIONS

From the discussion so far, we know that immediate reactions may occur despite premedication. Thankfully, serious reactions are rare. Equally important is to realize that mild reactions can progress to a severe reaction quickly. It is very important to recognize these reactions early. With early treatment, lower drug doses are used and this decreases the drug side effects as well.[22] Most of the serious reactions occur in the first 20 minutes after contrast injection. Hence, it becomes important to be on the lookout for them for at least 30 minutes after a procedure. Being prepared should be the dogma in the interventional suite. A well-stocked crash cart and having personnel certified in advanced cardiac life support (ACLS) and basic life support (BLS) is an essential requirement. It is useful to have laminated placards of common reactions with drug doses available for quick reference (Table 36-9). It is also useful to have big laminated placards of drug doses used to reverse conscious sedation in the suite as well. The procedure must be stopped immediately when a patient experiences a systemic reaction. Check vitals, oxygen saturation, and ensure oxygen flow. Rule out hypoglycemia. Talk to and reassure the patient. This will help in two ways: it will alleviate patient anxiety and assist the physician in evaluating signs and symptoms. Be calm yourself! Note the time to the reaction, the symptoms of the reaction, type, and amount of RCM given. Patients on nonselective β-blockers may pose a special situation. Epinephrine has both α and β agonist properties. β-Receptor sites need smaller doses of epinephrine than do the α-receptor regions. When given subcutaneously or slowly IV, the β agonist property predominates, while giving it rapidly IV and in larger doses, its α agonist property predominates.[22] Therefore, if the appropriate β-adrenergic response (bronchodilation) is not obtained, the physician may give more epinephrine, thereby producing unwanted α-adrenergic effects. Hence, it maybe better to use isoproterenol

TABLE 36–9

List of Common Immediate Reactions and Management

Clinical Diagnosis	Management[3,5,22,26,58]
Urticaria • Transient, scattered	• Observe (may progress to severe reaction) • Mark areas involved • Supportive care
• Protracted, scattered • Severe	• Diphenhydramine 25–50 mg IV/ IM, q 2–3 h • Diphenhydramine 25–50 mg IV/ IM, q 2–3 h • Cimetidine 300 mg IV, q 6–8 h • Adrenaline (1:1000) 0.1–0.3 mL (0.1–0.3 mg) SQ/IM*, q 6–8 h • Admit • Consult dermatologist and allergologist
Facial or Laryngeal edema	• Oxygen by mask (6–10 L/min) • Adrenaline (1:1000) 0.1–0.3 mL SQ/IM* • Airway suction • Call code team if severe • Admit • If facial edema is mild without progression, then observe only
Nausea, vomiting	• Diphenhydramine 25 mg IV/IM
Bronchospasm • Mild	• Oxygen by mask (6–10 L/min) • β2 adrenergic agonist nebulization q 4 h
• Severe	• Oxygen by mask (6–10 L/min) • β2 adrenergic agonist nebulization q 4 h • Adrenaline (1:1000) 0.1–0.3 mL IM*, q 10–15 min • Admit
Hypotension with bradycardia (Vagal reaction)	• Elevate patient's leg • Oxygen by mask (6–10 L/min) • IV fluids • Atropine 0.6–1 mg IV (repeat to a maximum does of 3 mg, q 3–5 min)
Generalized anaphylactoid reaction (severe bronchospasm, hypotension, laryngospasm, angioedema)	• Call code tam • Oxygen by mask (6–10 L/min) • Airway suction • Leg elevation • IV fluids • β2 adrenergic agonist nebulization • Diphenhydramine 25–50 mg IV/IM • Cimetidine 300 mg IV, q 6–8 h • Hydrocortisone 500 mg IV • Adrenaline (1:1000) 0.5 mL IM*
• For patients on β- blockers, instead of adrenaline use	• Glucagon 1–5 mg IV and then infusion 5–15 µg/min or • Isoproterenol (1:5000 solution, 0.2 mg/mL) IV (diluted to 10 mL normal saline). Give 1 mL/min (20 µg) increments.

*To give adrenaline IV (use 1:10,000 solution) 1 mL (0.1 mg) under ECG monitoring. Give slowly over 2–5 minutes, upto 3 mL/dose. Repeat in 5–30 minutes as needed.

(β1 and β2 agonist). Asthmatic patients who are on chronic β agonist medications will require larger doses of β agonist medications possibly secondary to desensitization.[22] Steroids generally have no role in an acute reaction except for reducing the severity of delayed symptoms.

Management of delayed reactions is symptomatic as the reactions are mostly mild and self-limiting. Localized reactions may need emollients and steroid creams. However, serious skin reactions will need systemic steroids and antihistaminics. Dermatological evaluation maybe warranted. Prophylaxis with steroids and diphenhydramine is recommended in those with a history of IL-2 therapy.[56] Prophylaxis is recommended for moderate-to-severe reactions along with the use of a structurally different agent.[5,31] Cross reactivity between different agents of the same group exists commonly (eg, different nonionic monomers)[57] but very rarely when considering agents between two different groups (eg, ionic versus nonionic).[31] However, reactions may still occur with prophylaxis.[34] Patients with a history of a delayed reaction do not appear to be at an increased risk for an immediate reaction and vice versa.[5]

RADIOCONRAST-INDUCED NEPHROPATHY

The administration of radiocontrast agents is a frequent cause of acute kidney injury. Radiocontrast-induced nephropathy (RCN) remains the third leading cause of hospital-acquired acute renal failure; accounting for up to 10% of all hospitalized patients.[59] This is very important information to know especially for interventional nephrologists who give contrast media on a routine basis when performing procedures. Patients who get these procedures often have advanced chronic kidney disease and are at higher risk RCN. Renal failure associated with contrast media carries increase risk of mortality.[59] This grave risk of mortality calls for a heightened awareness of the diagnosis and prevention of RCN.

RCN is defined as a sudden decline in renal function after radiocontrast administration. Typically, the serum creatinine level begins to increase by at least 0.5 mg/dL from baseline at 24–72 hours after the administration of contrast, peaks at 3–5 days, and requires another 3–5 days to return to baseline.[60] Significantly, contrast-induced renal failure is rare in patients with preserved renal function. Large doses and multiple injections of contrast media within 72 hours increase the risk of the patient's developing RCN.[60] The major risk factors for development of acute renal failure after radiocontrast administration include diabetic nephropathy, preexisting renal dysfunction, severe congestive heart failure, volume depletion, hypotension, elderly age group, multiple myeloma, concomitant treatment with angiotensin converting enzyme (ACE) inhibitors, NSAIDs, or exposure to other nephrotoxins.[61] Preexisting renal dysfunction is the most important risk factor for the development of RCN.[62]

RCN seems to be related to the agent's vasoactive effects on the kidney. In animal models, contrast injections initially cause vasodilatation of the renal circulation, followed by intense and persistent vasoconstriction. The persistent vasoconstriction causes tubular toxicity and renal medullary ischemia. The exact cause of the vasoconstrictive phase is not well defined. The proposed mechanism may include reduced production of vasodilator prostaglandins, enhanced endothelin release, or changes in intracellular calcium levels.[63] Clinical presentation of RCN is typically nonoliguric, but in severe cases one can see oliguria. The urine sediment is usually unremarkable and the fractional excretion of sodium is typically <1%, reflecting the prerenal component of injury described above. The injury may be mild, with transient reduction of renal dysfunction or severe enough to require hemodialysis. Strategies for the prevention of RCN include selection of contrast agents, volume of administration, pharmacologic therapy, hemodialysis or hemofiltration, and avoidance of concomitant nephrotoxins.

Selection of contrast agents will be discussed first in the prevention strategy. IOCM is least nephrotoxic followed by LOCM. In one large study of 1196 patients, it was shown that patients receiving diatrizoate (HOCM) were 3.3 times as likely to develop RCN as those receiving iohexol (LOCM).[64] Subsequent meta-analysis of 31 trials concluded that the use of LOCM rather than HOCM was beneficial to patients with preexisting renal failure.[65] Chalmers and Jackson[66] were first to suggest that there was a decreased incidence of RCN with iodixanol (IOCM). They looked at 124 consecutive patients with renal impairment (estimated C_{CR} <60 mL/min) undergoing renal angiography, peripheral angiography, or both (half of whom had diabetes) and found that iodixanol was 50% less nephrotoxic than iohexol (>10% increase in serum creatinine levels in 15% of the iodixanol group vs 30% in the iohexol group; $P < 0.05$). This was confirmed by a double-blind randomized controlled study of 129 patients by Aspelin et al in 2003,[65] which suggested that high-risk patients tend to develop less contrast nephropathy by using IOCM, as compared with an LOCM (odds were 11 times lower).[65] The effect of using high-volume IOCM on renal function in chronic kidney disease patients has also been investigated. A retrospective cohort study that looked at 117 patients with a creatinine clearance <60 mL/min (not on dialysis) concluded that volume did not affect the incidence of RCN when isoosmolar media was used.[67] The mean dose of contrast used was 84.3 ± 67 mL. The average dose of contrast used in interventional procedures in nephrology is less than 50 mL. Kian and Asif et al have shown that using <20 mL of LOCM during access salvage procedures and venography is associated with a low incidence (4%) of RCN.[68,69] The exact mechanism as to why IOCM are less nephrotoxic is not very well understood. It has been proposed that using IOCM causes less of a diuretic effect. HOCM enhance distal delivery of sodium, consequently increasing the work load of the renal medulla causing hypoxic injury in addition to volume depletion.[70]

MINIMIZING RADIOCONTRAST-INDUCED NEPHROPATHY

There are techniques proposed for minimizing the dose of RCM, one of which is digital subtraction angiography (DSA). This allows for one to see vascular structures more clearly. DSA achieves this by subtracting all the superimposed objects within the field to get a great image using low amounts of contrast. A second method of minimizing the dose of contrast media is by diluting the contrast agent by 50% with saline. Minimizing contrast use is particularly useful in patients with marginal renal function (CKD3-5) in whom contrast nephrotoxicity will result in the need for hemodialysis.

Several drug interventions have been tested in clinical trials for prophylaxis against the development of RCN. These will be discussed in the following section but have generated few significant positive results and are not widely used. At present, only IV hydration and avoidance of nephrotoxic agents are widely used to decrease the incidence of contrast-induced renal dysfunction.

Adequate hydration is the most cost-effective and simplest way of preserving renal function. High-risk patients should be given IV infusion of 0.9% saline at a rate of 1 mL/kg per hour. One must adjust appropriately with the patient's current volume status and cardiovascular condition. This treatment should be started 6–12 hours before the procedure and continued for up to 12–24 hours after the radiographic examination has been completed.[71] A retrospective nested cohort study conducted in 518 patients with impaired renal function (serum creatinine levels >1.9 mg/dL) reported that the 76 patients who developed RCN (defined as an increase in serum creatinine levels >0.5 mg/dL over 48 hours) had lower blood pressure before angiography and had less hydration before the procedure than 82 matched controls.[72] Similarly, results were seen in a smaller uncontrolled study of 25 patients with chronic renal insufficiency (serum creatinine levels >1.8 mg/dL), who received intraoperative hydration (550 mL/h of 0.9% saline) and did not developed renal dysfunction.[73]

Using IV bicarbonate as an alternative to normal saline has been studied in the prevention of RCN. A single-center randomized trial of 119 patients by Merten et al[74] showed that the use of sodium bicarbonate hydration was superior to sodium chloride. Rates of contrast-induced nephropathy were significantly lower in the sodium bicarbonate group (1.7%, $n = 1$) when compared with the sodium chloride group (13.6%, $n = 8$) when both cohorts were administered 154 mEq/L of either solution IV (mean difference, 11.9%; 95% CI: 2.6%–21.2%; $P = 0.02$). The study authors concluded that using bicarbonate ion is more efficacious than chloride and suggested that contrast-induced free-radical formation (which usually causes an acidic environment) was abrogated by the increased pH in the extracellular fluid induced by sodium bicarbonate. Repeat studies have failed to show any benefit in using sodium bicarbonate. A meta-analysis evaluating the value of sodium bicarbonate as a prophylaxis for contrast-induced nephropathy showed no significant benefit.[75]

There is some evidence that reactive oxygen species play a role in the renal damage caused by radiocontrast agents.[76] N-acetylcysteine (NAC), an antioxidant, can act as a free-radical scavenger. NAC increases nitric oxide (NO) formation by increasing the expression of NO synthase and also increases the biologic effects of NO by combining with NO to form S-nitrosothiol, which is a potent vasodilator.[77] NAC has been shown to reduce ischemic renal failure in animal models.[78] Tepel et al[79] found that the incidence of contrast nephropathy after CT in patients with chronic renal insufficiency was greatly decreased with NAC. Patients were given 1200 mg of NAC per day, orally in divided doses on the day before and the day of administration of the contrast agent. This prevented the expected decline in renal function in all patients with chronic renal insufficiency (mean serum creatinine level 2.4 ± 1.3 mg/dL; creatinine clearance <50 mL/min). However, the study was limited by its lack of power ($n = 83$) and long-term follow-up.

TABLE 36–10
Steps to Minimize RCN

Prior to procedure
 1. Withdraw potential nephrotoxic agents (NSAIDS, diuretics)
 2. Hydrate with normal saline (1 mL/kg per hour for 6–12 h) or increase salt and fluid intake if not contraindicated
 3. Use N-acetylcysteine (NAC) 600 mg PO bid
During procedure
 1. Use low or isoosmolar agents
 2. Use low volume of radiocontrast agents (< 20 mL)
  a. Dilute with normal saline when using LOCM (1:1 or 1:3 ratio)
  b. Use small puffs of contrast (1–3 mL)
  c. Utilize digital subtraction
Post procedure
 1. Continue hydration for 12–24 h
 2. Continue NAC
 3. Avoid repeat contrast study within 72 h
 4. Check creatinine in 2–3 days

A meta-analysis of the use of NAC for the prevention of RCN was conducted by Kelly in 2008 and showed only a mild benefit.[80] The usefulness of using NAC in clinical practice is a matter of some debate. However, given the association of renal dysfunction with increased mortality rates and in-patient hospital stays, the use of NAC seems reasonable to use in high-risk groups. An oral dose of 600 mg twice daily the day before and the day of procedure is the most commonly used regimen. IV doses of 150 mg/kg over half an hour before the procedure followed by 50 mg/kg administered over 4 hours can be used in critically ill patients or in those who are unable to take NAC orally.[81] Other agents have also been investigated such as mannitol, theophylline, furosemide, anaritide (the synthetic form of atrial natriuretic peptide), fenoldopam (dopamine agonist), and atorvastatin for prevention of RCN, but none of these have shown any benefit.

Removal of contrast media by hemodialysis and hemofiltration after the procedure in patients with preexisting renal failure has also been investigated. These studies have shown no effect on RCN and proven to be unwarranted as a routine clinical practice.[82, 83] Vogt et al[84] evaluated prophylactic hemodialysis to see if the contrast agent could be efficiently removed, thus reducing the concentration to which the kidneys were exposed, but this procedure showed no beneficial effect compared with using saline hydration alone. Table 36-10 summarizes the strategies for prevention of RCN.

CONCLUSION

Contrast media have well-recognized adverse events. While the majority of reactions are mild and self limiting, severe reactions contribute to morbidity and mortality in high-risk patients. It is therefore very important to recognize such patients early. Management includes being well versed with recognizing reactions early and giving appropriate treatment. Patients need to be informed of their reactions and such information must be noted in their charts as well. It may be helpful to refer them to an allergologist as well to evaluate for safer agents that can be used. RCN is another potential complication with contrast use in patients with chronic kidney disease. Hydration and the use of small doses of RCM along with isoosmolar agent use have been shown to be beneficial.

REFERENCES

1. Idee JM, Pines E, Prigent P, Corot C. Allergy-like reactions to iodinated contrast agents. A critical analysis. *Fundam Clin Pharmacol*. 2005;19:263–281.
2. Scherer K, Harr T, Bach S, Bircher AJ. The role of iodine in hypersensitivity reactions to radiocontrast media. *Clin Exp Allergy*. 2010;40:468–475.
3. ACR committee on drugs and contrast media. ACR manual on contrast media. Version 7, 2010;5–10.
4. Canter L. Anaphylactoid reactions to radiocontrast media. *Allergy Asthma Proc*. 2005;26:199–203.
5. Meth MJ, Maibach HI. Current understanding of contrast media reactions and implications for clinical management. *Drug Safety*. 2006;29(2):133–141.
6. Trcka J, Schmidt C, Seitz CS, Brocker EB, Gross GE, Trautman A. Anaphylaxis to iodinated contrast material: nonallergic hypersensitivity or IgE mediated allergy? *Am J Roentgenol*. 2008;190:666–670.
7. Laroche D, Namour F, Lefrancois C, Aimone-Gastin I, Romano A, Sainte-Laudy J, Laxenaire MC, Gueant JL. Anaphylactoid and anaphylactic reactions to iodinated contrast material. *Allergy*. 1999;54(suppl 58):13–16.
8. Lieberman PL, Seigle R. Reactions to radiocontrast material. *Clin Rev Allergy Immunol*. 1999;17:469–496.
9. Namasivayam S, Kalra MK, Torees WE, Small WC. Adverse reactions to intravenous iodinated contrast media: a primer for radiologists. *Emerg Radiol*. 2006;12:210–215.
10. Lang DM, Allpern MB, Visintainer PF, Smith ST. Increased risk for anaphylactoid reaction from contrast media in patients on B-adrenergic blockers or with asthma. *Ann Int Med*. 1991;115:270–276.
11. Lang DM, Allpern MB, Visintainer PF, Smith ST. Elevated risk of anaphylactoid reaction from radiographic contrast media is associated with both {beta}-blocker exposure and cardiovascular disorders. *Arch Intern Med*. 1993;153(17):2033–2040.
12. Rao VM, Rao AK, Steiner RM, Burka ER, Grainger RG, Ballas SK. The effect of ionic and nonionic contrast media on the sickling phenomenon. *Radiology*. 1982;144(2):291–293.
13. Aronson JK. *"Radiologic Contrast Media". Side Effects of Drugs Annual 27*. 1st ed, Amsterdam: Elsevier B.V; 2004.
14. Gueant-Rodriguez RM, Romano A, Barbaud A, Brockow K, Gueant JL. Hypersensitivity reactions to iodinated contrast media. *Curr Pharmaceut Design*. 2006;12:3359–3372.
15. Nygaard B, Nygaard T, Jensen LI, Court-Payen M, Soe-Jensen P, Nielson KG, Fugl M, Hansen JM. Iohexol: effects on uptake of radioactive iodine in the thyroid and on thyroid function. *Acad Radiol*. 1998;5:409–414.
16. Biad SK, Lai EW, Wesley RA, Ling A, Timmers HJLM, Adma KT, Kozupa A, Pacak K. Brief communication: radiographic contrast infusion and catecholamine release in patients with pheochromocytoma. *Ann Intern Med*. 2009;150(6):27–32.
17. Georgsen J, Rasmussen F, Antonsen S, Larsen ML. Influence of radiographic contrast media on granulocyte enzymes and complement during uncomplicated urographies. *Eur J Radiol*. 1991;12(1):63–66.
18. Rasmussen F, Antonsen S, Georgsen J. Granulocyte enzymes and complement after an anaphylactoid reaction to coronary angiography. *Eur J Radiol*. 1991;13(1):46–49.
19. Morcos SK. Effects of radiographic contrast media on the lung. *Brit J Radiol*. 2003;76:290–295.
20. Goldsmith SR, Steinberg P. Noncardiogenic pulmonary edema induced by nonionic low osmolality radiographic contrast media. *J Allergy Clin Immunol*. 1995;96:698–699.
21. Thomsen HS, Morcos SK. Radiographic contrast media. *BJU Int*. 2000;86(suppl. 1):1–10.
22. Bush WH, Swanson DP. Acute reactions to intravascular contrast media: types, risk factors, recognition and specific treatment. *Am J Roentgenol*. 1991;157:1153–1161.
23. Caro JJ, Trindade E, McGregor M. The risks of death and of severe nonfatal reactions with high vs. low osmolality contrast media: a meta-analysis. *Am J Roentgenol*. 1991;156:825–832.
24. Ansell G, Tweedie MCK, West CR, Evans P, Couch L. The current status of reactions to intravenous contrast media. *Invest Radiol*. 1980;15(6):532–539.
25. Katayma H, Yamaguchi K, Kozuka T, Takashima T, Seez P, Matsuura K. Adverse reactions to ionic and nonionic media. *Radiology*. 1990;175:621–628.
26. Morcos SK, Thomsen HS. Adverse reactions to iodinated contrast media. *Eur Radiol*. 2001;11:1267–1275.
27. Lang DM, Allpern MB, Visintainer PF, Smith ST. Increased risk for anyphylactoid reaction from contrast media in patients on B-adrenergic blockers or with asthma. *Ann Int Med*. 1991;115:270–276.
28. Lang DM, Allpern MB, Visintainer PF, Smith ST. Elevated risk of anaphylactoid reaction from radiographic contrast media is associated with both {beta}-blocker exposure and cardiovascular disorders. *Arch Intern Med*. 1993;153(17):2033–2040.
29. Greenberger PA, Meyers SN, Kramer BL, Kramer BL. Effects of beta-adrenergic and calcium antagonists on the development of anaphylactoid reactions from radiographic contrast media during cardiac angiography. *J Allergy Clin Immunol*. 1987;80(5):698–702.
30. Thomsen HS, Morcos SK, Management of acute adverse reactions to contrast media. *Eur Radiol*. 2004;14:476–481.
31. Christiansen C. Late-onset allergy-like reactions to X-ray contrast media. *Curr Opin Allergy Clin Immunol*. 2002;2:333–339.
32. Webb JAW, Stacul F, Thomsen HS, Morcos SK. Late adverse reactions to intravascular iodinated contrast media. *Eur Radiol*. 2003;13:181–184.
33. Sutton AGC, Finn P, Grech ED, Hall JA, Stewart MJ, Davies A, deBelder MA. Early and late reactions after the use of iopamidol 340, ioxaglate 320 and iodixanol 320 in cardiac catheterization. *Am Heart J*. 2001;141:677–683.
34. Christiansen C, Pichler WJ, Skotland T. Delayed allergy like reactions to the Xray contrast media: mechanistic considerations. *Eur Radiol*. 2000;10:1965–1975.

35. Mikkonen R, Kontkanen T, Kivisaari L. Acute and late adverse reactions to low osmolal contrast media. *Acta Radiol.* 1995;36:72–76.

36. Yoshikawa H. Late adverse reactions to nonionic contrast media. *Radiology.* 1992;183(3):737–740.

37. Baert AL. *"Adverse Reactions, Iodinated Contrast Media, Delayed".* Encyclopedia of Diagnostic Imaging. Vol. 2. Belgium: Springer; 2008.

38. Bohora S, Harikrishnan S, Tharakan J. Iodide mumps. *Int J Cardiol.* 2008;130:82–83.

39. Wyplosz B, Louet AL, Scotte F, Chevrot A. Recurrent iodide mumps after repeated administration of contrast media. *Ann Intern Med.* 2006;145(2): 155–156.

40. Park SJ, Hong HS, Lee HK, Joh JH, Cha JG, Kim HC. Ultrasound findings of iodide mumps. *Brit J Radiol.* 2005;78:164–165.

41. Beaty AD, Lieberman PL, Slavin R. Seafood allergy and radiocontrast media: Are physicians propagating a myth? *Am J Med.* 2008;121(2):158.e1–158.e4.

42. Schabelman E, Witting M. The relationship of radiocontrast, iodine and seafood allergies: A medical myth exposed. *J Em Med.* 2010;39(5): 701–707.

43. Shehadi WH. Adverse reactions to intravascularly administered contrast media. A comprehensive study based on a prospective survey. *Am J Roentgenol Radium Ther Nucl Med.* 1975;124:145–152.

44. Coakley FV, Panicek DM. Iodine allergy: An oyster without a pearl? *Am J Roentgenol.* 1997;169:951–952.

45. Shionoya H, Sugihara Y, Okano K, Sagami F, Mikami T, Katayama K. Studies on experimental iodine allergy: 2. Iodinated protein antigens and their generation from inorganic and organic iodine containing chemicals. *J Toxicol Sci.* 2004;29(2):137–145.

46. Boehm I. Letter to the Editor. Seafood allergy and radiocontrast media: Are physicians propagating a myth? *Am J Med.* 2008;121(8):e19.

47. Lierberman P. Anaphylactic reactions during surgical and medical procedures. *J Allergy Clin Immunol.* 2002;110: S64–S69.

48. Lasser EC, Berry CC, Talner LB, Santini LC, Lang EK, Gerber FH, Stolberg HO. Pretreatment with corticosteroids to alleviate reactions to intravenous contrast material. *N Engl J Med.* 1987;317:845–849.

49. Lasser EC, Berry CC, Mishkin MM, Williamson B, Zheutlin N, Silverman JM. Pretreatment with corticosteroids to prevent adverse reaction to nonionic contrast media. *Am J Roentgenol.* 1994;162(3):523–526.

50. Greenberger PA, Patterson R. The prevention of immediate generalized reactions to radiocontrast media in high risk patients. *J Allergy Clin Immunol.* 1991;87(4):867–872.

51. Dunsky EH, Zweiman B, Fischler E, Levy DA. Early effects of corticosteroids on basophils, leukocyte histamine, and tissue histamine. *J Allergy Clin Immunol.* 1979;63(6):426–432.

52. Morcos SK. Acute serious and fatal reactions to contrast media: our current understanding. *Brit J Radiol.* 2005;78:686–669.

53. Peachell PT, Morcos SK. Effect of radiographic contrast media on histamine release from human mast cells and basophils. *Brit J Radiol.* 1998;71:24–30.

54. Freed KS, Leder RA, Alexander C, DeLong DM, Kliewer MA. Breakthrough adverse reactions to low osmolar contrast media after steroid premedication. *Am J Roentgenol.* 2001;176:1389–1392.

55. Davenport MS, Cohan RH, Caoili EM, Ellis JH. Repeat contrast medium reactions in premedicated patients: frequency and severity. *Radiology.* 2009;253(2):372–379.

56. Zukiwski AA, David CL, Coan J, Wallace S, Gutterman JU, Mavligit GM. Increased incidence of hypersensitivity to iodine-containing radiographic contrast media after interleukin-2 administration. *Cancer.* 1990;65:1521–1524.

57. Scherer K, Harr T, Bach S, Bircher AJ. The role of iodine in hypersensitivity reactions to radio contrast media. *Clin Exper Allergy.* 2010;40:468–475.

58. Singh J, Daftary A. Iodinated contrast media and their adverse reactions. *J Nucl Med Technol.* 2008;36:69–74.

59. Tublin ME, Murphy ME, Tessler FN. Current concepts in contrast media-induced nephropathy. *Am J Roentgenol.* 1998;171:933–939.

60. Asif A, Preston RA, Roth D. Radiocontrast-induced nephropathy. *Am J Ther.* 2003;10:137–147.

61. Oliveira DB. Prophylaxis against contrast-induced nephropathy. *Lancet.* 1999;353:1638–1639.

62. Lindholt JS. Radiocontrast induced nephropathy. *Eur J Vasc Endovasc Surg.* 2003;25:296–304.

63. Briguori C, Tavano D, Colombo A. Contrast agent-associated nephrotoxicity. *Prog Cardiovasc Dis.* 2003;45:493–503.

64. Rudnick MR, Goldfarb S, Wexler L, Ludbrook PA, Murphy MJ, Halpern EF, Hill JA, Winniford M, Cohen MB, VanFossen DB. Nephrotoxicity of ionic and nonionic contrast media in 1196 patients: a randomized trial. The Iohexol Cooperative Study. *Kidney Int.* 1995;47:254–261.

65. Aspelin P, Aubry P, Fransson SG, Strasser R, Willenbrock R, Berg KJ, et al. Nephrotoxic effects in high-risk patients undergoing angiography. *N Engl J Med.* 2003;348(6):491–498.

66. Chalmers N, Jackson RW. Comparison of iodixanol and iohexol in renal impairment. *Br J Radiol.* 1999;72:701–703.

67. Tadros GM, Malik JA, Manske CL, Kasiske BL, Dickinson SE, Herzog CA, Wilson RF, Das G, Panetta CJ. Iso-osmolar radio contrast iodixanol in patients with chronic kidney disease. *J Invasive Cardiol.* 2005;17:211–215.

68. Kian K, Wyatt C, Schon D, Packer J, Vassalotti J, Mishler R. Safety of low dose radiocontrast for interventional AV fistula salvage in stage 4 chronic kidney disease patients. *Kidney Int.* 2006;69:1444–1449.

69. Asif A, Cherla G, Merrill D, Cipleu CD, Tawakol JB, Epstein DL, Lenz O. Venous mapping using venography and the risk of radiocontrast-induced nephropathy. *Semin Dial.* 2005;18(3):239–242.

70. Anto H, Chou SY, Porush J, Shapiro W. Infusion intravenous pyelography and renal function: effects of hypertonic mannitol in patients with chronic renal insufficiency. *Arch Intern Med.* 1981;141:1652–1656.

71. Gleeson TG, Bulugahapitiya S. Review of Contrast induced nephropathy. *Am J Radiol.* 2004;183:1673–1689.

72. Brown RS, Ransil B, Clark BA. Prehydration protects against contrast nephropathy in high risk patients undergoing cardiac catheterization. *J Am Soc Nephrol.* 1990;1:330A.

73. Eisenberg RL, Bank WO, Hedgock MW. Renal failure after major angiography can be avoided with hydration. *Am J Roentgenol.* 1981;136:859–863.

74. Merten GJ, Burgess WP, Gray LV, Holleman JH, Roush TS, Kowalchuk GJ, Bersin RM, Van Moore A, Simonton CA 3rd, Rittase RA, Norton HJ, Kennedy TP. Prevention of contrast-induced nephropathy with sodium bicarbonate: a randomized controlled trial. *J Am Med Assoc.* 2004;291:2328–2334.

75. Zoungas S, Ninomiya T, Huxley R, Cass A, Jardine M, Gallagher M, Patel A, Vasheghani-Farahani A, Sadigh G, Perkovic V. Systematic review: sodium bicarbonate therapy for contrast induced acute kidney injury. *Ann Intern Med.* 2009;151:631–638.

76. Love L, Johnson M, Bresler M, Nelson JE, Olson MC, Flisak ME. The persistent computed tomography nephrogram: its significance in the diagnosis of contrast-associated nephropathy. *Br J Radiol.* 1994;67:951–957.

77. Safirstein R, Andrade L, Vierira JM. Acetylcysteine and nephrotoxic effects of radiographic contrast agents: a new use for an old drug. (Editorial). *N Engl J Med.* 2000;343:210–212.

78. DiMari J, Megyesi J, Udvarhelyi N, Price P, Davis R, Safirstein R. N-acetylcysteine ameliorates ischemic renal failure. *Am J Physiol.* 1997;272: F292–F298.

79. Tepel M, Van Der Giet M, Schwarzfeld C, Laufer U, Liermann D, Zidek W. Prevention of radiographic-contrast-agent-induced reductions in renal function by acetylcysteine. *N Engl J Med.* 2000;343:180–184.

80. Kelly AM, Dwamena B, Cronin P, Bernstein SJ, Carlos RC. Meta-analysis of N-acetylcysteine for prevention of CIN. *Ann Intern Med.* 2008;48:284–294.

81. Baker C, Wragg A, Kumar S, De Palma R, Baker LR, Knight CJ. A rapid protocol for the prevention of contrast-induced renal dysfunction: the RAPID study. *J Am Coll Cardiol.* 2003;41:2114–2118.

82. Lehnert T, Keller E, Condolf K, Schaffner T, Pavenstadt H, Schollmeyer P. Effect of hemodialysis after contrast medium administration in patients with renal insufficiency. *Nephrol Dial Transplant.* 1998;13:358–362.

83. Younathan CM, Kaude JV, Cook MD, Shaw GS, Peterson JC. Dialysis is not indicated immediately after administration of nonionic contrast agents in patients with end-stage renal disease treated by maintenance dialysis. *Am J Roentgenol.* 1994;163:969–971.

84. Vogt B, Ferrari P, Schonholzer C, Marti HP, Mohaupt M, Wiederkehr M, Cereghetti C, Serra A, Huynh-Do U, Uehlinger D, Frey FJ. Prophylactic hemodialysis after radiocontrast media in patients with renal insufficiency is potentially harmful. *Am J Med.* 2001;111:692–698.

RADIOCONTRAST AND CARBON DIOXIDE ANGIOGRAPHY: ADVANTAGES AND DISADVANTAGES

TUSHAR J. VACHHARAJANI

LEARNING OBJECTIVES

1. To understand the physicochemical properties of radiocontrast agent.
2. To understand the role of iodinated agent versus carbon dioxide in interventional nephrology.

INTRODUCTION

A contrast agent is essential to define a vascular structure with imaging techniques involved in the practice of interventional nephrology. An ideal contrast agent should have several, if not all, of the following properties: water solubility, low viscosity, low or iso-osmolarity compared to human plasma, biologically inert with minimal toxicity, low cost, and a stable chemical compound.

Since 1950s, iodinated radiographic contrast media have been used to study various vascular beds in the human body. Despite major developments and chemical modifications of the basic iodinated benzene ring structure, an ideal contrast agent is still far from reality. Swick published the use of water-soluble iodinated intravenous contrast in urology[1] and continued to develop safer compound primarily for renal scintigraphy. Almen in 1960s developed the first nonionic monomer with lower osmolarity that was used primarily for myelography.[2] The continued research and developments have lead to the currently available contrast agents with varied physicochemical properties. The osmolarity and the ionic property of the radiocontrast agent have been modified to improve the side-effect profile of these agents.

CLASSIFICATION OF IODINATED RADIOCONTRAST AGENTS

1. Based on osmolarity: high-osmolar and low-osmolar agent.

   The osmolarity can range from 700 to 2100 mOsm/kg water for these agents. The low-osmolar agents have an osmolarity that is higher than that of plasma, but is low compared to the historic high-osmolar agents. The isoosmolar agents have an osmolarity that is closer to that of plasma (around 300 mOsm/kg water).

2. Based on chemical structure: ionic monomers, nonionic monomers, ionic dimers, nonionic dimers.

   Ionic monomeric agents have single tri-iodated benzene ring that form salts in plasma, ionic dimeric agents contain twice the number of iodine atoms per molecule and nonionic monomeric agents, the newest contrast materials, are essentially hydrophilic and less chemotoxic. The radiocontrast agents commonly used in US are listed in Table 37-1.

The radiocontrast agents have a long history of efficacy in clinical practice and serve as a standard for comparison with other contrast agents such as carbon dioxide. The efficacy in terms of vascular opacification is identical with high- and low-osmolar radiocontrast agents. However, the side-effect profile depends on the physicochemical properties of the specific contrast agent. Hemodynamic alterations due to the osmotic properties of a contrast agent include vasodilatation, hemodilution, endothelial damage, and changes in blood–brain barrier. The clinical changes seen as result of exposure to these agents include decrease in cardiac output, negative inotropic effect on

TABLE 37–1

Commonly Used Radiocontrast Agents in US

Generic Name (Trade Names)	Osmolarity
Ionic agents	
Iothalamate (Conray 60)	1400
Diatrizoate (Urografin)	2070
Nonionic agents	
Iopamidol (Isovue)	796
Ioversol (Optiray 300)	651
Iohexol (Omnipaque)	780
Iodixanol (Vispaque)	290
Iotrolan (Isovist)	320

the myocardium, renal vasoconstriction, osmotic diuresis, altered permeability of blood–brain barrier, and increased pulmonary arterial resistance.[3-5] Its effect on the red blood cells along with the endothelial damage and release of vasoactive substances (Table 37-2) can lead to changes in microcirculation.[5]

The high-osmolar radiocontrast agents are the oldest and have been associated with higher incidence of adverse events as compared to low-osmolar agents. In general, the low-osmolar nonionic contrast agents offer a better safety profile when compared to high-osmolar ionic contrast agents.[6]

ADVERSE REACTION TO IODINATED RADIOCONTRAST AGENTS

The safety profile of radiocontrast agent is superior relative to all other available drugs in the market. The fatal risk is low with a reported death rate of 1–3 events/100,000 contrast administrations.[7] The overall risk for adverse reactions is 4–12% with ionic (high-osmolar) radiocontrast agents and 1–3% with nonionic agents. The risk of severe adverse reaction with ionic and nonionic contrast agent is 0.16% and 0.03%, respectively.[7]

▶ Incidence

The frequency of adverse reactions is highest in 20–50-year-old adults and relatively rare in the pediatric

TABLE 37–2

Vasoactive Substances Released by Radiocontrast Agent

1. Histamine
2. Serotonin
3. Prostaglandins
4. Bradykinin
5. Complements
6. Kallikreins

population.[8] The overall risk of adverse reaction with radiocontrast agent is about 15%. Katayama et al reported the risk of adverse reactions in a large study, comparing ionic and nonionic contrast agent as 12.66% and 3.13%, respectively, while the risk of serious reaction as 0.22% and 0.04%, respectively.[9] The severe reactions included dyspnea, sudden hypotension, loss of consciousness, and death. In a retrospective review of more than 11,000 low-osmolality nonionic contrast administrations in children reported by Dillman et al, only 0.18% had acute allergic reactions with 80% categorized as mild, 5% as moderate, and 15% as severe.[10]

Severe adverse reactions have been found to be higher with high-osmolar compared to low-osmolar contrast agents. A meta-analysis published by Caro et al revealed risk of 0.157% versus 0.031% between the two types of agents with risk of death being identical with both types at 1 event/100,000 patients.[11]

Nephrotoxicity has been reported to be less frequent with low-osmolar agents.[12] Other side effects such as nausea and vomiting are less common with nonionic monomers compared to ionic dimers.[13]

▶ Risk Factors

Risk factors for idiosyncratic reactions include previous adverse reaction to contrast agent (3.9- to 6.9-fold), history of asthma (eightfold),[14] and history of atopy (fivefold).[9] The association between seafood allergy and increased risk of adverse reaction to radiocontrast agent has not been consistently reported in literature. Moreover, seafood allergy is rarely in response to iodine contained in the food.[8]

The presence of comorbid conditions such as cardiac disease, dehydration, hematological disorders predisposing to thrombosis, and preexisting renal disease has been known to increase the risk of adverse reactions.[15] Patients receiving β-blockers are more likely to experience an adverse reaction and frequently require hospitalization for their treatment.[14]

Contrast-induced nephrotoxicity is more likely in patients who are azotemic, diabetic, have history of class IV congestive heart failure, hyperuricemia, concomitant use of nonsteroidal anti-inflammatory agents, advanced age, and with large volume of contrast exposure.[16-18] The likelihood of developing nephrotoxicity was 3.3-fold more with high-osmolar agent compared to low-osmolar contrast agent.[19] The incidence of contrast-induced nephrotoxicity following interventional studies to salvage arteriovenous fistula in stage 4 chronic kidney disease patients has been reported to be 4% and 4.6%, 2 days and 1 week after contrast exposure, respectively.[20] Asif et al did not find any difference in the estimated glomerular filtration rate, 48 hours after venous mapping venography for permanent access placement in stages 4 and 5 chronic kidney disease patients.[21]

The incidence of adverse reactions has been reported to be higher in women. Lang et al reported 21/22 severe anaphylactoid reactions in 5264 consecutive CT-scans studies, occurring in women.[22] The risk of adverse reaction is identical with arterial and venous studies.[8]

▶ Classification

The adverse reactions can be classified as idiosyncratic and nonidiosyncratic.[3,23,24] Pathophysiologically these are related to the direct cellular effect, enzyme induction and activation of complement pathway, fibrinolytic, kinin, and other systems. The physicochemical properties of radiocontrast agent, the dose, and speed of injection can play a role in nonidiosyncratic reactions.

Idiosyncratic reactions are often referred to as allergic reactions and typically begin within 20 minutes of contrast administration. The idiosyncratic reaction is dose-independent and is mediated by complement activation and not via IgE. Thus it is not a true hypersensitivity reaction. They are also called anaphylactoid reaction as they are not IgE-dependent.[15,25,26]

Clinically these reactions can be classified as mild, moderate, and severe. Mild symptoms include nausea, vomiting, feeling of heat, sweating, itching, and pain. Moderate symptoms include dizziness, hypotension, prolonged vomiting, dyspnea, facial and laryngeal edema, chest pain, tachycardia or bradycardia, palpitation, and abdominal cramps. Severe symptoms include life-threatening arrhythmia, shock, seizures, severe bronchospasm, cardiac arrest, and death.

PROPHYLAXIS FOR ADVERSE REACTIONS

A radiocontrast study should be performed only when it is absolutely necessary. Patients at high risk should be considered for alternative noncontrast imaging studies. A proper history and review of available medical records can reduce the risk of adverse reactions in high-risk patients. Unfortunately there is no reliable predictive test that can be performed to identify patients who may develop severe reactions to radiocontrast agent. The incidence of idiosyncratic reactions is lower with nonionic agent and hence switching to these agents will decrease the chance of a reaction.

Several regimens using methylprednisolone (oral or intravenous) and diphenhydramine, H-2 blockers and H-1 antihistamines have been studied. Lasser et al studied methylprednisolone two oral doses of 32 mg each administered at 12 and 2 hours before contrast study reducing the incidence of all adverse reactions from 9% to 6.4%.[27] Marshall and Lieberman studied three different pretreatment regimens in 149 patients. Seven percent of the 149 pretreated patients developed reactions and the rate and severity of reaction was equal in all three groups.[28] The most widely practiced protocol in United States is prednisone 50 mg orally, 13, 7, and 1 hour before the procedure along with diphenhydramine 50 mg orally 1 hour prior to the procedure.

No pretreatment protocols have been shown to eliminate repeat reactions or significantly reduce the incidence

in high-risk patients. Greenberger et al showed a reduction in incidence of contrast-related adverse reaction from 9% to 7% in high-risk patients by using a premedication regimen with prednisone 50 mg orally 13, 7, and 1 hour along with diphenhydramine 50 mg orally 1 hour before the procedure.[29]

TREATMENT OF ADVERSE REACTIONS

The adverse reaction can vary in severity from mild to severe and physician responsible for administering radiocontrast should be able to recognize and treat these acute adverse events immediately. Availability of emergency equipment in the facility where these procedures are performed is essential. Most reactions occur within first 20–30 minutes following the administration of radiocontrast agent.

Minor symptoms such as urticaria, pruritus, or mild bronchospasm can be treated by immediate discontinuation of radiocontrast agent, if it is still being administered, followed by intravenous administration of H1 receptor blocker, diphenhydramine. If the symptoms persists then treatment with epinephrine 0.1–0.3 mL (1:1000) administered subcutaneously should be considered.

Hypotension, facial edema, and laryngeal spasms can quickly progress to life-threatening events and need to be recognized early and treated with supplemental oxygen and intravenous slow administration of epinephrine 1:10,000, 1 mL and repeated if necessary in 5–10 minutes. If patient continues to progress, intubation and full life support systems may be necessary.

▶ Severe Anaphylactoid Reaction

Early recognition of the problem and activating the advanced cardiac life support system is absolutely essential. Epinephrine is the mainstay therapy and should be administered intravenously as soon as possible and repeated if necessary. Airway management with supplemental oxygen support and intubation along with volume expansion is critical component of the therapy. The patient should be closely monitored for the subsequent 24 hours for any delayed recurrence of symptoms.

CARBON DIOXIDE AS A CONTRAST AGENT

Carbon dioxide (CO_2) is an alternate contrast agent that can be used in patients with history of life-threatening allergy to iodinated radiocontrast agent. Carbon dioxide use for angiographic studies has been widely reported in literature.[30-33] CO_2 has been used in all vascular bed except for cerebral and coronary circulation. CO_2 is a highly soluble gas and generates a negative image, whereas iodinated radiocontrast generates a positive radiographic image. The gas gets rapidly eliminated from the lungs and does not have the allergic reaction or nephrotoxic effect associated with iodinated radiocontrast agent.

► Advantages and Disadvantages of CO_2

CO_2 is an invisible, buoyant, nonviscous, and compressible gas. CO_2 does not mix with blood, unlike the iodinated radiocontrast agent and being buoyant can rise to the nondependent portion of the vessel. CO_2 is nonallergic, nonnephrotoxic and being of low viscosity can be easily delivered using smaller sized catheters. The CO_2 angiography is ideal in patient with allergic reaction to iodinated contrast and those with high risk of renal toxicity from conventional contrast agents. The major disadvantage is the need for a unique delivery system. The current delivery system has been largely developed over the past 20 years by Hawkins and Caridi.[34] Since the gas is invisible, there is a potential for contamination with room air. CO_2 angiography is absolutely contraindicated in cerebral and coronary circulation.

► Experience with CO_2 Angiography

CO_2 angiography has been used primarily in patients with renal dysfunction because it is not nephrotoxic. Animal studies in canines with selective renal arterial injection have been shown to be safe with no significant effects on renal function or histology.[35] As yet there are no published reports of CO_2-induced nephropathy in humans. CO_2 angiography has been used to study infradiaphragmatic arteries[36,37] and to effectively image the central veins and upper limb veins.[33,38]

CO_2 as a contrast agent to guide vascular intervention has been evaluated either as a single agent or in combination with gadolinium-based agents to prevent renal toxic effects in high-risk patients.[39,40] The strong association of nephrogenic systemic fibrosis with gadolinium-based contrast agents, this combination is definitely not a safe alternative in patients with renal failure.[41]

Eschelman et al performed 26 vascular interventions in 22 patients using combination of CO_2 and conventional radiocontrast agent. Of the various vascular beds that were evaluated, 80% were arterial interventions and remaining were venous including one study performed on a thrombosed lower extremity dialysis arteriovenous graft. Successful intervention was possible with CO_2 alone in 8 patients and 11 patients required less than 20 mL of supplemental radiocontrast agent. The CO_2 angiography was found to be unsatisfactory for intra-abdominal arteries.[39]

Heye et al prospectively compared the diagnostic performance of CO_2 venography to the conventional iodinated contrast venography for venous mapping for hemodialysis access creation in 22 patients (Figure 37-1). The degree of central vein stenosis was underestimated in 30% of cases. Overall CO_2 venography was 97% sensitive and 85% specific in assessing the upper limb and central veins as compared to the standard iodinated radiocontrast. The CO_2 venography was found to be a reproducible and reliable technique with independent observers.[38]

The clinical experience with CO_2 angiography in evaluating the hemodialysis access is limited. Ehrman et al compared the diagnostic accuracy of detecting stenosis in dialysis arteriovenous graft in 32 patients. Digital subtraction studies were performed in all patients using conventional radiocontrast agent and CO_2. The degree of stenosis was graded to be higher compared

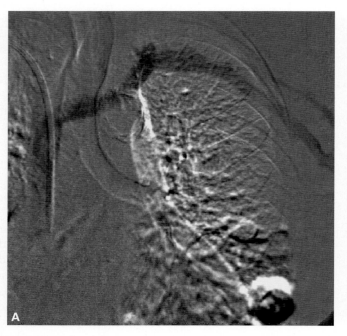
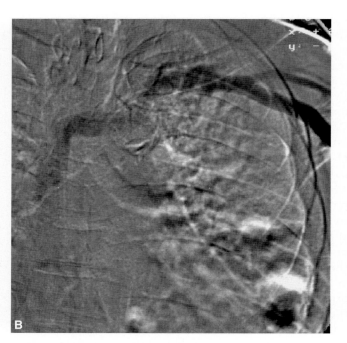

Figure 37-1. Venogram obtained in the same patient by CO_2 venography (**A**) and conventional iodinated contrast (**B**). (Images were kindly provided by Dr. S. Heye, from the department of radiology, University Hospitals Gasthuisberg, Leuven, Belgium.)

to iodinated contrast studies by two independent physicians. Even though CO_2 angiography was found to be safe, the specificity, sensitivity, and accuracy were 58%, 94%, and 75%, respectively.[42]

A recent study from Japan evaluated the efficacy of CO_2 angiography in failing hemodialysis access. CO_2 fistulography was performed in 115 of the 141 cases referred for access evaluation. CO_2 fistulography was not possible in thrombosed accesses or those with sluggish flow. Iodinated contrast agent had to be used in the event of vascular rupture or dissection. Serious complication due to reflux of CO_2 into the thoracic aorta during the procedure resulted in transient loss of consciousness in three patients.[43]

SUMMARY

A contrast agent is absolutely essential for imaging vascular structure. In clinical practice conventional iodinated radiocontrast agent, CO_2 gas and gadolinium-based agents have been used. The clinical experience with conventional iodinated radiocontrast agent is by far the most extensive when evaluating the hemodialysis access. The clinical experience with CO_2 fistulography remains limited and restricted to few centers.

REFERENCES

1. Swick M. Radiographic media in urology. The discovery of excretion urography: historical and developmental aspects of the organically bound urographic media and their role in the varied diagnostic angiographic areas. *Surg Clin North Am.* 1978;58(5):977–994.
2. Almen T. Contrast agent design. Some aspects on the synthesis of water soluble contrast agents of low osmolality. *J Theor Biol.* 1969;24(2):216–226.
3. Bush WH, Swanson DP. Acute reactions to intravascular contrast media: types, risk factors, recognition, and specific treatment. *AJR Am J Roentgenol.* 1991;157(6):1153–1161.
4. McClennan BL, Preston M. Hickey memorial lecture. Ionic and nonionic iodinated contrast media: evolution and strategies for use. *AJR Am J Roentgenol.* 1990;155(2):225–233.
5. Dawson P. New contrast agents. Chemistry and pharmacology. *Invest Radiol.* 1984;19(suppl 6):S293–S300.
6. Lawrence V, Matthai W, Hartmaier S. Comparative safety of high-osmolality and low-osmolality radiographic contrast agents. Report of a multidisciplinary working group. *Invest Radiol.* 1992;27(1):2–28.
7. Cochran ST. Anaphylactoid reactions to radiocontrast media. *Curr Allergy Asthma Rep.* 2005;5(1):28–31.
8. Lieberman PL, Seigle RL. Reactions to radiocontrast material. Anaphylactoid events in radiology. *Clin Rev Allergy Immunol.* 1999;17(4):469–496.
9. Katayama H, Yamaguchi K, Kozuka T, Takashima T, Seez P, Matsuura K. Adverse reactions to ionic and nonionic contrast media. A report from the Japanese Committee on the Safety of Contrast Media. *Radiology.* 1990;175(3):621–628.
10. Dillman JR, Strouse PJ, Ellis JH, Cohan RH, Jan SC. Incidence and severity of acute allergic-like reactions to i.v. nonionic iodinated contrast material in children. *AJR Am J Roentgenol.* 2007;188(6):1643–1647.
11. Caro JJ, Trindade E, McGregor M. The risks of death and of severe nonfatal reactions with high- vs low-osmolality contrast media: a meta-analysis. *AJR Am J Roentgenol.* 1991;156(4):825–832.
12. Kinnison ML, Powe NR, Steinberg EP. Results of randomized controlled trials of low-versus high-osmolality contrast media. *Radiology.* 1989;170(2):381–389.
13. Foord KD, Kaye B, Howard J, Cumberland DC. Comparison of the side-effects of low-osmolar contrast media in intravenous urography. *Clin Radiol.* 1985;36(4):379–380.
14. Lang DM, Alpern MB, Visintainer PF, Smith ST. Elevated risk of anaphylactoid reaction from radiographic contrast media is associated with both beta-blocker exposure and cardiovascular disorders. *Arch Intern Med.* 1993;153(17):2033–2040.
15. Hagan JB. Anaphylactoid and adverse reactions to radiocontrast agents. *Immunol Allergy Clin North Am.* 2004;24(3):507–519, vii–viii.
16. Asif A, Preston RA, Roth D. Radiocontrast-induced nephropathy. *Am J Ther.* 2003;10(2):137–147.
17. Lindholt JS. Radiocontrast induced nephropathy. *Eur J Vasc Endovasc Surg.* 2003;25(4):296–304.
18. Briguori C, Tavano D, Colombo A. Contrast agent—associated nephrotoxicity. *Prog Cardiovasc Dis.* 2003;45(6):493–503.
19. Rudnick MR, Goldfarb S, Wexler L, et al. Nephrotoxicity of ionic and nonionic contrast media in 1196 patients: a randomized trial. The Iohexol Cooperative Study. *Kidney Int.* 1995;47(1):254–261.
20. Kian K, Wyatt C, Schon D, Packer J, Vassalotti J, Mishler R. Safety of low-dose radiocontrast for interventional AV fistula salvage in stage 4 chronic kidney disease patients. *Kidney Int.* 2006;69(8):1444–1449.
21. Asif A, Cherla G, Merrill D, et al. Venous mapping using venography and the risk of radiocontrast-induced nephropathy. *Semin Dial.* 2005;18(3):239–242.
22. Lang DM, Alpern MB, Visintainer PF, Smith ST. Gender risk for anaphylactoid reaction to radiographic contrast media. *J Allergy Clin Immunol.* 1995;95(4):813–817.
23. Cutroneo P, Polimeni G, Curcuruto R, Calapai G, Caputi AP. Adverse reactions to contrast media: an analysis from spontaneous reporting data. *Pharmacol Res.* 2007;56(1):35–41.
24. Ansell G, Tweedie MC, West CR, Evans P, Couch L. The current status of reactions to intravenous contrast media. *Invest Radiol.* 1980;15(suppl 6):S32–S39.
25. Hong SJ, Wong JT, Bloch KJ. Reactions to radiocontrast media. *Allergy Asthma Proc.* 2002;23(5):347–351.
26. Greenberger PA. Contrast media reactions. *J Allergy Clin Immunol.* 1984;74(4 Pt 2):600–605.
27. Lasser EC, Berry CC, Talner LB, et al. Pretreatment with corticosteroids to alleviate reactions to intravenous contrast material. *N Engl J Med.* 1987;317(14):845–849.
28. Marshall GD, Jr., Lieberman PL. Comparison of three pretreatment protocols to prevent anaphylactoid reactions to radiocontrast media. *Ann Allergy.* 1991;67(1):70–74.
29. Greenberger PA, Patterson R, Radin RC. Two pretreatment regimens for high-risk patients receiving radiographic contrast media. *J Allergy Clin Immunol.* 1984;74(4 Pt 1):540–543.

30. Caridi JG, Hawkins IF, Jr. CO_2 digital subtraction angiography: potential complications and their prevention. *J Vasc Interv Radiol*. 1997;8(3):383–391.

31. Kerns SR, Hawkins IF, Jr. Carbon dioxide digital subtraction angiography: expanding applications and technical evolution. *AJR Am J Roentgenol*. 1995;164(3):735–741.

32. Kerns SR, Hawkins IF, Jr., Sabatelli FW. Current status of carbon dioxide angiography. *Radiol Clin North Am*. 1995;33(1):15–29.

33. Sullivan KL, Bonn J, Shapiro MJ, Gardiner GA. Venography with carbon dioxide as a contrast agent. *Cardiovasc Intervent Radiol*. 1995;18(3):141–145.

34. Hawkins IF, Jr., Caridi JG, Klioze SD, Mladinich CR. Modified plastic bag system with O-ring fitting connection for carbon dioxide angiography. *AJR Am J Roentgenol*. 2001; 176(1):229–232.

35. Hawkins IF, Jr., Mladinich CR, Storm B, et al. Short-term effects of selective renal arterial carbon dioxide administration on the dog kidney. *J Vasc Interv Radiol*. 1994;5(1):149–154.

36. Oliva VL, Denbow N, Therasse E, et al. Digital subtraction angiography of the abdominal aorta and lower extremities: carbon dioxide versus iodinated contrast material. *J Vasc Interv Radiol*. 1999;10(6):723–731.

37. Diaz LP, Pabon IP, Garcia JA, de la Cal Lopez MA. Assessment of CO_2 arteriography in arterial occlusive disease of the lower extremities. *J Vasc Interv Radiol*. 2000; 11(2 Pt 1):163–169.

38. Heye S, Maleux G, Marchal GJ. Upper-extremity venography: CO_2 versus iodinated contrast material. *Radiology*. 2006;241(1):291–297.

39. Eschelman DJ, Sullivan KL, Bonn J, Gardiner GA, Jr. Carbon dioxide as a contrast agent to guide vascular interventional procedures. *AJR Am J Roentgenol*. 1998;171(5):1265–1270.

40. Spinosa DJ, Angle JF, Hagspiel KD, Schenk WG, 3rd, Matsumoto AH. CO_2 and gadopentetate dimeglumine as alternative contrast agents for malfunctioning dialysis grafts and fistulas. *Kidney Int*. 1998;54(3):945–950.

41. Abu-Alfa AK. Nephrogenic systemic fibrosis and gadolinium-based contrast agents. *Adv Chronic Kidney Dis*. 2011;18(3):188–198.

42. Ehrman KO, Taber TE, Gaylord GM, Brown PB, Hage JP. Comparison of diagnostic accuracy with carbon dioxide versus iodinated contrast material in the imaging of hemodialysis access fistulas. *J Vasc Interv Radiol*. 1994;5(5):771–775.

43. Kariya S, Tanigawa N, Kojima H, et al. Efficacy of carbon dioxide for diagnosis and intervention in patients with failing hemodialysis access. *Acta Radiol*. 2010;51(9): 994–1001.

FLUOROSCOPY BASICS: THEORY, EQUIPMENT, AND USE IN VASCULAR ACCESS INTERVENTION

GERALD A. BEATHARD

LEARNING OBJECTIVES

Fluoroscopy and Radiation Exposure

1. Understand how X-rays are produced.
2. Understand the radiation exposure factors—milliamperage (mA) and kilovoltage (kVp).
3. Describe how mA and kVp are controlled when using a portable C-arm to perform fluoroscopy.
4. Discuss the two types of X-ray interactions with matter that are important to medicine.
5. Define the "inverse square law" and discuss its significance to preforming a fluoroscopic procedure.
6. Define the units of radiation.

Fluoroscopic Equipment

1. Discuss the major parts of a portable C-arm.
2. Discuss the differences between a 6-inch and a 12-inch image intensifier.
3. Discuss the use of magnification when using a portable C-arm for fluoroscopy.
4. Discuss the use of collimation and its value to fluoroscopy imaging.
5. Define "last image hold."

Imaging Techniques

1. Define pulse fluoroscopy.
2. Discuss the differences that would accrue from using a low pulse per second rate versus a high one when doing fluoroscopy.
3. Discuss digital subtraction angiography—how it is accomplished and its value to the interventionalist.

4. Discuss road mapping—how it is accomplished and its value to the interventionalist.
5. Discuss things that the interventionalist can do to improve image quality when doing a fluoroscopic examination.
6. Discuss factors that influence the amount of radiation that the patient receives when the interventionalist is doing a fluoroscopic examination.
7. Discuss the importance of source to tabletop distance when doing a fluoroscopic examination.
8. Discuss the importance of patient to image intensifier distance when doing a fluoroscopic examination.

RADIATION BASICS

Radiation is a form of energy. There are two basic types of radiation: particulate and electromagnetic. Particulate radiation involves fast-moving particles that have both energy and mass and is primarily produced by the disintegration of an unstable atom. This category includes alpha and beta particles. Electromagnetic radiation is pure energy with no mass. It exists as photons. It is composed of vibrating or pulsating waves of electrical and magnetic energy.

Light waves, radio waves, microwaves, X-rays, and gamma rays are examples of electromagnetic radiation. The basic difference between them is their wavelength and energy levels (Figure 38-1). X-rays are able to penetrate materials that light cannot because of their relatively short wavelength. X-rays and gamma rays differ only in their source of origin. X-rays are produced by an X-ray

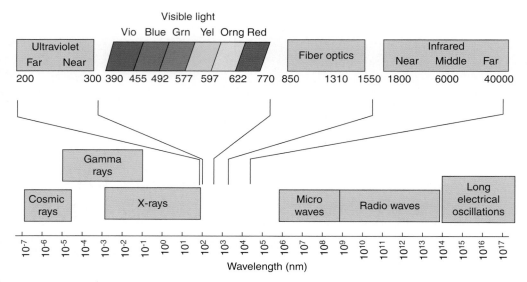

Figure 38-1. Electromagnetic radiation spectrum.

generator (manmade), while gamma radiation is the product of radioactive atoms (natural).

▶ Production of X-Rays

Medical X-ray photons are produced through a process referred to as *Bremsstrahlung* (from *bremsen* "to brake" and *Strahlung* "radiation," that is, "braking radiation" or "deceleration radiation"). This involves a change in the energy state of electrons. X-rays are generated when an electron is accelerated and then made to rapidly decelerate, usually due to interaction with another material. In an X-ray system (Figure 38-2), a large amount of electric current is passed through a tungsten filament (in a portable C-arm this is generally in the range of 30–150 kV), which heats the filament to several thousand degrees centigrade to create a source of free electrons. A large electrical potential is established between the filament (the cathode) and a target (the anode). The cathode and anode are enclosed

in a vacuum tube to prevent the filament from burning up and to prevent arcing between the cathode and anode. The electrical potential between the cathode and the anode pulls electrons from the cathode and accelerates them as they are attracted toward the anode or target, usually made of tungsten. The interaction of the electrons in the target results in the emission of X-rays from the target material. With most portable C-arms, the current flow is in the range of 0.5–5.0 mA. This can be pulsed on and off for on intervals measured in milliseconds. This enables consistent doses of X-rays, and taking "snapshots" of motion.

Once generated, X-rays are emitted in all directions in a relatively uniform manner. The lead housing surrounding the X-ray tube limits X-ray emission through a small opening or port. The resulting primary beam of useful radiation is shaped by additional lead shutters, or collimators, that can be adjusted to provide different beam shapes or sizes.

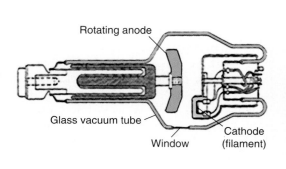

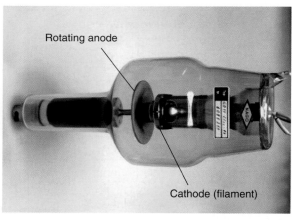

Figure 38-2. X-ray tube diagram.

In preforming a fluoroscopic procedure on a patient, there are dual goals that need to be considered: (1) diagnostic images of high quality should be obtained and (2) care should be exerted to reduce the radiation absorbed dose to the patient as much as possible. These goals are met by adjusting two factors: the mA and the kVp. The number of emitted X-ray photons, or dose, is adjusted by controlling the current flow (mA) and exposure time. The range of photonic energies emitted by the system can be adjusted by changing the applied voltage (kVp).

▶ Milliamperage

The quantity of electron flow, or current, in the X-ray tube is described in units of milliamperes (mA). With the types of procedures performed in the interventional lab using a portable C-arm, current in the range of 0.5–5 mA, usually 1–3 mA, is applied continuously (actually it is pulsed) as long as the fluoroscopy pedal is depressed. The X-ray output, and by definition the patient radiation dose, is directly proportional to the mA used. In simplistic terms, this variable can be thought of as the "quantity factor." The brightness of the image is directly proportional to the mA applied.

▶ Kilovoltage

The maximum kinetic energy of the accelerated electrons produced when the beam is activated is defined in terms of kilovolts peak potential (kVp). Producing a high-quality fluoroscopic examination largely depends upon proper selection of kVp. Proper selection of X-ray energy is required for maximum differential absorption by the tissue being examined. In simplistic terms, kVp can be thought of as the "quality factor." It determines the penetrating ability of the X-rays and the contrast of the image (Figure 38-3). Fluoroscopy tubes are designed for maximum kVp values of 125–150 kVp. With the types of procedures performed in the interventional lab using a portable C-arm, the kVp used rarely exceeds the 60–70 kVp range.

The rate of X-ray production is directly proportional to the electron flow. Higher mA values generate more electrons

to strike the tungsten target thereby producing more X-rays. The total number of X-rays produced at a set kVp depends directly on the product of the mA and exposure time and is directly proportional to these two variables.

Increasing kVp attracts more electrons from the filament, also increasing the rate of X-ray production. However, this relationship is not directly proportional; it is related to the square of the kVp. In obtaining a diagnostic image, there is a reciprocal relationship between mA and kVp. The brightness of the fluoroscopic image is directly proportional to the mA and proportional to the square of the kVp. Therefore if the kVp is increased from 80 to 88 kVp (a 10% change), a 100% change (doubling) of brightness occurs. This allows for the mA to be reduced by half to maintain the same standard output brightness. This has the effect of reducing the radiation dosage directed to the patient. It must be noted that there is a downside to this beneficial effect. The image contrast degrades as kVp is increased. Therefore if the system is operated at a high kVp and a low mA, the patient's radiation dosage will be reduced, but the image will not be as good. At lower kVp levels image contrast is enhanced, but because of the required increase in mA, the patient will receive more radiation. A balance between these two desirable effects must be made.

▶ Controlling the mA and kVp

Managing these factors, mA and kVp, seems like quite a challenge and it would be if not for the automatic brightness control (ABC) system that is incorporated into modern fluoroscopy machines. This system is a circuit that interfaces with the X-ray generator to adjust the kVp and mA in a fast feedback loop that keeps the light output of the image intensifier constant over variations in tissue thickness and density (patient attenuation) and system geometry. It allows for automatic changes in exposure factors under varying conditions and as conditions change during a procedure. It provides an optimum balance between mA and kVp to provide the best-quality image with the least radiation risk to the patient and personnel.

The mA/kVp ratio that is optimum to balance between the two goals of best possible image quality and lowest possible radiation absorbed dose to the patient is dependent upon the tissue type (Table 38-1) and thickness in the field. During a procedure, as one moves from the thickness of the chest with a large proportion of air-filled tissue to the shoulder with a greater ratio of bone and muscle to the arm with less thickness, a constant image quality is maintained due to the action of the ABC (Figure 38-4).

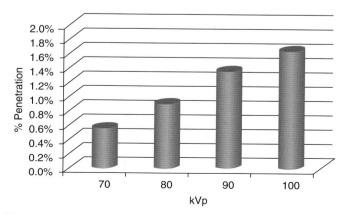

Figure 38-3. X-ray penetration versus kVp with 20 cm thickness.

TABLE 38–1	
Four Basic Tissue Types	
Air filled	Least dense
Fat	More dense
Muscle	More dense
Bone	Most dense

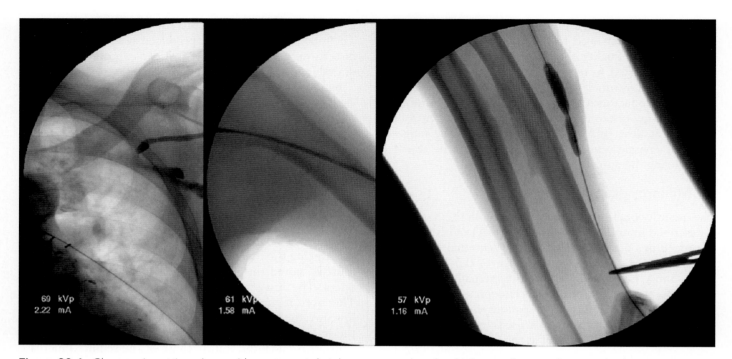

Figure 38-4. Changes in settings (arrows) by automatic brightness control as the thickness of target changes. As the image moves from the thorax to the shoulder and then the arm, both the mA and kVp are adjusted.

Interactions of X-Rays with Matter

Although all matter is comprised of atoms, subatomically it is made up of mostly empty space. Therefore, when electromagnetic waves pass through a material, they are primarily moving through free space. They may have a chance encounter with the nucleus or an electron of an atom.

Because the encounters of photons with atom particles are by chance, a given photon has a finite probability of passing completely through the medium it is traversing. Two factors have major effects on the likelihood of a photon encountering an atomic particle: the atomic number of the material (also referred to as its Z number—number of protons in nucleus) and its thickness. In other words, the more subatomic particles in a material, the greater the likelihood that interactions will occur. Similarly, the more material a photon must cross through, the more likely the chance of an encounter.

When a photon does encounter an atomic particle, it transfers energy to the particle and becomes attenuated. This results in a reduction in the number of X-ray photons in the beam, and a subsequent loss of energy. There are several types of interaction that can occur, but only two that are important to medical diagnostic applications such as fluoroscopy. These are photoelectric absorption and Compton scattering (Figure 38-5).

Photoelectric Absorption

Photoelectric absorption occurs when an X-ray photon interacts with an inner-shell electron of the nucleus of the matter being exposed. The incident X-ray photon ejects an electron from an inner shell resulting in the formation of an ionized atom and a free electron called a photoelectron. The incident photon is completely absorbed by this process. The photoelectron has mass as well as energy and therefore will not travel far. It is usually absorbed within 1 to 2 mm in soft tissue. The ionized atom is unstable with an inner shell electron missing. This vacancy is instantly filled by an electron from an outer shell. This process releases energy in the form of X-rays referred to as secondary radiation. Primary radiation is produced by energy bombardment of the target in the X-ray tube. Secondary radiation is produced by the energy released from irradiated matter by an electron shifting from an outer shell to an inner shell.

Radiography and fluoroscopy is useful medically because of the differential absorption of the tissues being examined. This differential absorption is due to the physics of photoelectric interactions. There are two important principles related to photoelectric absorption that are important to an understanding of the technical factors involved in image production:

1. A photoelectric absorption type of interaction is more likely to occur when the X-ray photon energy and the electron-binding energy that holds the electron in position within its shell are closer to one another. As photon energy increases, the chance of a photoelectric interaction decreases dramatically. This affects the penetration of the X-rays. With a low kVp, proton–matter interactions increase and there is less penetration and greater contrast. With a high kVp, fewer interactions occur and there is greater penetration with less contrast. This principle is very important in the selection of

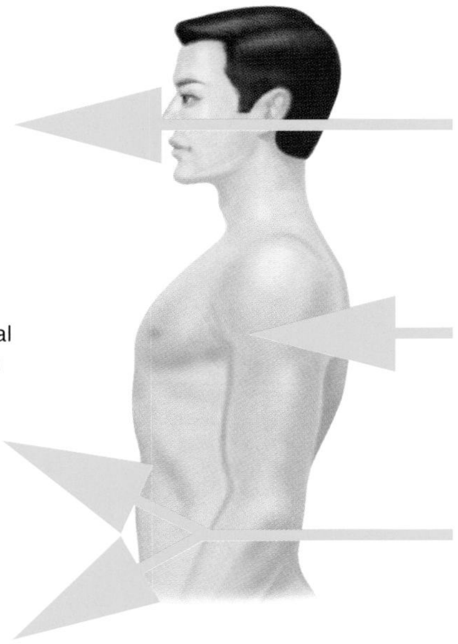

Complete penetration
No interaction, X-rays pass completely through tissue and into image recording device, the basis for the image

Photoelectric absorption
X-rays are absorbed by tissue, differentional absorption allows for tissue discrimination

Compton scattering
The resulting scattering of X-rays lead to image degradation and is the primary source of radiation exposure to personnel

Figure 38-5. X-ray attenuation (interactions).

appropriate technical factors for specific tissues. Basically, this means that bone will absorb X-rays and appear opaque at one kVp value, but if the kVp is increased it will fade as more photons escape absorption.

2. A photoelectric interaction is more likely to occur with an electron that is more tightly bound in its orbit. Binding energies of the electrons are greater in high atomic numbers elements than in low ones. The probability of photoelectric interaction increases dramatically as the atomic number of the matter increases. The relationship is approximately proportional to the third power of the atomic number. Since bone has a higher effective atomic number than that of soft tissue, photoelectric interactions are more likely to occur in bone than in soft tissue. Basically, this means that bone will appear more opaque than soft tissue. The effective atomic number of muscle, skin, and most body organs is approximately 7.42. The effective atomic number of bone is 13.80. The atomic number for aluminum is 13 and that for lead is 82. Dense materials like bone and contrast dye (high atomic number) attenuate more X-rays from the beam than less dense materials (muscle, fat, air). This differential rate of attenuation (proportional to the third power of the atomic number) provides the contrast necessary to form an image.

Compton Scattering

Compton scattering occurs when an incident X-ray photon interacts with a loosely bound outer-shell electron, removes the electron from its shell, and then proceeds in a different direction as a scattered electron. This scattered electron retains most of the energy. It is capable of reacting again and again. This energy is high enough to create a radiation hazard, and to impair image quality. In fact, scattered radiation emitted from the patient is the primary source of occupational radiation exposure to personnel involved with radiography and fluoroscopy.

Basis for Image

By examining Figure 38-3, one can see that with a 20-cm thickness and a kVp between 70 and 80 (usual maximum for portable C-arm) less than 1% of the X-rays actually emerge from the patient and reach the image recording device. It is these X-rays, sometimes referred to as remnant X-rays, that form the basis for the image. The remainder is attenuated either by photoelectric absorption or Compton scattering.

Divergent Nature of Radiation

The primary beam X-rays travel in a straight line but divergent directions as they exit the X-ray machine. The degree of divergence increases with distance from the X-ray origin. Consequently, the number of X-rays traveling through a unit area decreases with increasing distance. Likewise, radiation exposure decreases with increasing distance since exposure is directly proportional to the number of X-rays interacting in a unit area. This is the basis for the inverse square law, which states that "the intensity of radiation varies inversely with the square of the distance from the source." Examining Figure 38-6 illustrates that if one moves from a distance of 1 to 2 m, the radiation level decreases to ¼ of the intensity of the original distance. Moving to 3 m decreases it to 1/9.

Radiation Exposure

X-ray machine output is described in terms of entrance skin exposure (ESE) and is the amount of radiation delivered to the patient's skin at the beam's entrance point.

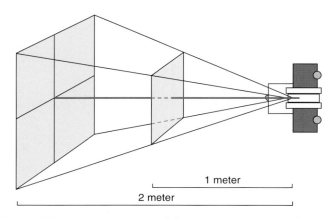

Figure 38-6. Demonstration of the inverse square law due to divergence of the X-ray beam.

This may also be described as "table-top dose." Most X-ray machine regulations are defined in ESE. The units of ESE are Roentgens per minute (R/min). You are more likely to hear the terms rad and rem used when referring to radiation dose and radiation exposure (see DAP below).

Rad

Rad is an acronym for radiation absorbed dose. Patient radiation exposure is described in terms of radiation dose. Radiation dose is the energy imparted per unit mass of tissue. The units used to express radiation dose is the rad. One rad is an absorbed dose of ionizing radiation equal to energy of 100 ergs/g of irradiated material. Immediate biological effects caused by radiation are described in terms of rad.

The quantity of radiation that is significant medically is not the amount of radiation passing through a point in air; rather, it is the amount of energy that is actually absorbed by the medium (tissue) at a particular point. In other words, it is the absorbed dose. The rad is of primary importance in radiation dosimetry. At the *Eleventh General Conference of Weights and Measures*, the Système Internationale d'Unités (SI) was defined and officially adopted. The SI unit for absorbed radiation dose was defined as the gray (Gy). One gray is equal to 100 rads. One rad is equal to 10 mGy. (Actually, the term rad has been abandoned in favor of gray, but we still use it.)

Rem

This is the acronym for radiation equivalent in man. Rems are synonymous with risk, with increasing rem being equivalent to increasing the probability of latent health effects. There are different kinds of radiation and some are more biologically active than others. Occupational dose equivalent limits are stated in terms of rems. Rem relates to the biological impact of the radiation; it is the equivalent dose. It is determined by multiplying the absorbed dose in rads by a quality factor which accounts for the biological effectiveness of the radiation. The quality factor for

X-rays is 1. Therefore an absorbed dose of 1 rad is equal to 1 rem. (The quality factor for alpha rays, for example, is 20, 1 rad absorbed dose would equal 20 rems). The SI unit for equivalent dose is defined as the sievert (Sv). One sievert is equal to 100 rems. One rem is equal to 10 mSv. (As with rad, the term rem has been abandoned in favor of sievert, but again, we still use it.)

DAP

In doing interventional procedures, the radiation dose delivered to the patient is an important variable and should be monitored as part of the facility's ongoing quality improvement program. The ESD is easy to measure, but it is not a good index for the amount of radiation delivered to the patient during fluoroscopy. During an interventional procedure using fluoroscopy, the beam size, the areas exposed, and the dose rate are constantly changing. This makes it impractical to determine the effective dose using ESD calculations. However, the fluoroscopic dose is very easily measured using a transmission ion chamber (DAP meter) covering the exit of the collimator. All of the radiation striking the patient must pass through the ion chamber. The collected ion current reading can easily be converted to the dose-area product (DAP). This is derived by multiplication of the radiation dose (expressed in Gy) and the area exposed (expressed in m^2). The S1 unit for expressing DAP is Gy/m^2 (or Gy/cm^2; simply multiply by 10 to convert). The reading from a DAP meter is approximately proportional to the amount of radiation the absorbed by the patient.

In actuality DAP is only a rough approximation of the patients radiation exposure, but it is currently the most convenient method of monitoring patient dosage. It reflects not only the dose within the radiation field but also the area of tissue irradiated. All modern fluoroscopy machines have DAP meters permanently installed making it easy to monitor this variable.

Uncomplicated dialysis vascular access procedures generally generate a DOP value of 0.02 (for angioplasty) to 0.05 (for thrombectomy) while complicated procedures generate values approximately 3 to 5 times higher. We view a DOP value of greater than 0.3Gy/m^2 as high in this setting. To place this into perspective, coronary angiography and coronary angioplasty procedures expose the patient to an average DAP in the range of 2.0 to 10.6 Gy/m^2 and 4.4 to 14.3 Gy/m^2 respectively.

FLUOROSCOPY EQUIPMENT

▶ Introduction

Fluoroscopy is defined as a radiological examination utilizing fluorescence for observation of a transient image. It is utilized primarily as a means of studying dynamic procedures. In order to perform most interventional procedures, it is necessary to use fluoroscopy. It allows one to see the anatomy in relation to what is being done and the device that is being manipulated. Relatively high-quality images are important. While a high-quality image does not assure a good result, a poor-quality image can definitely contribute to a poor result.

There are four important steps involved in a radiological or fluoroscopic procedure: (1) determining the need for the procedure, (2) performing the procedure, (3) interpretation of the result, and (4) providing documentation. In order to accomplish all these tasks, one must have a basic understanding of the principles of imaging and radiation safety.

▶ Portable C-Arm

Portable C-arm units (generally referred to simply as a "C-arm") have been developed that produce images that are of exceptional quality. Available features include digital images, multiple frame rates, image storage, road mapping, video playback, last image hold, and image magnification, both real-time and post-processing. The size and portability of these systems make them ideal for the work of the interventional nephrologist.

▶ Parts of the C-Arm

The C-arm has two components: the C-arm itself and the monitor console (Figure 38-7).

The C-arm component The C-arm has the configuration of a "C." It houses the X-ray tube (already described in detail above), the image intensifier, and the camera for the closed television system that generates the image seen on the monitor screen. It is connected to the monitor console by a heavy cable.

Image intensifier tube The image intensifier is the component that converts radiation energy into an image that is projected onto the screen of the monitor. The image intensifier is composed of several parts (Figure 38-8). The X-rays that have passed through the target and will

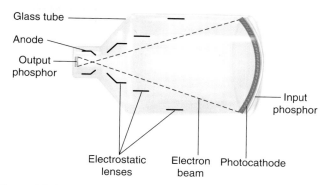

Figure 38-8. Diagram of image intensifier.

form the basis of the image first strike the input layer (phosphor, actually cesium iodide) that fluoresces to convert the X-ray photons into light photons proportional to the intensity of the X-ray beam. These light photons impact upon the photocathode causing electrons to be given off. The electrons are accelerated by an accelerating anode and focused by electrostatic lens onto an output layer (phosphor) that converts the focused electrons into visible light. This assembly is all contained within a vacuum tube.

The output image is several 1000 times brighter than the input image. This brightness gain is due to two factors intrinsic to the image intensifier: flux gain and minification gain (concentration of photons from a large input screen onto a small output screen). Flux gain is a measurement of the increase in light photons due to the conversion efficiency of the output screen. It generally varies from 50 to 150 depending upon the manufacturer's specifications.

Minification gain occurs as the result of the same number of electrons that were produced at the large input phosphor (screen) being compressed into the area of the small output phosphor (screen). It can be calculated as the ratio between the square area of the input and output screens. For example, if the input screen is 12 inches (as with a 12-inch image intensifier) and the output screen is 1 inch (which is usually the case):

$$\text{Minification gain} = \frac{(\text{Input screen})^2}{(\text{Output screen})^2} \quad \text{or} \quad \frac{(12)^2}{(1)^2} \quad \text{or} \quad 144$$

The total brightness gain can be calculated by multiplying the minification gain by the flux gain. For example if the minification gain is 144 (12 inch image intensifier) and the flux gain is 100, then the brightness gain is 144 × 100 or 14,400.

Brightness gain deteriorates a little each year due to the "aging" of the input and output phosphor, depending on how much the machine is used. Due to the automatic brightness control (ABC) built into the machine, this results in increased radiation dose being required to obtain a diagnostic image. Eventually, the tube will have to be replaced. For this reason a check of brightness should be made periodically. Actually, this frequency is controlled by state regulation. It is generally in the range of every 1–2 years.

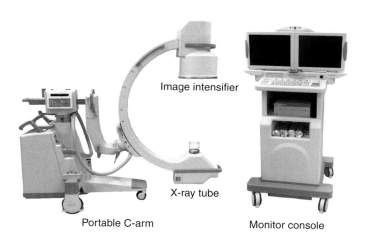

Figure 38-7. The components of the C-arm.

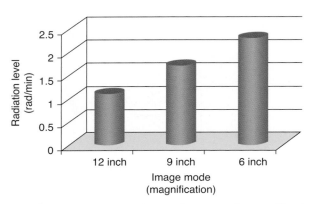

Figure 38-9. Increases in radiation dosage with magnification.

Automatic brightness control (ABC) system This device has already been discussed in the previous section. This system provides a consistent image of diagnostic quality during dynamic imaging by controlling mA and kVp levels in much the same way as an automatic exposure meter controls aperture and time of exposure in a digital camera.

Magnification C-arms are available with different size image intensifiers—6-, 9-, and 12-inch. The smaller the image intensifier the larger the object being viewed appears (and the smaller the field of view). When working with a larger image intensifier, switching to a smaller one (eg, going from 12 to 9 inch) will magnify the image because a smaller portion of the image from the input screen is being projected on the full output screen. This magnification is achieved by applying different voltages to the electrostatic lens of the image intensifier. It also causes an increase in the radiation dose delivered to the patient (Figure 38-9). Actually, a 6-inch image intensifier will produce more radiation than a 12-inch image intensifier.

Increased radiation dosage with magnification is due to the automatic brightness control mechanism that is built-in to the image intensifier. When the image is magnified, the minification gain is affected with a smaller number of electrons reaching the output screen. The automatic brightness control mechanism increases the X-ray output to maintain a constant level of brightness. The resulting increase in radiation dose can be calculated as follows:

$$\text{Increase dose} = \frac{(\text{normal mode size})^2}{(\text{magnification mode size})^2} \text{ or } \frac{(12)^2}{(9)^2}$$

$$\text{or } \frac{(144)}{(81)} \text{ or } 1.78\text{-fold increase}$$

Closed television system The image that is projected onto the monitor is the end product of the closed television system that is incorporated into the C-arm. It has three components: the camera, a camera control unit, and the monitor located within the console. The output phosphor (screen) of the image intensifier is optically linked to the television camera by a lens system. This system conveys the fluoroscopic image from the output screen of the image intensifier to the TV camera where it is converted into a video signal. This signal is then transmitted through the camera control unit where it is amplified and sent to the monitor via a cable connection. Because of the type of camera used, most systems have the problem of image lag. Lag is blurring of the image as the C-arm is moved rapidly during an imaging procedure. It occurs because of the time that is required for the image to build up and decay.

For good image visualization and to decrease the chance for excessive radiation to the patient, it is important that the brightness and contrast of the television monitor be properly adjusted. Once this is done, it should stay relatively stable.

Foot switch The C-arm is activated by means of a foot pedal that is movable for the convenience of the operator and connects to the monitor console by a cable. This is a dead-man type switch, meaning that it is active only with continuous pressure. In most cases, the foot switch mechanism is multifunctional. It has a right and left pedal which can be programed for different functions.

Radiation exposure during fluoroscopy is directly proportional to the length of time the unit is activated by the foot switch. Most C-arms also have some type of device to alert the operator when the X-ray tube is active. This is either a light or a noise generator (or both). This is an important feature because, with the activation switch under-foot, it is possible to activate the tube inadvertently.

Fluoroscopy machines are equipped with a timer and an alarm that sounds at the end of 5 minutes. The alarm serves as a reminder of the elapsed time and can then be reset for another 5 minutes. Most states have regulations that require total elapsed fluoroscopy time to be recorded for every procedure that is performed. Fluoroscopy time is also an important data point for the facility's CQI program.

Based upon a study of over 14,000 cases performed by interventional nephrologists,[1] the fluoroscopy time was found to be 12.7% of the total procedure time (Figure 38-10). The mean procedure time for these cases was 39.5 minutes (median 33 minutes). The mean fluoroscopy time was 5.9 minutes (median 4.2 minutes). The procedures performed included catheter placements and exchanges; fistula angioplasties and thrombectomies; and graft angioplasties and thrombectomies. Based upon this study, a fluoroscopy time of 15% or less than the procedure time seems reasonable for CQI purposes.

C-arm console The C-arm component also has a console built into it that allows for the entering of computer commands to control the imaging process. The C-arm, being portable, can be moved and positioned to best advantage for the individual procedure that is being performed.

Filtration The X-ray tube emits a spectrum of X-rays of differing energy levels. Only those of high energy are of value to the imaging process. However, even low-energy X-rays add to the patient's radiation exposure and contribute to X-ray scatter. Filtration is used to eliminate these low-energy X-rays. A filter, generally aluminum, is placed in the beam's path to preferentially absorb and eliminate the less penetrating X-rays before they reach the patient.

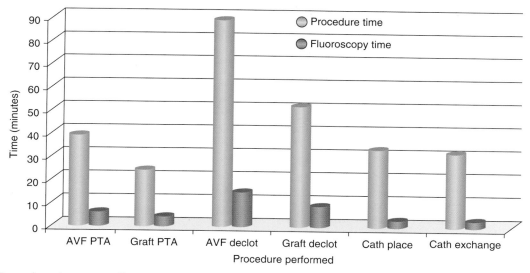

Figure 38-10. Procedure time versus fluoroscopy time. (Data from Beathard GA.[1])

Filtration serves to protect the patient's skin and decrease scatter; it also improves resolution of the image. Generally, the equivalent of 3 mm of aluminum is used as a filter. With modern fluoroscopy machines the filtration is built-in.

Collimation The collimator (Figure 38-11) is a piece of shielding, generally equivalent to 2 mm of lead, that acts as a shield to limit the size of the field of view and thus the size of the tissue that is exposed to radiation. Collimators may be linear, coming in from the sides (Figure 38-12) or circular like an iris diaphragm. These should be used to restrict the field to only the area of interest. Not only does this reduce the radiation dosage to the patient, it also improves the image quality by decreasing scattered radiation. This elimination improves image resolution.

Monitor console component The monitor console component has two television screens. The screen on the left is the active screen. This is the one that has the active image that is observed during the active part of the procedure. The machine can be operated in several different modes; the mode that is currently set is generally indicated at the bottom of the left screen. The right hand screen has a variety of uses.

Last image hold When the foot switch is released, the last active image remains frozen on the left screen until the foot switch is again activated. The last-frame-hold feature of the machine allows for very short exposure times. The switch can be activated to acquire an image, the exposure can be immediately terminated and the retained or frozen image can then be examined on the monitor with the X-ray beam off. Observing this principle will markedly reduce unnecessary radiation exposure.

Image swap An image being held on the left screen can be moved to the right one and held there until released. This allows for a comparison image to be available during the active portion of the procedure if desired.

Computer functions Most fluoroscopy machines are capable of a variety of computer functions. Post-procedure image manipulation is possible. Images saved during the procedure can be recalled and examined. The right screen serves as a computer monitor.

Printing of images Most fluoroscopy machines have an onboard printer, this is located in the monitor console and using the computer functions any of the saved images can be selected and printed.

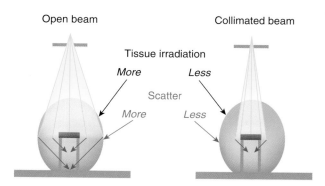

Figure 38-11. Collimation.

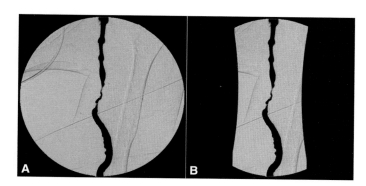

Figure 38-12. Collimated image: (**A**) without; (**B**) with.

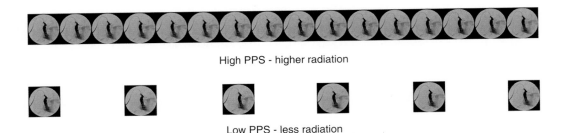

High PPS - higher radiation

Low PPS - less radiation

Figure 38-13. High versus low PPS.

Memory The typical fluoroscopy machine has considerable memory built-in. However, the storage of fluoroscopic images can take up a lot of memory. In most instances, all digital subtraction studies are entered into memory automatically. These are cine runs and often have as many as 80–100 images. In the standard fluoroscopy mode, images are not saved automatically. In order to save one of these images, it is necessary to do so manually. Standard fluoroscopy images are stored as singles. Once the machine's memory becomes full, it begins to drop the oldest images as new ones are added. This makes it important to have some mechanism for external storage to fulfil legal requirements for image retention and to serve as a record for later use. The period of time that images must be stored is determined by law.

IMAGING TECHNIQUES

In an interventional lab, specialized imaging techniques are frequently used to improve the acquisition of information or facilitate the performance of a procedure.

▶ Pulse Fluoroscopy

Although continuous fluoroscopy is possible, the equipment in common usage in the interventional lab utilizes a pulse technique in order to reduce radiation dosages to the patient. Pulse fluoroscopy is a dynamic imaging technique that uses short pulses of X-rays (5 milliseconds or less), synchronized to the video camera readout so that a single image will be acquired and digitalized in a digital image buffer memory where it is held until displaced by the next image. This gives the appearance of a continuous image unless the pulse rate is too low, then flickering will be apparent.

The pulse rate is referred to as pulses per second or PPS. Lower pulse rates (1, 2, 4, 8 PPS) can be obtained with most machines. The lower pulse acquisition rate results in decreased radiation dosage to the patient in comparison to continuous fluoroscopy (Figure 38-13). This is not completely proportional with all machines since in some, with a decreased pulse rate, the exposure time is slightly lengthened and the mA and kVp are different (Figure 38-14). The number of PPS required depends on the amount of

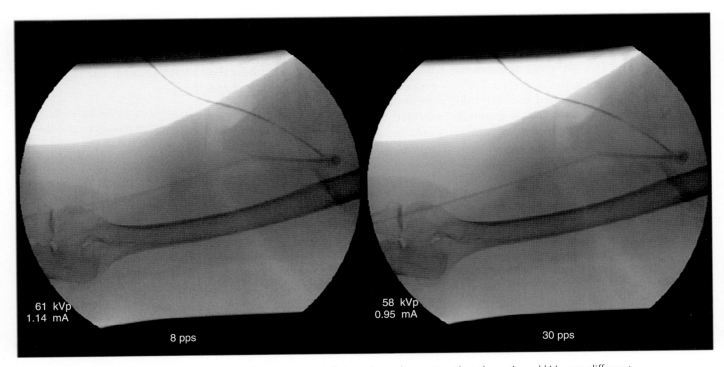

61 kVp
1.14 mA

8 pps

58 kVp
0.95 mA

30 pps

Figure 38-14. 8 PPS versus 30 PPS. Notice the image on left is grainy. Also notice that the mA and kVp are different.

movement in the object being imaged. If the PPS rate is too low, the image will appear to flicker if there is motion. Actually, 8 PPS is more than adequate for interventional procedures performed on dialysis vascular access and vascular mapping can be accomplished successfully with even less.

With most portable fluoroscopy machines, when fluoroscopy is in the normal mode, it is equivalent to 15–30 PPS. If this is changed to pulse mode at 8 PPS, the radiation level delivered to the patient is significantly reduced (approximately 70%). For this reason, it is important to do routine work with the lowest PPS that is practical. The resolution at a low PPS rate is not quite as good as at higher rates; however, this is not generally a problem and is barely noticeable, if at all. The image tends to be grainy (Figure 38-14) at a low PPS, which can affect the appearance of images if they are used for presentations or publications. Many interventionalists work at a low PPS rate during the routine portion of a procedure and then when they need to do something that might require better resolution or if they want an image for publication, they switch to a higher rate temporarily.

▶ Regular Fluoroscopy

When the fluoroscopy machine is used for standard fluoroscopic examination, the image seen is usually black and white. That is, dense objects appear black and less dense ones appear white. These images are not entered into the machines memory. If it is necessary to save a specific view, it must be done manually. Movement is possible; however, there may be some camera lag with movement resulting in temporary blurring. With some machines, as one moves from an area of one level of density to one of a significantly different density, the automatic brightness control does not immediately adjust. This can be remedied by simply releasing the foot switch and reactivating it.

At times tissue thickness is so great that it adversely affects the machine's ability to produce an adequate image. There is a high-level fluoroscopy (HLF) setting available. This increases the kVp to a higher range to provide greater penetration. The use of this setting should be limited since it increases the level of radiation delivered considerably.

It is possible to run standard fluoroscopy in a cine mode by adjusting the settings on the machine. This is sometimes useful for procedures that involve radiocontrast injection and movement such as vein mapping.

▶ Digital Subtraction Angiography

Images can be viewed and recorded in either a standard mode or a digital subtraction angiography (DSA) mode. In the standard mode, everything in the field of view is recorded according to the differential energy absorption of the object. Dense objects such as bone and radiocontrast absorb more energy. This allows them to be differentiated in the image. While this type of view has some advantages, it does not allow for fine discrimination due to the superimposition of objects within the field.

The computer within the C-arm generates the DSA image. First a mask is created. This is done by obtaining and recording a digitalized image which is subtracted from subsequently obtained images. After the mask is subtracted, the primary feature of the remaining image represents anything that was not present when the mask was created. This is generally the column of radiocontrast that is being injected. The actual mechanism by which this occurs involves the conversion of the normal negative image to a positive image which is then superimposed as a mask over all subsequent images. This mask image, referred to as a ghost image, can be adjusted to give very little background (or none) to much (or all) of the background. This ghost image is important for orientation. The net result of this superimposition is the subtraction of all structures that were present in the first image. For good DSA image quality, it is very important that neither the patient nor the field of view moves during imaging. DSA allows for easy discrimination of the vascular structures being studied. It is often critical to the success of the procedure being performed.

Employment of DSA also makes it possible to use diluted radiocontrast (50% or less) and still maintain good image quality even with a very small volume of radiocontrast. Both these attributes decrease the overall radiocontrast load received by the patient. Frequently, when imaging is not optimum, there is a tendency to repeat the image with additional radiocontrast; this is avoided using DSA. Image acquisition is continuous during the DSA study. Digital images are stored in a cineradiographic format. Representative images can be selected from those recorded to be printed for a hard copy record. Postprocedure image manipulation is also possible to enhance the image further.

A comparison of the image obtained between regular fluoroscopy and digital subtraction reveals some definite differences. With standard fluoroscopy, electron dense objects such as bone and radiocontrast absorb more energy and therefore appear white on a black background (Figure 38-15A). Generally, however, this white on black image is not what is seen. It is artificially reversed to black on white so that the standard view will look like the digital view (Figure 38-15B). This is helpful. With the standard mode, structures are superimposed; this interferes with fine discrimination. With digital subtraction the colors are reversed, and electron dense objects such as radiocontrast appear black on a white background (Figure 38-15C). Because of the subtraction, there is no superimposition of images; only a ghost background is seen. This allows for easy discrimination. (Note: With most fluoroscopy machines, you can reverse the black to white image.)

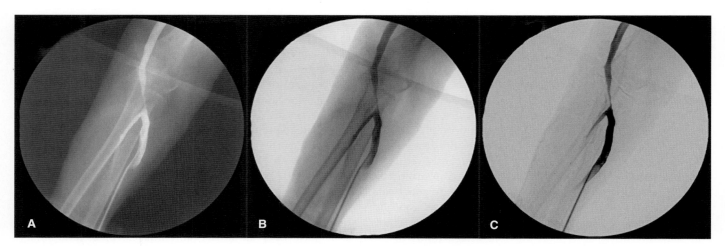

Figure 38-15. Comparison of modes: (**A**) standard fluoroscopy (white on black); (**B**) standard fluoroscopy (black on white); (**C**) digital subtraction (black on white with ghost background).

▶ Road Mapping

Road mapping is a feature on digital C-arms units that permits real-time guidewire guidance (Figure 38-16). An active fluoroscopic image is superimposed on a previously constructed digital angiographic mask (reversed) of the target that is obtained during a radiocontrast injection. Subsequent images are automatically subtracted. The result allows for passage of a device such as a guidewire through the area of interest with the visual impression of opacification of the surrounding vascular structures. The movement of the guidewire is active; the angiographic ghost image is static.

Road mapping is useful in (1) finding and marking the vessel origin during selective catheterization, (2) passing through a tortuous segment, and (3) crossing a stenosis. Road mapping is an extra step and is only worth the time when undertaking specific tasks. The road map mask also degrades with motion so the image quality slowly deteriorates during usage. For the technique to be successful, it

is essential that any movement be avoided following the creation of the road map.

IMAGE QUALITY

Image quality of the image intensifier system is affected by four basic factors: contrast, resolution, distortion, and quantum mottle. Each of these should be understood.

▶ Contrast

Contrast is the difference between the darkest and the lightest parts of an image. Overall contrast in the image is dependent upon subject contrast and detector contrast. Subject contrast is simply the intrinsic contrast of the subject being examined. Detector contrast is determined by the characteristics of the image intensifier and the TV system. There are things that can and should be done that will improve contrast such as selection of appropriate kVp, collimation, and filtration. In addition to this, the TV monitor should be adjusted to give optimum contrast.

▶ Resolution

Resolution refers to the ability of the system to differentiate small objects positioned closely together as separate images (Figure 38-17). The resolution available in the standard systems used in the interventional lab is quite adequate for the procedures performed.

▶ Distortion

Electron focusing is not uniform across the entire field of an image intensifier; those at the center are more accurately focused than those at the periphery. This results in some degree of distortion. The amount of distortion is greater with large intensifiers because the further an electron is from the center, the more difficult it is to

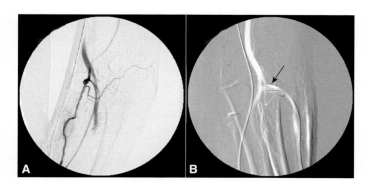

Figure 38-16. Road mapping: (**A**) digital subtraction angiogram; (**B**) road map, notice the angiogram mask with the guidewire visible (arrow), this allows real-time manipulation of the guidewire.

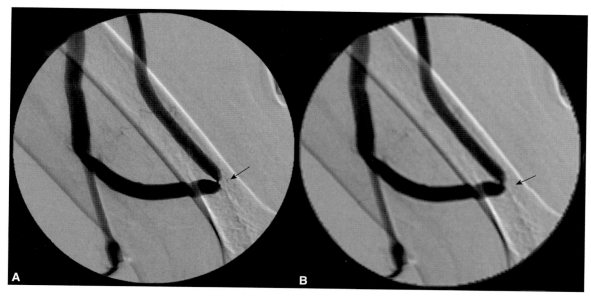

Figure 38-17. Resolution. (**A**) Good resolution, anastomotic stenosis is evident (arrow); (**B**) Poor resolution, anastomosis is not clearly seen (arrow).

focus. Additionally, the input screen is curved while the output screen is flat; this results in some degree of distortion. Lag or blurring of the image with rapid camera movement during an imaging procedure can also result in distortion.

▶ Quantum Mottle

This refers to a grainy appearance in an image caused by too few X-ray photons reaching the input screen of the image intensifier. If the intensity of the beam is turned lower and lower, the image eventually begins to deteriorate and appear grainy—quantum mottle. The patient receives less radiation, but the image is not adequate. This is corrected by increasing the exposure factors (mA and kVp). Proper exposure is critical to a good image. Fortunately this is handled by the built-in ABC system.

IMPROVING IMAGE QUALITY

The quality of the image produced will materially affect your ability to make an appropriate interpretation. The highest quality image possible under any given circumstance is the obvious goal of fluoroscopy. There are several things, which can improve the quality of the image (Table 38-2). In some instances, one must balance the desirable effects of a given variable on image quality and its adverse effect on radiation dosage.

Proper positioning of both the patient and the C-arm, getting as much of the target area in the field are important to getting the best possible image. This also minimizes the need for multiple views. Most of the imaging that is done in connection with dialysis access management

is performed on the extremity where motion resulting from the patient's respiration is not an issue. However, when viewing central structures, having the patient hold their breath during imaging, may make the difference between a sharp image with good resolution and one that is less than optimum due to movement. Images taken in different projections are frequently important. An oblique view of the extremity can be obtained by rotation of the arm; however, the C-arm is also capable of rotation in both horizontal and vertical planes. This feature should be used when appropriate for an optimum image.

TABLE 38–2
Improving Image Quality
• Include as much of the area of interest in one field as possible
• Position the patient and the image intensifier before imaging is begun
• Initiate filming in the best projection (ie, an oblique view) for a given vessel
• Minimize motion especially with DSA (breath-holding sedation, restraint)
• Use collimation
• Use magnification to enhance detail in a specific area of interrogation
• Move the image intensifier closer to the patient to reduce scatter
• Increase the resolution of DSA by using a higher PPS
• Use full strength radiocontrast rather than dilute
• Inject radiocontrast as close to the target site as is safe

Collimation should always be used. As previously stated, this will improve image quality by reducing scatter. Magnification is an important feature of the fluoroscopy machine and is very helpful when very small features are difficult to adequately visualize. The resultant increase in radiation must be kept in mind when this is used.

Resolution can be improved by shifting to a higher PPS setting on the fluoroscopy machine if one is working with a lower setting while doing routine viewing. Again, the increase in radiation dose that is delivered to the patient when this is done should be kept in mind.

When using DSA, dilute radiocontrast works quite well under most circumstances. Its use obviously decreases the total dose of radiocontrast employed for the procedure. In instances in which radiocontrast is being injected at a site on the distal extremity and the image being sought is in the central circulation, considerable dilution takes place because of the distance. If a better image is needed, changing to undiluted radiocontrast or inserting a vascular catheter and administering the dosage closer to the target may resolve the problem.

FACTORS INFLUENCING RADIATION DOSAGE TO PATIENT

There are multiple factors that can either directly or indirectly influence the dosage of radiation directed at the patient (Table 38-3). These should be understood by any individual who uses fluoroscopy equipment. One should also keep in mind that any maneuver that reduces the patient's radiation will have a direct and proportional effect in reducing the potential for personnel exposure. The two most important of the variables, mA and kVp, have already been discussed. Collimation and filtration are also important and have been presented above. Both mA and kVp are automatically controlled by the ABC. Filtration is not generally variable on the portable C-arm. Collimation, however, is optional and must be set by the staff at the direction of the operator. It should always be used unless impractical in an individual situation.

TABLE 38–3
Factors Influencing Radiation Dosage to Patient
• Optimizing exposure factors (mA, kVp)
• Collimation use
• Filtration use
• Minimize exposure time
• Proper X-ray tube position
• Maximize source to table top distance
• Minimize patient to image intensifier distance
• Minimize use of magnification
• Minimize use of alternate projections (oblique views)
• Optimize room illumination

▶ Exposure Time

The radiation dosage delivered to the patient and the operator is directly related to the duration of the exposure. Doubling the time of exposure doubles the radiation dose. It is very important that a fluoroscopy operator restrict the time that the X-ray beam is activated as much as is practical. Significant reductions can be realized by:

- not exposing the patient while not viewing the monitor image;
- preplanning images; an example would be to ensure correct patient positioning before imaging to eliminate unnecessary "planning";
- avoiding redundant views; and
- operator awareness of the 5-minute time alarm notifications.

Human eye integration time or recognition time of a fluoroscopy image is approximately 0.2 seconds. Therefore, short "looks" usually accomplish the same as a continuous exposure. Prolonged observation will not improve the image brightness or resolution. Use the last-frame-hold feature for prolonging review of an area of interest.

▶ X-Ray Tube Position

All fluoroscopy examinations should be performed with the X-ray tube beneath the examination table. Having the C-arm rotated so that the X-ray tube is above the patient will result in a considerable increase in operator exposure from scatter (Figure 38-18). Additionally, whenever possible, the operator should avoid the X-ray tube side of the table when imaging oblique or lateral images.

Source to tabletop distance

The radiation dosage decreases with increased distance due to loss of low-energy X-rays and decreased energy intensity as determined by the inverse square law. For this reason having the X-ray tube (source) as far below the patient (table top) as is practical is important (Figure 38-19). In general, this should be no less than 12 inches and optimally it should be 18 inches. Remember that less than 3%, often less than 1%, of the X-rays actually penetrate the subject to form the basis of the image. With some fluoroscopy machines, there is a clear acrylic spacer on top of the X-ray tube; this should not be removed.

Patient to image intensifier distance

Since only a very small portion of the X-rays penetrate the patient, the image intensifier needs to be as close to the patient as possible. Because of the automatic brightness control mechanism, moving the image intensifier away from the patient will increase the radiation dosage. As fewer X-ray photons are intercepted by the image intensifier because of the increased distance and the inverse square law, the ABC will increase the intensity of

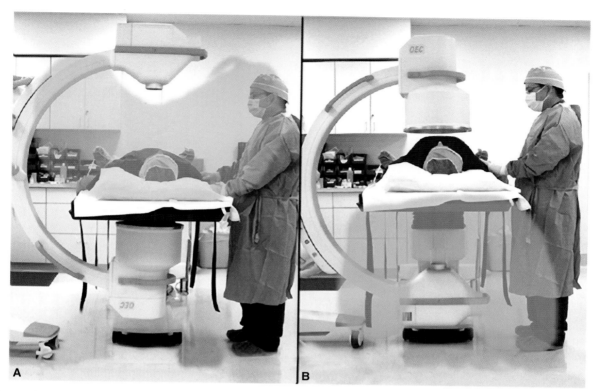

Figure 38-18. Illustration of difference in radiation scatter based upon position of X-ray tube. (**A**) Above table; (**B**) below table.

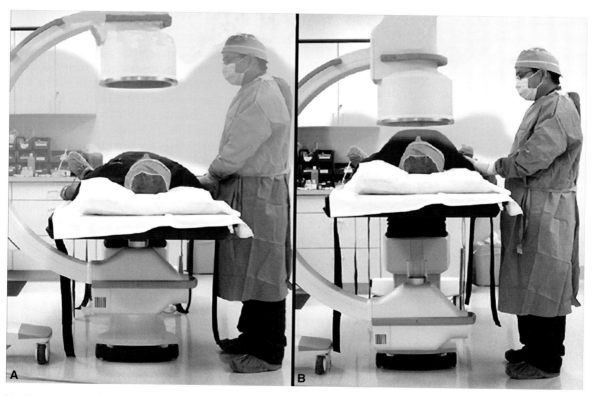

Figure 38-19. Source to tabletop and image intensifier to patient distance. (**A**) Short source to table top and long image intensifier to patient distance; (**B**) long source to table top and long image intensifier to patient distance.

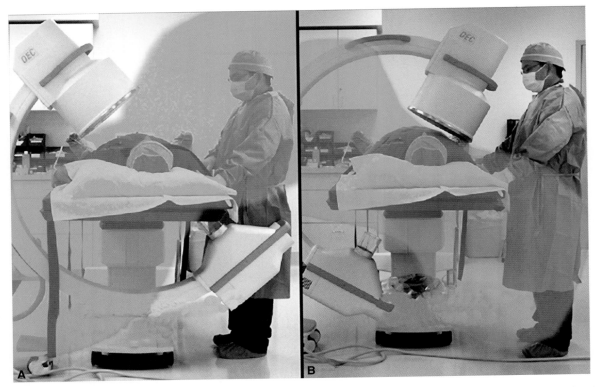

Figure 38-20. Radiation pattern with oblique view. (**A**) X-ray tube on same side as operator; (**B**) X-ray tube on opposite side.

the X-ray beam to maintain a constant level of brightness. Increasing the distance between the patient and the image intensifier will also enhance geometric magnification. The objects will appear larger with increasing gap size. Additionally, larger patient to image intensifier distances have a tendency to increase scatter. This can adversely affect image quality by decreasing resolution. Therefore a minimum patient to image intensifier distance should be maintained (Figure 38-19).

Since with the C-arm the distance between the X-ray tube housing (source) and the image intensifier is fixed, when one is positioned optimally, the other will be as well (Figure 38-9).

Operator height Unfortunately, the linearly challenged (short) operator is at a disadvantage. Due to the fact that for such an individual, the table will be lower than otherwise, there is a limit to how far the X-ray tube can be moved downward before the limit of the floor. These individuals will have higher levels of radiation exposure to the patient (due to ABC) and themselves (scatter).

▶ Use of Magnification

Use of magnification significantly increases radiation exposure to patient, operator, and staff. Going from the normal mode (II equivalent of 12 inch) to a magnification mode (II equivalent to 9 inch) will increase the radiation level that is delivered by a factor of 1.78. Magnification modes should be employed only when the increased resolution of fine detail is necessary.

▶ Use of Alternative Projections (Oblique Views)

Steeply angled oblique images are typically associated with increased radiation exposure. With an oblique view, X-rays must pass through more tissue before reaching the image intensifier. The ABC system compensates for X-ray loss caused by this increased attenuation by generating more X-rays. Steep oblique angles are typically associated with increased X-ray tube to image intensifier distances. Again, the ABC compensates for brightness loss caused by inverse square law effects by generating more X-rays. Additionally, oblique views may bring the X-ray tube closer to the operator side of the table, increasing radiation exposure from scatter (Figure 38-20). For this reason, the physician should relocate himself when oblique views are being used. (Note: Oblique views are also referred to as orthogonal views.)

▶ Room Illumination

Provisions should be made to eliminate extraneous light that can interfere with the fluoroscopic examination. The level of illumination or lighting in the fluoroscopy room will also have a tendency to affect the radiation dosage. To be effective, the operator's eyes must adapt to perceiving images that may be dim. Excessive light decreases the ability of the eye to resolve detail on the TV screen of the monitor. Measures taken to improve detail often involve increasing patient/staff exposure.

It is important that lighting in the procedure room be installed so that it can be dimmed when needed. The luminance of the monitor (brightness and contrast of the TV screen) must also be adjusted properly for the same reason.

REFERENCE

1. Beathard GA, Litchfield T. Physician operators forum of RMS Lifeline, Inc: effectiveness and safety of dialysis vascular access procedures performed by interventional nephrologists. *Kidney Int.* 2004;66:1622–1632.

FLUOROSCOPY CLINICAL: RADIATION EXPOSURE AND SAFETY

GERALD A. BEATHARD

Radiation Protection

1. Discuss the factors related to operator protection during fluoroscopy.
2. Discuss the various types of shielding that might be used for radiation protection.
3. Discuss the various types of dosimeter badges that are available and their use.
4. Discuss the proper wearing of a dosimeter badge to measure total body radiation, hand radiation.
5. Define radiation dose limits as they relate to whole body, hand, and eye radiation exposure.
6. Discuss radiation exposure of the pregnant worker.

Radiation Biology

1. Discuss the determinants of cell sensitivity to radiation.
2. Define stochastic effect to radiation exposure.
3. Define deterministic effect to radiation exposure.

RADIATION PROTECTION

▶ Basic Principle

Concern over the biological effect of ionizing radiation began shortly after the discovery of X-rays in 1895. Over the years, numerous recommendations regarding occupational exposure limits have been developed by the International Commission on Radiological Protection (ICRP) and other radiation protection groups. In general, the guidelines established for radiation exposure have had two principle objectives: (1) to prevent acute exposure and (2) to limit chronic exposure to "acceptable" levels.

Current guidelines are based on the conservative assumption that there is no safe level of exposure. In other words, even the smallest exposure has some probability of causing a stochastic effect. This assumption has led to the general philosophy of not only keeping exposures below recommended levels or regulation limits but also maintaining all exposure "as low as reasonable achievable" (ALARA). ALARA is a basic requirement of current radiation safety practices. It means that every reasonable effort must be made to keep the dose to workers and the public as far below the required limits as possible. This is a basic principle that permeates all medical use of ionizing radiation—using all possible measures to minimize exposure that are reasonable achievable while accomplishing the task at hand. It also includes the appropriate application of principles of radiation protection. To use fluoroscopy, one must be completely familiar with the principles and practice of ALARA.

▶ Operator Exposure

The chief danger to the operator during a fluoroscopic examination is exposure to scattered radiation emanating primarily from the patient and to a lesser degree, other scattering materials such as the tabletop and the X-ray tube housing. The operator must keep in mind that his/her radiation dose from scattered radiation is directly proportional to the patient's radiation dosage. Anything that is done to affect that level will have a similar and proportional effect on the operator's exposure.

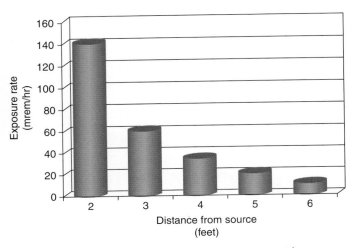

Figure 39-1. Decrease in radiation exposure rate with increasing distance.

▶ Operator Protection

The factors related to operator protection during fluoroscopy can be distilled into three principles: time, distance, and shielding.

Time

The importance of time in determining the radiation dosage has already been discussed. Remember that the absorbed dose of radiation relates to intensity over time. Decreasing the time of exposure has a direct and proportional effect on absorbed dose.

Basic principle is to keep the time of X-ray exposure as short as possible. For each individual, determine if their presence during the procedure is needed.

Distance

This principle has also been discussed (Figure 39-1). The intensity of radiation varies inversely with the square of the distance from the source.

Basic principle is to keep the distance between the source of radiation (X-ray tube, or any scattering medium such as the patient) and the exposed individual as great as is practical.

Shielding

Materials are available that can block X-rays. These materials can be utilized as a shield in clothing or as a barrier to prevent radiation exposure. This is one of the most important principles for radiation protection. Shielding refers to the different means used to block radiation and prevent exposure.

Basic principle is to always wear protective clothing (lead garments). Never allow anyone in the fluoroscopy room during X-ray use unless they are wearing such protection.

Protective shielding. When an X-ray beam is directed at a patient, most of the photons interact with body tissue and less than 3% emerge unaffected. These unaffected photons

are the portion of the beam that creates the image that is viewed fluoroscopically. When an X-ray photon interacts with matter it is either absorbed and removed from the beam or is scattered. Factors that result in an increase in scattered radiation are the use of a higher kVp, large field size, and a thick body part being exposed. In fluoroscopy the patient (body part being examined) is the main source of scattered radiation. This scattered radiation creates a medical hazard for all individuals in the immediate vicinity and the need for protective shielding.

There are several basic points that should be kept in mind concerning shielding:

- Persons outside of the shadow cast by the shield are not protected. The same is true for parts of the body.
- A wall or partition is not necessarily a safe shield for persons on the other side. It depends upon its construction (construction material).
- Radiation can bounce around corners (it can be scattered).

The absorption of X-ray photons is determined by the elemental composition of the material. Higher atomic number materials will absorb more X-rays than those with lower effective numbers. The atomic number for aluminum is 13 and that for lead is 82.

Shielding falls into two categories: barrier shields and protective clothing. While in the past protective clothing was constructed of lead, today most are not. They are made of alloys that provide the equivalent of lead. Lead garments in particular are heavy and somewhat fragile—they crack easily. If the integrity of the material is lost because of a crack or a hole, then there is no protection at that point.

Barrier shields. Many fluoroscopy systems contain side-table drapes or similar types of lead shielding. Use of these items can significantly reduce operator exposures. With the types of procedures being performed for dialysis vascular access management, a side-table drape type of shield is not practical. The X-ray tube is not under the table most of the time; it is under the arm board. However, it has been found that using an arm board barrier shield (Figure 39-2) is very effective in reducing the radiation exposure. This is ideally suited for the type of procedures usually performed by interventional nephrologists. A study was conducted using such a shield in which a 2-mm copper plate was used as the target. The radiation dose was measured 12 inches from the arm board and 5 inches above it, the usual position of the operator. It was found that without the shield, the dose was 230 mrad/h. With the barrier in place, the dose was reduced to 0.05 mrad/h.[1] This is a marked reduction produced by this safety device.

Protective clothing. The basis for personnel protection in the fluoroscopy room is the use of protective clothing or lead (equivalent) garments. Use of this apparel substantially reduces radiation exposure by protecting specific body regions.

Lead apron. At a kVp of 75, an apron having a lead equivalent of 0.25 mm will eliminate 96% of the

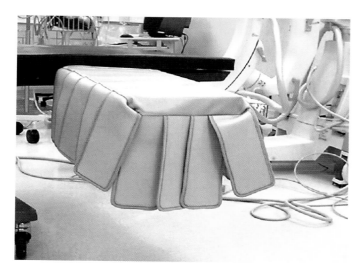

Figure 39-2. Cotar arm board barrier shield.

radiation. An apron with 0.5 mm of lead equivalent will eliminate 99%. At 100 kVp, these numbers drop slightly to 91% (for 0.25 mm) and 95.3% (for 0.5 mm). All personnel should wear an apron of no less than 0.25 mm lead equivalent. One with 0.5 mm is optimum. New alloys are available that significantly decrease the weight of the apron. Most states require an apron with 0.5 mm of lead equivalent.

The lead apron comes in two styles: the front cover and the wrap around (Figure 39-3). The latter style is usually designed as a two-piece unit. The choice of which of these two to use is individual. The front cover has the advantage of being lighter, easier to put on, and cooler (lead aprons

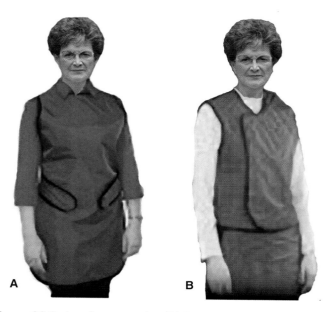

Figure 39-3. Lead apron styles: (A) Front cover; (B) wrap around.

can get quite hot). There is the potential for more weight on the shoulders; however, most of these aprons have wide elastic Velcro belt closures that when tight, place most of the weight on the hips. The front cover apron configuration offers no protection when your back is turned to the radiation source; however, for the types of procedures performed in vascular access labs, back protection is really not needed for the operator.

Although heavier overall, the wrap around apron does place much of the weight on the hips. It is harder to put on and not as cool to wear. However, it does offer protection to the back of the individual. Individuals who are at risk of turning their back to the radiation source during the procedure should wear this type of protection.

Since the weight of the apron represents a very real occupational hazard for the individual who spend several hours each day wearing it, the lighter the apron the better as long as adequate protection is afforded. As stated previously "lead aprons" today are not constructed of lead. They are made of a much lighter and more durable alloy. However, even these aprons can crack with time. When this occurs, it creates a "hot spot" at which there is no protection. Each facility should have a policy of checking all aprons on an annual basis. This is done by simply placing the apron under the fluoroscopy beam and looking for defects. If an apron is cracked, it should be replaced.

It is also critical that the apron fits properly. A poorly fitting apron can result in excessive back fatigue and back pain. It can also increase radiation exposure. If the shoulders are too wide, the apron can slip off rendering that area unprotected.

Thyroid shield. The sensitivity of tissue to ionizing radiation varies. The thyroid is one of the more sensitive organs. It should be protected. A thyroid shield is a better alternative than the discomfort of an apron with a high neck. This shield should offer the same level of protection as the apron, that is, the equivalent of 0.5 mm of lead.

Leaded glasses. Radiation can cause cataracts. This injury is dose dependent. Acute doses of 200 rem and lifetime-accumulated doses of 500 rem are associated with cataracts. It is unlikely that an interventional nephrologist would ever achieve this level of exposure making leaded glasses not essential; however, these devices are not expensive and unlike the past, they are not particularly uncomfortable to wear. Eye protection against fluid splash is important. Leaded glasses can serve a dual purpose. It is possible to get leaded glasses with one's eyeglass prescription if needed.

▶ **Personnel Dosimetry Monitoring**

All individuals who routinely perform image acquisition procedures requiring the use of ionized radiation or those whose work requires them to be in locations where sources of radiation are in use must participate in a dosimeter-monitoring program. Law requires this. This program is under the direction of the Radiation Safety Officer of the facility and must be operated in accordance with federal and state regulations. This involves the wearing of a personal dosimeter monitor. There are three types of personal dosimeter monitors: the film badge, the thermoluminescent dosimetry badge, and the optically stimulated luminescent dosimetry badge.

Film badge

The personal dosimeter most commonly used in the past was the film badge. These are composed of film sensitive to radiation (as well as to heat and moisture) of the types used in image acquisition. The film is sensitive to a wide range of radiation sources that include microwaves produced by cooking ovens and cable television substations, video monitors such as television sets and computer monitors, as well as natural environmental sources. In order to preserve the integrity of the radiation monitoring program, and thereby personal safety, the dosimeter badges should not be taken outside of the facility.

When only a single film badge is worn, it is recommended that they be worn outside the lead apron at the level of the collar. Film badges are capable of measuring exposures over a range of approximately 10 mrem to 2000 rem and are most commonly used to measure total body radiation exposure. Readings of less than 10 mrem are generally not detectable. These are not widely used today being largely replaced by other types of dosimeters.

Thermoluminescent dosimeter (TLD) badge

Personal dosimeter devices using thermoluminescent monitors are similar in appearance to the film badge. Instead of using film to measure the radiation exposure, they use small chips of thermoluminescent material, usually lithium fluoride. When exposed to radiation, these chips store energy within their crystalline structure. If the chip is then heated, the energy is released as visible light. The amount of light released is proportional to the absorbed radiation. The sensitivity of the TLD badge is approximately the same as the film badge. However, because of their small size, they are commonly used for monitoring exposure to the extremities in the form of a ring badge (Figure 39-4).

Ring badge dosimeters are worn to monitor the radiation exposure to the hand. It is important when using this type of dosimeter to realize that the sensing surface of the device should be toward the palm side of the hand. If it is worn facing the opposite direction (back of the hand), it is measuring X-rays that have passed through the hand.

Optically stimulated luminescent dosimeter

The optically stimulated luminescent (OSL) dosimeter (Figure 39-5) measures the radiation that passes through a thin layer of aluminum oxide. A laser is used to stimulate the aluminum oxide, which becomes luminescent in proportion to the amount of radiation it has received.

The advantage of the OSL dosimeter over either the film badge or the TLD badge is its sensitivity and accuracy. It can detect doses from as low as 1 mrem with a precision of 1 mrem. It also has excellent long-term and environmental

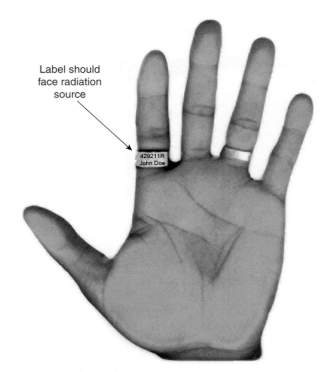

Figure 39-4. Thermoluminescent dosimeter (TLD) badge.

(temperature and humidity) stability. The OSL badge can undergo reanalysis to confirm the accuracy of a radiation dose measurement. This has become the most commonly used type of personal dosimeter monitor today. In many facilities two badges are worn. These badges are coded to distinguish them (Figure 39-5). One is worn outside the lead apron at the neck external to the thyroid shield and the other beneath the apron at the waist. Readings taken at the level of the neck are recorded as the whole body irradiation dosage (if two are worn calculations are based on a formula that uses the readings of both badges).

Care of dosimetry badges

All dosimetry badges should be stored in a designated area. They should never be left in the procedure room where they will be exposed to radiation that is not related to

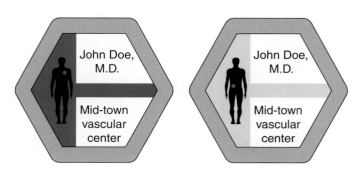

Figure 39-5. OSL dosimetry badges. The dot on the human image indicates the site where the badge is to be worn.

the individual to whom they are assigned. Likewise, one should never wear someone else's badge. In order to avoid other sources of radiation or damage, they should not be removed from the facility.

Film badges are generally changed at monthly intervals. Dosimetry readings become part of the individual's permanent record. Elevated or unusual dosimeter readings should be reported to the monitored individual and the facility administration so that corrective action can be taken to avoid undue risks.

Dose limits

Radiation exposure limits pertinent to the protection of radiation workers are known as dose limits and are specified for both whole body exposure and for exposure to certain tissues and organs. Prior to 1987, the term used to refer to dose limits was "maximum permissible dose." This is no longer considered acceptable terminology because no dose is considered permissible. Dose equivalent limit (DEL) is considered a better term.

Currently recommended values for occupational DEL are shown in Figure 39-6. These reflect the recommendations of the National Council on Radiation Protection and Measurements.

Radiation exposure to any area of the body above the knees and above the elbows, including the head and neck, is interpreted as whole body irradiation. Monitoring using a badge attached outside of the lead apron at the level of the neck is taken to measure the whole body dose of radiation. The primary objective of a monitoring program is to keep the radiation dose of occupationally exposed individuals well below a level at which adverse effects are likely to be observed during their lifetime.

Whole body radiation should be limited to no more than 5 rems per year for individuals over the age of 18. For individuals under 18, the dose should be limited to 10% of this level. The total accumulative dose limit is determined by multiplying the individual's age by 1 rem. In other words, an individual who is 35 years of age would have a DEL of 35 rems. Extremity radiation as measured with a ring badge should not be allowed to exceed 50 rems per year. Radiation to the lens of the eye should not exceed 15 rems per year (Figure 39-6).

Pregnant worker radiation exposure

A pregnant worker can continue working in an X-ray department as long as there is reasonable assurance that the fetal dose can be kept below 0.5 rem during the pregnancy.[2] One rem is approximately the dose that all persons receive annually from penetrating natural background radiation. Fluoroscopy procedures do not result in high exposures to the fetus. Consequently, radiologic technologists can continue their work assignments in fluoroscopy and special procedures throughout pregnancy. However, she should monitor her film-badge readings carefully and report any unusual reading to the radiation safety officer.

In order to be considered a pregnant radiation worker, the woman must declare her pregnancy to her employer. The declaration of pregnancy must be voluntary, in writing, dated, and including an estimated month of conception. She has the right to choose whether or not to declare her pregnancy. This is currently interpreted as including the right to revoke her declaration at any time. In addition, a female worker can legally declare pregnancy without medical proof and there is no limit on how often or for how long a duration a woman can declare that she is pregnant.[3]

Effective, fair management of pregnant employees exposed to radiation requires the balancing of three factors: (1) the rights of the expectant mother to pursue her career without discrimination based on sex, (2) the protection of the fetus, and (3) the needs of the employer. The facility should establish a realistic policy that addresses these three concerns.[4]

The Nuclear Regulatory Commission regulations state that the dose equivalent to the embryo/fetus during the entire pregnancy, due to occupational exposure of a declared pregnant woman, cannot exceed 0.5 rem.[2] Further, exposure should not exceed a limit of 0.05 rem per month.

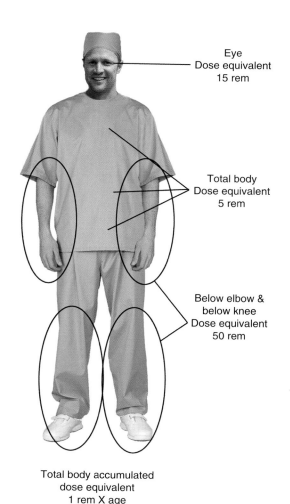

Eye
Dose equivalent
15 rem

Total body
Dose equivalent
5 rem

Below elbow &
below knee
Dose equivalent
50 rem

Total body accumulated
dose equivalent
1 rem X age

Figure 39-6. Dose limits for radiation exposure.

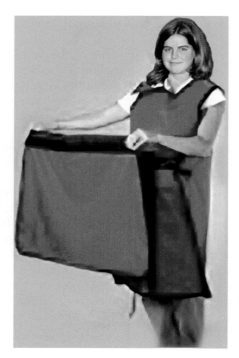

Figure 39-7. Pregnancy apron.

The pregnant individual should wear two badges. The primary badge should continue to be positioned on the collar; the second monitor should be worn at the waist beneath the apron. The deep dose equivalent at the waist is used to estimate the dose to the fetus. Each month the result of this fetal monitoring should be recorded. Special "pregnancy aprons" are available (Figure 39-7).

Calculation of dose

Using data derived from dosimetry badges, the radiation dose can be calculated more than one way. With the standard method, a single dosimeter is worn outside the lead apron at the level of the collar. What the dosimeter reads is the "Assigned Deep Dose" or whole body dose (the control dosimeter reading is subtracted). This technique does not take into account the fact that most of body is covered by a lead apron.

A more reasonable way to calculate exposure is to use a technique that takes into account the fact that a lead apron is being worn. The most common approach of this type involves the wearing of two dosimeter badges. One is worn at the neck outside of the lead apron, and the other at the waist beneath the apron. A formula is then used to determine an "Assigned Dose."

▶ Biological Effects of Radiation

As previously discussed, photons that interact with atomic particles can transfer their energy to the material and break chemical bonds in materials. This interaction is known as ionization and involves the dislodging of one or more electrons from an atom of a material. This creates electrons, which carry a negative charge, and atoms without electrons, which carry a positive charge. Ionization in industrial materials is usually not a big concern. In most cases, once the radiation ceases the electrons rejoin the atoms and no damage is done. However, ionization can disturb the atomic structure of some materials to a degree where the atoms enter into chemical reactions with each other. In living tissue ionization can be very detrimental to cells. Ionization of living tissue causes molecules in the cells to be broken apart. This interaction can kill the cell or cause them to reproduce abnormally.

Damage to a cell can come from direct action or indirect action of the radiation. Cell damage due to direct action occurs when the radiation interacts directly with a cell's essential molecules. The radiation energy may damage cell components such as the cell walls or the deoxyribonucleic acid (DNA). Cell damage due to indirect action occurs when radiation interacts with the water molecules, which are roughly 80% of a cell's composition. The energy absorbed by the water molecule can result in the formation of free radicals. Free radicals are molecules that are highly reactive due to the presence of unpaired electrons, which result when water molecules are split. Free radicals may form compounds, such as hydrogen peroxide, which may initiate harmful chemical reactions within the cells. As a result of these chemical changes, cells may undergo a variety of structural changes which lead to altered function or cell death.

Various possibilities exist for the fate of cells damaged by radiation. A damaged cell can

- completely and perfectly repair itself with the body's inherent repair mechanisms,
- die during its attempt to reproduce, or
- repair itself imperfectly and replicate the imperfect structure of damaged DNA.

Large doses of radiation may kill many cells causing noticeable damage such as erythema or epilation following skin exposure. Low doses do not cause such significant changes but may eventually produce a malignant change. Germ cells can be damaged and produce effects that may not be apparent until much later.

▶ Cell Radiosensitivity

The term radiosensitivity refers to the relative susceptibility of cells or tissues to the injurious action of radiation. Radiosensitivity is highest in undifferentiated and actively proliferating cells, proportionate to the amount of mitotic and developmental activity that is occurring and the length of time that the cells of the tissue remain in active proliferation. For example, bone marrow is much more sensitive to radiation than nerve cells, which have an extremely long cell cycle. Table 39-1 lists cell types in diminishing order of radiosensitivity.[5] Hemopoietic tissue is the most sensitive.

▶ Determinants of Biological Effects

The occurrence of particular health effects from exposure to ionizing radiation is complicated and involves the interaction of a number of factors.

TABLE 39–1
Cell Radiosensitivity

High Radiosensitivity
　Lymphoid organs, bone marrow, blood, testes, ovaries, intestines
Fairly High Radiosensitivity
　Skin and other organs with epithelial cell lining (cornea, oral cavity, esophagus, rectum, bladder, vagina, uterine cervix, ureters)
Moderate Radiosensitivity
　Optic lens, stomach, growing cartilage, fine vasculature, growing bone
Fairly Low Radiosensitivity
　Mature cartilage or bones, salivary glands, respiratory organs, kidneys, liver, pancreas, thyroid, adrenal, and pituitary glands
Low Radiosensitivity
　Muscle, brain, spinal cord

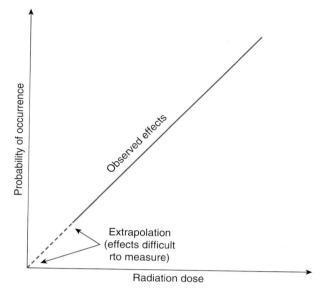

Figure 39-8. Dose–response curve for stochastic radiation effect.

Size of dose received

The higher the dose of radiation received, the higher the likelihood of health effects. There is a very small probability of an individual receiving an acute injury from the level of radiation used for the typical dialysis vascular access procedure. In general, up to 25 rads of radiation can be absorbed without any indication of injury using ordinary laboratory or clinical techniques. The lethal dose (LD50) in humans from acute, whole body radiation exposure is approximately 450 rads (4.5 Gy).

Rate of the dose received

Tissue can better tolerate receiving a larger dosage over a longer period of time. If the dosage occurs over a number of days or weeks, the results are often not as serious if a similar dose was received in a matter of minutes.

Part of the body exposed

Extremities such as the hands or feet are able to receive a greater amount of radiation with less resulting damage than blood-forming organs housed in the torso.

▶ Effects of Ionizing Radiation

The effects of ionizing radiation upon humans are often broadly classified as being either stochastic or deterministic (nonstochastic).

Stochastic effects

Stochastic effects are those that occur by chance. They demonstrate a nonthreshold linear response to the dose–effect relationship (Figure 39-8). The identical problems occur randomly within the general, unexposed population. Their incidence increases with radiation exposure; however, regardless of the dose, some will experience an effect.

As dose goes up, the chance of experiencing an effect also goes up. Stochastic effects often show up years after exposure and consist primarily of cancer and genetic effects. However, at no time, even for high doses, is it certain that cancer or genetic damage will result. Because stochastic effects can occur in individuals that have not been exposed to radiation above background levels, it can never be determined for certain that an occurrence of cancer or genetic damage was due to a specific exposure.

Carcinogenic effects. Cancer risk estimates from lower radiation exposures are difficult to determine because of the high incidence of malignancy in the general, unexposed population. However, the U.S. National Council of Radiation Protection and Measurements (NCRP 1987) estimated that an exposure of 1 rem to 1 million persons would result in an increase in cancer deaths from 190,000 (the expected background incidence) to 190,400—an increase of 0.2%. The types of cancer associated with radiation exposure are shown in Figure 39-9.

While it cannot be determined conclusively, it is often possible to estimate the probability that radiation exposure will cause a stochastic effect. The total risk to an individual

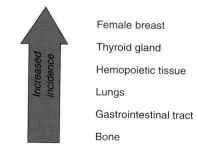

Frequency of radiation induced cancer

Female breast
Thyroid gland
Hemopoietic tissue
Lungs
Gastrointestinal tract
Bone

Increased incidence

Figure 39-9. Frequency of radiation induced cancer.

TABLE 39–2

Cancer Risk Over Working Lifetime (30 Years)

Annual Dose (rem)	30-Year Total Dose (rem)	Incremental Fatal Cancer Risk (%)
0.5	15	0.6
1	30	1.2
2	60	2.4
5	150	6

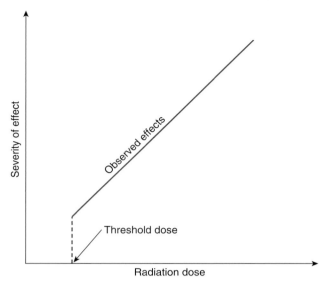

Figure 39-10. Dose–response curve for deterministic radiation effect.

continually increases with increasing radiation exposure. For radiological workers, small savings in radiation exposure realized by altering technique can result in significant reductions in personal risk when integrated over a working lifetime. Table 39-2 illustrates the effects of various levels of radiation exposure magnified over a 30-year period. Note that the first entry represents the annual maximal allowable limit for occupational exposure.

Genetic effects. Radiation-induced hereditary effects have not been observed in human populations, yet they have been demonstrated in animals. If the germ cells that are present in the ovaries and testes and are responsible for reproduction were modified by radiation, hereditary effects could occur in the progeny of the individual. Exposure of the embryo or fetus to ionizing radiation could increase the risk of leukemia in infants and, during certain periods in early pregnancy, may lead to mental retardation and congenital malformations if the amount of radiation is sufficiently high.

Deterministic effects

Unlike stochastic effects, deterministic (nonstochastic) effects are characterized by a threshold dose below which they do not occur (Figure 39-10). In other words, these occurrences have a clear relationship between the exposure and the effect. In addition, the magnitude of the effect is directly proportional to the size of the dose. Deterministic effects typically result when very large dosages of radiation are received in a short amount of time. Although the dose has to be high to demonstrate the effect, once that dose is achieved, the probability of demonstrating the effect is very high (Table 39-3). These effects will often be evident within hours or days. Examples include erythema (skin reddening), skin and tissue burns, cataract formation, sterility, radiation sickness, and death. Each of these effects differs from the others in that both its threshold dose and the time over which the dose was received cause the effect (ie, acute vs chronic exposure). These so-called deterministic effects are usually divided into tissue-specific local changes and whole body effects, which lead to acute radiation syndrome.

Skin effects. Local skin changes secondary to radiation exposure include erythema, epilation, and necrosis. Erythema can be temporary at doses of 200 rad or permanent

at doses greater than 600 rad. Dermal necrosis can occur if levels approximately threefold greater than this are experienced.

Cataractogenic effects. Cataract induction should be of special interest to fluoroscopy operators since the lens of eye often receives the most significant levels of radiation (provided a lead apron is used). Radiation is known to induce cataracts in humans from single doses of 200 rad. Higher exposures can be tolerated when accumulated over time. Cumulative exposures of up to 750 rads have resulted in no evidence of cataracts. Personnel exposed to the maximum levels each year would accumulate only 450 rems over 30 years. As such, the risk for cataracts is likely to be small.

Bone marrow suppression. Because of its number of undifferentiated cells and the degree of mitotic activity present, hematopoietic tissue is one of the tissues most sensitive to radiation exposure. Above 50 rad, a decrease in leukocyte counts can be detected within days.

TABLE 39–3

Deterministic Effects of Radiation*

- 0–25: No injury evident, first detectable blood change at 5 rem
- 25–50: Definite blood change at 25 rem, no serious injury
- 50–100: Some injury possible
- 100–200: Injury and possible disability
- 200–400: Injury and disability likely, death possible
- 400–500: Median lethal dose (MLD) 50% of exposures are fatal
- 500–1000: Up to 100% of exposures are fatal
- 1000 and over: 100% likely fatal

*Dosages are in Roentgen equivalent man (Rem).

► ## Radiation Exposure Associated with Interventional Nephrology Procedures

Although radiation exposure should never be taken lightly and radiation safety should be considered mandatory, the actual amount of radiation that one can expect to receive in a year doing procedures on dialysis vascular access is rather small. The material described above relates to much different types of situations. It is unusual for someone performing dialysis access procedures full-time to exceed (or even approach) the annual limit of 5 rem when the basic protection measures are followed.

REFERENCES

1. Henry Cotar, Lifeline Vascular Access. (Personal observation.)
2. Available at: http://www.access.gpo.gov/nara/cfr/waisidx_00/10cfr20_00.html. Accessed Sept. 6, 2011.
3. www.nrc.gov/reading-rm/doc-collections/reg-guides/occupational-health/active/8-13v. Accessed Sept. 6, 2011.
4. Hedrick WR, Feltes JJ, Starchman DE, Berry GC. Managing the pregnant radiation worker: a realistic policy for hospitals today. *Radiol Manage.* 1986;8:28.
5. Rubin P, Casarett GW. *Clinical Radiation Pathology,* Philadelphia: W. B. Saunders; 1968.

COMPLICATIONS OF ENDOVASCULAR DIALYSIS ACCESS PROCEDURES

GERALD A. BEATHARD

LEARNING OBJECTIVES

1. List the primary complications of catheter insertion.
2. Discuss the major determinants of complications associated with catheter insertion.
3. Understand the variability in the position and presence of an internal jugular vein in dialysis patients.
4. Describe the management of a pneumothorax.
5. Describe the management of an air embolus.
6. Discuss the major determinates of infectious complications associated with catheter placement.
7. Discuss the major complications of catheter removal.
8. Describe the classification system for extravasation associated with angioplasty of a vein and the management of the various categories.
9. Discuss the major factors relating to the occurrence of an arterial embolus complication a thrombectomy procedure.
10. Discuss the management of an arterial embolus complicating a thrombectomy procedure.
11. Understand the importance of CQI as it relates to complications of procedures.

INTRODUCTION

Endovascular procedures have become the standard of care for the management of dysfunctional problems associated with dialysis vascular access. As with any type of medical procedure, these techniques result in procedure-related complications. In general, a procedure-related complication for any given procedure is an adverse event that can be expected to occur. The rate at which it can be expected to occur varies with the individual procedure. The actual rate observed can be affected by external factors such as the manner in which the procedure is performed. A background occurrence rate is expected; however, the rate should not exceed a defined acceptable norm. An excessive complication rate suggests the need for critical evaluation of techniques and procedures.

Since the performance of endovascular procedures in the dialysis vascular access facility generally involves the need for sedation/analgesia, complications associated with the procedures fall into two categories—those related to the procedure itself and those related to sedation/analgesia. We will discuss only the major complications that are procedure related.

DIALYSIS CATHETER PROCEDURES

Dialysis catheters can be classified as either tunneled or untunneled; these are also referred to, because of customary usage, as chronic and acute. The procedure-related complications that are associated with these two categories of devices are, in general, the same, but may differ in incidence because the conditions of placement are frequently quite different.

There are three basic procedures related to dialysis catheters—placement, exchange, and removal. Although complications are most likely to occur with placement, they can occur with any of the three. These adverse events when they occur, can be classified as either mechanistic or infectious.

▶ Catheter Insertion

Mechanical complications

Most adverse events associated with dialysis catheter placement occur with cannulation of the vein. A variety of complications can occur at the time of catheter placement, especially with blind cannulation (cannulation based only upon anatomical land marks). Even in the hands of experienced surgeons in the operating room, blind cannulation of central veins can result in complication rates as high as 5.9%.[1,2] In one small series, a complication rate of 58% was reported.[3] These complications include[1,2,4–12] air embolism (up to 1.8%), hematoma formation (up to 8.4%), pneumothorax (up to 4.3%), hemothorax (up to 0.6%), hemomediastinum (up to 1.2%), recurrent laryngeal nerve palsy (up to 1.6%), and carotid puncture (up to 8%) including bleeding requiring re-exploration and/or transfusion (up to 4.7%).

Additionally, inability to cannulate the internal jugular vein may occur in up to 19.4% of cases.[13] With difficulty cannulating the vein requiring additional attempts, the incidence of complications rises. One report found that after three or more attempts at insertion, mechanical complications increase sixfold compared with a single attempt.[14]

A major issue that jeopardizes the success of blind internal jugular vein cannulation is the variability that exists in the vein's position (Figure 40-1).[11,15,16] In one study, 80 sequential patients requiring central vein access were examined with ultrasound to determine the size, patency, and location of the right internal jugular vein before puncture.[15] The anatomy of the right internal jugular vein was typical in only 57 (71%) patients. In another 13 patients

(16%), sonography showed a medial position of the right internal jugular vein, anterior to the common carotid artery. In three other patients (4%), the right internal jugular vein was positioned laterally by more than 1 cm. In the remaining seven patients (9%), the vein was thrombosed.

In the dialysis patient, the situation is complicated by the fact that frequently the patients have had multiple prior procedures resulting in a significant incidence of central vein pathology ranging from stenosis to complete loss of major veins.[17,18] In a review of ultrasound findings in 79 hemodialysis patients,[18] significant abnormalities were present in 28 patients (35%). Findings included total occlusion ($n = 18$), nonocclusive thrombus ($n = 11$), stenosis ($n = 5$), and anatomic variation ($n = 1$). These required a change in access approach in 21 patients.

Due in part to these variations and co-morbid anomalies, accidental arterial puncture is the most frequent complication of central vein cannulation and may occur in up to 8% of cases performed blindly based upon landmarks.[19] The use of ultrasound-guided cannulation has resulted in a substantial decrease in procedural complications[11,19–25] including carotid puncture[24,26] and is strongly recommended.[27] Many consider it mandatory.

In a series of 250 catheter placements performed using real-time ultrasound guidance,[28] the complication rate was limited to 2 cases (0.8%) of clinically silent air embolism. In a second series in which 220 temporary internal jugular vein hemodialysis catheters were placed in normal and high-risk patients under ultrasound guidance,[29] only 9 (4%) minor complications were encountered. Inadvertent carotid artery puncture without sequelae occurred in four procedures (1.8%), oozing of blood around the catheter in three procedures (1.4%), a small hematoma in one procedure (0.4%), and puncture through the pleura without development of pneumothorax (0.4%) in one procedure. Oozing of blood was seen only in patients with a disorder of hemostasis.

A review of 1765 ultrasound and fluoroscopy-guided catheter placements performed by 29 different interventional nephrologists operating in 11 freestanding outpatient interventional facilities[30] showed a success rate of 98.24%. There were 25 (1.42%) adverse events, 23 (1.30%) cases had delayed bleeding requiring medical management, 1 had a reaction to medication, and 1 case experienced a pneumothorax.

Avoidance of mechanical complications

The primary approach, which is very successful, in avoiding complications with dialysis catheter insertion is the use of ultrasound and fluoroscopy for an image-guided placement. Ultrasound usage, especially with added fluoroscopic guidance, should reduce the incidence of catheter placement complications to almost nil.[19–25,30] The use of these devices[11,19,21,22] and the experience of the operator[13,31] are the major determinants for problems at the time of catheter insertion. The vein being cannulated also can

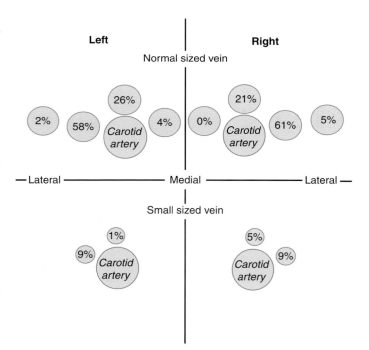

Figure 40-1. Variability in location of internal jugular vein. (Adapted from Lin B. et al.[16])

affect the incidence of complications, these adverse events being more common with subclavian and left internal jugular catheter placements.

Even with the use of imaging devices, experience is important. In a series of 486 cases[32] where the catheters were primary inserted by surgical trainees and were ultrasound- and fluoroscopy-guided, complication occurred in 41 (8.4%). Of these, 38 were arterial punctures and pneumothorax occurred in 3 patients. This underscores the importance of experience in use as well as the availability of the devices. As previously stated, with difficulty cannulating the vein requiring additional attempts, the incidence of complications rises.[14]

A meta-analysis[33] of eight randomized-controlled trials found that ultrasound guidance significantly decreased internal jugular and subclavian catheter placement failure (relative risk 0.32; 95% confidence interval 0.18 to 0.55), decreased complications during catheter placement (relative risk 0.22; 95% confidence interval 0.10 to 0.45), and decreased the need for multiple catheter placement attempts (relative risk 0.60; 95% confidence interval 0.45 to 0.79) when compared with the standard landmark placement technique.

The use of fluoroscopy has been emphasized for facilitating proper catheter tip placement in order to maximize blood flow.[34–36] However, its use can also serve to decrease complications associated with placement.[37] Insertion of a tunneled catheter involves the use of graduated dilators passed over a guide wire. If this is not done carefully, it can be a major problem. If one of the large dilators is passed into the internal jugular vein unguided (the dilator and guide wire moving together), it can perforate the brachiocephalic vein or superior vena cava, often with a disastrous result. Observing this part of the procedure under fluoroscopy can be a major help in avoiding this complication.

The leading complications are carotid artery puncture, hematoma formation, pneumothorax, air embolism, and hemomediastinum. It is important to consider techniques that might help in decreasing the chances of one of these adverse events occurring.

Carotid artery puncture—When doing ultrasound-guided internal jugular cannulation, the carotid artery and its relationship to the vein should be readily apparent. The internal jugular vein lies lateral to the common carotid and slightly more superficial in its normal configuration. However, there is significant variability in this position (Figure 40-1).[11,15,16] One must rely on observing the pulsatility of the artery or using color flow Doppler for its identification. In instances in which the vein lies immediately above the artery and a double wall puncture is unavoidable due to collapse of the vein by the pressure of the needle, the use of ultrasound allows detection of the problem and also permits the use of an angled approach from a slightly more lateral site to avoid the problem.

Review of published series reveals that arterial puncture still occurs despite real-time ultrasound guidance. Although accidental arterial penetration with the cannulating needle

may occur occasionally with little harm, actual arterial dilation and line placement may result in serious complications including death.[38–40] The inability to maintain visualization of the needle tip during ultrasound guidance may contribute to this complication. Traditionally, the ultrasound probe is placed along the short axis of the vein to visualize and direct needle placement. Since the ultrasound image is only two-dimensional, this view has the limitation of being unable to visualize the needle tip in many instances. Some practitioners place the ultrasound probe in the long axis of the vessel to direct needle placement[39,41,42] allowing better visualization of the needle entering the vein, but this does not allow visualization of other relevant anatomic structures.

Other practitioners have recommended an oblique positioning of the probe.[43] They feel that this view allows better visualization of the needle shaft and tip but also offers the safety of being able to visualize all relevant anatomically significant structures at the same time and in the same plane. This orientation is halfway between the short and long axis of the vessel, allowing visualization of the needle as it enters the vessel. This capitalizes on the strengths of the long axis while optimizing short-axis visualization of important structures during intravenous line placement.

The use of a Micro-puncture needle (Micropuncture® Introducer—Cook Medical, Inc., Bloomington, IN) may also affect not only the incidence but the consequence of a carotid artery puncture. This needle being sharper and of smaller diameter (21 gage), it is easier to insert and manipulate than a standard 18 gage introducer needle. Additionally, arterial puncture is less likely to be associated with an adverse sequela due to the smaller hole that is created.

Hematoma formation—Hematoma formation has been reported in up to 8.4% of cases of central vein cannulation.[11,13,44] Most of these are related to inadvertent carotid artery puncture. Measures taken to decrease the incidence of this event will also be reflected in a decreased incidence of hematoma formation. If an inadvertent arterial puncture does occur, pressure should be applied for 10–15 minutes to prevent bleeding. Then site should be observed over the next 20–30 minutes to assure that delayed bleeding does not occur.

It is also possible to get a hematoma from the venous puncture. If a patient has a severe paroxysm of coughing, especially a patient with a high venous pressure, a hematoma can result. This eventuality is hard to prevent, but should be watched for; firm pressure over the site during the coughing may prevent or at least minimize the problem.

Many patients who come to the vascular access facility are on anticoagulant medications and there is always a concern that they will be disposed to bleeding complications or hematoma formation. In a review of 1765 cases of catheter placement using both ultrasound and fluoroscopy guidance, no problems related to anticoagulation were noted.[30] In another report involving nontunneled catheters, the effects of catheter placement in patients who had altered coagulation were tabulated.[45] Patients were considered to have a hemostatic disorder if they had a prothrombin time more than 1.2 times normal or activated partial thromboplastin time more than 1.2 times normal and/or platelet count less than 150,000/mm³. Patients were considered to be at high risk for bleeding if they had a prothrombin time and partial thromboplastin time more than 2.2 times normal and/or a platelet count less than 50,000/mm³. One hundred twenty-two catheters were inserted in patients who had hemostatic disorders including 45 patients considered to be at high risk for bleeding. All catheters were successfully placed with no major complications such as bleeding. No patient underwent any correction for an abnormal coagulation profile.

Hemomediastinum—Hemomediastinum can occur as a complication of arterial bleeding resulting from an inadvertent puncture of the carotid artery. This is more likely to occur if the hole left by the puncture is large as from a large gage needle or if the artery has been torn. The issues previously discussed to decrease the incidence of inadvertent arterial puncture will also serve to decrease the incidence of hemomediastinum.

Hemomediastinum can also occur from the puncture of the brachiocephalic vein or superior vena cava by a dilator if improper technique is used. Insertion of a tunneled catheter involves the use of graduated dilators passed over a guide wire. If one of the large dilators is passed into the internal jugular vein unguided (the dilator and guide wire move together), it can go where it will and can perforate the vein leading to a hemomediastinum or worse.

It is important that the operator exert special care to allow the dilator to track over the guide wire during its insertion. Additionally, this process can be facilitated, enhancing its safety greatly, if it is directly observed with fluoroscopy.

If mediastinal bleeding is large, it can interfere with other mediastinal structures and lead to serious problems and even death.[39] Patients who have hemomediastinum need to be carefully observed; hospitalization for observation with a surgical consult is appropriate.

Pneumothorax—The incidence of pneumothorax (Figure 40-2) with blind attempts at cannulation of the central vein has been reported to be as high as 4.3%.[12] The occurrence of this adverse event is more common with subclavian cannulation that with internal jugular due to the proximity of the apex of the lung and the inherent difficulty with sonographic visualization of the vein.[25] Patients with bullous lung disease are at increased risk. Careful visualization of the vein and the associated structures that lie in close proximity will help to minimize the possibility of this adverse event. One should also recognize a moratorium on subclavian catheterization for dialysis catheters; this too will decrease the incidence of this problem.

A small pneumothorax may be tolerated without any treatment; however, the patient should be carefully

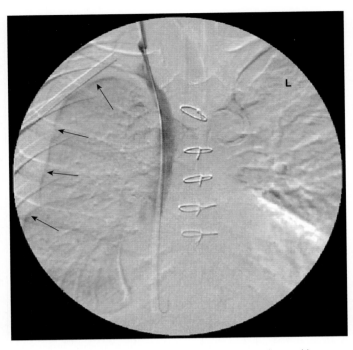

Figure 40-2. Pneumothorax. Collapsed lung indicated by arrows.

observed for any evidence of deterioration that would indicate the need for a chest tube. The risk of a tension pneumothorax should be considered. Facilities performing catheter insertion should be prepared to place either a chest tube or some type of thoracic vent device should such an eventuality materialize.

Air embolism—There are several opportunities for air in sufficient quantities to be introduced into the vein to result in an air embolus (Figure 40-3). This can occur anytime a pressure gradient develops that favors the ingress of air into the venous system. Air is transported to the right atrium and ventricle and on to the pulmonary arteries. Small amounts of air do not produce symptoms because the air is broken up and absorbed from the circulation; however, large volumes of air can block blood flow presenting a medical emergency requiring quick action to prevent death of the patient.

Any device that is open to air while inserted into a central vein is a possible risk—needle, sheath, dilator, and catheter with clamp not closed. In addition, many dialysis patients have sleep apnea.[46,47] This can result in marked snoring when the patient is sedated. Inspiratory effort exerted against a partially obstructed respiratory passage results in a marked decrease in intrathoracic pressure. If this occurs while there is an open passage for air to enter the circulation, for example, a catheter with an open clamp, a large volume of air can be introduced. Patients who are dyspneic, un-cooperative, or have a language barrier may also be at a greater risk for the development of an air embolus due to their inability to either understand or to cooperate.[25]

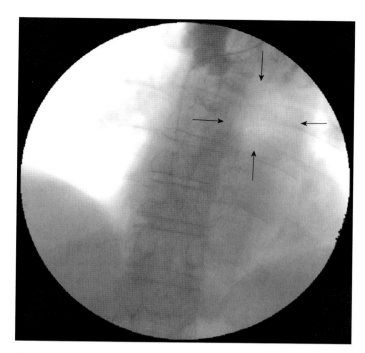

Figure 40-3. Air embolus (arrows). Can be seen better on real-time fluoroscopy with the active movement.

Classical teaching[48] states that more than 5 mL/kg of air (350 mL for 70 kg) is required for significant injury (including shock and cardiac arrest); however, patient complications secondary to as little as 20 mL of air have been reported.[49]

The primary treatment of a symptomatic air embolus is 100% oxygen.[48–50] This can be accomplished using a nonrebreather mask. Increasing the oxygen tension of the patient's blood reduces bubble size by increasing the gradient for nitrogen (the major component of the bubble) to move out decreasing its size. The response is generally rapid, occurring within 2–3 minutes unless the embolus is very large. Obviously, an important part of the patient's management is assuring that the source of air entry into the circulation is stopped. If the response to 100% oxygen administration seems delayed, placing the patient in a left lateral decubitus, Trendelenburg position is of some value.[48,49] In severely symptomatic cases, cardiovascular-pulmonary resuscitation (CPR) may be required to maintain cardiac output.[48,49] This also has the potential of breaking larger air bubbles into smaller ones and forcing air out of the right ventricle into the pulmonary vessels.

Infectious complications

Infection associated with a chronic dialysis catheter is a major problem. However, the vast majority of these are not complications of the placement procedure; they are a complication of usage. Problems associated with catheter insertion should be suspected in any case in which catheter-related bacteremia occurs within the first 72 hours.[51] The likelihood of this being the culprit diminishes markedly as time extends beyond this initial period.

It is essential that all TDCs be placed under conditions of maximal sterile barrier precautions. This means an operating room type of environment.[51] The use of a surgical cap and mask, sterile gown, sterile gloves, and a large sterile drape during the insertion of a TDC substantially reduces the incidence of infection compared with standard precautions with only sterile gloves and small drapes.[52,53]

It has been proposed that ultrasound-guided catheter insertion increased the incidence of infection. It was proposed that the additional equipment and manipulation associated with the ultrasound method might have an adverse effect. Apparently, this concern was ignoring the requirement for a sterile technique and the use of maximal sterile barrier precautions. Where the data has been obtained, the incidence of infection has actually been found to be lower when ultrasound-guided placement was used in comparison with blind placement based upon landmarks.[54,55]

▶ Catheter Removal

Catheter removal is not normally associated with procedure-related complications. However, there are two that can occur and although rare, can cause concern—catheter adherence to the vessel wall and retention of cuff material.

Catheter adherence to the vessel wall preventing easy removal can occur. It has been reported primarily in cases in which the catheter has been in place for a prolonged period, in the range 1–10 years before removal was attempted.[56,57] It has been suggested that there is tissue growth encasing the catheter fixing it in place, preventing direct removal. In earlier cases where this has occurred, the catheters were either removed surgically or simply left in place where they did not appear to cause any problem in the short term.[56,57] There is concern that these in situ catheters might eventually result in venous stenosis. More recently, the laser technique that is used to remove pacemaker/implantable cardioverter defibrillator leads has been used successfully to remove these tethered catheters.[58]

The authors of these reports[56,57] raise the question as to whether central venous access catheters should be routinely replaced to prevent this complication. They suggest an interval of 2 years.

Retained cuff

Polyester cuff retention to a variable degree can occasionally occur and is of little clinical consequence in all but a handful of patients.[59,60] Occasionally, it can inhibit healing of the site, become infected, or become cosmetically objectionable.[61–63] It is recommended that retained polyester cuffs be left behind unless they are associated with a problem.[60] The benefits of avoiding a cut down outweigh the small risk of subsequent infection or extrusion of the cuff. When a retained cuff becomes problematic for whatever reason, it is easily removed.

Removal of nontunneled catheter

A special mention should be made related to the removal of nontunneled (acute) dialysis catheters. If it has been in place for more than a few days, it can create a tract that will allow for the aspiration of air once the catheter has been removed. This is particularly a problem if the catheter is removed with the patient in a sitting position. These devices should always be removed with the patient in a supine position.

▶ Catheter Exchange

The catheter exchange procedure is a composite of catheter removal followed by catheter insertion at the same site. As such, the complications associated with catheter removal may be expected to occur. In addition, catheter-related bacteremia as a procedure-related complication may occur. Catheter exchange is performed for two indications: infection and dysfunction. In either instance, the removal of an old catheter over a guide wire creates the possibility for contamination of a new catheter that is placed at that site.

Published studies have shown that exchange of a catheter over a guide wire using the same venous entry site does not result in an increased incidence of infection.[64–67] In doing this, it is critical that maximum sterile barrier protection be utilized. In a series of 2262 cases of tunneled catheter exchange in which 98.4% were successful,[30] there were no instances of catheter-related bacteremia in the immediate post-procedure period (72 hours). In this series, the guide wire was cleansed after the removal of the old catheter by wiping it three times with betadine-soaked gauze, followed by three times with sterile saline soaked gauze before the new catheter was inserted.

Many physicians feel that a de novo access is required when converting temporary hemodialysis catheters to long-term or permanent catheters. However, others feel that since vascular access sites are at a premium in the dialysis patient, it is important to preserve existing central venous catheters and conserve future access sites. Consistent with this philosophy, there are times when an exchange is performed by removing a temporary untunneled catheter and inserting a tunneled catheter. Reports in the literature indicate that this is not associated with an increased infection rate,[68,69] as long as appropriate sterile technique with maximum barrier protection is used.

Another variant of catheter exchange is the placement of a new catheter through an existing tunnel that has just recently become vacated by a pre-existing catheter that has fallen out. In a report of 10 cases of catheters that had been in place for 2–6 months, a new catheter was inserted over a guide wire that had been introduced through the old tunnel using sterile technique.[70] The time elapsed after catheter extrusion ranged from 6–72 hours. None of the patients demonstrated any evidence of infection for up to 4 weeks follow-up.

These observations suggest that although infection is a possible procedure related complication with catheter exchange and its variants, it can be avoided with appropriate technique.

ARTERIOVENOUS ACCESS PROCEDURES

Basically, there are two procedures that are commonly performed that can result in adverse events—angioplasty and thrombectomy. The most frequent procedure-related complication seen in association with angioplasty that dictates the need for intervention is tearing of the vein or vein rupture. In addition to this adverse event, arterial embolization may also be seen as a complication of thrombectomy. Although rare, symptomatic pulmonary embolism can occur[71] and paradoxical embolization associated with a thrombectomy has been reported.[72]

▶ Venous Rupture

The most frequent procedure related complication seen in association with angioplasty that dictates the need for intervention is tearing of the vein or vein rupture. Although some investigators have reported an alarmingly high incidence of vein rupture in association with angioplasty treatment of autologous fistulae,[73,74] in other reports the occurrence has been relatively low,[30,75–78] generally 2% or less. In a series of 1222 cases with dysfunctional hemodialysis grafts, angioplasty-induced vascular ruptures occurred in 24 (2.0%).[77] In another report of 1796 angioplasty procedures an overall complication rate of 2.4% (44 cases) was seen. This series was composed of 73% synthetic grafts (1311 cases with a 1.8% overall complication rate) and 27% autologous fistulae (485 cases with a 4.1% overall complication rate). Seventy percent of these complications (34 cases) were vein rupture of some degree.[30]

Venous rupture appears to be more commonly associated with the treatment of fistulas than with grafts.[73,79] In a series of 75 instances of vein rupture in 1985 hemodialysis interventions,[79] it was found that this problem occurred in 5.6% of fistulas (693 treated) and in 2.8% of grafts (1292 treated). When only nontransposed fistulas were compared to grafts, there was no difference. Transposed fistulas were more problematic (10.7% of 187) than nontransposed ones (3.8% of 506). The terminal arch of the cephalic vein is especially susceptible to rupture.[73,75,80] It has been reported that the incidence is higher in female patients than in males, one study finding a 2:1 ratio.[79]

The clinical significance of this complication is variable, ranging from none to a loss of the access. The difference lies in the severity of the tear and the success of the management. The presence of this complicating event is heralded by the extravasation of radiocontrast, blood, or both. Small extravasations are of no clinical significance. It is not unusual to observe a small ecchymosis over the treated site the day following therapy making it obvious

TABLE 40–1

Extravasation Classification

Subclinical extravasation of contrast
   No associated hematoma*
   Only evident on fluoroscopy
Grade 1 hematoma
   Does not interfere with flow*
     Size variable
     Requires no therapy
     Stable*
Grade 2 hematoma
   Slows or stops flow*
   Size variable
   Therapy required
   Stable*
Grade 3 hematoma (vein disruption)
   Large extravasation or hematoma
   Size variable, generally large
   Continues to expand may be rapid*
   Pulsatile*

*Denotes defining feature.

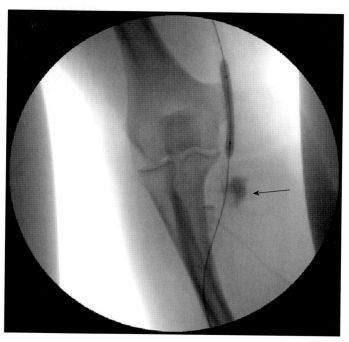

Figure 40-4. Subclinical extravasation of radiocontrast (arrow).

that a small, subclinical extravasation of blood has occurred. There may be tenderness at the site as well. These are of no consequence and may be totally missed except by the patient who may not mention it. Nothing need be done except to reassure the patient.

Clinical problems can occur when the extravasation is associated with the formation of a hematoma. This occurs when blood has extravasated and accumulated in a significant amount although its clinical consequence may range from minimal to major. The amount of extravasated radiocontrast associated with the hematoma may be minimal or absent. A classification system has been devised for extravasation (Table 40-1). This is based primarily on clinical significance of the hematoma.[81]

When a hematoma is noted, one must make two determinations—(1) is it stable or continuing to enlarge and (2) does it affect flow. It is advisable in all cases of venous rupture that the access be manually occluded immediately upon recognition that the event has occurred until the situation can be properly evaluated. This serves to minimize the degree of extravasation in cases where its control is critical.

Subclinical extravasation of radiocontrast

Occasionally, during the course of an angioplasty procedure, a blush of radiocontrast adjacent to the vein at the site of the dilatation is observed but there is no associated hematoma (Figure 40-4, Table 40-1). As is the case with extravasated blood, this small amount of radiocontrast is subclinical in that it is asymptomatic and only obvious on fluoroscopy. It takes on significance only because it is immediately obvious on the fluoroscopic image. Specific treatment is not required (Table 40-2).

Grade 1 hematoma

A grade 1 hematoma is stable, not continuing to grow, and does not affect flow (Figure 40-5, Table 40-1). If it is not stable, it can rapidly progress to a more problematic situation. Although the grade 1 situation causes concern on the part of the operator and the patient, it is of no real consequence to the outcome of the procedure and requires no specific treatment (Table 40-2). This is true regardless of its size. In general, a hematoma that remains stable over 30 minutes to an hour period will continue to behave in this manner as long as the downstream vascular drainage is patent. This is the most common complication associated with venous angioplasty. In the large angioplasty series mentioned previously,[30] 68% of the total complications (30 cases of 1796) fell within this category.

TABLE 40–2

Managing Extravasation

Subclinical extravasation of radiocontrast
   No treatment required
Grade 1 hematoma
   Symptomatic management of symptoms
Grade 2 hematoma
   Restore lumen with prolonged balloon dilatation
     (primary)
   Endovascular stent (secondary)
Grade 3 hematoma (vein disruption)
   Endovascular stent (primary)
   Occlude access (secondary)

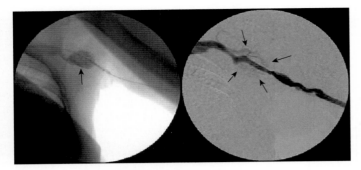

Figure 40-5. Grade 1 hematoma.

Grade 2 hematoma

If a hematoma is stable but affects flow, it is classified as a grade 2 hematoma (Figure 40-6, Table 40-1). This is the only feature that distinguishes it from a grade 1. Most of these lesions stabilize very quickly after they are formed. If they do not, they can progress rapidly. These cases require treatment in order to restore flow. If treatment is unsuccessful, the access may be lost if surgical revision is not possible. In the

series mentioned previously,[30] 1.9% of the total complications (2 cases of 1796) fell within this category.

With a grade 2 hematoma, there is a possibility for two mechanisms that can obstruct flow—first, the tear in the wall of the vessel may be displaced into the former lumen resulting in its obstruction, and second, the hematoma can compress the vessel obstructing its lumen. The goal of treatment is to press the vessel wall and the tear outward to open the lumen and restore flow (Table 40-2). If the lumen is opened with an angioplasty balloon (Figure 40-6c), the pressure of the balloon will generally stabilize the situation after a few minutes and allow for the restoration of flow. This treatment requires that a guide wire be positioned across the lesion. For this reason, it is important that the guide wire never be removed after an angioplasty until the treated lesion has been evaluated for complications. To treat the problem, the angioplasty balloon is passed over the guide wire and positioned across the site of the tear. Once in position, the balloon should then be inflated with a low pressure, only the amount necessary to fully expand the balloon should be applied.

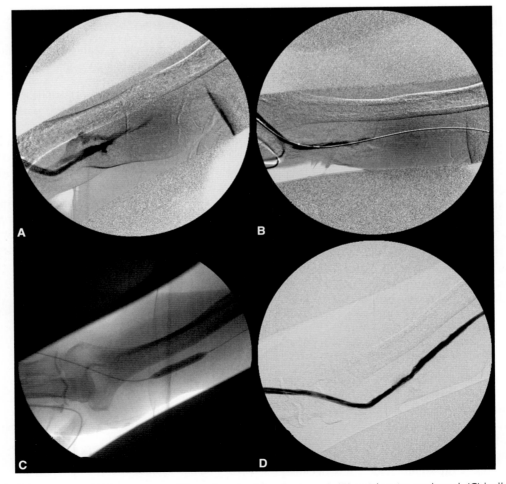

Figure 40-6. Grade 2 hematoma. (**A**) hematoma with no flow (guide wire is out), (**B**) guide wire replaced, (**C**) balloon tamponade, (**D**) restoration of flow.

The inflated balloon should be left in place for 4–5 minutes. This is done to plaster the torn endothelial surfaces against the wall and to displace the compressing hematoma. After the required time, deflate the balloon and remove it gently. The site should then be checked using a puff of radiocontrast to see if flow has been restored. If flow appears normal or relatively so and the hematoma is stable, nothing further needs to be done. If flow continues to be significantly affected, insertion of an endovascular stent should be considered.[82-85]

Grade 3 hematoma

The defining feature of a grade 3 hematoma is that it is unstable. It continues to progress. Hematoma formation generally occurs very rapidly. The size of the hematoma, however, is quite variable. It depends on how quickly the condition is recognized and controlled.

When a grade 3 hematoma occurs, there is a risk of losing the access. The primary goal in the management of a grade 3 hematoma is to arrest its progression. This is critical to limit the size of the hematoma and the volume of blood lost. The hematoma begins, expands rapidly, and is pulsatile. Arterial blood is being pumped directly into the tissue surrounding the area. Early recognition is critical, but not always easy. It can be diagnosed by palpating the area just dilated. A rapidly expanding, pulsatile mass (Figure 40-7, Table 40-1) will generally be readily evident. In addition, it may be painful.

As soon as the situation is recognized, the access should be manually occluded to arrest further extravasation.[86] A stent graft (Table 40-2) should be attempted and may be

successful.[75,87] If it is not, the graft should be thrombosed. To accomplish this, simply inflate the angioplasty balloon to a low pressure within the access below the site of rupture and leave it in position until the access is thrombosed. This generally necessitates an overnight admission for observation. Emergency surgery is not necessary. However, the patient will need a dialysis access for both the short and long term.

Prevention

It is not clear that venous rupture can be totally prevented. For an angioplasty to be effective, there has to be a disruption of the physical integrity of the vein. When this occurs, precise control of the degree of injury (tear) is not possible. One needs to be careful in sizing the balloon that is used for the treatment. It is suggested that the size of the angioplasty balloon that is used to treat stenosis be 20–30% larger than the vessel size. However, this should not be overdone. A "one size fits all" approach is sure to be accompanied by an increase in adverse events and should be avoided.

▶ Arterial Embolization

Arterial embolization is a complication of thrombectomy and can occur regardless of the method used, mechanical or surgical. It is actually as frequent during surgical thrombectomy of hemodialysis grafts than during percutaneous procedures.[88] Additionally, the reported incidence for mechanical methods is about the same regardless of the method used.[71]

The occluded graft contains two types of thrombus, a firm arterial plug and a variable amount of soft thrombus. Most of the clot is of the latter type. This is poorly organized red thrombus that is friable and disintegrates easily. The arterial plug consists of a firm, laminated, organizing thrombus of variable size.[89] It is found just downstream (antegrade) from the arterial anastomosis. This thrombus generally has a concave surface and forms a plug that is firmly attached to the wall of the graft at the point of maximum turbulence from the arterial inflow. It has been reported to be present (discoverable) in up to 73% of cases[90] treated percutaneously and has been reported to be resistant to enzyme lysis.[90,91] Any thrombotic material within the access has the potential for giving rise to an embolus; however, it is usually the arterial plug that is involved, or at least a piece of it.

The volume of actual clot that is present within a graft is generally rather small. It has been determined from surgical specimens that the total clot volume for grafts measuring 30 to more than 50 cm (mean, 42 cm) averages only 3.2 mL in volume; this includes the arterial plug.[89] The volume of thrombus associated with a fistula is small in most cases; however, some fistulas can have large clot loads. This is more likely to be the case with upper arm fistulas and with large, dilated, aneurysmal fistulas (mega-fistula). Arterial emboli are more commonly associated with the

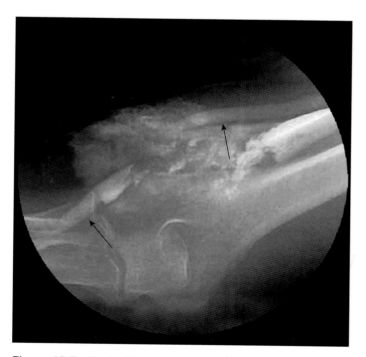

Figure 40-7. Grade 3 hematoma, vessel below and above disruption indicated by arrows.

thrombectomy of a graft than with a fistula, but can occur with either.[30] Although the reasons for this are not clear, it should be noted that the thrombus present in a fistula is mildly inflammatory and tends to become attached to the vessel wall.

Residual thrombi are present following an endovascular thrombectomy even after the graft is flowing.[92] These can be washed or pushed back across the arterial anastomosis and into the artery. Over injection (injection of saline or radiocontrast into the graft in an amount that exceeds the graft volume) can promote this occurrence, especially if there is a downstream obstruction. Just the passage of a catheter or guide wire across the arterial anastomosis can result in this complication.

Frequency

When one considers the frequency of arterial embolization, it is important to define what is meant by the term. What is actually being reported in most series is the incidence of symptomatic arterial emboli. The true incidence is much higher that has been documented because most are asymptomatic and are recognized only radiographically. These do not require treatment.[88] In fact, the attempted treatment of an asymptomatic embolus may cause more problems than it solves. In one series, postoperative angiograms were obtained following surgical thrombectomy. Emboli were found in 12% of 67 cases. Only one of these was symptomatic. Even after a mean follow-up of 14 months, no other patient had developed hand or digital ischemia.

Since most emboli are recognized only if they are symptomatic, they tend to be larger and as such lodge in the upper portion of the arterial tree downstream from the arterial anastomosis. This means that in a brachial artery associated access, the embolus generally stops just before the bifurcation. However, the offending thrombotic material can move more distally, even into much smaller arterial branches. These emboli are less likely to be symptomatic and are therefore more likely to go undetected. In a series of 1176 cases of thrombosed grafts treated by endovascular means, only 4 cases of symptomatic arterial emboli were seen.[93]

Symptoms

The symptoms are those of hand ischemia. The hand, especially the fingers, turns cold and takes on a bluish discoloration that becomes mottled (Figure 40-8). These symptoms generally come on with the sudden onset of pain. In evaluating a patient's hand for a suspected embolus, it is important to compare it with the opposite hand. If both are cold and mottled, it is not likely that the hand in question reflects an acute problem. The pulses at the wrist are generally absent or considerably diminished a change that can be appreciated only if the patient was carefully evaluated prior to having the thrombectomy procedure. A Doppler signal is generally present over the arteries at the wrist although frequently diminished. If nothing is

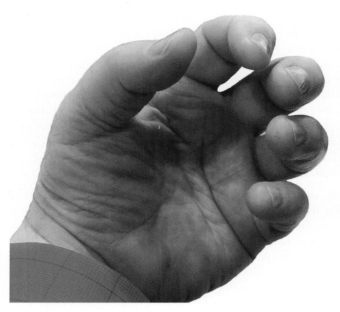

Figure 40-8. Ischemic hand. Mottled coloration is evident.

detected with Doppler examination, the urgency for immediate treatment to avoid tissue damage is even greater.

Symptomatic emboli must be treated in a timely fashion in order to prevent permanent sequelae. Treatment is urgent and is directed at restoring flow to the ischemic hand as quickly as possible in order to relieve the patient's pain and preserve hand function by avoiding secondary muscle ischemia and necrosis. Outcomes and prognosis largely depend on the rapidity of diagnosis and initiation of appropriate and effective therapy.[94] There are several approaches to the therapy of asymptomatic peripheral artery emboli.

Treatment

The treatment of an acute arterial embolization following a dialysis access thrombectomy can be divided into percutaneous and surgical (Table 40-3). Further, the percutaneous approach can be subdivided into mechanical and pharmacological.

Percutaneous mechanical—There are three different percutaneous mechanical techniques for the treatment of an arterial embolus in this situation that have been described.

TABLE 40–3
Treatment Modalities for Arterial Emboli

Percutaneous—mechanical
    Balloon catheter embolectomy
    Catheter thromboaspiration
    Back-bleeding
Percutaneous—pharmacological
    Thrombolysis
    Surgical embolectomy

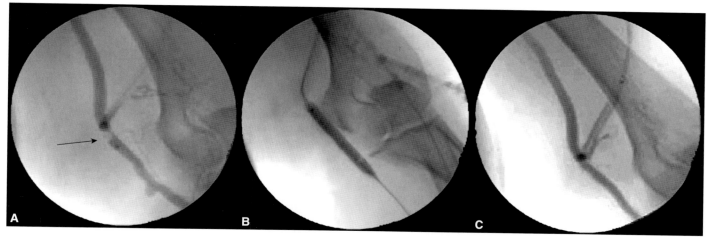

Figure 40-9. Balloon catheter embolectomy. (**A**) Embolus in brachial artery, (**B**) angioplasty balloon beyond site, (**C**) result of embolus removal.

Balloon catheter embolectomy—This technique (Figure 40-9, Table 40-4) is one that has been used by surgery for many years. The only difference here is that it is done percutaneous. As usually performed,[86,87] this technique involves the passage of a guide wire beyond the embolus once it has been identified and localized angiographically. Then a balloon, either an occlusion balloon (Boston Scientific, Natick MA) or an angioplasty balloon, is passed over the guide wire to a level below the embolus, inflated and withdrawn to extract the clot.

Catheter thromboaspiration—The percutaneous aspiration thrombectomy technique uses a large bore catheter connected to a syringe to aspirate clot from the vessel (Figure 40-10, Table 40-5). With this technique,[95,96] after the embolus is identified and localized angiographically, a 7 or 8 French catheter is passed down to a point that it is in contact with the embolus. Suction is then applied with a large syringe to secure the clot to the end of the catheter. The catheter is then withdrawn along with the clot as continuous suction is applied.

Back-bleeding—The back-bleeding technique (Table 40-6)[97] is dependent upon the fact that, except in the face of severe peripheral artery disease, when the distal brachial artery is occluded, there is enough blood flow to the distal extremity through other vessels to still provide adequate perfusion. Success of this procedure is dependent upon the presence of this persistent perfusion, which allows blood to flow retrograde in the artery below the arterial anastomosis and push the clot upward and into the graft relieving the obstruction. Firstly, the artery above the anastomosis is occluded with a balloon catheter. The patient is then instructed to exercise their hand for 1 minute. A repeat angiogram is performed to check the result.

Percutaneous pharmacological—The technique that is used is actually selective regional intraarterial infusion.[94] Firstly, the occluded arterial segment is selectively catheterized using a vascular catheter. Then the catheter shaft is positioned just proximal to the embolus and a lytic agent is infused. Tissue plasminogen activator (t-PA) is the agent generally used which is a very effective fibrinolytic agent and has the additional advantage of an extremely short half-life (5.0 ± 1.8 minutes).

Since this technique takes a longer period of time to effect, it is usually reserved as a backup in the event of failure of one or more of the other percutaneous techniques. Additionally, these cases are more likely to be referred to the hospital for the procedure; this involves additional delay in obtaining resolution. Patients with evidence of severe ischemia should not be treated with this technique because catheter-based thrombolytic therapy

TABLE 40–4
Balloon Catheter Embolectomy
• Document the presence and location of the embolus • Pass a guide wire (a hydrophilic guide wire has a potential advantage) past the blockage • Insert a balloon catheter, angioplasty or occlusion balloon, beyond embolus • Inflate and pull back to retrieve the clot • Document the final appearance of the vessel angiographically

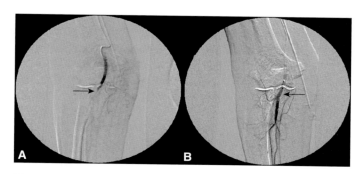

Figure 40-10. Thromboaspiration. Arrow indicates site of embolus, (**A**) before and (**B**) after.

TABLE 40–5

Catheter Thromboaspiration

- Document the presence and location of the embolus angiographically
- Pass a guide wire beyond the clot fragment and insert a 7 or 8F catheter
- Position the catheter just above the embolus and in contact with it
- Apply strong manual aspiration pressure using a 50 mL Luer-Lok syringe attached to the catheter as it is slowly withdrawn
- Check the aspirate to see if the clot has been removed
- Repeated the angiogram with a small volume of radiocontrast to document the result

---

often takes several hours and threatened ischemic changes may become irreversible over the course of treatment. These patients should be treated surgically on an emergent basis.[94] Additionally, the arterial plug is generally the clot that results in an embolus and it is somewhat resistant to fibrinolysis. The reasons for this are not totally clear. It is a dense fibrin plug and it has been shown that clots composed of dense fibrin networks have reduced permeability to the lytic agent making them more resistant to lysis.

As with all thrombolytic therapy, absolute and relative contraindications should be observed.[94,98] A significant number of patients will be found to fall within this category.[99] If these cases cannot be managed with mechanical means, surgical management is indicated.

Surgical embolectomy—A surgical thrombectomy generally consists of opening the exposed artery and extracting the clot with an embolectomy balloon. This procedure is facilitated considerably by localizing the exact site of the embolus angiographically prior to beginning. Clot resistance plus the fact that thrombolysis is not rapid has led some to feel that prompt surgical treatment may have an advantage. This is especially true in cases of severe ischemia requiring emergent reperfusion.[94] The obvious

---

TABLE 40–6

Back-Bleeding

- Document the presence and location of the embolus angiographically
- Occlude the distal brachial artery central to the anastomosis using a balloon—Fogarty catheter or an angioplasty balloon
- Instructed the patient to exercise their hand vigorously for approximately one minute
- This increases blood flow to the hand and enhances the back flow up the artery
- After the occluding balloon has been deflated, perform an arteriogram to document the result

---

problem with both of these in-hospital techniques is the availability of facilities.

Prevention of arterial embolization

Although the occurrence of small asymptomatic and therefore inconsequential emboli may be unavoidable when doing a thrombectomy procedure, it is important to take measures to avoid the introduction of large clot fragments across the arterial anastomosis. Fluids (saline, radiocontrast, medications) are commonly introduced into the access during a thrombectomy procedure; care should be exerted to avoid doing it too rapidly and never doing it if the outflow is obstructed. The volume of a graft is actually rather small, injected fluid has to go somewhere. If the outflow is not open, it will generally go retrograde due to pressurization of the graft lumen refluxing thrombotic material across the arterial anastomosis. This is true even after the thrombectomy procedure is completed. One should never occlude the access and do a retrograde injection to visualize the anastomosis and adjacent artery following a thrombectomy. Even if the graft looks clean angiographically, clot fragments may still be present. Additionally, care must be used in passing devices across the arterial anastomosis as part of the thrombectomy procedure. It is possible to push material into the artery resulting in a problem.

▶ Antegrade Embolization

Antegrade embolization associated with thrombectomy of an arteriovenous dialysis access occurs and is probably unavoidable. This generally goes to the lungs, but therein some patients there is a potential for paradoxical embolization.

Pulmonary embolization

There are reports of patients experiencing acute cardiopulmonary distress and even dyspnea and chest pain soon after dislodgement of the arterial plug in the thrombectomy procedure. This temporal relationship strongly suggests that dislodgement of the arterial plug, and subsequent embolization of thrombotic material to the pulmonary arteries, is the cause of these clinical symptoms.[71,100–103] There is no doubt that during a thrombectomy procedure there is some degree of embolization to the lungs of the patient. Even during dialysis, there is microembolization to the lungs.[104–106]

Clinical studies have demonstrated that the entire contents of a thrombosed hemodialysis graft can be safely embolized to the pulmonary circulation.[93,107–109] Although the majority of patients tolerate iatrogenic pulmonary emboli, the long-term consequence of these "silent" emboli has raised concern.[110] A high incidence (40–52%) of pulmonary hypertension as detected by Doppler echocardiography has been reported in patients receiving chronic hemodialysis therapy via arterial–venous access.[111,112] A relationship between this and both microembolization[105]

TABLE 40–7

Complications of Tunneled Catheter Placement

Event	Threshold
Adverse reaction to medication	3%
Hemorrhage requiring transfusion	0%
Hemorrhage treated medically	10%
Infection occurring within 72 h	0%
Pneumothorax	0%
Oxygen saturation <90% requiring therapy	0%
Referrals to surgery	
As a complication of procedure	0%
Aborted procedure*	10%
Death	0%

*Procedure failure—not a procedure-related complication, but should be tracked.

and embolization from recurrent access thrombectomy[112] has been suggested.

Several different investigators have utilized ventilation and perfusion lung scans to evaluate post-thrombectomy pulmonary embolization.[93,113–115] Some of these studies have shown no problems.[114] However, in other series, the incidence of abnormal perfusion scans following percutaneous thrombectomy of hemodialysis grafts have been high even though patients remained asymptomatic.[93,115] This is thought to be related to the fact that the quantity of thrombus present in a thrombosed access is generally small.[89] However, death from acute pulmonary embolism in this setting has been reported.[113] Patients with severe cardiopulmonary disease are at higher risk for complications during a percutaneous thrombectomy procedure. The clinical significance of pulmonary embolization is not entirely based upon the volume of thrombus.[110] Even smaller emboli can result in the release of vasoactive substances that cause constriction of the pulmonary arterioles and an acute elevation of pulmonary arterial pressure. Patients with preexisting heart failure may not be able to tolerate this additional increase in pulmonary arterial pressure. Patients with a large clot load associated with large dilated, aneurysmal fistulas are at much greater risk of serious effects from embolized thrombus.

Paradoxical emboli

Approximately 20% of the "normal" population has a probe-patent foramen ovate. This means that if, at autopsy, a probe is used to explore the foramen ovale, it is found to be open. These individuals do not have right to left shunts under normal conditions. However, they are at risk for its development. In dialysis patients with severe pulmonary hypertension, shunting from right to left can occur. These individuals are at risk of developing paradoxical emboli.[116,117] A fatality due to a paradoxical embolism that occurred during a hemodialysis graft thrombectomy procedure has been reported.[118]

Prevention of major embolization

Some embolization associated with thrombectomy of an arteriovenous dialysis access occurs and is probably unavoidable. Although there has been concern that it might contribute to the pulmonary hypertension that affects many of these patients, these emboli do not appear to have any discernable immediate acute affect. This paucity of adverse effects is undoubtedly related to the small volume of clot associated with most thrombosed accesses and the efficiency of the lungs thrombolytic defenses. However, there are cases in which the clot load can be large. It is felt advisable, for safety sake, that before doing endovascular thrombectomy, the case be evaluated for the size of the thrombotic material that is present. If this appears to be large, as in a dilated aneurysmal fistula (mega-fistula), the case should be referred to surgery if it is to be done. In some instances, the patient would be better served if this type of access was replaced.

TABLE 40–8

Complications of Angioplasty Treatment of Venous Stenosis

Event	Threshold
Adverse reaction to medication	3%
Hemorrhage requiring transfusion	0%
Class 1 hematoma	2%
Class 2 hematoma	1%
Class 3 hematoma	0%
Oxygen saturation <90% requiring therapy	0%
Referrals to surgery:	
As a complication of procedure	0%
Not amenable to angioplasty*	10%
Death	0%

*Procedure failure—not a procedure-related complication, but should be tracked.

TABLE 40–9

Complications of Percutaneous Thrombectomy

Event	Threshold
Adverse reaction to medication	3%
Hemorrhage requiring transfusion	0%
Subclinical extravasation of contrast	2%
Class 1 extravasation	2%
Class 2 extravasation	1%
Class 3 extravasation	0%
Arterial embolism	0%
Clinical pulmonary embolism	0%
Oxygen saturation <90% requiring therapy	0%
Referrals to surgery:	
As a complication of procedure	0%
Not amenable to treatment*	10%
Death	0%

*Procedure failure—not a procedure-related complication, but should be tracked.

CONTINUOUS QUALITY IMPROVEMENT

It is critical that all interventional facilities and even individual interventionalist collect data on the procedures that they perform. Part of this process involves collecting data on complications. A certain frequency of background complications is to be expected with all endovascular procedures. The only way to completely avoid a complication is to not do any procedures. A facility that reports no complication has a serious problem with data collection. The incidence of any given complication serves two purposes. First, if the frequency of even minor adverse events is too high, it should be cause for investigation. Second, there are some complications that, even though they have a single occurrence, should be cause for a review. The goal is to improve performance and be constantly vigilant for ways to minimize the chances of an adverse event occurring.

Tables 40-7 through 40-9 are some suggested thresholds for the major procedures that are performed in the interventional facility dealing with hemodialysis access.

REFERENCES

1. Bour E, Weaver A, Yang H, Gifford, R. Experience with the double lumen Silastic catheter for hemoaccess. *Surg Gynecol Obstet.* 1990;171:33.
2. McDowell DE, Moss AH, Vasilakis C, et al. Percutaneously placed dual-lumen silicone catheters for long-term hemodialysis. *Am Surg.* 1993;59:569.
3. Dennis MJ, Hunter AE, Ryan JJ. Long-term indwelling silastic central venous catheters: clinical audit leading to improved surgical technique. *J R Soc Med.* 1990;83:620.
4. Blake PG, Huraib S, Wu G, Uldall PR. The use of dual lumen jugular venous catheters as definitive long term access for haemodialysis. *Int J Artif Organs.* 1990;13:26.
5. Schwab, SJ Buller, GL McCann, RL, et al. Prospective evaluation of a Dacron cuffed hemodialysis catheter for prolonged use. *Am J Kidney Dis.* 1988;11:166.
6. Moss A, Vasilakis C, Holley J, et al. Use of a silicone dual-lumen catheter with a Dacron cuff as a long-term vascular access for hemodialysis patients. *Am J Kidney Dis.* 1990; 16:211.
7. Tesio, F De Baz, H Panarello G, et al. Double catheterization of the internal jugular vein for hemodialysis: indications, techniques, and clinical results. *Artif Organs.* 1994;18:301.
8. Uldall R, DeBruyne M, Besley M, et al. A new vascular access catheter for hemodialysis. *Am J Kidney Dis.* 1993; 21:270.
9. Shusterman N, Kloss K, Mullen J. Successful use of double-lumen, silicone rubber catheters for permanent hemodialysis access. *Kidney Int.* 1989;35:887.
10. Mosquera, DA Gibson, SP Goldman, MD. Vascular access surgery: a 2-year study and comparison with the Permcath. *Nephrol Dial Transplant.* 1992;7:1111.
11. Karakitsos D, Labropoulos N, De Groot E, et al. Real-time ultrasound-guided catheterisation of the internal jugular vein: a prospective comparison with the landmark technique in critical care patients. *Crit Care.* 2006;10:R162.
12. Nelson BE, Mayer AR, Tseng PC, Schwartz PE. Experience with the intravenous totally implanted port in patients with gynecologic malignancies. *Gynecol Oncol.* 1994;53:98.
13. Sznajder JI, Zveibil FR, Bitterman H, et al. Central vein catheterization. Failure and complication rates by three percutaneous approaches. *Arch Intern Med.* 1986;146:259.
14. Lee AC, Thompson C, Frank J, et al. Effectiveness of a novel training program for emergency medicine residents in ultrasound-guided insertion of central venous catheters. *Canadian J Emerg Medical Care.* 2009;11:343.
15. Caridi JG, Hawkins IF, Jr., Wiechmann BN, et al. Sonographic guidance when using the right internal jugular vein for central vein access. *AJR Am J Roentgenol.* 1998;171:1259.
16. Lin B, Kong C, Tarng D, et al. Anatomical variation of the internal jugular vein and its impact on temporary haemodialysis vascular access: an ultrasonographic survey in uraemic patients. *Nephrol Dial Transplant.* 1998;13:134.
17. Taal MW, Chesterton LJ, McIntyre CW. Venography at insertion of tunnelled internal jugular vein dialysis catheters reveals significant occult stenosis. *Nephrol Dial Transplant.* 2004;19:1542.
18. Forauer AR, Glockner JF. Importance of US findings in access planning during jugular vein hemodialysis catheter placements. *J Vasc Interv Radiol.* 2000;11:233.
19. Conz PA, Dissegna D, Rodighiero MP, La Greca, G. Cannulation of the internal jugular vein: comparison of the classic Seldinger technique and an ultrasound guided method. *J Nephrol.* 1997;10:311.
20. Gordon AC, Saliken JC, Johns D, et al. US-guided puncture of the internal jugular vein: complications and anatomic considerations. *J Vasc Interv Radiol.* 1998;9:333.
21. Lameris JS, Post PJ, Zonderland HM, et al. Percutaneous placement of Hickman catheters: comparison of sonographically guided and blind techniques. *AJR Am J Roentgenol.* 1990;155:1097.
22. Mallory DL, McGee WT, Shawker TH, et al. Ultrasound guidance improves the success rate of internal jugular vein cannulation. A prospective, randomized trial. *Chest.* 1990;98:157.
23. Hayashi H, Amano, M. Does ultrasound imaging before puncture facilitate internal jugular vein cannulation? Prospective randomized comparison with landmark-guided puncture in ventilated patients. *J Cardiothorac Vasc Anesth.* 2002;16:572.
24. Farrell J, Gellens, M. Ultrasound-guided cannulation versus the landmark-guided technique for acute haemodialysis access. *Nephrol Dial Transplant.* 1997;12:1234.
25. Docktor BL, Sadler DJ, Gray RR, et al. Radiologic placement of tunneled central catheters: rates of success and of immediate complications in a large series. *AJR Am J Roentgenol.* 1999;173:457.
26. Froehlich CD, Rigby MR, Rosenberg ES, et al. Ultrasound-guided central venous catheter placement decreases complications and decreases placement attempts compared with the landmark technique in patients in a pediatric intensive care unit. *Crit Care Med.* 2009;37:1090.
27. NKF-DOQI Clinical Practice Guidelines for Vascular Access. Guideline 2: selection and placement of hemodialysis access.
28. Trerotola SO, Johnson MS, Harris VJ, et al. Outcome of tunneled hemodialysis catheters placed via the right

internal jugular vein by interventional radiologists. *Radiology*. 1997;203:489.

29. Oguzkurt L, Tercan F, Kara G, et al. US-guided placement of temporary internal jugular vein catheters: immediate technical success and complications in normal and high-risk patients. *Eur J Radiol*. 2005;55:125.

30. Beathard GA, Litchfield, T. Effectiveness and safety of dialysis vascular access procedures performed by interventional nephrologists. *Kidney Int*. 2004;66:1622.

31. Beathard, G (ed). *Complications of Vascular Access*. New York: Marcel Dekker, Inc., 2000.

32. Hameeteman M, Bode AS, Peppelenbosch AG, et al. Ultrasound-guided central venous catheter placement by surgical trainees: a safe procedure? *J Vasc Access*. 2010;11:288–292.

33. Randolph AG, Cook DJ, Gonzales CA, Pribble CG. Ultrasound guidance for placement of central venous catheters: a meta-analysis of the literature. *Crit Care Med*. 1996;24:2053.

34. Sotirakopoulos N, Skandalos L, Tsitsios T, et al. The incorrect placement of hemodialysis catheters in veins. The necessity for urgent x-ray evaluation for its position. *Ren Fail*. 2001;23:127.

35. Work, J. Chronic catheter placement. *Semin Dial*. 2001; 14:436.

36. Schnabel KJ, Simons ME, Zevallos GF, et al. Image-guided insertion of the Uldall tunneled hemodialysis catheter: technical success and clinical follow-up. *J Vasc IntervRadiol*. 1997;8:579.

37. Gebauer B, El-Sheik M, Vogt M, Wagner HJ. Combined ultrasound and fluoroscopy guided port catheter implantation—high success and low complication rate. *Eur J Radiol*. 2009;69:517.

38. Matsushita T, Huynh AT, James, A. Misplacement of hemodialysis catheter to brachiocephalic artery required urgent sternotomy. *Interact Cardiovasc Thorac Surg*. 2006;5:156.

39. Blaivas, M. Video analysis of accidental arterial cannulation with dynamic ultrasound guidance for central venous access. *J Ultrasound Med*. 2009;28:1239.

40. Fangio P, Mourgeon E, Romelaer A, et al. Aortic injury and cardiac tamponade as a complication of subclavian venous catheterization. *Anesthesiology*. 2002;96:1520.

41. Blaivas M, Adhikari S. An unseen danger: frequency of posterior vessel wall penetration by needles during attempts to place internal jugular vein central catheters using ultrasound guidance. *Crit Care Med*. 2009;37:2345.

42. Stone MB, Moon C, Sutijono D, Blaivas, M. Needle tip visualization during ultrasound-guided vascular access: short-axis vs long-axis approach. *Am J Emerg Med*. 2010;28:343.

43. Phelan M, Hagerty D. The oblique view: an alternative approach for ultrasound-guided central line placement. *J Emerg Med*. 2009;37:403.

44. Denys BG, Uretsky BF, Reddy PS. Ultrasound-assisted cannulation of the internal jugular vein. A prospective comparison to the external landmark-guided technique. *Circulation*. 1993;87:1557.

45. Della Vigna P, Monfardini L, Bonomo G, et al. Coagulation disorders in patients with cancer: nontunneled central venous catheter placement with US guidance—a single-institution retrospective analysis. *Radiology*. 2009;253:249.

46. DeLoach SS, Berns JS. Impact of obstructive sleep apnea in hemodialysis patients. *Semin Dial*. 2009;22:308.

47. Kraus MA, Hamburger RJ. Sleep apnea in renal failure. *Adv Perit Dial*. 1997;13:88.

48. Mirski MA, Lele AV, Fitzsimmons L, Toung TJ. Diagnosis and treatment of vascular air embolism. *Anesthesiology*. 2007;106:164.

49. Moon, R. Air or gas embolis. *Hyperbaric Oxygen Committee Report*, 2003:5.

50. Muth CM, Shank ES. Gas embolism. *N Engl J Med*. 2000; 342:476.

51. Beathard GA, Urbanes, A. Infection associated with tunneled hemodialysis catheters. *Semin Dial*. 2008; 21:528.

52. Mermel LA, McCormick RDS, S.R., Maki DG. The pathogenesis and epidemiology of catheter-related infection with pulmonary artery Swan-Ganz catheters: a prospective study utilizing molecular subtyping. *Am J Med*. 1991;91(suppl):S197.

53. Raad II, Hohn DC, Gilbreath BJ, et al. Prevention of central venous catheter-related infections by using maximal sterile barrier precautions during insertion. *Infect Control Hosp Epidemiol*. 1994;15:231.

54. Subhan I, Jain A, Joshi, M. Asepsis in ultrasound guided central venous access: a new technique. *Ann Emerg Med*. 2009;54:S100.

55. Shabbir J, Kallimutthu SG, O'Sullivan JB, et al. An audit of ultrasound-assisted catheter insertion in patients receiving chemotherapy. *Surgeon*. 2005;3:32.

56. Hassan A, Khalifa M, Al-Akraa M, et al. Six cases of retained central venous haemodialysis access catheters. *Nephrol Dial Transplant*. 2006;21:2005.

57. Liu T, Hanna N, Summers D. Retained central venous haemodialysis access catheters. *Nephrol Dial Transplant*. 2007;22:960.

58. Carrillo RG, Garisto JD, Salman L, et al. A novel technique for tethered dialysis catheter removal using the laser sheath. *Semin Dial*. 2009;22:688.

59. Bjeletich J, Hickman RO. The Hickman indwelling catheter. *Am J Nurs*. 1980;80:62.

60. Kohli MD, Trerotola SO, Namyslowski J, et al. Outcome of polyester cuff retention following traction removal of tunneled central venous catheters. *Radiology*. 2001; 219:651.

61. Ruppel LJ, Brown RA, Borson RA, Whitman ED. Retained Hickman catheter cuff as an infection source following allogeneic bone marrow transplant. *Bone Marrow Transplant*. 1994;14:169.

62. al-Wali WI, Wilcox MH, Thickett KJ, et al. Retained Hickman catheter cuff as a source of infection. *J Infect*. 1993;26:199.

63. Fisher WB. Complication of a Hickman catheter. Cutaneous erosion of the Dacron cuff. *JAMA*. 1985; 254:2934.

64. Duszak R, Jr., Haskal ZJ, Thomas-Hawkins C, et al. Replacement of failing tunneled hemodialysis catheters through pre-existing subcutaneous tunnels: a comparison of catheter function and infection rates for de novo placements and over-the-wire exchanges. *J Vasc Interv Radiol*. 1998;9:321.

65. Garofalo RS, Zaleski GX, Lorenz JM, et al. Exchange of poorly functioning tunneled permanent hemodialysis catheters. *AJR Am J Roentgenol*. 1999;173:155.

66. Janned'Othee B, Tham JC, Sheiman RG. Restoration of patency in failing tunneled hemodialysis catheters: a comparison of catheter exchange, exchange and balloon disruption of the fibrin sheath, and femoral stripping. *J Vasc Interv Radiol.* 2006;17:1011.

67. Casey J, Davies J, Balshaw-Greer A, et al. Inserting tunnelled hemodialysis catheters using elective guidewire exchange from nontunnelled catheters: is there a greater risk of infection when compared with new-site replacement? *Hemodial Int.* 2008;12:52.

68. Falk A, Prabhuram N, Parthasarathy, S. Conversion of temporary hemodialysis catheters to permanent hemodialysis catheters: a retrospective study of catheter exchange versus classic de novo placement. *Semin Dial.* 2005;18:425.

69. Van Ha TG, Fimmen D, Han L, et al. Conversion of non-tunneled to tunneled hemodialysis catheters. *Cardiovasc Intervent Radiol.* 2007;30:222.

70. Asif A. Insertion of accidentally extruded catheters by interventional radiologists. *Semin Dial.* 2008;21:586.

71. Vesely TM. Complications related to percutaneous thrombectomy of hemodialysis grafts. *J Vasc Access.* 2002;3:49.

72. Bentaarit B, Duval AM, Maraval A, et al. Paradoxical embolism following thromboaspiration of an arteriovenous fistula thrombosis: a case report. *J Med Case Reports.* 2010;4:345.

73. Turmel-Rodrigues L, Pengloan J, Baudin S, et al. Treatment of stenosis and thrombosis in haemodialysis fistulas and grafts by interventional radiology. *Nephrol Dial Transplant.* 2000;15:2029.

74. Turmel-Rodrigues, L. Diagnosis and endovascular treatment for autologous fistula-related stenosis. In: Gray R, Sand J, eds. *A Multidisciplinary Approach for Hemodialysis Access.* New York: Lippincott Williams & Wilkins; 2002;170–183.

75. Raynaud AC, Angel CY, Sapoval MR, et al. Treatment of hemodialysis access rupture during PTA with Wallstent implantation. *J Vasc Interv Radiol.* 1998;9:437.

76. Beathard GA. The treatment of vascular access graft dysfunction: a nephrologist's view and experience. *Adv Ren Replace Ther.* 1994;1:131.

77. Pappas JN, Vesely TM. Vascular rupture during angioplasty of hemodialysis raft-related stenoses. *J Vasc Access.* 2002; 3:120.

78. Beathard GA. Percutaneous transvenous angioplasty in the treatment of vascular access stenosis. *Kidney Int.* 1992;42:1390.

79. Kornfield ZN, Kwak A, Soulen MC, et al. Incidence and management of percutaneous transluminal angioplasty-induced venous rupture in the "fistula first" era. *J Vasc Interv Radiol.* 2009;20:744.

80. Rajan DK, Clark TW, Patel NK, et al. Prevalence and treatment of cephalic arch stenosis in dysfunctional autogenous hemodialysis fistulas. *J Vasc Interv Radiol.* 2003;14:567.

81. Beathard GA. Angioplasty for arteriovenous grafts and fistulae. *Semin Nephrol.* 2002;22:202.

82. Bittl JA. Venous rupture during percutaneous treatment of hemodialysis fistulas and grafts. *Catheter Cardiovasc Interv.* 2009;74:1097.

83. Funaki B, Szymski GX, Leef JA, et al. Wallstent deployment to salvage dialysis graft thrombolysis complicated by venous rupture: early and intermediate results. *AJR Am J Roentgenol.* 1997;169:1435.

84. Rundback JH, Leonardo RF, Poplausky MR, Rozenblit, G. Venous rupture complicating hemodialysis access angioplasty: percutaneous treatment and outcomes in seven patients. *AJR Am J Roentgenol.* 1998;171:1081.

85. Rajan DK, Clark TW. Patency of Wallstents placed at the venous anastomosis of dialysis grafts for salvage of angioplasty-induced rupture. *Cardiovasc Intervent Radiol.* 2003; 26:242.

86. Beathard GA. Management of complications of endovascular dialysis access procedures. *Semin Dial.* 2003;16:309.

87. Sofocleous CT, Schur I, Koh E, et al. Percutaneous treatment of complications occurring during hemodialysis graft recanalization. *Eur J Radiol.* 2003;47:237.

88. Trerotola SO, Johnson MS, Shah H, et al. Incidence and management of arterial emboli from hemodialysis graft surgical thrombectomy. *J Vasc Interv Radiol.* 1997;8:557.

89. Winkler TA, Trerotola SO, Davidson DD, Milgrom ML. Study of thrombus from thrombosed hemodialysis access grafts. *Radiology.* 1995;197:461.

90. Valji K, Bookstein JJ, Roberts AC, et al. Pulse-spray pharmacomechanical thrombolysis of thrombosed hemodialysis access grafts: long-term experience and comparison of original and current techniques. *AJR Am J Roentgenol.* 1995;164:1495.

91. Kumpe DA, Cohen MA. Angioplasty/thrombolytic treatment of failing and failed hemodialysis access sites: comparison with surgical treatment. *Prog Cardiovasc Dis.* 1992;34:263.

92. Vesely TM, Hovsepian DM, Darcy MD, et al. Angioscopic observations after percutaneous thrombectomy of thrombosed hemodialysis grafts. *J Vasc Interv Radiol.* 2000;11:971.

93. Beathard GA, Welch BR, Maidment HJ. Mechanical thrombolysis for the treatment of thrombosed hemodialysis access grafts. *Radiology.* 1996;200:711.

94. Rajan DK, Patel NH, Valji K, et al. Quality improvement guidelines for percutaneous management of acute limb ischemia. *J Vasc Interv Radiol.* 2005;16:585.

95. Sniderman KW, Bodner L, Saddekni S, et al. Percutaneous embolectomy by transcatheter aspiration. Work in progress. *Radiology.* 1984;150:357.

96. Turmel-Rodrigues LA, Beyssen B, Raynaud A, Sapoval, M. Thromboaspiration to treat inadvertent arterial emboli during dialysis graft declotting. *J Vasc Interv Radiol.* 1998;9:849.

97. Trerotola SO, Johnson MS, Shah H, Namyslowski, J. Backbleeding technique for treatment of arterial emboli resulting from dialysis graft thrombolysis. *J Vasc Interv Radiol.* 1998;9:141.

98. Thrombolysis in the management of lower limb peripheral arterial occlusion—a consensus document. Working Party on Thrombolysis in the Management of Limb Ischemia. *Am J Cardiol.* 1998;81:207.

99. Results of a prospective randomized trial evaluating surgery versus thrombolysis for ischemia of the lower extremity. The STILE trial. *Ann Surg.* 1994;220:251.

100. Dolmatch BL, Casteneda F, McNamara TO, et al. Synthetic dialysis shunts: thrombolysis with the Cragg thrombolytic brush catheter. *Radiology.* 1999;213:180.

101. Vorwerk D, Schurmann K, Muller-Leisse C, et al. Hydrodynamic thrombectomy of haemodialysis grafts and fistulae: results of 51 procedures. *Nephrol Dial Transplant.* 1996;11:1058.

102. Sofocleous CT, Cooper SG, Schur I, et al. Retrospective comparison of the Amplatz thrombectomy device with modified pulse-spray pharmacomechanical thrombolysis in the treatment of thrombosed hemodialysis access grafts. *Radiology.* 1999;213:561.

103. Barth KH, Gosnell MR, Palestrant AM, et al. Hydrodynamic thrombectomy system versus pulse-spray thrombolysis for thrombosed hemodialysis grafts: a multicenter prospective randomized comparison. *Radiology.* 2000;217:678.

104. Bischel MD, Scoles BG, Mohler JG. Evidence for pulmonary microembolization during hemodialysis. *Chest.* 1975;67:335.

105. Droste DW, Kuhne K, Schaefer RM, Ringelstein EB. Detection of microemboli in the subclavian vein of patients undergoing haemodialysis and haemodiafiltration using pulsed Doppler ultrasound. *Nephrol Dial Transplant.* 2002;17:462.

106. Rolle F, Pengloan J, Abazza M, et al. Identification of microemboli during haemodialysis using Doppler ultrasound. *Nephrol Dial Transplant.* 2000;15:1420.

107. Trerotola SO, Lund GB, Scheel PJ, Jr., et al. Thrombosed dialysis access grafts: percutaneous mechanical declotting without urokinase. *Radiology.* 1994;191:721.

108. Middlebrook MR, Amygdalos MA, Soulen MC, et al. Thrombosed hemodialysis grafts: percutaneous mechanical balloon declotting versus thrombolysis. *Radiology.* 1995;196:73.

109. Soulen MC, Zaetta JM, Amygdalos MA, et al. Mechanical declotting of thrombosed dialysis grafts: experience in 86 cases. *J Vasc Interv Radiol.* 1997;8:563.

110. Dolmatch BL, Gray RJ, Horton KM. Will iatrogenic pulmonary embolization be our pulmonary embarrassment? *Radiology.* 1994;191:615.

111. Yigla M, Nakhoul F, Sabag A, et al. Pulmonary hypertension in patients with end-stage renal disease. *Chest.* 2003;123:1577.

112. Harp RJ, Stavropoulos SW, Wasserstein AG, Clark TW. Pulmonary hypertension among end-stage renal failure patients following hemodialysis access thrombectomy. *Cardiovasc Intervent Radiol.* 2005;28:17.

113. Swan TL, Smyth SH, Ruffenach SJ, et al. Pulmonary embolism following hemodialysis access thrombolysis/thrombectomy. *J Vasc Interv Radiol.* 1995;6:683.

114. Petronis JD, Regan F, Briefel G, et al. Ventilation-perfusion scintigraphic evaluation of pulmonary clot burden after percutaneous thrombolysis of clotted hemodialysis access grafts. *Am J Kidney Dis.* 1999;34:207.

115. Kinney TB, Valji K, Rose SC, et al. Pulmonary embolism from pulse-spray pharmacomechanical thrombolysis of clotted hemodialysis grafts: urokinase versus heparinized saline. *J Vasc Interv Radiol.* 2000;11:1143.

116. Briefel GR, Regan F, Petronis JD. Cerebral embolism after mechanical thrombolysis of a clotted hemodialysis access. *Am J Kidney Dis.* 1999;34:341.

117. Yu AS, Levy E. Paradoxical cerebral air embolism from a hemodialysis catheter. *Am J Kidney Dis.* 1997;29:453.

118. Owens CA, Yaghmai B, Aletich V, et al. Fatal paradoxic embolism during percutaneous thrombolysis of a hemodialysis graft. *AJR Am J Roentgenol.* 1998;170:742.

KIDNEY BIOPSY

STEVEN WU

1. To understand indications, contraindications, and risk stratification prior to kidney biopsy.
2. To review patient preparation and strategies for reduction of bleeding risk.
3. To emphasize the technique of ultrasonography-guided kidney biopsy.
4. To understand postbiopsy management and complications.

INTRODUCTION

Percutaneous kidney biopsy with a needle aspiration technique was first performed by a Swedish nephrologist, Nils Alwall, in 1944,[1,2] and then first described by Iversen and Brun in 1951.[2,3] The cutting needle technique was introduced in 1954.[4] The procedure is now commonly performed by nephrologists and radiologists worldwide. In the modern era, kidney biopsy can be safely performed with relatively low complication rates using imaging guidance, such as ultrasonography,[5-7] or CT.[8] Coinciding with the rapid growth of interventional nephrology and the availability of high-quality portable ultrasonographic equipment, kidney biopsy will likely become an increasingly common procedure within the practice of nephrology.

Kidney biopsy provides tissue samples for accurate diagnosis and better estimation of prognosis of renal and other systemic disease. It allows for an in-depth understanding of pathogenesis and disease processes at the cellular and molecular levels, and is the cornerstone of current general and transplant nephrology. The information gleaned from renal biopsy specimens has an approximately 45–50% chance of directly impacting patient management decisions.[9-11]

Although kidney biopsy can be performed for focal lesions (such as tumor or cyst) and can also be performed under CT-guidance or via a transjugular approach, this chapter will mainly focus on the ultrasonography-guided nonfocal biopsy of native and transplant kidneys.

INDICATIONS AND CONTRAINDICATIONS

▶ Indications

Indications for kidney biopsy are broad. In general, any acute or chronic kidney disease (CKD), which requires elucidation of the disease process, has a clinical course deviating from that which is expected, or must establish a definitive prognosis relies on tissue diagnosis. In the setting of renal transplant, biopsy is usually indicated for ruling out acute or chronic allograft rejection, allograft dysfunction, or for diagnosis of de novo kidney disease. Beyond primary renal diseases, kidney biopsy may also provide diagnosis of certain systematic disorders that involve the kidney. In these conditions, renal biopsy may be preferable to other forms of diagnosis because of the proven safety profile of the procedure and easy accessibility to the kidneys.[12,13]

Although most nephrologists would consider biopsy in patients with microhematuria or proteinuria with otherwise normal renal function, there are some exceptions.[14,15] In the setting of diabetes, proteinuria with normal or slightly enlarged kidneys is likely indicative of diabetic nephropathy and biopsy would only be necessary if the clinical course deviates significantly from the expected course.[16,17] In the setting of chronic renal disease, kidney size is a major determinant of the need for and utility of biopsy. Shrunken, atrophic kidneys are typically representative of nonreversible disease, with little value added to clinical care by tissue sampling.

However, the specific incidence, indications, and timing of kidney biopsy vary among practicing nephrologists. There is uncertainty with regard to proceeding to biopsy in patients with chronic nonnephrotic proteinuria and preserved renal function.[14] Similarly, the appropriate timing of biopsy for evaluation of acute kidney injury is controversial, with some nephrologists preferring to sample at the onset of the acute process, but others waiting and basing further decisions on the trend of renal function.[18]

► Contraindications

Contraindications to renal biopsy include uncorrectable coagulopathy or bleeding diatheses and obesity or body habitus that prevent adequate visualization of the kidneys.[15] Uncooperative patients are also a contraindication.[15] However, these are all considered relative contraindications, with the urgency of the clinical situation often overruling the potential risks of biopsy. The available alternative approaches, including transjugular or CT-guided biopsy, and the availability of conscious sedation or general anesthesia has made renal biopsy feasible in almost any clinical scenario.[19,20] Kidney biopsy is also a safe and well-tolerated procedure in the elderly population and will usually affect management, often revealing advanced kidney disease.[21–23]

PREBIOPSY PREPARATION

► Clinical Assessment and Risk Stratification

Prior to kidney biopsy, a detailed clinical assessment of bleeding risks should be performed. The factors associated with bleeding include anticoagulation therapy (warfarin, heparin, low-molecular-weight heparin (LMWH), antiplatelet agents, glycoprotein IIb/IIIa inhibitors), NSAIDS usage, uncontrolled hypertension, uncooperative patients, obesity, platelet reduction, and/or dysfunction due to uremia, cirrhosis, bone marrow diseases, and other hematologic and oncological disorders. Patients can be simply divided into low-risk and high-risk groups as below (see Table 41-1). The low-risk group patients may receive kidney biopsy with minimal preparation. The high-risk

TABLE 41–1

Bleeding Risk Stratification Prior to Biopsy

Low Risk Group	High Risk Group
Young	Elderly
Normal blood pressure	Uncontrolled blood pressure
Not on antiplatelet agents or NSAIDs	On Aspirin, clopidogrel, or NSAIDS
Not on anticoagulation therapy; if yes, INR $\leq$ 1.5	On anticoagulation therapy or INR >1.5
Platelet >50,000	Platelet <50,000
	Obesity
	Uncooperative patients
	Severe anemia
	Cirrhosis, sever liver failure, uremia, or other hematological or oncology disorders leading to bleeding tendency

patients should undergo further management to reduce the risks of bleeding.

► Management of High-Risk Patients

Anticoagulation therapy

Warfarin Ideally, warfarin should be held for 3–5 days[24] until international normalization ratio (INR) is less than 1.5. Heparin may be used to bridge the period of anticoagulation therapy if indicated based on cardiovascular risk factors.[25] If warfarin cannot be held or kidney biopsy needs to be performed as a medical emergency, the warfarin anticoagulation effect can be temporally reversed with vitamin K and/or fresh frozen plasma (FFP). In a medical emergency, the sooner a patient receives the first dose of vitamin K and FFP, the quicker the INR value will respond.[26] Interestingly, at least in one study, dosing of vitamin K and FFP had no effect on reversal time of INR.[26] INR should be closely monitored after administering vitamin K and/or FFP. INR <1.5 is usually required for a safe kidney biopsy although INR $\leq$ 2.0 is recently recommended.[24] While correcting coagulopathy with FFP, one should also keep in mind that there is an imperfect correlation between mild elevations in the INR and subsequent bleeding tendency. Furthermore, FFP transfusion may not always be sufficient to achieve targeted INR values.[27–29]

Heparin or low-molecular-weight heparin and argatroban Many patients now commonly receive unfractionated heparin or low-molecular-weight heparin (LMWH) for prophylaxis of deep vein thrombosis, for bridging therapy while warfarin is held, or for cardiac diseases such as atrial fibrillation. Some patients receive argatroban, a direct thrombin inhibitor, for treatment of heparin-induced thrombocytopenia (HIT). Given the short half-life of unfractionated heparin (1.5 hours), LMWH (2–4 hours), and argatroban (50 minutes), these agents can be discontinued on the day of kidney biopsy.

NSAIDs and other antiplatelet agents Patients on antiplatelet agents such as clopidogrel, aspirin, nonsteroidal anti-inflammatory drugs (NSAIDs), or glycoprotein IIb/IIIa inhibitors should be properly prepared prior to kidney biopsy. Discontinuing these agents for 5–7 days prior to the procedure is acceptable. If emergency biopsy is required, transfusion of fresh platelets may be helpful. However, even so, relatively higher risks of bleeding seen with these medications are concerning.

Medical diseases associated with high risks of bleeding

Cirrhosis or severe liver dysfunction Many coagulation factors are synthesized in the liver. End-stage liver disease such as cirrhosis and severe liver dysfunction such as acute hepatitis may greatly compromise coagulation capacity. In addition, splenomegaly secondary to portal hypertension/cirrhosis can result in depletion of platelets from the peripheral circulation. Replacement of certain coagulation factors using FFP is helpful in this situation. Factor VII has the shortest half-life (4–6 hours) among all the liver-related coagulation factors, and timing of FFP transfusion prior to kidney biopsy is important in order to give the maximal protective effect during and immediately after the biopsy. Although most practitioners will transfuse the patient if the platelet number is less than 50,000, recent studies have demonstrated that invasive procedure can be safely performed with a platelet number >25,000.[24] However, this threshold may need to be individualized in cirrhotic patients with reduced coagulation factors. When correction of coagulopathy is inadequate or impossible, the alternative approach of transjugular biopsy is a more advisable option.

Chronic kidney diseases Acute and/or CKD, particularly the uremic stage, is associated with increased bleeding tendency secondary to platelet dysfunction. Toxins in the bloodstream of these patients inhibit the release of von Willebrand's factor and cause platelet dysfunction. Certain treatment regimens may restore, at least partially, the platelet function. Estrogen and desmopressin (1-deamino-8-D-arginine vasopressin [DDAVP]) have been used in this clinical situation although their efficacies remain to be determined. The common dosing of estrogen and DDAVP are as the follows:

> Conjugated estrogen: 0.6 mg/kg intravenously over 30–40 minutes once daily for five consecutive days.[30–32] DDAVP: 0.3 μg/kg to 0.4 μg/kg intravenously or subcutaneously as a single injection.[33,34]

Hematologic, oncologic disorders and other medical conditions Many other medical conditions such as hematologic and oncologic disorders can cause reduction of platelet numbers and platelet dysfunction. Chemotherapy may also destroy bone marrow and result in coagulation problems. In these more complicated clinical scenarios, consultation and recommendations from hematology/oncology are a recommended strategy prior to biopsy planning.

Thrombocytopenia

There are many causes of thrombocytopenia, from drug-induced to bone marrow disorder-related. Regardless of underlying etiology, as mentioned previously, most interventionalists will consider fresh platelet transfusion if platelet number is less than 25,000–50,000.[24]

Uncontrolled hypertension

Uncontrolled hypertension is believed to increase the bleedings risk after kidney biopsy. It is ideal if blood pressure can be managed to 130/80 mm Hg prior to the procedure.

Uncooperative patients

For uncooperative patients due to poor mental status or anxiety related to the procedure, use of conscious sedation or general anesthesia offers a safe alternative.

Obesity

If the kidneys are not well-visualized under ultrasonography due to obesity, other modalities, such as CT-guided biopsy, can be considered.

▶ Reassessment on the Day of Biopsy

On the day of the procedure, it is crucial to reassess the risks of bleeding. The reassessment should include the following: (1) confirm that antiplatelet or anticoagulation agent(s) is discontinued as instructed; (2) coagulation tests such as platelet number, PTT, PT/INR; (3) hemoglobin and hematocrit; (4) blood bank sample, and type and cross in case blood transfusion is needed; (5) appropriate arrangement of postbiopsy observation including possible admission is made; and (6) postbiopsy tissue process team is informed.

ULTRASOUND-GUIDED KIDNEY BIOPSY

▶ Rationale

Direct visualization of the kidney along with observation of the biopsy needle position is considered a major advantage contributing to the excellent safety profile of modern kidney biopsy procedures. Ultrasound is able to produce clear images of the kidneys without ionizing radiation exposure. Sonography is also useful for its ability to be able to detect other potential causes of renal dysfunction such as hydronephrosis secondary to urinary tract obstruction. When the biopsy needle is well-aligned longitudinally with an ultrasound transducer, the sonographic beam will reflect back from the needle, leading to clear visualization on the screen. With reasonable training and practice, one should be able to coordinate the hand holding the transducer and the hand inserting the biopsy needle. The goal is to find satisfactory alignment between transducer and needle, allowing the needle to be inserted through a clear pathway to the targeted renal cortex under direct and real-time observation. An alternative to the freehand approach involves use of a needle guide that can be mounted to the transducer. The guide assures perfect alignment between the needle and ultrasound beam for easy visualization of the needle.

▶ Selection of Correctly Sized Biopsy Device

The most commonly used biopsy devices are spring-loaded, automated, and cutting needle based. The diameter of commonly used biopsy devices varies from 14G to 18G. Although 18G devices are associated with lower risks of bleeding, the better safety profile is at the expense of tissue sample quality. The inner diameter of an 18G biopsy needle is 300–400 μm, which is just above the size of average glomeruli (200–250 μm). Samples obtained through 18G biopsy needles may not be adequate due to damaged glomeruli and disturbed cellular structure. In order to obtain decent tissue samples, 14G (900–1000 μm) or

16G (600–700 µm) biopsy devices are recommended for adults. 16G or 18G devices are preferred in children under 8 years of age.

Numbers of Passes

The more passes the biopsy needle makes into the cortex, the better the chance of high quality tissue samples being obtained. However, more passes will also increase the risk of bleeding. Most clinicians are comfortable with one or two passes, but the number of glomeruli obtained is the final arbiter of tissue quality. It is sometimes possible to adequately arrive at a diagnosis with 6–10 glomeruli, and occasionally even with 1 glomerulus, but 10–15 glomeruli are ideal. Having a pathologist or pathology assistant in the procedure room to examine the collected specimens using dissecting microscopy will assure good quality samples and avoid unnecessary passes.

Target Areas of Kidney

For native kidney biopsy, the left kidney is preferred. The lower pole is easier to access and is better visualized. The upper pole or the cortex of the interpolar area can be used as well if it can be clearly visualized. The biopsy needle should avoid aiming toward the medulla (pyramid) or the hilum. This will avoid unnecessary traversal of vital structures, including the renal arteries, veins, and pelvis. For transplant kidneys, any easily accessible cortex away from medulla or hilum is an acceptable biopsy site.

Sedation Versus Local Anesthesia

Kidney biopsy can be performed safely under local anesthesia. Conscious sedation, and occasionally general anesthesia, may be used to facilitate the procedure based on different institutions' policies. Anxious or uncooperative patients may require conscious sedation or general anesthesia. These patients should have nothing-by-mouth (NPO) after midnight the day prior to the procedure.

Positions

For native kidney biopsy, a prone position with a pillow, a rolling towel or cushion underneath the upper abdominal area to position the kidney posteriorly is a preferred position. The biopsy device is inserted from the back avoiding pelvic rim and the lower rib. For a transplant kidney biopsy, a supine position is ideal since the kidney is typically superficial in the right or left pelvic fossa (see Figure 41-1).

Detailed Steps of the Native Kidney Biopsy

1. Patient is consented and understands the steps of procedure.
2. A thorough ultrasound examination of both kidneys, renal vasculatures, and urinary tract system should be performed and documented prior to the biopsy.
3. Patient is then placed in a prone position with a pillow or a rolling towel or a cushion underneath upper abdomen to push the kidney posterior.

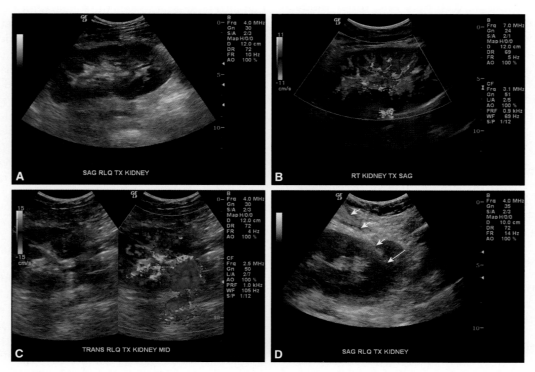

FIGURE 41-1. (**A**) Sagittal view of transplant kidney. (**B**) Doppler evaluation of transplant kidney (sagittal view). (**C**) Transverse view of transplant kidney with and without Doppler. (**D**) Biopsy gun firing moment with the gun aiming the cortex of the lower pole (short arrows: biopsy gun needle viewed under ultrasound; long arrow: the tip of the biopsy gun).

4. The right or left kidney is selected for biopsy based on accessibility at deep breathing and holding position.

5. Patient is asked to practice deep breathing and holding technique, and expect to hear firing sounds of biopsy gun.

6. The target kidney is reassessed using ultrasound and an incision site with a potential trajectory is determined at deep breathing and holding position.

7. The patient is then prepped and draped in a sterile fashion.

8. Ultrasound transducer is gelled and wrapped with a sterile cover. A sterile ultrasound guide can be mounted to the transducer if the guide is used.

9. The incision site is anesthetized with 1% lidocaine, and a small incision is made using a scalpel.

10. Under ultrasound guidance, 1% lidocaine is injected through the planed trajectory using a 20G spine needle all the way to kidney capsule. It is important to visualize the needle during the injection.

11. A right-sized, loaded biopsy gun was inserted from the incision and passed through the trajectory to near the kidney capsule. The needle avoids pointing to hilum or medulla, but cortex of such as lower pole.

12. At this point, patient is asked to take a deep breath and hold. The tip of biopsy gun needle is inserted 1–2 mm into renal parenchyma, and the gun fires. The ultrasound image of gun firing is recorded and documented.

13. The gun is quickly removed, and the biopsy needle is re-open while the gun is reloaded.

14. The core of tissue is carefully transferred to a gauze moistened with normal saline, and the core is then examined by a qualified pathologist or pathology assistant using a dissecting microscopy.

15. If another core is required, steps 11–14 are repeated.

16. The kidney is assessed for hematoma; images are recorded and documented.

17. A sterile bandage was applied to the incision.

18. Patient is transferred in supine position with a pillow underneath the biopsy side.

▶ Detailed Steps of Transplant Kidney Biopsy

1. Patient is consented and understands the steps of procedure.

2. A thorough ultrasound examination of the transplant kidney, renal vasculatures, and urinary tract system should be performed and documented prior to the biopsy.

3. Patient is then placed in a supine position.

4. The transplant kidney is reassessed using ultrasound and an incision site with a potential trajectory is determined based on accessibility of needle and avoidance of bowels and adjacent organs.

5. The patient is then prepped and draped in a sterile fashion.

6. Ultrasound transducer is gelled and wrapped with a sterile cover. A sterile ultrasound guide can be mounted to the transducer if the guide is used.

7. The incision site is anesthetized with 1% lidocaine, and a small incision is made using a scalpel.

8. Under ultrasound guidance, 1% lidocaine is injected through the planed trajectory using a 20G spine needle all the way to kidney capsule. It is important to visualize the needle during the injection.

9. A right-sized, loaded biopsy gun was inserted from the incision and pass through the trajectory to near the kidney capsule. The needle avoids pointing to hilum or medulla, but cortex of such as lower or upper pole.

10. At this point, the tip of biopsy gun needle is inserted 1–2 mm into renal parenchyma, and the gun fires. The ultrasound image of gun firing is recorded and documented.

11. The gun is quickly removed, and the biopsy needle is re-open while the gun is reloaded.

12. The core of tissue is carefully transferred to a gauze moistened with normal saline, and the core is then examined by a qualified pathologist or pathology assistant using a dissecting microscopy.

13. If another core is required, steps 9–14 are repeated.

14. The kidney is assessed for hematoma; images are recorded and documented.

15. A sterile bandage was applied to the incision.

16. Patient is transferred in supine position with a weight bag on the biopsy side.

POSTBIOPSY CARE

▶ Postbiopsy Orders and Monitoring

The patient is instructed to undergo bed rest for 6 hours. Vital signs are monitored every 15 minutes for 2 hours, then every 30 minutes for 2 hours, and then hourly. It is critical to encourage the patient to void after the biopsy. If gross hematuria is observed, serial urine sample saving and monitoring of color change would be an acceptable method of evaluating whether bleeding is resolving or worsening. After discharge to home, the patient should be instructed to avoid vigorous activities for 1 month.

▶ Same-Day Discharge Versus Overnight Observation

There is no evidence to favor either same-day discharge or overnight observation after kidney biopsy. The decision is highly variable from practice to practice and from one subspecialty to another subspecialty. Although longer observation is theoretically safer to ensure delayed bleeders are identified, actual safety benefit versus cost remains to be determined. Most physicians simply follow their own training and institutional policies to determine this. Most interventional radiologists would prefer the same-day discharge, likely due to their busy procedure schedule and practice settings. Most nephrologists appear to favor the overnight observation approach.

COMPLICATIONS AND TREATMENT

▶ Bleeding

Although kidney biopsy is a safe procedure, clinically insignificant bleeding is common. Bleeding and/or hematoma can be confined within Gerota's capsule, which typically is self-limiting due to the confined anatomic space. Occasionally, bleeding can extend into the retroperitoneal space and the pelvis. Hematuria occurs in up to 35% of patients and perinephric hematoma in up to 65% of patients. The majority of patients with hematuria and/or hematoma are clinically stable, and only 1% will require blood transfusion. Less than 0.1% of patients eventually lose their kidneys due to uncontrolled bleeding. Death is very rare.

▶ Infection

Infection is a rare complication. The biopsy is performed under sterile conditions, and the occurrence of infection at incision site or kidney is indeed very rare. If the patient has any symptoms and/or signs of urinary tract infection, biopsy should be postponed until the infection is adequately treated.

▶ Pneumothorax

Injury to the lung is a rare potential complication of renal biopsy. This is associated with accessing the upper pole for sampling, which may lead to an inadvertent transpleural approach. When it occurs, it may require close monitoring with the possibility of chest tube placement and hospital admission.

▶ Injury to Adjacent Organs

The liver, bowel, and spleen are organs in close proximity to the kidney. Kidney biopsy may potentially injure these organs. Direct visualization of the kidney and biopsy needle and careful planning of the sampling trajectory are key to limiting the incidence of this kind of complication.

▶ Arteriovenous Fistula and Pseudoaneurysm

The development of AVFs and pseudoaneurysms following renal biopsy are related to trauma to the renal vasculature during biopsy. Clinically significant lesions are rare, but there is likely a high percentage of undocumented insignificant AVFs and pseudoaneurysms. When clinically significant, these lesions are identified due to persistent symptoms such as back pain occasionally renal dysfunction. Endovascular intervention with coiling and/or stent placement is curative.

SUMMARY

Percutaneous kidney biopsy is a widely performed procedure by nephrologists. In most instances, it can be accomplished under ultrasound guidance, with occasional cases requiring CT-guidance or a transjugular approach. It is crucial to assess bleeding risks prior to biopsy. With risk reduction strategies, renal biopsy can be performed safely with minimal complications.

REFERENCES

1. Alwall N. Aspiration biopsy of the kidney including i.a. a report of a case of myloidosis diagnosed through aspiration biopsy of the kidney in 1944 and investigated at an autopsy in 1950. *Acta Medica Scandinavica.* 1952; 143:430–435.
2. Cameron JS, Hicks J. The introduction of renal biopsy into nephrology from 1901 to 1961: a paradigm of the forming of nephrology by technology. *Am J Nephrol.* 1997;17 (3–4):347–358.
3. Iversen P, Brun C. Aspiration biopsy of the kidney. *Am J Med.* 1951;11:324–330.
4. Kark RM, Muehrcke RC. Biopsy of kidney in prone position. *Lancet.* 1954;266:1047–1049.
5. Pollack HM, Goldberg BB, Kellermann E. Ultrasonically guided renal biopsy. *Arch Intern Med.* 1978;138:355–356.
6. Backman U, Lindgren PG. Percutaneous renal biopsy with real time ultrasonography. *Scand J Urol Nephrol.* 1982;16: 65–67.
7. Patel MD, Phillips CJ, Young SW, Kriegshauser JS, Chen F, Eversman WG, Silva AC, Lorans R. US-guided renal transplant biopsy: efficacy of a cortical tangential approach. *Radiology.* 2010;256:290–296.
8. Haaga JR, Alfidi R. Precise biopsy localization by computed tomography. *Radiology.* 1976;118:603–609.
9. Paone DB, Meyer LE. The effect of biopsy on therapy in renal disease. *Arch Intern Med.* 1981;141:1039–1041.
10. Andreucci VE, Fuiano G, Stanziale P, Andreucci M. Role of renal biopsy in the diagnosis and prognosis of acute renal failure. *Kidney Int Suppl.* 1998;66:S91–S95.
11. Amann K, Haas CS. What you should know about the work-up of a renal biopsy. *Nephrol Dial Transplant.* 2006; 21:1157–1161.
12. Cohen SD, Kimmel PL. Renal biopsy is necessary for the diagnosis of HIV-associated renal diseases. *Nat Clin Pract Nephrol.* 2009;5:22–23.
13. Seshan SV, Jennette JC. Renal disease in systemic lupus erythematosus with emphasis on classification of lupus glomerulonephritis: advances and implications. *Arch Pathol Lab Med.* 2009;133:233–248.
14. Fuiano G, Mazza G, Comi N, Caglioti A, De Nicola L, Iodice C, Andreucci M, Andreucci VE. Current indications for renal biopsy: a questionnaire-based survey. *Am J Kidney Dis.* 2000;35:448–457.
15. Geddes CC, Baxter GM. Renal biopsy: how to do it. *Imaging.* 2008;20:20–22.
16. Biesenbach G, Bodlaj G, Pieringer H, Sedlak M. Clinical versus histological diagnosis of diabetic nephropathy—is renal biopsy required in type 2 diabetic patients with renal disease? *QJM.* 2011;104(9):771–774.

17. Serra A, Romero R, Bayés B, Lopez D, Bonet J. Is there a need for changes in renal biopsy criteria in proteinuria in type 2 diabetes? *Diabetes Res Clin Pract.* 2002;58:149–153.

18. McQuarrie EP, Mackinnon B, Young B, Yeoman L, Stewart G, Fleming S, Robertson S, Simpson K, Fox J, Geddes CC, Scottish Renal Biopsy Registry. Centre variation in incidence, indication and diagnosis of adult native renal biopsy in Scotland. *Nephrol Dial Transplant.* 2009;24:1524–1528.

19. Thompson BC, Kingdon E, Johnston M, Tibballs J, Watkinson A, Jarmulowicz M, Burns A, Sweny P, Wheeler DC. Transjugular kidney biopsy. *Am J Kidney Dis.* 2004;43:651–662.

20. Stiles KP, Yuan CM, Chung EM, Lyon RD, Lane JD, Abbott KC. Renal biopsy in high-risk patients with medical diseases of the kidney. *Am J Kidney Dis.* 2000;36:419–433.

21. Moutzouris DA, Herlitz L, Appel GB, Markowitz GS, Freudenthal B, Radhakrishnan J, D'Agati VD. Renal biopsy in the very elderly. *Clin J Am Soc Nephrol.* 2009;4:1073–1082.

22. Kohli HS, Jairam A, Bhat A, Sud K, Jha V, Gupta KL, Sakhuja V. Safety of kidney biopsy in elderly: a prospective study. *Int Urol Nephrol.* 2006;38:815–820.

23. de Oliveira CM, Costa RS, Vieira Neto OM, Dantas RA, Moysés Neto M, Romão EA, Barros-Silva GE, Coelho EB, Dantas M. Renal diseases in the elderly underwent to percutaneous biopsy of native kidneys. *J Bras Nefrol.* 2010;32:379–385.

24. O'Connor SD, Taylor AJ, Williams EC, Winter TC. Coagulation concepts update. *AJR.* 2009;193:1656–1664.

25. Kaatz S, Paje D. Update in bridging anticoagulation. *J Thromb Thrombolysis.* 2011;31:259–264.

26. Goldstein JN, Thomas SH, Frontiero V, Joseph A, Engel C, Snider R, Smith EE, Greenberg SM, Rosand J. Timing of fresh frozen plasma administration and rapid correction of coagulopathy in warfarin-related intracerebral hemorrhage. *Stroke.* 2006;37(1):151–155.

27. West KL, Adamson C, Hoffman M. Prophylactic correction of the international normalized ratio in neurosurgery: a brief review of a brief literature. *J Neurosurg.* 2011;114(1):9–18.

28. Abdel-Wahab OI, Healy B, Dzik WH. Effect of fresh-frozen plasma transfusion on prothrombin time and bleeding in patients with mild coagulation abnormalities. *Transfusion.* 2006;46(8):1279–1285.

29. Holland LL, Brooks JP. Toward rational fresh frozen plasma transfusion: the effect of plasma transfusion on coagulation test results. *Am J Clin Pathol.* 2006;126(1):133–139.

30. Livio M, Mannucci PM, Vigano G, Mingardi G, Lombardi R, Mecca G, Remuzzi G. Conjugated estrogens for the management of bleeding associated with renal failure. *N Engl J Med.* 1986;315:731–735.

31. Vigano G, Gaspari F, Locatelli M, Pusineri F, Bonati M, Remuzzi G. Dose-effect and pharmacokinetics of estrogens given to correct bleeding time in uremia. *Kidney Int.* 1988;34(6):853–858.

32. Heistinger M, Stockenhuber F, Schneider B, Pabinger I, Brenner B, Wagner B, Balcke P, Lechner K, Kyrle PA. Effect of conjugated estrogens on platelet function and prostacyclin generation in CRF. *Kidney Int.* 1990;38(6):1181–1186.

33. Mannucci PM, Remuzzi G, Pusineri F, Lombardi R, Valsecchi C, Mecca G, Zimmerman TS. Deamino-8-D-arginine vasopressin shortens the bleeding time in uremia. *N Engl J Med.* 1983;308(1):8–12.

34. Kohler M, Hellstern P, Tarrach H, Bambauer R, Wenzel E, Jutzler GA. Subcutaneous injection of desmopressin (DDAVP): evaluation of a new, more concentrated preparation. *Hemostasis.* 1989; 19(1):38–44.

42

RENAL ULTRASONOGRAPHY

EDGAR V. LERMA

1. Understand the history and development of ultrasonography, from the pre-War to the modern era.
2. Understand the basic physics of ultrasonography.
3. Understand normal kidney anatomy and its relations to bordering structures and organs.
4. Discuss the indications and limitations of renal ultrasonography.
5. Discuss the role of ultrasonography in the evaluation of renal allografts.
6. Understand the techniques involved in the performance of a complete ultrasound evaluation of the kidneys, ureters, and bladder.
7. Identify normal anatomical variants and abnormal findings on ultrasonography.

INTRODUCTION

Ultrasound refers to a medical technique that uses a special device, referred to as a transducer, to bounce high-frequency sound waves off tissues. The echoes are then converted into images of soft tissues, internal organs, and body cavities. The image is referred to as a sonogram, and the technique is referred to as ultrasonography. Typical diagnostic ultrasound devices, referred to as scanners, operate at a frequency of 2–18 MHz (abbreviation for megahertz, one MHz represents one million cycles per second).

The evolution of the science of ultrasonography can be appreciated by comparing the results obtained with the early versions of the static B-mode scanner with the detailed imaging possible today with B-mode scanning. In early versions of the static B-mode scanner, the image was created on a direct viewing storage cathode ray tube. On such a tube, the image could be viewed for 10 minutes before it disappeared. The storage tubes had a very limited ability to display shades of gray; some of them could only show black and white. Today's scans are very detailed, with a wide gray-scale range displayed in high resolution, providing detailed information. These changes can be attributed to developments in engineering and computer technology.

APPLICATIONS, ADVANTAGES, AND LIMITATIONS

Ultrasonography is widely used in virtually all fields of medicine, facilitating the performance of a wide array of diagnostic and therapeutic procedures. It is especially ideal for imaging various soft tissues. When imaging any specific tissue, there are two issues of concern—resolution and penetration. These variables are determined by the ultrasound frequency that is used for the examination. Frequencies ranging from 2 to 18 MHz are used. Ultrasound cannot detect objects that are smaller than its wavelength, and therefore higher frequencies of ultrasound produce better resolution. On the other hand, higher frequencies of ultrasound have short wavelengths and are absorbed easily and therefore are not as penetrating. For this reason, high frequencies (7–18 MHz) are used for scanning areas of the body close to the surface (vascular access, muscle, and breast) and low frequencies (2–6 MHz) are used for areas that are deeper in the body (liver, kidney, and gallbladder).

Renal ultrasonography offers distinct advantages over other radiological imaging procedures. It is a portable, fast, and noninvasive imaging modality that can be used to detailed information about the kidneys and the urinary tract. In particular, it avoids the attendant risks associated with ionizing radiation and exposure to intravenous radiocontrast material (anaphylactic reaction and contrast nephropathy). It can be easily performed at the bedside. It provides good differentiation between cortex and medulla and shows the renal contour as well as perinephric space. It is sensitive for demonstrating perirenal fluid collections, AND pyelocalyceal dilatation; it can differentiate cysts versus solid masses, and it provides adequate renal imaging regardless of renal function; that is, it is safe to use EVEN in those with significant azotemia.

Ultrasound techniques can be used to provide "live" or real-time images allowing for the performance of other diagnostic or therapeutic procedures such as ultrasound-guided biopsies, injections, or drainage of abscesses. Additionally, it is more economical than the other commonly used imaging modalities such as computed tomography scanning or magnetic resonance imaging.

However, renal ultrasonic imaging does have some potential disadvantages. Although it provides excellent anatomical detail of the kidneys and the urinary tract, it cannot assess renal function. The images tend to be suboptimal when there is overlying gas or subcutaneous fat between the probe and tissue of interest or when there are superimposed bony structures. Image quality can be significantly compromised in obese subjects, making these examinations particularly difficult. Renal ultrasonography is limited in showing fine pyelocalyceal detail or the entire "normal" ureter. Ureteral calculi and small renal calculi can be easily missed on routine ultrasound examination. In the presence of early obstructive uropathy in the volume-depleted state, hydronephrosis may not be readily appreciated giving a false-negative impression.

INDICATIONS

An ultrasound evaluation is indicated for a wide array of problems that can affect the kidneys and urinary system. These include the evaluation of acute and chronic renal failure, renal colic, hydronephrosis, acute kidney injury, postsurgical status of kidney and/or ureter, acute renal vein thrombosis, renal masses, and calculi and renal trauma. It is also useful in the detection and assessment of renal anatomical variants such as duplication of the kidney, ectopic kidneys, and horseshoe kidneys. Ultrasonography is especially useful in the diagnosis and evaluation of cysts, both simple and compound. Screening for autosomal dominant polycystic kidney disease (ADPKD) has become the standard of practice using well-defined criteria (Table 42-1). Interventional procedures performed on the kidney, percutaneous renal biopsy, and cyst aspiration are greatly facilitated by the use of ultrasound.

Ultrasonography occupies a major role in the evaluation of the transplanted kidney. Any change in real function can be viewed as an indication for evaluation using this noninvasive modality. Conditions such as hematomas, lymphoceles, urinomas, and vascular complications that can occur in the postoperative period can be detected. The evaluation of suspected rejection should include renal ultrasound.

Bladder ultrasonography is also useful in measuring postvoid residual and in the evaluation of other diseases involving the bladder such as bladder tumors, diverticuli, blood clots, calculi, foreign bodies, and even prostate enlargement.

TABLE 42–1				
Revised Unified Diagnostic Ultrasound Criteria for Autosomal Dominant Polycystic Kidney Disease[1,*]				
Age	**Ultrasound Findings**	**PKD 1**	**PKD 2**	**Unknown ADPKD Gene Type**
15–29	≥3 cysts, unilateral or bilateral	PPV = 100% Sen = 94.3%	PPV = 100% Sen = 69.5%	PPV = 100% Sen = 81.7%
30–39	≥3 cysts, unilateral or bilateral	PPV = 100% Sen = 96.6%	PPV = 100% Sen = −94.9%	PPV = 100% Sen = 95.5%
40–59	≥2 cysts in each kidney	PPV = 100% Sen = 92.6%	PPV = 100% Sen = 88.8%	PPV = 100% Sen = 90%
Revised Ultrasound Criteria for Exclusion of Autosomal Dominant Polycystic Kidney Disease[29]				
15–29	≥1 cyst	NPV = 99.1% Spec = 97.6%	NPV = 83.5% Spec = 96.6%	NPV = 90.8% Spec = 97.1%
30–39	≥1 cyst	NPV = 100% Spec = 96%	NPV = 96.8% Spec = 93.8%	NPV = 98.3% Spec = 94.8%
40–59	≥1 cyst	NPV = 100% Spec = 93.9%	NPV = 100% Spec = 93.7%	NPV = 100% Spec = 93.9%

*For at risk subjects ≥60 years of age, 4 or more cysts pert kidney have a sensitivity and specificity of 100%, whether in PKD 1 or PKD 2 (and therefore of unknown gene type as well).

Abbreviations: PPV = positive predictive value; Sen = sensitivity; NPV = negative predictive value; Spec = specificity.

HISTORY OF ULTRASONOGRAPHY

In 1794, Spallanzini[2] demonstrated that bats relied on their hearing capability (as opposed to vision) in navigating through their habitat and capturing their prey. Jacques and Pierre Curie[2] together with Charles Friedel published their studies and observations on the physical characteristics of various types of crystals in 1881. Their work centered on "pyroelectricity," a phenomenon whereby electrical charges appeared on certain crystals when exposed to increased temperatures. Eventually, this led to the discovery of "piezoelectricity" (the ability of certain crystals to produce a voltage when subjected to mechanical stress. They also demonstrated that when an alternating electrical field was applied to quartz and tourmaline crystals, the piezoelectric plates of the two substances underwent expansion or contraction, leading to the production of sound waves of very high frequency. From this concept came the idea for the Galton dog whistle, which produced a sound that is audible to dogs but not to man.

When the Titanic sunk in 1912, it was not expected to have a major influence on medicine. However, the public outcry to detect icebergs following this major disaster had a major effect on the development of ultrasound technology. The world's first patent for an underwater echo ranging device was filed at the British Patent Office a month after the sinking of the Titanic. During World War I the need to navigate and detect submarines underwater prompted more research into the use of sound and ultimately led to the development of SONAR (Sound Navigation and Ranging).

With technological advancements after World War II, came the ability to amplify low-amplitude electrical signals and display them on the screen of a cathode ray oscilloscope. In the postwar era, in 1947, Douglass Howry, a radiologist from Denver, Colorado, first used ultrasound to visualize soft-tissue structures by displaying echoes from different tissue interfaces. Two years later, in 1949, he worked with William Roderic Bliss, an engineer, and they developed a pulse-echo system that could record echoes from tissue interfaces. They utilized the principle of "compound scanning," that consisted of two or more movements of the transducer, such that the transducer was continuously looking at tissue interfaces from various angles or perspectives. The advent of such "compounding" is believed to have paved the way for eventual real-time scanning. These early scans required cumbersome water-immersion techniques in which a variety of huge water containers such as laundry tub and even the gun turret tank of a B-29 airplane were used.

The first applications of ultrasound in the medical field took advantage of its heating and disruptive effects applied to therapy. In the 1940s, Karl Theo Dussik was the first to apply this technology to diagnosis. Dussik, a neurologist/psychiatrist at the University of Vienna, Austria, and his brother Friederich, a physicist, attempted to locate brain tumors by sending an ultrasound beam through the skull which produced an A-mode image. The amplitudes seen on the image showed both sides of the skull and the midline of the brain. If a midline shift was seen, a conclusion was made that there was either a tumor or a bleed. The "image" was recorded photographically on heat-sensitive paper. Dussik published the first paper on medical ultrasonics in 1942.

John Wild, a surgeon at the University of Minnesota, was interested in using ultrasound to diagnose gastrointestinal (GI) and breast tumors, and in doing so he made significant observations about distinguishing malignant from nonmalignant tumors in the breast. Wild joined forces with an electrical engineer named John Reid and developed an "echograph" and later a linear B-mode instrument that led the way to real-time scanning. In 1951, Wild and Donald Neal, an electrical engineer,[3] published work suggesting the potential of ultrasound to distinguish normal and diseased tissues by A-mode display. For this seminal work, Wild has been considered by many to be the "father of medical ultrasound (2009)."

In 1952, Wild collaborated with Reid[4] and published two-dimensional scans, which included a normal kidney. They were also credited as the first to demonstrate the diagnostic application of ultrasound in urology, with their screw-type rectal scanner. This was used a transducer that was inserted rectally, rotated, and then withdrawn in a planned scanning pattern. He also constructed a double transducer scanner for the study of the heart.

During that same time, Howry and Bliss[5] published two-dimensional ultrasonic tomograms using a sector scan of various tissues in vitro and of the forearm in vivo. Howry called his device a "somoscope" since it was most effective in studying soft tissues. Howry is also known for his initial work with applying mechanical sector scanners to the body surface. This eventually led to the development of the handheld system with the ability to scan in different planes.

In 1955, Shigeo Satomura collaborated with two cardiologists from the Osaka University Hospital, T Yoshida and Yasaharu Nimura, as they attempted to apply ultrasonic techniques to the measurement of the pulsations of cardiac, peripheral, and ocular vasculatures. Later that year, he published his first paper on the subject entitled "A new method of the mechanical vibration measurement and its application," where he demonstrated that Doppler signals can be retrieved from cardiac muscular movements when insonated with 3 MHz ultrasonic waves. Four years later, he published his seminal paper "Study of the flow pattern in peripheral arteries by ultrasonics."

In 1957, a group of Japanese scientists led by Yoshimitsu Kichuchi[6] demonstrated the use of the reflection technique and showed that it was possible to elicit echoes from abnormal growths or tumors through the intact skull. Much of the work on ultrasound during this time focused its application to the neurological system.

In 1962, Joseph H. Holmes, a nephrologist from the University of Colorado, in collaboration with William Wright and Ralph (Edward) Meyerdirk, developed one of the earliest versions of the real-time compound B-scanner. The latter two were later credited for developing the first commercial handheld articulated arm compound contact B-mode scanner in 1963. This paved the way for the design of modern day ultrasound scanners.[7]

In 1964, Werner Buschmann, an ophthalmologist, described the Doppler technique, also referred to as "carotid echography," at that time. In 1968, Somer described an electronic scanner developed for the purpose of ultrasonic diagnosis, and it produced a "real-time" image.

The 1970s era witnessed a marked improvement in the resolution of real-time scanners and the development of portable sector scanners. The introduction of the gray-scale presentation in 1971 became a prelude to the widespread clinical application of ultrasound. Through the development of a scan converter, high and low level echoes were displayed as various shades of gray. Three years later, in 1973–1974, ultrasound visualization of the liver and kidneys became a common thing.

One of the modern developments in the field is the "phased array" principle, developed by Thurstone and von Ramm[8] in 1974. Ultrasound probes using a pulsed array are used today in doing diagnostic studies. These probes consist of many small ultrasonic elements, each of which can be pulsed individually. By varying the timing, for instance by pulsing the elements one by one in sequence along a row, a pattern of constructive interference is set up that result in a beam at a set angle. The beam is swept like a searchlight through the tissue or object being examined, and the data from multiple beams are put together to make a visual image showing a slice through the object.

BASIC PHYSICS OF ULTRASONOGRAPHY

Ultrasounds are consist longitudinal waves of variable frequency, which cause particles to oscillate back and forth, and produce a series of compressions and rarefactions (Figure 42-1).

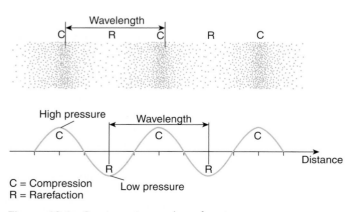

C = Compression
R = Rarefaction

Figure 42-1. Compression and rarefraction.

This phenomenon can be harnessed for diagnostic purposes. These sound waves are produced and detected using an ultrasound transducer (pulse-echo principle). These are devices that are capable of sending out an ultrasound and then the same transducer can detect the reflected sound and convert it to an electrical signal that is then converted to an image.

The basic principle at work is referred to as the piezoelectric effect, defined as the conversion of electrical energy to mechanical energy by a piezoelectric crystal. When an electrical current is applied across a piezoelectric crystal, it grows and shrinks (vibrates) depending on the voltage that is being applied. An alternating current causes the crystal to vibrate at a high speed and to produce an ultrasound. When this sound wave is directed toward a tissue being examined, sound waves bounce back toward the crystal that also acts as a receiver. The piezoelectric effect works in reverse. The mechanical energy produced from the reflected sound vibrates the crystal and is converted into electrical energy. By measuring the time between when the sound was sent and received, the amplitude of the sound and the pitch of the sound, a computer can produce images, calculate depths and calculate speeds.

Sound travels through materials under the influence of sound pressure. Because molecules or atoms of a solid material such as tissue are bound elastically to one another, the excess pressure results in a wave propagating through the solid. There is a tendency for any solid material to resist the passage of the sound wave, a phenomenon referred to as impedance or more precisely acoustical impedance. This causes some of the sound to be reflected back toward its source. Different tissues have differing degrees of acoustical impedance determined by their density and the velocity of the sound wave (acoustic velocity); therefore, they reflect differing amounts of the sound wave. These differences allow for differentiation between tissues. This allows for the distinction between tissues of varying density. Based upon differences in acoustic impedance, there are three basic components of the human body, namely: gas, soft tissue (fat, muscle, etc.), and bone. The higher the difference in acoustic impedance (impedance mismatch) between two adjacent tissues, the more the sound waves will be reflected at the interface between the tissues. It is this impedance mismatch that forms the basis for diagnostic ultrasound.

▶ Technological Advances

A major limitation to image formation in conventional real-time ultrasonography is the presence of artifacts, for example, shadowing, refraction, and speckling (graininess of image). Many of the improvements in ultrasound technology have sought to minimize artifacts and improve image quality, thus improving its diagnostic acuity.

An important advance in ultrasound technology has been the introduction of real-time spatial compound sonography or simply compound scanning. With conventional ultrasound, the target is viewed (insonated) at a singular constant angle. By combining ultrasound information obtained from multiple angles, real-time compound ultrasound improves the image quality of B-mode scans. This results in better delineation of margins, decreased image artifacts and noise, as well as enhancement of image contrast.[9,10,11,12] It has been shown to suppress speckling, thereby decreasing the "grainy appearance" of images. Additionally, it improves signal-to-noise ratio, which potentially helps in delineating certain structural lesions.

This technique was initially available for use on linear array transducers only (see Table 42-3), but nowadays it is available for use with curved array transducers as well, that is, abdominal and pelvic sonographic studies.

Another new gray-scale sonographic technique is called tissue harmonic sonography.[13] This technique is based on the nonlinear interaction of an acoustic signal as it propagates through tissue. It was originally developed for detecting nonlinear vibrations of micro-bubble contrast agents. As compared to conventional ultrasonography, the images obtained with tissue harmonic sonography are noted to have significantly reduced artifacts, hence improved image contrast and quality, thereby potentially increasing diagnostic accuracy.[14]

A detailed discussion of compound and tissue harmonic sonography is beyond the scope of this chapter.

Doppler ultrasonography

Whereas the use of gray-scale ultrasonography is limited to the evaluation of kidney structure and anatomy, Doppler ultrasonography has been used to assess the renal arteries, for example, renal artery stenosis. Peak renal artery velocities in the main renal and intrarenal arteries, intrarenal lobar arteries are obtained, and the resulting waveforms can be analyzed.[15]

The normal duplex waveform from an intrarenal artery has a sharp systolic upstroke, a gradual decrease in velocity of flow in later systole, and low-velocity forward flow throughout diastole. In the investigation of intrarenal arteries, the presence of a small amplitude waveform with a prolonged systolic rise (slow upstroke) is considered to be indicative of a proximal stenosis such as a renal artery stenosis, and this is referred to as "parvus-tardus effect."

In the presence of normal velocity and morphology of the waveform, it may be possible to exclude significant renal artery stenosis, that is, reduction in luminal diameter $\geq 80\%$ or more. This makes it an option in the evaluation of suspected renal artery stenosis in patients at high risk for contrast nephropathy, for example, underlying kidney disease. While some studies suggest a good correlation between renal Doppler scanning and conventional renal angiographic studies, particularly in the evaluation of renovascular disease, there are also some limitations that need to be taken into consideration, such as, being highly operator dependent, technical difficulties due to the subjects body habitus (obesity), as well as in the presence of multiple renal arteries and

TABLE 42–2	
Different Modes of Ultrasonography	
A-Mode (amplitude)	A short ultrasound pulse is emitted and propagated through tissue; the reflected echoes are displayed on a graph as vertical deflections along a time axis
B-Mode (brightness)	A short ultrasound pulse is emitted and propagated through tissue; the reflected echoes are displayed as shades of gray
M-Mode (motion)	Used to display moving structures; a gray-scale modulated image line is produced

even distal arterial stenosis, which can lead to false negative diagnoses.

Despite its limitations, this technique is particularly useful in the evaluation of transplant renal artery stenosis (see below).

MODES OF ULTRASONOGRAPHY

There are different modes of ultrasound as depicted in Table 42-2. For purposes of this discussion, we will focus on B-mode ultrasonography.

SAFETY

Renal ultrasonography is generally considered to be a safe imaging modality. According to the World Health Organization technical report series, "Diagnostic ultrasound is recognized as a safe, effective, and highly flexible imaging modality capable of providing clinically relevant information about most parts of the body in a rapid and cost-effective fashion."

EQUIPMENT

Figures 42-2 and 42-3.

▶ The Ultrasound Machine

A basic ultrasound machine has the following parts:

- Transducer probe—probe that sends and receives the sound waves.
- Computer—Central processing unit (CPU) that does all of the calculations and contains the electrical power supplies for itself and the transducer probe.
- Transducer pulse controls—changes the amplitude, frequency, and duration of the pulses emitted from the transducer probe.
- Display—displays the image from the ultrasound data processed by the CPU.

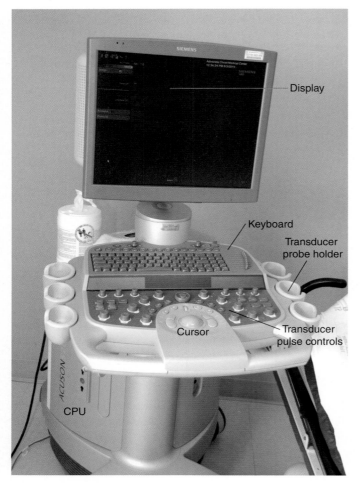

Figure 42-2. Typical ultrasound machine.

- Keyboard/cursor—inputs data and takes measurements from the display.
- Disk storage device (hard, floppy, and CD)—stores the acquired images.
- Printer—prints the image from the displayed data.

► Transducer

The transducer probe (see Figure 42-4) is the main part of the ultrasound machine. It is the device that makes the sound waves and receives the echoes. The probe also has a sound absorbing substance to eliminate back reflections from the probe itself and an acoustic lens to help focus the emitted sound waves. Transducer probes come in a variety of shapes and sizes. The shape of the probe determines its field of view, and the frequency of emitted sound waves determines how deep the sound waves penetrate and the resolution of the image. In interventional nephrology, frequencies ranging from 2 to 18 MHz are generally used, generated by one of two types of probes or transducers—the linear array transducer and the curved or curvilinear array transducer.

► Linear Array Transducer

This is an ultrasound transducer with crystals arranged in a line. It gives a rectangular field of view. Since the transducer's array element is narrow, it diverges after it has traveled only a few millimeters. These transducers come with a variety of face sizes, the smaller the face the more divergent the beam. The beam can be focused, and the depth of focus can be changed during scanning

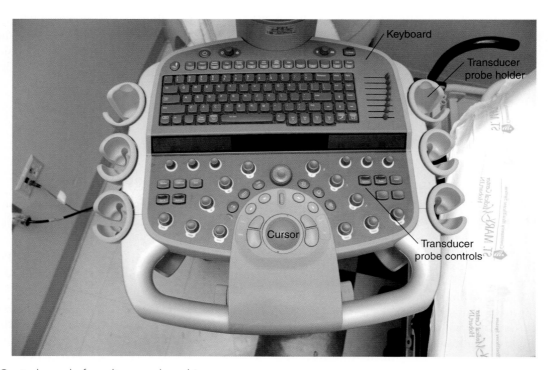

Figure 42-3. Control panel of an ultrasound machine.

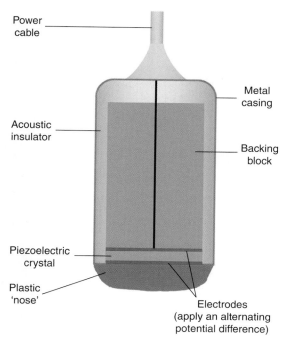

Power cable

Metal casing

Acoustic insulator

Backing block

Piezoelectric crystal

Plastic 'nose'

Electrodes (apply an alternating potential difference)

Figure 42-4. Schematic of ultrasound transducer.

to improve resolution. The linear transducer has greater skin contact than other types, making it more difficult to reach organs between ribs.

▶ Curved Array Transducer

A curved or curvilinear array transducer is similar to a linear array except that the image created has a sector-type format. A curvilinear array gives a large footprint and near field with a wide sector. Additionally, they have a wider field of view from the transducer face. Sector scanners are most especially useful for examinations where the beam is directed between the ribs for imaging (Table 42-3).

NORMAL ANATOMY

▶ The Kidneys

The kidneys (see Figure 42-5) are a pair of bean-shaped organs located underneath the diaphragm, in the retroperitoneal area, on each side of the vertebral column. Each kidney is located anterior to the psoas and quadratus lumborum muscles, medial to the transverse rectus abdominis muscles, and lateral to the quadratus lumborum muscles.

TABLE 42–3

Principal Transducer Designs[3]

		Advantages	Disadvantages
Sector transducer	US beam is moved through a fan-shaped sector	• Small footprint • Can scan through small acoustic window • Can scan between ribs • Clear definition of structures at greater depths	• Poor resolution of structures near the transducer
Linear transducer	Multiple parallel elements are arranged in a straight line, producing a rectangular image field	• Good resolution of structures near the transducer • Used for studies of vascular structures	• Large footprint • Cannot scan through a small acoustic window close to the transducer (not ideal for abdominal imaging)
Curved array	The crystals are lined up on a convex surface, producing a fan-shaped image which is wider in the near field	• Compromise between a sector and a linear transducer • Used for abdominal scanning	• Line density decreases with depth

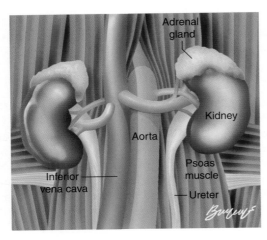

Figure 42-5. The kidneys and bordering structures. (Illustration by Bashar Ericsoossi, MD.)

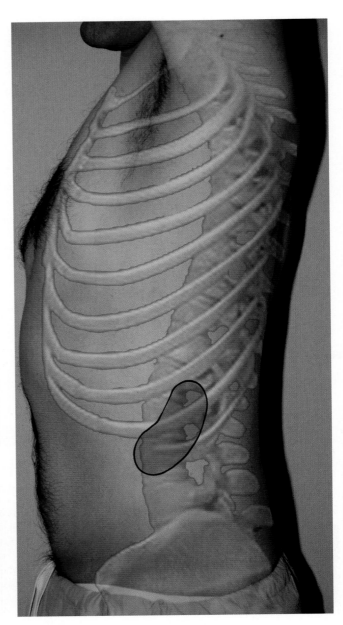

Figure 42-7. Lateral view of the left kidney and its relation to the left subcostal margin and the lumbar vertebrae.

Grossly, each kidney measures approximately 9–12 cm in length, 4–5 cm in width, and 2–3 cm in height. Each kidney is enveloped by a smooth, transparent, and fibrous membrane, the renal capsule. It is this transparent capsule that gives the kidney a "glistening" appearance. The left kidney is slightly higher than the right, which is displaced inferiorly by the liver.

The superior pole of both kidneys is tilted slightly medially and posteriorly (oblique lie) (see Figures 42-6 and 42-7).

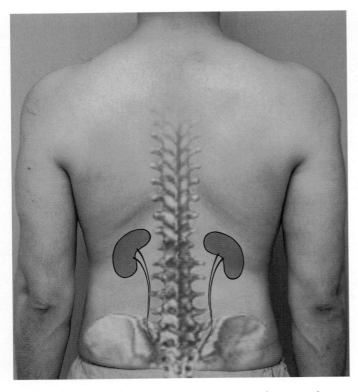

Figure 42-6. Posterior view of the kidneys in relation to the thoracolumbar vertebrae.

Each kidney has a convex lateral border and a concave medial border, the renal hilum, from which the ureter leaves the kidney and the other structures, for example, blood vessels, lymphatic vessels, and nerves enter/leave the kidney.

Lying on the superomedial aspect of the kidneys (see Figure 42-5) are the adrenal glands. The right adrenal gland is somewhat triangular, while the left adrenal gland is a bit more rounded, and crescentic. Both the kidneys and adrenal glands are enclosed in the Gerota's fascia.

The superior pole of each kidney lies opposite the 12th thoracic vertebra and above the costal margin, while the inferior pole of each kidney extends opposite the 3rd lumbar vertebra, (see Figures 42-6 and 42-7) just corpuscles), the cortex, and a darker reddish-brown inner region (consisting of the loops of Henle and collecting ducts), the medulla. The medulla is divided into approximately 8–18 striated renal pyramids, each of which is triangular or conical in configuration. The apex of each renal pyramid lead to a renal papilla, which merges with each other, forming the renal pelvis (also called "renal sinus"), which further leads to the ureter. The renal pelvis is divided into the major calyces and minor calyces.

▶ The Urinary Bladder and Ureters

The ureters (see Figure 42-5) are muscular tubular structures (measuring about 30 cm in length) each of which leave the kidneys through the renal hilum and drain toward the urinary bladder. The ureters enter the bladder base posterolaterally and (with the urethra) form the trigone of the bladder.

The urinary bladder is a hollow, muscular receptacle or reservoir that is collapsible. Inside the bladder is a lining consisting of heavily folded, thick muscular walls, particularly in the nondistended state. When filled with urine, these walls can be stretched. A completely full bladder measures approximately 12.7 cm and can accommodate over 1000 mL of urine.

In males, the urinary bladder is superior to the prostate gland and is situated behind the lower abdominal wall and the symphysis pubis. It is posteriorly bounded by the rectum.

In females, the urinary bladder is posteriorly bounded by the uterus, which causes an invagination.

▶ The Prostate

Just inferior to the urinary bladder and posterior to the symphysis pubis is the fibromuscular and glandular prostate, through which course the posterior urethra. Traditionally, it is grossly divided (Lowsley) into five lobes namely: anterior, posterior, median, right lateral, and left lateral.

PREPARATION OF THE PATIENT

Preparation of the patient (fasting) is usually unnecessary. Ideally, the examination should be performed in a warm, dark room with the patient initially assuming the supine position. Having the patient assume the prone position is only done when performing a percutaneous renal biopsy, because of suboptimal visualization of the kidney through the psoas muscles.

Neither sedation nor anesthesia is required during diagnostic ultrasonography. In fact, the patient may need to be fully conscious during the procedure particularly when he/she is asked to assume various positions or take deep breaths to help with optimizing visualization of the kidneys (see below).

For ultrasound examination of the bladder, patients are advised to drink 8–16 ounces of water, at least 60 minutes before the study. This allows the distention of the urinary

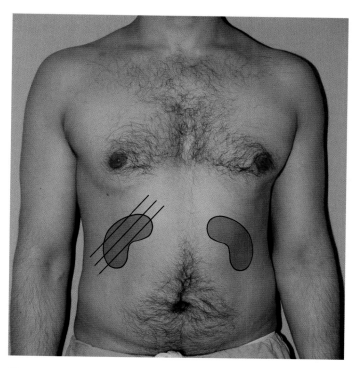

Figure 42-8. Anterior view of the kidneys with their 'oblique' lie.

below the costal margin. As previously noted, each kidney has an oblique lie, such that the long axis of each kidney lies at an approximately 20° angle, in relation to the sagittal plane (see Figure 42-8).

On cross-section (see Figure 42-9), each kidney has a pale homogenous outer region (consisting of the glomeruli and proximal and distal convoluted tubules and renal

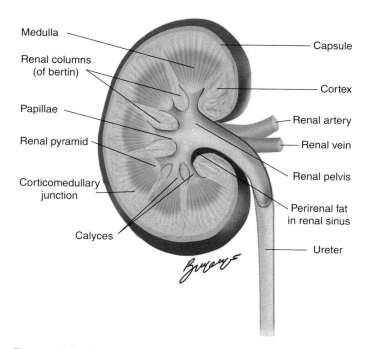

Figure 42-9. Cross sectional anatomy of the kidney. (Illustration by Bashar Ericsoossi, MD.)

bladder, thereby facilitating identification of anatomical abnormalities within the bladder lumen. Patients are allowed to urinate after the study.

TECHNIQUE

With the use of a 3.5–5-MHz transducer, a longitudinal and transverse view of each kidney is obtained. A complete examination consists of the following:

1. A longitudinal view demonstrating both superior and inferior poles of each kidney. Occasionally, the liver and/or spleen can also be visualized and used as acoustic windows for comparison. This is obtained by rotating the transducer obliquely along the lie of the kidney.

   In the longitudinal view, the kidney appears as "football-shaped" (see Figure 42-10).

2. A transverse view showing the renal hilum, (see Figures 42-11A, 42-11B, and 42-11C). This is obtained by rotating the transducer 90° from the longitudinal

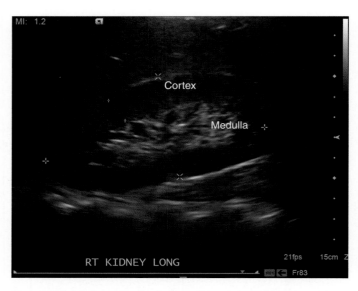

Figure 42-10. Longitudinal view of the right kidney showing 'corticomedullary differentiation'. The central echogenic part of the kidney (sinus) is composed of the pelvis, the calyces, blood and lymphoid vessels, and interposed adipose tissue.

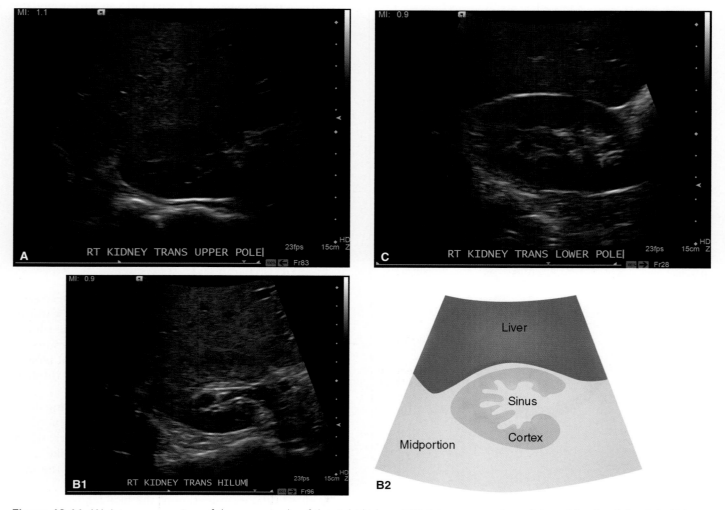

Figure 42-11 (**A**) A transverse view of the upper pole of the right kidney. (**B1**) A transverse view of the mid-pole of the right kidney. (**B2**) A schematic diagram showing a transverse view of the right kidney, using the liver as an 'acoustic window.' (Illustration by Bashar Ericsoossi, MD.) (**C**) A transverse view of the lower pole of the right kidney.

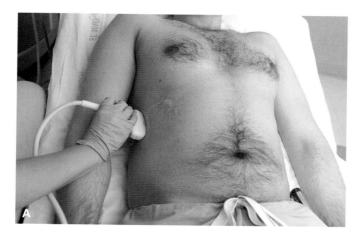

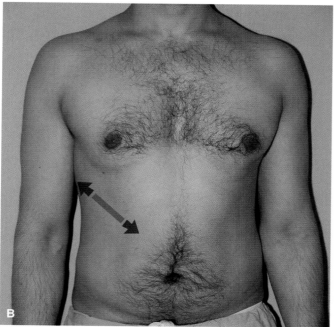

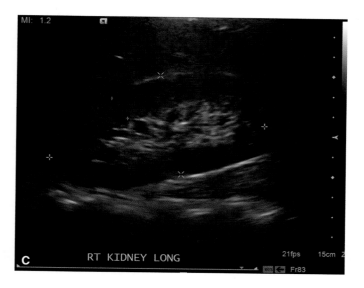

Figure 42-12. (**A**) Initially, the transducer is placed over the inferior and lateral edge of the right costal margin, in the mid-axillary line. (**B**) In the longitudinal plane, the transducer is moved medially and inferiorly until the right kidney is visualized. (**C**) Longitudinal view of the right kidney.

view. The transducer is then moved superiorly and medially to visualize the superior pole of the kidney and inferiorly and laterally to view the inferior pole of the kidney. Renal contour irregularities, for example, masses or tumors can oftentimes be identified in this view.

In the transverse view, the kidney appears as "C-shaped" (see Figures 42-11A, 42-11B, and 42-11C).

▶ Right Kidney

The right kidney is best viewed with the patient lying supine. The main barriers to visualizing the right kidney are the 11th and 12th ribs as well as occasional bowel gas. Anterior to the right kidney is the right lobe of the liver.

Initially, the transducer is placed over the inferior and lateral edge of the right costal margin, in the mid-axillary line (see Figure 42-12A). In the longitudinal

plane, the transducer is moved medially and inferiorly (see Figure 42-12B) until the right kidney is visualized (see Figure 42-12C). Once identified, the transducer should be rotated obliquely according to the lie of the kidney, thereby enabling visualization of the entire length of the kidney.

At times, it may be helpful to have the patient take deep breaths, as the kidneys tend to move superiorly and inferiorly (approximately 4–5 cm) with inspiration and expiration, respectively. Although not specific, the absence of such normal mobility may be suggestive of abnormal fixation to surrounding structures, for example, inflammatory states, pyelonephritis, and so on.

In thin individuals, it may be possible to view the right kidney from an anterior approach.

The right kidney is usually easier to visualize than the left because the adjacent liver acts as an excellent acoustic window (see Figures 42-13A1 and 42-13A2).

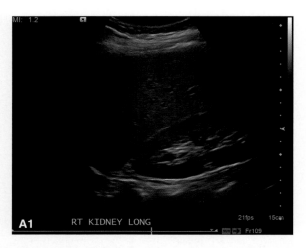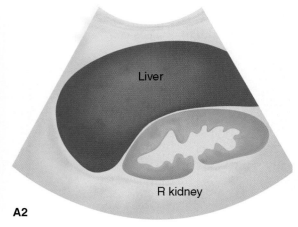

Figure 42-13. (**A1**) The right kidney is usually easier to visualize than the left because the adjacent liver acts as an excellent acoustic window. (**A2**) A schematic diagram showing a longitudinal view of the right kidney, using the liver as an 'acoustic window.' (Illustration by Bashar Ericsoossi, MD.)

▶ Left Kidney

The left kidney is best viewed with the patient lying in the right lateral decubitus position. At times, it may be ideal to put a rolled blanket or towel under the patients left side (so-called scoliosis position) or have the patient raise the left upper extremity (to widen the intercostal spaces) to help with the imaging. The main barriers to visualizing the kidney are the 11th and 12th ribs as well as occasional bowel gas. The spleen lies antero-lateral to the left kidney.

Initially, the transducer is placed mid-axillary line, just above the left superior iliac crest. In the longitudinal plane, the transducer is moved inferiorly and superiorly until the left kidney is visualized (see Figures 42-14A, 42-14B, and 42-14C).

Once identified, the transducer should be rotated obliquely according to the lie of the kidney, thereby enabling visualization of the entire length of the kidney.

As compared to the right kidney, sometimes it is more difficult to visualize the left kidney because it is closer to the transducer, and there is no adjacent organ that can act as an acoustic window. Occasionally, an enlarged spleen may function as such (see Figure 42-15A1 and 42-15A2).

Organ details

Size, shape, and volume In the longitudinal plane, the normal kidney has a "football-shaped" configuration and measures 10–12 cm in length, which varies with the patient's height.[16,17]

Estimation of renal size by ultrasonography can be performed by measuring renal length and cortical thickness, and determining the renal volume. A good correlation has been demonstrated between both glomerular filtration rate (GFR) and estimated renal plasma flow (ERPF) and total renal parenchymal volume as well as renal parenchymal area.[18]

However, there is so much intraobserver and interobserver variation in these measurements, in particular renal volume (calculated with a water delay ultrasonographic device) which can be especially cumbersome.

Therefore, renal length measurement is preferred to renal volume estimation, especially when comparing repeated measurements.[16]

Echogenicity The normal renal cortex appears hypoechoic as compared to the highly echogenic fat-containing renal sinus. The echogenicity of the cortex is compared to the liver or spleen[17] either of which is used as acoustic windows (see Figures 42-13A1 and 42-13A2, Figures 42-14D1 and 42-14D2). Although nonspecific, increased cortical echogenicity is suggestive of parenchymal renal disease. The histopathological correlate of increased echogenicity is "tubular atrophy".[19]

Decreased echogenicity is seen in acute pyelonephritis and acute renal vein thrombosis.

Renal parenchyma and renal sinus In the longitudinal view, the renal sinus appears as a homogenous ovoid structure, which is centrally located and appears to be hyperechoic as compared to the adjacent cortex (as noted above).

In some disease states, for example, pyelonephritis, there is "loss of corticomedullary differentiation," brought about by the kidney becoming more hyperechoic secondary to parenchymal edema.

The medullary pyramids (see Figure 42-14C2) (composed of the urine-filled collecting tubules and loops of Henle) are hypoechoic (not anechoic) triangular or conical structures seen between the cortex and renal medulla.

They appear to be more prominent and more distinguishable in infants and younger children, as well as in well-hydrated subjects.

The cortical thickness of the kidney is the distance between the renal capsule and the external margin of the medullary pyramid. Such measurement (minimum of 1 cm) varies in between individuals and within individual kidneys. With advancing age, advanced stages of chronic kidney disease, and in those with atrophic kidneys, such distance tends to decrease, hence, referred to as "cortical thinning." Some studies have showed no correlation between cortical thickness and body mass

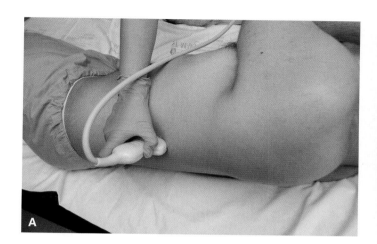
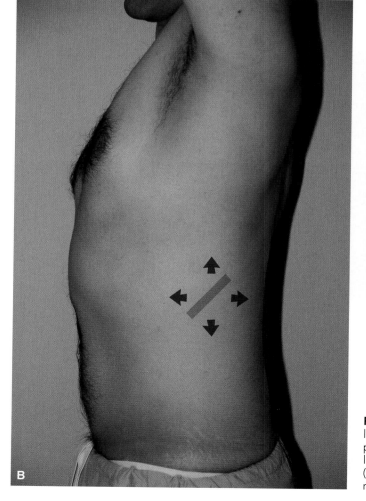
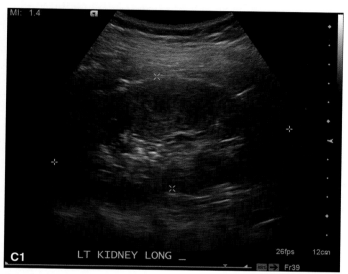
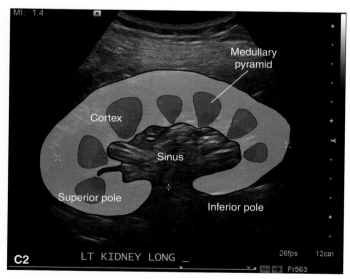

Figure 42-14. (**A**) Initially, the transducer is placed mid-axillary line, just above the left superior iliac crest. (**B**) In the longitudinal plane, the transducer is moved inferiorly and superiorly until the left kidney is visualized (**C1**) Longitudinal view of the left kidney. (**C2**) A longitudinal view of the left kidney showing schematic representation of the medullary pyramids.

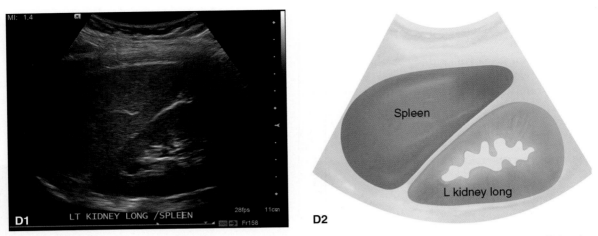

Figure 42-14. (*continued*) (**D1**) A longitudinal view of the left kidney, using the liver as an 'acoustic window.' (**D2**) A schematic diagram showing a longitudinal view of the left kidney, using the spleen as an 'acoustic window.' (Illustration by Bashar Ericsoossi, MD.)

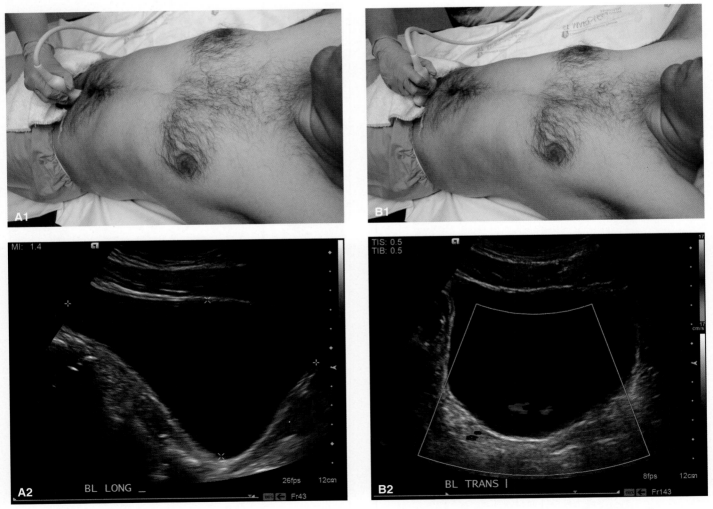

Figure 42-15. (**A1**) In the longitudinal view, the transducer is placed in the mid-hypogastric area, just above the symphysis pubis. (**A2**) Longitudinal view of the urinary bladder. (**B1**) In the transverse view, he transducer is angled slightly caudally, until the echo-free lumen of the urinary bladder is identified. (**B2**) Transverse view of the urinary bladder (Note the presence of bilateral ureteral jets).

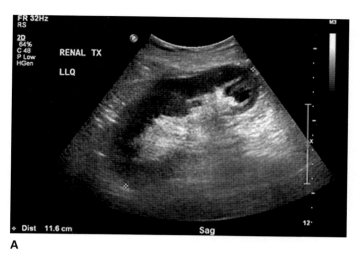

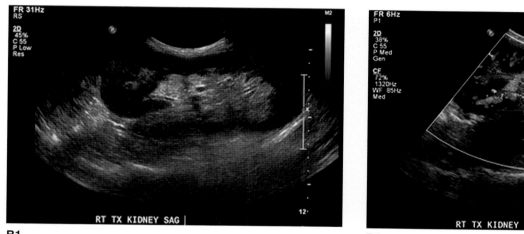

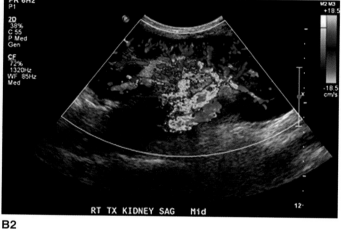

Figure 42-16. (**A**) Longitudinal view of transplanted kidney. (**B1**) Transverse view of transplanted kidney. (**B2**) Transverse view of transplanted kidney with color flow imaging showing 'increased vascularity' of the kidney.

index or weight.[20] Interestingly, some suggest that when compared to renal length, renal cortical thickness in pre-dialysis patients may actually correlate better with estimated GFR.[21]

▶ Ureters

The ureters are not visualized in a normal ultrasound examination. However, in cases of obstructive uropathy, for example, hydronephrosis, it may be possible to see the proximal portion of the ureter.

▶ Urinary Bladder and Prostate

With a full bladder, in the longitudinal view, (see Figures 42-15A1 and 42-15A2) the transducer is placed in the mid-hypogastric area, just above the symphysis pubis. It is then angled slightly caudally, (see Figures 42-16B1 and 42-16B2) until the echo-free lumen of the urinary bladder is identified. Posterior to the urinary bladder is the hypoechoic prostate gland.

▶ Transplanted Kidney

Most transplanted kidneys are positioned in the anterior right or left iliac fossa in front of the psoas and iliacus muscles. Such superficial positioning allows for excellent evaluation by ultrasonography. The renal sinus appears hyperechoic, while the renal cortex appears hypoechoic. The medullary pyramids may be prominent, and occasionally, even the arcuate vessels may be demonstrable. It is not uncommon to observe a small amount of fluid collection[22] surrounding a renal allograft, particularly in the immediate postoperative period, and this usually undergoes spontaneous resolution/resorption. Fluid collections seen in the immediate postoperative period include hematomas, seromas, or urinomas. In the later periods, abscesses and lymphoceles[23] may be observed.

From the longitudinal view, the transducer can be rotated at an angle of 90° to get the transverse view. In the immediate posttransplant period, it is not unusual to observe a small amount of perirenal fluid, which commonly resolves spontaneously (see Figure 42-16).

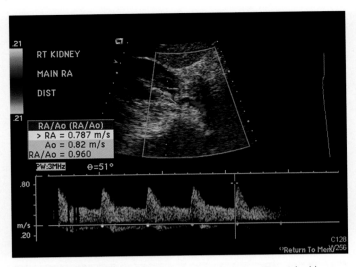

Figure 42-17. Duplex US of main renal artery. (Provided by Dr. Sangarappillai Asokan, Department of Radiology, Advocate Christ Medical Center, Oak Lawn, IL.)

Doppler ultrasonography

The value of Doppler ultrasonography is that it is noninvasive, yet it permits early diagnosis of transplant renal artery stenosis (TRAS). It is however limited, such that, optimal Doppler sampling of the transplant renal artery is oftentimes difficult and time consuming. Similarly, it is highly operator dependent and requires great skill and experience. Discussion of this modality is beyond the scope of this chapter.

Resistive index Also referred to as "Pourcelot's index," the resistive index (RI),[24] is derived as the ratio of peak systolic and end-diastolic velocity, obtained from Doppler spectrum of the renal vessels (see Figure 42-17). It is used as a measurement of the resistance to arterial inflow within the renal vascular bed. This is commonly used in the evaluation of renal allografts (Table 42-4).

Caution must be exercised in the interpretation of the RI values, as they have to be taken in the context of time of onset of renal dysfunction, clinical presentation, as well as laboratory values. With the sensitivities ranging between 58% and 100% and specificities between 87% and 100%, such indices are touted as not very useful by some experts.[25]

Recently, a comprehensive meta-analysis attempted to compare the capabilities of various duplex sonography parameters to detect renal artery stenosis in known hypertensive patients with angiography proven diseases. Looking at the peak systolic velocity, acceleration time, acceleration index, and renal–aortic ratio, the study showed that these parameters had only moderate accuracy in detecting renal artery stenosis, with peak systolic velocity being the most accurate and acceleration index the least accurate. Even when combined with peak systolic velocity, the above sonographic indices there was no improvement in its predictive power.[26]

Unfortunately, this procedure is greatly limited by its dependence on operator skills. In some institutions, the acceleration time, acceleration index, and resistance index are measured without actually interrogating the renal artery and may be less cumbersome than trying to measure the peak systolic velocity (see Figure 42-17).

ANATOMICAL VARIANTS

▶ Horseshoe Kidney

See Figures 42-18A1, 42-18A2, 42-18B1, and 42-18B2.

▶ Hypertrophied Column of Bertin

See Figures 42-19A1, 42-19A2, 42-19B1, and 42-19B2.

▶ Dromedary Hump

See Figure 42-20A1 and 42-20A2.

▶ Fetal Lobulation

See Figure 42-21.

TABLE 42–4		
Resistive Indices		
Resistive index (RI)		
<0.7	Normal	Can be seen during tachyarrythmias, due to earlier timing of systolic peak
0.7–0.8	Indeterminate	A value <0.7–0.8 in renal allografts is considered abnormal.[10,13]
>0.8	Abnormal	• Acute tubular necrosis • Pyelonephritis • Acute transplant rejection • Renal vein thrombosis • Ureteral obstruction • Toxic nephropathies or drug toxicities (immunosuppressive agents) • Graft compression (commonly seen in renal allografts)

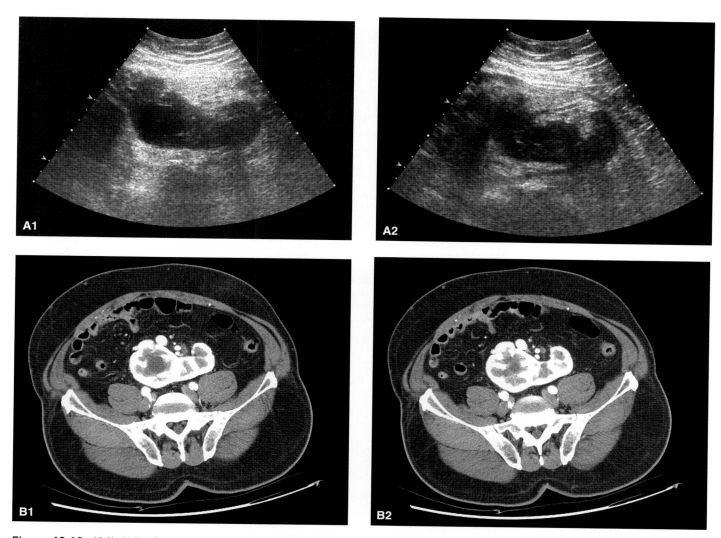

Figure 42-18. (**A1**)–(**A2**) Ultrasound showing fusion of both mid-poles of the kidneys with a parenchymal or connective tissue bridge (isthmus). (**B1**)–(**B2**) CT Scan showing fusion of both mid-poles of the kidneys with a parenchymal or connective tissue bridge (isthmus). (Provided by Dr. Sangarappillai Asokan, Department of Radiology, Advocate Christ Medical Center, Oak Lawn, IL.)

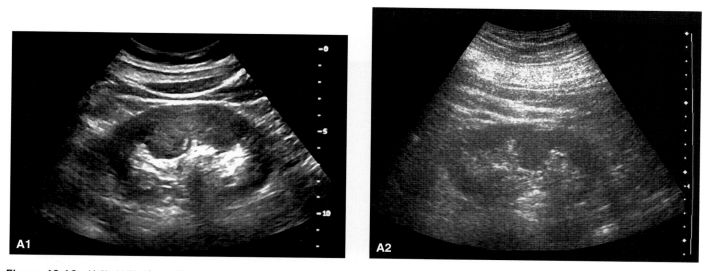

Figure 42-19. (**A1**)–(**A2**) Also called as a 'renal pseudotumor,' a hypertrophied column of Bertin is a normal extension of the cortical tissue that separates the pyramids. Its main importance is that it can often be mistaken for a renal mass. (Provided by Dr. William Simpson, Department of Radiology, Mount Sinai School of Medicine, New York, NY.)

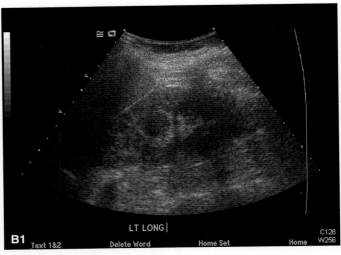

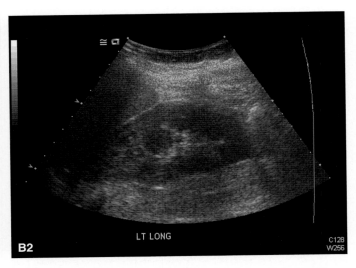

Figure 42-19. (*continued*) (**B1**)–(**B2**) Also called as a 'renal pseudotumor,' a hypertrophied column of Bertin is a normal extension of the cortical tissue that separates the pyramids. Its main importance is that it can often be mistaken for a renal mass. (Provided by Dr. Sangarappillai Asokan, Department of Radiology, Advocate Christ Medical Center, Oak Lawn, IL.)

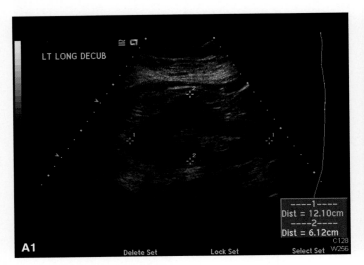

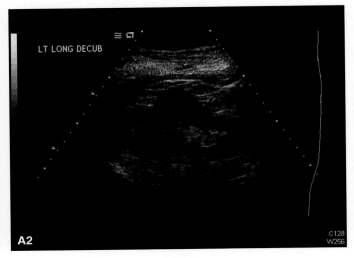

Figure 42-20. (**A1**)–(**A2**) A longitudinal view showing a dromedary hump that is a prominent focal bulge on the lateral border of the left kidney; a normal variant of renal contour, it is usually caused by the splenic impression on the superolateral aspect of the left kidney. (Provided by Dr. Sangarappillai Asokan, Department of Radiology, Advocate Christ Medical Center, Oak Lawn, IL.)

Figure 42-21. A persistent fetal lobulation is a normal variant often seen in adult kidneys, when there is incomplete fusion of the developing renal lobules. (Provided by Dr. Anil Agarwal, Department of Nephrology, Ohio State University Medical Center, OH.)

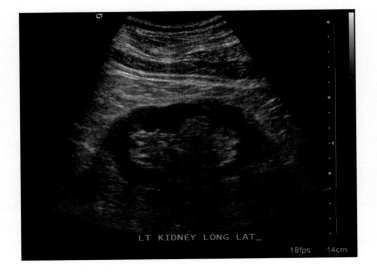

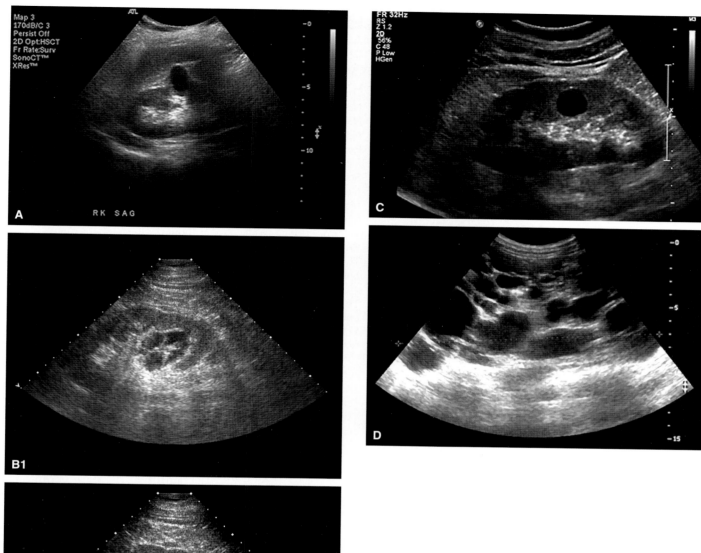

Figure 42-22. (**A**) Simple (exophytic) cyst. (Provided by Dr. William Simpson, Department of Radiology, Mount Sinai School of Medicine, New York, NY.) (**B1**)–(**B2**) Parapelvic cysts. It is important to distinguish parapelvic cysts from hydronephrosis. (Provided by Dr. Sangarappillai Asokan, Department of Radiology, Advocate Christ Medical Center, Oak Lawn, IL.) (**C**) Cortical cyst. (Provided by Dr. William Simpson, Department of Radiology, Mount Sinai School of Medicine, New York, NY.) (**D**) Polycystic kidney. (Provided by Dr. Sangarappillai Asokan, Department of Radiology, Advocate Christ Medical Center, Oak Lawn, IL.)

CYSTS

Simple renal cysts (see Figure 42-22A) are usually benign and asymptomatic, unless they are large enough to cause distortion of normal anatomy, thereby causing mechanical compression of adjacent structures causing obstructive symptoms or when they bleed, causing pain. They may appear either as solitary or multiple, unilateral or bilateral. Peripelvic cysts (see Figures 42-22B1 and 42-22B2.) are located in the region of the renal pelvis, whereas parapelvic cysts are located in the region of the renal hilum. Those on the cortex are referred to as cortical cysts (see Figure 42-22C).

Simple cysts are characterized by several things, namely: anechoic appearance, round or oval shape, has a thin-well-defined (hyperechoic) capsule and smooth margins, and has posterior acoustic enhancement. At times, the presence of blood or infectious debris within the cyst's cavity can lead to the appearance of low-level echoes within the cyst. Such cysts are referred to as complex cysts and may require additional imaging studies to

TABLE 42–5

Bosniak Classification and Evaluation of Simple and Complex Renal Cysts

Classification		Ultrasound Findings	CT Scan Findings
Type I	Simple cyst	• Anechoic • Thin-walled	• Thin-walled • No septations • No calcifications • No contrast enhancement
Type II	Minimally complicated	• Mural calcification • Thin septations	• Few hairline thin septations • Fine calcification in the wall • Sharp margin • No contrast enhancement
Type IIF	Complicated	• Coarse calcification • Thick septations • Mural nodules	• More hairline thin septations • Minimal thickening of septation or wall • Thick or nodular calcification without contrast enhancement • Well-marginated
Type III	Indeterminate	• Calcification • Septations • Mural nodules	• Thickened irregular walls or septations in which contrast enhancement can be seen
Type IV	Malignancy	• Mural nodules • Neovascularization	• Thickened irregular walls or septations in which contrast enhancement can be seen • Enhancing soft-tissue components

Source: Data from Bosniak MA. Difficulties in classifying cystic lesions of the kidney. *Urol Radiol.* 1991:91–93 and Bosniak MA. Problems in the radiologic diagnosis of renal parenchymal tumors. In: S. I. Olsson CA, eds. *Urologic Clinics of North America.* Philadelphia, PA: WB Saunders; 1993:217–230.[27,28]

rule out other more alarming causes, for example, tumors. Multiloculated cysts are noted for the appearance of distinct septations.

The presence of calcifications may also be indicative of a malignant process (Table 42-5).

The number of cysts tends to increase with age. Although their etiology remains unclear, it is not uncommon to observe them in those with decreased renal function. In patients who have been on renal replacement therapy, or dialysis, the appearance of multiple cysts may suggest an "acquired cystic disease of the kidneys," which can potentially undergo malignant transformation. There is a direct correlation between the number of cysts and the length of time on dialysis.

MASSES

▶ Benign

Angiomyolipoma

Commonly found incidentally on routine ultrasonographic studies, angiomyolipomas appear as solitary and tend to be asymptomatic. They are usually well-defined and hyperechoic (in contrast to cysts), containing vascular strictures, as well as muscle and fatty tissues. Similarly, when compared to carcinomas, angiomyolipomas tend to be smaller, and more echogenic and associated with shadowing.[29] Oftentimes, a CT scan is recommended to differentiate angiomyolipomas from carcinomas, by virtue of their fat content. It must be noted however, that approximately <5% of angiomyolipomas may have no fat content (see Figure 42-23).[30]

▶ Malignant

Renal cell carcinoma (hypernephroma)

Often referred to as "the internist's tumor," renal cell carcinomas (adenocarcinomas) (see Figures 42-24A1 and 42-24A2, AND 42-24B1 and 42-24B2) are commonly incidentally discovered on ultrasonographic studies for other reasons. A renal cell carcinoma usually appears as a heterogeneous mass that can enlarge and mechanically

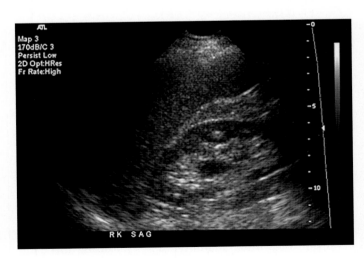

Figure 42-23. Angiomyolipoma. There is a small echogenic structure in the mid kidney completely surrounded by cortex and separate from the sinus fat. The diagnosis of angiomyolipoma was confirmed with CT showing fat in the lesion. (Provided by Dr. William Simpson, Department of Radiology, Mount Sinai School of Medicine, New York, NY.)

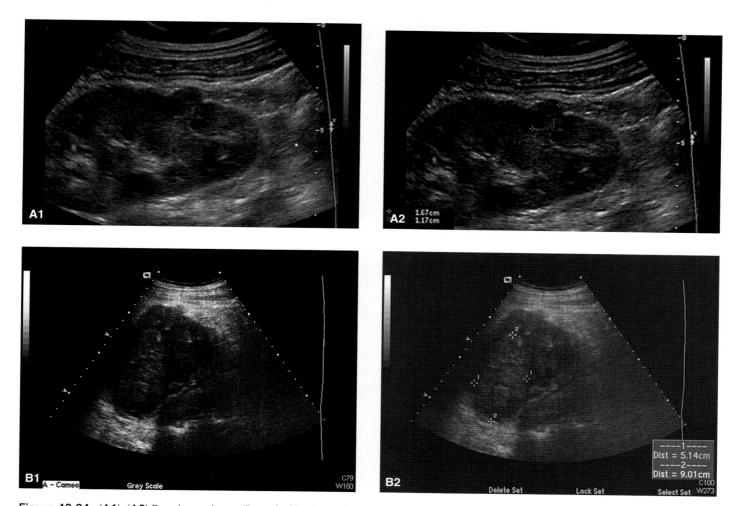

Figure 42-24. (**A1**)–(**A2**) Renal neoplasm. (Provided by Dr. William Simpson, Department of Radiology, Mount Sinai School of Medicine, New York, NY.) (**B1**)–(**B2**) Renal neoplasm. (Provided by Dr. Sangarappillai Asokan, Department of Radiology, Advocate Christ Medical Center, Oak Lawn, IL.)

distort normal renal anatomy. The mass may contain areas of cystic degeneration and/or calcifications. One has to be wary of its particular tendency to involve the renal vein and inferior vena cava.

Such masses also tend to be highly vascularized (neo-vascularization), which may be well-appreciated on Color Doppler studies. The walls are usually ill-defined. With larger masses, a search for adjacent and distant lymphadenopathies, for example, adrenals and liver, is warranted.

OBSTRUCTIVE UROPATHY

The most common causes of obstructive uropathy are listed in Table 42-6.

Along the course of the ureter, there are three distinct narrowings, where obstruction can potentially occur namely: the ureteropelvic junction, the point at which the iliac vessels cross the ureter (where the ureter crosses the pelvic brim), and at the ureterovesical junction.

According to Webster's Online Dictionary, "hydronephrosis" refers to the distention and dilation of the renal pelvis, usually caused by obstruction of the free flow of urine from the kidney.[32]

On ultrasonographic imaging, fluid-containing areas within the renal sinus (conforming to the renal collecting system) are demonstrated. The main important finding is the thinning of the renal parenchyma secondary to pyelocalyceal dilatation (see Table 42-7A[33] and 42-7B[33] and Figure 42-25[34]).

As previously noted, at times, even in the presence of early obstructive uropathy in the volume depleted state, hydronephrosis may not be readily appreciated giving a false negative impression. This gives credence to performance of serial ultrasonographic studies after adequate fluid hydration, particularly in those with where obstruction is highly suspected. Other causes of false negative and false positive ultrasound readings in obstructive uropathy are listed in Table 42-8.[35,36]

It is important to emphasize that the presence of hydronephrosis does not always indicate the presence of

TABLE 42–6

Causes of Obstructive Uropathy

	Intrinsic	Extrinsic	Functional
Ureter	• Ureteropelvic junction stricture • Ureterovesical junction obstruction • Papillary necrosis • Ureteral folds • Ureteral valves • Ureterovesical reflux • Ureteral stricture (iatrogenic) • Blood clot • Benign fibroepithelial polyps • Ureteral tumor • Fungus ball • Ureteral calculus • Ureterocele • Endometriosis • Tuberculosis • Retrocaval ureter	• Retroperitoneal lymphoma • Retroperitoneal sarcoma • Cervical cancer • Prostate cancer • Retroperitoneal fibrosis • Aortic aneurysm • Inflammatory bowel disease • Ovarian vein syndrome • Retrocaval ureter • Uterine prolapse • Pregnancy • Ureteral ligation (iatrogenic) • Ovarian cysts • Diverticulitis • Tubo-ovarian abscess • Retroperitoneal hematoma • Lymphocele • Pelvic lipomatosis • Radiation fibrosis • Urinoma	Gram-negative septicemia Neurogenic bladder
Bladder	• Bladder cancer • Bladder calculii • Bladder neck contracture • Cystocele • Primary bladder neck hypertrophy • Bladder diverticula	• Pelvic lipomatosis	• Neurogenic bladder • Vesicoureteric reflux
Urethra	• Urethral stricture • Urethral valves • Urethral diverticula • Urethral atresia • Labial fusion • Hypospadias and epispadias	• Benign prostatic hypertrophy • Prostate cancer • Urethral and Penile cancer • Phimosis	

Source: Reprinted with permission from Medscape.com, 2012. Available at: http://emedicine.medscape.com/article/436259-overview.[31]

obstruction, for example, reflux nephropathy, during pregnancy, postobstructive dilatation, papillary necrosis, and congenital megacalyces.

At times, the dilated proximal ureter may also be visualized in the presence of obstructive uropathy (see Figures 42-26C, 42-26D1, and 42-26D2).

Calculi

Renal calculi or stones are the most common cause of obstructive uropathy. They are characteristically well-circumscribed hyperechoic structures with distal acoustic shadowing. When located in the similarly hyperechoic renal sinus, smaller stones may be difficult to differentiate and clearly identify. The presence of acoustic shadowing with stones is the main differentiation. One of the advantages of ultrasonography over conventional X-rays is that even noncalcified stones (uric acid and cystine) can be identified because of the acoustic shadowing.

Obviously, demonstration of larger stones tends to be a bit more straightforward (see Figures 42-27A, 42-27B1 and 42-27B2).

Nephrocalcinosis

Nephrocalcinosis usually has bilateral renal involvement and is manifested by hyperechoic appearance of the medullary pyramids (see Figure 42-28).

TABLE 42–7a

Grading Classification of Hydronephrosis

	Renal Pelvis	Calyces	Parenchymal Thickness
Grade I	Dilated	Normal	Normal
Grade II	Dilated	Dilated	Thinned
Grade III	Cystic dilatation noted	Enlarged	Significantly thinned
Grade IV			Parenchyma is no longer demonstrated

Source: Data from Block B. Kidneys.[33]

TABLE 42–7b

Grading Classification of Hydronephrosis

		Calyceal Dilatation	Other Features
Grade I	Mild	Slight	
Grade II	Moderate	Extensive	• Thinned renal pelvis
			• Splaying of calyces (bear claw)
Grade III	Severe	Massive	• Loss of renal parenchyma
			• Resistive index < 0.7

Source: Data from Block B. Kidneys.[33]

TABLE 42–8

Limitations of Ultasonography in Obstructive Uropathy[35,36]

False Negatives	False Positives
Acute urinary tract obstruction	Novice sonographer
Volume depleted state	Multiple cysts involving the kidneys
Retroperitoneal fibrosis from any cause, leading to restrictive encasement of one or more ureters	
Staghorn calculi	

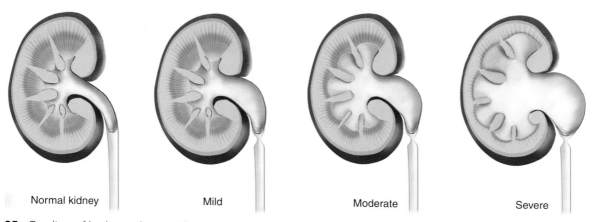

Normal kidney   Mild   Moderate   Severe

Figure 42-25. Grading of hydronephrosis. (Illustration by Bashar Ericsoossi, MD.)[34]

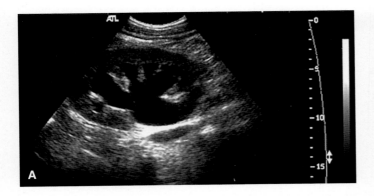

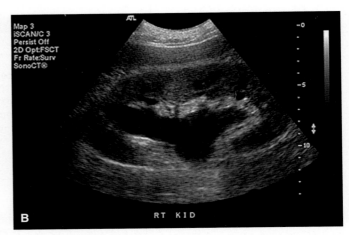

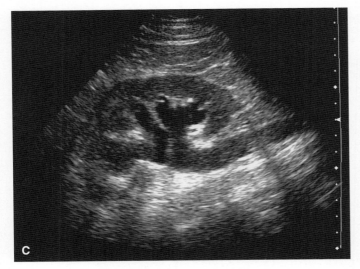

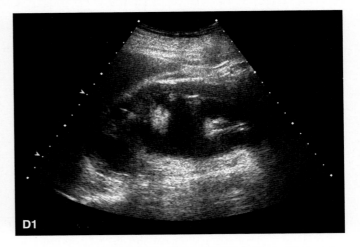

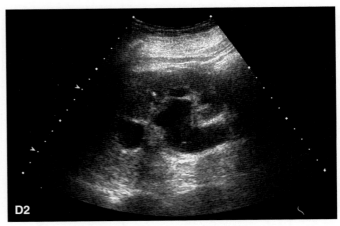

Figure 42-26. (**A**) Hydronephrosis (Provided by Dr. William Simpson, Department of Radiology, Mount Sinai School of Medicine, New York, NY.) (**B**) mild hydronephrosis (**C**) moderate hydronephrosis with dilated proximal ureter (**D1**)–(**D2**) severe hydronephrosis. (Provided by Dr. Sangarappillai Asokan, Department of Radiology, Advocate Christ Medical Center, Oak Lawn, IL.)

INFECTIONS

In acute pyelonephritis, the involved kidney may be enlarged and hypoechoic. Whereas the findings tend to be subtle and nonspecific, the contrast between the involved kidney and the acoustic windows (liver or spleen) tend to be a bit exaggerated due to overlying edema.

In chronic pyelonephritis, due to the recurrent nature of the inflammation, the kidney tends to be smaller in size (shrunken appearance), with a significantly thinned and hyperechoic cortex.

ACUTE KIDNEY INJURY

In acute kidney injury, the kidneys appear normal ultrasonographically, for example, size, shape, echogenicity, to name a few.

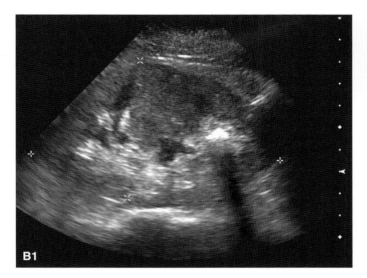

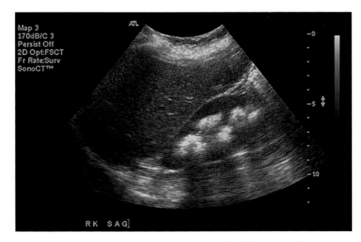

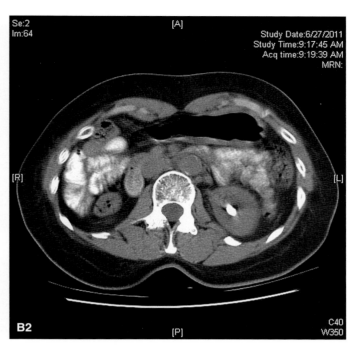

Figure 42-27. (**A**) 'Left kidney with calculus showing 'acoustic shadowing.' (Provided by Dr. William Simpson, Department of Radiology, Mount Sinai School of Medicine, New York, NY.) (**B1**) Ultrasound showing calculus with 'acoustic shadowing.' (Provided by Dr. Sangarappillai Asokan, Department of Radiology, Advocate Christ Medical Center, Oak Lawn, IL.) (**B2**) CT scan of the same patient showing renal calculus. (Provided by Dr. Sangarappillai Asokan, Department of Radiology, Advocate Christ Medical Center, Oak Lawn, IL.)

Figure 42-28. Nephrocalcinosis. (Provided by Dr. William Simpson, Department of Radiology, Mount Sinai School of Medicine, New York, NY).

ABNORMALITIES IN THE RENAL ALLOGRAFT

Approximately 50% of renal transplants may be associated with some form of fluid collection or peri-renal fluid.[37] The ultrasound is very useful in following up these fluid collections, especially when deciding whether or not, some form of percutaneous intervention may be indicated. From the imaging standpoint alone, it is difficult to differentiate the various fluid collections from each other. One has to correlate the findings on sonography with the appropriate clinical presentation and timing of appearance of the fluid collection in question.

▶ **Hematoma**

This is commonly observed in the immediate postoperative period, as an ill-defined hyperechoic area, and usually resolves spontaneously as the blood collection is eventually resorbed (the margins become more

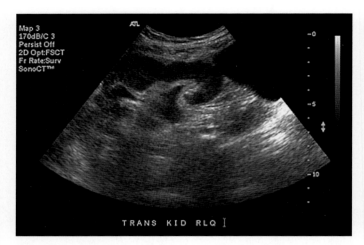

Figure 42-29. Transplanted kidney with urinoma. This shows the TXP with hydronephrosis (dilated calyces) and a fluid collection (urinoma) adjacent and medial to the lower pole.

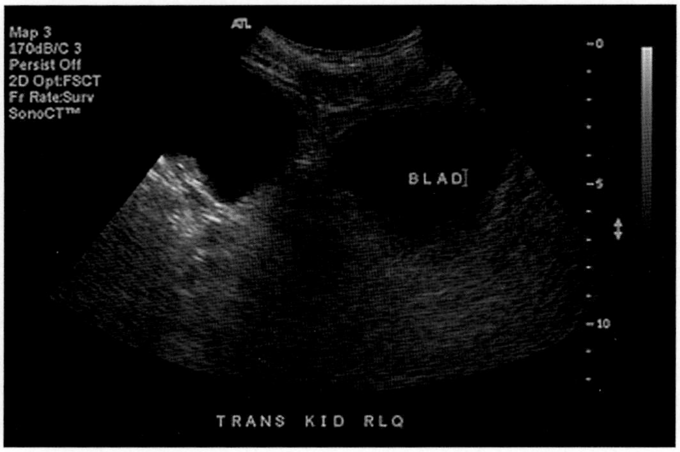

Figure 42-30. Transplanted kidney with urinoma. This shows the urinoma to the right of the superior aspect of the bladder (BLAD).

defined while the center becomes more anechoic). In rare instances, it can be secondary to an anastomotic leak at the main artery or vein and may grow to a large enough size that can cause extrinsic compression of the renal vasculature, for example, ischemia, thrombosis, to name a few.

▶ Urinoma

Also observed in the immediate postoperative period, urinomas occur secondary to an anastomotic leak in the surgically implanted ureter. In extreme circumstances, they can progress to urinary ascites (see Figures 42-29 and 42-30).

▶ Lymphocele

This is the most common peri-renal fluid collection observed in renal transplants. In contrast to hematomas and urinomas, they usually develop several weeks to months after the transplantation procedure. Although they usually resolve spontaneously, they may also increase in size, to the point of causing extrinsic compression of the kidney and its vasculature, and may also require percutaneous drainage at times.

On ultrasonography, lymphoceles appear anechoic, but may contain loculations or septations.

Any of the perirenal fluid collections can become secondarily infected, especially in light of the patient's immunosuppressed state. Abscesses are characterized by having hyperechoic debris within the fluid collection, and usually require percutaneous drainage.

PERFORMING A PERCUTANEOUS RENAL BIOPSY

Please refer Chapter 41 for a detailed discussion.

BILLING, TRAINING, AND CERTIFICATION

Please refer Chapters 7 and 9.

REFERENCES

1. Pei Y, Watnick T. Diagnosis and screening of autosomal dominant polycystic kidney disease. *Adv Chronic Kidney Dis*. 2010 Mar;17(2):140–152. Review.
2. Martin, JF. History of ultrasound. In: Resnick MI, Sanders RC, eds. *Ultrasound in Urology*. Baltimore: Williams & Wilkins; 1984:1.
3. Wild J, Neal D. Use of high frequency ultrasonic waves for detecting changes of texture in living tissues. *Lancet*. 1951 Mar 24;1(6656):655–657.
4. Wild J, Reid J. Application of echo-ranging techniques to the determination of structure of biological tissues. *Science*. 1952;115(2983):226–230.
5. Howry DH, Bliss WR. Ultrasonic visualization of soft tissue structures of the body. *J Lab Clin Med*. 1952 Oct;40(4):579–592.
6. Kikuchi Y, Uchida R, Tanaka K, Wagai T, Hayashi S. Early cancer diagnosis through ultrasonics. *J Acoust Soc Am*. 1956;28(4):779 (1 page)
7. Woo J. A short history of the development of ultrasound in obstetrics and gynecology. Available at: http://www. ob-ultrasound.net/history1.html.
8. Thurstone F, Von Ramm O. A new ultrasound imaging technique employing two-dimensional electronic beam steering (for medical diagnosis). International Symposium on Acoustical Holography and Imaging, 5th, Palo Alto, California, United States, 18–20 July 1973;1974:249–259.
9. Berson A, Roncin M, Pourcelot L. Compound scanning with an electrically steered beam. *Ultrason Imaging*. 1981;3(3):303–308.
10. Carpenter DA, Dadd MJ, Kossoff G. A multimode real time scanner. *Ultrasound Med Biol*. 1980;6(3):279–284.
11. Jespersen SK, Wilhjelm JE, Sillesen H. Multi-angle compound imaging. *Ultrason Imaging*. 1998;20(2):81–102.

12. Shattuck DP, Olaf T, von Ramm O. Compound scanning with a phased array. *Ultrason Imaging.* 1982;4(2):93–107.

13. Burns PN, Powers JE, Hope Simpson D, Uhlendorf V, Fritzsch T. Harmonic imaging: principles and preliminary results. *Angiology.* 1996;47:63–73.

14. Desser T, Jeffrey R, Lane M, Ralls P. Tissue harmonic imaging: utility in abdominal and pelvic sonography. *J Clin Ultrasound.* 1999;27(3):135–142.

15. Richardson D, Foster J, Davison A, Irving H. Parvus tardus waveform suggesting renal artery stenosis—remember the more proximal stenosis. *Nephrol Dial Transplant.* 2000;15(4):539–543.

16. Emamian S, Nielsen M, Pedersen J. Intraobserver and interobserver variations in sonographic measurements of kidney size in adult volunteers: a comparison of linear measurements and volumetric estimates. *Acta Radiol.* 1995;36(4):399–401.

17. Miletic D, Fuckar Z, Sustic A, Mozetic V, Stimac D. Sonographic measurement of absolute and relative renal length in adults. *J Clin Ultrasound.* 1998;26(4):185–189.

18. Troell S, Berg U, Johansson B, Wikstad I . Comparison between renal parenchymal sonographic volume, renal parenchymal urographic area, glomerular filtration rate and renal plasma flow in children. *Scand J Urol Nephrol.* 1988;22(3):207–214.

19. Hricak H, Cruz C, Romanski R, Uniewski M, Levin N, Madrazo B, Sandler M, Eyler W. Renal parenchymal disease: sonographic-histologic correlation. *Radiology.* July 1982;144(1);141–147.

20. Adibi A, Emaimi Nani A, Salehi H, MatinpourM. Renal cortical thickness in adults with normal renal function measured by ultrasonography. *Iran J Radiol.* 2008;5(3):163–166.

21. Beland M, Walle N, Machan J, Cronan J. Renal cortical thickness measured at ultrasound: is it better than renal length as an indicator of renal function in chronic kidney disease? *Am J Roentgenol.* 2010;95(2):146–149.

22. Irving H, Kashi S. Complications of renal transplantation and the role of interventional radiology. *J Clin Ultrasound.* 1992;20(8):545–552.

23. Richard HM. Perirenal transplant fluid collections. Semin *Intervent Radiol.* 2004;21(4):235–237.

24. Don S, Kopecky K, Filo R, Leapman S, Thomalla J, Jones J, Klatte E. Duplex Doppler US of renal allografts: causes of elevated resistive index. *Radiology.* 1989;171(3): 709–712.

25. O'Neill WC, Baumgarten DA. Ultrasonography in renal transplantation. *Am J Kidney Dis.* 2002;39(4):663–678.

26. Riehl J, Brandenburg VM. Which is the best duplex sonographic parameter to use when screening for renal artery stenosis? *Nat Clin Pract Nephrol.* 2007;414–415.

27. Bosniak MA. Difficulties in classifying cystic lesions of the kidney. *Urol Radiol.* 1991;13(1):91–93.

28. Bosniak MA. Problems in the radiologic diagnosis of renal parenchymal tumors. In: S. I. Olsson CA, eds. *Urologic Clinics of North America.* Philadelphia, PA: WB Saunders; 1993:217–230.

29. Siegel C, Middleton W, Teefey S, McClennan B. Angiomyolipoma and renal cell carcinoma: US differentiation. *Radiology.* 1996;198(3):789–793.

30. Prasad S, Surabhi V, Menias C, Raut A, Chintapalli K. Benign renal neoplasms in adults: crosssectional imaging findings. *Am J Roentgenol.* 2008;190(1):158–164.

31. Lusaya DG, Lerma EV. Hydronephrosis and hydroureter. Available at: http://emedicine.medscape.com/ article/436259-overview. Accessed May 22, 2011.

32. Webster's Online Dictionary. (n.d.). Available at: http:// www.websters-online-dictionary.org/definitions/ hydronephrosis?cxpartner-pub0939450753529744% 3Av0qd01-tdlq&cofFORID%3A9&ieUTF-8&qhyd ronephrosis&saSearch#922. Accessed May 22, 2011.

33. Block B. Kidneys: organ details. In: *The Practice of Ultasound: A Step-by-Step Guide to Abdominal Scanning.* New York: Thieme; 2004:212.

34. Ovel S. *Mosby's Comprehensive Review for General Sonography Examinations.* St. Louis: Mosby Elsevier; 2009.

35. Webb JA. Ultrasonography in the diagnosis of urinary tract obstruction. *BMJ.* 1990;301:944–946.

36. Rascoff J, Golden R, Spinowitz B, Charytan C. Nondilated obstructive nephropathy. *Arch Intern Med.* 1983;143(4):696–698.

37. Tublin M, Dodd G. Sonography of renal transplantation. *Radiol Clin North Am.* 1995 May;33(3):447–459.

43

EMERGING ROLE OF VASCULAR ULTRASOUND IN ARTERIOVENOUS DIALYSIS ACCESS

MARKO MALOVRH

INTRODUCTION

Vascular access for hemodialysis is the "life line" for patients with end-stage renal disease (ESRD) on chronic hemodialysis (HD). An ideal access delivers a flow rate adequate for the dialysis prescription, has a long life span, and has a low rate of complications. Although no current type of access (arteriovenous fistula (AVF), arteriovenous graft (AVG), and central vein catheter (CVC)) fulfills all of these criteria, the native AVF comes closest to doing so. The first AVF was constructed by Appel, Cimino, and Brescia in 1965.[1] The problems connected with the construction of AVFs have increased since that time. Currently, the most frequent problems with AVFs are primary failure, unsuccessful maturation, and an inability to cannulate the fistula, resulting in inadequate blood flow during HD treatment. For radiocephalic AVFs, a meta-analysis[2] estimated modest primary (63%) and secondary (66%) patencies at 1 year.

An assessment of the vessels of the upper extremity is mandatory prior to fistula creation. Physical examination is important and many times is a valuable tool in the work-up of patients awaiting vascular access surgery, but it should be recognized that it is challenging and of limited value in obese, older patients, and diabetics. Malovrh[3] found that physical examination failed to identify suitable veins for AVF creation in over half of all patients undergoing dialysis access surgery ($n = 62/116$ or 54%). A majority (77%) of these 62 patients showed an adequate vein on duplex ultrasound (DUS).

One of the most important predictors of successful AVF maturation is the ability of the arterial and venous vessels to dilate under the influence of the increased shear stress, resulting in vessels remodeling. Over the last decade, there has been increase of interest in preoperative ultrasonography for dialysis vascular access. Routine use of upper extremity DUS identifies many patients with veins that are suitable for use and also determines which arteries have optimal arterial inflow for successful AFV creation which serves to reduce AVF failures, especially in risk groups of patients with co-morbid conditions such as diabetes and vascular disease. This approach was initially stimulated by the ease and safety of ultrasonography.

Access complications are a major determinant of morbidity in patients receiving hemodialysis. The most common complications are nonmaturation, access failure caused by thrombosis, due to the development of vascular stenosis, aneurysm or pseudoaneurysm, and steal syndrome. Clinical monitoring DUS can be used effectively for primary radiological evaluation of a malfunctioning AVF or AVG.

This chapter will provide the nephrologists, radiologists, and vascular access surgeons with an overview of the clinical role, merits, and shortcomings of DUS which enable information both on the morphology and on the function of vessels in the preoperative work-up of patients awaiting surgical creation of vascular access for HD, in the routine monitoring of AVFs or AVGs to detect, localize, and characterize vascular access complications and in placement of CVC for hemodialysis.

ULTRASOUND TECHNIQUE

Ultrasound allows for noninvasive and safe imaging with low cost and avoids the need for radiocontrast agents. It does, however, require that time be spent conducting the scan as well as skill and experience on the part of the operator. Additionally, knowledge of the changes in local vasculature hemodynamics after AVF creation and of the pathophysiological mechanisms behind access complications is needed in order to interpret the DUS image adequately.[4]

Ultrasound is sound above the audible range with frequency above 20,000 MHz. The ultrasound machine should allow examination with B-mode (black and white brightness) and Doppler mode (color and spectral analyses). B-mode allows visualization of structures as being black (blood, fluid, etc), grey (solid organs), or white (vessel, calcification, graft wall). The three main types of Doppler imaging used in vascular access ultrasound are color Doppler imaging, pulsed wave Doppler, and power Doppler which gives the information both acoustically and on the screen as the blood velocity changes during cardiac cycle.[5] Appropriate for most vessels are linear array probes with a frequency of 7–12 MHz or higher for B-mode, and 5 MHz or higher for Doppler. When conducting the examination, the ultrasound gel used should be warmed. The patient should be placed in a supine position and in stable ambient conditions.[6,7]

DUS enables assessment of vessel parameters such as patency, diameter, and quality of the vein and arterial wall—intima-media thickness (IMT), measurement of hemodynamic characteristics: flow velocities, calculation of blood flow, and resistive index (RI).[7–9] The internal diameter is measured in longitudinal or transverse sections in the radial, ulnar, or brachial artery. In the longitudinal section, the probe is aligned to show the intimal layers at the near and far walls to measure the distance from intima to intima perpendicular to the arterial wall. Systolic–diastolic diameter variation due to arterial pulsatility occurs. With M-mode, a point of the artery may be insonated over time and the diameter may be measured at the desired point of the cardiac cycle. M-mode measurement is useful when the small error due to arterial pulsatility could become relevant, for instance in small caliber arteries.[10] The arterial diameter correlates well with the diameter measured at surgery.[11]

We recommend measurement of volume flow of native fistulas in the feeding brachial artery, which correlates very well with access flow rates. Blood flow in AVG can be investigated by DUS along the entire access. Flow calculations in the venous outflow tract are often difficult because of curves, bifurcations, variations in vessel diameter, turbulent flow, and vibrations due to the superficial localizations and arterializations of the veins. The calculation of the flow volume is based on the measurement of internal diameter and time-averaged velocity integral of the mean velocity. Using the mean maximal velocity to calculate the volume should not be done because this will overestimate the access flow. Modern ultrasound devices usually have special software for calculating blood flow after the input of appropriate data. Due to inherent errors of measurement, the mean of three consecutive flow volume measurements should be used.[4] RI is calculated by dividing the difference between the peak systolic velocity (PSV) and the end diastolic velocity (EDV) by the PSV.[12]

In doing the DUS examination, the forearm and upper arm veins should be distended by placing a tourniquet. Often, the more central veins cannot be assessed directly.[13] This scan yields an anatomic vein map and may identify an outflow obstruction that could result in AVF failure.

PREOPERATIVE EXAMINATION

Vascular mapping to assess the presence of vessels suitable for creation of an AVF or AVG is obligatory in all patients approaching dialysis. Preoperative vascular examination has recently been shown to predict AVF outcome.[4,7,8,14,15] Basic physical examination usually yields more information from venous than arterial assessment. In contrast, DUS gives relatively more information about the artery than the vein.[10] Wong et al[8] compared the accuracy of predicting AVF failure from the preoperative evaluation of the forearm cephalic vein. The positive predictive value was better with DUS than for physical vein palpation. AVF failure occurred for all veins that were abnormal on the DUS.

▶ Arterial Assessment

A good caliber artery is needed for adequate arterial inflow to allow fistula maturation and prevent "steal" syndrome. Preoperative DUS examination should include assessment of the arteries from infraclavicular subclavian artery down to the radial artery at the wrist.[13] Ultrasound identifies anatomical variations, such as a proximal origin (high bifurcation) of the radial and ulnar arteries in the upper arm. Ultrasound measurements of the vessel diameter and time-averaged velocity allow calculation of blood flow. However, blood flow estimates in a small-caliber radial artery are often inaccurate. Therefore, the suitability of the radial artery for AVF formation must be determined by other

TABLE 43–1

Minimum Vessel Diameter for Successful Creation of Radiocephalic Fistula

Minimum Internal Diameter of the Radial Artery

Author	Radial Artery Internal Diameter (mm)	Year of Publication
Wong et al	1.6	1998
Silva et al	2.0	1998
Malovrh	1.5	2002
Parmar et al	≥1.5	2007

Minimum Internal Diameter of the Cephalic Vein

Author	Cephalic Vein Internal Diameter	Year of Publication
Wong et al	1.6	1998
Silva et al	2.5	1998
Malovrh	1.6	2002
Mendes et al	2.0	2002
Brimble et al	2.6	2002

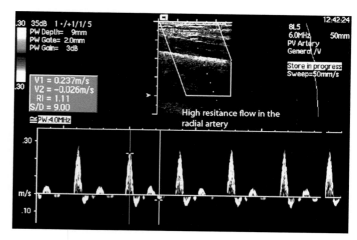

Figure 43-1. High-resistance Doppler waveform in the artery.

criteria, including the diameter, wall morphology, and the hyperemic response.[3,11] Arterial diameters smaller than 1.5 have been associated with increased nonmaturation rates of AVFs.[3,8,16–19] One analysis of prospectively collected data found the greatest 1 year patency of radiocephalic fistulae with preoperative radial artery diameters between 2.1 and 2.5 mm.[18] While the authors concluded that a single radial artery cut-off cannot be recommended, these results highlight the importance of including other factors in conjunction with radial artery diameter in predicting success. The ideal cut-off point for the arterial diameter in terms of AVF maturation and adequacy for dialysis is not known, probably because other factors such as the presence of arterial disease may also play an important role.[7,10]

The internal arterial diameter has been used in several studies to predict the outcome of radiocephalic AVF (Table 43-1). Wong et al[8] observed either thrombosis or non-maturation in all AVFs created with a radial artery diameter less than 1.6 mm. Malovrh[3] found an immediate patency rate of 92% and a patency rate of 83% after 12 weeks in AVFs created with arteries whose diameter was >1.5 mm. When an arterial diameter <1.5 mm was used, the patency rates were 45% and 36%.

During AVF maturation, AVF blood flow increases with dilatation of the feeding artery, but this may not occur in a diseased artery. Morphologic information on the thickness and structure of the arterial wall (smoothness of the intima, wall thickening, and calcification) can be obtained with B-mode ultrasound. Using high-resolution ultrasound, IMT may be quantified on the far wall of a longitudinal section of the distal radial artery. Heavy calcification, identified in B-mode, may make surgery difficult.[3,8]

In addition to diameter, assessing the artery's propensity to dilate in response to reactive hyperemia is a diagnostic maneuver that may be helpful.[3,11] After ischemia has been induced by clenching a fist, reactive hyperemia is observed immediately after release. This results from low resistance flow from the radial artery. Doppler evaluation of the distal radial artery shows a triphasic high-resistance waveform during ischemia; this changes to a monophasic low-resistance waveform with an overall increased velocity during reactive hyperemia (Figures 43-1 and 43-2).[3] The spectral waveform change may be quantified by the RI or by the difference in peak systolic velocity. This same phenomenon occurs after AVF construction, when arterial flow is directed toward the low-resistance venous compartment (Figure 43-3). The greater the hyperemic response of the artery, the lower the RI will be, or the greater the peak velocity difference.[3,11,20] Wall et al[20] measured both hyperemic resting peak velocity and posthyperemia peak velocity and calculated the differences. The results they called the hyperemic response. A reduced or absent hyperemic response was found to be an independent predictor of access failure. The RI is less prone to error because it is less dependent on the Doppler angle.

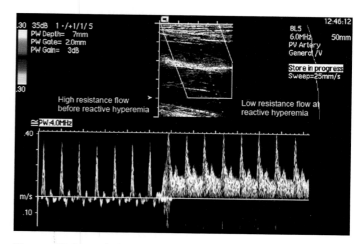

Figure 43-2. Radial artery high resistance flow with clenched fist and low resistance flow during reactive hyperemia after releasing the fist.

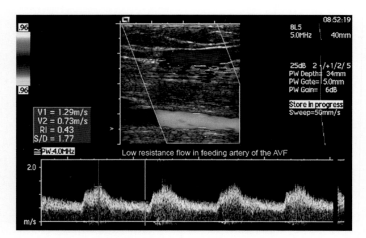

Figure 43-3. Normal Doppler wave-form of the AVF feeding artery—low resistance flow with a low resistive index.

Malovrh[3] found that the critical cut for access failure was a RI of 0.7 or more. In his study, a feeding artery baseline flow of 54.5 mL/min was increased with reactive hyperemia to 90.9 mL/min in the group of successful constructed AVFs (66% of cases) compared to a baseline of 24.1 mL/min, increasing at reactive hyperemia to 33.1 mL/min in the group of unsuccessful AVFs (35% of cases). For the AVFs patent at 24 hours, it was shown that blood flow in the feeding artery increased significantly more in the AVFs with preoperative hyperemic response (close to 500 mL/min) compared to those without it (300 mL/min) by 12 weeks. Lockhart et al[21] suggested that this test was less predictive in women compared to men. Despite conflicting study results, this type of provocative test is extremely interesting.[3,11,21] It remains to be established whether a combination of parameters might enable better prediction of vascular access function and minimize early failure and nonmaturation. Currently, at the University Medical Centre Ljubljana, Slovenia, Malovrh and his coworkers are using preoperatively DUS in all patients in need of vascular access for HD. It is our view that for the final decision before surgery, a combination of the various DUS morphological and functional arterial parameters is important.

▶ Venous Assessment

The superficial venous system of the upper extremity is easily assessable by DUS and results in the detection of more veins when compared to physical examination.[3] In conducting the examination, the forearm cephalic vein should be distended by placing a tourniquet downstream. The cephalic vein should be followed to the point of its drainage into the deep venous system. Patency is assessed by frequent intermittent compression of the distended vein with the probe placed in the transverse section. If a suitable cephalic vein is not found, the basilic vein should be examined in the same manner. The deep venous system beyond the drain point should be followed to the subclavian vein.[22]

Criteria used to determine the suitability of a vein for AVF formation include appearance, diameter, distensibility, shape of Doppler venous waveform, phenomena of respiratory filling, and suitability for cannulation. The diameter and depth should be measured at points throughout the upper limb. In doing this, it is important to avoid direct pressure on the vein by using sufficient gel and resting the probe to the side of the vein. Diameters can be measured in the longitudinal or transverse section.[22,23]

Multiple studies have assessed vein size as a predictor of fistula outcome, with larger vein diameter associated with improved outcome and thresholds ranging from 1.6 to 3.0 mm (Table 43-1).[3,8,16,24–28] Recent information concerning the reproducibility of ultrasound vein imaging to assess distensibility of individual vein indicates improvements and standardizations are needed for these tests to be used routinely in clinical practice.[27,28] To assess venous distensibility (the percentage increase in venous diameter), venous diameter should be measured before and 2 minutes after the application of a tourniquet or a blood pressure cuff inflated to more than 40 mm Hg.[3,24,26–29]

The vein considered for AVF creation should have sufficient length for future needle placement, at least 20 cm and should lay less than 6 mm deep.[24] Some studies have found an association between the presence and size of venous side branches and AVF nonmaturation.[8,27] In a normal vein, spectral Doppler shows spontaneous flow. Local venous hemodynamic can be assessed by observing the typical shape of the Doppler vein signal and Doppler signal changes during deep inspiration (Figure 43-4). The absence or diminished vein flow velocities or no change in flow-velocities due to deep inspiration is associated with a higher risk of vascular access early failure and nonmaturation.[23]

▶ Preoperative Ultrasound Use and Vascular Access Outcomes

Many investigators have demonstrated a marked improvement in fistula placement with the use of vascular mapping. Allon et al[30] found a huge increase in arteriovenous fistula

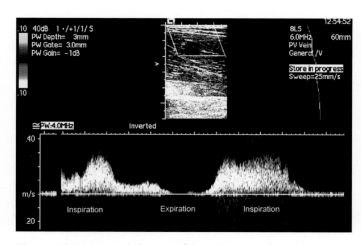

Figure 43-4. Normal change of Doppler wave-form during respiration.

creation when preoperative vascular mapping using ultrasonography was employed compared with clinical examination (preoperative clinical examination: 34% fistula creation; preoperative sonographic vascular mapping: 64% fistula creation). Silva[18] found a significant improvement in arteriovenous fistulae creation (from 14% to 63%), reduction in graft placement (from 62% to 30%), and reduction in tunneled hemodialysis catheters insertion (from 24% to 7%) when preoperative mapping of the arteries and veins was performed by DUS. Practice changes other than ultrasound may have contributed to the increase in AVF creation.[10]

More important than an increase in arteriovenous fistula creation is the influence of preoperative DUS examination on outcomes of AVF. Different outcomes of AVF have been reported in studies examining the effect of preoperative evaluation. Silva et al[18] reported good AVF outcomes (8% early failure, 83% functional primary patency at 1 year) if a venous minimum diameter of 2.5 mm with tourniquet and a minimal arterial diameter threshold of 2.0 mm was used. Malovrh[3] used duplex ultrasonography to examine forearm arteries and veins before the creation of AVFs. The AVF primary patency rate (successfully constructed AVFs) was 80.2% in the group whose mean value of artery internal diameter was 2.6 mm, the RI with reactive hyperemia was less than 0.5 and the feeding artery baseline mean artery blood flow 54.5 ml/min was increased with reactive hyperemia to 90.9 mL/min (66% increase). The author concluded that DUS helped identify the optimal location for successful creation of vascular access and the time necessary for its development.

Three studies have examined the preoperative response to reactive hyperemia and related this to AVF outcomes. These studies are heterogeneous and difficult to compare but suggests that the hyperemic response may be a useful adjunct in evaluating arteries of borderline quality or caliber.[3,10,20,21] Clinical examination alone is insufficient in a considerable proportion (25–50%) of patients.[3,21] Some studies have provided evidence to suggest that patients with insufficient veins determined by clinical examination benefit from ultrasound, while ultrasound is not needed when adequate vessels are defined by clinical examination.[31–34] Another study[35] showed that a strategy of routine ultrasound, compared to one of the exclusive physical examination without imaging, could reduce early AVF failure (immediate patency 95% vs 75%). Ferring et al[15] reported a prospective randomized study investigating the influence of physical examination compared to routine preoperative vasculature ultrasound on AVF outcome. From 218 included patients, 106 had clinical examination and 112 had ultrasound assessment of the vessels before surgery. Immediate failure of AVF was significantly higher in the clinical group (13.3%) versus the ultrasound group (3.6%). Primary AVF survival at 1 year was 56% for the clinical group and 65% for the ultrasound group (not statistically significant). The assisted primary survival at 1 year was significantly better for the ultrasound group (80% vs 65%). This trial demonstrated a benefit of routine preoperative ultrasound in AVFs outcomes. DUS resulted

in less immediate failure, less early AVF thrombosis, and better assisted primary AVF survival.

It is well recognized that AVFs as access for hemodialysis are less prevalent among patients of older age, of female gender, among patients with obesity, diabetes, or cardiovascular disease.[36] In these groups of patients, who are at higher risk of AVF failure, physical examination alone is not sufficient. Since the exclusive application of clinical assessment without an option for imaging is not the usual clinical practice, the benefit of routine ultrasound may appear greater than it would be if ultrasound had been used selectively in these clinical groups.

ULTRASOUND FOR EVALUATION OF A MALFUNCTIONING ARTERIOVENOUS FISTULA OR GRAFT

Access complications are major determinants of morbidity and multiple hospital admission of patients receiving hemodialysis. The most common complications observed are maturation failure of a fistula and access failure (AVF or AVG) caused by stenosis, thrombosis, infection, and aneurysm or pseudoaneurysm formation. After clinical examination, DUS is frequently used for primary evaluation of a malfunctioning hemodialysis fistula or graft.[37] In doing this evaluation, the entire vascular access tree should be examined, including the feeding artery.

Nonmaturation of AVF is a growing problem. The most important determinant of fistula maturation is the response of the feeding artery and the drainage vein to the increase blood flow following the creation of an arteriovenous anastomosis. There is a dramatic increase in the arterial inflow that is evident by the first postoperative day and reaches a maximum (>10-fold increase) by about 8 weeks.[3] Won et al[38] found a significant increase in blood flow from an average of 20.9 mL/min in the radial artery to an average of 174 mL/min in the fistula only 10 minutes after creation of anastomosis.

The identification of an immature AVF is possible by physical examination; however, DUS has been shown to be a valuable diagnostic modality. Stenosis of the feeding artery and outflow stenosis are the most frequent causes of nonmaturation. Stenosis in an AVF tends to be located more centrally in the outflow tract and is caused by bifurcations of the vein, by scarring of puncture sites or by venous valves. Graft stenosis usually develops in the venous outflow tract at the site of the anastomosis between the graft and the vein.[39] Unfortunately, there is no general agreement on the diagnostic criteria of hemodynamically significant stenosis.[12] Generally, the measured diameter of the residual lumen at the point of maximal narrowing in a vascular segment is simply compared with the measured diameter at a normal point in that segment. Stenosis is considered to be significant if narrowing of 50% or more is observed on B-mode scan.[40]

Peak systolic velocities should be recorded; both at the site of a stenosis and at an adjacent normal vascular segment, a pronounced aliasing phenomenon will be observed. The perivascular space should also be investigated since functional stenosis may be the result of extra luminal compression of the access by abscess, hematoma, or seroma.[37] DUS has been demonstrated to be an accurate technique for detecting, locating, and characterizing vascular access complications, with a sensitivity of 90% for the detection of access site stenosis and outflow stenosis.[40] However, DUS criteria for more centrally located arterial stenosis are not well established. Indirect characteristics at the feeding brachial artery such as high resistance Doppler waveform and reduction in access flow volume can be detected. It is proposed that an inflow stenosis may be considered if the DUS examination shows a combination of a peak systolic velocity ratio ≥2 and a luminal diameter reduction of 50% or more.[12,41]

The most common cause of vascular access failure is thrombosis. Once AVFs are fully matured, thrombosis is rare. DUS is the most accurate noninvasive method for direct detection of thrombus formation in AVFs and grafts. The localization and extension of an acute thrombosis is evaluated easily by DUS since fresh thrombotic material may still have the same echogenicity as blood. Older thrombotic material shows an increased echogenicity and therefore facilitates B-mode imaging of the thrombus. An inability of manual compression of the vein with the linear transducer is not sufficient to diagnose access thrombosis using B-mode imaging.

Aneurysms and pseudoaneurysms usually develop at sites of vessel destruction after repeated cannulation (segmental overutilization). DUS flow imaging can easily distinguish pseudoaneurysms from hematoma, showing the so-called to-and-from sign, a typical waveform characterized by the backflow of blood from the aneurysmatic sac into the original vessel lumen during diastole.

Because of low resistance in the venous outflow, the fistula sucks not only the antegrade flow into the feeding artery but also steals retrograde flow from the hand via the palmar arch, which jeopardizes adequate perfusion of the hand. Usually, the steal phenomenon is clinically silent and the patient remains asymptomatic. Preoperatively, the Doppler spectrum, especially with reactive hyperemia, is useful to predict the risk of low flow steal. Absent or low diastolic flow correlates with impaired capacity of the palmar arch arteries to vasodilate. Steal syndrome is access-induced ischemia with pain during dialysis or at night, pale and cold finger, neurologic deficit, gangrene, and/or ulceration. In this situation, the diagnosis can be made on clinical criteria alone. However, a diagnostic challenge arises when the clinical presentation is less pronounced and the clinician is faced with uncertainty as to whether an intervention will be beneficial. DUS has been proposed as a noninvasive tool in the evaluation of peripheral ischemia. DUS enables measurement of the blood flow through the AVF and, in addition, can evaluate the peripheral and collateral blood vessels for occlusions and stenosis. The direction of flow is very easy to demonstrate by DUS. If ultrasound shows a change in flow direction (reversal), a steal situation is documented.[44]

ULTRASOUND-GUIDED CENTRAL VENOUS CATHETER PLACEMENT

CVCs are widely used to create a temporary or long-term vascular access for hemodialysis treatment. The usual site for CVC insertion is the internal jugular vein (IJV). The right side is preferred because of the straight course to the right atrium. Other veins for CVC placement include the subclavian vein, the femoral vein, and the external jugular vein. CVC placement in these veins, however, may be associated with a high incidence of complications. Visualization of the veins by ultrasound facilitates locating and judgment of the accessibility of the vein and thereby reduces the number of failed punctures and placement complications.[42,43] B-mode ultrasound imaging allows for detailed evaluation of vascular anatomy and structural characteristics and has been employed to outline the vascular system and locate blood vessels. As a real-time imaging modality, ultrasound allows the operator to visualize vessel compliance and observe changes in vessel caliber when variable pressure is applied to the overlying tissue what is helpful to distinguish between arterial and venous images.[44]

A 7.5 MHz linear transducer is most often used for ultrasound-guided CVC placement. Mechanical guides are manufactured to help the operator position and advance the needle when attempting vascular access under ultrasound guidance. The short-axis view provides visualization of the vessel in the transverse plane. When this view is obtained correctly, the vein with its corresponding artery should appear circular or oval in shape. After local anesthesia is injected, the needle is advanced toward the target vessel and ideally, the operator should directly visualize entrance of the needle into the vessel. Typically, the IJV lies anterior and slightly lateral to the carotid artery (Figure 43-5). However, anatomic variations have been reported to occur in up to 5.5% of patients.[45] In one sonographic study of vessels of the neck, it was found that the IJV was located in a position

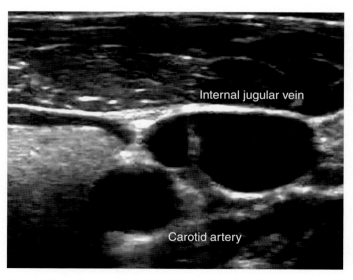

Figure 43-5. Position of internal jugular vein and carotid artery estimated by ultrasound before insertion of CVC.

to overlay the carotid artery in 54% of cases.[46] In a 6-year prospective study of ultrasound-assisted central vein catheterization in dialysis patients, a 100% success rate and an arterial puncture of 2.9% was reported.[6]

CONCLUSION

The number of patients requiring renal replacement therapy by hemodialysis is rising rapidly. The percentage of high-risk patients, elderly, diabetics, and patients with different vascular diseases is also increasing. Construction of an appropriate vascular access is a challenge to nephrologists and vascular surgeons. The clinical success of an AVF is jeopardized by high early failure and high failure to mature rates. Guidelines recommend the use of various diagnostic modalities to enable tailored vascular access creation for individual patients to avoid these complications.[47–50] Medical history and physical examination are basic. Physical examination can be carried out rapidly at no extra cost or equipment. This diagnostic modality yields more information from the venous than the arterial assessment. Unfortunately, its utility is less than optimal, especially in the high-risk group of patients. In this group and whenever the results of clinical examination are uncertain, ultrasound as an additional diagnostic modality should be used because of its noninvasive nature, ease of performance, and safety.

Various preoperative parameters determined by ultrasound are associated with an increased risk of vascular access early failure and nonmaturation. To better predict vascular access a combination of arterial, venous, and cardiac parameters should be used instead of a single parameter. Preoperative mapping should ideally be carried out close to the operation date and by a skilled person with understanding of the goal of vascular access for hemodialysis. Since 1995, in our department three nephrologists have performed preoperative vessels evaluation by ultrasound routinely at all patients. One of them is also a vascular access surgeon. Before a final decision is made, a combination of different clinical and ultrasound parameters is considered. Otherwise, two dedicated nephrologists from our department perform vascular access surgery. In 2008, 82% (1107/1343) of prevalent patients in Slovenia had a native arteriovenous fistula as their permanent vascular access.[51]

Central venous catheter placement under ultrasound guidance is widely supported in current nephrological practice. This technique has been shown to ensure safe and timely catheter placement and to reduce many of the potential complications associated with landmark methods.

REFERENCES

1. Brescia MJ, Cimino JE, Appel K, Hurwich BJ. Chronic hemodialysis using venipuncture and a surgically created arteriovenous fistula. *N Engl J Med.* 1966;275:1089–1092.
2. Rooijens PP, Tordoir JH, Stijnen T, Burgmans JP, Smet de AA, Yo TI. Radiocephalic wrist arteriovenous fistula for hemodialysis: meta-analysis indicates a high primary failure rate. *Eur J Vasc Endovasc Surg.* 2004;28:583–589.
3. Malovrh M. Native arteriovenous fistula: preoperative evaluation. *Am J Kidney Dis.* 2002;39:1218–1225.
4. Malik J, Tuka V, Tesar V. Local hemodynamic for the vascular access for hemodialysis. *Kidney Blood Press Res.* 2009;32:59–66.
5. Bonnin PH, Fressonnet R. Principles of hemodynamics and sonographic techniques for the evaluation of arteries. *J Radiol.* 2005;86:615–626.
6. Wiese P, Nonnast-Daniel B. Colour Doppler ultrasound in dialysis access. *Nephrol Dial Transplant.* 2004;19:1956–1963.
7. Malovrh M. The role of sonography in the planning of arteriovenous fistulas for hemodialysis. *Semin Dial.* 2003;16:299–303.
8. Wong V, Ward R, Taylor J, Selvakumar S, How TV, Bakran A. Factors associated with early failure of arteriovenous fistulae for haemodialysis access. *Eur J Vasc Endovasc Surg.* 1996;12:207–213.
9. Ku YM, Kim YO, Kim JI, Choi YJ, Yoon SA, Kim YS, Song SW, Yang CW, Kim YS, Chang YS, Bang BK. Ultrasonographic measurement of intima–media thickness of radial artery in pre-dialysis uraemic patients: comparison with histological examination. *Nephrol Dial Transplant.* 2006;21:715–720.
10. Ferring M, Henderson J, Wilmink A, Smith S. Vascular ultrasound for the pre-operative evaluation prior to arteriovenous fistula formation for haemodialysis: review of the evidence. *Nephrol Dial Transplant.* 2008;23:1809–1815.
11. Malovrh M. Non-invasive evaluation of vessels by duplex sonography prior to construction of arteriovenous fistulas for haemodialysis. *Nephrol Dial Transplant.* 1998;13:125–129.
12. van Hooland S, Malik J. Hemodialysis vascular access ultrasonography: tips, tricks, pitfalls and a quiz. *J Vasc Access.* 2010;11:255–262.
13. Zwiebel WJ. Technique for extremity venous ultrasound examination. In: Zwiebel W, Pellerito J, eds. *Introduction to Vascular Ultrasonography*. Philadelphia, PA: Elsevier Saunders; 2005:431–447.
14. Parmar J, Aslam M, Standfield N. Pre-operative radial artery diameter predicts early failure of arteriovenous fistula (AVF) for haemodialysis. *Eur J Vasc Endovasc Surg.* 2007;33:113–115.
15. Ferring M, Claridge M, Smith SA, Wilmink T. Routine preoperative vascular ultrasound improves patency and use of arteriovenous fistulas for hemodialysis: a randomized trial. *Clin J Am Soc Nephrol.* 2010;5:2236–2244.
16. Tordoir J, Mickley V. European guidelines for vascular access: clinical algorithms on vascular access for haemodialysis. *EDTNA ERCA J.* 2003;29:131–136.
17. Allon M, Bailey R, Ballard R, , Deierhoi MH, Hamrick K, Oser R, Rhynes VK, Robbin ML, Saddekni S, Zeigler ST. A multidisciplinary approach to hemodialysis access: prospective evaluation. *Kidney Int.* 1998;53:473–479.
18. Silva MB, Jr., Hobson RW, 2nd, Pappas PJ, Jamil Z, Araki CT, Goldberg MC, Gwertzman G, Padberg FT, Jr. A strategy for increasing use of autogenes hemodialysis access procedures: impact of preoperative noninvasive evaluation. *J Vasc Surg.* 1998;27:302–307.
19. Korten E, Toonder IM, Schrama YC, Hop WCJ, van der Ham AC, Wittens CHA. Dialysis patency and preoperative diameter ultrasound measurements. *Eur J Vasc Endovasc Surg.* 2007;33:467–471.

20. Wall LP, Gasparis A, Callahan S, van Bemmelen P, Criado E, Ricotta J. Impaired hyperemic response is predictive of early access failure. *Ann Vasc Surg.* 2004;18: 167–171.

21. Lockhart ME, Robbin ML, Allon M. Preoperative sonographic radial artery evaluation and correlation with subsequent radiocephalic fistula outcome. *J Ultrasound Med.* 2004;23:161–168.

22. Robbin ML, Lockhart ME. Ultrasound assessment before and after hemodialysis access. In: Zwiebel W, Pellerito J, eds. *Introduction to Vascular Ultrasonography.* Philadelphia, PA: Elsevier Saunders; 2005:325–340.

23. Malovrh M. The role of sonography in the planning of arteriovenous fistulas for hemodialysis. *Semin Dial.* 2003;16:299–303.

24. Malovrh M. Update on pre-operative assessment. In: Tordoir J, ed. *Vascular Access.* Turin: Edizioni Minerva Medica; 2009:15–20.

25. Mendes RR, Farber MA, Marston WA, Dinwiddie LC, Keagy BA, Burnham SJ. Prediction of wrist arteriovenous fistula maturation with preoperative vein mapping with ultrasonography. *J Vasc Surg.* 2002;36:460–463.

26. Brimble KS, Rabbat Ch G, Treleaven DJ, Ingram AJ. Utility of ultrasonographic assessment prior to forearm arteriovenous fistula creation. *Clin Nephrol.* 2002;58:122–127.

27. Planken RN, Tordoir JH, Duijm LE, de Haan MW, Leiner T. Current techniques for assessment of upper extremity vasculature prior to hemodialysis vascular access creation. *Eur Radiol.* 2007;17:3001–3011.

28. Van der Linden J, Lameris TW, van den Meiracker AH, de Smet AAEA, Blankestijn PJ, van den Dorpel MA. Forearm venous distensibility predicts successful arteriovenous fistula. *Am J Kidney Dis.* 2006;47:1013–1019.

29. Planken RN, Keuter XHA, Kessels AGH, Hoeks APG, Leiner T, Tordoir JHM. Forearm cephalic vein cross-sectional area changes at incremental congestion pressures: towards a reproducible and standardized vein mapping protocol. *J Vasc Surg.* 2006;44:353–358.

30. Allon M, Lockhart ME, Lilly RZ, Gallichio MH, Young CJ, Barker J, Deierhoi MH, Robbin ML. Effect of preoperative sonographic mapping on vascular access outcomes in hemodialysis patients. *Kidney Int.* 2001;60:2013–2020.

31. Robbin ML, Gallichio MH, Deierhoi MH, Young CJ, Weber TM, Allon M. Use vascular mapping before hemodialysis access placement. *Radiology.* 2000;217:83–88.

32. Wells AC, Fernando B, Butler A, Huguet E, Bradley JA, Pettigrew GJ. Selective use of ultrasonographic vascular mapping in the assessment of patients before haemodialysis access surgery. *Br J Surg.* 2005;92:1439–1443.

33. Parmley MC, Broughan TA, Jennings WC. Vascular ultrasonography prior to dialysis access surgery. *Am J Surg.* 2002;184:568–572.

34. Nursal TZ, Oguzkurt L, Tercan F, Torer N, Noyan T, Karakayali H, Haberal M. Is routine preoperative ultrasonographic mapping for arteriovenous fistula creation necessary in patients with favorable physical examination findings? Results of a randomized controlled trial. *World J Surg.* 2006;30:1100–1107.

35. Mihmanli I, Besirli K, Kurugoglu S, Atakir K, Haider S, Ogut G, Numan F, Canturk E, Sayin AG. Cephalic vein and hemodialysis fistula: surgeon's observation versus color Doppler ultrasonographic findings. *J Ultrasound Med.* 2001;20:217–222.

36. Pisoni R, Young E, Dykstra D, Greenwood RN, Hecking E, Gillespie B, Wolfe RA, Goodkin DA, Held PJ. Vascular access use in Europe and the United States: results from the DOPPS. *Kidney Int.* 2002;61:305–316.

37. Wiese P, Nonnast-Daniel B. Colour Doppler ultrasound in dialysis access. *Nephrol Dial Transplant.* 2004;19: 1956–1963.

38. Won T, Jang JW, Lee S, Han JJ, Park YS, Ahn JH. Effects of intraoperative blood flow on the early patency of radiocephalic fistulas. *Ann Vasc Surg.* 2000;14:468–472.

39. Besarab A, Sullivan KL, Ross RP, Moritz MJ. Utility of intra-access pressure monitoring in detecting and correcting venous outlet stenoses prior to thrombosis. *Kidney Int.* 1995;47:1364–1373.

40. Doelman G, Duijm LE, Liem YS, Froger CL, Tielbeek AV, Donkers-van Rossum AB, Cuypers PW, Douwes-Draaijer P, Buth J, van den Bosch HC. Stenosis detection in failing hemodialysis access fistulas and grafts: comparison of color Doppler ultrasonography, contrast-enhanced magnetic resonance angiography and digital subtraction angiography. *J Vasc Surg.* 2005;42:739–746.

41. Yo LS, Duijm LE, Planken RN, et al. Dysfunctional haemodialysis fistulas and grafts: detection of arterial inflow stenos with colour Doppler ultrasonography. *Eur Radiol.* 2009;19(suppl 1):S290.

42. Gallieni M. Central vein catheterization of dialysis patients with real time ultrasound guidance. *J Vasc Access.* 2000;1:10–14.

43. Hameeteman M, Bode AS, Peppelenbosch AG, van der Sande FM, Tordoir JHM. Ultrasound-guided central venous catheter placement by surgical trainees: a safe procedure? *J Vasc Access.* 2010;11:288–292.

44. Rose SC, Neslson TR. Ultrasonographic modalities to assess vascular anatomy and disease. *J Vasc Interv Radiol.* 2004;15:25–38.

45. Denys BG, Uretsky BF. Anatomical variations of internal jugular vein location: impact of central venous access. *Crit Care Med.* 1991;19:1516–1519.

46. Troianos CA, Jobes DR, Ellison N. Ultrasound-guided cannulation of the internal jugular vein. A prospective randomized study. *Anesth Anal.* 1991;72:823–826.

47. Duijm LE, Caris R. Imaging techniques of vascular access. In: Tordoir J, ed. *Best Practice in Vascular Access.* Turin: Edizioni Minerva Medica; 2010:29–37.

48. III. NKF-K/doqi Clinical Practice Guidelines for Vascular Access: update 2000. *Am J Kidney Dis.* 2001;37:S137–S181.

49. Clinical practice guidelines for vascular access. *Am J Kidney Dis.* 2006;48(suppl 1):S176–S247.

50. Tordoir J, Canaud B, Haage P, Konner K, Basci A, Fouque D, Kooman J, Martin-Malo A, Pedrini L, Pizzarelli F, Tattersall J, Vennegoor M, Wanner C, ter Wee P, Vanholder R. EBPG on vascular access. *Nephrol Dial Transplant.* 2007;22(suppl 2):ii88–ii117.

51. Buturović-Ponikvar J, Adamlje T, Arnol M, et al. *Slovenian Renal Replacement Therapy Registry 2007&2008 Annual Report.* Ljubljana: The Slovenian Society of Nephrology; 2010:50.

44

PERITONEAL DIALYSIS CATHETER INSERTION

MARY BUFFINGTON, ADRIAN SEQUEIRA, BHARAT SACHDEVA, & KENNETH ABREO

LEARNING OBJECTIVES

1. Understand the role of nephrologists in placing peritoneal dialysis (PD) catheters.
2. Describe the types of PD catheters, with emphasis on most commonly used types.
3. Understand issues involved in preoperative evaluation for PD catheter placement.
4. Describe the techniques used to percutaneously place PD catheters.
5. Understand the complications that arise following PD catheter placement.

INTRODUCTION

Peritoneal dialysis (PD) has many advantages and should be encouraged for all appropriate end-stage renal disease (ESRD) patients. However, it is an underutilized mode of dialysis with only 7.2% prevalence among ESRD patients.[1] Increased utilization of PD is an important goal, and nephrologists should make an effort to increase the number of patients on PD. Since the function of the PD catheter is critical to the patient's ability to initiate and continue peritoneal dialysis, providing and maintaining peritoneal access is an important part of successful and lasting use of the PD modality. Involvement of interventional nephrologists in the placement of PD catheters has been shown to increase utilization of PD. Benefits of nephrologists placing catheters percutaneously under fluoroscopic or peritoneoscopic guidance with conscious sedation also include avoiding delays associated with scheduling a surgical procedure and avoiding the risks associated with general anesthesia. This chapter describes the role of the nephrologist in catheter insertion, the types of catheters available, and preoperative preparation. Techniques of PD catheter placement using two percutaneous methods, fluoroscopically guided and peritoneoscopic, are reviewed. Finally, this chapter also reviews postoperative complications and percutaneous placement in comparison with surgical techniques.

▶ Role of Nephrologists

Studies have shown that involvement of interventional nephrologists in the placement of PD catheters improves the utilization of PD.[2-4] Factors that cause underutilization of PD include lack of a pre-ESRD educational program, late patient referral for dialysis, limited presentation of choice of dialysis modality to patients, and poor infrastructure for PD training and research. Other factors are the lack of nephrologists' experience in PD during fellowship training and physician bias toward hemodialysis (HD). An interventional nephrology PD access program was developed and incorporated into a pre-existing CKD patient education structure in one center; this led to an increase in the number of PD patients from a baseline of 43 to 80 patients over the course of 18 months.[4] Using a peritoneoscopic method under local or light conscious sedation, the nephrologists were able to avoid delays associated with referral to surgery with associated scheduling issues and clearance for general anesthesia. Often the patient can avoid HD altogether and avoid the risks associated with general anesthesia.

A retrospective analysis of interventional nephrologists placing PD catheters at three centers reinforced this point.[2] The three centers with ongoing interventional nephrology programs saw an increase in their PD population. Center 1 had an increase from baseline of 20–43 patients to 101 patients and center 2 from 70–78 patients to 125 patients. The third center saw an increase from 20–30 patients to 97 patients, but the program was suspended when they were unable to maintain their procedure time in the operating suite. Following suspension, the PD population in center 3 declined from 97 patients to 25 patients. PD utilization increased in these centers because dialysis modality advantages and disadvantages were presented to the patients by nephrologists and nurse educators. When a patient chooses PD, the interventional nephrologists can quickly place a PD access and avoid or limit time on HD. Early placement is especially important considering that catheter placement should occur at least 2 weeks prior to starting PD.[5] Nephrologists are in the best position to judge when the patient will need dialysis. Limiting delays in catheter placement gives the nephrologist more control over initiation of dialysis and avoids unnecessarily early catheter placement. In addition, catheter insertion by nephrologists generates enthusiasm for PD through patient education and stimulates interest in PD in general.

The techniques described herein are applicable to PD catheter placement in the outpatient setting. In a recent study, one center moved away from a surgical technique because of delays in scheduling and lengthy hospital stays to a radiologic technique that performed outpatient PD catheter placement at the same level of convenience as obtaining a tunneled dialysis catheter. This facilitated a more planned outpatient PD initiation for most patients in their study and resulted in meeting best practice guidelines for a timely start of PD.[6] Radiological insertion plus assistance from a dedicated nurse coordinator allowed patients to have both PD catheter insertion and PD training without a hospital admission.

According to Center for Medicare and Medicaid Services data for 2007, 2.3% of PD catheters are placed by nephrologists, compared to 5.3% by interventional radiologists and 87.2% by surgical specialties.[7] A recent study examined the residency training of surgeons in placing peritoneal dialysis catheters based on the response to a questionnaire by residency program directors.[8] Most residents placed only two to five PD catheters during their training. The major obstacle to more experience in PD catheter placement according to program directors in this study was lack of referrals from nephrologists.

Patients started on PD each year belong to programs of varying sizes. Eighty percent of PD centers in the cohorts analyzed by Mujais and Story[9] had fewer than 20 patients. The number of new patients per year correlated with center size with 55% of centers starting less than five patients per year. Another 22% of PD programs start between 5 and 10 patients annually. Thus, 77% of PD programs initiate 10 or fewer patients per year on PD. These data indicate that proficiency in PD catheter placement for the majority of centers, whether for surgeons or interventionalists, may be limited by a paucity of placement opportunities. The referral of more patients for PD benefits not only the patients, but also improves the proficiency of all practitioners who place the catheters.

▶ Types of Peritoneal Dialysis Catheters

It is important to note that the method of catheter placement has a greater impact on the outcome of PD than does choice of catheter.[10,11] None of the most commonly used catheters are free from complications. Conditions other than catheter design contribute to complications, especially the care directed to the exit site and the technique used for catheter placement.[11] PD catheters are made of either silicone or polyurethane, with most being made of silicone. Only one type of catheter, the Cruz catheter, is actually made of polyurethane. Silicone has the advantage of being less irritating to the peritoneum and more flexible over a wide range of temperatures. Polyurethane catheters are thinner but have a tendency to break if alcohol or polyethylene glycol is applied to them.[12] Additionally, the glue that holds the cuff to the polyurethane catheter can fail within 2 years resulting in leaks and infections.[13]

The intraperitoneal segment of the catheter comes in four basic designs (Figure 44-1): straight (Tenckhoff), coiled (Tenckhoff), straight with silicone discs (Toronto Western Hospital, TWH), and T-fluted (Ash Advantage®).[13] Variations in the intraperitoneal segment have been designed in an attempt to diminish outflow obstruction either by preventing the peritoneal surfaces from occluding the side holes (coiled Tenckhoff) or by preventing omental entrapment (TWH, Ash Advantage), tip migration (coiled Tenckhoff), and outward migration of the catheter (Ash Advantage). Additionally, coiled catheters cause less discomfort by minimizing the jet effect caused by rapid inflow of dialysate. Studies suggest that coiled catheters do

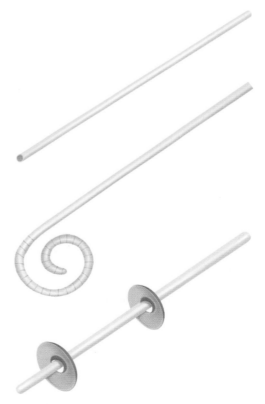

Figure 44-1. Intraperitoneal catheter design from top: straight Tenckhoff, coiled Tenckhoff, Toronto-Western Hospital catheter with silicone discs.

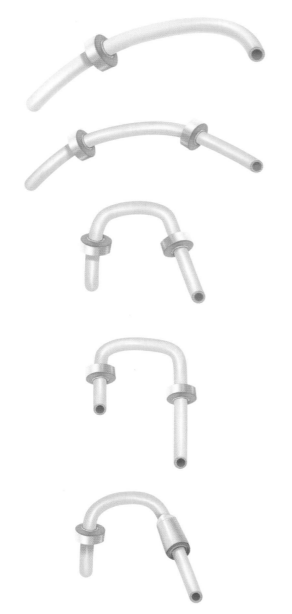

Figure 44-2. Extra-peritoneal catheter design from top: straight with single cuff, straight with double cuff, swan neck with two cuffs; Cruz catheter with pail handle design; swan neck with Moncrief-Popovich modification of elongated superficial cuff.

better than straight catheters in terms of minimizing tip migration (leading to drainage failure) and are associated with better catheter survival.[14,15]

The extraperitoneal segment of the catheter has either a Dacron cuff or a disc bead with or without a second Dacron cuff (Figure 44-2). These serve to hold the catheter in position. The cuff induces a mild local inflammatory response with subsequent fibrosis that serves to anchor the catheter and prevent leaks. It also prevents bacterial migration either from the exit site or from the peritoneum into the subcutaneous tunnel. Double cuffed catheters have been shown to minimize exit site/tunnel infections and peritonitis;[10,11,13,16] however, the single cuff catheter can have good

results when that cuff is placed in a deep (within the rectus muscle) rather than a superficial position. When placed in this manner, the outcomes are essentially comparable to the two cuffed straight Tenckhoff catheters.[12,17]

The subcutaneous segment (between rectus muscle and exit site) of the extra-peritoneal segment has been generally designed to direct the catheter in a lateral or downward direction toward the exit site thereby minimizing exit site infection. There are three basic shapes for this portion of the catheter: straight, "swan neck" with a 150° bend, and "pail handle" with two 90° bends (Cruz catheter).[10] Studies suggest that there is no difference in exit site infections between the swan-neck and straight catheters[18]; however, the swan neck catheter appears to have a lower incidence of cuff extrusion and pericatheter leakage.[19] The swan-neck catheter can be extended using a titanium connector to exit onto the chest wall, an advantage in obese patients, those with abdominal stoma, children with recurrent exit site infections and those in diapers.

▶ **Preoperative Evaluation**

The preoperative assessment should include a history, physical exam, and laboratory evaluation (CBC, blood group, PT/PTT, INR). Previous abdominal surgeries or attempts at catheter placement should raise the question of whether the patient has anatomic barriers to percutaneous placement. Those patients with an extensive history of abdominal surgeries should be referred for laparoscopic placement of the catheter. The physical exam should focus on the presence of abdominal hernias or abdominal wall weakness. Careful attention should be paid to hepatosplenomegaly, an enlarged bladder, or a pelvic mass such as that caused by uterine fibroids.

With the patient supine and wearing clothing so as to identify the belt line, select and mark the exit site to be used for the catheter with a marker that will not be removed by the surgical preparation (Figure 44-3). The exit site should be either above or below the belt line and away from scars. Observe the patient sitting and standing to identify folds of the abdominal wall or sites where pressure might be applied during daily activity. The exit site should be directed laterally and downward when using a swan-neck catheter or laterally when the catheter does not have a preformed bend. It should never be directed in an upward direction; this will increase the risk for exit site infection. The exit site should be easily visualized by the patient. Obese patients or those with stomas or excessive abdominal folds may be better served with a presternal catheter that places the exit site onto the chest.

Anticoagulant therapy (low-molecular-weight heparin, warfarin) should be held for 24 hours prior to catheter placement. When this is done, a bleeding rate of only 2% has been reported.[20] PD catheter placement can be safely performed in patients on low dose aspirin therapy.[21,22] Screening for nasal colonization of methicillin-resistant staphylococcus aureus (MRSA) allows identification of carriers and treatment in order to reduce the rate of exit

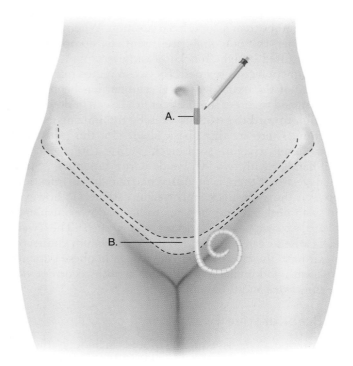

Figure 44-3. Locate insertion site by placing the tip of the catheter at pubic symphysis and extending deep cuff lateral to umbilicus. Mark at deep cuff for incision. (Modified from Crabtree.[38])

site and tunnel infections.[23,24] Some physicians prefer to insert a Foley catheter into the bladder the morning of the procedure to prevent urinary retention from incomplete voiding and assist with early detection of inadvertent placement of the PD catheter into the bladder. However, this is considered optional. There are reports of percutaneous PD catheters being placed without complication in absence of bladder catheterization. Bowel evacuation has been recommended.[12] The use of prophylactic antibiotics with a first- or second-generation cephalosporin reduces the risk of peritonitis and exit site infections.[12,24,25] Routine use of vancomycin should be avoided to prevent the development of vancomycin-resistant enterococcus (VRE).[12] The patient should shower the morning of the procedure. Abdominal hair should be clipped if present.

▶ **Placement of the Catheter**

Choice of insertion site

The risk of a catheter leak can be minimized by observing two issues: insertion of the deep cuff in the paramedian position relative to the umbilicus and insuring that the deep cuff is tunneled into the rectus muscle. The left side of the abdomen is usually selected for convenience because most operators are right handed. Peristaltic movements can cause migration of the catheter into the right upper quadrant, a complication seen in 15–30% of insertions. This is more likely to happen when the catheter tip

is positioned in the right iliac fossa.[3,26,27] Some studies have shown that when a catheter with an exit site on the right side of the abdomen has its tip implanted in the left iliac fossa, there is a decreased tendency for it to migrate.[27]

Commonly, a site 2–4 cm to the left of and either below (caudal) or above (cephalad) the level of the umbilicus is selected for catheter insertion.[28–33] The optimal location can be determined in reference to the pubic symphysis. This has been confirmed laparoscopically to be a reliable landmark for positioning the catheter tip within the true pelvis.[34,35] With the tip of the catheter at the pubic symphysis, place the deep cuff 2–4 cm to the left of the umbilicus and mark this site as the point for the incision, as shown in Figure 44-3.

Incision and blunt dissection

After infiltrating the skin and underlying tissue with 2% lidocaine with epinephrine, make a horizontal incision 3–4 cm long to expose the subcutaneous tissue (obese individuals may need an appropriately longer incision). Open the subcutaneous tissue using blunt dissection until the shiny anterior rectus sheath is seen. All bleeding vessels must be ligated or cauterized. Infiltrate the rectus sheath, rectus muscle, and peritoneum with local anesthetic (aspirate the needle as it is withdrawn to ascertain that the epigastric artery is not in its path).

The above steps are common to the fluoroscopic and peritoneoscopic techniques of catheter placement. The steps unique to each technique are described below.

Fluoroscopic catheter insertion Materials needed for catheter insertion under fluoroscopic guidance include sequential dilators from 10 French to 16 French, an 18 French dilator with a peel-away sheath (Figure 44-4), an 18 gauge blunt tip needle and a double-cuffed swan-neck PD catheter with a coiled tip (Figure 44-5). Additionally, we use components of a Y-TEC® pac, which

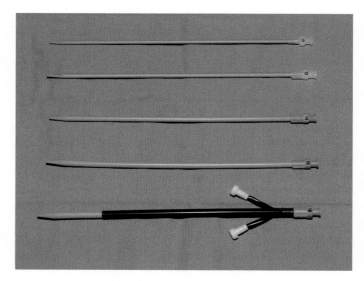

Figure 44-4. Cook 20-cm dilators used in PD Catheter implantation. Diameter is 10 French to 18 French. The 18 French dilator has the Peel-Away® Introducer.

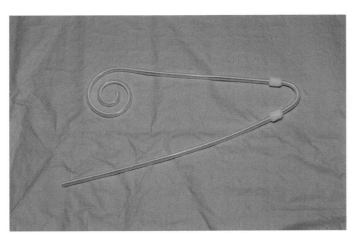

Figure 44-5. Photograph of 62.5-cm double-cuffed swan-neck peritoneal dialysis catheter with coiled tip.

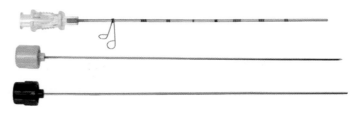

Figure 44-7. Hawkins™ blunt needle by Angiotech.

Angiotech is 18 gauge × 10 cm that comes with a blunt tip stylette is ideal for this purpose (Figure 44-7).

After the optimal site has been selected and the incision has been made as described above, insert the blunt needle with stylette in place at an angle of not more than 45°, directed toward the lower pelvis (Figure 44-8). It is important that the needle enter the peritoneal cavity 2–3 cm caudal to (below) the entry into the rectus sheath. Tunneling the catheter within the rectus sheath at this angle helps to minimize catheter migration within the pelvis (Figure 44-9). Confirm the location of the needle within the peritoneal cavity by removing the stylette and injecting 3–5 mL of radiocontrast. If the needle is placed correctly, radiocontrast will be observed lining the outer contour of the bowel (Figure 44-10). A smudge at the needle tip indicates that the needle tip is still within the rectus sheath and not the peritoneal cavity. In this case, the stylette should be replaced and the needle advanced further. Observation of a scaffolding pattern (bowel lumen pattern) with the radiocontrast injection indicates that the needle tip has penetrated the bowel lumen. Perforation of the bowel with the blunt needle has minimal risk of peritonitis; however, if perforation is observed or suspected the best option is to abandon the procedure and administer broad-spectrum antibiotics for 24 hours.

When the radiocontrast image indicates that the needle tip is correctly positioned within the peritoneum, insert a 0.035 inch (150 cm length) guide wire through the needle while observing its course under fluoroscopy. The goal is to insert enough guide wire to create a large loop within the pelvis (Figure 44-11). The formation of this loop

includes the Quill® guide assembly, a small and large dilator, a Tunnelor® tool, and a Cuff Implantor® (Figure 44-6). A 62-cm stylette passed within the catheter can aid in implanting the cuff in the rectus muscle.

When performing fluoroscopic catheter insertion, gaining access to the peritoneal cavity is facilitated by utilizing real-time ultrasound guidance.[31,32] This allows one to measure the distance from the skin to the peritoneal cavity. Color Doppler can be used to locate the epigastric and hypogastric vessels, minimizing the risk of injury to these vessels.[31]

Use of either a small (21 gauge) or blunt needle to access the peritoneum minimizes the risk of bowel perforation.[28] We feel that an 18 gauge blunt tip needle is optimal. With this device, a "pop and give" can be felt upon entry into the peritoneal space. Additionally, this needle's size allows for the standard guide wire (0.035 inch) to be passed directly into the peritoneal cavity. This precludes the necessity of using a micropuncture needle and guide wire as an intermediary step. The Hawkins™ blunt needle made by

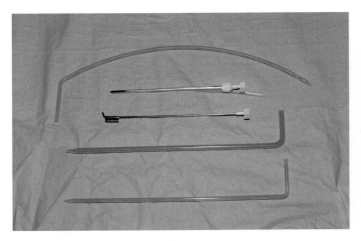

Figure 44-6. Y-TEC® pac contains from top to bottom: Tunnelor® tool, Quill® guide assembly, cuff implantor®, large dilator, small dilator.

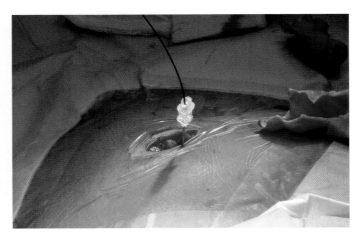

Figure 44-8. Blunt tipped needle in rectus sheath with a wire.

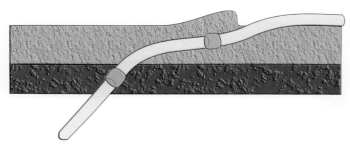

Figure 44-9. Deep cuff of catheter in rectus sheath and 2–3 cm of catheter tunneled in rectus to maintain tip in pelvis.

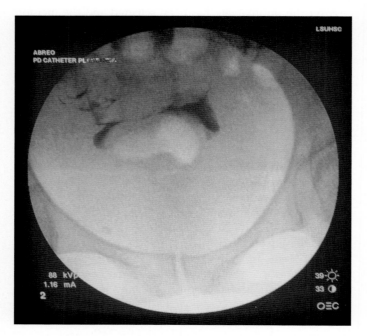

Figure 44-10. Fluoroscopy image of radiocontrast lining the outer contour of the bowel.

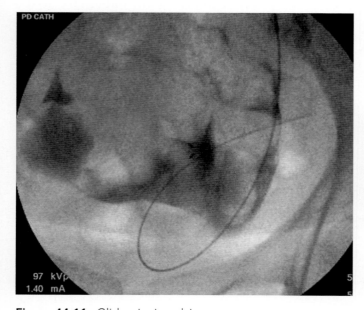

Figure 44-11. Glide wire in pelvis.

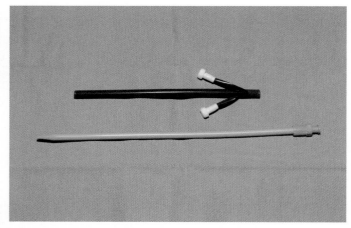

Figure 44-12. Detail of Cook 18-French dilator with Peel-Away® Introducer.

demonstrates that the guide wire is lying free within the peritoneal cavity.

The next step is to sequentially dilate the rectus sheath, rectus muscle, deep fascia and the peritoneal membrane using 10 French to 18 French dilators passed over the guide wire. The final dilator (18 French) is inserted along with a peel-away sheath (Figure 44-12) which is left in place when this dilator is removed (Figure 44-13). Advance the PD catheter over the guide wire through the peel-away sheath. A radio-opaque line on the PD catheter allows for confirmation of its position in the lower pelvis (Figure 44-14). By watching this line, one can also be assured that the catheter is not twisted during insertion. The catheter can be rotated and moved at this point to ensure that the "pigtail" portion is located within the pelvis. After removal of the guide wire, radiocontrast can be injected into the catheter for better visualization. Infuse 1 L of PD fluid into the abdomen through the catheter and then allow it to drain in order to evaluate its function. Inflow should be rapid and pain free and outflow should be a fast drip or stream that increases with deep inspiration. If necessary, the catheter can be repositioned using a metal stylette until optimum function is achieved.

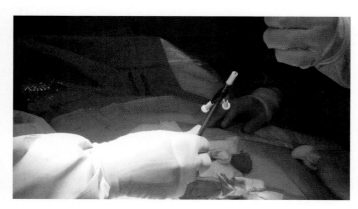

Figure 44-13. Dilator with a peel away sheath in place.

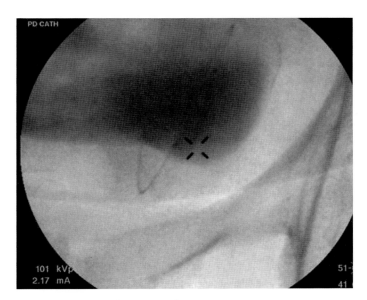

Figure 44-14. Catheter in pelvis.

Bury the deep cuff into the rectus muscle using the Cuff Implantor® while stabilizing the catheter on the stylette.[30] Alternatively, a set of nontraumatic forceps can be used to push the cuff through the rectus sheath into the muscle. Withdraw the peel-away sheath slowly, ensuring that the cuff stays within the rectus muscle.[31,32] Holding the cuff in place with the blunt forceps, while the peel-away sheath is removed, helps prevent its dislodgement. Removing the sheath then manipulating the cuff into the rectus muscle is also an effective way to implant the cuff. Some operators place an absorbable suture through the deep cuff and the outer rectus sheath and subcutaneous tissues once the cuff is buried in the rectus muscle to anchor the cuff.[29,33]

Peritoneoscopic catheter placement The Y-TEC® System itself is composed of reusable instruments (2.2 mm diameter endoscope, fiberoptic light guide, sterilization tray, and a fiberoptic light source) and a choice of two disposable catheter implantation kits, referred to as "pacs" by Y-Tec. This system and procedure can be used to implant almost all PD catheters including the Flex-Neck®, Swan-Neck™, and conventional catheters. (The Toronto Western™ and Missouri Swan-Neck™ catheters cannot be implanted with this technique.)

Peritoneoscopic placement is performed under local anesthesia using a single puncture site for the Quill® Catheter Guide[36] through which the scope is inserted; this later becomes the pathway for insertion of the catheter. The Quill® Catheter Guide is an assembly consisting of three parts: a trocar that is fitted and locked into a metal cannula and an outer sheath (the Quill sheath).

In order to perform the procedure, firstly select the optimal site as described above and make the incision. Once the rectus sheath is identified, infiltrate the muscle with more lidocaine. Ask the patient to tighten his/her abdominal muscles in preparation for inserting the Quill® Catheter

Guide assembly. Just as with the fluoroscopic catheter placement, it is important to orient the catheter toward the pelvis. The catheter guide assembly should enter the rectus sheath at a 30 degree directed toward the coccyx. Peritoneal entry should be felt with a giveaway sensation at entry into the peritoneal cavity. Remove the trocar and place the patient in a Trendelenburg position. At this point, 700–1200 mL of air should be injected into the peritoneal cavity using a large syringe (comes in the kit) to allow optimal visualization with the peritoneoscope.

Bowel perforation has been described in <1% of trocar insertions into the peritoneal cavity using the technique as described. Although not generally done, insufflating the peritoneal cavity with air prior to trocar insertion can decrease the incidence of this complication even further. This can be achieved by introducing a blunt tip needle or Veress® insufflation needle into the peritoneal cavity followed by injection of air prior to trocar use.[28,37]

The Y-TEC® modified optic scope for peritoneoscopic catheter insertion, should be passed into the cannula, locked, the light guide snapped onto the scope and its location within the peritoneum should be visually confirmed. Every time the scope is passed into the cannula, it should be locked to the cannula prior to visualizing the peritoneal cavity. The goal of peritoneoscopy is twofold: first, to identify adhesions and omentum that would interfere with catheter function, and second, to advance the Quill guide assembly into the peritoneal cavity until the distal end is in the lower quadrant of the abdomen in an appropriate position for the tip of the dialysis catheter.

Peritoneoscopic examination of the peritoneal cavity ensures that one has entered the peritoneal cavity. It is very important that bowel surface be seen and its movement observed in conjunction with respiration to verify that the scope is within the peritoneal cavity. If there is no movement, the scope should be withdrawn slowly while asking the patient to take deep breaths until back-and-forth bowel movement is observed; this confirms that the Quill guide is in the proper intraperitoneal position. Once the placement is confirmed, withdraw the scope from the cannula and inject air (if not done earlier). Distending the abdomen with air is necessary to separate the abdominal wall from the viscera and provide space for visualization with the peritoneoscope. Approximately 1.5 L of air is considered optimal. Once the abdomen has been appropriately distended, replace the scope and lock it to the cannula with the light source attached. Reactivate the light source and slowly advance the scope along with the Quill guide in a caudal direction under direct visualization through the scope. This allows for adhesions or other intra-abdominal features that might affect catheter function to be avoided. Once the assembly has been advanced to the point desired for catheter tip placement, remove the scope leaving the Quill assembly in place. The patient can now be returned to the normal supine position.

The next step is to remove the cannula, leaving the Quill sheath in place. The Quill sheath and the cannula are attached with a wrapping of tape. To remove the cannula, the plastic tab of the Quill is grasped with a pair of hemostats and a second pair of hemostats is used to remove the tape using a winding motion. While continuing to grasp the tab of the Quill sheath, remove the cannula using a slight twisting/rotating motion. The Quill sheath must be maintained in the same location where the scope had directed it. After each has been lubricated with gel, insert the dilators into the Quill sheath starting with the smaller 4.8 mm one followed by the 6.4 mm dilator.

Choose a stylette of appropriate length and prepare the catheter for insertion by placing it onto the stylette using sterile gel or saline. The tip of the catheter should be even with that of the stylette for proper insertion. The catheter is marked with a white (radio-opaque) line that runs its entire length. This line should be used for catheter orientation during insertion. The line should be aligned to assure that the catheter is not twisted or rotated on its axis as it is advanced. Carefully insert the catheter with the stylette through the Quill sheath while it is carefully anchored in position using the attached hemostats. A catheter should have its white stripe at the 12 o'clock position when placed on the left and at the 6 o'clock when placed on right. It is important for the catheter to follow the Quill sheath through the rectus muscle and into the desired location while its tip is maintained in the desired position within the peritoneal cavity. Once the catheter has advanced through the Quill sheath to the desired position, carefully withdraw (only partially) the stylette releasing the catheter into the peritoneal cavity. The tip of the stylette should be kept within the abdomen to help place the catheter cuff through the rectus muscle. The operator should make certain that the catheter does not appear doubled on itself, kinked, or twisted when viewed on fluoroscopy.

To bury the internal cuff, position the Y-TEC® Cuff Implantor® parallel with and over the catheter between the two cuffs. Gently advance the catheter and Cuff Implantor simultaneously through the Quill sheath until the inner cuff has passed through the sheath and into the rectus muscle. This determination can be made by direct observation of the cuff. While maintaining the position of the cuff within the muscle, gently retract the Quill sheath using the attached hemostats until it is out. While carefully holding the catheter in position, slide the Cuff Implantor upward toward the outer cuff and remove it from the catheter. Gently remove the stylette from the catheter while anchoring the catheter in place with the opposite hand.[23,31]

At this point, 500–1500 mL of PD fluid can be infused into the abdominal cavity to test catheter function. There should be no pain on infusion, no entry of PD fluid into the Foley bag, and no diarrhea to suggest perforation of the bladder or colon respectively. PD fluid should return briskly as a stream or rapid drip from the external end of the catheter.

Exit site and superficial cuff (both techniques)

The location of the exit site should be determined as described above. The swan neck catheter is best suited for the location of the exit site on the lower abdomen and the straight catheter for exit sites on the upper abdomen. Patients who are obese, have abdominal stomas, are incontinent of urine or feces, or who desire to take a deep tub bath will benefit from an extended catheter system that allows for an exit site located on the upper abdomen or chest, as shown in Figure 44-15.[38,39]

After local anesthesia, make a stab wound at the site selected for the catheter exit. Insert a tunneling device or a Kelly clamp into the stab incision and tunnel through the subcutaneous tissue toward the earlier incision to engage or grasp the catheter tip. Pull the catheter through the tunnel and out the exit site.[28,30,31] The external cuff should be located in the subcutaneous tissues approximately 2 cm from the exit site.

Wound closure

Close the subcutaneous tissue of the primary incision with absorbable sutures and the skin with nonabsorbable

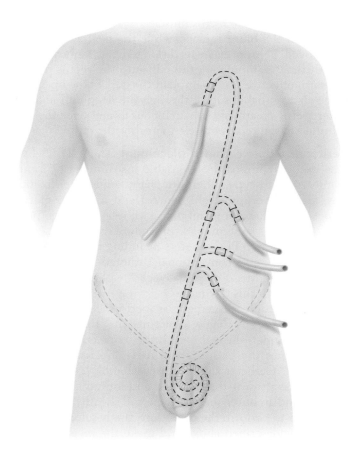

Figure 44-15. Potential exit sites for Tenckhoff catheter. (Modified Reference 38.)

sutures.[30] The exit site should not be sutured, as this may lead to an exit site infection.[29] The two cuffs provide sufficient anchoring to prevent the catheter from being dislodged. Heparin (7000 units) should be instilled into the catheter after the connectors have been attached.

▶ Postoperative Management

After catheter placement, the patient's vital signs should be monitored to assure their stability. Some centers perform this procedure on an outpatient basis with the patient returning home 4–6 hours postprocedure, whereas others prefer to observe the patient in the hospital overnight.[40] The exit site and surgical incision should be covered with sterile gauze and a nonocclusive dressing. Advise the patient to minimize contact with the catheter and surgical incisions until the wounds have healed and the tunnel has matured. The catheter should be taped securely and remain immobile when not in use. After discharge, a PD nurse should evaluate the patient each week and perform a low volume exchange with 1 L of 1.5% dextrose (Dianeal) to test the function of the catheter. Patient education concerning PD and appropriate catheter use should begin. Full volume exchanges can begin in 2–3 weeks after catheter placement.[41] Patients should avoid baths that immerse the exit site and swimming in lakes, rivers, or public baths.[41]

Beginning PD before the deep cuff has matured increases the risk of leakage. If the patient requires dialysis immediately following the procedure, low volume exchanges are preferred. This will spare the patient the need for a central venous catheter. However, the patient should remain supine during catheter use to avoid pericatheter leakage.[41]

▶ Complications of Catheter Placement

The incidence of complications following PD catheter insertion depends largely upon the skill and experience of the operator. Current clinical practice guidelines for peritoneal access recommend a yearly audit of PD catheter insertion with a view toward achieving a 1 year patency rate of >80%.[5,12] The percutaneous method of catheter placement has low complication rates when performed by experienced operators (Table 44-1).

Complications after PD catheter placement may be defined as either early, those occurring less than 30 days after surgery or late, those occurring more than 30 days after catheter placement.

Early complications

Early complications include bowel perforations, bleeding, leakage of dialysate, catheter dysfunction, and infection. Although not common, it is important that these be recognized and managed appropriately.

Bowel and bladder perforations are not common; a number of studies report no occurrences. With the percutaneous technique, it is possible to perforate the bowel with the micro-puncture needle if this device is used. This will generally become apparent immediately and in this instance, the needle should be withdrawn and the patient given broad spectrum antibiotics intravenously overnight. No further therapy is indicated since the small diameter of the needle will not leave a defect and the muscular wall closes over this puncture very quickly.[50] If the patient remains afebrile, the procedure can be attempted again the following day.

The occurrence of small tears in the bowel wall caused by larger instruments during placement is infrequent, but the consequences of perforation are serious and could potentially require surgery. Perforations are generally small and can spontaneously seal on their own.[50,51] Conservative treatment of these tears is generally adequate to prevent overt peritonitis.[51–53] The signs of perforation during a procedure include the emanation of foul smelling gas from the needle or cannula, return of bowel contents through the cannula, and peritoneoscopic visualization of the bowel lumen. In one retrospective study of 750 PD catheter placements over a period of 12 years, the authors found only six incidents of bowel perforation.[52] Five of these were managed conservatively and four of these were discharged home after 3 days. One case developed signs of peritoneal irritation, fever, and peritonitis and required surgery. The final patient developed peritonitis the day after the procedure and also required surgery.

When a perforation is suspected, the patient should be made NPO to keep the bowel at rest. Broad-spectrum antibiotics such as vancomycin, gentamicin, and metronidazole covering gram positive, gram negative, and anaerobic organisms should be administered. The patient should be followed with serial abdominal examinations. If the patient is clinically stable without signs of peritonitis, then on the second day, a clear liquid diet can be started. If the patient does not have signs of peritonitis on the third day, the patient can be discharged home on oral antibiotics for 10 days. If during the 3 days following the procedure the patient deteriorates clinically, surgery should be consulted.[52]

Bleeding is rarely a significant problem after catheter implantation and usually occurs at the exit site. Blood may be present initially in the effluent drained, owing to the trauma of insertion, but the drainage should return to normal within few days. Manual pressure or additional suturing can stop persistent bleeding. Hematomas and bleeding can occur when the epigastric vessels are perforated. Using ultrasound to visualize these vessels significantly reduces the risk of this complication.[26]

Leakage of dialysate occurs when the deep cuff either is displaced or does not form a fibrotic reaction within the rectus muscle. Treatment of leakage involves resting the peritoneum for 2 days–3 weeks while the patient is temporarily on hemodialysis, if necessary. Alternatively, the patient can undergo low volume exchanges immediately after catheter placement, preferably with the patient in the supine position. Leakage occurred in 3–8% of percutaneous placements, with one study showing a 23% leakage rate (see Table 44-1).

TABLE 44–1

Summary of Complications of Catheter Placement

Source	No. of Catheters	Infection	Drainage Problem	Migration	Leak	Perforation	Success
Fluoroscopy/ Percutaneous							
Moon[42]	134 caths/ 114 pts	Early peritonitis 2.2%	1.5%	1.5%	3%	0	1 yr. 80% 2 yr. 74.9% 5 yr 71.1%
Zaman[30]	36 caths	0	2.9%	3%	3%	0	1 m. 100%; 3 m. 97%; 1 yr. 89%
Vaux[32]	209	Early exit site 6.5%; Early peritonitis 1.5%	5%	7%	5%	0	1 yr 77%; 2 yr 61%; 5 yr 31%
Maya[31]	32	0		3%	0	3%	27 mos. 90.6%
Jacob[28]	45	Total peritonitis 7%	13.3%	11%	9%	4.4%	
Peritoneoscope							
Goh[3]	91	1 in 93.7 pt mos	17.6%	9.8%			1 yr 86.4%
Gadallah[43]	76	Early peritonitis 2.6% Late infection 48.7%	Early 7.9% Late 7.9%		Early 1.3%	Colon 1.3%	1 yr 77.5% 2 yr 63% 3 yr 51.3%
Percutaneous							
Henderson[44]	283	Early peritonitis 4% (30 days)	21%		6%		1 mo 87%; 6 mo. 83%
Perakis[45]	86	Early peritonitis 4.3 per 1000 pt mo.; early exit site 1.6 per 1000 pt mo.	23.2% (10.7 per 1000 pt mo)	15.1%	23%	0	1 yr 89.5%; 2 yr 83.7%; 3 yr 83.7%
Ozener[46]	133	Early cath related Infection 3%	11.2%	8.2%	8.3%	0	1 yr 90% 2 yr 82%
Surgery/ Laparoscopy							
Henderson[44]	150	Early peritonitis 13% (30 days)	23%		10%		
Maio[47]	100		6%	6%	13%		1 yr 97% 2 yr 95% 3 yr 91%
Perakis[45]	84	Early peritonitis 10.1 per 1000 pt mo; early exit site 6.3 per 1000 pt mo	29.7% (7.9 per 1000 Pt mo)	28.6%	13%		1 yr 91.1%; 2 yr 80.7%; 3 yr 73.2%
Crabtree[35]	200		0.5%		2%		
Keshvari[48]	175		8.5%	1.7%	7.4%	0	1 yr 92.7% 2 yr 91.3%
Ataluri[49] (advanced technique)	129		4.6%	0	0.51%	0	1 yr 100%
Surgery/ Dissection							
Ozener[46]	82	Early cath related Infection 2%	19.5%	13.4%	6.1%		1 yr 73% 2 yr 60%
Gadallah[43]	72	Early Peritonitis 12.5% Late Infection 48.6%	Early 8.3% Late 11.1%		Early 11.1%	Bladder 1.4%	1 yr 62.5% 2 yr 41.5% 3 yr 36%

Catheter dysfunction may occur early. This entails drainage problems due to migration of the catheter, omental wrapping, or obstruction. Placing the catheter by the percutaneous method using fluoroscopic guidance can result in obstruction by omentum or adhesions. The laparoscopic technique offers an advantage in this regard because the omentum in the pelvis can be tacked to the abdominal wall or removed and adhesions can be lysed. Migration of the catheter tip is caused by peristaltic movement of the bowel that moves the catheter tip into the right upper quadrant. One report noted that placement of the catheter on the right side of the abdomen with the tip in the left iliac fossa reduced the incidence of catheter migration.[27] With migration, the dialysate will easily fill the peritoneum but will not drain. This has occurred in up to 15% of percutaneous procedures and up to 28% in laparoscopic procedures.[45] Migration can be related to constipation, and initial treatment should be laxatives to stimulate the bowel. Other treatments for migration are fluoroscopic manipulation, catheter replacement, or surgical salvage procedures.[54] Some research has shown that the swan-neck catheter design reduces the incidence of tip migration.[12] Inflow dysfunction is often related to fibrin or clot in the catheter. This can be treated with forceful infusion of dialysate followed by thrombolytics if necessary.

Leakage of dialysate can be deducted with fluid drainage from the exit site or with the appearance of a bulge underneath the entrance site. Causes of leaks may be due to hernia at the entrance site as a result of very large incision, positioning of the proximal cuff on the rectus muscle, and trauma. Catheter rest without dialysate instillation for some weeks is most likely to solve this problem. Temporary HD treatment is usually required.

The reported incidence of early peritonitis ranged from 1.5% to 4%.[32,42–44] If this complication is due to poor surgical technique, it should be seen within the first 2 weeks following catheter placement.[5] If the peritoneal fluid becomes cloudy, associated with pain, then the dialysate should be cultured and appropriate antibiotics must be administered. Eradication of nasal staphylococcus carriers by mupirocin and antibiotic prophylaxis with vancomycin may substantially decrease the rate of early peritonitis.[55]

Late complications

Late complications (>30 days) include exit-site infection, tunnel infection, cuff protrusion, outflow failure, and dialysate leaks or hernias.

An exit site infection is culture positive inflammation external to the cuff and is characterized by some combination of induration, erythema, and drainage from the site where the catheter exits the skin. This is one of the most frequent complications of PD catheters in general. Studies have reported a rate of early exit site infections ranging from 0% to 6.5% using the percutaneous method.[30–32] Directing the exit site laterally or inferiorly has been shown to reduce its occurrence. Additionally, use of an antibiotic cream at the exit site, either mupirocin to prevent gram-positive infections or gentamicin to prevent gram-positive and gram-negative infections, will reduce the occurrence of both exit site infections and peritonitis.[56,57] Modifying the swan-neck catheter to a presternal exit site location has shown an increase in access survival up to 95% at 2 years and also a decrease in both exit site infections and peritonitis.[58]

Outflow failure beyond 30 days is frequently due to constipation and may be relieved by administering a laxative. Leaks and hernias may occur and become symptomatic because of the increased intra-abdominal pressure, secondary to the dialysate. Leaks can also result from umbilical hernias or the presence of a patent processus vaginalis, resulting in scrotal edema. Surgical repair of hernias or processus vaginalis may be indicated with a temporary shift to HD for adequate wound healing.

Infection is the most serious and frequently occurring complication associated with a PD catheter in this late period. This may be classified as an exit site infection, tunnel infection, or peritonitis. The exit site infection is as has been described above. These must be treated promptly to avoid extension of the infection into the tunnel and the possibility of eventually leading to peritonitis.

Tunnel infection is characterized by erythema, edema, and tenderness over the subcutaneous tract of the PD catheter. This may co-exist with an exit site infection. If the internal cuff is also involved, catheter removal may be necessary. Detection of the presence and the extent of this infection may be aided by the use of ultrasound examination. Fluid around the catheter and fluid around the internal cuff is diagnostic given the typical signs of inflammation. Early diagnosis and prompt treatment with appropriate antibiotics based upon cultures is critical.

Peritonitis is a major problem for patients on PD and the primary complication leading to the patients needing to switch to HD. Peritonitis often results from contamination with skin bacteria. In addition, gram-negative bacteria, associated with diarrhea or diverticulitis, may be the problem. The clinical picture of the patient with PD-associated peritonitis is typical. Patients complain of abdominal pain, sometimes accompanied with fever. The PD fluid white blood cell counts and cultures may reveal leucocytes and bacteria. Systemic or intraperitoneal antibiotics, according to the cultured organisms, should be administered. In most cases, the peritonitis resolves after proper treatment; however, with persistent infection, catheter removal and shift to HD for 4–6 weeks may be required.

▶ Comparison with Surgical Techniques

Current laparoscopic placement procedures allow surgical correction of visualized defects during the placement procedure. The surgeon can repair hernias, perform adhesiolysis, and minimize contact with redundant omentum by performing omentopexy. Both laparoscopic and percutaneous procedures have low complication rates when performed by experienced operators. Patients should be referred for laparoscopic catheter placement when they are obese, have had complicated abdominal surgery, or have had repeated episodes of peritonitis that would cause adhesions. Some have argued that comparing complication rates between the two procedures is flawed because there is a selection bias in favor of less challenging subjects for the percutaneous approach. The results of the laparoscopic procedure should be viewed in light of the fact that in some studies the laparoscopic subjects are more challenging.[59] Overall, the complication rate is lower for the percutaneous method. The 1-year survival rate of catheters is lowest for catheters placed surgically by the dissection method, but highest for catheters placed by the laparoscopic method. The 1-year survival for laparoscopic placement is slightly better than that of the percutaneous method (Table 44-1).

Embedded Peritoneal Dialysis Catheters

Typically, the catheter is exteriorized at the time of implantation and the patient undergoes a 2-week "break-in" period in which the device is flushed weekly. By allowing 2 weeks for the cuffs to mature, dialysate leakage and periluminal migration of bacteria are minimized. However, it is difficult to judge the appropriate time to implant the catheter in order to allow for this 2-week period before it is time for the patient to start dialysis. This problem can be avoided by embedding or burying the catheter at the time of implantation and then exteriorizing it when it is time to start dialysis, a technique first described by Moncrief et al.[60]

This embedding technique was accomplished by first making a 2–3-cm incision at the exit site and a creating a pouch created under the skin at the time of catheter implantation. The catheter was tied off with silk suture, coiled, and then placed into the pouch. The incision was then closed, to be opened in order to exteriorize the free end of the catheter for PD when needed. This allowed the cuffs to mature and was shown to reduce the incidence of leakage and peritonitis.[60] Episodes of peritonitis were reduced with occurrence of one episode per 29.4 patient months, compared to one episode per 9 patient months in historical controls (using a spike-bag exchange system). However, episodes of exit site infections occurred more frequently that had been observed in historical controls at a rate of one episode per 12.57 patient months. Although exit site infections were not decreased, this technique has been subsequently shown to lower rates of catheter infection and peritonitis as well as provide longer catheter life.[13,61] The benefit of reduced peritonitis may not be realized in centers that have lower peritonitis rates overall, likely from using the double bag Y connect system.[62]

Catheters embedded using a modified Y-Tec procedure or modified Moncrief-Popovich method in which the free end of the catheter is not coiled, but is subcutaneously embedded in a linear fashion have shown better results.[13] In one study, the first 30 catheters placed using this technique were all functional upon exteriorization after a period ranging from 3 to 12 months. This technique allows for placement of the PD catheter in patients with CKD 4 followed by a period of maturation in a manner very similar to that used for fistulas. Additionally, the patient is not required to maintain the exit site and catheter until the catheter is exteriorized at the discretion of the nephrologist.[13]

The University of Ottawa used a modified Moncrief technique to implant and embed PD catheters in a series of patients who were referred 3–6 months before their anticipated initiation on dialysis.[63] In this modified technique, a double-cuffed coiled catheter with an arcuate bend was placed laparoscopically. Then, an incision was made 2 cm longer than the length of the external portion of the catheter. The tunneling device was used to pull the catheter through the subcutaneous tissue, and the tip of the tunneler was left to plug the catheter. The skin was closed and the catheters remained embedded for at least 4 weeks. Exteriorization was performed by the nephrologist when dialysis was needed and training started.

Exteriorization involved making a 3–4 mm incision approximately 2 cm distal to the superficial cuff. Using blunt dissection, the catheter was exteriorized. It was then clamped; the distal end was removed and fitted with a titanium adapter. Using this technique, 304 catheters were embedded. The median time to exteriorization was 92 days, 85% had good initial flow, and 15% had obstruction with primary nonfunction observed in 7%. Exit site leaks occurred in 3%. Six percent had poor initial function that required salvage procedures.

The early placement of PD catheters should lead to improved utilization of PD by avoiding the bridging period of hemodialysis when renal function unexpectedly declines.

CONCLUSION

Patients who are obese, with a history of abdominal surgery, or with a history of repeated episodes of peritonitis should be referred to a capable surgeon for the laparoscopic placement of the catheter. For patients without these risk factors, percutaneous placement of peritoneal dialysis catheters by interventional nephrologists should be attempted. The complication rates for the percutaneous method are similar to those of laparoscopic procedures. This chapter summarizes the catheter types, preprocedure work-up, catheter placement technique, postprocedure care, and complications. Additionally, having an interventional nephrologist involved in the placement of PD catheters increases utilization of this modality of dialysis.

REFERENCES

1. U.S. Renal Data System, USRDS 2009 Annual Data Report: Atlas of chronic kidney disease and end-stage renal disease in the United States, National Institutes of Health, National Institute of Diabetes and Digestive and Kidney Diseases, Bethesda, MD, 2009. The data reported here have been supplied by the United States Renal Data System

(USRDS). The interpretation and reporting of these data are the responsibility of the authors and in no way should be seen as an official policy or interpretation of the U.S. government.

2. Asif, A, Pflederer TA, Vieira CF, Diego J, Roth D, Agarwal A. Does catheter insertion by nephrologists improve peritoneal dialysis utilization? A multicenter analysis, *Semin Dial.* 2005;18:157–160.

3. Goh BL, Ganeshadeva YM, Chew SE, Dalimi MS. Does peritoneal dialysis catheter insertion by interventional nephrologists enhance peritoneal dialysis penetration? *Semin Dial.* 2008;21:561–566.

4. Asif A. Peritoneal dialysis underutilization: the impact of an interventional nephrology peritoneal dialysis access program. *Semin Dial.* 2003;16:266–271.

5. Figueiredo A, Goh BL, Jenkins S, et al. Clinical practice guidelines for peritoneal access. *Perit Dial Int.* 2010;30: 424–429.

6. Brunier G, Hiller JA, Drayton S. A change to radiological peritoneal dialysis catheter insertion: three-month outcomes. *Perit Dial Int.* 2009;30:528–533.

7. Crabtree JH. Who should place peritoneal dialysis catheters? *Perit Dial Int.* 2010;30:142–150.

8. Wong LP, Liebman SE, Wakefield KA, Messing S. Training of surgeons in peritoneal dialysis catheter placement in the United States: a national survey. *Clin J Am Soc Nephrol.* 2010;5:1439–1446.

9. Mujais S, Story K. Peritoneal dialysis in the US: evaluation of outcomes in contemporary cohorts. *Kidney Int.* 2006;70:S21–S26.

10. Aquila RD, Chiaramonte S, Rodighiero MP, et al. Rational choice of peritoneal dialysis catheter. *Perit Dial Int.* 2007;27(S2):S119–S125.

11. Gokal R, Alexander S, Ash S, et al. Peritoneal catheters and exit site practice: toward optimum peritoneal access. *Perit Dial Int.* 1998;18:11–33.

12. Flanigan M, Gokal R. Peritoneal catheters and exit site practices toward optimum peritoneal access: a review of current developments. *Perit Dial Int.* 2005;25:132–139.

13. Ash SR. Chronic peritoneal dialysis catheters: overview of design, placement and removal procedures. *Semin Dial.* 2003;16(4):323–334.

14. Ates K, Karatan O, Erturk S, Erbay B, Duman N, Nergisoglu G, Ertug AE. Comparison between straight single cuff and curled double cuff catheters in patients on continuous ambulatory peritoneal dialysis. *Nephrol Dial Transplant.* 1996;11:914.

15. Nielsen PK, Hemmingsen C, Friis SU, Ladefoged J, Olgaard K. Comparison of straight and curled Tenckhoff peritoneal dialysis catheters implanted by percutaneous technique: a prospective randomized study. *Perit Dial Int.* 1995;15:18–21.

16. Thodis E, Passadakis P, Lyrantzopoou016 N, Panagoutsos S, Vargemezis V, Oreopoulos D. Peritoneal catheters and related infections. *Int Urol Nephrol.* 2005;37:379–393.

17. Eklund BH, Honkanen EO, Kyllonen LE, Salmela K, Kala AR. Peritoneal dialysis access: prospective randomized comparison of single cuff and double cuff straight Tenckhoff catheters. *Nephrol Dial Transplant.* 1997;12:2664–2666.

18. Eklund BH, Honkanen EO, Kyllonen LE. Peritoneal dialysis access: prospective randomized comparison of the Swan Neck and Tenckhoff Catheters. *Perit Dial Int.* 1995;15: 353–356.

19. Hwang T-L, Huang C-C. Comparison of Swan Neck catheter with Tenckhoff catheter for CAPD. *Adv Perit Dial.* 1994;10:203–205.

20. Mital S, Fried LF, Piraino B. Bleeding complications associated with peritoneal catheter insertion. *Perit Dial Int.* 2004;24:478–480.

21. Shpitz B, Plotkin E, Spindel Z, et al. Should aspirin therapy be withheld before insertion and/or removal of a permanent peritoneal dialysis catheter? *Am Surg.* 2002;68:762–764.

22. O'Connor SD, Taylor AJ, Williams EC, Winter TC. Coagulation concepts update. *Am J Roentgenol.* 2009;193:1656–1764.

23. Mupirocin Study Group. Nasal mupirocin prevents *Staphylococcus aureus* exit site infection during peritoneal dialysis. *J Am Soc Nephrol.* 1996;7:2403–2408.

24. Bonifati C, Pansini F, Torres DD, Navaneethan SD, Craig JC, Strippoli GF. Antimicrobial agents and catheter-related interventions to prevent peritonitis in peritoneal dialysis: using evidence in the context of clinical practice. *Int J Artif Organs.* 2006;29:41–49.

25. Wikdahl AM, Engman U, Stegmayr BG, Sorenssen JG. One dose cefuroxime i.v. and i.p reduces microbial growth in PD patients after catheter insertion. *Nephrol Dial Transplant.* 1997;12:157–160.

26. Goh, BL, Yudistra MG, Lim TO, Establishing learning curve for Tenckhoff catheter insertion by interventional nephrologist using CUSUM analysis: how many procedures and in which situation? *Semin Dial.* 2009;22:199–203.

27. Twardowski ZJ, Nolph KD, Khanna R, Prowant BF, Ryan LP, Nichols K. The need for a "swan neck" permanently bent, arcuate peritoneal dialysis catheter. *Perit Dial Bull.* 1985;5:219–223.

28. Jacobs IG, Gray RR, Elliott DS, Grosman H. Radiologic placement of peritoneal dialysis catheters: preliminary experience. *Radiology.* 1992;182:251–255.

29. Savader SJ, Geschwind JF, Lund GB, Scheel PJ. Percutaneous radiological placement of peritoneal dialysis catheters: long-term results. *J Vasc Interv Radiol.* 2000;11:965–970.

30. Zaman F, Pervez A, Atray NK, Murphy S, Work J, Abreo KD. Fluoroscopically-assisted placement of peritoneal dialysis catheters by nephrologists. *Semin Dial.* 2005;18:247–251.

31. Maya I. Ultrasound/fluoroscopy-assisted placement of peritoneal dialysis catheters. *Semin Dial.* 2007;20:611–615.

32. Vaux EC, Torrie PH, Barker LC, Naik RB, Gibson MR. Percutaneous fluoroscopically guided placement of peritoneal dialysis catheters: a 10-year experience. *Semin Dial.* 2008;21:459–465.

33. Rosenthal MA, Yang PS, Liu IA, Sim JJ, Kujubu DA, Rasgon SA, Yeoh HH, Abcar AC. Comparison of outcomes of peritoneal dialysis catheters placed by the fluoroscopically guided percutaneous method versus directly visualized surgical method. *J Vasc Interv Radiol.* 2008;19:1202–1207.

34. Twardowski ZJ. Peritoneal catheter placement and management. In: Massry SG, Suki WN, eds. *Therapy of Renal Disease and Related Disorders.* Dordrecht: Kluwer Academic; 1997:953–979.

35. Crabtree JH, Fishman A. A laparoscopic method for optimal peritoneal dialysis access. *Am Surg.* 2005;71:135–143.

36. Y-Tec Instructions: Laparoscopic & Peritoneoscopic Placement of Peritoneal Dialysis Catheters. © 2007 Available

at: http://www.medigroupinc.com/choosing-the-right-implantation-method-y-tec-system/y-tec-pd-catheter-implantation

37. Asif A, Tawakol J, Khan T, et al. Modification of the peritoneoscopic technique of peritoneal dialysis catheter insertion: experience of an interventional nephrology program. *Semin Dial.* 2004;17:171–173.

38. Crabtree JH. Selected best demonstrated practices in peritoneal dialysis access. *Kidney Int.* 2006;70:S27–S37.

39. Sreenarasimhaiah VP, Margassery SK, Martin KJ, Bander SJ. Percutaneous technique of presternal peritoneal dialysis catheter placement. *Semin Dial.* 2004;17:407–410.

40. Maya ID. Ambulatory setting for peritoneal dialysis catheter placement. *Semin Dial.* 2008;21:457–458.

41. Gokal R, Ash SR, Helfrich B, et al. Peritoneal catheters and exit-site practices: toward optimum peritoneal access. *Perit Dial Int.* 1993;13:29–39.

42. Moon J-Y, Sebin S, Jung K-H, et al. Fluoroscopically guided peritoneal dialysis catheter placement: long-term results from a single center. *Perit Dial Int.* 2008;28:163–169.

43. Gadallah MF, Pervez A, El-Shahawy MA, et al. Peritoneoscopic versus surgical placement of peritoneal dialysis catheters: a prospective randomized study on outcome. *Am J Kidney Dis.* 1999;33:118–122.

44. Henderson S, Brown E, Levy J. Safety and efficacy of percutaneous insertion of peritoneal dialysis catheters under sedation and local anaesthetic. *Nephrol Dial Transplant.* 2009;24:3499–3504.

45. Perakis KE, Stylianou KG, Kyriazis JP. Long-term complication rates and survival of peritoneal dialysis catheters: the role of percutaneous versus surgical placement. *Semin Dial.* 2009;22:569–575.

46. Ozener C, Bihorac A, Akoglu E. Technical survival of CAPD catheters: comparison between percutaneous and conventional surgical placement techniques. *Nephrol Dial Transplant.* 2001;16:1893–1899.

47. Maio R, Figueiredo N, Costa P. Laparoscopic placement of Tenckhoff catheters for peritoneal dialysis: a safe, effective, and reproducible procedure. *Perit Dial Int.* 2008;28:170–173.

48. Keshvari A, Najafi I, Jafari-Javid M, Yunesian M, Chaman R, Taromlou MN. Laparoscopic peritoneal dialysis catheter implantation using a Tenckhoff trocar under local anesthesia with nitrous oxide gas insufflation. *Am J Surg.* 2009;197:8–13.

49. Ataluri V, Lebeis C, Brethauer S, et al. Advanced laparoscopic techniques significantly improve function of peritoneal dialysis catheters. *J Am Coll Surg.* 2010;211:699–704.

50. Birns MT. Inadvertent instrumental perforation of the colon during laparoscopy: nonsurgical repair. *Gastrointest Endosc.* 1989;35:54–56.

51. Rubin J, Oreopoulos DG, Lio TT, Matthews R, deVeber GA. Management of peritonitis and bowel perforation during chronic peritoneal dialysis. *Nephron.* 1976;16:220–225.

52. Asif A, Byers P, Vieira CF, Merrill D, et al. Peritoneoscopic placement of peritoneal dialysis catheter and bowel perforation: experience of an interventional nephrology program. *Am J Kidney Dis.* 2003;42:1270–1274.

53. Kahn SI, Garella S, Chazan JA. Nonsurgical treatment of intestinal perforation due to peritoneal dialysis. *Surg Gynecol Obstet.* 1973;136:40–42.

54. Santos CR, Branco PQ, Martinho A, et al. Salvage of malpositioned and malfunctioning peritoneal dialysis catheters by manipulation with a modified Malecot introducer. *Semin Dial.* 2010;23:95–99.

55. Gadallah MF, Ramdeen G, Mignone J, et al. Role of preoperative antibiotic prophylaxis in preventing postoperative peritonitis in newly placed peritoneal dialysis catheters. *Am J Kidney Dis.* 2000;36:1014–1019.

56. Wong S, Chu K, Cheuk A, et al. Prophylaxis against gram-positive organisms causing exit-site infection and peritonitis in continuous ambulatory peritoneal dialysis patients by applying mupirocin ointment at the catheter exit site. *Perit Dial Int.* 2003;23(S2):S153–S158.

57. Bernardini J, Bender F, Florio T, Sloand J, PalmMontalbano L, Fried L, Piraino B. Randomized double-blind trial of antibiotic exit site cream for prevention of exit site infection in peritoneal dialysis patients. *J Am Soc Nephrol.* 2005;16:539–545.

58. Twardowski ZJ, Prowant BF, Nichols WK, Nolph KD, Khanna R. Six-year experience with swan neck presternal peritoneal dialysis catheter. *Perit Dial Int.* 1998;18:598–602.

59. Crabtree JH. Fluoroscopic placement of peritoneal dialysis catheters: a harvest of the low-hanging fruits. *Perit Dial Int.* 2008;28:134–137.

60. Moncrief JW, Popovich RP, Broadrick LJ, He ZZ, Simmons EE, Tate RA. The Moncrief-Popovich catheter: a new peritoneal access technique for patients on peritoneal dialysis. *ASAIO J.* 1993;39:62–65.

61. Asif A. Peritoneal dialysis access-related procedures by nephrologists. *Semin Dial.* 2004;17:398–406.

62. Danielsson A, Blohme L, Tranaeus A, Hylander B. A prospective randomized study of the effect of a subcutaneously "buried" peritoneal dialysis catheter technique versus standard technique on the incidence of peritonitis and exit-site infection. *Perit Dial Int.* 2002;22:211–219.

63. McCormick BB, Brown PA, Knoll G, et al. Use of the embedded peritoneal dialysis catheter: experience and results from a North American center. *Kidney Int.* 2006;70:S38–S43.

45

COMPLICATIONS OF PERITONEAL DIALYSIS CATHETER PROCEDURES

LOAY SALMAN & ARIF ASIF

LEARNING OBJECTIVES

1. Understand the complication profile related to PD catheter.
2. Describe the manifestations of various PD catheter complications.
3. Describe the management strategies of various PD catheter complications.
4. Describe the PD catheter removal procedure.

INTRODUCTION

While peritoneal dialysis PD catheters are called the "good" catheters, they have their own special noninfectious spectrum of complications and problematic issues. Difficult scenarios such as PD fluid leaks, outflow failure, cuff extrusion, bowel perforation and bleeding can all be encountered and result in cessation of peritoneal dialysis therapy. These complications can occur during the catheter insertion procedure and can also be encountered later. Of these, visceral perforation is the most feared complication of PD catheter placement. Fortunately, it is not observed commonly. Catheter migration is a relatively common condition leading to outflow failure.[1,3] PD catheter cuff extrusion is an uncommon complication that exposes the cuff to the external environment and can result in catheter loss.[2] Multiple reports have highlighted noninfectious complications associated with catheter insertion, their management and the catheter removal procedure.[1-46] Herein, we highlight some of the complications associated with peritoneal dialysis catheter insertion. Because management of some of these complications requires the knowledge of catheter removal, the steps of removal of a peritoneal dialysis catheter are also highlighted in this chapter.

Peritonitis is an important complication that is associated with increased morbidity and mortality. Although we will not discuss infectious complications in this chapter, it is vital for the interventionalist to have a complete knowledge of the infectious-related indications for PD catheter removal. Briefly, peritonitis and other infectious complications can be frequently treated successfully with appropriate antibiotic therapy. There are occasions when the PD catheter needs to be removed. The official recommendations[4-6] suggest that PD catheter be removed in conditions of relapsing peritonitis defined as another episode of peritonitis with the same organism within 4 weeks period of the previous peritonitis after a complete course of therapy, refractory peritonitis defined as no response after 5 days of appropriate antibiotics, refractory PD catheter exit site and tunnel infections and fungal peritonitis. PD catheter removal can also be considered in cases of fecal peritonitis or peritonitis in the settings of intra-abdominal pathology and conditions of relapsing peritonitis with no obvious cause. Special considerations need to be given to cases of repeat peritonitis, mycobacterial peritonitis, and cases of peritonitis with multiple organisms.

PD CATHETER COMPLICATIONS
NONINFECTIOUS VISCERAL PERFORATION

Bowel perforation is the most feared complication of PD catheter placement and probably is the single most important factor that keeps nephrologists from performing this procedure. Although the risk of bowel perforation following a PD catheter placement is low, interventionalists performing this procedure should be well aware of it and versed in diagnosing this complication promptly and managing the patient effectively.

The most common reason for bowel complication is the PD catheter placement procedure itself. However, it can occur during the lifetime of the PD catheter. This may be due to the constant irritation of the catheter with the surrounding tissue. The true incidence of bowel perforation with the peritoneoscopic technique is unknown. We have evaluated 750 peritoneoscopic PD catheter insertions performed by nephrologists and found the incidence of this complication to be 0.8%.[1] It is worth mentioning that procedure-related bowel perforation can be treated successfully with conservative management using bowel rest and intravenous antibiotics.[1] In one study, six cases suffered bowel perforation out of a total of 750 PD catheter insertions. Diagnosis was established by direct peritoneoscopic visualization of bowel mucosa, bowel contents or hard stool, return of fecal material, or emanation of foul smelling gas through the cannula in a great majority of the patients. Once the diagnosis was established, all of the patients were maintained NPO and given intravenous triple antibiotic therapy. Four patients recovered with conservative treatment while two eventually needed surgical interventions. Of the two patients who required surgery, one was a lung transplant recipient and heavily immunosuppressed. In the second patient, the bowel rest and the antibiotics were not initiated until the next day. The initial introduction of the needle or Trocar diameter 2.2 mm into the abdominal cavity is likely responsible for bowel injury when a PD catheter is inserted using the fluoroscopic or peritoneoscopic technique.[1] The mechanism is akin to bowel injuries that occur due to the introduction of insufflations needles, trocars, rigid catheters, and colonoscopic examinations.[4–7] A majority of these perforations are usually small and have a good chance in sealing spontaneously.[8,9] The likelihood of healing within 24–48 hours is based on the fact that these perforations are "mini-perforations" will close most likely secondary to omental adherence.[8,9,11] Indeed, during surgical explorations, Simkin and Wright[9] have directly observed sealed bowel perforations that were sustained during PD catheter insertion 12–16 hours earlier. This finding provided direct evidence of the self-sealing nature of bowel perforations sustained during PD catheter insertion. We have modified the peritoneoscopic technique by using Veress needle instead of a trocar to gain access to the abdominal cavity in an attempt to further minimize/avoid the risk of bowel perforation.[10] In contrast to the sharp tip of the trocar, the Veress needle has a blunt, self-retracting end. In addition, the Veress needle is only 14-gauge as opposed to the 2.2 mm diameter of the trocar. Veress needle can be utilized once the anterior rectus sheath is identified and local anesthesia infiltrated. At this point, a Veress insufflation needle Ethicon Endo-Surgery Inc., Cincinnati, OH, is introduced into the abdominal cavity at the site chosen for trocar insertion. Two distinct "pops" are discerned similar to the cannula and trocar of the peritoneoscopic technique. Four to five hundred cubic centimeters of air are infused into the abdominal cavity through the needle using the insufflation device

provided by the Y-Tech Kit Medigroup, Naperville, IL, to create an air-filled space between the parietal and visceral peritoneal layers. The Veress needle is then removed. At this point, the trocar and cannula are introduced into this space in the abdominal cavity. The remainder of the steps is similar to the traditional steps of the peritoneoscopic insertion technique. Veress needle insertion adds 2–3 minutes to the procedure time. In our hands, Veress needle has decreased bowel perforation rate significantly.[10]

While bowel perforation is the most feared complication, it is still relatively uncommon. It can be diagnosed by the operator during the procedure by utilizing the peritoneoscope or subsequently by various clinical manifestations nausea, vomiting, abdominal pain, rigid abdomen, and so on. While surgical consult is essential, a majority of these patients can be successfully managed conservatively with close monitoring of vital signs, serial abdominal examination, bowel rest, and the administration of broad spectrum intravenous antibiotics.[1] Surgical intervention may be needed in patients with clinical deterioration and signs of peritoneal irritation.

▶ Peritoneal Dialysis Catheter Outflow Failure

Outflow failure is a relatively common problem. By definition, it is the inability to recover the whole amount of the infused dialysate fluid. While constipation is a common cause of outflow failure, there are other culprits such as catheter migration, intraluminal occlusion, that is, thrombus, extraluminal occlusion, that is, omentum, adhesions, and the like, and catheter kinking. Constipation can be treated with laxatives with good results. Intraluminal occlusion can be treated with heparin, urokinase, or alteplase instilled into the catheter. PD catheter migration can be easily diagnosed by a simple abdominal X-ray but its management can be fairly challenging. A variety of techniques have been used to combat migration with long-term success rates ranging from 27% to 70%.[3,12–15,41] A recent progressive study evaluated the success of Fogarty catheter manipulation for the migrated PD catheter in 232 patients.[3] The incidence of migration was found to be 15%. In this study, a Fogarty catheter was advanced into the PD catheter to a premarked point at which the end of the Fogarty catheter was near the end of the intraperitoneal portion of the PD catheter. The Fogarty catheter was then inflated with 0.5 mL of sterile saline and manipulation was performed by tugging movement until the proper positioning of the catheter into the pelvis was suspected (Figure 45-1). Four to five attempts were made. Technical success can be evaluated by abdominal X-ray and functional success can be evaluated by checking dialysis inflow and outflow. Overall, the procedure was successful in 70% of the patients. In contrast, in our hands, Fogarty catheter manipulation corrected only 1/10 10% of the migrated catheters.[4] It is important to mention that migrated PD catheter can also be manipulated under Fluoroscopic guidance with technical success of 85% and clinical success of 45–55%.[15,41]

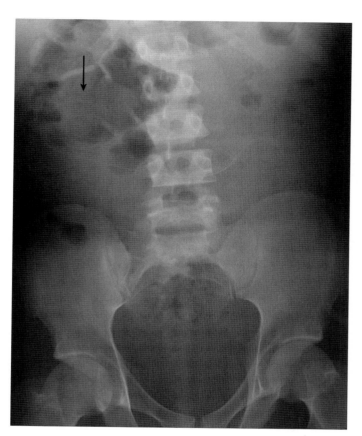

Figure 45-1. A mal-positioned catheter is shown. Note that the catheter had migrated to the right upper quadrant (arrow) leading to catheter dysfunction.

▶ Peritoneal Dialysate Fluids Leaks

For the most part, the peritoneal cavity is a closed space and as such dialysate fluid is expected to be contained within this space. However, there are specific anatomical locations that will make the membrane subject to weakness. Additionally, when placing a peritoneal dialysis catheter a peritoneal hole is induced by the operator in order to be able to pass the catheter into the peritoneal cavity. These areas can allow dialysate fluids to leak from the preferred peritoneal cavity space to the other not preferred locations such as PD catheter tunnel, abdominal wall, genital and scrotal area, pleural space, and the like. The increase intraabdominal pressure that is associated with the infusion of dialysate fluids is an important additional factor. Intraabdominal pressure increases proportional to the amount of dialysate fluids infused and can reach 10–12-cm H_2O. Incidence of dialysate leaks can vary between 5% and 40% based on the technique used to place the catheter and the definition used to describe the condition.[18] Leaks can be divided into early leaks less than 30 days postcatheter placement and late leaks greater than 30 days postcatheter placement. This definition helps to guide treatment and prognosis of leaks.

There are multiple factors that increase the risk for developing leaks. Technique of PD catheter placement can be

an important factor in inducing leaks. It has been observed that percutaneous placement demonstrates less leaks as compared to the traditional surgical approach.[18] Logically, one could expect more leaks with early start less than 14 days after catheter placement of peritoneal dialysis with large volume exchanges compared to late start more than 14 days after PD catheter placement and gradual increase of dialysate volume. Abdominal wall weakness, that is, previous abdominal surgeries, multiple pregnancies, long-term therapy with steroids, hernias, heavy straining, abdominal obesity, and so on, is another important factor.[42]

Dialysate leaks manifest with outflow failure and signs and symptoms of fluid accumulation in the affected area, that is, fluids leaks around the catheter from the exit site, abdominal wall edema, genital edem, pleural effusion, and the like.

Diagnosis can be easily established by checking the sugar level in the fluids if obtaining fluid was possible leaks from the exit site, and the like; however, if the fluids cannot be collected, a CT scan of the abdomen with pelvis or chest CT, if clinically indicated after infusing dialysate fluid with contrast material into the peritoneal cavity, would disclose the etiology. Intraperitoneal injection of radioisotope technetium tagged macroaggregated albumin followed by peritoneal scintigraphy can also be undertaken to help establish the diagnosis.[43]

Treatment of dialysate leaks can be difficult. Conservative management has been more successful in early leaks as compared to late leaks. First step of treating early leaks after catheter placement should be peritoneal dialysis interruption for 2 weeks to allow for appropriate healing of the deep cuff. Late leaks treatment is more challenging and requires surgical treatment in higher percentage. However, there has been success in treating late dialysate leaks with peritoneal dialysis interruption and changing the peritoneal dialysis technique to automated PD. This makes it advisable to attempt it on every patient with dialysate leaks.[42,44,45]

▶ Previous Abdominal Surgeries

Previous abdominal surgery could result in significant intraperitoneal adhesions and has been repeatedly highlighted as a relative contraindication to peritoneal dialysis.[16,17] While previous abdominal surgeries can add additional challenges to the PD catheter placement itself, catheter insertion should not be a contraindication and a thorough evaluation should be undertaken in these patients. In our experience, PD catheter placement can be successfully accomplished in this population.[1] Furthermore, a prior history of abdominal surgery does not necessarily increase the risk of bowel perforation compared to those with no previous abdominal surgeries. A multicenter study found that of the 326 peritoneoscopic catheter insertions performed in patients with prior abdominal surgery, 324 received a PD catheter successfully.[1] In this study, four perforations occurred in 424 peritoneoscopic insertions in patients without prior abdominal surgery as compared to only two perforations that occurred in the 326 patients with a history of previous abdominal surgery. Based on these information patients with multiple previous abdominal surgeries should still be considered as candidates for PD catheter placement and appropriately evaluated. Patients with a history of prior abdominal surgery should not be routinely denied this modality because PD catheter insertion can be successfully performed in this population with a high success rate >95%.[1,18]

▶ Catheter and Superficial Cuff Extrusion and Superficial Abscess

Other problems that can be observed in patients with peritoneal dialysis catheters are catheter extrusion, extruded superficial cuff, and superficial abscess. These issues can lead to the loss of PD access and transfer of the patient to hemodialysis. Recent information has emphasized that these problems could be successfully managed on an outpatient basis.[2] PD catheters with these complications can be salvaged by the application of elementary surgical procedures such as wound cleaning saline, hydrogen peroxide, betadine, debridement, and creation of a subcutaneous pocket, a catheter tunnel, and a catheter exit site. Fortunately, these procedures can be easily performed on an outpatient basis and under local anesthesia.

Sonographic assessment to ascertain the possibility of infection involving the tunnel or superficial or deep cuff has been reported by many investigators.[19-22] Infection of the tunnel or catheter cuff significantly increases the risk of catheter loss.[19,20,22] Consequently, sonographic examination of the catheter becomes a critical tool in decision-making regarding management. Sonographic evidence of fluid collection at the catheter tunnel or cuff has been documented to be a useful predictor of catheter loss.[21] Indeed, in one study,[20] 11 of 25 patients with a positive ultrasound examination lost their catheters due to infectious complications, while no patient with a negative ultrasound examination underwent surgery for infectious reasons $P < 0.01$. Additionally, although adequate for an exit site infection, physical examination does not optimally assess the status of tunnel or cuff infection, particularly at an early stage.[22] Therefore, infectious involvement of the catheter tunnel and cuffs must be determined prior to the application of salvage procedures.

PD CATHETER REMOVAL

Many of the PD catheter associated complications require removal of the catheter and insetion of a new one. In this context, removal procedure is as important as the insertion of a PD catheter. All Tenckhoff-type PD catheters that are placed by interventionalists can also be removed safely without significant discomfort by same operator and under local anesthesia. This procedure can be performed in the interventional suite using sedation and analgesia and using standard precautions for infection control.

The steps of a peritoneal dialysis catheter removal procedure are not extensive (Figure 45-2). Briefly, local anesthetic is infiltrated at the site of the primary incision and the subcutaneous tissue. Dissection is then carried down to the subcutaneous tissue and the catheter tunnel aiming to free the PD catheter. Using blunt dissection, a portion

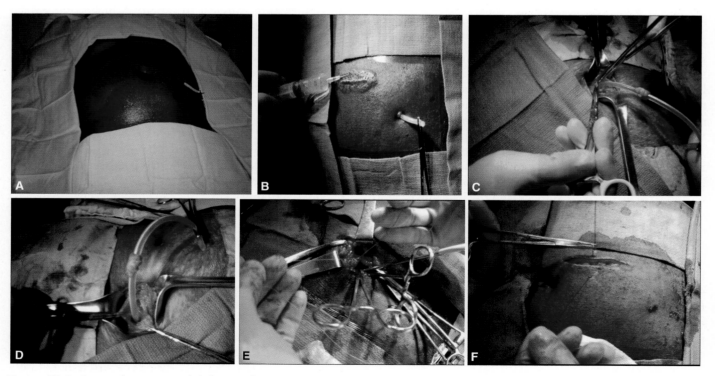

Figure 45-2. Steps of a peritoneal dialysis catheter are shown (**A**)–(**F**). The procedure is performed under local anesthesia.

of the tunnel is separated from the surrounding tissue. The catheter is then lifted by passing a curved hemostat under it. The tunnel layers are cut in a longitudinal direction in order to expose the catheter. The catheter is clamped with hemostats and a nylon suture is applied through the catheter just lateral to the hemostat's clamped area. The catheter then is cut just outside the hemostat remaining inside the nylon tag suture. At this point, using Metzenbaum scissors, dissection is performed toward the deep cuff. Once the deep cuff is identified local anesthetic is infiltrated around it. Generally, the longer the catheter has been in place the harder it will be to release the cuff. Peritoneal dialysis catheters that have been in place for less than 1 month are relatively easy to remove compared to those that have been in place for a longer period. Therefore, catheters that have been in place for less than a month, blunt dissection using hemostats is all that is required to free the superficial and the deep cuff. On the other hand, catheters that have been in place for more than a month, sharp dissection using Metzenbaum scissors and rarely a scalpel is needed. Once the deep cuff is freed, the intraperitoneal portion of the catheter is withdrawn. The defect created at the entry point anterior rectus sheath of the catheter is then closed with a purse string suture. At this point, the dissection is performed in the direction of the superficial cuff. Once the superficial cuff is free, this portion of the catheter can be easily removed through the primary incision site or the exit site. The wound is then close in layers. The skin in sutured using nylon. The exit site is not sutured. The procedure should be performed only in the usual sterile fashion and in a surgical ready room. It is important to mention that catheter removal is based upon the type of the catheter used and placement technique. In general, a catheter that was inserted using the surgical technique should be removed by the surgeon.

In summary, peritoneal dialysis catheter can be associated with multiple complications. While some can be management conservatively, others require invasive maneuvers. At times, these complications require catheter removal. An interventionalist must be versed in not only catheter insertion but also the management of complications and catheter removal procedure.

REFERENCES

1. Asif A, Byers P, Vieira CF, et al. Bowel perforation peritoneoscopic placement of peritoneal dialysis catheter and bowel perforation: experience of an interventional nephrology program. *Am J Kidney Dis.* 2003;426:1270–1274.
2. Asif A, Gadalean F, Vieira CF, et al. *Semin Dial.* 2006;19:180–183.
3. Gadallah MF, Aurora N, Arumugam R, et al. Role of Fogarty catheter manipulation in management of migrated, nonfunctional peritoneal dialysis catheters. *Am J Kidney Dis* 2000;35:301–305.
4. Asif A, Byers P, Gadalean F, et al. Peritoneal dialysis underutilization: the impact of an interventional nephrology peritoneal dialysis access program. *Semin Dial.* 2003;16:266–271.
5. Reich H. Laparoscopic bowel injury. *Surg Laparosc Endosc.* 1992;2:74–78.
6. Birns MT. Inadvertent instrumental perforation of the colon during laparoscopy: nonsurgical repair. *Gastrointes Endosc.* 1989;35:54–56.
7. Nomura T, Shirai Y, Okamoto H, et al. Bowel perforation caused by silicone drains: a report of two cases. *Surg Today.* 1998;28:940–942.
8. Christie JP, Marrazzo J 3rd. "Mini-perforation" of the colon—not all postpolypectomy perforations require laparotomy. *Dis Colon Rectum.* 1991;34:132–135.
9. Simkin EP, Wright FK. Perforating injuries of the bowel complicating peritoneal catheter insertion. *Lancet.* 1968;1:64–66.
10. Damore LJ II, Rantis PC, Vernava AM III, et al. Colonoscopic perforations. Etiology, diagnosis, and management. *Dis Colon Rectum.* 1996;39:1308–1314.
11. Asif A, Tawakol J, Khan T, et al. Modification of the peritoneoscopic technique of peritoneal dialysis catheter insertion: experience of an interventional nephrology program. *Semin Dial.* 2004;17,171–173.
12. Gadallah MF, Mignon J, Torres C, et al. The role of peritoneal dialysis catheter configuration in preventing catheter tip migration. *Adv Perit Dial.* 2000;16:47–50.
13. Siegel RL, Nosher JL, Gesner LR. Peritoneal dialysis catheters: repositioning with new fluoroscopic technique. *Radiology.* 1994;190:899–901.
14. Kappel JE, Ferguson GM, Kudel RM, et al. Stiff wire manipulation of peritoneal dialysis catheters. *Adv Perit Dial.* 1995;11:202–207.
15. Simons ME, Pron G, Voros M, et al. Fluoroscopically-guided manipulation of malfunctioning peritoneal dialysis catheters. *Perit Dial Int.* 1999;19:544–549.
16. Nkere UU. Postoperative adhesion formation and the use of adhesion preventing techniques in cardiac and general surgery. *ASAIO J.* 2000;46:654–656.
17. Brandt CP, Franceschi D. Laparoscopic placement of peritoneal dialysis catheters in patients who have undergone prior abdominal operations. *J Am Coll Surg.* 1994;178:515–516.
18. Gadallah MF, Pervez A, EI-Shahawy MA, et al. Peritoneoscopic versus surgical placement of peritoneal dialysis catheters: a prospective randomized study on outcome. *Am J Kidney Dis.* 1999;33:118–122.
19. Domico J, Warman M, Jaykamur S, et al. Is ultrasonography useful in predicting catheter loss? *Adv Perit Dial.* 1993;9:231–232.
20. Holley JL, Foulks CJ, Moss AH, et al. Ultrasound as a tool in the diagnosis and management of exit-site infections in patients undergoing continuous ambulatory peritoneal dialysis. *Am J Kidney Dis.* 1989;14:211–216.
21. Plum J, Sudkamp S, Grabensee B. Results of ultrasound-assisted diagnosis of tunnel infections in continuous ambulatory peritoneal dialysis. *Am J Kidney Dis.* 1994;23:99–104.
22. Korzets Z, Erdberg A, Golan E, et al. Frequent involvement of the internal cuff segment in CAPD peritonitis and exit-site infection—an ultrasound study. *Nephrol Dial Transplant.* 1996;11:336–339.
23. Ash SR, Handt AE, Block R. Periotoneoscopic placement of Tenchoff catheter: further clinical experience. *Perit Dial Bull.* 1983;3:8–12.

24. Handt AD, Ash SR. Longevity of Tenckhoff catheters placed by the y-tec® Peritoneoscopic technique. *Perspect Peritoneal Dial.* 1984;2:30–33.

25. Cruz C, Faber M, Melendez A. Peritoneoscopic implantation of Tenckhoff catheters for CAPD: effect on catheter function, survival and tunnel infection. *Perit Dial Int Abstr.* 1989;9:S1.

26. Adamson AS, Kelleher JP, Snell ME, et al. Endoscopic placement of CAPD catheters: a review of one hundred procedures. *Nephrol Dial Transplant.* 1992;7:855–857.

27. Chadha I, Mulgaonkar S, Jacobs M, et al. Outcome of laparoscopic Tenckhoff catheter insertion LTCI versus surgical Tenckhoff catheter insertion STCI: a prospective randomized comparison. *Perit Dial Int Abstr.* 1994;14:S89.

28. Swartz DA, Sandroni SE, Moles KA. Laparoscopic Tenckhoff catheter placement: a single center's experience. *Perit Dial Int Abstr.* 1993:S31.

29. Scott PD, Bakran A, Pearson R, et al. Prospective randomized trial of 3 different peritoneal catheters—preliminary report. *Perit Dial Int.* 1994;14:289–290.

30. Copley JB, Lindberg JS, Back SN, et al. Peritoneoscopic placement of Swan neck peritoneal dialysis catheters. *Perit Dial Int.* 1996;16:S330–S32.

31. Vaux EC, Torrie PH, Barker LC, et al. Percutaneous fluoroscopically guided placement of peritoneal dialysis catheters—a 10-year experience. *Semin Dial.* 2008;21:459–465.

32. Moon JY, Song S, Jung KH, et al. Fluoroscopically guided peritoneal dialysis catheter placement: long-term results from a single center. *Perit Dial Int.* 2008;28:163–169.

33. Rosenthal MA, Yang PS, Liu IL, et al. Comparison of outcomes of peritoneal dialysis catheters placed by the fluoroscopically guided percutaneous method versus directly visualized surgical method. *J Vasc Interv Radiol.* 2008;19:1202–1207.

34. Jacobs IG, Gray RR, Elliott DS, et al. Radiologic placement of peritoneal dialysis catheters: preliminary experience. *Radiology.* 1992;182:251–255.

35. Zaman F, Pervez A, Atray NK, et al. Fluoroscopy-assisted placement of peritoneal dialysis catheters by nephrologists. *Semin Dial.* 2005;18:247–251.

36. Savader SJ, Geschwind JF, Lund GB, et al. Percutaneous radiologic placement of peritoneal dialysis catheters: long-term results. *J Vasc Interv Radiol.* 2000;11:965–970.

37. Maya ID: Ultrasound/fluoroscopy-assisted placement of peritoneal dialysis catheters. *Semin Dial.* 2007:20:611–615.

38. Crabtree JH, Burchette RJ. Effective use of laparoscopy for long-term peritoneal dialysis access. *Am J Surg.* 2009;198:135–141

39. Crabtree JH, Fishman A. A laparoscopic method for optimal peritoneal dialysis access. *Am Surg.* 2005;71:135–143.

40. Crabtree JH. Who should place peritoneal dialysis catheters? *Perit Dial Int.* 2010;30:142–150.

41. Dobrashian RD, Conway B, Hutchison A, et al. The repositioning of migrated Tenckhoff continuous ambulatory peritoneal dialysis catheters under fluoroscopic control. *Br J Radiol.* 1999;72857:452–456.

42. Leblanc M, Ouimet D, Pichette V. Dialysate leaks in peritoneal dialysis. *Semin Dial.* 2001;141:50–54.

43. Kopecky RT, Frymoyer PA, Witanowski LS, et al. Complications of continuous ambulatory peritoneal dialysis: diagnostic value of peritoneal scintigraphy. *Am J Kidney Dis.* 1987;102:123–132.

44. Holley JL, Bernardini J, Piraino B. Characteristics and outcome of peritoneal dialysate leaks and associated infections. *Adv Perit Dial.* 1993;9:240–243.

45. Gokal R, Alexander S, Ash S, et al. Peritoneal catheters and exit-site practices toward optimum peritoneal access: 1998 update. Official report from the International Society for peritoneal dialysis. *Perit Dial Int.* 1998;18(1):11–33.

46. Li, PK, Szeto, CC, Piraino, B, et al. Peritoneal dialysis-related infections recommendations: 2010 update. *Perit Dial Int.* 2010;30:393.

46

PERITONEAL DIALYSIS CATHETER REMOVAL

BHARAT SACHDEVA

LEARNING OBJECTIVES

1. Maintenance of peritoneal dialysis (PD) access may require PD catheter removal or replacement.

2. Review the common complications seen with PD catheters and identify the situations where PD catheter needs to be replaced or removed.

3. Common techniques used to remove PD catheters are explained to understand the steps involved in removing a PD catheter.

4. Timely action on a malfunctioning PD catheter can avoid morbidity and mortality associated with PD.

INTRODUCTION

Underutilization of PD in end-stage renal disease (ESRD) patients has been long recognized.[1-5] One of the several factors identified has been the inability of the surgeons to provide timely insertion of the PD catheter in a patient initiating renal replacement therapy.[6-9] Success and safety of PD catheter insertion by nephrologists have been well documented.[9-19] Catheters in peritoneal cavity can be placed using a variety of techniques each with pros and cons. As nephrologists get actively involved in placement of PD catheters, it brings the responsibility of managing, maintaining, and ensuring functionality of the catheter placed.[11,20,21]

This chapter provides a review of PD catheter removal procedures with emphasis on practice principles, techniques, and critical issues of peritoneal dialysis catheter removal.

INDICATIONS FOR PD CATHETER REMOVAL

Most common indication for removal of a PD catheter is infection of the peritoneal cavity or a tunnel infection (Table 46-1). Removal of catheter after a successful renal transplantation accounts for the second most common indication for removal of PD catheter.[21] Together these two indications make up for nearly 4/5 (80%) of all catheter removals. Less common indications for catheter removal include; patients preference to do hemodialysis, abdominal pathology requiring catheter removal, poor catheter function/flows, poor compliance on PD, to name a few.

Exit-site infection is defined by the presence of purulent drainage, with or without erythema of the skin at the catheter–skin interface.[22] Early infection of the exit site may present as erythema alone without any drainage. It will be important to mention here that erythema can commonly be seen after initial catheter placement and clinical judgment will be required to follow the patient or to start antibiotic treatment. Swab cultures from the exit site should be sent to identify the organisms, *Staphylococcus aureus* and *Pseudomonas aeruginosa* being the most common isolates.[22] Treatment for exit-site infection is empirical antibiotics initially targeting *S. aureus* and *P. aeruginosa* with swab culture. Specific antibiotic should then be continued for 3 weeks (Double antibiotic for *P. aeruginosa* due to high antibiotic resistance). Catheter exchange is indicated if the exit site fails to respond to antibiotics at end of 3 weeks of therapy. Simultaneous removal and placement of PD catheter can be done for persistent exit-site infection provided there is no evidence of peritonitis/tunnel infection (see below).

Tunnel of PD catheter, area of catheter between the proximal and distal cuff of a commonly used double cuff PD catheter can get infected usually with an exit-site

TABLE 46–1

Organisms Associated with Dialysis Associated Peritonitis and Indications for Catheter Removal

Organism Isolated	Comments
Coagulase-negative Staphylococcus and other Gram+ve Cocci	Relapsing infection or peritonitis with exit-site or tunnel infection
Enterococcus/ Streptococcus	Peritonitis with exit-site or tunnel infection
Staphylococcus aureus	Peritonitis with exit-site or tunnel infection may prove to be refractory (failure to respond in 5 days)
	Catheter removal should be seriously considered
	Allow a minimum rest period of 3 weeks before reinitiating PD
Culture negative	If no clinical improvement in 5 days, remove catheter
Pseudomonas species	No clinical improvement by 5 days on appropriate antibiotics, remove catheter
E. coli, Proteus, Klebsiella	No clinical improvement by 5 days on appropriate antibiotics, remove catheter
Polymicrobial Peritonitis	With exit-site or tunnel infection, remove catheter
Fungal Peritonitis	Remove catheter (within 24 h)
Mycobacteria Peritonitis	Removal in refractory cases

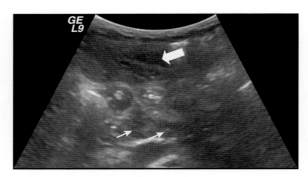

Figure 46-2. Ultrasound of anterior abdominal wall with PD catheter in the rectus sheath. Thick arrow: shows rectus muscle with PD catheter surrounded by radiolucent area. Short arrow: shows bowel gas in peritoneum.

infection, occasionally as an isolated catheter infection (Figure 46-1). Infected tunnel may present as erythema, edema, or tenderness over the subcutaneous pathway but is often clinically occult, and seen only by sonographic studies.[31,32] Fluid collection around the external cuff (>1 mm) and or involvement of the proximal cuff are signs of tunnel infection and a poor catheter outcome to antibiotic therapy alone (Figure 46-2). Sonography of the tunnel should be used in evaluation of the extent of infection along the tunnel and also the response to therapy.[31,32] Catheter removal should be considered earlier for exit-site infections associated with a tunnel infection. Concomitant exit-site infection with peritonitis with the same organism usually will require catheter removal.

Infection in the peritoneal cavity increases the risk of damage to the peritoneal membrane and every effort should be made to eradicate the infection and not to save the catheter. Early identification with initiation of antibiotics is key to prevent injury to the peritoneal membrane. Refractory peritonitis, defined as failure of the effluent to clear after 5 days of appropriate antibiotics can cause irreversible injury to peritoneal membrane. A recent retrospective study showed that peritoneal dialysate white cell count $\geq 1090/mm^3$ on day 3 was an independent prognostic marker for treatment failure and suggested removal of catheter for these patients.[23]

Infection caused by the same organism within 4 weeks of the last infection (relapsing), despite adequate antibiotic treatment or when the infection occurs within 4 weeks after treatment but with a different organism (recurrent); are at high risk for treatment failure and should be considered for catheter removal.[22] All effort should be made to identify the causative organism. Readers are encouraged to review the recent update of peritoneal dialysis catheter infections for a list of organisms that are related to a high risk of failure of conservative treatment and require catheter removal for eradication of infection.[22]

The only absolute indication for catheter removal after peritonitis associated with catheter in a peritoneal dialysis patient remains fungal infection (Table 46-2). Fungal peritonitis is one infection with the risk of death being very high and evidence suggests that prompt catheter removal may lower risk of death.[24,25]

Simultaneous replacement for exit-site infections is indicated to prevent the catheter infection from spreading intraperitoneally.[22] Catheter replacement as a single procedure should also be entertained for relapsing peritonitis if the effluent can first be cleared. Colonization of the intraabdominal portion of the catheter with biofilm (Figure 46-3) is seen more commonly in some infections than others and is best treated by replacing the catheter (*Staphylococcus epidermidis, Escherichia coli, Klebsiella*, or *Proteus*).

Catheter malfunction (Figure 46-4) is not only frustrating for patient and physicians; is also frequently the cause of PD catheter removal and shift to hemodialysis often against the desires of the patient. Attempts to salvage the

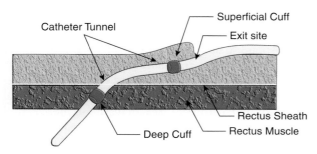

Figure 46-1. Diagram of double cuff PD catheter. Relation of the two cuffs with exit site and the rectus muscle/sheath.

TABLE 46-2

Indications for Catheter Removal for Peritoneal
Dialysis-Related Infections

Refractory peritonitis: Failure of the effluent to clear after
    5 days of appropriate antibiotics
Relapsing peritonitis: Repeat infection by the same organism
    within 4 weeks of completion of therapy
Repeat peritonitis: Repeat infection by the same organism
    more than 4 weeks after completion of therapy
Recurrent peritonitis: Repeat infection with a different
    organism within 4 weeks of completion of therapy
Refractory exit-site and tunnel infection
Fungal peritonitis
Catheter removal should also be considered for
    Repeat peritonitis
    Mycobacterial peritonitis
    Multiple enteric organisms

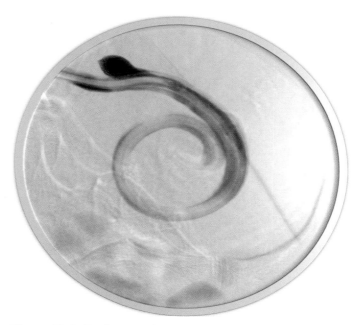

Figure 46-4. Dysfunctional peritoneal dialysis catheter, poor flows, peritoneogram suggests omentum wrap requiring removal and reinsertion of catheter.

catheter prior to removal have been described and succeed in keeping patient on peritoneal dialysis.[26–29] Removal/replacement of the catheter should be considered only after thorough evaluation and after exhausting conservative techniques of catheter rescue have failed.

Peritoneal dialysis catheter removal after renal transplantation is often delayed till good function of the graft kidney is noted. This provides for continuation of peritoneal dialysis when needed in patients with delayed graft function after renal transplantation. If PD catheter is removed at time of transplantation, uncommon outcome of early transplant failure requires a new peritoneal catheter be placed along with transplant nephrectomy.

STEPS OF CATHETER REMOVAL

▶ Preparation

History of the current illness and the indication of removal of PD catheter should be carefully evaluated. Operative note of the original placement and all subsequent revisions should be noted. PD catheters are placed by varied practitioners using a variety of techniques. Knowledge of the

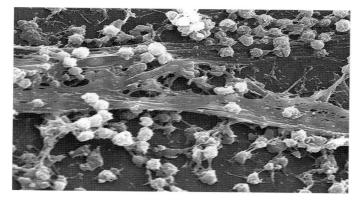

Figure 46-3. Electron microgram of a catheter showing biofilm impregnated with Staphylococcus bacteria. (Source Wikimedia.)

type of catheter (Figure 46-5) being removed is also important to determine the approach and dissection required to remove the anchoring cuff.

Patient can eat normally if no conscious sedation is anticipated (acute catheter removal). Acute catheters do not have any retaining cuff and are removed after removing the suture at the exit site. Chronic PD catheter removal requires dissection of fibrous adhesions anchoring the catheter to surrounding tissue.

Patient should be counseled of the risks, expectations, answer any questions, and have a consent form signed. PD catheter removal can be safely performed by nephrologists without significant discomfort under local anesthesia. Procedure can be performed in a procedure room using standard precautions for infection control.

Un-cuffed catheters (acute) can be removed after removing the anchoring suture holding the catheter. Catheter is simply pulled out and exit-site occlusive dressing is placed.

The following description describes removal of double cuff catheter with a deep cuff placed below the rectus sheath and the superficial cuff placed in the subcutaneous tunnel. Several variations are noted in catheter design and it is important for nephrologists to familiarize with the catheter design and modify approach based on the catheter type.

Conscious sedation will be required if deep blunt dissection is anticipated (catheter in place for greater than a month). Six hours of fasting is recommended for all patients requiring conscious sedation prior to catheter removal.

▶ Deep Cuff

Under sterile condition, the area of catheter entry and exit site is cleaned and draped. Local anesthetic, 2% lidocaine

Peritoneal catheters

Combinations of intraperitoneal and extraperitoneal designs

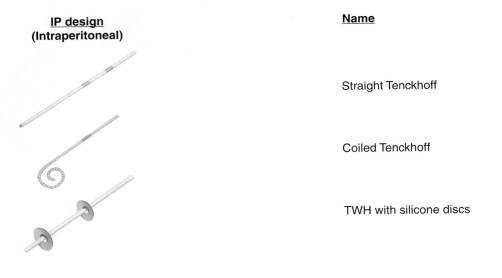

IP design **(Intraperitoneal)**	**Name**
	Straight Tenckhoff
	Coiled Tenckhoff
	TWH with silicone discs

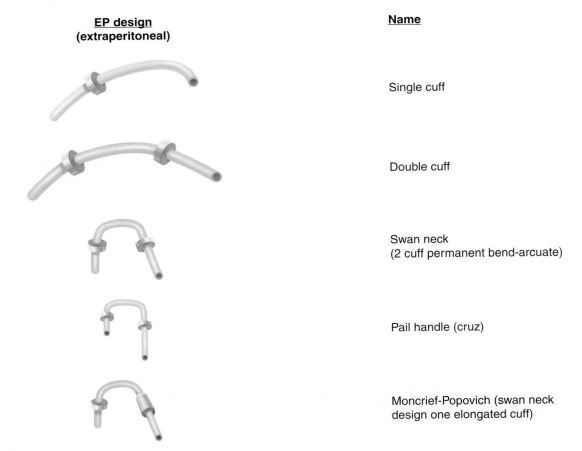

EP design **(extraperitoneal)**	**Name**
	Single cuff
	Double cuff
	Swan neck (2 cuff permanent bend-arcuate)
	Pail handle (cruz)
	Moncrief-Popovich (swan neck design one elongated cuff)

Figure 46-5. Combination of varied catheter deigns and shapes.

with epinephrine, is infiltrated at the site of the primary incision (position of deep cuff) and the subcutaneous tissue (Figure 46-1). Dissection is then carried down to the subcutaneous tissue and the subcutaneous tunnel harboring the catheter is identified. Using blunt dissection, a portion of the tunnel is separated from the surrounding tissue.

The tunnel (Figure 46-1) is then lifted by passing a curved hemostat under tunnel and the catheter within. Using toothed forceps and Metzenbaum scissors, the tunnel layers are cut in a longitudinal direction and the catheter is exposed. The catheter is clamped with blunt tube clamp. A variation of catheter design may have a connector in the tunnel (Flex-Neck ExxTended Catheter; Medigroup Inc., Oswego, IL, USA; Curl Cath Catheter [abdominal segment] with a Swan Neck Presternal Catheter [extension segment]; Covidien AG, Mansfield, MA, USA). Clamp the two-part catheter superficial to titanium connector.

Using Metzenbaum scissors, dissection is extended, exposing tissue in the direction of the deep cuff. Local anesthetic is then infiltrated around the deep cuff. For catheters that have been in place for less than a month, blunt dissection using hemostats and a sustained pull on the catheter is all that is required to free the deep cuff. When that catheter is firmly anchored below the rectus sheath, dissection is carried down to expose the anterior rectus sheath and a sharp incision made adjacent to the catheter entry into the rectus muscle. The ingrown rectus muscle is now cut from the catheter cuff. Once free, the intraabdominal part of the catheter is removed by gently pulling on the catheter.[11,30]

The abdominal opening is closed by Prolene® 2-0 (Ethicon, Somerville, NJ) and the rectus sheath opening also approximated using the above suture.[11,30]

Absorbable suture material, such as Vicryl® 2-0 (Ethicon, Somerville, NJ), is used to close the subcutaneous tissue and Ethilon® 2-0 (Ethicon, Somerville, NJ) is used to close the skin.

Inspection of the tunnel should be done at time of removal for signs of infection. If tunnel is infected, the incision site is packed after through irrigation of tunnel and primary incision and closure by secondary healing is achieved.

▶ Superficial Cuff

Presternal catheter position

The parasternal insertion is opened after local anesthetic is infiltrated into skin and subcutaneous tissue. Blunt dissection is done to dissect both the cuffs from surrounding tissue. The abdominal portion of the catheter (with the deep cuff out of the rectus sheath) is now cut above the tube clamp. The subcutaneous area of catheter can now be retrieved from the presternal exit site by pulling the catheter cephalad.[11,30] The exit site is not sutured.

Abdominal catheter exit site

Once the deep cuff is out, catheter is cut superficial to the tube clamp. The cut surface of the outer catheter segment

is dissected in the direction of the superficial cuff. Once the superficial cuff is free, this portion of the catheter can be easily removed through the primary incision site or the exit site.[11,30] The exit site is again not sutured.

▶ Postoperative Instructions

Pressure dressing should be placed at the wound for 48 hours and care should be taken not to get the dressing wet. After 2 days, the dressing is removed; incision site is washed with plain soap and water and dressed with dry gauze. Superficial sutures are removed upon 2-week follow-up.

Patients are instructed to call interventional unit for:

I. Temperature higher than 101°F (38.6°C)
II. Redness or warmth around the catheter removal site.
III. If noted to have a lot of drainage coming from where the catheter was taken out.

▶ Complications Associated with PD Catheter Removal

Removal procedure is done as an outpatient procedure and several authors have reported minimal complications. Kahveci et al[21] recently reported their experience with 42 PD catheter removal and none of the patients required preoperative or postoperative surgical evaluation. No major complications were noted. Three of 42 (7%) had minor complications. Two of 42 (5%) had minor bleeding from the subcutaneous tunnel, not requiring blood transfusion. Both cases were conservatively managed with pressure dressing. One of 42 (2%) had infection of the wound requiring short-term oral antibiotics.

Occasionally, infection in the tunnel persists after catheter is removed, this can present as pain at the catheter tunnel site along with cellulites at the superficial skin with drainage at exit/insertion site. A thorough abdominal examination should be done to determine the depth and extension of the fluid collection if any in the tunnel. Computerized tomography imaging (Figure 46-6) is required to rule out extension into the rectus sheath/muscle. Exploration of the tunnel may be required to drain any fluid collection and wound should be packed for secondary healing.

"PULL AND JERK" TECHNIQUE FOR PD CATHETER REMOVAL

The conventional surgery for removal of peritoneal dialysis catheter as described above requires the surgeon to either go through the same incision or make a parallel incision close to the previous scar. Shroff et al described "Pull and Jerk" technique for catheter removal involving a small incision and sustained pull and with some jerks for the removal of the catheter. The technique was used from 1997 to 2006 on 41 patients for catheter removal with a success rate of 95%.[33]

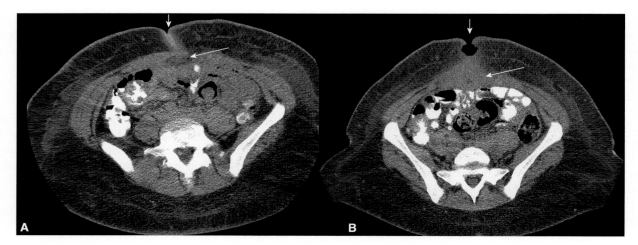

Figure 46-6. **(A)** Increased attenuation within the subcutaneous fat suggesting inflammation or edema and fluid pocket (long arrow), catheter tunnel site (short arrow). **(B)** Increased attenuation within the subcutaneous fat suggesting inflammation or edema (long arrow), open skin wound for drainage (short arrow).

After infiltration of local anesthetic to the exit site, a sustained traction is applied on the catheter till the external cuff comes out. After this, the catheter is regripped and pulled as one gives a sustained traction the inner cuff may give way and the catheter thereafter slips out.

If the catheter has been kept for long duration, the inner Dacron cuff can become part of the tissues and it does not come out but yields in such a way that the silicon catheter comes out leaving behind the Dacron cuff. A retained cuff can be source of infection or a granulation reaction after the catheter is removed. This will present as pain at the catheter insertion site and/or drainage/fluid collection in the abdominal wall. Ultrasound imaging of the abdominal wall will identify the cause of pain/drainage as a fluid collection at the position of deep cuff. Removal of deep cuff will require dissection insertion site with resection of the Dacron cuff.

SIMULTANEOUS INSERTION AND REMOVAL OF PD CATHETER: PD CATHETER EXCHANGE

Catheter-related infections and malfunction result in high patient morbidity, the need for temporary hemodialysis. Posthuma et al described a protocol for the simultaneous peritoneoscopic insertion and removal of peritoneal catheters in patients with catheter-related infections.[34] All patients had dialysate leukocyte count below 100/mm³ before replacing catheter and exchange was performed under antibiotic therapy. The old catheter was removed after the new catheter had been inserted in the opposite abdominal region. Authors reported few minor complications: position-dependent outflow problems and dialysate leakage occurred in two patients. Two patients developed peritonitis within the first 30 days after surgery, one of which was procedure related. Remarkably 38/40 (95%) procedures were successful

and the patients could continue peritoneal dialysis with night low volume dwell and dry day for 2 weeks.

For refractory bacterial and fungal peritonitis, simultaneous catheter replacement is not recommended. Optimal time period between catheter removal and reinsertion of a new catheter is not clear. A minimum period of 2–3 weeks between catheter removal and reinsertion of a new catheter is recommended,[22] with a longer interval recommended for catheter insertion after a fungal peritonitis. A useful predictor of full recovery from acute peritonitis is a rising serum albumin level, a low level seen with acute infection.

A review of current literature by Mitra et al noted 20 publications on simultaneous catheter placement at time of PD catheter removal.[35] Replacement of catheter for exit-site infection and tunnel infection had a 93% success rate with an overall success of 88%. Authors recommended simultaneous removal and replacement an acceptable and safe procedure for recurrent peritonitis or peritonitis associated with exit-site/tunnel infection when staphylococcal species are the causative organism but insufficient evidence to support the use of replacement in peritonitis associated with *Pseudomonas* or other gram-negative organisms. Fungal, mycobacterial, and enteric infections were noted not suitable for a replacement procedure and require the catheter to be removed.

Replacement of catheter after a peritonitis that required removal of PD catheter should only be done once complete resolution of symptoms has occurred. The optimal time period between catheter removal for infection and reinsertion of a new catheter is not known. Two- to three-week interval between catheter removal and reinsertion of a new catheter is recommended (opinion). Most patients on PD wish to return to home dialysis therapy rather than stay on in center hemodialysis and a final decision for returning to PD should be individualized.

Postperitonitis, PD catheter reinsertion may pose a challenge due to change in peritoneal cavity architecture and it is proposed that replacement be the attempted using an open or laparoscopic technique.[36] This would allow visual information on adhesions or compartments within the peritoneal cavity and placement of catheter with adhesion lysis if needed.

CONCLUSION

Peritonitis is a serious complication of PD and one of the most common causes of technique failure in PD. Only a fraction of patients who loose catheter to peritonitis return to PD. Severe peritonitis complicated by catheter removal is usually associated with significantly higher mortality rates[37,38] than those reported for PD-related peritonitis overall.[39,40] In the United States, 18% of the infection-related mortality in PD patients is secondary to peritonitis.[37] A episode of peritonitis is a direct contributing factor to the death of 16% of PD patients.

Removal of PD catheter within 24 hours of diagnosis of peritoneal infection not will help reduce the membrane failure and adhesions, but reduce risk of death by 40% for fungal infections when catheter is removed within 24 hours versus delayed removal.[41]

REFERENCES

1. Gokal R, Blake PG, Passlick-Deetjen J, Schaub TP, Prichard S, Burkart JM. What is the evidence that peritoneal dialysis is underutilized as an ESRD therapy? *Semin Dial.* 2002;15:149–150.
2. Blake PG. What is the evidence that peritoneal dialysis is underutilized as an ESRD therapy? *Semin Dial.* 2002;15:151–153.
3. Passlick-Deetjen J, Schaub TP. What is the evidence that peritoneal dialysis is underutilized as an ESRD therapy? *Semin Dial.* 2002;15:153–155.
4. Prichard S. What is the evidence that peritoneal dialysis is underutilized as an ESRD therapy? *Semin Dial.* 2002;15:155–157.
5. Burkart JM. What is the evidence that peritoneal dialysis is underutilized as an ESRD therapy? *Semin Dial.* 2002;15:157–161.
6. Blake PG, Finkelstein FO. Why is the proportion of patients of doing peritoneal dialysis in North America declining? *Perit Dial Int.* 2001;21:107–114.
7. Mehrotra R, Blake P, Berman N, Nolph KD. An analysis of dialysis training in the United States and Canada. *Am J Kidney Dis* 2002;40:152–160.
8. Nissenson AR, Prichard SS, Cheng IKP, Gokal R, Kubota M, Maiorca R, Riella MC, Rottembourg J, Stewart JH. ESRD modality selection into the 21st century, the importance of non medical factors. *ASAIO J* 1997;43:143–150.
9. Asif A, Byers P, Gadalean F, Roth D. Peritoneal dialysis underutilization: the impact of an interventional nephrology peritoneal dialysis access program. *Semin Dial.* 2003;16:266–271.
10. Gadallah MF, Ramdeen G, Torres-Rivera C, Ibrahim ME, Myrick S, Andrews G, Quin A, Fang C, Crossman A. Changing the trend: a prospective study on factors contributing to the growth rate of peritoneal dialysis programs. *Adv Perit Dial.* 2001;17:122–126.
11. Ash SR. Chronic peritoneal dialysis catheters: procedures for placement, maintenance and removal. *Semin Nephrol* 2002;22:221–236.
12. Ash SR. Who should place peritoneal catheters? A nephrologist's view. *Nephrol News Issues* 1993;7:33–34.
13. Ash SR. Bedside peritoneoscopic peritoneal catheter placement of Tenckhoff and newer peritoneal catheters. *Adv Perit Dial.* 1998;14:75–79.
14. Ash SR, Handt AE, Bloch R. Peritoneoscopic placement of the Tenckhoff catheter: further clinical experience. *Perit Dial Bull.* 1983;3:8–12.
15. Pastan S, Gassensmith C, Manatunga AK, Copley JB, Smith EJ, Hamburger RJ. Prospective comparison of peritoneoscopic and surgical implantation of CAPD catheters. *Trans Am Soc Artif Organs.* 1991;37: M154–M156.
16. Gadallah MF, Pervez A, El-Shahawy MA, Sorrells D, Zibari G, McDonald J, Work J. Peritoneoscopic versus surgical placement of peritoneal dialysis catheters: a prospective randomized study on outcome. *Am J Kidney Dis.* 1999;33: 118–122.
17. Zaman F, Pervez A, Atray NK, Murphy S, Work J, Abreo K. Fluoroscopy-assisted placement of peritoneal dialysis catheters by nephrologists. *Semin Dial.* 2005;18:247–251.
18. Moon JY, Song S, Jung KH, Park M, Lee SH, Ihm CG, et al. fluoroscopically guided peritoneal dialysis catheter placement: long-term results from a single center. *Perit Dial Int.* 2008;28:163–169.
19. Alejandro C. A, Loay S. Peritoneal dialysis catheter insertion by interventional nephrologists. *Am J Kidney Dis.* 2009;6:378–385.
20. Gadallah MF, Aurora N, Arumugam R, Moles K. Role of Fogarty catheter manipulation in management of migrated, nonfunctional peritoneal dialysis catheters. *Am J Kidney Dis.* 2000;35:301–305.
21. Kahveci A, Ari E, Asicioglu E, Arikan H, Tuglular S, Ozener C. Peritoneal dialysis catheter removal by nephrologists: technical aspect from a single center. *Perit Dial Int.* 2010;30:570–572.
22. Li PK, Szeto CC, Piraino B, Bernardini J, Figueiredo AE, Gupta A, Johnson DW, Kuijper EJ, Lye WC, Salzer W, Schaefer F, Struijk DG. Peritoneal dialysis-related infections recommendations: 2010 update. *Perit Dial Int.* 2010;30:393–423.
23. Chow KM, Szeto CC, Cheung KK, Leung CB, Wong SS, Law MC. Predictive value of dialysate cell counts in peritonitis complicating peritoneal dialysis. *Clin J Am Soc Nephrol.* 2006;1:768–73.
24. Prasad KN, Prasad N, Gupta A, Sharma RK, Verma AK, Ayyagari A. Fungal peritonitis in patients on continuous ambulatory peritoneal dialysis: a single centre Indian experience. *J Infect.* 2004;48:96–101.
25. Wang AY, Yu AW, Li PK, Lam PK, Leung CB, Lai KN. Factors predicting outcome of fungal peritonitis in peritoneal dialysis: analysis of a 9-year experience of fungal peritonitis in a single center. *Am J Kidney Dis.* 2000;36:1183–1192.
26. Asif A, Gadalean F, Vieira CF, Hogan R, Leon C, Merrill D, Ellis R, Amador A, Broche O, Bush B, Contreras G, Pennell

P. Salvage of problematic peritoneal dialysis catheters. *Semin Dial*. 2006;19(2);180–183.

27. Santos CR, Branco PQ, Martinho A, Gonçalves MS, Gaspar A, Messias H, Barata JD. Salvage of malpositioned and malfunctioning peritoneal dialysis catheters by manipulation with a modified Malecot introducer. *Semin Dial*. 2010;23:95–99.

28. Faintuch S, Salazar GM. Malfunction of dialysis catheters: management of fibrin sheath and related problems. *Tech Vasc Interv Radiol*. 2008;11:195–200.

29. Goh YH. Omental folding: a novel laparoscopic technique for salvaging peritoneal dialysis catheters. *Perit Dial Int*. 2008;28:626–631.

30. Khanna R, Krediet R *Nolph and Gokal's Textbook of Peritoneal Dialysis. Springer Science + Business Media*, 3rd edition, Berlin: *Springer Science + Business Media*, LLC; 2009:435–436.

31. Plum J, Sudkamp S, Grabensee B. Results of ultra sound assisted diagnosis of tunnel infections in continuous ambulatory peritoneal dialysis. *Am J Kidney Dis*. 1994;23: 99–104.

32. Vychytil A, Lorenz M, Schneider B, Horl WH, Haag-Weber M. New criteria for management of catheter infections in peritoneal dialysis patients using ultrasonography. *J Am Soc Nephrol*. 1998;9:290–296.

33. Shroff S, Pandey S, Abraham G, Soundarrajan P. A simple closed 'Pull and Jerk' technique for CAPD catheter removal. Online at http://www.medindia.net/articles/capd-catheter-removal.asp#ixzz1mtvLUwRi. Accessed May 1, 2011.

34. Posthuma N, Borgstein PJ, Eijsbouts Q, ter Wee PM. Simultaneous peritoneal dialysis catheter insertion and removal in catheter-related infections without interruption of peritoneal dialysis. *Nephrol Dial Transplant*. 1998;13: 700–703.

35. Mitra A, Teitelbaum I. Is it safe to simultaneously remove and replace infected peritoneal dialysis catheters? Review of the literature and suggested guidelines. *Adv Perit Dial*. 2003;19:255–259.

36. Pérez FM, Rodríguez-Carmona A. Peritoneal catheter removal for severe peritonitis: landscape after a lost battle. *Perit Dial Int*. 2007;27:155–158.

37. Bloembergen WE, Port FK. Epidemiological perspective on infections in chronic dialysis patients. *Adv Ren Replace Ther*. 1996;3:201–207.

38. Mujais S. Microbiology and outcomes of peritonitis in North America. *Kidney Int*. 2006;70(suppl 103):S55–S62.

39. Pérez FM, Rodríguez-Carmona A, García-Naveiro R, Rosales M, Villaverde P, Valdés F. Peritonitis-related mortality in patients undergoing chronic peritoneal dialysis. *Perit Dial Int*. 2005;25:274–284.

40. Fried LF, Bernardini J, Johnston JR, Piraino B. Peritonitis influences mortality in peritoneal dialysis patients. *J Am Soc Nephrol*. 1996;7:2176–2182.

41. Chang TI, Kim HW, Park JT, Lee DH, Lee JH, Yoo TH, Kang SW. *Perit Dial Int*. 2011;31(1):60–66.

47

ANTIBIOTIC PROPHYLAXIS FOR DIALYSIS ACCESS INTERVENTIONS

RAJIV K. DHAMIJA, LOAY SALMAN, ARIF ASIF, & GERALD A. BEATHARD

LEARNING OBJECTIVES

1. Understand the historical perspective on the role of antibiotic prophylaxis for dialysis access procedures.
2. Understand the role of antibiotic prophylaxis for hemodialysis access procedures.
3. Understand the role of antibiotic prophylaxis for peritoneal dialysis procedures.
4. Under the timing of administration, duration, and concerns for antibiotic prophylaxis.

Any invasive procedure carries a potential risk of procedure-related infection. Such infections can range from local phenomena requiring minimal actions to catastrophic systemic involvement requiring major interventions to minimize morbidity and mortality. Surgeons have been the pioneers in conducting research in preventing procedure-related infection; however, cardiologists and interventional radiologists have played a central role in antibiotic prophylaxis during percutaneous interventions. Multiple reports have documented a beneficial effect of antibiotic prophylaxis in reducing postoperative infection for many minimally invasive procedures. Nevertheless, there is a lack of established guidelines regarding the use of prophylactic antibiotics for dialysis access procedures. Practice patterns for the use of prophylactic antibiotics demonstrate a wide variation among interventionalists. Many use them routinely for the insertion of tunneled central venous catheters, while others perform this procedure without any coverage. While the use of prophylactic antibiotics can potentially limit the development of subsequent infection, their use can also be associated with severe allergic reactions, the development of drug resistance and increased costs.

For many years, antibiotic prophylaxis has been advocated for the prevention of infection during many surgical and percutaneous interventions. The goal of such therapy has been to limit the development of postoperative infection and reduce patient's morbidity and mortality.[1-9] However, the validity of this practice and these concerns should be examined and our intent is to do so. The use of preoperative antibiotics for any given situation must be based upon evidence of its effectiveness in limiting postoperative infection. The question is, are they really medically indicated and does their use expose the patient to additional risks rather than reduce the chances of an adverse event? While antibiotics can prevent infection, their use can be associated with adverse events, some of which are serious, such as anaphylaxis, the development of drug resistance and increased costs. The validity of their use in association with dialysis access interventions where very limited information exists is of particular concern.

HISTORICAL PERSPECTIVE

The occurrence of significant bacteremia following cardiac catheterization was documented in several early reports.[6,10,11] The reported incidence ranged from 4–18%.[10,11] This finding coupled with the concern that bacteremia could potentially lead to increased patient morbidity and mortality led to the routine application of antibiotic prophylaxis for cardiac catheterization. This practice pattern persisted even though controlled studies performed at the time found no benefit in favor of antibiotics compared to the placebo group.[5,11]

With the advent of percutaneous transluminal balloon coronary angioplasty (PTCA) for the management of coronary stenosis, procedure-related bacteremia again became the subject of investigation. In a prospective study designed to evaluate the incidence of bacteremia associated with

PTCA, 164 cases were evaluated.[12] Unlike diagnostic cardiac catheterization, this procedure involves the use of an indwelling arterial sheath after completion of the procedure. Blood cultures were drawn from the femoral catheter at the completion and 30 minutes later from the indwelling catheter. Additionally, temperature was monitored for 36 hours after the procedure. Patients currently receiving antibiotics or demonstrating active infection were excluded from the study. Skin antisepsis was obtained by using povidone-iodine. Only a single case of bacteremia was documented (*Staphylococcus aureus*). The authors concluded that the overall risk of bacteremia after coronary angioplasty was low and, therefore, antimicrobial prophylaxis was not warranted.

In a subsequent larger prospective report, 960 cases were evaluated.[13] In this study, three blood cultures were drawn—first, immediately after the arterial puncture, second, at the conclusion of the procedure, and the third, 4 hours after the completion of the procedure. The first two cultures were performed from the femoral sheath while the last one was drawn from a peripheral vein. The authors distinguished between clinically significant and nonsignificant bacteremia. Clinically significant bacteremia was defined as the presence of bacteria in ≥ 1 blood culture in the presence of sign or symptoms of infection. This was encountered in only four cases (0.4%) and all were related to the presence of an intravenous line; none were related to the procedure itself. The authors concluded that prophylactic antibiotics were not needed for this procedure.

ENDOVASCULAR DIALYSIS ACCESS PROCEDURES

In contrast to coronary interventions, the incidence of procedure-related bacteremia in patients undergoing dialysis access interventions has not been studied in a prospective fashion. The only information available is derived from published studies on dialysis access procedures and from practical experience gained by performing large numbers of these procedures. The presence of local or systemic signs and symptoms such as erythema, tenderness, fever, chills, malaise, and leukocytosis within 72 hours of a procedure is generally accepted as an indicator for a related clinical infection, even before culture confirmation. However, once a clinical infection is suspected, the diagnosis should be confirmed by obtaining blood cultures. Not only is this confirmatory, it also serves as a guide for selecting appropriate antibiotic treatment.

In a recent study, prospectively collected data on 3162 consecutive percutaneous interventions performed on hemodialysis and peritoneal dialysis (PD) patients were reviewed.[14] The procedures included percutaneous balloon angioplasty (arterial and venous) ($n = 2,052$ [AVF $= 1300$; AVG $= 752$]), venography for vascular mapping ($n = 110$), endovascular stent insertion ($n = 26$), intravascular coil placement ($n = 31$), thrombectomy for an arteriovenous fistula ($n = 106$), thrombectomy for an arteriovenous graft ($n = 110$), tunneled hemodialysis catheter (TDC) insertion and exchange ($n = 283$), TDC removal ($n = 160$), and insertion of accidentally extruded TDC through the existing exit site ($n = 9$). There were 260 PD catheter insertions and 15 repositioning procedures. Only patients undergoing TDC insertion for accidentally extruded catheter and PD catheter placement received prophylactic antibiotics 1–2 hours before the procedure. A gram of cefazolin was given to the TDC cases and a gram of vancomycin was administered to the PD cases. One patient (0.04%) postangioplasty and one patient (0.3%) after tunneled catheter placement developed clinical infection manifested by fever, chills, and malaise within 24 hours of the procedure. Both required hospitalization and demonstrated positive blood cultures for *S. aureus*. The patient with angioplasty was diabetic with an arteriovenous graft, while TDC insertion was performed in a patient with advanced HIV. Based on this experience demonstrating such a low incidence of infection, it is difficult to endorse the routine use of prophylactic antibiotics for these procedures.

In a cohort of 12,896 cases that included percutaneous balloon arterial and venous angioplasty ($n = 5228$), thrombectomy for an arteriovenous fistulas ($n = 371$), thrombectomy for an arteriovenous graft ($n = 3941$), TDC insertion ($n = 1050$), and TDC removal ($n = 2306$), prospectively collected data concerning complications were examined.[15] Monthly verification of the electronic record was performed against each individual procedure room log for quality assurance purposes. Individual patient data was then randomly selected for verification against the medical record and the physician procedure note using a random number generator. Patient follow-up data was collected by review of patient records at individual dialysis facilities. Antibiotic prophylaxis was not used. Only three instances of infection were recorded within 72 hours following the associated procedure in the cohort of cases. All of these were *S. aureus*.

Combining these two series, one can see that in a total of 16,058 cases representing the spectrum of cases normally seen in a dialysis vascular access facility, only five cases (0.03%) of infection were noted. Based on this experience demonstrating such a low incidence of infection, it is difficult to endorse the routine use of prophylactic antibiotics for these procedures.

Because it involves skin penetration by a foreign device that is left in place, prophylactic antibiotic coverage for catheter insertion has been an issue of particular concern (3.16–17). However, randomized studies[16,17] dealing with single lumen catheters have shown that, although there was a significant incidence of infection, it was not reduced by the administration of periprocedural antibiotics. It is important to note that the incidence of infection with tunneled catheters is significantly lower than that seen with nontunneled catheters. Nevertheless, both types of catheters are associated with a serious risk of infection. Despite this fact, there has been a lack of randomized studies to evaluate the use of prophylactic antibiotics for either short or

TABLE 47–1

Antibiotic Prophylaxis for a Variety of Dialysis Access Procedures

Procedure Type	Comments	Suggestion
Angioplasty	Venous	No routine antibiotic
	Arterial	No routine antibiotic
Thrombectomy	Fistulae and grafts	No routine antibiotic
Stent placement		No routine antibiotic
Coil placement		No routine antibiotic
Catheter procedures	New placement	No routine antibiotic
	Exchange for catheter dysfunction	No routine antibiotic
	Accidentally extruded catheters*	Consider intravenous cefazolin (1 gm)/vancomycin 500 mg if penicillin allergy
Peritoneal dialysis catheter insertion		Intravenous vancomycin (1 gm)

*NOTE: For accidentally extruded catheters that are placed through the existing exit, tunnel and venotomy site prophylactic antibiotic coverage can be considered.

long-term catheter placement. A large series of tunneled dialysis catheter insertion was reported by Trerotola et al.[18] These investigators performed 250 TDC catheter insertions in 175 patients. Although this was not a randomized controlled study evaluating the effect of prophylactic antibiotics, these agents were not used and clinical infection in the post operative period was not observed. Based on the above information, it is difficult to support the use of prophylactic antibiotics in for the insertion of a tunneled hemodialysis catheter.

The replacement of an accidentally extruded catheter through the existing tunnel is a somewhat unique situation. Intuitively, it seems that this might be an exception where prophylactic antibiotics would be warranted. Unfortunately, the situation has never been studied in a randomized clinical trial. In the reports in which this procedure has been performed[19–22] prophylactic antibiotics, both cefazolin and vancomycin, have been used without the support offered by data confirming efficacy. In a recent report, data on 49 patients who underwent 57 replacements of accidentally dislodged catheters were presented.[22] Intravenous cefazolin or vancomycin (for penicillin allergic patients) was used as prophylactic agents. None of the patients had procedure-related infection for up to 48 hours. The infection rate observed in this series was within the upper limit of results of de novo placement and over-the-wire exchange of catheters in the literature. Conclusions concerning the use of prophylactic antibiotics in this situation must await the availability of appropriately derived data.

Given the similarities of the percutaneous balloon angioplasty for dialysis access to the coronary angioplasty one might assume that the risk of infection might be similar in dialysis access angioplasty to that observed in coronary interventions. One clinical infection experienced in 2052 consecutive dialysis access angioplasty procedures in the above-cited experience testifies to the validity of this assumption. Multiple reports published on routine

angioplasty, stent, and coil insertion or thrombectomy procedures for dialysis access in well-established journals did not use antibiotic prophylaxis for these interventions.[23–30] In addition, significant clinical infections in the postoperative period have not been reported by these studies. In the presence of low incidence of clinical infection, prophylactic use of antibiotics cannot be endorsed in percutaneous balloon angioplasty, endovascular stent insertion, intravascular coil insertion, and thrombectomy procedures (Table 47-1).

PERITONEAL DIALYSIS CATHETER INSERTION

Peritoneal catheters can be placed by surgeons or interventional nephrologists.[31] In contrast to endovascular procedures, the use of prophylactic antibiotics has been more accepted in the area of peritoneal catheters.[32–36] The first published report that evaluated the role of prophylactic antibiotics was performed by Lye et al[32] in 1992. The study revealed that the prophylactic regimen of a single dose of cefazolin and gentamicin did not reduce the number of peritonitis events. Subsequent, studies by Bennet-Jones[33] and Wikdahl[34] showed that antibiotic use significantly reduced the risk for early peritonitis (<1 month from catheter insertion) but not the risk for exit-site or tunnel infection. In view of these conflicting data, Gadallah and colleagues[35] undertook a prospective randomized study of 254 peritoneal dialysis catheter insertion procedures. Patients were randomized to prophylactic intravenous vancomycin, cefazolin, or no antibiotics. The results showed that single-dose vancomycin was superior to single-dose cefazolin in reducing the risk for postoperative peritonitis and that the no prophylactic antibiotics group was associated with the highest risk of postoperative infection (vancomycin = 1%, cefazolin = 7%, no antibiotics = 12%;

$P = 0.02$).[35] The development of peritonitis is not only associated with catheter loss, but also inflicts the risk of peritoneal membrane damage. Based on this information, antibiotic prophylaxis is warranted in patients with peritoneal dialysis catheters.

TIMING, DURATION, AND CONCERNS FOR ANTIBIOTIC PROPHYLAXIS

Although their use is common in many procedures, multiple complicating issues such as timing of administration, duration of prophylaxis as well as adverse reactions associated with the medication continue to surround the use of prophylactic antibiotics. The role of antibiotic administration and its timing in limiting infection was first investigated over half a century ago.[37] In an elegant study, Miles et al[37] tested the concept of the decisive period regarding the suppression of infection after the administration of antibiotics.

Using the intracutaneously inoculation of bacteria in guinea pigs a model, three groups were studied—in one group, antibiotics (penicillin and streptomycin) were administered 0–1 hour before bacterial injection, in a second group, the antibiotic administration was delayed for 3–5 hours after bacterial injection and a third group received a placebo. The results disclosed a significant reduction in local infection in the animals that received antibiotics 0–1 hour before bacterial injection compared to the placebo group. Local infections induced by bacterial administration that were 3–5 hours old did not respond to the type and dose of antibiotics that were effective against the same bacteria when given 0–1 hour before the bacterial inoculation. This was the first report that provided the basis to the timing of prophylactic antibiotics used today. These findings were later confirmed by Burke, who also demonstrated that antibiotics administered more than 3 hours before the procedure actually increased the incidence of infection and adverse events fivefold.[38]

For the most part, the timing of preoperative administration of antibiotic for prophylaxis has been established. However, the duration of therapy has not been standardized. In 1977, Strachan[39] randomized 201 patients into no treatment group, single preoperative dose of the cefazolin group and single preoperative dose with five postoperative doses of the cefazolin group. The authors found that a single preoperative dose was superior to no treatment and at least as effective as prolonged treatment.[39] This finding was later confirmed in follow-up studies.[40,41] It is for this reason that many interventionalists utilize a single dose of prophylactic antibiotic for percutaneous interventions.[4]

While the use of prophylactic antibiotics in certain situations is valid, the development of resistance against antibiotics has been a major concern for decades.[42–44] Mutation and transfer of resistance-encoding genetic material from one bacterium to another is thought to be one of the mechanisms of the development of bacterial resistance. Misuse as well as overuse of antibiotics has a major impact on the spread of antibiotic resistant bacterial species.[42] Increased numbers of immunocompromised patients and not following appropriate infection control practices are also other important factors for bacterial resistance. The development of multidrug-resistant virulent organisms, such as methicillin-resistant *S. aureus* (MRSA), vancomycin-resistant enterococcus (VRE), and extended-spectrum beta-lactamase (ESBL) producing Gram-negative bacilli, has created an alarming situation.

The National Nosocomial Infections Surveillance System (NNIS) has reported that while there has been little change in the incidence and distribution of the pathogens isolated from infections during the last decade, more of these pathogens show antimicrobial-drug resistance. This has raised a serious concern and triggered the urgency and pressure to reevaluate the use of empiric protocols in all specialties.[43]

Published information on the incidence adverse events associated with the use of prophylactic antibiotics has shown a great deal of variation. A large prospective study reported that 3.2% of cases demonstrated true penicillin allergy of which 0.2% were anaphylactic in nature.[45] In contrast, another prospective study found the rate of adverse events to be 22%.[46] Allergic reactions associated with the prophylactic use of antibiotics is a cause of great concern, especially when one considers the fact that many patients require repeated procedures during the period they are on dialysis. Many of these reactions are mild, requiring only minimal intervention, but some can be serious and even life-threatening. It is imperative that this concern be taken into account when evaluating the use of antibiotics in this manner.

CONCLUSION

For the most part antibiotic prophylaxis for hemodialysis access-related procedures is not warranted. However, preoperative antibiotic administration has been for reinsertion of an accidentally extruded tunneled hemodialysis catheter when performed through the same exit site. There is evidence that peritoneal dialysis catheter insertion should be performed under preoperative antibiotic cover to minimize the development of subsequent infection. While the abovementioned suggestions are justifiable at present, large scale, multicenter studies with appropriate designs are needed to establish guidelines for the use of prophylactic antibiotics in patients undergoing percutaneous vascular access procedures.

REFERENCES

1. Classen DC, Evans RS, Pestotnik SL. The timing of prophylactic administration of antibiotics and the risk of surgical wound infection. *N Engl J Med.* 1992;326:281.
2. Spies JB, Rosen RJ, Lebowitz AS. Antibiotic prophylxis in vascular and interventional radiology: a rational approach. *Radiology.* 1988;166:381–387.

3. Ryan JM, Ryan BM, Simth TP. Antibiotic prophylaxis in interventional radiology. *J Vasc Interv Nephrol.* 2004;15:547.

4. Beddy P, Ryan JM. Antibiotic prophylaxis in interventional radiology—anything new? *Tech Vasc Interventional Rad.* 2006;9:69.

5. Gould L, Lyon AF. Penicillin prophylaxis in cardiac catheterization. *JAMA.* 1976;202:210.

6. Sande MA, Levinson ME, Lukas DS, Kaye D. Bacteremia associated with cardiac catheterization. *N Engl J Med.* 1969;281(13):1104.

7. Shawker TH, Kluge RM, Ayella RJ. Bacteremia associated with angiography. *JAMA.* 1974;229:1090.

8. Shea KW, Schwartz RK, Gambino AT, Marzo KP, Cunha BA. Bacteremia associated with percutaneous transluminal coronary angioplasty. *Cathet Cardiovasc Diagn.* 1995;36:5.

9. Banai S, Selitser V, Keren A, Benhorin J, Shitrit OB, Yalon S, Halperin E. Prospective study of bacteremia after cardiac catheterization. *Am J Cardiol.* 2003;92:1004.

10. Marshall MD, Kreidberg B, Harvey MD, Chernoff L. Ineffectiveness of penicillin prophylaxisin cardiac catheterization. *J Pediatr.* 1965;66:286.

11. Clark H. An evaluation of antibiotic prophylaxis in cardiac catheterization. *Am Heart J.* 1969;77:767.

12. Shea KW, Schwartz RK, Gambino AT, Marzo KP, Cunha BA. Bacteremia associated with percutaneous transluminal coronary angioplasty. *Cathet Cardiovasc Diagn.* 1995;36:5.

13. Banai S, Selitser V, Keren A, Benhorin J, Shitrit OB, Yalon S, Halperin E. Prospective study of bacteremia after cardiac catheterization. *Am J Cardiol.* 2003;92:1004.

14. Salman L, Asif A. Antibiotic prophylaxis: is it needed for dialysis access procedures? *Semin Dial.* 2009;22:297.

15. Beathard GA, Litchfield T. Physician Operators Forum of RMS Lifeline, Inc: effectiveness and safety of dialysis vascular access procedures performed by interventional nephrologists. *Kidney Int.* 2004;66:1622.

16. Ranson MR, Oppenheim BA, Jackson A, Kamthan AG, Scarffe JH. Double-blind placebo controlled study of vancomycin prophylaxis for central venous catheter insertion in cancer patients. *J Hosp Inf.* 1990;15:95.

17. McKee R, Dunsmuir R, Whitby M, Garden OJ. Does antibiotic prophylaxis at the time of catheter insertion reduce the incidence of catheter-related sepsis in intravenous nutrition? *J Hosp Inf.* 1985;6:419.

18. Trerotola SO, Johnson MS, Harris VJ, et al. Outcome of tunneled right internal jugular hemodialysis catheters placed via the right internal jugular vein by interventional radiologists. *Radiology.* 1997;203:489.

19. Lin BH, Funaki B, Szymski GX. A technique for inserting inadvertently removed tunneled hemodialysis catheters using existing subcutaneous tracts. *Am J Roentogenol.* 1997;169:1157.

20. Atray N, Asif A. New tunneled hemodialysis catheter placement through the old exit site. *Semin Dial.* 2008; 21:97.

21. Sombolos K, Bamichas G, Gionanlis L, Fragidis S, Veneti P, Natse T. Placement of a new hemodialysis catheter through the old exit site without the use of a guidewire. *Semin Dial.* 2008;21:371.

22. Saad NE, Saad WE, Davies MG, Waldman DL. Replacement of inadvertently discontinued tunneled jugular high-flow central catheters with tract recannulation: technical results and outcome. *J Vasc Interv Radiol.* 2008;19:890.

23. Beathard GA, Arnold P, Jackson J, Litchfield T. Physician operators forum of RMS lifeline. Aggressive treatment of early fistula failure. *Kidney Int.* 2003;64:1487.

24. Beathard GA, Litchfield T. Physician Operators Forum of RMS Lifeline, Inc. Effectiveness and safety of dialysis vascular access procedures performed by interventional nephrologists. *Kidney Int.* 2004;66:1622.

25. Beathard GA. Angioplasty for arteriovenous grafts and fistulae. *Semin Nephrol.* 2002;22:202.

26. Beathard GA. Gianturco self-expanding stent in the treatment of stenosis in dialysis access grafts. *Kidney Int.* 1993;43:872.

27. Vesely TM. Use of stent grafts to repair hemodialysis graft-related pseudoaneurysms. *J Vasc Interv Radiol.* 12005; 6:1301.

28. Vesely TM, Amin MZ, Pilgram T. Use of stents and stent grafts to salvage angioplasty failures in patients with hemodialysis grafts. *Semin Dial.* 2008;21:100.

29. Chan MR, Bedi S, Sanchez RJ, Young HN, Becker YT, Kellerman PS, Yevzlin AS. Stent placement versus angioplasty improves patency of arteriovenous grafts and blood flow of arteriovenous fistulae. *Clin J Am Soc Nephrol.* 2008;3:699.

30. Maya ID, Allon M. Outcomes of thrombosed arteriovenous grafts: comparison of stents vs angioplasty. *Kidney Int.* 2006;69:934.

31. Asif A. Peritoneal dialysis catheter insertion. *Minerva Chir.* 2005;5:417.

32. Lye WC, Lee EJ, Tan CC. Prophylactic antibiotics in the insertion of Tenckhoff catheters. *Scand J Urol Nephrol.* 1992;26:177.

33. Bennet-Jones DN, Martin J, Barratt AJ, Duffy TJ, Naish PF, Aber GM. Prophylactic gentamicin in the prevention of early exit-site infections and peritonitis in CAPD. *Adv Perit Dial.* 1998;4:147.

34. Wikdahl AM, Engman U, Stegmayr G, Sorensen JG. One-dose cefuroxime i.v and i.p. reduces microbial growth in PD patients after catheter insertion. *Nephrol Dial Transplant.* 1997;12:157.

35. Gadallah MF, Ramdeen G, Mignone J, Patel D, Mitchell L, Tatro S. Role of preoperative antibiotic prophylaxis in preventing postoperative peritonitis in newly placed peritoneal dialysis catheters. *Am J Kidney Dis.* 2000;36:1014.

36. Strippoli G, Tong A, Johnson D, Schena F, Craig JC. Antimicrobial agents to prevent peritonitis in peritoneal dialysis: a systematic review of randomized controlled trials. *Am J Kidney Diseases.* 2004;44:591.

37. Miles AA, Miles EM, Burke J. The value and duration of defense reactions of the skin to primary lodgment of bacteria. *Br J Exp Pathol.* 1957;38:79.

38. Burke JF. The effective period of preventive antibiotic action in experimental incisions and dermal lesions. *Surgery.* 1961;50:161.

39. Strachan CJ. Prophylactic use of cefazolin against sepsis after cholecystectomy. *BMJ.* 1977;1:1254.

40. Classen DC, Evans RS, Pestotnik SL. The timing of prophylactic administration of antibiotics and the risk of surgical wound infection. *N Engl J Med.* 1992;326:281.

41. DiPiro JT, Cheung RP, Bowden TA. Single dose systemic antibiotic prophylaxis of surgical wound infections. *Am J Surg.* 1986;152:552.

42. Dzidic S, Bedekovic V. Horizontal gene transfer-emerging multidrug resistance in hospital bacteria. *Acta Pharmacol Sin.* 2003;24:519.

43. National nosocomial infections surveillance (NNIS) system report: Data summary from January 1992–April 2000. *Am J Infect Control.* 2000;28:429.

44. Rossolini GM, Mantengoli E. Antimicrobial resistance in Europe and its potential impact on empirical therapy. *Clin Microbiol Infect.* 2008;6:2–8.

45. International Rheumatic Fever Group. Allergic reactions to long-term benzathine penicillin prophylaxis for rheumatic fever. *Lancet.* 1991;337:1308.

46. Macpherson RD, Willcox C, Chow C, et al. Anaesthetist's response to patients' self-reported drug allergies. *Br J Anaesth.* 2006;97:634.

SECTION IV
Surgical Aspects of Vascular Access

SECTION IV

48

SITES AND TYPES OF ARTERIOVENOUS FISTULAE

KLAUS KONNER, RICK MISHLER, & JEFFREY PACKER

LEARNING OBJECTIVES

1. Learn the history of vascular access (VA).

2. Describe the trends in demographics and comorbidities of hemodialysis patients as it relates to VA in the modern era.

3. Understand the pathophysiology of arteriovenous fistulae (AVF).

4. Describe the benefit of preoperative diagnostic evaluations.

5. Describe different options for placement of AVF with regard to type and site.

6. Understand indications for different types and sites of AVF.

7. Learn the necessary steps to creation of arteriovenous fistulae that are functional.

8. Learn to aim at an individualized, patient-specific approach to VA.

9. Learn to establish VA surgery as a part of an interdisciplinary VA team.

INTRODUCTION

Access to the circulation is required to successfully perform repeated "chronic" hemodialysis therapy (HD) throughout a patient's life or until renal transplantation is performed.

Although HD equipment was available in the late 1950s, long-term access to the circulation that is required to perform HD continued to prove challenging. In 1960, Dr. Scribner, from Seattle, WA, introduced the Scribner arteriovenous shunt, thus, initiating the era of arteriovenous access for chronic HD.[1] In 1966, Brescia, Cimino, and colleagues published the first results of their arteriovenous fistulae (AVF), thus ushering in an era of a pathologic, non-physiological, vascular construct that functions as a lifesaving tool.[2]

In the early 1970s, various synthetic and biologic graft materials came into use. The abundant use of these conduits since 1975 brought about increasing rates of patient morbidity and mortality as well as a substantial rise in financial expenditures. In the 1980s, central venous catheters (CVC) entered the scene, followed by interventional radiological procedures. Later, two-dimensional (2D) and Doppler ultrasound techniques were developed as an integral part of preoperative vascular access (VA) planning and postoperative VA surveillance. Despite the presence of these diagnostic and therapeutic tools, the rates of use of autologous AVF in the United States end stage renal disease (ESRD) population has lagged behind Europe and Japan for decades. As a result of these problems, in the mid-1990s a series of guidelines such as NKF-KDOQI (1997, 2002, and 2006) were published.[3]

In 2012, there is an agreement in the literature that AVF is the preferred VA for hemodialysis compared to arteriovenous synthetic grafts (AVG) and CVC. Autologous AVF are superior to other accesses with respect to VA complication rates, access-related morbidity and mortality, quality of life, and financial costs. Although superior to other accesses, AVF are far from being trouble free. Recently, interest has focused mainly on high early failure rates of AVF.

▶ Is an AVF a Pathologic Entity a Priori?

The "surgically created arteriovenous fistula" as titled in the original article by Brescia, Cimino, and Appel in 1966[2] is a nonphysiological construct. The purpose of intentionally creating this abnormal situation is to achieve a high blood flow volume of approximately 1000 mL/min that will allow a blood flow through the dialyzer of

300–500 mL/min that is required for an adequate dialysis treatment and that can be repeatedly cannulated. Why is the AVF considered to be a nonphysiological entity?

These high blood flow volumes are to be provided by a peripheral artery with an original average diameter of 2–2.5 mm and a baseline flow of ~20–30 mL/min (in the case of the radial artery),[4] delivered to a tiny, thin-walled vein constructed by nature for a flow of ~5–10 mL/min. Today, we know that initial flow rates immediately after creation of the arteriovenous anastomosis reach 400 mL/min, a multifold level of the original flow volume on both, arterial as well as venous sides of the AV fistula.[5]

After anastomosis is created, a process of remodeling is initiated. Reliable cannulation of the vein is only possible after it is "arterialized"; later in this process, a moderate elongation of the vein is also observed. With increasing experience in the beginning of 1970s, we learned that this venous dilatation exclusively happens as a consequence of arterial dilatation. The AV anastomosis causes a fall in peripheral resistance, thus favoring high flow volumes. Even today, mechanisms such as flow velocity, peak flow velocity, shear stress, increase in diameter and other factors involved in the maturation process are not fully understood. Dr. Corpataux's observations are of particular interest in understanding this process.[6]

What has Changed Over Time?—The Pivotal Role of the Feeding Artery

As a young nephrologist in the early 1970s the author (KK) witnessed the restriction of renal replacement therapy to those patients less than 40 years of age. As a result, VA, exclusively Scribner shunts and AVF, were placed in these young patients; problems of arterial vascular disease were unknown among this dialysis cohort at that time. Since then, the demographics of incident hemodialysis patients have dramatically changed worldwide. In 2012, we have a predominance of old, diabetic, and hypertensive patients with a high rate of cardiovascular disease due to damage of the arterial vasculature.[7] The frequent presence of these comorbidities requires a much more structured approach to AVF creation than has been necessary in the past.

Preoperative diagnostic procedures start with a careful, meticulous clinical examination, ultrasound vascular mapping has become mandatory in the modern era of access planning. Beyond venous anatomy and arterial diameter, visual analysis of the inflow and outflow vascular systems may address arterial characteristics such as calcifications of different types and stiffness of the arterial wall resulting in impaired arterial distension capacity. In addition, Dr. Malovrh introduced the resistance index as a functional parameter for arterial capacity and recommends that the operator should: "select a segment of artery with greater diameter, less wall structural changes and best functional characteristics."[8] Few years ago, severe calcifications were noted by one of the authors (KK) in the peripheral radial artery wall in many patients and these were less pronounced along the proximal segments of the radial artery or the distal brachial artery.

The time has passed when the radial artery AVF at the wrist should be considered *the* "gold standard" for VA in every patient. The K-DOQI guideline that distal AV access is necessarily better is an antiquated concept. The challenge in 2012 is to find the *best* arterial segment for placement of the initial AV fistula; careful clinical and ultrasound guided examination of the arterial vasculature will assist in this task.

Early care by nephrologists and early referral to a VA surgeon have a clear benefit for the incident hemodialysis patient in achieving a timely initial access creation so that the VA can be used at initiation of HD therapy.[9] Every patient *is* a candidate for an AV fistula; good reasons should be present for *nonacceptance* of any patient for creation of an AVF. Medical history, meticulous clinical evaluation, and ultrasound analysis of arteries and veins contribute to the choice of the best artery and best vein for successful initial AV fistula placement.

Today careful documentation has become a mandatory medical practice. With regard to VA creation, it starts with the clinical history, followed by the results of the ultrasound study. Sketches of the superficial veins and arteries are very beneficial, giving rapid, clear information that often is more direct and more precise than words alone.

At Which Site Should the Initial AVF be Created?

Historically, it was recommended that the nondominant arm was preferred for creation of an initial AVF. Based on the authors' experience, this may be misleading today. It seems that the first AVF should be placed in the arm with the better venous *and* arterial vasculature as determined by the preoperative diagnostic clinical and ultrasound evaluations.

Any segment of the radial or ulnar artery in the forearm can be used to create an arteriovenous anastomosis (Figure 48-1). The choice is dependent on the quality of arteries and veins. Determinants of quality include absence of severe arterioatherosclerosis, absence of calcifications, maintenance of arterial distension capacity, and an adequate arterial diameter. To use the arterial diameter as the sole parameter with which to describe a "good" artery is inadequate; the functional parameters as mentioned earlier are an integral part of a "good," a suitable artery with which to construct an AV fistula. AV fistula maturation will not be possible without an optimal arterial inflow volume.

Currently more patients with severe pathology of peripheral arteries are developing ESRD. This change in patient comorbidities often requires a more proximal access to arterial vasculature in order to create a viable AVF. If a peripheral (distal) anastomosis is not feasible, many authors recommend using the upper arm vessels above the elbow for a brachio-basilic or brachio-cephalic AV fistula. This choice may sacrifice numerous valuable

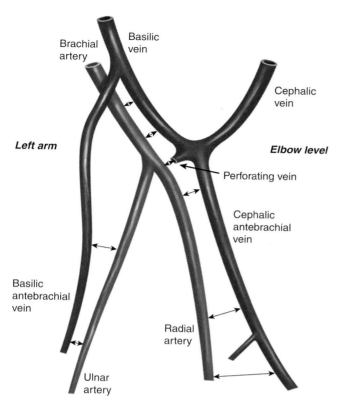

Figure 48-1. Options for creation of arteriovenous fistulae in the arm. Notice the multiple choices of sites within the gap between the commonly cited limitations of "wrist fistula" and "brachiobasilic/cephalic fistula."

options for placing an AV fistula at sites between the wrist and the upper arm (Figure 48-1). The author's (KK) experience with >2000 consecutive primary autologous AV fistulae demonstrates that ~60% of these operations were performed along this so-called gap between the wrist and antecubital fossa.[10]

▶ Anastomotic Techniques

Vessel anastomoses may be of three different types. One way to describe them is to name the anastomotic type based on the direction of blood flow from the artery to the vein with the anatomic description following:

1. side-to-side anastomosis (SSA);
2. end-to-end anastomosis (EEA);
3. artery-side-to-vein-end anastomosis (SEA).

The classical radial artery AV fistula at the wrist, as introduced by Brescia, Cimino, and Appel (the surgeon!) is an artery-side-to-vein-side anastomosis connecting the radial artery and the closely adjacent cephalic vein.[2] Over time, we have learned to ligate the arterialized vein just distal to the anastomosis in order to prevent distal venous hypertension from occurring. This action results in a functional artery-side-to-vein-end anastomosis (Figure 48-2).

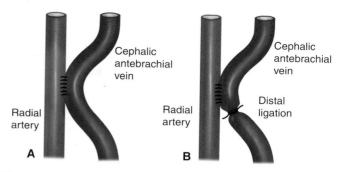

Figure 48-2. (**A**) Peripheral radial artery side-to-side arteriovenous fistulae with predominant venous drainage and subsequent obliteration of the proximal venous limb. (**B**) Ligation of the peripheral venous limb leads to a functional artery-side-to-vein-end anastomosis.

Many surgeons are accustomed to placing sutures at the apices of the arteriotomy to properly position the vessels for anastomosis; as a result, a high level of skill is required to evert the edges of artery and vein on the back wall that is required for proper stitch placement. Dr. Tellis published a variation on this common practice that is easy to accomplish. By placing an initial suture in the mid-portion of the back wall, the vessels are thus maintained in a proper and stable position for the anastomotic work. So, the suture can be performed utmost controlled (Figure 48-3).[11]

Studies of this configuration demonstrate that, in approximately 25% of patients, retrograde arterial inflow into the anastomosis from the ulnar artery through the palmar arch is observed that can be seen as a "physiologic steal phenomenon."[12]

One year after the initial report of the "Cimino" AVF, in 1967, Sperling et al introduced the artery-end-to-end-vein technique.[13] In this procedure, the most distal portion of the artery is occluded and then transected so that it can be curved proximally and positioned adjacent to the vein for anastomosis. The suturing technique is more demanding as compared to the side-to-side procedure. In the majority of patients, a difference in arterial and venous

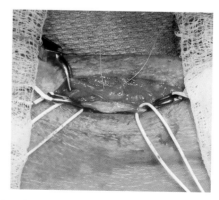

Figure 48-3. Photograph depicting Tellis technique: placing an initial suture in the mid-portion of the back wall of the vessel, thus, maintaining the vessels in a proper and stable position for the anastomotic work.

diameter is observed that can cause technical problems in achieving an adequately functioning AV anastomosis; several tricks were introduced over the years to overcome these obstacles.

Today, the end-to-end technique is not the preferred method of anastomosis in initial AV fistula operations given the risk of occluding an artery in a highly morbid, old, and often diabetic HD patient. Less risky options such as artery-end-to-end-vein technique are available. However, despite the perceived risks, there are single, very experienced centers that favor the end-to-end technique even today.

In 1968, Röhl and colleagues published an artery-side-to-vein-end anastomotic technique that was useful in situations when there is a larger distance between the target artery and vein.[14] The distal portion of the vein is cut and then mobilized while avoiding any tension or torsion. The length of the mobilized venous segment should not be too long; otherwise there is a risk of torsion that may cause the venous wall to form a stenosis and become obstructed. In the author's experience (KK), these risks are greater in initial AVF operations when a "fresh, virgin" vein is being used.

The length of a side-artery-to-vein-end anastomosis varies depending on the angle between artery and the approaching vein. In the case of a right angle approach of the vein, an arteriotomy (or anastomotic length) equal to the diameter of the vein is required. In the case of an acute angle, a longer arteriotomy is used. In practical terms, position the vein near its final position with respect to the artery. Then cut the vein in a parallel direction with regard to the axis of the artery (Figure 48-4); the length of the venous cut will determine the length of the arteriotomy (and thus the anastomosis).

One final note: in case of a right angle approach of the vein to the artery, the final, mobilized segment of the vein should undergo an outward directed rotation up to 90° to minimize the risk of torsion (Figure 48-5).

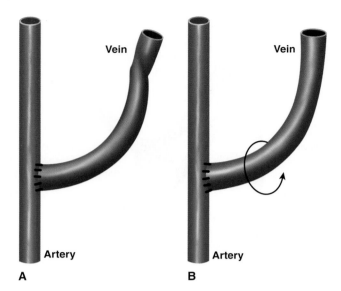

Figure 48-5. In case of a right angle approach of the vein to the artery, the final, "free" venous segment should undergo an outward rotation of up to 120° in order to avoid torsion of the vein and subsequent kinking and stenosis.

▶ **Options for Creation of AV Fistula in the Forearm**

1. *The Tabatière AV fistula*: The most peripheral option for VA is the *Tabatière AV fistula* (or so-called snuff box fistula). Since the anastomosis is constructed distal to the wrist, the entire length of the cephalic vein is available for use as the AVF conduit, thus, providing a wide cannulation area and offering multiple potential sites for subsequent revisions. Currently, this technique seems to be used in some younger patients. The Tabatière AV fistula has never enjoyed widespread use.

2. *The radial artery AV-fistula at the wrist*: Dr. Tellis proposed in 1971 a new variant to construct a side-to-side anastomosis: the suture starts in the mid-portion of the back wall and allows an optimal accuracy particularly when sewing the angles as well as a consequent eversion of the suture.[11]

In the 1970s, the end-to-end variant was the preferred type of anastomosis but was technically demanding due to different arterial and venous lumina and differing thickness of arterial and venous vessel wall; this technique was abandoned for the most part due to the high risk of hand ischemia when ligating a radial or an ulnar artery in the patients with multiple comorbidities such as age and diabetes as well as advanced peripheral arterial occlusive disease (PAOD) (Figure 48-6).

In patients where the distal cephalic vein lies some distance from the radial artery, the technique of choice may be the artery-side-to-vein-end anastomosis. Construction of a side-to-end anastomosis in these patients may avoid tension on the vein thus preventing early failure and thrombosis of the AVF. If torsion on the vein is not avoided, the risk of AVF failure is high. Special attention

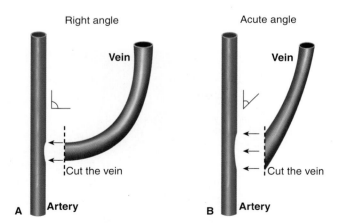

Figure 48-4. (A) With a 90 degree artery-vein angle, the diameter of the arteriotomy should be equal to the diameter of the vein. **(B)** With an acute artery-vein angle, the vein should be transected parallel to the artery, which will necessitate a longer arteriotomy and anastomosis.

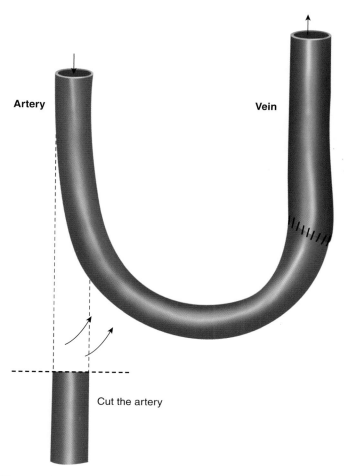

Figure 48-6. When creating an end-to-end anastomosis it is mandatory to form a complete 180 degree turn with the arterial segment and avoid any torsion. Atherosclerotic plaques may cause a kinking phenomenon. If this is the case, abandon this technique and select another type of anastomosis.

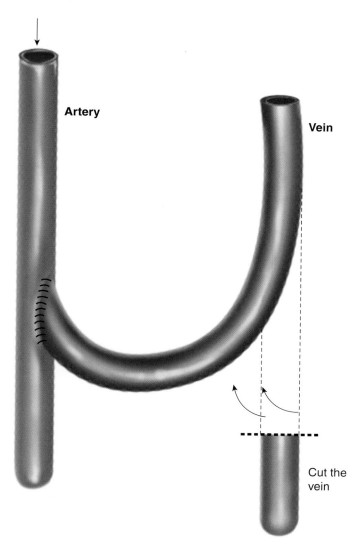

Figure 48-7. "Smooth loop" artery-side-to-vein-end anastomosis—theoretically brilliant and conclusive, but not functional in reality.

is required when mobilizing the vein in this situation. It is very important to avoid a small radius in mobilizing the vein as proposed by Karmody et al in 1973[15] (Figure 48-7). Dr. Karmody's idea was theoretically brilliant and logical, but did not work in reality.

When using side-artery-to-end-vein anastomosis, it is also important to understand that with maturation, the arterialized vein will predictably undergo longitudinal elongation. Therefore, the anastomosis must be created without any extra length in the venous segment.

3. *The ulnar artery—AV fistula*: In a patient where the radial artery/cephalic vein anatomy does not allow for the placement of an AV fistula, the conditions for creation of an ulnar artery/basilic vein anastomosis should be evaluated. The use of this configuration of AVF creation is not common and may be used in only ~2–5% of initial AVF creations. Construction of an anastomosis between the ulnar artery and the basilic antebrachial vein may be demanding. Dissection of the ulnar artery is often a challenge since its position may be quite deep when

compared to the radial artery; preoperative ultrasound examination and a thorough physical examination are helpful in determining its location and size. In addition, the wall of the antebrachial basilic vein is often quite thin, thus, making it an extremely vulnerable structure. The friability of this vein is comparable to that of the two brachial deep veins accompanying the brachial artery in the upper arm. Due to the fragile character of the venous wall, maturation may take a longer time and the initial cannulation may be challenging. It is important to avoid a hematoma that may be caused by high venous pressure (eg, use a cuff inflated to a maximum of 60 mmHg). For some patients, it may be difficult to tolerate the unusual positions of the arm that are required with the dialysis cannulae placed on the medial aspect of the forearm. Nevertheless, ulnar artery/basilic vein AVF may be a valuable option in a few patients.

4. *The mid-forearm AV fistula*: The mid-forearm region covers the space between the wrist and the forearm below the antecubital fossa offering a wide range of sites in which to create an AV anastomoses. When adequate vessels are not present at the wrist as determined by the availability and quality of the arteries and veins, one should examine the more proximal vasculature with careful clinical and ultrasound examination. In rare patients, a venography maybe required for adequate evaluation of the vein. Arteriography may be required if there is any doubt about the quality of the arterial vasculature beyond the ultrasound findings.

An additional challenge is the superficial position of the vein and the deep position of the radial artery. As a consequence, a more extensive dissection of the radial artery is required in many patients. The result is an arterial superficialization that brings the artery up to the level of the more superficial vein: the artery is mobilized and fixed superficially by connecting the dissected tissue layers. The type of the anastomosis used in this area is determined by the distance between artery and vein and their relative positions; sometimes, a top-artery to bottom-vein anastomosis (a variant of a side to side anastomosis) is required. In summary, the wide range of options available in this mid-forearm requires improvisation and creativity from the operator (Figure 48-8).

In many patients, VAs in the mid-forearm region may provide a sustained period of function. Cannulation of the vein can sometimes be extended to the upper arm cephalic vein depending on the patient's anatomy. If the cephalic vein is not available, the distal portion of the basilic vein below or in the elbow region may be cannulated. In some patients superficialization of the more proximal basilic vein may be required.

5. *The proximal forearm AV fistula*: In the author's experience (KK) the proximal forearm region, located about 1 in (~25.4 mm) distal to the antecubital fossa is a potential goldmine for successful initial AV fistula placement.

Placing the AV anastomosis at this site allows arterialization of both the basilic *and* the cephalic veins offering cannulation options in both veins close to the elbow joint. This is sometimes the only option in extremely obese patients unless these patients undergo an additional venous superficialization procedure. If the latter is required, it is most often performed with the basilic vein. Less frequently, it may be necessary to elevate the cephalic vein (see Section "*Venous Superficialization*" below).

There are numerous options for placement of an arteriovenous anastomosis at the proximal forearm location: the brachial artery, having passed the elbow, branches into the radial, ulnar, and interosseous vessels. The latter is not used in access surgery. The luminal diameter of the ulnar artery is usually substantially (up to twofold) greater than the diameter of the radial artery lumen. In addition, approximately 10% of all patients have a bifurcation of the brachial artery that is well proximal to the elbow in the upper arm

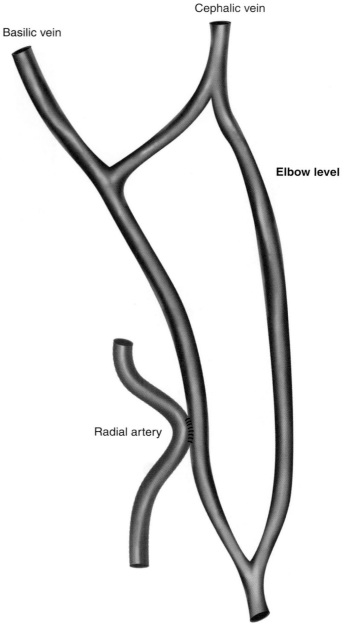

Figure 48-8. Side-to-side anastomosis located in the mid-forearm. Superficialization of the radial artery may be required given its deeper position relative to the vein. Notice the "arterialization" of the complete venous vasculature.

("high bifurcation"). This condition can be diagnosed by preoperative ultrasound analysis. The presence of a "high bifurcation" of the brachial artery is pertinent information for the operating surgeon since a small radial artery at the level of the elbow may not deliver adequate blood flow for maturation of the AVF. Thus, it may be necessary to use the ulnar artery for the AVF creation. Surgical strategies at any site often require a change during the operation given the anatomic variations of patients.

The superficial venous vasculature in the proximal forearm is also characterized by a pronounced variation from patient to patient. In the classical configuration, the

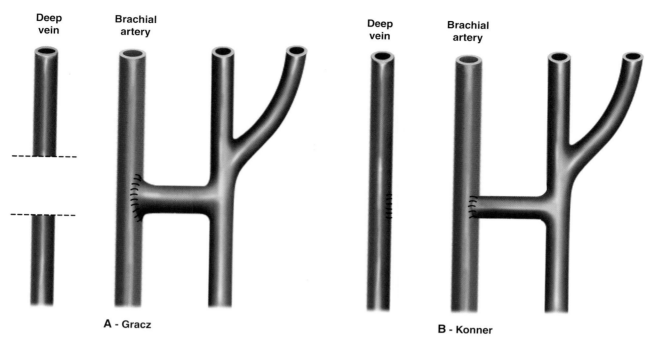

Figure 48-9. (**A**) Original technique of the Gracz-perforating vein fistula; resection of the deep vein to form a trumpet like venous end, resulting in a length of the anastomosis of ~8 mm. (**B**) The Konner version of the perforating vein arteriovenous fistula: preservation of the deep vein, length of the anastomosis 3–5 mm = diameter of the vein.

cephalic antebrachial vein branches into the Y-like shape of the basilic and cephalic upper arm veins; approximately 5–10% of all patients have either a basilic or a cephalic vein but not both. The overarching challenge of this proximal forearm region is the superficial position of the venous vasculature and the deeply hidden arterial system that may require significant dissection for proper anastomosis.

In this location, a widely forgotten, neglected treasure is the perforating vein AV fistula, first published by Dr. Gracz from Chicago in 1977.[16] One of the authors of this article (KK) introduced a modification of the original technique that aims to reduce the length of the anastomosis and to preserve the continuity of the deep venous vasculature (Figure 48-9). Most of the perforating vein anastomoses are sutured to the brachial artery in an artery-side (top)-to-vein-end fashion. If this is not feasible due to anatomical limitations, the ulnar artery would be preferred to the radial artery because of the larger diameter when compared to the radial artery as mentioned before. It is essential to limit the length of the anastomosis in order to lower the risk of access-related peripheral ischemia leading to steal syndrome; the length of the anastomosis should not exceed the diameter of the artery involved by any significant amount, for example, an anastomosis length of 3–5 mm is used in most instances.

The author's experience (KK) with >900 AV fistulae of the modified Gracz type have proven that this procedure is a useful technique, which can be effective in providing elderly, diabetic, and hypertensive patients with a functioning AV access. In the author's series, many of these patients had few if any episodes of malfunction or complications.[10] Reducing the length of the anastomosis is important in reducing the risk of a steal syndrome. Additionally, controlling the blood flow volume by limiting the anastomotic size may have a protective effect on the heart by limiting the changes in cardiac output that can result from AVF creation.

▶ **Options for Creation of AV Fistulae in the Elbow/Upper Arm**

6. *Brachio-basilic and brachio-cephalic AV fistulae:* First, in many patients where an upper arm fistula is planned, it is preferable to place the AV fistula alternatively within or just below the elbow. This allows in many patients to cannulate the beginning of the basilic vein and/or the cephalic vein over years without basilic or cephalic vein superficialization. If the anastomosis only can be created within the elbow region, a great variety of anastomoses are feasible depending upon anatomical conditions.

Generally, it is important to preserve the continuity of the venous triangle: if the cephalic antebrachial vein is cut distal to the basilic-cephalic vein branching, the "natural" fixation of both upper arm draining veins is interrupted. This means there may be an increased risk of venous kinking due to elongation induced by the process of maturation. In the majority of patients the AV anastomoses in the elbow region or along the beginning basilic (or cephalic) vein should be performed as side-to-side anastomosis to care for a venous drainage via both big upper arm veins.

There are good reasons to aim at an arterialization of the basilic *and* the cephalic vein:

- the cephalic upper arm vein can be cannulated without superficialization (except in extremely obese patients);
- if an outflow obstruction develops along *one* of these veins, then the alternative vein offers good cannulation conditions as long as the basilic vein will undergo superficialization.

A fundamental error made by surgeons operating in this anatomic region is the conclusion that these larger diameter vessels need a big, long anastomosis. Such an approach may substantially increase the risk of peripheral ischemia due to steal syndrome. The author's experience is that the length of the anastomosis should not exceed the diameter of the feeding artery, here mostly the brachial artery. This will lower the risk of steal syndrome, although it cannot be avoided completely. It may be mentioned that it is technically much easier to create a big than a small anastomosis. In some patients, an extreme difference in the arterial and venous wall thickness complicates sewing of the anastomosis.

In highly comorbid patients with pronounced PAOD, it may be justified to connect only one upper arm vein to the artery but these cases are rare exceptions. More often it makes sense to allow primary arterialization of both veins; if ligation of one upper arm vein should become necessary it can be easily done later using local anesthesia or performed percutaneously using interventional tools.

When creating the first AV fistula, a long distance venous transposition should be avoided. Any subcutaneous superficialization of the basilic or cephalic vein is better performed as a two-stage or second-step procedure (see the next paragraph).

Particularly in very tiny individuals, great care should be used when canulating even a well palpable basilic vein. Even in this setting, there is a high risk of injury to the brachial artery and the median nerve, since both are often in close proximity to the vein.

7. *Brachial artery to brachial vein AV fistula*: This rarely used variant (even more rarely mentioned in the literature), may, nevertheless, provide a real benefit for a few patients.[17] There are situations where the superficial veins of the arm are too tiny or have been exhausted by other uses. In these patients, nature uses the deep brachial veins, the "twin companions" of the brachial artery, for venous drainage thus resulting in an increased diameter.

When creating an anastomosis between the brachial artery and one of the deep concomitant brachial veins attention should be paid to some special aspects:

- The wall of these deep brachial veins is extremely thin and sometimes transparent, a type of venous wall that is only found in the arm with the basilic antebrachial vein.
- When suturing the anastomosis, extreme caution and skill is needed not to harm the tiny venous wall.

- Preferably, a side-to-side anastomosis should be placed; ligation of the distal venous limb will result in a functional side-to-end anastomosis.

These AV fistulae never will become suitable for cannulation due to the deep position and the close relationship with the brachial artery; any attempt to cannulate would presumably result in an uncontrolled hematoma with subsequent emergency surgical repair. So, in any case, it is mandatory to wait a couple of weeks for maturation as manifested by an increase in blood flow volume and by an increase in arterial as well as venous diameters, and then to superficialize the vein to allow for cannulation. Palpation, auscultation, and ultrasound examination indicate good function before this second-step or second-stage procedure. Ultrasound can describe the amount of blood flow and diameter of the vessels involved: arterial diameter 4–5 mm, venous diameter 5–6 mm, and flow rate ~600 mL/min.

There are two options for the second-step procedure:

- the superficialization of the brachial vein and
- the insertion of a graft, preferably an ePTFE-type graft using the now mature brachial vein as a target for the venous anastomosis.

A few factors make it difficult to superficialize a brachial vein. There may be communicating or bridging veins from one to the other brachial vein like staves of a ladder. Careful ligation may escalate into a time consuming procedure. However, superficialization of the brachial vein is the preferred technique in nonobese patients. Sometimes, the brachial vein can only superficialized over a short length but this may still allow successful cannulation for years. Alternatively, in obese patients, the remodeled and dilated brachial artery and the arterialized deep brachial vein can be used to insert a, for example, 6 mm ePTFE loop graft, preferably a thin-walled version, thus, paying attention to the tiny venous wall. Due to the deep positioning of all structures involved—artery, both deep veins and median nerve—any dissection and surgical manipulation require extreme caution and instinctive feeling.

▶ Venous Superficialization

Any creation of an AV fistula aims at a mature vein with a diameter exceeding 6 mm and a blood flow rate of 600–1000 mL/min or even more. In addition, repeated cannulation, normally six cannulae per week, requires an optimal subcutaneous position of the arterialized vein. A venous position that is too deep requires superficialization of the vein.

Different techniques were described since the publication by Dr. Dagher and colleagues in 1976,[18] mostly concerning the basilic vein. These techniques range from full length open dissection to key-hole minimally invasive surgical techniques. As is often the case in surgery, there is no technique that has been shown to be superior to another. Personal preferences, the operator's experience and number of operations play a role. The main determinants are a low rate of complications (hematoma, bleeding, infection, and outflow stenosis), conditions amenable to good cannulation for adequate HD therapy and long-term functional access survival.

Superficializations are more often done with the (i) basilic vein at the inner aspect of the upper arm and less frequently performed, (ii) cephalic antebrachial (forearm) vein, or (iii) cephalic vein along the upper arm. These later two procedures are more common in extremely obese patients. The very rare superficialization of the deep brachial vein was described before.

i.   *Basilic vein superficialization*: The deeply hidden natural position of the basilic vein prevents routine cannulation for blood sampling, infusions, and transfusions. If there is an indication for a primary brachial artery to basilic vein anastomosis, venous superficialization should be preferably done as a second-step procedure. This means that one should first place the AV anastomosis, and then wait for maturation. Once there is a strong thrill, often in as little as 2 weeks, ultrasound analysis will reveal an increase of venous diameter up to 6 or more mm and a blood flow volume of >600 mL/min, both average target values. After a 4–6 week maturation period one can proceed with the second-stage superficialization or transposition.

After a series of >200 basilic vein superficializations over a time of more than three decades and analysis of the literature over this time, the clear preference of the author (KK) is the complete open dissection. This technique is simple; it allows optimal control of intraoperative bleeding, lowers the rate of postoperative bleeding complications, makes ligation of side branches easier, and provides safe care for big communicating branches to the deep veins that may require a vascular suture where a ligation is not sufficient. The open dissection technique also allows patching procedures, if necessary. Meticulous, well-controlled efforts for a "dry" wound will reduce postoperative hematoma formation.

Technically, one dissects the arterialized basilic vein, elevates the vessel and closes the deep fat layer covering now the former bed of that basilic vein. Then, the operator creates a pocket in the subcutaneous fatty layer toward the region of the cephalic vein and transposes the basilic vein into this pocket in a bow-shaped subcutaneous position. Special attention is paid to the position of the vein leaving the new course neither too superficial, nor too deep under the skin. Dermal necrosis is a potential serious complication.

There is only one situation when a basilic vein superficialization should be performed during a primary brachio-basilic AV fistula operation. If the patient has a tiny arm with a reduced fatty layer combined with a large-diameter basilic vein and a big feeding brachial artery, a primary superficialization might be pursued. In this situation, a high-flow primary fistula will mature very early avoiding a second operation.

The second-stage transposition can be done a number of ways. Some surgeons elect to ligate the AV anastomosis

and to cut the basilic vein at this level. Then a tunnel for the new course of the vein is formed and the basilic vein guided back through the tunnel to be reanastomosed to the brachial artery. It works in the hands of very experienced and skilled access surgeons although it is time consuming and the tunneling procedure requires special attention to avoid torsion of the basilic vein. An alternative approach is to cut the proximal basilic vein, to transpose it through a tunnel in the cephalad direction and to perform a veno-venous end-to-end anastomosis; tunneling a basilic vein "under pressure" lowers the risk of torsion.

ii. *Superficialization and transposition*: Even a superficialized basilic vein may be difficult to cannulate if it remains in the original position along the inner aspect of the upper arm. In most of these basilic vein superficializations the author aimed at a simple open transposition without the need to construct a new anastomosis. In this circumstance, an additional venous length of 2–3 cm will be needed when deciding where to place the initial anastomosis (Figure 48-10). Then, transposition of the isolated vein into a position close to the cephalic vein makes sense. Now, cannulation can be done easily and in a safer, more

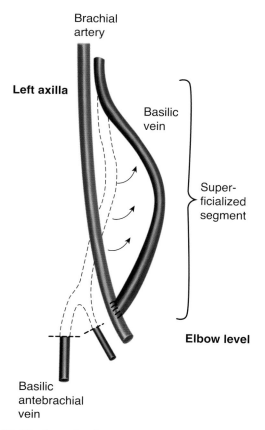

Figure 48-10. Superficialization and transposition of the basilic vein (only for demonstration: one sketch for the two-step procedure). Notice the use of the basilic antebrachial vein in order to obtain additional length.

reliable manner allowing for comfort of the patient. Respectively, the tunnel will be placed at an identical position.

Although not a part of primary AV fistula operations, it should be mentioned that in patients with a history of forearm or elbow AV fistulae and an exhausted, not suitable cephalic upper arm vein, a *one-step* procedure, anastomosing the basilic vein to the brachial artery and superficialization/transposition, can easily be performed. Here, the perfectly remodeled "mature" basilic vein is easily to handle, resistant to the trauma of dissection and transposition/superficialization as well as to potential compression by hematoma.

iii. *Superficialization of the antebrachial cephalic vein*: A few extremely obese patients, mostly of a younger age, present with a suitable artery and vein allowing the easy performance of a forearm AV.[19] However, the deeply hidden position under the subcutaneous fatty layer prevents repetitive safe dialysis cannulation. If auscultation, palpation and ultrasound evaluation signal good fistula function, superficialization of the vein can be easily done as a second-step procedure. In most of these patients, it is sufficient to resect a portion of the fatty tissue covering the vein.

This is a very simple procedure although some attention is required to create the best position for the arterialized vein. There is no risk of torsion and kinking. Meticulous care to prevent bleeding is mandatory.

This technique is less a true superficialization than a type of lipo-resection to reduce the distance between vein and skin surface by reducing the tissue covering the vein.

iv. *Superficialization of the cephalic upper arm vein*: The indications for this procedure and the technical aspects are essentially identical those described above for the superficialization of the antebrachial cephalic vein. Here, too, superficialization via lipo-resection provides a well-functioning VA that can be cannulated easily.

Special attention should be given to the cannulation strategy of these accesses. It is strongly recommended to use the rope ladder technique, thus changing the site of cannulation with every HD session. Otherwise, formation of an aneurysm(s) will occur in many patients, often combined with stenoses.[20] What starts as an even mild to moderate narrowing will progress to a clinically significant stenotic lesion; there is no exception. Besides these cannulation-related complications, the most critical point of any superficialized vein is the outflow segment, specifically at the transition from the superficialized to the nonsuperficialized venous section. Stenoses and/or kinking phenomena are often observed at this location.

▶ Venous Transposition

In first AV fistula operations, transposition of a mobilized vein to bridge a longer distance to meet the artery for placing the AV anastomosis should be an exception. The main risk is that the process of remodeling does *not* result in venous dilatation but in a transformation of that venous segment into a scar tube, a functional long distance stenosis. Many reasons were/are discussed. All we know is that there may be several factors contributing to this pathologic result. It is identical to the situation known as "swing stenosis" along the first postanastomotic venous segment in primary wrist AV fistulae. In contrast, a "matured" vein that has dilated, has developed wall thickening, and has adapted to high flow conditions, is an ideal material for transposition or even for use as a (short) interposition graft or for patching a stenotic segment.

▶ Venous Ligation

During the initial placement of AV fistulae, the author's (KK) experience with >2000 primary autologous AVF's clearly states: never ligate a draining vein during first operation! The reason is that even with careful preoperative clinical, ultrasound, and/or venographic evaluation, one cannot predict the subsequent pattern of blood flow under the conditions of remodeling. High-flow volume rates via the AV anastomosis, high-flow velocity, high shear stress, high intravenous pressure and so on may occur. Therefore, "blind" ligation may be risky: ligation of a "good" *accessory* vein in presence of an undiagnosed slight narrowing in the main vein, now revealed as a stenosis under high flow conditions, could harm the patient if the ligation was performed without a real need for action.

Beyond the fundamental statement that a good arterial inflow will feed two or even three draining veins, it seems a responsible attitude to wait under most circumstances a couple of weeks after the first operation before ligating branches. The indication for venous ligation is not given by speculations during the first operation but exclusively by clinical needs as observed during vein maturation or even later. Then, ligation can be performed within a few minutes, either surgically or percutaneously with interventional techniques.

SUBSEQUENT TREATMENT OF ACCESSORY VEINS

It is well known that a "normal" fistulogram never shows side branches. If an "accessory" vein can be visualized angiographically it is most likely that the flow in the main vein is impaired. Ligation of the "accessory" vein in this situation means one will close the really working venous drainage. Therefore, it seems logical to check the anatomic situation carefully and critically by clinical, ultrasonic, and angiographic tools. Ligation should only be performed based on a clear clinical indication.

▶ The Role of Grafts in First VA Operations

After a large series of consecutive autologous primary AV fistulas, the authors feel that using a graft as the first VA operation should be an absolute exception. Grafts need both a good arterial inflow *and* a good venous outflow.

Over many years, a frequent and even published conclusion has been that in a patient with no suitable vessels to place an AV fistula, a graft is needed. Mostly, this has referred to the elderly, the hypertensive, the diabetic and the highly comorbid patients who actually represent the majority of incident hemodialysis patients worldwide today. Placing an AV graft in many of these patients means one would use a stiff-walled artery with a small lumen that would only allow a limited arterial inflow into a tiny vein with a functional outflow obstruction. The fate of such a construction is well known. In this situation, the challenge is to create an AV anastomosis with autologous vessels as they are, only aiming at (and waiting for!) a high flow maturation to dilate both, the artery *and* the vein. A few weeks later, the insertion of a graft could be done with far more success. This procedure was once described by Dr. Keoghane.[21]

THE INTERDISCIPLINARY VA TEAM

Patients suffering from chronic kidney disease are treated by nephrologists. As these patients approach HD, the question of VA must be considered. The challenge is to start hemodialysis therapy with a well-functioning VA, preferably with an AV fistula thus avoiding catheter use.[9] Here, the nephrologist should contact an experienced VA surgeon. Both disciplines should reach agreement regarding preoperative evaluations such as a clinical vascular examination and a standardized ultrasound examination. The best approach is to meet at the bedside with the patient and come to a common decision about the type, side and site of the first VA, which may require additional preoperative studies like a venogram or even an arteriogram.

TABLE 48–1

How to Place a Primarily Well-Working First Arteriovenous Fistula: A Personal Approach

- We do not know *the best* vascular access; we have to aim at the *best* vascular access for *this* patient at *that* time.
- Individualize all your decisions along the patient's specific conditions.
- Adapt your skills and techniques to the patient's individual vasculature.
- Every patient is a candidate for an arteriovenous fistula.
- You have to look for good reasons *not* to place an arteriovenous fistula in *single* patients.
- Preoperatively, start with the patient's medical vascular history and a careful clinical examination of the arterial and venous vasculature in *both* arms.
- A color-Doppler ultrasound evaluation is mandatory to detect arterial calcifications, to measure blood flow volume at the brachial artery, and to clarify venous topography including the perforating vein below the elbow. Surgery appreciates three-dimensional information.
- Select the arm with the best conditions for a first arteriovenous fistula. *Dominant* or *nondominant* arm are only secondary parameters for consideration.
- Summarizing all clinical and ultrasound findings, a team-based decision is needed regarding the side, site and type of first arteriovenous fistula. It is fundamentally beneficial to include the patient into this decision. Even the vascular access surgeon should know his patient in advance.
- This policy encourages shared responsibilities, allowing all the disciplines involved to learn from each other, to build up respect and confidence amongst each other.
- Strive for a *well-cooperating team* to provide the best care.
- Use an optimal, not too short skin incision and perform sufficient dissection to achieve good visualization and an exact control of any bleeding, of arterial and venous structures, and of nerves.
- Avoid any tension, any torsion, and any sharp curve when transposing the isolated vein to the artery.
- A professional, meticulous dissection achieved with patience will transfer a complex anatomical situation into a clear condition.
- A sharp angle between artery and vein does not harm.
- Use a simple, soft, and small lumen catheter to test the continuity of the proximal vein. Inject 0.9% saline against digital pressure to dilate the vein before sewing the anastomosis.
- Hand stitching allows an operator to achieve the best individual results, placing any stitch at the optimal position, while always respecting the mandatory everting character of vascular suture.
- Use anastomosis types and techniques that allow for the best visualization and that give optimal results.
- An aesthetic arteriovenous fistula will work.
- Having completed the anastomosis, palpate along all proximal veins, look for the feeling of "electricity" with your fingertips. A hard, filled vein means a cephalad obstruction.
- Press the main draining vein for a few seconds to completely interrupt the blood flow; no bleeding at the anastomosis should be noticed as a proof of a safe suture technique.
- To close the skin, use nontraumatic techniques as far as possible.
- Postoperatively, evaluate arteriovenous fistula function by auscultation. It is mandatory to confirm a strong characteristic two-phase noise with a long diastolic section.
- Immobilization of the arm for a limited time favors good healing.
- Respecting these remarks may bring you closer to success.
- Any patient has a right to receive a successful operation. Your patients will be grateful.

Responsibilities are shared in the success *and* failure of the VA. These decisions are far better discussed by the team paying attention to the present complex nature of CKD patients concerning age, vascular damage by diabetes, hypertension and a high incidence of different comorbidities, life-expectancy, and so on; surgical techniques have to be adapted to this challenging situation. Furthermore, over time, an atmosphere of better understanding will grow, including the appreciation of and a knowledge of the specific requirements and thought processes of each other's disciplines. Substantial medical *and* organizational work can be achieved by a VA coordinator, who may be a nurse or be a technician.

It is very important to document all that happens with the patient from the first presentation to the placement of the AV fistula. The operation should be documented not only by a text, but by a sketch. Such a drawing can be helpful to the experienced staff who do nearly all cannulation work. The drawing remains the best tool of communication, and this may then be converted by way of digital techniques for electronic transmission. Nowadays, we have excellent tools—why not use them? A well-working system of communication is a real benefit for all people involved in VA, but mostly for the patient (Table 48-1).

Different models of VA teams/centers are working around the world, from university hospitals to small private institutions. Quality standards may be achieved in small institutions because the size and short distances make communication easier. Big academic facilities may be equipped with best technologies, but may require more effort motivating interdisciplinary cooperation and continuity amongst co-workers.

Finally, as scientists and clinicians, we must remember that all patients have the right to get the best VA.

REFERENCES

1. Scribner BH, Buri R, Caner JEZ, Hegstrom R, Burnell JM. The treatment of chronic uremia by means of intermittent hemodialysis: a preliminary report. *Transact Am Soc Artif Intern Organs.* 1960;6:114–122.
2. Brescia MJ, Cimino JE, Appel K, Hurwich BJ. Chronic hemodialysis using venipuncture and a surgically created arteriovenous fistula. *N Engl J Med.* 1966;275:1089–1092.
3. National Kidney Foundation. KDOQI Clinical Practice Guidelines and Clinical Practice Recommendations for 2006 Updates: vascular access. *Am J Kidney Dis.* 2006;48(suppl 1):S176–S317.
4. Wedgwood KR, Wiggins PA, Guillou PJ. A prospective study of end-to-side vs. side-to-side arteriovenous fistulas for haemodialysis. *Brit J Surg.* 1984;71:640–642.
5. Wiese P. Personal communication.
6. Corpataux J-M, Haesler E, Silacci P, Ris HB, Hayoz D. Low-pressure environment and remodelling of the forearm vein in brescia-cimino haemodialysis access. *Nephrol Dial Transplant.* 2002;17:1057–1062.
7. Goodkin DA, Pisoni PL, Locatelli F, Port FK, Saran R. Hemodialysis vascular access are the key to improved access outcomes. *Am J Kidney Dis.* 2010;56:1032–1042.
8. Malovrh M. Native arteriovenous fistula: preoperative evaluation. *Am J Kidney Dis.* 2002;39:1218–1225.
9. Mendelssohn DC, Curtis B, Yeates K, Langlois S, Macrae JM, Semeniuk LM, Camacho F, McFarlane P. for the STARRT Study investigators. Suboptimal initiation of dialysis with and without early referral to a nephrologist. *Nephrol Dial Transplant.* 2011;26:2659–2665.
10. Konner K, Hulbert-Shearon TE, Roys EC, Port FK. Tailoring the initial vascular access for dialysis patients. *Kidney Int.* 2002;62(1):329–338.
11. Tellis VA, Veith FJ, Sobermann RJ, Freed SZ, Gliedman ML. Internal arteriovenous fistula for hemodialysis. *Surg Gynecol Obstet.* 1971;132:866–870.
12. Sivanesan S, How TV, Bakran A. Characterizing flow distributions in AV fistulae for haemodialysis access. *Nephrol Dial Transplant.* 1998;13:3108–3110.
13. Sperling M, Kleinschmidt W, Wilhelm A, Heidland A, Klütsch K. Die Subkutane Arteriovenöse Fistel zur Intermittierenden Hämodialyse-Behandlung. *Dtsch Med Wschr.* 1967;92:425–426.
14. Röhl L, Franz HE, Möhring K, Ritz E, Schüler HW, Uhse HG, Ziegler M. Direct arteriovenous fistula for hemodialysis. *Scand J Urol Nephrol.* 1968;2:191–195.
15. Karmody AM, Lempert N. Smooth loop arteriovenous fistulas for hemodialysis. *Surgery.* 1974;75:238–242.
16. Gracz KC, Ing TS, Soung L-S, Armbruster KFW, Seim SK, Merkel FK. Proximal forearm fistula for maintenance hemodialysis. *Kidney Int.* 1977;11:71–74.
17. Greenberg JI, May S, Suliman A, Angle N. The Brachial artery-brachial vein fistula: expanding the possibilities for autogenous fistulae. *J Vasc Surg.* 2008;48:1245–1250.
18. Dagher FJ, Gelber RL, Ramos EJ, Sadler JH. Basilic vein to brachial artery fistula: a new access for chronic hemodialysis. *South Med J.* 1976;69:1438–1440.
19. Weyde W, Krajewska M, Letachowicz W, Klinger M. Superficialization of the wrist native arteriovenous fistula for effective hemodialysis vascular access construction. *Kidney Int.* 2002;61:1170–1173.
20. Krönung G. Plastic deformation of cimino fistula by repeated puncture. *Dial Transplant.* 1984;13:635–638.
21. Keoghane SR, Kar LC, Gray DWR. Routine use of arteriovenous fistula construction to dilate the venous outflow prior to insertion of an expanded polytetrafluoroethylene (PTFE) loop graft for dialysis. *Nephrol Dial Transplant.* 1993;8:154–156.

49

CREATION OF ARTERIOVENOUS FISTULAE BY NEPHROLOGISTS

RICK MISHLER, JEFFREY PACKER, & SHOUWEN WANG

LEARNING OBJECTIVES

1. Understand the historical context of arteriovenous fistula creation in the United States.

2. Describe the early experience related to AVF creation for hemodialysis vascular access.

3. Understand the key elements of the modern era of AVF creation by nephrologists in the world.

4. Understand the general techniques required for successful AVF creation.

5. Understand the past, current, and future roles of US interventional nephrologists in vascular access creation within the context of nephrology practice in the world.

INTRODUCTION

Since the development of hemodialysis, vascular access has been considered by many to be the Achilles' heel of this life saving therapy.[1] In the early years, venous–venous cannulation was employed. Venous cannulation of an arm as well as a vein in the lower extremity was preferred. Distal venous cannulation of an extremity with return of blood to a venous cannulation proximal to a lightly inflated blood pressure cuff also was utilized.[2] Faced with daunting challenges in achieving adequate dialysis therapy due to inadequate vascular access, four physicians, Michael Brescia, James Cimino, Kenneth Appel, and Baruch Hurwich from the Bronx Veterans Administration Hospital, published the sentinel article in the field of hemodialysis vascular access. In 1966, they described the radial-cephalic fistula that was created using a side-to-side anastomosis between a distal radial artery and cephalic vein as is depicted in Figures 49-1 and 49-2.[3] Even though much of the developmental work in nonhuman subjects for this novel approach to dialysis access was achieved by the nephrologists, the actual creation of autologous arteriovenous fistulae (AVF) in humans as reported by Brescia et al was performed by a surgeon, Dr. Appel (personal communication from Dr. Brescia). Despite numerous advances in dialysis technology since that time, this basic vascular configuration remains the standard for hemodialysis vascular access in 2011. Although, nephrologists outside of the United States have been creating AVF for many years, only a few nephrologists within the United States have engaged in arteriovenous fistula (AVF) creation in the ensuing years.[4,5] Reports from some of the most active European centers indicate very favorable outcomes when fistula surgeries are performed by experienced nephrologists.[4–7] Based on the excellent out comes from outside of the United States, Anel et al[8] well as Asif et al[9] proposed that US interventional nephrologists should become active in AVF creation in order to increase AVF use in the dialysis population of the United States. The purpose of this chapter is to describe the past and current role of US nephrologists in vascular access creation within the context of vascular access creation by nephrologists in other parts of the world.[9,10]

▶ What is in a Name?

The term "interventional nephrologist" was coined in the United States more than a decade ago as the discipline of endovascular therapy as performed by nephrologists for vascular access malfunction was being developed. In publications from Europe, the term "operating nephrologist" has emerged as a moniker with which to identify those nephrologists that perform AVF creation and other vascular access surgery. This seems to be an appropriate name but perhaps

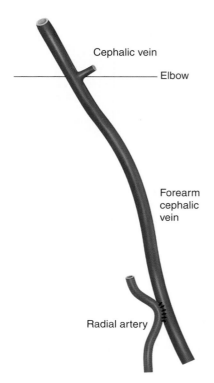

Figure 49-1. Distal radial artery to median antebrachial vein, side-to-side anastomosis. (Diagram courtesy of Klaus Konner, MD.)

lacks some specificity. If it is necessary to distinguish those nephrologists who perform access surgery from others, an appropriate option might to be that of *nephrologist-access surgeon*. Surgeons by definition are physicians who specialize in performing surgeries and those who perform dialysis access creation surgeries are called access surgeons. These physicians historically have come from backgrounds of vascular surgery, cardiothoracic surgery, transplant surgery, general surgery, urology, and other specialties.[10] Nephrologists from many countries who specialize in dialysis access creation are among these access surgeons. No one is a born surgeon, but individuals are trained to be surgeons

and nephrologists have been trained to become surgeons as well. Nephrologists pioneered dialysis access surgeries and well-trained nephrologist-access surgeons may be among the most qualified physicians to create dialysis accesses. Like the newly emerged interventional nephrologists, nephrologist-access surgeons can play a crucial role in the care of the dialysis access because of their understanding of dialysis therapy and their close interactions with CKD and dialysis patients. A review of representative published AVF outcomes from around the world follows.

North America (United States): During his distinguished career over several decades, Peter Ivanovich, MD, has been prolific in his contributions to dialytic therapy through the Society of Artificial Organs as well as many other organizations. He has historically been very active in performing and teaching the art of AVF creation in the university environment and may be the only academic nephrologist to have done so. Early in his career he was a nephrology fellow with Belding Scriber, MD, and was an early active participant in the placement of the Scribner Shunt. Many of these Scribner Shunts were later converted to secondary radial artery-cephalic vein fistulae in chronic dialysis patients as depicted in Figure 49-3. Having developed his surgical skills during these experiences, he became active in AVF creation over several decades. Subsequently, Professor Ivanovich became proficient in the use of a stapling tool that facilitated creation of radial artery to cephalic vein fistulae using an end-to-end anastomosis.[11] Dr. Ivanovich's experience represents one of the earliest attempts by US nephrologists to become active in the creation of dialysis vascular access for their patients.

Europe (Germany): Among the most prolific centers in terms successful nephrologist-managed procedures and publications are those in Italy and Germany. In 2002,

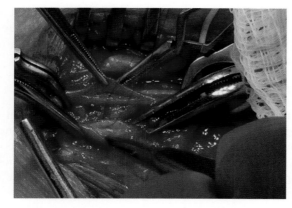

Figure 49-2. Preparation of a side-to-side anastomosis. (Picture courtesy of Rick Mishler, MD.)

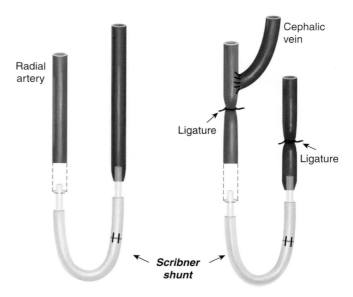

Figure 49-3. Scribner Shunt conversion to secondary radial artery-cephalic vein fistula. (Diagram courtesy of Klaus Konner, MD.)

Klaus Konner and others published outcomes of fistula creation in 748 consecutive patients with ESRD from 1993 to 1998.[12-14] Of these patients, 24% were diabetic and 42% were greater than 65 years of age, yet none of these patients required synthetic graft material for placement of their arteriovenous access. The investigators demonstrated no statistical difference in primary access survival at 1 and 2 years when comparing patients older than 65 years (77%, 68%) and younger patients (77%, 65%) nor was there any significant difference in secondary access survival at 1 and 2 years for younger patients (95%, 90%) and patients older than 65 years (93%, 90%). Dr. Konner has performed more than 5000 vascular access surgical procedures during his more than 30-year career and is among the most prolific authors in disseminating the technical aspects of successful AVF creation.

Europe (Italy): Pietro Ravani et al reported 197 consecutive patients from 1995 to 2001 that received a fistula as a first permanent access even though almost 60%, initiated dialysis therapy using a dialysis catheter.[6] These results were achieved even though 22% of the patients were diabetic, 50% had vascular disease, and 15% had neoplasm as comorbid conditions. Primary patency including early failures within 7 days at 1 and 2 years was 64% and 55%, respectively. The secondary patency at 1 and 2 years was 72% and 64%, respectively.

In 2010, Stanziale, Lodi, et al analyzed end-to-end (ETEa) and the end-to-side (ETSa) anastomosis in patients starting hemodialysis by means of radio-cephalic arterio-venous fistulae (AVF). They reported early failure (EF), late thrombosis (LT), stenosis, steal syndrome, and primary patency (PP), in two groups of hemodialysis incident patients that had an AVF placed by means of ETEa or ETSa. The observation period lasted 24 months for each of the two types of AVF, initially from October 2005 to September 2007 for ETEa and subsequently from October 2007 to September 2009 for ETSa. One hundred forty patients were included in the study. The authors of the manuscript were the nephrologist access surgeons and performed 99 AVF creations at the wrist or at the third distal of the forearm, in 70 patients by means of ETEa and 82 AVF creations in the same anatomical places in 70 patients by means of ETSa. The patients with ETEa had a mean age of 64.4 ± 14.6 years, males were 65.8% and the access age at the end of observation was 10.4 ± 5.7 months. Those with ETSa had a mean age of 65.9 ± 15.5 years and the males were 62.9%, the access age at the end of observation was 9.2 ± 5.5 months. The statistical study was performed by means of the χ chi-square and Fisher's exact test. They observed more late thrombosis (10% vs 4.1%) and stenosis (21.4% vs 2.7%) in ETEa than in ETSa. The number of early thrombosis was similar in the two types of anastomosis. The primary patency 1-year rate was better, though not significantly, in the ETSa (80% vs 85.7%) Their outcomes compared very favorably with the best centers in the world and their data seemed to indicate that ETSa provides, overall better results, both regarding the complications and primary survival than ETEa.[7]

India and China (Asia-Pacific Rim): Dr. Modi presented his AVF creation outcomes in India at the American Society of Nephrology meeting on more than one occasion. His outcomes seem to be on par with the other world literature. However, the prevalence of AVF creation by nephrologists in India as whole is uncertain.[5] Based on knowledge that is disseminated at nephrology meetings in China, many nephrologists-access surgeons are known to be creating AV fistulae in that populous nation. However, citable scientific publications are difficult to find. Therefore, it is difficult to access the clinical outcomes and prevalence of the practice (personal communication Dr. Wang).

North America (Phoenix, USA): the emergence of Interventional Nephrology as a discipline during the past decade has changed dialysis access maintenance care substantially.[15] It has been demonstrated that many vascular access maintenance procedures can be done in an outpatient facility and therefore providing better patient care as well as comparable outcomes.[16,17] By leveraging interventional nephrology skills, it might seem reasonable that interventional nephrologists can be trained to create dialysis accesses.[9,10,18] Since 2004, four interventional nephrologists from Arizona Kidney Disease and Hypertension Centers (AKDHC), Phoenix, AZ, have been among the few US nephrologists who currently perform vascular access surgery.

In these few years, the cumulative experience of the AKDHC physicians has increased both in terms of numbers and spectrum of the procedures performed. Dr. A has created more than 1300 fistulae since 2004. Dr. B has created over 800 fistulae since 2007. Dr. C has created over 400 fistulae since 2008. Dr. D has recently completed training in June 2010 and has begun operating independently. Dr. A was trained in fistula creations by a United States vascular surgeon and heavily influenced by subsequent work with Dr. Klaus Konner (KK). Dr. B was trained by Dr. A and KK. Dr. C was trained by Drs. A , B and KK. Dr. D was trained by the three nephrologist access surgeons. With the exception of Dr. C, all were classically trained nephrologists with no previous surgical experience beyond the usual rotations that occur during medical school, residency and fellowship training. Dr. C is an international medical graduate and previously trained in orthopedic surgery prior to becoming a United States nephrologist.

The array of procedures currently performed by the group is as follows:

- Forearm and upper arm fistula creations including primary and subsequent accesses (Figure 49-4).
- Fistula revisions and neoanastomosis.
- Basilic vein transposition, two-stage technique is preferred (Figures 49-5, 49-6, 49-7).
- Deep fistula conduit superficialization.
- Cephalic vein turn-down for resistant cephalic arch stenosis.

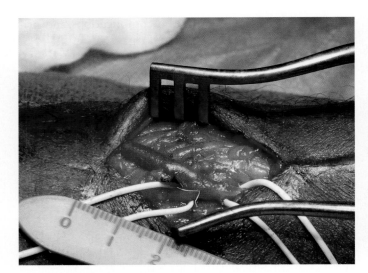

Figure 49-4. Secondary radial artery-cephalic vein fistula, end to side anastomosis. (Picture courtesy of Jeffrey Packer, DO.)

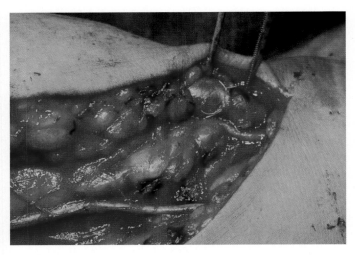

Figure 49-6. Re-anastomosis of the basilic vein during transposition. (Picture courtesy of Shouwen Wang, MD.)

- Fistula/graft banding for steal syndrome.
- Fistula and graft aneurysm repair using both open, endovascular and combined techniques including use of a pneumatic tourniquet.
- All endovascular interventions needed to promote maturation and maintain potency.
- Use of prosthetic material for primary and secondary access placement as well as patch angioplasty for resistant stenoses.

All surgeries take place in an ambulatory surgery center (ASC) or a vascular access center (VAC) and are performed using sedation and analgesia (s/a) with midazolam and fentanyl. Use of s/a has been proven to be safe when used by interventional nephrologist during thousands of endovascular procedures.[19] Anecdotally, the doses given and complications recorded by the AKDHC group during vascular access surgery approximate those described by the

Lifeline vascular access group during endovascular intervention.[17] Of note is that all of the vascular access surgeries reported by Dr. Konner in 2002 were performed using only local anesthesia.[12] Undergirding the surgical aspects of care is a comprehensive system of dialysis access care at AKDHC that consists of the following.

1. Focused effort to create fistula in patients who are dialyzing with tunneled dialysis catheters.
2. CKD care and dialysis education.
3. Elective ultrasound vessel mapping (VM) for limb protection with estimated GFR <30 mL/min.
4. Preoperative ultrasound VM of all patients.
5. All VM are reviewed by these four nephrologist-access surgeons.
6. Selected arm veins are protected.

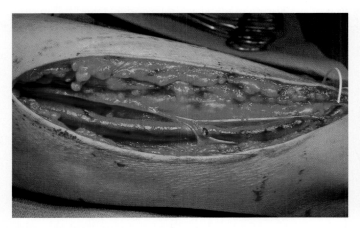

Figure 49-5. Basilic vein dissection during transposition. (Picture courtesy of Shouwen Wang, MD.)

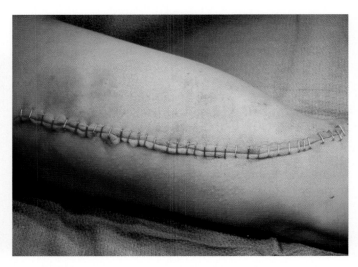

Figure 49-7. Basilic vein transposition incision closed with skin staples. (Picture courtesy of Shouwen Wang, MD.)

7. Fistulae are created in suitable patients when eGFR <20 mL/min.

8. Prosthetic access when needed if the patient is not a candidate for AVF.

9. Systematic follow-up with physical examination and ultrasound surveillance.

10. Endovascular interventions and/or surgical revisions as needed.

Early outcomes data from the AKDHC center is as follows.

One hundred and five ($n = 105$) patients were referred to a single center with a single operator over a 1-year period and were initially included in the database. Seven patients were excluded from analysis for missing data fields with 98 patients available for follow up. An AVF was placed in 100% of patients referred for vascular access. Two complications were identified (one steal syndrome and one infection) for a rate of 1.9%. The patient demographics included 38.7% female, age 63.6 ± 14.8, 50.0% diabetic, 66.0% hypertensive, with 65.1% of patients being on hemodialysis (HD) using a tunneled dialysis catheter (TDC) at time of AVF placement. Average target artery diameter was 4.09 ± 1.16 mm while average target vein diameter was 3.66 ± 1.20. Twenty-one AVF were placed in the forearm (19.8%) with the remainder being placed in the upper arm vessels. Eighteen patients (18.56%) failed to mature at 6 weeks. Sixty-four patients (65.98%) required revision or intervention of their AVF between 12 weeks postoperatively and the end-point of the study. Eighty patients (84.21%) had patent AVF at an average follow-up of 286.2 ± 98.14 days. No identifiable risk factors among those listed above were associated with a significant impact on AVF outcomes. This AVF outcomes data compares favorably to those of our European colleagues and demonstrates the safety and efficacy that can be achieved by US Interventional Nephrologists.[20,21,22] A preliminary analysis of 462 consecutive AVF created by Dr. B over a 30-month period noted that his patient cohort achieved a patency rate of 79%, an outcome that is comparable with those previously reported.[23,24]

Further analysis was performed in order to access the impact of the AKDHC fistula program in dialysis units. Two dialysis units in rural Arizona communities were chosen due to reports from ESRD Network 15 that these dialysis units had undergone a significant increase in the use of AVF and a significant reduction in tunneled dialysis catheters and were exceeding NKF:KDOQI goal of 66% AVF[25–27] use in prevalent dialysis patients. The total population of the two dialysis units was 160 patients and all were included in the analysis. During the 19 months between October 2008 and May 2010, the rate of AVF use in prevalent dialysis patients increased from 56% to 76%. During the same time period, TDC use decreased from 26% to 12%. The percentage of prosthetic grafts remained stable at 12%. Overall, 56% of the fistulae were created by

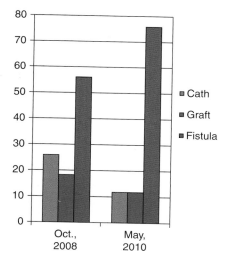

Figure 49-8. Percentage TDC, AVG, and AVF in October 2008 and May 2010. (Courtesy of Rick Mishler, MD.)

AKDHC IN and tended to be those that were constructed more recently[28] (Figure 49-8). These data compare very favorably with the Fistula First goal of 66% prevalent AVF by the end of 2009.

While early data from this single center seems favorable when compared to the best outcomes from outside of the United States, many barriers remain to be overcome if AVF creation by US interventional nephrologists is to become commonplace.[29] Among these are training, malpractice insurance and a safe environment in which to perform these operations. Given the difficulties of establishing interventional nephrology training centers in some university settings, it seems unlikely that training for fistula creation will be widespread in university communities anytime soon. However, in certain private practice settings, training for vascular access surgery may be possible. Several interventional groups in the United States already collaborate closely with surgeons who perform vascular access work for their patients in the setting of ambulatory surgical centers. These same surgeons might be amenable to teaching an experienced interventionist the skills of access creation. It might also be possible to establish a collaborative relationship with our European colleagues that would allow American nephrologists to experience fistula creation on the continent over an extended period of time such as was reported by Sreenarasimhaiah and Ravani in 2005.[30]

What are the barriers to obtaining malpractice coverage for surgical procedures? At the AKDHC ASC malpractice coverage has not been difficult to obtain. The same carrier that provides coverage for interventional privileges will also provide insurance for surgical cases at no extra charge after the physician has completed 25 supervised surgical cases as the primary operator. Finally, an environment in which it is suitable for the nephrologist to perform these procedures already exists. Dr. Konner performed more than 5000 access procedures in an out-patient procedure room near a dialysis unit. It seems that the very vascular access centers and ambulatory surgical centers that have provided excellent vascular access care for our dialysis patients over the past decade are venues that are very well suited for vascular access creation and revision. More than 2100 vascular surgeries performed by four AKDHC interventional nephrologists since 2004 also attest to the safety and efficacy of this model.[18,22,30] Finally, many opportunities exist for research in the area of AVF creation. Some of the questions to be answered may include: What is the optimal timing of AVF placement in a CKD patient? What is the best method for postoperative follow-up of the access? How can the AVF blood flow be optimized in the intraoperative and immediate postoperative periods through pharmacological or mechanical interventions?

Over the past several years, we as nephrologists were challenged by our colleagues from around the world to become more involved in AV fistula creation.[4,5,6,9,10] As the more recent data discussed above seems to suggest, there is reason to believe that the many elements are aligning to favor fistula creation by certain United States nephrologist access surgeons. Most of this activity seems to be centered within the interventional nephrology community and there may be good reason for this. The skill set and knowledge base that are developed by an experienced interventional nephrologist seem to be well aligned with those needed to perform vascular access creation and tools such as a thorough physical examination, fluoroscopic guidance, and Doppler ultrasound surveillance are readily available. Another potential advantage of fistula creation in the interventional nephrology setting is that many CKD and dialysis patients may become acquainted with the facilities and physicians and staff through previous appointments and procedures. This familiarity may obviate the need for obtaining a consultation with a new physician at a new center and perhaps facilitate scheduling a vascular access creation in a timely manner. In addition to pre-emptive AV fistula placement, these same interventional centers will likely be key elements in the postoperative care that may entail duplex Doppler surveillance and possible endovascular therapy in certain situations. It is on this foundation of continuity of patient care that US interventional nephrologists will likely continue to expand their roles in the care of dialysis patients by engaging in vascular access surgery.[18]

REFERENCES

1. Schwab SJ. Hemodialysis vascular access: the Achilles' heel remains. *Kidney Int.* 2007;72:665–666.
2. Cimino J, Brescia M. Simple venipuncture for hemodialysis. *N Engl J Med.* 1962;267:608–609.
3. Brescia M, Cimino J, Appel K, et al. Chronic hemodialysis using venipuncture and a surgically created arteriovenous fistula. *N Engl J Med.* 1966;275:1089–1092.
4. Bonucchi D, D'Amelio A, Capelli G, et al. Management of vascular access for dialysis: an Italian survey. *Nephrol Dial Transplant.* 1999;14:2116–2118.
5. Modi G. Interventional nephrology and vascular access management-AV fistulae creation by the nephrologist. *J Am Soc Nephrol.* 2008;19:470A.
6. Ravani P, Marcelli D, Malberti F. Vascular access surgery managed by renal physicians: the choice of native arteriovenous fistulas for hemodialysis. *Am J Kidney Dis.* 2002;40:1264–1276.
7. Stanziale R, Lodi m, D'Andrea E, et al. Arteriovenous fistula: end-to-end or end-to-side anastomosis? *Hemodial Int* 2011;15:100–103.
8. Anel R, Yevzlin A, Ivanovich P. Vascular access and patient outcomes in hemodialysis: questions answered in recent literature. *Artif Organs.* 2003;27:237–241.
9. Asif A, Leclercq B, Merrill D, Bourgoignie J, Roth D. Arteriovenous fistula creation: should US nephrologists get involved? *Am J Kidney Dis.* 2003;42:1293–1300.
10. Van Glabeke E, Belenfant X, Barrou B, et al. Surgical learning curve for creation of vascular accesses for haemodialysis: value of medico-radio-surgical collaboration. *Prog Urol.* 2005;15:339–343.
11. Ivanovich P, Kahan B, Bergan J, Someya S, Ono K, Inokuchi K. Stapler for A-V anastomosis: simplified, immediate vascular access. *Trans Am Soc Artif Intern Organs.* 1977;23:716–718.
12. Konner K, Hulbert-Shearon T, Roys E, Port F. Tailoring the initial vascular access for dialysis patients. *Kidney Int.* 2002;62:329–338.
13. Konner K, Nonnast-Daniel B and Ritz E. The arteriovenous fistula. *J Am Soc Neph.* 2003;14:1669–1680.
14. Konner K. The initial creation of native arteriovenous fistulas: surgical aspects and their impact on the practice of nephrology. *Semin Dial.* 2003;16:291–298.
15. O'Neill WC. The new nephrologist. *Am J Kidney Dis.* 2000;35:978–979.
16. Mishler R, Sands J, Ofsthun N, Teng M, Schon D, Lazarus J. Dedicated outpatient vascular access center decreases hospitalization and missed outpatient dialysis treatments. *Kidney Int.* 2006;69:393–398.
17. Beathard GA, Litchfield T. Physician operators forum of RMS lifeline, inc. effectiveness and safety of dialysis vascular access procedures performed by interventional nephrologists. *Kidney Int.* 2004;66:1622–1632.
18. Mishler R. Global vascular access surgery by nephrologists. *Semin Dial* 2005;18:540–541.
19. Beathard G, Urbanes A, Litchfield T, Weinstein A. The risk of sedation/analgesia in hemodialysis patients undergoing interventional procedures. *Semin Dial.* 2011;24:97–103.
20. Mishler R, Outcomes of arteriovenous fistulae creation by a US interventional nephrologist. *J Am Soc Nephrol.* 2008;19:471A.
21. Mishler R. AV fistula creation by a US interventional nephrologist. *Adv Perit Dial.* 2006;22:2–210.
22. Mishler R, Yevzlin A. Outcomes of arteriovenous fistulae creation by a US interventional nephrologist. *Semin Dial.* 2010;23:224–228.
23. Packer J. Fistula creation—the next generation. Poster presented at American Society of Diagnostic and Interventional Nephrology Annual Scientific Meeting 2008. *Semin Dial.* 2008;21:109.
24. Packer J. Unconventional fistula creation—Is KDOQI misleading? Poster presented at American Society of

Diagnostic and Interventional Nephrology Scientific Meeting 2010. *Semin Dial.* 2010;23:341–342.

25. End Stage Renal Disease Network 15 Data, May 2010.

26. National Kidney Foundation: NKF-DOQI Clinical Practice Guidelines for Vascular Access, 1997. *Am J Kidney Dis.* 1997;30:S137–S191.

27. National Kidney Foundation: KDOQI Clinical Practice Guidelines for Vascular Access, update 2006. *Am J Kidney Dis.* 2006;48(suppl):S176–S247.

28. Mishler R. How nephrologists can safely create arterial-venous access in an outpatient center. *J Vasc Access.* 2010; 11:205–206.

29. Georgiadis G, Polychronidus A. Access surgery and the role of nephrologists. *Am J Kidney Dis.* 2003;41:1126–1127.

30. Sreenarasihaiah V, Ravani P. Arteriovenous fistula surgery an American perspective from Italy. *Semin in Dial.* 2005; 18:542–549.

50

SECONDARY ARTERIOVENOUS FISTULA

LARRY SPERGEL & ARIF ASIF

LEARNING OBJECTIVES

1. Describe the four basic steps important in a well-designed SAVF strategy.
2. Define a type-I SAVF.
3. Define a type-II SAVF.
4. Describe how candidates for an SAVF can be identified.
5. Describe the basic protocol that should be used to determine the timing for conversion to an SAVF.
6. How does the primary patency of a SAVF compare in general to that for a primary AVF.
7. Describe factors that might affect the patency rates that are seen in SAVF series.
8. Describe the factors that determine whether or not a dialysis catheter may be required for period after the creation of a SAVF.

INTRODUCTION

Much of the focus on maximizing the use of arteriovenous fistulas (AVFs) has emphasized the early identification of chronic kidney disease (CKD) patients, early referral to nephrology, and the timely placement of an AVF prior to initiating hemodialysis. The goal of such efforts is to minimize the use of arteriovenous grafts (AVGs) and tunneled dialysis catheters (TDCs) in order to reduce the morbidity, mortality, and costs associated with such vascular accesses. An equally important strategy to maximize the use of AVFs is the creation of secondary fistulas (SAVFs). Both the fistula first initiative and the NKF-KDOQI vascular access guidelines emphasize the importance of SAVFs.[1,2] KDOQI guideline 2.1.4 states, "patients should be considered for construction of a primary fistula after failure of every dialysis AV access." Fistula first change concept # 6

is entitled "Secondary AVFs in AVG patients." This change concept lists four important points.

- Nephrologists should evaluate every AVG patient for possible SAVF conversion, including mapping as indicated, and document the plan in the patient's record.
- Dialysis facility staff and/or rounding nephrologists should examine the outflow vein of all AVG patients ("sleeves up") during dialysis treatments (minimum frequency, monthly) and identify patients who may be suitable for elective SAVF conversion in the upper arm and inform nephrologists of a suitable outflow vein.
- During an intervention for AVG failure, interventionalists should examine and report on suitability of outflow vein(s) for a planned SAVF.
- Nephrologists should refer candidates to a surgeon for placement of a SAVF before the AVG is abandoned.

The goal of nephrologists should clearly be to transition AV graft patients to an AVF to the maximum degree possible and break the graft—graft failure, catheter, and new graft cycle.

DEFINITIONS

Although historically in the hemodialysis literature, a SAVF has been considered to be one that is constructed utilizing the outflow vein of an AVG, the definition has been expanded to refer to any AVF constructed following another access. Whereas the classic, direct SAVF utilizes an outflow vein of an AVG (type-I SAVF), other SAVFs utilize the many other autogenous access opportunities when the existing access venous outflow will not permit the standard direct SAVF conversion (type-II).[3]

▶ Type-I SAVF

A type-I SAVF is defined as an AVF that is created following an existing access using the outflow veins of that access. The strategy of converting the mature, arterialized outflow

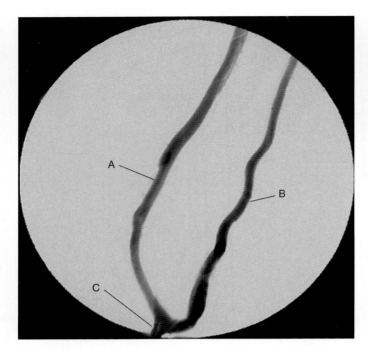

Figure 50-1. Angiogram of veins draining forearm AVG. (**A**) Basilic vein, (**B**) cephalic vein, and (**C**) graft and anastomosis.

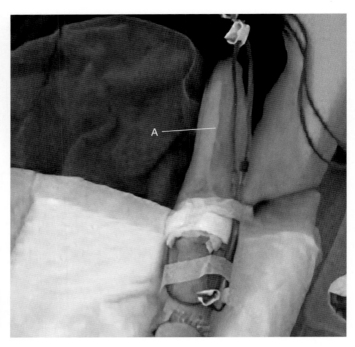

Figure 50-2. Appearance of patient's upper arm with "sleeves up." (**A**) Prominent cephalic vein.

vein of an existing access to a type-I SAVF is most often applicable to forearm AVGs. The outflow vein options in the upper arm are the cephalic, basilic, and brachial veins (Figure 50-1). In patients with an established forearm AV graft, the veins of the upper arm undergo the same process of maturation as is seen with AVF development and for the same reasons.[4–8] In most instances this will involve the creation of either a brachial-cephalic or a brachial-basilic AVF. Even when one of these veins is not suitable, there may be an adequate vein in the forearm that can be utilized as a retrograde-flow middle-arm SAVF, after disrupting one or more valves.[9]

When an AVG has to be placed in a patient, it should be done with a dual purpose in mind—firstly, providing an access for hemodialysis and secondly, as a means of maturing veins in the upper arm for a type-I SAVF. Utilization of the AVG outflow vein to construct a type-I SAVF is, in essence, the equivalent of the second stage of a two-stage procedure resulting in an autogenous AVF.

▶ Type-II SAVF

A type-II SAVF is defined as an AVF constructed following an existing access that does not utilize the outflow drainage of that access, but one of the other autogenous access opportunities detected by vascular mapping. In cases where mapping fails to reveal a suitable outflow vein on imaging of the ipsilateral arm, the patient should be scheduled for vascular mapping of the contralateral extremity.

IDENTIFICATION OF SAVF CANDIDATES

Every patient receiving dialysis via an AV graft should be viewed as a potential candidate for a secondary AVF. To identify the patient some mechanism for visualizing the veins of the upper arm is necessary. This is most easily accomplished by simply having the patient roll up their sleeve. In fact this can be easily accomplished while making dialysis rounds. It is surprising how many patients with an AV graft have large veins easily visible in the upper arms (Figure 50-2) that have gone unnoticed (ignored). With any type of procedure to treat AVG dysfunction, angiographic studies can be used to identify optimal candidates for a secondary AVF if the operator is alert to this issue. Actually, the procedure used to treat AVG dysfunction captures most of the data required for mapping related to SAVF creation. In a study of the angiograms that was performed as part of either an angioplasty or a thrombectomy procedure, 75% of the patients with lower arm grafts were found to have one or both upper arm superficial veins that were optimal for AVF conversion[6] (Figure 50-3). It should be noted that even in patients with an upper arm AVG, a type-I SAVF may still be possible (Figure 50-4).

TIMING OF SAVF CONVERSION

The appropriate timing of conversion of an AVG to a SAVF is somewhat controversial—should it be done early or should wait until late. If it is done while the AVG is still functioning, thereby sacrificing the AVG, some of the

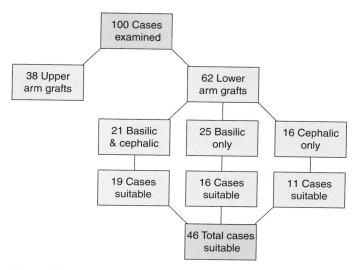

Figure 50-3. Results of evaluation of 100 consecutive cases presenting with AVG dysfunction.[6]

potential use-life of the access will be forfeited. On the other hand if the conversion is delayed too long, certainly if salvage procedures are performed in order to extend the use-life of the access, the opportunity may be lost.[10,11] Additionally, if the procedure is delayed until the AVG has to be abandoned, a mandatory period of catheter usage will be incurred. Even if started immediately, the process leading to a functional SAVF generally takes months to complete (referred to as fistula hurdles).[12] The prolonged use of a CVT is associated with significant risk of morbidity and even mortality that would be better avoided if possible.

The use of an endovascular stent-graft at the venous anastomosis of an AVG has been recommended[13,14]; however, it should be obvious that this is not consistent with the recommended SAVF strategy. There are both medical and economic reasons for advocating the conversion of an AVG to a SAVF. Placing stents of any type to prolong the use-life of an AVG is counterintuitive.

The recommendation of fistula first[2] represents a balance between the early and late options. It starts with an anticipation of the need to create a SAVF by recommending that a center-based plan be in place as a part of a CQI program. This program should assure that when a dysfunctional AVG (venous stenosis or thrombosis) is referred for the first intervention, the imaging study that is performed should evaluate the condition of the outflow vein(s) and central vasculature in preparation for SAVF surgery. Certainly, decisions regarding the timing for surgery will need to be individualized based on the circumstances and angiographic findings at the time of AVG intervention. The approach to transitioning to an SAVF should be based upon the status of the draining vein(s) relative to the creation of an AVF (Figure 50-5).

▶ **Suitable Draining Vein(s)**

If the outflow vein is suitable, creation of type-I SAVF should be considered at that time or on recurrent AVG

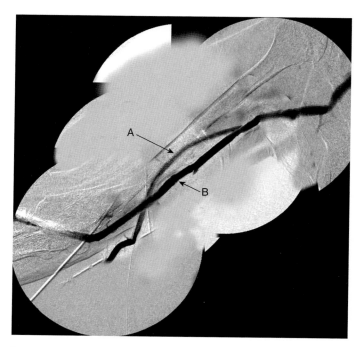

Figure 50-4. Montage of angiograms of upper arm showing an AVG with a basilic vein candidate for an SAVF. (**A**) AVG and (**B**) basilic vein.

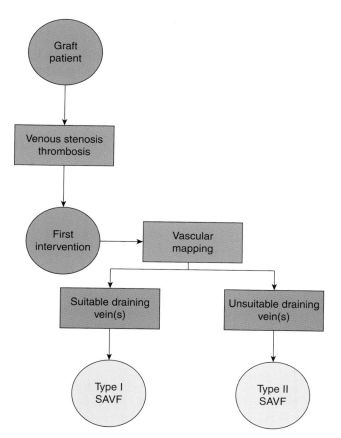

Figure 50-5. Algorithm for timing of SAVF conversion.

failure, depending on the angiographic findings, condition of the AVG, and the outcome of intervention. If angioplasty produces a good result, then conversion to a SAVF should be planned following the second episode of dysfunction or thrombosis (Figure 50-5).

▶ Unsuitable Draining Vein(s)

If the outflow vein is not suitable, a new vein is going to be required for SAVF construction. In that case, the creation of a type-II SAVF should be seriously considered at that time, or at least not later than the first recurrent AVG failure, as it can be expected to take at least 3–4 months from the time the decision is made until there is a usable AVF. It is more important to have a fistula in place a few months early to avoid a catheter, allow for a longer maturation period that many AVFs require (fistula hurdles), and avoid the risk of losing an important AVF opportunity rather than waiting until the AVG is lost.

KEYS TO SUCCESS

Three things are critical to the success of this SAVF strategy. Firstly, vascular access education is an essential component for converting a patient to a SAVF.[15] It is often difficult for the patient to understand and accept the creation of a new access when they have an old access (AVG or TDC) that they perceive as still being functional. Patients with AVGs and TDCs must be educated regarding the superiority of AVFs and then be given the opportunity to select the best available vascular access.

Secondly, it is crucial that there be ongoing collaboration between the nephrologist, interventionalist, and surgeon, so that the opportunity is not lost.

Thirdly, it is crucial that a protocol be in place to assure that there is an AVF evaluation and plan established well before permanent loss of an AVG in order to provide suitable patients with the opportunity to have an AVF as their next access and to avoid the need for long-term and recurrent catheter use. This protocol should be overseen by the vascular access coordinator (VAC), or equivalent, in the dialysis clinic.

SAVF SERIES

Patency rates for SAVF series have varied and often differ significantly from those for primary AVF series.[16–18] When examining these data one should keep in mind that the patient populations are not necessarily comparable. Several different types of patient may be included in a series of cases with SAVFs. All patients will have had a previous access failure; this alone differentiates them from cases with primary AVFs. However, some may have had multiple access failures. Others had vascular mapping and received an AVG because a suitable vein was not detected. Some may have had the placement of a graft without any preliminary vascular mapping.

In one study,[16] 71 type-II SAVFs were created over a 30-month period. These consisted of 40 brachial-cephalic (BCAVF) and 22 brachial-basilic (BBAVF) AVFs. In this study, 29 of the BCAVFs and 16 of the BBAVFs had previously undergone placement of an AVF while 20 of the BCAVFs and six of the BBAVFs had prior placement of an AVG. The study concluded that patency rates for these type-II SAVFs were inferior to primary AVFs with 1- and 2-year primary patency of 58% and 22%, respectively. The 1- and 2-year primary patency rate for primary upper arm AVFs were 75% and 61%, respectively.

In another report two separate groups of patients were presented.[17] In the first group, 40 consecutive patients who were transitioned from an AV graft to a SAVF were analyzed. The patients had 1–22 previous access operations (mean = 3). Twenty-six of the 40 patients had a forearm AVG and the remaining 14 had an upper arm AVG. Of the 26 forearm AVGs, 22 (84.6%) were converted to type-I SAVFs, with the remaining four undergoing type-II SAVF constructions because outflow veins were considered to be unsuitable for a type-I SAVF. Of the 22 type-I conversions, 13 utilized the basilic vein in the arm as a transposition, six utilized the cephalic vein in the arm, one utilized the brachial vein in the arm as a transposition, and two were direct antecubital constructions resulting in retrograde flow into the forearm to create an access. Of the 15 transpositions, 10 were based on the brachial artery and five on the proximal radial artery.

Of the 40 patients who underwent SAVF construction, 37 underwent SAVF surgery prior to abandonment of the AV graft. Twenty-two patients required a catheter. Seventeen of the catheters were short-term (<10 days). No catheter was required for more than 12 weeks. Follow-up was 5–53 months (mean = 20 months). The primary and cumulative patency rates for these 40 SAVF operations (types I and II) were 82.5% and 92.5% at 1 year, and 60.0% and 87.5% at 2 years. Cumulative patency for type I SAVFs was 95.5% at 2 years.

In the second group of this report,[17] 102 consecutive patients were transitioned from an AVG to a SAVF. These patients had 1–50 previous access operations (mean = 3). Forty-four individuals had one or more AVGs in both arms and seven had additional thigh grafts. Eighty-three of the 102 patients had at least one forearm AVG and the remaining 19 had only upper arm AVG(s). Of the 83 patients with at least one forearm AVG, only 16 (19.3%) were referred with a patent AVG or suitable outflow vein for conversion to a type-I SAVF. The remaining patients required type-II SAVF constructions because of thrombosed AVGs with outflow veins that were either obliterated or considered to be unsuitable for a type-I SAVF. Of the 16 type-I conversions, four utilized the basilic vein in the arm as a transposition, 10 utilized the cephalic vein in the arm, and two were direct antecubital constructions with limited distal valve disruption, which depended primarily upon retrograde flow into the forearm to maintain adequate access.

Follow-up was 2–44 months (mean = 14 months). The primary and cumulative patency rates for these 108 SAVF operations were 55.5% and 94.4% at 1 year, and 50.5% and 91.6% at 2 years. Cumulative patency for type-I SAVFs was 100% at 2 years. Individual catheter time was not recorded for this group but as 86 (84.3%) individuals had a SAVF created without a functioning AVG for access, it is clear that prolonged catheter use was common.

In this combined series of 141 cases, all patients with upper arm AVGs underwent type-II SAVFs. All individuals had a SAVF created with no patient requiring a new AVG. The combined type-I SAVF cumulative patency for both groups was 97.4% at 2 years.

In another study, 62 SAVFs were studied.[18] Of these, 35 were type I and 27 were type-II. The primary patency rates for types-I and II-SAVF at 6 and 12 months were 87% and 14% (type-I) and 71% and 11% (type-II), respectively. The secondary patency rates for type-I at 12, 24, and 36 months were 100%, 100%, 83%, respectively, and for type-II were 92%, 88%, 83%, respectively. The primary and secondary patency rates between the groups were not statistically significant. The cumulative patency rates for type-I at 12, 24, and 36 months were 100%, 100%, 94%, respectively, and for type-II were 96%, 96%, and 91%, respectively. Type-I required 1.4 procedures/year, and type-II needed 1.5 procedures/year (p = nonsignificant). Tunneled dialysis catheters were required in 21 patients with type-I and all 27 patients with type-II SAVF.

TDC REQUIREMENT AFTER SAVF

The need for a catheter after a SAVF conversion is variable. As has been mentionable in the series listed above, many cases do not require a catheter. Slayden et al[17] noted that the need for a TDC was dramatically less in the patients with an established SAVF conversion plan. This certainly appears to be an important issue in TDC avoidance. The type of SAVF created is also an important determining factor. Patients who are transitioned to a type-II SAVF can be expected to be catheter dependent until the AVF matures adequately for use.[17,18] With a type-I SAVF, the use of a catheter varies with the type of fistula that is created. Of the 40 patients in the first group reported by Slayden et al,[17] none of the patients with a cephalic vein AVF in the upper arm required a catheter. As is the case with primary AVFs, vein transposition SAVFs require a catheter. Another issue that is an important TDC determining factor is whether the patient is seen for SAVF creation prior to the loss of the existing access. In these cases, a period of catheter dependency is to be expected.

In patients with a forearm graft and a well-developed upper arm cephalic vein, it is reasonable to begin cannulating the vein prior to conversion to a SAVF. When the conversion occurs, it is just a matter of continuing what has already been initiated.

REFERENCES

1. National Kidney Foundation. K/DOQI clinical practice guidelines in vascular access: 2006 update. *Am J Kidney Dis.* 2006;48(suppl 1):S176.
2. http/www.fistulafirst.org. Accessed 2011.
3. Spergel LM, Ravani P, Asif A, et al. Autogenous arteriovenous fistula options. *J Nephrol.* 2007;20:288.
4. Nguyen VD, Treat L, Griffith C, Robinson K. Creation of secondary AV fistulas from failed hemodialysis grafts: the role of routine vein mapping. *J Vasc Access.* 2007;8:91.
5. Beathard GA. Strategy for maximizing the use of arteriovenous fistulae. *Semin Dial.* 2000;13:291.
6. Beathard GA. Interventionalist's role in identifying candidates for secondary fistulas. *Semin Dial.* 2004;17:233.
7. Hemphill H, Allon M, Konner K, et al. How can the use of arteriovenous fistulas be increased? *Semin Dial.* 2003;16:214.
8. Asif A, Unger SW, Briones P, et al. Creation of secondary arteriovenous fistulas: maximizing fistulas in prevalent hemodialysis patients. *Semin Dial.* 2005;18:420.
9. Jennings WC. Creating arteriovenous fistulas in 132 consecutive patients: exploiting the proximal radial artery arteriovenous fistula: reliable, safe, and simple forearm and upper arm hemodialysis access. *Arch Surg.* 2006;141:27.
10. Spergel L. Vascular access conundrum. *Semin Dial.* 2005; 18:161.
11. Asif A, Leon C, Merrill D, et al. Optimal timing for secondary arteriovenous fistula creation: devastating effects of delaying conversion. *Semin Dial.* 2006;19:425.
12. Lee T, Barker J, Allon M. Tunneled catheters in hemodialysis patients: reasons and subsequent outcomes. *Am J Kidney Dis.* 2005;46:501.
13. Maya ID, Allon M. Outcomes of thrombosed arteriovenous grafts: comparison of stents vs angioplasty. *Kidney Int.* 2006;69:934.
14. Haskal ZJ, Trerotola S, Dolmatch B, et al. Stent graft versus balloon angioplasty for failing dialysis-access grafts. *N Engl J Med.* 2010;362:494.
15. Asif A, Cherla G, Merrill D, et al. Conversion of tunneled hemodialysis catheter-consigned patients to arteriovenous fistula. *Kidney Int.* 2005;67:2399.
16. Ascher E, Hingorani A, Yorkovich W. *Techniques and Outcomes after Brachiocephalic and Brachiobasilic Arteriovenous Fistula Creation.* Philadelphia: Lippincott Williams & Wilkins; 2002;84–92.
17. Slayden GC, Spergel L, Jennings WC. Secondary arteriovenous fistulas: converting prosthetic AV grafts to autogenous dialysis access. *Semin Dial.* 2008;21:474.
18. Salman L, Alex M, Unger SW, et al. Secondary autogenous arteriovenous fistulas in the "fistula first" era: results of a longterm prospective study. *J Am Coll Surg.* 2009;209:100.

51

SURGICAL OPTIONS FOR ARTERIOVENOUS ACCESS IN PATIENTS WITH EXHAUSTED VEINS

ERIC S. CHEMLA

LEARNING OBJECTIVES

1. Describe surgical alternatives that are available for the placement of an arteriovenous access in a patient without peripheral veins but with a patent superior vena cava.

2. Describe surgical alternatives that are available for the placement of an arteriovenous access in a patient without peripheral veins whose superior vena cava is occluded.

3. Describe surgical alternatives that are available for the placement of an arteriovenous access in a patient without peripheral veins in whom both the superior and inferior vena cava are occluded.

INTRODUCTION

A native arteriovenous autogenous fistula is the preferred long-term vascular access for hemodialysis. However, in patients who have exhausted all their native veins and when neither peritoneal dialysis nor transplantation is an option, creation of an access using either a synthetic or biological graft should be considered. The population undergoing dialysis has grown by 9% over the past 10 years in the USA and the profile of this population has evolved considerably. Patients are older and while diabetes and hypertension remain the most commonly reported causes of end-stage renal failure, end-stage atherosclerotic renovascular disease seems to be on the rise in older patients.[1] The net result is that over the past years there has been a change in the dialysis population to one that is frailer population with a poorer vasculature in need of dialysis for a longer period of time as there is no age limit to enter a dialysis program.

Several complex procedures for patients with no native arteriovenous options have been described in the literature.[2,3] We would like here to describe our personal approach in considering different types of clinical features and also to propose a flow chart establishing that what we feel are the best indications for each type of clinical presentation.

PATIENTS WITH A PATENT SUPERIOR VENA CAVA (SVC)

A significant proportion of patients, especially the diabetic and obese patients, will present to access clinics with no native arteriovenous options even for their first access. Some arrive at this situation even without any previous catheter insertion.[4] It is extremely important to ponder what type of access to perform in these cases, bearing in mind that peritoneal dialysis and transplantation will never be a potential solution if they run out of access. Here is what we currently propose for these patients in hierarchical order.

▶ Brachio-Axillary Artery Bypass Graft

This would be our first proposal when confronted with no native arteriovenous options, but a patent SVC. A polytetrafluoroethylene (PTFE) 6 mm (diameter) and 40 cm (length) internally reinforced and coated with heparin (Propaten, Gore Ltd®, Flagstaff, AZ, USA) is our preferred option, unless the patient needs immediate dialysis through the graft when no central lines can be used. If such were the case, then a Flixene® (Atrium Medical, Hudson, NH,

USA or Acuseal Gore Ltd Flagstaff, AZ, USA) would be preferred. This can be cannulated after only 12 hours.

In order to create this access, the patient is positioned in a decubitus position and fully anesthetized. Two incisions are performed—one at the elbow crease level and the other on the medial aspect of the arm below the axilla. This lower incision is made 4 cm in length while the upper one is 7–8 cm. Both the brachial artery and axillary–brachial vein are dissected free and a subcutaneous tunnel is created. After having injected 2000 IU of heparin intravenously, the graft is inserted into the tunnel and anastomosed end to side to the vein and the artery. The arterial anastomosis will be measured at 6 mm long, while the venous one will strive to be up to 40 mm long depending upon the local anatomy. The lower one is small so as to avoid steal syndrome that could be induced by a much too high inflow, while the upper one is very long so as to mitigate the potential for myointimal hyperplasia.

▶ Axillary–Axillary Necklace Bypass Graft

The axillary-axillary necklace graft (Figure 51-1) represents our last upper body attempt before contemplating a lower limb fistula. When brachio-axillary grafts are not possible or have been exhausted or when there is a past medical history of severe steal syndrome a necklace graft is indicated.

We currently use the same type of grafts, as previously described. After obtaining consent, the patient is fully anesthetized and positioned in a decubitus position. A support is placed underneath their shoulders while the head is in extension. Incisions are made 1 cm below the lateral third of each clavicle. The pectoralis muscles are dissected free and split. The clavi-pectoro-axillary fascia is dissected and the artery and contralateral vein are mobilized on a sling. A subcutaneous tunnel is created with the help of one of our access nurse coordinators who usually comes to the operating room to indicate what would suit best the patient for future cannulation of the graft. The shape of the tunnel depends upon the patient's anatomy and their body habitus. It could be straight or slightly curved either very close or further away from the manubrium. Heparin is injected

and the anastomoses are conducted as previously described and respecting the same length.

We have previously reported a series of 18 consecutive patients[5] with an axillary–axillary necklace graft. In this series, 50% were diabetic. They had a primary patency rate at 73% while secondary patency was 89% at 1 year. Five cases needed surgical revision for thrombosis or stenosis and only one could not be rescued and had to be abandoned.

We advocate the use of a straight graft rather than a loop on the chest wall as described by another team[6] as it seems easier to cannulate (as expressed by our dialysis nurses) and to rescue when introducing embolectomy catheters and dilators. This also allows the possibility of creating a loop at another time if the straight graft fails.[7] When a patient needs immediate dialysis through the graft either because of an infected or poorly working central venous catheter, we dialyze them with in and out of sheaths for a couple of days, leaving them "plastic free" for at least 48 hours before performing a necklace operation using a early cannulation grafts that is cannulated within 12 hours. We have operated successfully on a series of 13 patients with a median delay to first cannulation of 24 hours only.

This type of access is also advocated in cases with a previous history of upper limb fistulas involving the brachial artery with steal syndrome that was severe enough to contraindicate any type of regular access contralaterally. As it is a proximal anastomosis, it prevents quite well further steal syndrome as reported by several teams that prefer a proximalization or a distalization of the anastomosis rather than a DRIL or a banding when treating or preventing steal syndrome usually triggered by a fistula anastomosed to the brachial artery.[8,9] Being very superficial, this type of access is easy to cannulate regardless of the body habitus of the patient and is well accepted both by patients and by dialysis staff.

SVC OCCLUDED OR CENTRAL VEINS OCCLUDED BILATERALLY

If an occluded SVC or bilaterally occluded central veins is established before the patient is referred for surgery or is discovered during the work-up for an access, it always triggers a discussion with our interventional radiologists to examine a potential endovascular recanalization. If possible and successful, our attitude in case of exhaustion of all veins is as described above. If impossible or unsuccessful we then propose either a superficial femoral vein transposition to the popliteal artery above the knee or a complex bypass.

▶ Superficial Femoral Vein Transposition to the Popliteal Artery

A popliteal–femoral transposition is a native fistula with excellent results as long as properly indicated and performed.[10,11] The length of vein available is relatively short, the profunda vein should be left intact to ascertain a

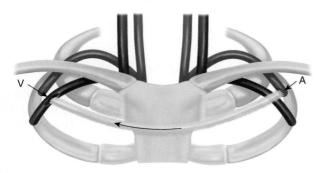

Figure 51-1. Necklace graft shown with a straight subcutaneous tunnel performed just at the level of the manubrium sternum with a 6–40 early cannulation PTFE graft.

proper venous return for the lower limb and avoid chronic edema. The popliteal vein should be ligated above the knee so as to protect the venous drainage of the leg and therefore avoid ischemic complications. Once the vein is dissected between these two landmarks, it is tunneled sub-cutaneously toward the popliteal artery to which it is anastomosed end to side again on a limited length (6 mm). If the patient is obese, then the short length of vein available contraindicates the technique as the segment available to cannulation in the subcutaneous tunnel will be very short and therefore unrealistic. Similarly, if the patient is diabetic, often with a poor leg run off, then any anastomosis to the popliteal artery will be at high risk of steal syndrome.[12]

One author has reported his experience to overcome these difficulties by extending the available vein with a PTFE graft (6 mm in diameter) that would be anastomosed end to end to the vein and then to the artery end to side either to the popliteal artery in case of obesity or to the femoral artery in case of high risk of steal thus realizing a proximalization of the anastomosis.[9,12] When such contraindications are present, it is on a case-to-case basis that we either propose a very complex bypass or extend the vein with a PTFE graft.

▶ Axillary Artery to Popliteal Bypass Graft

The axillary artery to popliteal bypass graft (Figure 51-2) overcomes serious obstacles encountered in the most extreme patients (obese or severe diabetic) for whom access is paramount and where there are no other options for their renal replacement therapy. This access prevents steal as it arises from the axillary artery, is not limited in length, and bypasses the femoral triangle which is very prone to infection and wound break down.

In order to create this access, the patient is fully anesthetized and positioned in a decubitus position with a support underneath the shoulder and the lower limb involved. Half the body is draped in the operating field. The axillary artery is dissected through an incision immediately underneath the clavicle while the popliteal vein is mobilized via an incision through the medial aspect of the lower thigh. A very long subcutaneous tunnel is created with a relay incision in regard of the anterosuperior iliac spine. A 6 mm–80 cm PTFE graft is used; it might be extended with another 6 mm–40 cm PTFE graft if too short. The graft is anastomosed end to side to the eatery and the vein, again with a short incision on the artery (6 mm) and very long on the vein (up to 40 mm). The graft then needs 2 weeks before cannulation can start.[13]

▶ Femoral Artery to Femoral Vein Crossover Bypass Graft

Although rarely indicated, the operation to create this access is easy and quick to perform and could even be carried out under local anesthetics. The patient is placed in a supine position and the common femoral vein and artery are dissected free through two very small groin incisions

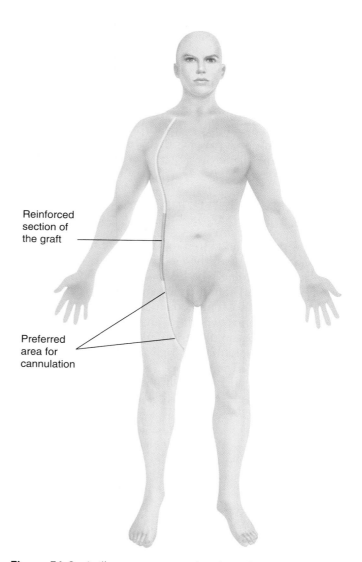

Reinforced section of the graft

Preferred area for cannulation

Figure 51-2. Axillary artery to popliteal vein bypass graft.

following the inguinal fold over 4–5 cm. A 6 mm–40 cm PTFE graft is then tunneled subcutaneously on the lower abdominal wall and both anastomoses are conducted end to side. This operation is contraindicated in obese patients as it is impossible to cannulate the graft even if tunneled very superficially and in case of heart failure as the graft develops high blood flow quickly. An early cannulation graft could be used allowing cannulation within 12 hours. This access is usually proposed to patients suitable for a superficial femoral vein transposition but who are reluctant either because of body image concerns or by sheer fear of an important operation.[14]

▶ Superficial Femoral Artery to Popliteal Vein Bypass Graft

In order to create this access, the patient is either fully anesthetized or under local anesthetics and positioned in a decubitus position with support underneath the operated limb. The femoral artery is dissected through an upper thigh incision below the femoral triangle. The popliteal vein is dissected through an incision above the knee in the medial aspect of the thigh. The graft is a 6 mm–40 cm PTFE graft that could be early cannulation; it is tunneled subcutaneously describing a gentle curve on the medial–anterior aspect of the thigh. This procedure is contraindicated in case of peripheral vascular disease or diabetes as the risk of steal syndrome is high in these cases. It is performed only in obese patients that would not be suitable for a general anesthetic.

SVC AND IVC OCCLUDED OR BILATERAL ILIAC VEINS OCCLUDED

In these very rare and extreme cases where no options are left to dialyze a patient, then a careful discussion needs to take place to examine whether dialysis should be discontinued or if there is an alternate method of dialysis such as peritoneal dialysis. If hemodialysis should continue then the only option left is to perform an access that will involve the right appendage in the atrium. We would normally recommend a brachial artery to right appendage bypass but in our very limited experience (only one patient) both brachial arteries had been used for previous accesses and were not suitable for any further surgery. We therefore did use and would recommend a femoral artery to right atrium (appendage) bypass using a 6–80 Intering (Gore Tex®; Flagstaff, AZ, USA) tunneled subcutaneously and then in between two ribs. We did at that time perform a sternotomy but would rather envisage, if today confronted with a similar case, a much less invasive mini-thoracotomy through the second intercostal space. Our patient was recovered in the cardiac ICU for 24 hours and was then dialyzed successfully through the graft for 6 months after which he decided to discontinue dialysis.[15]

In all the interventions described above, heparin is given intravenously during surgery and anticoagulation is organized but only for the patients that will receive a graft. Our target INR is established between two and three. All patients, regardless of their surgery, have the same follow-up organized by the access coordinator. Nurse led clinics happen on a regular basis (at least six times per annum) where transonic measurements are taken four times at different moments during a dialysis shift. In case of an inflow below 600 mL per minute, a drop of inflow by 20% in between two sets of measurements or a recirculation rate above 5%, an ultrasound scan is obtained and a decision to intervene or not surgically or by endovascular means is taken by the surgeon and the access team in a multidisciplinary meeting.

When a patient who has exhausted their entire venous anatomy is referred, they enter into our complex access program where, before any surgery, two consultations with the surgeon and access coordinator with a week interval in between are organized. A visit to our nephrologist during the week between the two surgical visits is also recommended. This allows our patients to understand fully the pros and cons as well as the intended benefits and potential complications of our complex approach.

We routinely ask for a full cardiac review with a cardiology consultation, an Electrocardiogram (EKG), and a stress echocardiogram. All prescribed antihypertensive drugs are reviewed and sometimes discontinued as low blood pressure is a major risk of failure in these cases. Peritoneal dialysis as well as urgent transplant are always envisaged and preferred to a complex vascular access whenever possible. Unfortunately, it has proven extremely difficult to switch to these treatments for any of our complex patients and only a small proportion (less than 10%) have been successfully steered toward peritoneal dialysis, while none could have an urgent transplant.

When dialysis through a temporary catheter, while waiting for a graft or a native fistula to be ready (2 weeks for any PTFE grafts and 5–6 weeks for a femoral vein transposition) is impossible, we tend to propose an early cannulation graft specifically in a necklace position if the SVC is patent. We propose a cross-over femoral artery to femoral vein bypass or femoral artery to popliteal vein bypass if the SVC is obstructed. We have sometimes had to use a temporary dual lumen catheter in the femoral artery in order to dialyze some of our patients adequately prior to performing a complex graft of fistula. In these cases (we reported 13 successfully), there are no veins to insert a temporary catheter, the internal jugular, subclavian, or femoral veins are occluded or have proven impossible to cannulate.[16] Our experience shows that it is extremely important to dialyze these patients properly before any operation; this avoids a potentially very difficult recovery period with low blood pressure spells that usually jeopardize the patency of any newly created access. We normally do not send these patients to ICU after surgery. We manage their fluid balance very carefully preferring blood products in case of depletion while keeping track of their potassium level. We normally start cannulating early cannulation grafts after 12 hours, regular grafts after 2 weeks, and native accesses within 4–6 weeks.

SUMMARY

The need for complex accesses in a context of complete native option exhaustion will continue to increase and there are no clear established pathways or flowcharts widely agreed upon by the medical community for these patients. In case of native option exhaustion with a patent SVC, our first choice will be a necklace axillary artery to axillary vein bypass. Although well described in the literature[5] very few long-term results are available.[2,17] In individual cases, good results and usually uneventful follow up have been observed[17,18]; our series of 18 patients has shown the same favorable results at 1 year. The axillary loop has also been reported successfully[6] but it seems, in our opinion, to be less accessible to a potential rescue when compared to a straight graft. It also generated numerous complaints from our dialysis nurses when we used to perform them about the difficulty they constantly encountered with cannulation. We therefore now keep an indication for loop configurations for rare cases of occlusion of both axillary artery and vein on the same side or for a rescue of a thrombosed straight necklace where an occlusion of the vein downstream the anastomosis is responsible for the failure.[7]

In case of SVC obstruction we have omitted in our proposed flowchart long saphenous vein fistulae (LSVF) as well as femoral loop grafts necessitating extensive dissection of the femoral triangle. It is widely acknowledged that LSVF yield poor results[10,14] and we firmly believe that a femoral triangle dissection should be avoided specifically in diabetic and/or obese patients because of an increased risk of wound breakdown, infection, steal syndrome, or very high inflow. We therefore recommend either a superficial femoral vein transposition or an axillary artery to popliteal vein bypass graft. The former if the patient is neither diabetic nor obese so that enough vein length could be tunneled subcutaneously to allow safe cannulation. The latter is indicated for any obese diabetic patient with an SVC stenosis or obstruction. In any case a very low systolic blood pressure or a history of cardiac failure would contraindicate these surgeries and render the patients' catheter ridden for the rest of their hemodialysis history. These operations being complex, before proposing them to our patients we always examine the possibility of switching to peritoneal dialysis or organizing an urgent transplant. This multidisciplinary process involving the access nurse coordinator, the nephrologists, the anesthetist, and the surgeon in constant liaison with the patients and their family has allowed us to avoid any misunderstanding or complaints regardless of the surgical outcome.

Our experience is now 9-year long and it seems that the best model of care is to have a multidisciplinary approach with nephrologists, access coordinators, and dedicated access surgeons. This approach has transformed our practice and has permitted better dialysis to a group of patients who would have been catheter bound in the past. Access surgery has now become a specialty per se and we would advise large centers in large hospitals to recruit at least two dedicated access surgeons among their vascular team, with a good knowledge and experience in complex vascular access formation and management.

REFERENCES

1. Foley RN, Collins AJ. End-stage renal disease in the United States: an update from the United States Renal Data System. *J Am Soc Nephrol.* 2007;18:2644.
2. McCann RL. Axillary grafts for difficult hemodialysis access. *J Vasc Surg.* 1996;24:457.
3. Hazinedaroglu S, Karakayali F, Tuzuner A, et al. Exotic arteriovenous fistulas for hemodialysis. *Transplant Proc.* 2004;36:59.
4. Murphy GJ, Nicholson ML. Autogeneous elbow fistulas: the effect of diabetes mellitus on maturation, patency, and complication rates. *Eur J Vasc Endovasc Surg.* 2002;23:452.
5. Morsy MA, Khan A, Chemla ES. Prosthetic axillary–axillary arteriovenous straight access (necklace graft) for difficult hemodialysis patients: a prospective single-center experience. *J Vasc Surg.* 2008;48:1251.
6. Jean-Baptiste E, Hassen-Khodja R, Haudebourg P, et al. Axillary loop grafts for hemodialysis access: midterm results from a single-center study. *J Vasc Surg.* 2008;47:138.
7. Frampton AE, Hossain M, Hamidian Jahromi A, et al. Rescue of an axillary–axillary arteriovenous graft not amenable to endovascular intervention by formation of an axillary loop: a case report. *J Vasc Access.* 2009;10:55.
8. Gradman WS, Pozrikidis C. Analysis of options for mitigating hemodialysis access-related ischemic steal phenomena. *Ann Vasc Surg.* 2004;18:59.
9. Minion DJ, Moore E, Endean E. Revision using distal inflow: a novel approach to dialysis-associated steal syndrome. *Ann Vasc Surg.* 2005;19:625.
10. Chemla ES, Korrakuti L, Makanjuola D, Chang AR. Vascular access in hemodialysis patients with central venous obstruction or stenosis: one center's experience. *Ann Vasc Surg.* 2005;19:692.
11. Gradman WS, Cohen W, Haji-Aghaii M. Arteriovenous fistula construction in the thigh with transposed superficial femoral vein: our initial experience. *J Vasc Surg.* 2001;33:968.
12. Gradman WS, Laub J, Cohen W. Femoral vein transposition for arteriovenous hemodialysis access: improved patient selection and intraoperative measures reduce postoperative ischemia. *J Vasc Surg.* 2005;41:279.
13. Calder FR, Chemla ES, Anderson L, Chang RW. The axillary artery-popliteal vein extended polytetrafluoroethylene graft: a new technique for the complicated dialysis access patient. *Nephrol Dial Transplant.* 2004;19:998.
14. Chemla ES, Morsy M, Anderson L, Makanjuola D. Complex bypasses and fistulas for difficult hemodialysis access: a prospective, single-center experience. *Semin Dial.* 2006;19:246.
15. Suckling R, Morsy M, Chemla ES. Right superficial femoral artery to superior vena cava graft using a polytetrafluroethylene graft: a new technique in a complicated dialysis access patient. *Nephrol Dial Transplant.* 2007;22:970.
16. Frampton AE, Kessaris N, Hossain M, et al. Use of the femoral artery route for placement of temporary catheters for emergency haemodialysis when all usual central venous access sites are exhausted. *Nephrol Dial Transplant.* 2009;24:913.
17. Ono K, Muto Y, Yano K, Yukizane T. Anterior chest wall axillary artery to contralateral axillary vein graft for vascular access in hemodialysis. *Artif Organs.* 1995;19:1233.
18. Dracon M, Watine O, Pruvot F, et al. Axillo-axillary access in hemodialysis. *Nephrologie.* 1994;15:175.

52

HEMODIALYSIS ACCESS-INDUCED DISTAL ISCHEMIA (HAIDI): SURGICAL MANAGEMENT

PIERRE BOURQUELOT

1. Understand the pathophysiology of hemodialysis access-induced distal ischemia.

2. Be able to diagnose the four stages of ischemia.

3. Be able to diagnose ischemic monomelic neuropathy.

4. Describe the technical evaluation of a patient suspected of having hemodialysis-induced access ischemia.

5. Describe the importance of proximal artery stenosis to dialysis access related ischemia.

6. Describe the MILLER procedure and explain when it might be appropriate.

7. Describe the differences between the RUDI procedure and the DRIL procedure.

8. Describe the DRAL procedure and explain when it might be appropriate.

9. Describe the Scheltinga Classification of hemodialysis access-induced distal ischemia and explain how it might be used in making decisions related to therapy.

INTRODUCTION

Distal ischemia is occasionally observed in the upper limb when there is no arteriovenous angioaccess, especially in diabetic patients. Distal ischemia following access creation (Figure 52-1) may be related to steal of blood flow from the arterial system by the arteriovenous access (AVA), in association with artery disease. Most publications refer to "steal syndrome" but the term "hemodialysis access induced distal ischemia" (HAIDI)[1] would be more

appropriate as the physiopathology of ischemia is not restricted to steal.

After fistula creation, the flow that is increased in the proximal artery, above the anastomosis, is totally or partially diverted into the low-pressure venous system, instead of flowing down into the main artery or into collaterals to supply the distal extremity. The flow in the distal artery below the anastomosis will simultaneously decrease and may even become retrograde, running to the fistula, being supplied by collateral arteries. This retrograde flow is observed physiologically in >90% of distal AVAs and very frequently in proximal AVAs. Finally, when associated with arterial lesions preventing normal compensation by collateral flow, both antegrade and retrograde flow diversion can result in insufficient blood supply to peripheral tissues and lead to clinical manifestations of distal ischemia (1–10% of patients). Surgical or percutaneous treatment (see the percutaneous section on HAIDI) may be necessary to treat ischemia and preserve an AVA, if possible.

PATHOPHYSIOLOGY

An arteriovenous anastomosis creates a communication between the high-pressure arterial system and the low-pressure venous system.[2,3] The blood velocity then increases, inducing vasodilatation, due to a release of nitric oxide (NO) by the endothelium and to vascular structural adaptation associated with modifications of the vessel wall matrix by metalloproteinases.[4] The main consequences are a progressive increase in fistula flow and "steal." High flow and ischemic symptoms thus occur earlier and more frequently after creation of a proximal AVA on large arteries in the elbow or thigh compared to forearm distal AVAs. Limitation of fistula flow when creating the arteriovenous anastomosis might be possible for "small" fistulas by reducing

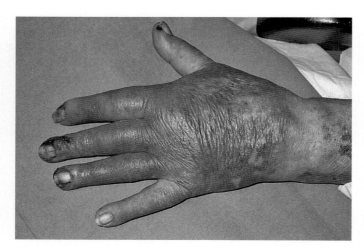

Figure 52-1. Hemodialysis access induced distal ischemia (HAIDI) 1 month after first-stage brachial basilic autogenous arteriovenous angioaccess (AVA).

the length of the anastomosis, but this carries an increased risk of early postoperative thrombosis. For "large" and permanent anastomoses (more than 75% of the diameter of the inflow artery), the flow is in fact independent of the fistula diameter and mainly dependent on the diameter of the artery and its ability to dilate postoperatively.[5,6] Although frequently recommended in scientific publications, there is no published evidence that limitation of the length of the anastomosis for elbow and femoral vein fistulas would be effective for prevention of high-flow and ischemia. Finally, it has been reported[7] that the use of 4–7-mm tapered forearm loop grafts did not reduce the incidence of steal.

Nevertheless, in spite of the reduction in distal perfusion pressure resulting from steal from the main artery flow, sufficient flow is usually supplied by collateral arteries to the distal tissues in the absence of artery disease. The main arterial disorders responsible for HAIDI are atherosclerosis, diabetes, and uremia-related medial calcinosis.[8] Old age, female gender, smoking, and obesity are frequently related, as are an angioaccess in the same limb and a previous angioaccess-related ischemia in the opposite limb. Tynan-Cuisinier and Berman,[9] who performed a prospective evaluation of extremity perfusion, stated that measurement of the digital-brachial index (DBI) at the time of access surgery may help to distinguish at-risk patients when the DBI is <0.45. A striking and markedly increased incidence of severe steal was noted in female patients with intraoperative DBIs of <0.45 at the time of upper arm arteriovenous loop graft placement (68%).

Lower limb HAIDI warrants special mention. In their original report[10] of 25 arteriovenous access constructions in the thigh with transposed superficial femoral vein (tSFV) or composite PTFE-tSFV loop arteriovenous access (mean age 52 years, diabetes 60%), Gradman et al showed good functional 2-year primary (73%) and secondary (86%) patency rates, but an alarming incidence of ischemic complications requiring reoperation. Eight patients

required a second operation to alleviate symptomatic steal syndrome. One acute anterior compartment syndrome was not promptly recognized and required successively a fasciotomy, stenting of an unexpected iliac artery stenosis, a femoral-popliteal bypass graft, and an above-knee amputation. One symptomatic case of foot ischemia and foot drop was associated with complete loss of peroneal nerve function. The other six reoperative procedures for symptomatic ischemia included three above-knee femoral-popliteal bypass grafts, one femoral-tibial bypass graft, one fistula ligation, and one conversion of a tSFV to a composite PTFE-tSFV loop arteriovenous access. Interval ligation was not performed with any bypass graft. Finally three amputations (12%) were necessary. In an additional publication,[11] Gradman et al reported 22 adult patients (mean age 48 years) with tSFV. Steal prophylaxis was combined in 14 patients (tapering the SFV to 5 mm at its takeoff from the femoral artery). However, patients with significant distal occlusive disease, and old and frail patients were not offered a tSFV access. None of these 14 patients required a remedial procedure to correct ischemia. Two-year secondary functional access patency was 94%. Our personal experience with tSFV-associated HAIDI is similar to Gradman's and we always exclude patients with diabetes and occlusive arterial disease. On the other hand, we are skeptical about the efficacy of "tapering" to prevent HAIDI, especially in the absence of any reported flow measurements by Gradman et al.[10] Antoniou et al[12] recently systematically reviewed and analyzed the available literature regarding lower extremity vascular access. They noted that HAIDI was a commonly described complication associated with lower extremity vascular access construction, especially in the elderly, in diabetic patients, and in patients with long-standing end-stage renal disease. However, some of the studies reviewed had failed to provide adequate information regarding the severity of the steal syndrome, thus complicating the grading process. Ischemic complication rates were found to be higher in femoral vein transposition compared to prosthetic arteriovenous grafts (21% vs 7%, $P < 0.05$). The amputation rates as a result of creation of lower extremity arteriovenous accesses ranged between 0% and 7%.

Venous hypertension-related ischemia is pathophysiologically different from HAIDI. Blood stagnation, responsible for retrograde venous flow, limb edema, cyanosis, and skin ulceration, is induced by down-flow vein stenosis, frequently related to a previous central vein catheter.

In children, although high-flow fistulas are not infrequent, HAIDI is rare. One case was recently observed (unpublished data) in a 3-year-old child after an upper-arm basilic vein transposition, associated with distal pain and decreased fistula flow (Figure 52-2). There was also catheter-induced innominate vein thrombosis, without major limb edema. The artery stenosis was effectively treated with percutaneous transluminal angioplasty (PTA). One case reported by Shemesh et al[13] in a 3-year-old child with a brachial basilic PTFE graft was treated by banding.

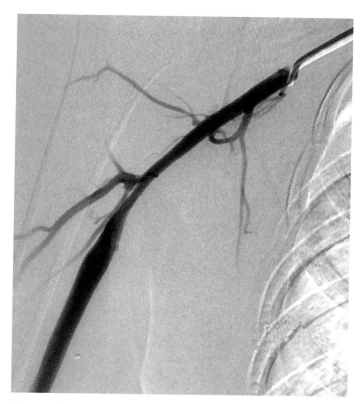

Figure 52-2. Brachial artery stenosis in a 3-year-old child 1 year after basilic vein superficialization.

TABLE 52–1
Clinical Classification of Hemodialysis Access Induced Ischemia
Stage I: Pale/blue and/or cold hand without pain
Stage II: Pain during hemodialysis
Stage III: Rest pain
Stage IV: Ulcer/necrosis/gangrene.

Source: Data from Tordoir.[14]

The clinical symptoms of HAIDI may be acute, especially after an autogenous or graft elbow AVA that may develop early postoperative high-flow due to the large caliber of the vessels. Acute HAIDI may also be observed after imprudent or unnecessary percutaneous angioplasty (Figure 52-3). Most frequently,[16] symptoms are mild and recede within days or weeks under strict surveillance. Lazarides et al[17] prospectively measured the systolic pressure index (SPI; postoperative forearm systolic pressure divided by contralateral forearm systolic pressure) in 69 consecutive patients. Ninety-four percent of these patients had an SPI below 0.8, and the mean SPI 24 hours after fistula creation was 0.55. However, most of these patients were asymptomatic, and by 11 months after access creation the mean SPI had risen to 0.74. This gradual improvement in SPI is the result of compensatory distal artery vasodilatation and the progressive development of a rich artery collateral network around the fistula. On the other hand, symptoms may be more threatening or may worsen rapidly, and urgent explorations (DU and angiography) are needed.

Ischemic monomelic neuropathy (IMN)[14,15,18–19] is a rare and potentially disastrous form of HAIDI. Typically, the symptoms appear immediately after the creation of an elbow access in a patient with long-standing insulin-dependent diabetes complicated by neuropathy. Severe dysfunction of distal nerves (ulnar, radial, and median) is

CLINICAL PRESENTATION

Four stages are identified in the usual classification of ischemia, which derives from Fontaine's peripheral obstructive arterial disease of the lower limbs[14] (Table 52-1). A classification of HAIDI, including symptoms, signs, and a therapeutic approach for each stage, was recently proposed by Scheltinga et al[15] (Table 52-2).

TABLE 52–2
Classification of Hemodialysis Access Induced Ischemia (HAIDI), Including Symptoms, Signs, and Treatment
HAIDI Grade 1. No clear symptoms but discrete signs of mild ischemia may be observed (slight cyanosis of nail beds, mild coldness of skin of hand, reduced arterial pulse at wrist, reduced systolic finger pressures). Conservative treatment may be indicated.
HAIDI Grade 2a. Complaints mentioned during dialysis sessions or intense use of hand: *tolerable* pain, cramps, paresthesia, numbness, or uncomfortable coldness of fingers or hand. Conservative treatment is indicated.
HAIDI Grade 2b. Complaints mentioned during dialysis sessions or use of hand: *intolerable* pain, cramps, paresthesia, numbness or uncomfortable coldness of fingers or hand. Treatment combining conservative and invasive treatment (endovascular or surgical) is indicated.
HAIDI Grade 3. Rest pain or motor dysfunction of fingers or hand. Urgent invasive treatment supported by conservative measures is indicated.
HAIDI Grade 4a. Limited tissue loss (ulceration, necrosis). Clinically significant hand function is probably maintained if ischemia is reversed. Urgent invasive treatment supported by conservative measures is indicated.
HAIDI Grade 4b. Irreversible tissue loss to the hand or proximal parts of the extremity. Impossible to preserve clinically significant hand function. Amputation is required.

Source: Data from Scheltinga.[15]

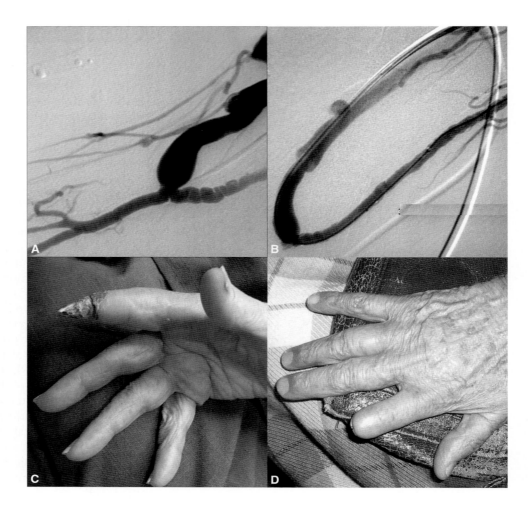

Figure 52-3. HAIDI after unnecessary PTA. (**A**) Before PTA; (**B**) after PTA; (**C**) hand after PTA; (**D**) hand after DRIL.

observed, with major pain, sensory loss, and severe distal weakness of the limb, and without obvious coolness of the extremity and skin or muscle necrosis. A pulse distal to the access may be palpable and pressure indices may be above critical values, but mild distal ischemia may also be present. IMN may also occur after an acute thrombosis of a major upper arm artery, independently of ESRD and hemodialysis. It is thought to be related to a reduction in the blood flow in the *vasa nervorum*, causing irreversible nerve damage, whereas the other tissues would resist more effectively. EMG shows motor and sensory nerve axon loss, chiefly distally. IMN has possible medico-legal implications as, despite the severe disability, it may not be recognized for weeks. Once recognized, it may be wrongly attributed to the surgical procedure or anesthetic technique (axillary nerve block). Immediate ligation of the fistula, as suggested by many authors, might not result in any improvement in motor function and/or limb causalgia. Occasionally, a mature AV fistula, with no distal tissues loss, may be preserved in spite of the irreversible neurologic deficit.

The chronic form of HAIDI appears progressively, weeks to years after access creation. It may be confused or associated with diabetes or uremic distal neuropathy and carpal tunnel syndrome. Chronic HAIDI is infrequent in distal ulnar to basilic autogenous AVA, probably due to the low flow related to the small diameter of the artery and to the preservation of the radial artery, which serves as a collateral artery preventing deterioration of digital blood pressure and flow. It is also occasionally observed in prosthetic AVA, probably because of the early flow reduction related to stenosis of the venous anastomosis stenosis which almost always occurs.

TECHNICAL EVALUATION

Technical examinations are necessary to evaluate the respective responsibility of steal (flow diversion) and arterial lesions.

All patients with significant clinical symptoms of ischemia should undergo duplex ultrasonography (DU) with determination of access blood flow in the brachial artery, estimation of possible retrograde flow in the juxta-anastomosis distal artery, and diagnosis of obstructive disease from axillary to digital arteries. It is necessary to evaluate finger pressures and waveforms, with and without compression of the access, using a digital cuff placed at the base of the finger and a photoplethysmographic sensor placed on the fingertip (Figure 52-4). Digital pressures and waveforms on the dialysis access side are uniformly lower than the nonaccess extremity, or below 50 mm Hg, flat or even nonrecordable in severe cases of steal. Compression of the

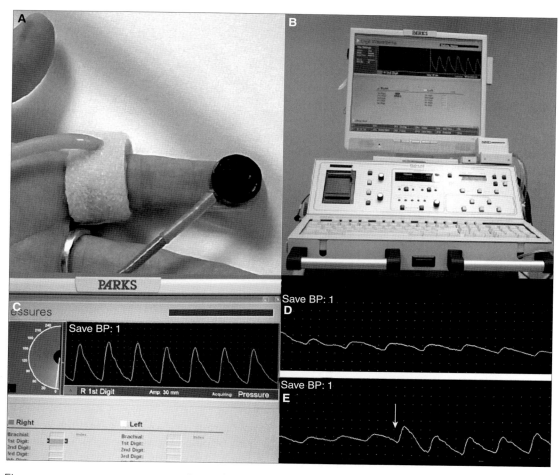

Figure 52-4. Finger pressure measurements and waveform evaluations with permission from J. Malik et al.[21] (**A**) Blood pressure cuff and photoplethysmographic sensor; (**B**) recording equipment; (**C**) normal digit waveforms; (**D**) lower pressure and digit waveforms on the dialysis access side; (**E**) compression of the dialysis access (at arrow) improves the waveforms.

dialysis access will improve the waveform or return it to similar to that of the nonaccess extremity.[20,21,22]

Digital angiography is indicated whenever ischemia requires active treatment. Direct puncture of the brachial artery, possibly complemented by retrograde catheterization, is often sufficient. Angiography after fistula compression may identify dilatation or stenosis of proximal and distal arteries, from the aortic arch to the fingers. This may confirm the direction of flow (antegrade, retrograde or both) in the artery below the anastomosis, and possible early bifurcation of the brachial artery (15% of the population). Angiography can identify any down-flow vein stenosis and any residual persistent distal fistula. Finally, it provides the opportunity for immediate percutaneous treatment of any possible proximal inflow lesion (see the percutaneous section on HAIDI). Unlike duplex examination and digital angiography, magnetic resonance imaging and computerized tomographic angiography are rarely indicated.

SURGICAL TREATMENT OPTIONS

Surgical treatment is indicated for patients with severe limb-threatening ischaemia, including rest pain, major distal weakness, and gangrene.[23] Proximal artery inflow

stenoses can be cured by standard, mainly percutaneous, interventions (see the percutaneous section on HAIDI). It appears at the moment that not only the proximal but also some distal artery stenoses may be responsible for AVA-related distal ischemia and might be even treated with prudent percutaneous angioplasty.

When there is no proximal artery stenosis, several surgical and hybrid techniques have been published, from access ligation to banding (including MILLER), revision using distal inflow (RUDI), distal revascularization-interval ligation (DRIL) and proximalization of the arterial inflow (PAI) for proximal accesses, and proximal radial artery ligation (PRAL) and distal radial artery ligation (DRAL) for distal accesses. All these techniques that are reported to improve the perfusion pressure of distal arteries have one common outcome, which is reducing fistula flow (except PAI, and to a lesser extent DRIL). Finally associated distal finger amputation may be necessary.

▶ Correction of Artery Stenosis

With a few exceptions, upper limb artery disease is usually asymptomatic prior to AVA creation (Figure 52-5). Proximal artery inflow stenosis has been demonstrated to be present

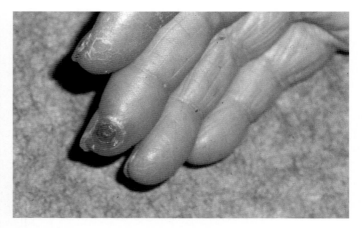

Figure 52-6. Gracz fistula-related HAIDI.

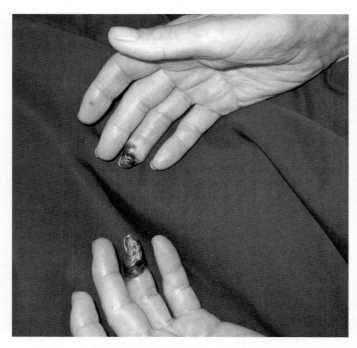

Figure 52-5. Bilateral ischemia in a diabetic patient before angioaccess construction.

in 25–50% of patients with access-related ischemia[24–25]. Such stenoses should have been ruled out with a good preoperative evaluation (systematic DU) prior to access creation. The best treatment is the minimally invasive percutaneous balloon angioplasty that can be easily performed on an outpatient basis. Surgical bypass may be necessary after failure of percutaneous treatment or after early restenosis.

Stenosis of distal arteries associated with brachial AVA is usually diffuse and may not be accessible to PTA. However Raynaud et al[26] recently reported one case of radial cephalic autogenous access complicated by distal ischemia, which was successfully treated by ulnar artery dilatation, preserving both AVA maturation and hand blood supply.

▶ Access Ligation

Access ligation with placement of a central vein catheter is indicated for low-flow associated HAIDI or after failure of conservative treatment, mainly for proximal fistula ischemia. Further creation of a more distal fistula is rarely possible. A proximal AVA placed in the opposite limb would be almost certainly complicated by an ischemic syndrome. Ligation of an associated residual distal fistula in the same limb may occasionally be sufficient to cure low-grade ischemia.

If ischemia is related to a side-to-side fistula at the elbow (Gracz fistula),[27,28] which is prone to very high flow, the ligation of every vein connected to the artery but one may be successful (Figure 52-6).

▶ Banding

Banding is a popular technique. It consists of producing stenosis in the vein or graft, close to the artery anastomosis. A long enough (2 cm), considerable (>80%), and precise

reduction of caliber would be necessary to reduce flow in the fistula in order to increase perfusion to the extremity. Unfortunately our personal experience with this technique, even with intraoperative flowmetry, has been poor, reinforced by the failure of banding performed by other surgeons in many patients then referred to us. Such banding proved to be either too tight, resulting in access thrombosis, or too loose and therefore ineffective. These disappointing results were in agreement with two publications (Odland et al[29] and DeCaprio et al[30]) reporting poor secondary patency rates of 38% and 9%, respectively, at 1 year.

Recent publications have reported more favorable results of banding procedures. Zanow et al[31] achieved flow reduction using a spindle-like narrowing suture near the anastomosis and final placement of a polytetrafluoroethylene strip in 78 patients with ischemia and 12 with cardiac failure. The mean preoperative access flow was 1469 ± 633 mL/min in patients with ischemia and 2084 ± 463 mL/min in patients with cardiac failure. The flow was reduced to 499 ± 175 mL/min for autogenous accesses and to 676 ± 47 mL/min for prosthetic accesses. The mean follow-up was 25 months (range = 1–73 months). Complete long-term relief of symptoms was observed in 86% of patients with ischemia and in 96% of patients with cardiac failure. Banding significantly increased the digital-brachial index (0.41 ± 0.12 vs 0.74 ± 0.11; $P < .05$) and the mean distal arterial pressure (47 ± 17 mm Hg vs 79 ± 21 mm Hg; $P < .05$) in patients with ischemia. Primary patency rates were significantly better for autogenous accesses compared to prosthetic accesses (91% ± 4% vs 58% ± 12% at 12 months; 81% ± 6% vs 41% ± 14% at 36 months; $P < .001$). The low patency of prosthetic accesses was probably related to the high risk of thrombosis with accesses that have a flow <700 mL/min.

Thermann et al[32] performed banding by longitudinal tailoring combined with circular narrowing with a nonresorbable suture. The aim of banding was to reduce the flow to approximately 50% of the initial measured flow. Twenty-one patients (20 brachial accesses, 1 wrist access) developed symptoms (eg, coldness, severe stress-induced pain) without distal ulceration or gangrene. Three of these patients also had neurologic deficiency as proved by electromyography.

Nine patients had diabetes (43%). Seventeen patients developed clinical symptoms 17 ± 11 days (1–30 days) after access creation; in two patients this period was 2 years and in one patient 3 years. Fistula flow was high in all patients (1375 ± 690 mL/min). Immediate banding was performed in 17 (78.5%) patients, while closure of the angioaccess was necessary in four patients owing to concomitant cardiac failure. Symptoms disappeared after the banding procedure and the angioaccess could be successfully used for dialysis in all 17 cases. Revision was necessary in one patient for early thrombosis after banding. In two patients, a second banding procedure was necessary (at 4 and 8 months, respectively) after the first because of recurrence of the ischemic symptoms. Primary patency after 1 year was 94%. Among 34 patients who had developed distal ulceration, banding was unsuccessful in 8/8 patients. However, such improved outcome of banding in selected patients (absence of distal necrosis) needs to be confirmed by other teams since, in our experience, flow rate monitoring might not be very reliable in patients under regional or general anesthesia and because of spasm caused by surgical dissection.

The MILLER procedure (minimally invasive limited ligation endoluminal-assisted revision) is a hybrid variety of banding. It was described by US interventional nephrologists[33] in 2006 for the treatment of access-induced steal syndrome and high-output cardiac overload. In the radiology unit, the access vein/graft is exposed after blunt dissection near the artery, through a limited skin incision. A 2-0 monofilament ligature of Prolene is pulled around the access and tied over an angioplasty balloon (3–5 mm diameter) introduced percutaneously into the vein. A second publication[34] reported the results of a multicenter retrospective study involving 183 patients, of which 114 presented with hand ischemia (HAIDI) and 69 with clinical manifestations of pathologic high access flow such as congestive heart failure. Overall, 183 patients underwent 229 bandings with technical success achieved in 225. Three cases of access bleeding during the procedure were treated with manual compression of the injured area until bleeding subsided, and this led to abandonment of the procedure. Three patients developed postoperative infection, resulting in access ligation and vein/graft removal; the protocol was then successfully modified to include antibiotic prophylaxis. Complete symptomatic relief (clinical success) was reported in 109 steal patients and in all high-flow patients. The primary access patency for steal and high-flow patients was 52% and 63% at 3 months, with a secondary access patency of 90% and 89% at 24 months, respectively. Unfortunately, these two publications might be criticized for the absence of pre- and postoperative flow measurement reports, the predefined diameter and short length reduction, the danger of blunt surgical dissection, and the poor primary patency rates.

▶ RUDI

The revision using distal inflow (RUDI) procedure replaces a proximal by a distal artery anastomosis (Figure 52-7A–C). The caliber reduction and the length extension of the

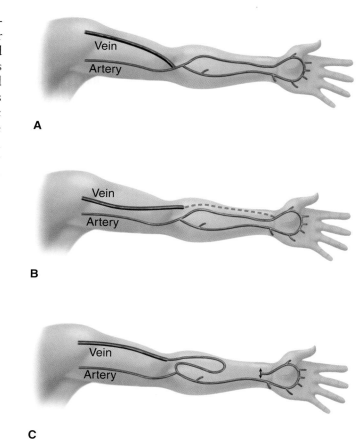

Figure 52-7. Revision using distal inflow (RUDI). (**A**) Proximal AVA; (**B**) PTFE distalization; (**C**) transposition of the radial artery.

access reduce high access flow, increasing perfusion of distal extremity arteries. The RUDI procedure has two variants.

Distalization of the arterial anastomosis. This procedure was described by Bourquelot et al[35] in 1989 for reduction in high fistula flow. The mean flow reduction rate in this series of 35 patients was $60 \pm 18\%$. The technique involves replacing the inflow of a proximal AVA from the brachial artery by the inflow from one of its smaller caliber distal branches. The original arteriovenous anastomosis is closed at the elbow; a bridge graft (e-PTFE, thin wall, stretch, 6-mm-diameter) is connected between the radial or the ulnar artery at the wrist and the outflow tract (vein or prosthesis) at the elbow, the patency of both distal arteries being checked preoperatively. In a few cases, this method was impossible, due to diabetes-related distal artery calcifications. When the high flow related ischemia occurred after the first stage of a brachial basilic vein transposition (elbow AVA), the graft was placed subcutaneously to allow for puncture in the forearm. The drawback of this technique is the risk of secondary stenosis at the graft-vein anastomosis.

A variant of this technique was published by Minion et al[36] in 2005 reporting a short distalization to the proximal radial or ulnar artery approximately 2–3 cm distal to the brachial artery bifurcation in four patients. Unfortunately the length of the distalization may have been too short, and pre- and postoperative flow rates were not reported.

Transposition of the radial artery (TRA). TRA was described by Bourquelot et al in 2009.[37] This technique, eliminating the use of a PTFE graft, is also a RUDI-procedure to reduce excessive blood flow in a proximal AVA. After ligation of the original fistula at the elbow, the brachial artery is replaced by the radial artery. For this purpose, the radial artery is first dissected from the forearm as a single block with its two concomitant veins in order to minimize arterial spasm, divided at the wrist and then turned upward to reach the vein at the elbow. A surgical microscope is used for creation of the new arteriovenous anastomosis, which is preferably end-to-side from the artery to the vein. Patency is checked intraoperatively using a sterile Doppler probe. The intervention is practicable even with moderately calcified arteries. Forty-seven consecutive patients with brachial artery to elbow vein AVA underwent TRA. The indications were hand ischemia ($N = 4$), cardiac failure ($N = 13$), concerns about future cardiac dysfunction ($N = 23$), and chronic venous hypertension resulting in aneurysmal degeneration of the vein ($N = 7$). Mean fistula age before flow reduction was 2.5 years. Technical success was 91%. The mean flow rate reduction was 66% ± 14%. All four patients with hand ischemia were cured, with no recurrence during follow up. Primary patency rates at 1 and 3 years were 61% ± 7% and 40% ± 8%, respectively, and secondary patency rates at 1 and 3 years were 89% ± 5% and 70% ± 8%, respectively.

These two RUDI procedures are effective to reduce high fistula flow. They provide a good alternative to banding in high flow associated HAIDI (Figure 52-8).

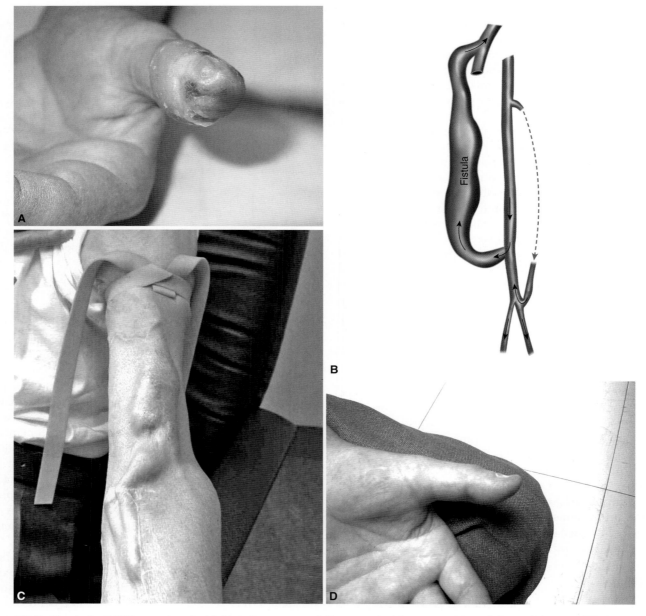

Figure 52-8. Grade 4a HAIDI associated with high flow, successfully treated with transposition of the radial artery (TRA). (**A**) Preoperative; (**B**) duplex; (**C,D**) postoperative.

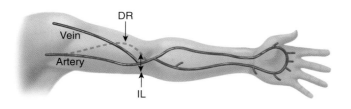

Figure 52-9. Distal revascularization–interval ligation (DRIL).

▶ DRIL

The distal revascularization and interval ligation (DRIL) procedure was described by Schanzer et al in 1988 (Figure 52-9). The retrograde flow into the fistula, considered by the author as the pathophysiological principle of distal ischemia, is suppressed by ligation of the brachial artery distal to the access. A bypass (saphenous vein rather than PTFE) is combined with this from the artery proximal to the arteriovenous anastomosis to the artery distal to the ligation (length 5–7 cm).

In 1996 Haimov et al[38] demonstrated improvement in all 23 patients undergoing the DRIL procedure, with a bypass patency rate of 95% at 2 years. Katz and Kohl,[39] and Lazarides,[17] subsequently published small series of six to seven patients treated with revascularization and interval ligation with similar success rates. In 2002 Knox et al[20] reported 47 of 52 (90%) patients demonstrating significant or complete symptomatic improvement. All patients with tissue loss had healed or were currently healing their

lesions, and the 12-month actuarial primary patency rate of prosthetic arteriovenous grafts was nearly 85%. In 2004, Sessa et al[40] reported 18 patients with 100% clinical success and 94% primary patency rates at 1 year for both DRIL bypass and autogenous access. Excellent results were also reported by Diehl et al,[41] Korzets et al,[42] Mwipatawy et al,[43] and Walz et al.[44] In 2006, Tynan-Cuisinier and Berman[9] reported an 80% DRIL primary patency rate at 48 months (life-table method) and thus proved that DRIL was a long-term reliable procedure to improve distal perfusion without significantly reducing fistula blood flow. Similarly, in 2008 Huber et al[45] reported a series of 64 patients with primary and secondary DRIL patency rates (Kaplan-Meier) of 77%, 75%, and 71% at 1, 3, and 5 years, respectively.

Because there is no topological alteration in anatomy after DRIL (Figure 52-10), it was unclear as to why the procedure was effective. In a prospective study, Illig et al[46] (Figure 52-11) used intraoperative measurements of pressure and flow in nine patients undergoing DRIL for symptomatic steal to determine the impact of the operation on access flow. They observed that the increase in flow to the forearm as a result of the DRIL procedure was due to increased pressure at the point where flow splits to supply the forearm and the access. This increase in pressure at the "split point" is due to the increased resistance of the fistula created by interposing the arterial segment between the original anastomosis (AV anastomosis) and the new anastomosis (proximal anastomosis). This implies that the length between the beginning of the new bypass and the existing AV anastomosis will potentially determine

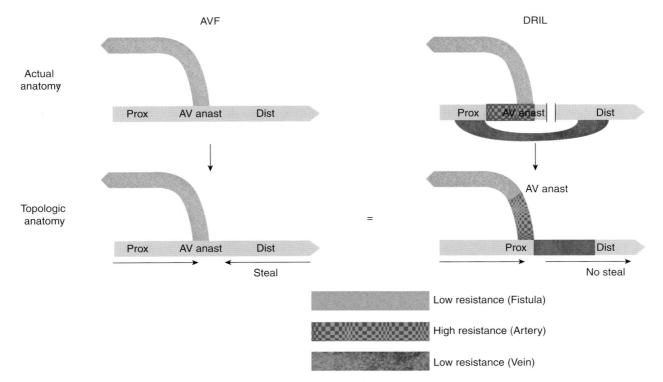

Figure 52-10. Schematic views of the AVA, with ischemia, and final DRIL. The segments have been labeled to emphasize changes in resistance and resulting change in the direction of flow in the forearm. (**A**) Original AVF; (**B**) arm following DRIL. (Modified from Ref. 46.)

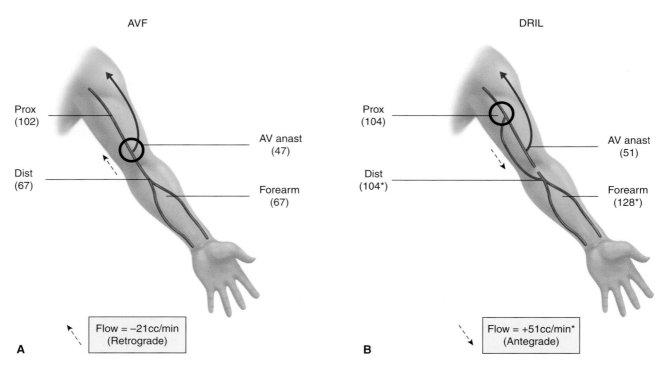

Figure 52-11. Diagram of measurement sites and systolic pressures at each site. Asterisks (Dist and Forearm pressures and Dist flow) denote significant differences. (**A**) Original AVF; (**B**) arm following DRIL. Black circles implies split points. (Modified from Ref. 46.)

success. Perfusion to the distal arm was improved without degradation of fistula performance. This was not surprising because, at the range of blood flow needed to supply the arm (50 mL/min in their experience) compared to within these fistulas (4–600 mL/min), a small alteration in extremity perfusion would not have decreased fistula flow enough to cause problems.

A variant of DRIL, that is, "interval distal artery ligation without bypass," has been suggested. In one patient reported by Blaji et al,[47] an increase in the distal brachial artery pressure from 22 to 60 mmHg was observed after distal artery ligation while both saphenous veins were found to be unusable, and the evolution was favorable despite the absence of an associated bypass. No other case has been published to date, to our knowledge. It has not been demonstrated whether simply eliminating retrograde flow, with a modest increase in distal pressure, might be adequate. The opposite variant, that is, "bypass alone without ligation," has also been suggested by Knox,[20] although no results have been published. The benefit of this method would be to decrease the resistance to the hand, by substituting a vein for an artery.

The DRIL procedure has been shown to result in immediate relief of signs and symptoms of ischemia in the great majority of patients, and it provides excellent long-term patency rates for both vein bypasses and accesses. DRIL seems to be the ideal treatment for steal-related ischemia but there are several disadvantages. DRIL is a rather complex and time-consuming procedure, which is possible only when a suitable vein can be harvested. As the reduction in the fistula flow is small, the procedure may

not be appropriate for high flow fistula associated ischemia. Finally, only a very few DRIL procedures have been reported for treatment of lower limb HAIDI.

▶ PAI (PAVA)

Proximalization of the arterial inflow (PAI) (Figure 52-12), also called "more proximal arteriovenous anastomosis" (PAVA), was proposed by Gradman and Pozrikidis in 2004.[48]

The first clinical experience was reported by Zanow et al[49] in 2006. The original elbow AV anastomosis is ligated and a small caliber (4–5 mm, or 4–7 tapered graft) interposition graft is used to connect the access vein or graft with the proximal brachial or even the axillary artery access. The various procedures performed by these authors between January 1999 and May 2005 to treat HAIDI in 133 patients were reported (Figure 52-13). PAI was performed only in the 30 patients with severe HAIDI who had a flow rate of <800 mL/min in native AV fistulas and <1000 mL/min in AV grafts. Complete relief of ischemic symptoms

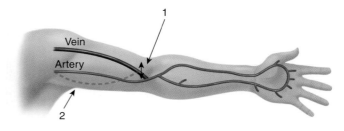

Figure 52-12. Proximalization of the arterial inflow (PAI).

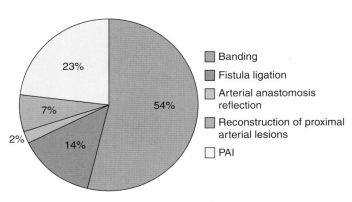

Figure 52-13. Various surgical procedures to treat HAIDI in 133 patients. (Data from Zanow.[49])

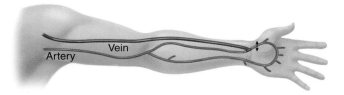

Figure 52-14. Distal radial artery ligation (DRAL).

was achieved in 84% of patients, with excellent long-term results: the primary and secondary patency rates were 87% and 90% at 1 year, and 67% and 78% at 3 years, respectively. No other results have been reported to date, although according to Mickley the procedure is widely used.

In 2010 Thermann et al[50] reported a multicenter experience totalizing 40 PAI operations (regular or heparinized PTFE). Four patients had acute pain and sensorimotor dysfunction with no lesions, 33 had small acral lesions, and 3 had extensive lesions following the creation of autogenous fistulas. In 36 cases (90%), PAI was clinically successful. Primary patency was 62% after 12 months and secondary patency was 75% after 18 months. In three of the four patients with large acral lesions, graft explantation was necessary due to infection or failing success. The results were poor in cases of extensive limb necrosis/gangrene.

As with the RUDI procedure, PAI increases the flow to the forearm by increasing the pressure at the point where flow is split between the arm and the access. Although this concept is supported by the mathematical model reported by Gradman et al,[48] clinical experience with this approach is limited. Moreover, in the experimental flow model reported by the same author, DRIL had the greatest increase in distal arm flow.

The benefits of PAI over the DRIL procedure are that the anastomoses are easy to suture on large and nonovercalcified vessels, there is no need to harvest a saphenous vein, and there is no ligation of the main upper arm artery (with potential future ischemia issues). The drawbacks are the risk of PTFE-related infection or stenosis of the venous anastomosis, and the risk of increasing the fistula flow far too much must not be underestimated. Finally, as stated by Mickley,[51] PAI could be the best if not the only option to preserve both the access and the extremity in low flow associated steal syndrome.

▶ DRAL and PRAL for Distal AVA

For distal AVA distal radial artery ligation (DRAL) (Figure 52-14), first reported by Bussell et al,[52] is the equivalent of "interval-ligation" DRIL for proximal AVA.

They both ligate the retrograde distal artery. Although the AVA flow reduction is not great, the adjunction of an arterial bypass is not necessary as long as the ulnar artery and palmar arches are patent.

Juxta-anastomosis proximal radial artery ligation (PRAL) (Figure 52-15) provides greater AVA flow reduction. This technique was recently reported by Bourquelot et al[53] as a simple, safe, and effective surgical technique for reduction in excessive blood flow in radial cephalic autogenous AVA. The prospective study included 37 consecutive patients (29 adults) who underwent PRAL of high-flow radial cephalic autogenous AVAs. Mean preoperative flow in adults was 1739 mL/min ± 526 (1000–3000). Anatomical prerequisites were a side-to-end anastomosis fistula and a retrograde flow in the distal radial artery. The success rate was 92% (34/37). The three failures included one excessive and two insufficient reductions of flow (<33%). Mean flow reduction rates were 50% in children and 53% in adults. Primary patency rates (life-table method) at 1 and 2 years were 88% and 74%, respectively. Secondary patency rates were 88% and 78%, respectively. The two patients with ischemia were cured.

In cases of HAIDI related to radial cephalic autogenous AVAs, the usual treatment is ligation of the distal (DRAL), not the proximal radial artery (PRAL), to suppress the steal related to the retrograde flow.[9,40] Both surgical techniques are equally simple, and DRAL might even be tested and achieved percutaneously.[54] However, the problem of concomitant high flow has never been discussed in publications referring to distal radial artery ligation.[55] We achieved reduction in the high flow in several ischemic patients and this suppression of the proximal radial artery antegrade steal to the brachial artery by PRAL also meant disappearance of the clinical steal to the hand. However, any definitive recommendations would be premature.

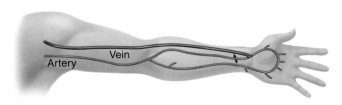

Figure 52-15. Juxta-anastomosis proximal radial artery ligation (PRAL).

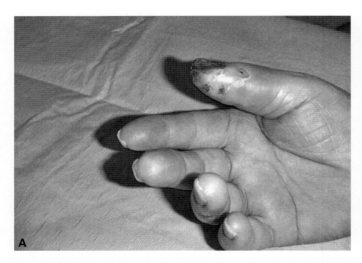
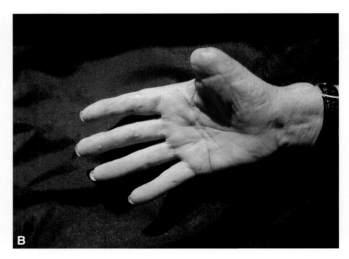

Figure 52-16. Radial-cephalic AVA. Before (**A**) and after (**B**) AVA ligation and amputation.

CONCLUSION

HAIDI is a serious complication of hemodialysis access related to the steal of arterial flow associated with artery disease, and is increasing as the numbers of patients who are ageing increase. Prevention of distal ischemia is difficult. Because there is less risk of ischemia an AVA must be created as distally as possible, even in elderly patients, and patients with occlusive disease of distal arteries must definitely be excluded from performing an autologous lower limb access.[56] When present, proximal artery stenosis is best

treated percutaneously. For brachial artery accesses DRIL is the gold-standard technique for increasing flow and pressure in the distal arteries, and DRAL is the most frequently used procedure for distal accesses. When associated with a high-flow AVA, ischemia may be treated effectively with surgical flow reduction techniques, as transposition of the radial artery or PTFE-distalization of the arterial anastomosis for proximal access, and PRAL for distal AVA, while the favorable results of two recently reported series using banding await confirmation. Although it results in access loss, fistula ligation may be necessary in some patients with distal ischemia (Figure 52-16). Finally, we proposed an algorithm (Figure 52-17) for the surgical treatment of HAIDI.[57]

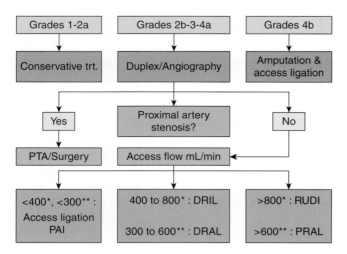

Figure 52-17. Algorithm for treatment of hemodialysis access induced ischemia (HAIDI): a proposal for proximal and distal accesses, and various access flows (Grades refer to Sheltinga Classification[15]).
* Proximal access
**distal access. PAI, proximalization of the arterial inflow; DRIL, distal revascularization interval ligation; DRAL, distal radial artery ligation; RUDI, revision using distal inflow; PRAL, juxta-anastomosis proximal radial artery ligation. With the collaboration of Frank Le Roy and Mélanie Hanoy (CHU, Rouen).

REFERENCES

1. Scheltinga MR, Hoek van F, Bruyninckx CM. Surgical banding for refractory hemodialysis access-induced distal ischemia (HAIDI). *J Vasc Access*. 2009;10:43–49.
2. Barnes RW. Hemodynamics for the vascular surgeon. *Arch Surg*. 1980;115:216–223.
3. Wixon CL, Mills JL. Hemodynamic basis for the diagnosis and treatment of angioaccess-induced steal syndrome. *Adv Vasc Surg*. 2000;8:147–159.
4. Tronc F, Mallat Z, Lehoux S, Wassef M, Esposito B, Tedgui A. Role of matrix metalloproteinases in blood flow-induced arterial enlargement: interaction with NO. *Arterioscler Thromb Vasc Biol*. 2000;20:E120–E126.
5. Wixon CL, Hughes JD, Mills JL. Understanding strategies for the treatment of ischemic steal syndrome after hemodialysis access. *J Am Coll Surg*. 2000;191:301–310.
6. Sumner DS. Arteriovenous fistula. In: Strandness DE, Sumner DS, eds. *Hemodynamics for Surgeons*. 1st ed. New York: Grune & Stratton; 1975:621–664.
7. Dammers R, Planken RN, Pouls KP, Van Det RJ, Burger H, Van Der Sande FM, Tordoir JH. Evaluation of 4-mm to 7-mm versus 6-mm prosthetic brachial-antecubital forearm loop access for hemodialysis: results

of a randomized multicenter clinical trial. *J Vasc Surg.* 2003;37:143–148.

8. Ackerman F, Levy A, Daugas E, Schartz N, Riaux A, Derancourt, Urena P, Lebbé C. Sodium thiosulfate as first-line treatment for calciphylaxis. *Arch Dermatol.* 2007;143:1336–1337.

9. Tynan-Cuisinier GS, Berman SS. Strategies for predicting and treating access induced ischemic steal syndrome. *Eur J Vasc Endovasc Surg.* 2006;32:309–315.

10. Gradman WS, Cohen W, Haji-Aghaii M. Arteriovenous fistula construction in the thigh with transposed superficial femoral vein: our initial experience. *J Vasc Surg.* 2001;33:968–975.

11. Gradman WS, Laub J, Cohen W. Femoral vein transposition for arteriovenous hemodialysis access: improved patient selection and intraoperative measures reduce postoperative ischemia. *J Vasc Surg.* 2005;41:279–284.

12. Antoniou GA, Lazarides MK, Georgiadis GS, Sfyroeras GS, Nikolopoulos ES, Giannoukas AD. Lower-extremity arteriovenous access for haemodialysis: a systematic review. *Eur J Vasc Endovasc Surg.* 2009;38(3):365–372.

13. Shemesh D, Olsha O, Mabjeesh NJ, Abramowitz HB. Dialysis access induced limb ischemia corrected using quantitative duplex ultrasound. *Pediatr Nephrol.* 2001;16:409–411.

14. Tordoir JMH, Dammers R, van der Sande FM. Upper extremity ischemia and hemodialysis vascular access. *Eur J Vasc Endovasc Surg.* 2004;27:1–5.

15. Scheltinga MR, van Hoek F, Bruijninckx CMA. Time of onset in haemodialysis access-induced distal ischaemia (HAIDI) is related to the access type. *Nephrol Dial Transplant.* 2009:24:3198–3204.

16. van Hoek F, Scheltinga MR, Kouwenberg I, Moret KEM, Beerenhout CH, Tordoir JHM. Steal in hemodialysis patients depends on type of vascular access. *Eur J Vasc Endovasc Surg.* 2006;32:710–717.

17. Lazarides MK, Staramos DN, Panagopoulos GN, Tzilalis VD, Eleftheriou GJ, Dayantas JN, et al. Indications for surgical treatment of angioaccess-induced arterial "steal." *J Am Coll Surg.* 1998;187:422–426.

18. Wilbourn AJ, Furlan AJ, Hulley W, Ruschhaup TW. Ischemic monomelic neuropathy. *Neurology.* 1983;33: 447–451.

19. Riggs JE, Moss AH, Labosky DA, Liput JH, Morgan JJ, Gutmann L. Upper extremity ischemic monomelic neuropathy: a complication of vascular access procedures in uremic diabetic patients. *Neurology.* 1989;39:997–998.

20. Knox RC, Berman SS, Hugues JD, Gentile AT, Mills JL. Distal revascularization-interval ligation: a durable and effective treatment for ischemic steal syndrome after hemodialysis access. *J Vasc Surg.* 2002;36:250–256.

21. Malik J, Tuka V, Kasalova Z, Chytilova E, Slavikova M, Clagett P, Davivson I, Dolmatch B, Nichols D, Gallieni M. Understanding the dialysis access steal syndrome. A review of the etiologies, diagnosis, prevention and treatment strategies. *J Vascular Access.* 2008;9:155–166.

22. Schanzer H, Eisenberg D. Management of steal syndrome resulting from dialysis access. *Semin Vasc Surg.* 2004;17:45–49.

23. Lazarides MK, Staramos DN, Kopadis G, Maltezos C, Tzilalis VD, Georgiadis GS. Onset of arterial "steal" following proximal angioaccess: immediate and delayed types. *Nephrol Dial Transplant.* 2003;18:2387–2390.

24. DeCaprio JD, Valentine RJ, Kakish HB, et al. Steal syndrome complicating hemodialysis access. *Cardiovasc Surg.* 1997;5:648–653

25. Asif A, Leon C, Merrill D, et al. Arterial steal syndrome: a modest proposal for an old paradigm. *Am J Kidney Dis.* 2006;48:88–97.

26. Raynaud A, Novelli L, Rovani X, Carreres T, Bourquelot P, Hermelin A, Angel C, Beyssen B. Radiocephalic fistula complicated by distal ischemia: treatment by ulnar artery dilatation. *Cardiovasc Intervent Radiol.* 2010;33:223–225.

27. Gracz KC, Ing TS, Soung LS, Armbruster KF, Seim SK, Merkel FK. Proximal forearm fistula for maintenance hemodialysis. *Kidney Int.* 1977;11(1):71–75.

28. Vascular Access 2006 Work Group. Clinical practice guidelines for vascular access. *Am J Kidney Dis.* 2006;48:S176–S247.

29. Odland MD, Kelly PH, Ney AL, et al. Management of dialysis-associated steal syndrome complicating upper extremity arteriovenous fistulas: use of intraoperative digital photoplethysmography. *Surgery.* 1991;110:664–669.

30. DeCaprio JD, Valentine RJ, Kakish HB, et al. Steal syndrome complicating hemodialysis access. *Cardiovasc Surg.* 1997;5:648–653.

31. Zanow J, Petzold K, Petzold M, et al. H. Flow reduction in high-flow arteriovenous access using intraoperative flow monitoring. *J Vasc Surg.* 2006;44:1273–1278.

32. Thermann F, Wollert U, Dralle H, Brauckhoff M. Dialysis shunt-associated steal syndrome with autogenous hemodialyis accesses: proposal for a new classification based on clinical results. *World J Surg.* 2008;32: 2309–2315.

33. Goel N, Miller GA, Jotwani MC, Licht J, Schur I, Arnold WP. Minimally invasive limited ligation endoluminal-assisted revision (MILLER) for treatment of dialysis access associated steal syndrome. *Kidney Int.* 2006;70:765–770.

34. Miller GA, Goel N, Friedman A, Khariton A, Jotwani MC, Savransky Y, Khariton K, Arnold WP. Preddie DC. The MILLER banding procedure is an effective method for treating dialysis-associated steal syndrome. *Kidney Int.* 2010;77:359–366.

35. Bourquelot P, Corbi P, Cussenot O. Surgical improvement of high-flow arteriovenous fistulas. In: Sommer BG, Henry ML, eds. *Vascular Access for Hemodialysis.* Hong Kong: Pluribus Press; 1989:124–130.

36. Minion DJ, Moore E, Endean E. Revision using distal inflow: a novel approach to dialysis-associated steal syndrome. *Ann Vasc Surg.* 2005;19:625–628.

37. Bourquelot P, Gaudric J, Turmel-Rodrigues L, Franco G, Van Laere O, Raynaud A. Transposition of radial artery for reduction of excessive high-flow in autogenous arm accesses for hemodialysis. *J Vasc Surg* 2009;49:424–428.

38. Haimov M, Schanzer H, Skladani M. Pathogenesis and management of upper-extremity ischemia following angio-access surgery. *Blood Purif.* 1996;14:350–354.

39. Katz S, Kohl RD. Treatment of hand ischemia by arterial ligation and upper extremity bypass after angioaccess surgery. *J Am Coll Surg.* 1996;183:239–242.

40. Sessa C, Riehl G, Porcu P, Pichot O, Palacin P, Maghlaoua M, Magne J-L. Treatment of hand ischemia following angioaccess surgery using the distal revascularization interval-ligation technique with preservation of vascular access: description of an 18-case series. *Ann Vasc Surg.* 2004;18:685–694.

41. Diehl L, Johansen K, Watson J. Operative management of distal ischemia complicating upper extremity dialysis access. *Am J Surg.* 2003;186:17–19.

42. Korzets A, Kantarovsky A, Lehmann J, Sachs D, Gershkovitz R, Hasdan G, et al. The "DRIL" procedure—a neglected way to treat the "steal" syndrome of the hemodialysed patient. *Isr Med Assoc J.* 2003;5:782–785.

43. Mwipatayi BP, Bowles T, Balakrishnan S, Callaghan J, Haluszkiewicz E, Sieunarine K. Ischemic steal syndrome: a case series and review of current management. *Curr Surg.* 2006;63:130–135.

44. Walz P, Ladowski JS, Hines A. Distal revascularization and interval ligation (DRIL) procedure for the treatment of ischemic steal syndrome after arm arteriovenous fistula. *Ann Vasc Surg.* 2007;21:468–473.

45. Huber TS, Brown MP, Seeger JM, Lee WA. Midterm outcome after the distal revascularization and interval ligation (DRIL) procedure. *J Vasc Surg.* 2008;48:926–933.

46. Illig KA, Surowiec S, Shortell CK, Davies MG, Rhodes JM, Green RM. Hemodynamics of distal revascularization-interval ligation. *Ann Vasc Surg.* 2005;19:199–207.

47. Balaji S, Evans JM, Roberts DE, Gibbons CP. Treatment of steal syndrome complicating a proximal arteriovenous bridge graft fistula by simple distal artery ligation without revascularization using intraoperative pressure measurements. *Ann Vasc Surg.* 2003;17:320–322.

48. Gradman WS, Pozrikidis C. Analysis of options for mitigating hemodialysis access-related ischemic steal phenomena. *Ann Vasc Surg.* 2004;18:59–65.

49. Zanow J, Kruger U, Scholz H. Proximalization of the arterial inflow: a new technique to treat access-related ischemia. *J Vasc Surg.* 2006;43:1216–1221.

50. Thermann F, Ukkat J, Wollert U, Dralle H, Brauckhoff M. Dialysis shunt-associated steal syndrome (DASS) following brachial accesses: the value of fistula banding under blood flow control. *Langenbecks Arch Surg.* 2007;392:731–737.

51. Mickley V. Steal syndrome-strategies to preserve vascular access and extremity. *Nephrol Dial Transplant.* 2008;23:19–24.

52. Bussell JA, Abbott JA, Lim RC. A radial steal syndrome with arteriovenous fistula for hemodialysis. Studies in seven patients. *Ann Intern Med.* 1971;75:387–394.

53. Bourquelot P, Gaudric J, Turmel-Rodrigues L, Franco G, Van Laere O, Raynaud A. Proximal radial artery ligation (PRAL) for reduction of flow in autogenous radial cephalic accesses for haemodialysis. *Eur J Vasc Endovasc Surg.* 2010;40:94–99.

54. Chemla E, Raynaud A, Carreres T, Sapoval M, Beyssen B, Bourquelot P, Gaux JC. Preoperative assessment of the efficacy of distal radial artery ligation in treatment of steal syndrome complicating access for hemodialysis. *Ann Vasc Surg.* 1999;13:618–621.

55. Duncan H, Ferguson L, Faris I. Incidence of the radial steal syndrome in patients with Brescia fistula for hemodialysis: its clinical significance. *J Vasc Surg.* 1986;4:144–147.

56. Bourquelot P, Rawa M, Van Laere O, Franco G. Long-term results of femoral vein transposition for autogenous arteriovenous hemodialysis access. *J Vasc Surg* (in press).

57. Bourquelot P, Le Roy F. Flow reduction: revision using distal inflow (RUDI) and juxta-anastomosis proximal radial artery ligation (PRAL). In: Jean-Pierre Becquemin, Yves S. Alimi et Jean-Luc Gérard, eds. *Controversies and Updates in Vascular Surgery 2010.* Torino, Italy: Edizioni Minerva Medica; 2010:174–178.

53

ETIOLOGY AND MANAGEMENT OF CEPHALIC ARCH STENOSIS

RAMANATH DUKKIPATI, KAVEH KIAN, & ARIF ASIF

In patients with brachiocephalic fistulas, the cephalic arch region is particularly vulnerable to the development of stenosis.[1,2] This vulnerability is felt to be due to its anatomic location and hemodynamic factors.[3,4] Although percutaneous balloon angioplasty has generally been the initial option for the treatment of vascular access stenosis, the results of this treatment for lesions in the cephalic arch area have been less than optimal.[1]

This chapter focuses on cephalic arch stenosis (CAS). It discusses the unique anatomical relationships of this vascular structure and they are thought to be the etiology of this problem. Endovascular and surgical treatment options are reviewed.

The cephalic vein is part of the superficial venous system of the upper extremity.[5,6] It ascends on the anterolateral side of the forearm to the anterior aspect of the elbow where it communicates with the basilic vein through the median antecubital vein. It then ascends along the lateral surface of the biceps to the pectoralis major muscle, entering the deltopectoral groove (a triangular space located between the anteromedial border of the deltoid muscle and the lateral border of the pectoralis major muscle). It passes beneath the clavicle and turns sharply to pierce the clavipectoral fascia. It then terminates in the axillary vein. The cephalic arch is the term given to the final arch of the cephalic vein before it joins the axillary vein to form the subclavian vein.

There are anatomic variants of the terminal portion of the cephalic vein.[3] A single channel that joins the axillary vein to form the subclavian vein is the most common; however, a double (bifid) arch is occasionally encountered. A bifid arch is one that bifurcates, and both limbs may drain into the axillary vein or one limb joins the axillary vein and the other joins the external or internal jugular veins. The arch can also directly drain into the external, internal jugular, or subclavian vein.

Veins generally have valves for the purpose of preventing blood reflux.[4,7] The distribution of valves is both "vein-specific" and "region-specific." The cephalic vein has valves throughout its route, but it is most common in the final portion of the cephalic vein (cephalic arch). There are at least twice as many valves in this region of the cephalic vein compared to any similar portion of the cephalic vein. There is on average two valves in the cephalic arch in most individuals.[5,6] As valves commonly exist immediately distal to the venous route, the single most common location of valves in the cephalic vein (92%) is just (3 mm) distal to the orifice where it drains into the axillary vein.[3,5,6]

Whether a small-sized arch will have difficulty dilating after the creation of a brachiocephalic fistula is not known. Insight into the potential impact of vessel diameter on maturation can be gleaned from the cardiology literature. Chen et al[8] examined the cephalic arch in 82 consecutive patients undergoing pacemaker implantation procedure. Using color Doppler ultrasonography, venous diameter, depth, flow velocity, and morphology were evaluated. Comparisons were made between the successful and failed pacemaker implantations. Pacemaker implantation was successful in 68 (83%) of the cases. Venous diameter was found to be the only independent predictor for implantation failure. The best cutoff value of cephalic venous diameter to predict unsuccessful cephalic venous approach was equal to or less than 2.2 mm. The impact that this particular size cutoff may have on arteriovenous fistulas (AVF) maturation rates remains unclear, but is certainly a potential avenue of future investigation.

ETIOLOGY OF CAS

Little is known as to the origin and progression of venous stenosis in this region. It is known that the cephalic vein of patients with renal failure shows wall thickening and intimal hyperplasia compared with the cephalic vein in normal subjects.[9] However, this does not explain the high occurrence of cephalic arch stenoses as compared to the more distal segments of the vein. Multiple hypotheses have been put forward to explain this observation. First, the course of the vein in the deltopectoral groove may be of significance, as the turbulence and shear stress related to the curve may lead to intimal injury. The structure of the arch may give rise to turbulent flow. This provides an environment of low wall shear stress that, in turn, promotes endothelial proliferation, vasoconstriction, and platelet aggregation.[10,11] Second, the presence of higher number of valves in this region, especially just distal to the orifice of axillary vein, may be of great significance. These valves can potentially hypertrophy in the presence of high blood flows and reduce the lumen diameter significantly.[12] Third, the precreation venous diameter may be of great significance. As pointed out above, the arch diameter can vary in size and may impact subsequent enlargement. Finally, of critical importance is the concept of vascular remodeling (the capacity of this vein to dilate) in the presence of high flow rates through the fistula. The distal part of the vein dilates significantly in response to higher flows, but the cephalic arch may be limited in its ability to undergo the transformations necessary to support an AVF.

The clavipectoral fascia is a very dense membrane through which the cephalic arch must pass along with the thoracoacromial artery and vein, and lateral pectoral nerve. The density of this fascial membrane and the fact that it is accompanied by other structures of significant size as it passes through the foramen may prove problematic when this vein is called upon to dilate with the increased flow associated with a functioning dialysis access.

Failure of a vessel to dilate in the face of intimal hyperplasia will result in luminal narrowing and obstruction to flow.[13] It is difficult to say whether there is a single mechanism that causes CAS. Perhaps, a combination of the factors mentioned above contributes to the problems seen in this portion of the cephalic vein.

PREVALENCE OF CAS

One of the earliest reports documenting the existence of the phenomenon of CAS was by Glanz et al[12] over two decades ago. These investigators hypothesized that the lesion is caused by the presence of hypertrophied valves. Over the last decade, numerous studies have been published describing the patency of fistulas and outcomes of angioplasty. Very few, however, have specifically addressed lesions in the cephalic arch area.[1,2,14] In one study, Rajan et al[1] investigated 177 upper arm and forearm dysfunctional fistulas. The results disclosed a 39% prevalence of CAS for brachiocephalic and 2% for radiocephalic fistulas. These investigators reported, in another study of 155 malfunctioning fistulas, that the rate of CAS was 30% for brachiocephalic fistulas and 0% for the radiocephalic fistulas.[14] While it is unclear if the same patients were included in both reports, it is evident that CAS is a major component of malfunctioning brachiocephalic fistulas.

The reason for the discrepancy between the CAS prevalence in brachiocephalic and radiocephalic fistulas is thought to be related to differences in blood flow. Typically, the brachiocephalic access, with its brachial artery connection, has higher flow than an access associated with the smaller radial artery. Additionally, all the access blood flow associated with a brachiocephalic fistula courses through the cephalic arch. With a radiocephalic fistula, the blood flow is frequently distributed to both the cephalic and basilic veins at the level of the elbow because of cross-connections at that level. In fact, it is not unusual to see a radiocephalic fistula in which the majority of the upper arm flow is via the basilic vein, which is larger and has less resistance than the cephalic. In summary, based on the available information, CAS is a frequent occurrence in patients with brachiocephalic AVF.

MANAGEMENT OF CAS

▶ Percutaneous Balloon Angioplasty

Percutaneous transluminal balloon angioplasty (PTA) has been established as the current standard of care for the treatment of venous stenosis in patients with an arteriovenous access (Figure 53-1). A few reports have made reference to angioplasty of the cephalic arch. Turmel-Rodrigues and colleagues[2] presented a large series of 1118 procedures performed in fistulas and grafts. There were 74 upper arm fistulas. More than half (55%) of lesions in the upper arm fistulas were present in the outflow vein. Lesions resistant to angioplasty occurred in 4.8% of the upper arm fistulas and most of these were within the cephalic arch. This compared to 1.3% of forearm fistulas. A rupture rate of 14.9% was observed in the upper arm, and again most of these were within the final arch of cephalic vein. This contrasted to 8.3% rupture rate in forearm angioplasties. Intravascular stents were needed to salvage 13% of forearm versus 23% of upper arm ruptures.

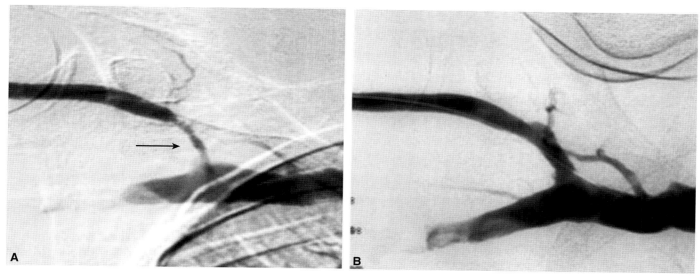

Figure 53-1. The arrow demonstrates the presence of cephalic arch stenosis (**A**). The stenosis has been successfully dilated using the percutaneous balloon angioplasty procedure (**B**).

In another study, Rajan et al[1] specifically studied the CAS. A total of 177 failing fistulas were retrospectively investigated. Most, 116 (66%), were in the forearm and 61 (34%) in the upper arm. As pointed out above, 39% of brachiocephalic fistulas had a CAS compared to 2% of radiocephalic fistulas. In this analysis, brachiocephalic fistulas were 37 times more likely to have CAS than radiocephalic fistulas. Fifty angioplasties were performed in the 26 fistulas. Anatomic success was 76%, while clinical success was 98%. Higher inflation pressures (>15 atm) were needed in 58% of the cases. Rupture occurred in 6% of cases (3/50), one of which led to fistula loss. The other two cases were salvaged with prolonged balloon inflation or stenting. Primary patency was 42% at 6 months and 23% at 1 year (median primary patency of 5 months). Primary-assisted patency was 83% at 6 months and 75% at 1 year (median 3 years). An average of 1.6 procedures a year was required per fistula. Of note, the 6-month primary patency of 42% falls below the Dialysis Outcome Quality Initiative (DOQI) guideline of 50%.[15] Additionally, CAS is often resistant to PTA, frequently requiring high-pressure balloons and being vulnerable to rupture (6%).[1,2,16]

The higher complication rate of PTA in the treatment of CAS as well as the disappointing primary patency highlights the importance of finding alternate avenues of intervention for this problem.

▶ Intravascular Stent Insertion

Suboptimal angioplasty outcomes have led to a search for alternative means of salvaging failing brachiocephalic fistulas with CAS. Ideally, a study comparing angioplasty alone versus stent placement for recurrent CAS would be required to endorse the superiority of one intervention over the other. Nevertheless, stents are being used to treat CAS. If a stent is placed at the arch, a few important factors

should be considered. Optimally, the device should not cross the confluence of the cephalic arch and axillary vein.[16] A stent placed across the cephalic arch that advances into the subclavian vein will jeopardize future use of the basilic and axillary vein for fistula creation or for drainage of an upper arm access (Figure 53-2). However, if the stenosis is at the point of confluence, the only way to ensure successful stenting is to achieve full coverage of the lesion, and therefore some part of the stent will protrude into the

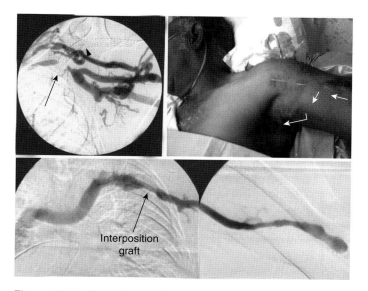

Interposition graft

Figure 53-2. An endovascular stent is shown in the cephalic arch (upper left). Note the stent has moved into the confluence of cephalic arch and the axillary vein (upper left; arrow). Also notice the fracture of the stent (upper left; arrowhead). In this patient, the stent was surgically removed (upper right; shoulder scar) and the fistula surgically rerouted through the basilic system (lower panel). Note that a small piece of graft was used to connect the fistula to the subclavian vein.

axillary/subclavian vein. In this context, jeopardizing the basilic axillary system to salvage a failing brachiocephalic fistula might not be appropriate in the long term.

Falk and Gelbfish[17] refrained from placing stents into the subclavian vein after two CAS ruptures during thrombectomy procedures. The author emphasized that the basilic axillary system could be used for new access creation rather than risking abandoning the entire arm from subsequent occlusion of the subclavian vein by the intravascular stent. It is worth mentioning that the cephalic arch overlies the glenohumeral joint. In this scenario, there is potential for kinking, crushing, and migration of the stent on movement of the shoulder.[18]

Recently, stent-grafts have been employed for the management of CAS. In this context, a randomized study evaluating the role of the stent-graft versus bare stent provided rather interesting observations.[19] In this investigation, 25 patients with recurrent CAS (within 3 months of successful balloon angioplasty) were randomized to receive angioplasty plus deployment of either stent-graft or bare metal stent. Only patients with brachiocephalic fistulae were included and demographic characteristic of the study groups showed no difference. Twelve patients received bare stents, while 13 had stent-grafts. The average follow-up for this study was 13.7 months (range 1.7–21.6 months). At 3 months, angiography was performed to assess the degree of stenosis. At this point, two patients in the bare stent and two in the stent-graft group were lost to the study. Of the 21 patients remaining, significant stenosis ($\geq$50%) was found in 7/10 (70%) bare stents and 2/11 (18%) stent-grafts ($P = 0.024$, 95% confidence interval: 1.03%–14.38%). During the follow-up period, 12 additional patients were lost to the study, 4 in the bare stent group and 8 in the stent-graft group, and 1 patient in the bare stent group thrombosed. The 6-month primary patency for stent-graft and bare stent was 81.8% and 39.1%, respectively. One-year primary patency for stent-graft and bare stent was 31.8% and 0.00%, respectively ($P = 0.002$). The authors concluded that restenosis rates in recurrent cephalic arch restenosis were significantly better for stent-grafts compared with bare stents. The investigators further suggested that in patients where intimal hyperplasia is a possibility, stenting should be limited to the use of stents completely covered with polytetrafluoroethylene (PTFE) material.

While the above-mentioned study purportedly demonstrated the value of stent-grafts in the management of CAS, it has several problems. It does not meet the basic requirements of a randomized controlled trial. The sample size was too small to have the power necessary for such a study. Secondly, primary patency analysis included protocol angiograms and duplex ultrasound rather than clinical indications for a repeat angiogram. While important, from a practical standpoint these parameters might not be considered clinically meaningful endpoints. Lastly, one has to question the cost–benefit ratio of using multiple stents to treat a problem that might have more economical

alternatives. Nevertheless, stent-graft insertion does provide an obvious approach to the management of CAS.

Cutting balloons

As venous PTA is a traumatic event resulting in damage of the vascular wall, it may itself lead to the development of neointimal hyperplasia at the site of vascular injury. Indeed, CAS can be recurrent and resistant, which would support the notion that even though PTA results in initial success in dilating the stenosis, the high recurrence rate may be due to the injury induced by the initial intervention. Peripheral cutting balloons create microsurgical incisions in the vascular wall with the least amount of radial force, thereby reducing trauma to the vessel wall.[20] However, despite the theoretical benefit, these balloons have so far failed to show an increase in patency rates of fistulas. No studies have been designed specific to CAS; however, in a large randomized study, Vesely and Siegel[20] failed to show superior 6-month patency rates compared to angioplasty by conventional balloons. The cutting balloons resulted in higher rate of venous rupture and dissections. Based on the available information, their use cannot be endorsed over that of conventional angioplasty balloons for the treatment of CAS.

Flow reduction

Since it has been postulated that CAS is linked to high flow, flow reduction has been attempted as a therapeutic maneuver. In a retrospective study of 33 patients who had undergone two or more instances of CAS, banding of the fistula to reduce the blood flow rate using a balloon-assisted technique was evaluated.[21] Angioplasty rates for CAS were calculated for the pre- and postbanding periods. At 3, 6, and 12 months postbanding, the cephalic arch primary lesion patency was 91%, 76%, and 57%, respectively. The cephalic arch intervention rate was reduced from 3.34 to 0.9 per access-year ($t = 7.74$, $P < .001$). The average follow-up time was 14.5 months (range 4.8–32).

▶ Surgical Interventions

Surgical interventions have also been attempted for the management of CAS. One such approach, described by Chen et al, involves surgical revision to redirect the blood flow to the adjacent patent veins.[22] The cephalic vein is dissected as proximal as possible to ensure adequate length. A second incision in the axilla exposes the axillary vein. The cephalic vein is then transposed through a subcutaneous tunnel and anastomosed to the upper basilic/axillary vein in an end-to-side manner. In their report, 9 patients with brachiocephalic fistula having a median age of 14 months underwent surgical revision. Seven fistulas underwent cephalic vein transposition (transferring the cephalic vein to the axillary–basilic vein) and two had basilic vein transpositions (moving the proximal basilic vein to the cephalic vein). Primary patencies of 70% at 6 months and 60% at 12 months were achieved. While stenosis may recur at the site of reanastomosis, this was infrequent. Perhaps more importantly, patency rates were superior to those reported for angioplasty of CAS.[1] It is worth mentioning that a cephalic vein that has been anastomosed to the axillary–basilic vein may jeopardize the creation of a basilic vein fistula in the future. This situation must be considered and discussed among the patient, interventionalist, and the surgeon.

Another surgical study of patients with recurrent CAS provides a good comparison to the stent-graft study presented above.[23] Thirteen patients with frequently recurring CAS were referred for surgical intervention. The surgical procedure entailed transecting the healthy portion of the cephalic vein distal to the stenotic segment in the shoulder area, moving and connecting it to the veins in the inner part of the upper arm (basilic/axillary vein)—a procedure that has come to be referred to as outflow relocation (Figure 53-2). Following surgical revision, development of access dysfunction was treated with percutaneous balloon angioplasty. Patency rates for angioplasty before and after the surgical revision were evaluated. Primary patency rates for angioplasty before the surgical revision were 23%, 8%, and 0% at 3, 6, and 12 months, respectively. Following surgical revision, all patients needed an angioplasty procedure. However, primary patency increased to 92%, 69%, and 39% at 3, 6, and 12 months, respectively ($P = 0.0001$). Secondary patency before the surgical revision at 3, 6, and 12 months was 100%, 39%, and 8%, respectively, compared with 92% at 3, 6, and 12 months postsurgical revision ($P = 0.0003$). The results of this study demonstrated that outflow relocation surgery of the cephalic vein in frequently recurring CAS was a viable option and yields better patency rates for future angioplasty procedures. No stent-grafts or bare stents were used in this study. Nevertheless, the 1-year primary patency (39%) for conventional angioplasty (without stents) observed by Kian et al[23] after surgical revision of recurrent CAS compared favorably to that obtained by Shemesh et al[19] for the stent-graft (1-year primary patency = 31.8).

Another novel surgical approach is a cutdown and patch angioplasty of the arch at the area of stenosis (Surrender Shenoy, personal communication). During a 66-month follow-up period of seven cases, one patient did not require any angioplasty, five patients needed one angioplasty each, and one patient required two angioplasty procedures. No procedure-related complications were noted. A disadvantage of this approach is that the procedure can be challenging due to the location of the lesion. It has the advantage, however, that surgical outflow relocation can always be done at a later stage.

While further studies are needed to conclusively establish the superiority of surgical intervention, based on the available information, surgical treatment for recurrent and resistant CAS may lead to improved long-term patency. Additionally, this may be more economical than the use of multiple stents.

SUMMARY

The cephalic arch is a unique anatomical structure. While multiple options are available, the application of an intervention must take into consideration the evidence, invasiveness, patency outcomes, and cost-to-benefit ratio. The management of CAS must include the patient, nephrologist, interventionalist, and the surgeon. A team approach will only improve patient care.

REFERENCES

1. Rajan DK, Clark TWI, Vatel NK, Stavropoulos SW, Simons ME. Prevalence and treatment of cephalic arch stenosis in dysfunctional autogenous hemodialysis fistulas. *J Vasc Interv Radiol.* 2003;14:567.
2. Turmel-Rodrigues L, Pengloan J, Baudin S, et al. Treatment of stenosis and thrombosis in hemodialysis fistulas and grafts by interventional radiology. *Nephrol Dial Transplant.* 2000;15:2029.
3. Lau EW, Liew R, Harris S. An unusual case of the cephalic vein with a supraclavicular course. *PACE.* 2007;30:719.
4. Iimura A, Nakamura Y, Itoh M. Anatomical study of distribution of valves of the cutaneous veins of adult's limb. *Ann Anat.* 2003;185:91.
5. Hallock GG. The cephalic vein in microsurgery. *Microsurg.* 1993;14:482.
6. Au FC. The anatomy of cephalic vein. *Am Surgeon.* 1989; 55:638.
7. Harmon JV, Edwards WD. Venous valves in subclavian and internal jugular veins. *Am J Card Pathology.* 1987;1:51.
8. Chen JY, Chang KC, Lin KH, Lin YC, Lee JD, Huang SKS. Ultrasonographic predictors of unsuccessful cephalic vein approach during pacemaker or defibrillator lead implantation. *PACE.* 2006;29:706.
9. Wali MA, Eid RA, Dewan M, Al-Homrany MA. Intimal changes in the cephalic vein of renal failure patients before arterio-venous fistula (AVF) construction. *J Smooth Muscle Res.* 2003;4:95.
10. Van Tricht I, De Wachter D, Tordoir J, Verdonck P. Hemodynamics and complications encountered with arteriovenous fistulas and grafts as vascular access for hemodialysis: a review. *Ann Biomed Eng.* 2005;33:1142.
11. Paszkowiak JJ, Dardik A. Arterial wall shear stress: observations from the bench to the bedside. *Vasc Endovascular Surg.* 2003;37:47.
12. Glanz S, Bashist B, Gordon DH, Butt K, Adamsons R. Angiography of upper extremity access fistulas for dialysis. *Radiology.* 1982;143:45.
13. Roy-Chaudhury P, Sukhatme VP, Cheung AK. Hemodialysis vascular access dysfunction: a cellular and molecular viewpoint. *J Am Soc Nephrol.* 2006;17:1112.
14. Rajan DK, Bunston S, MIsra S, Vinto Ruxandra, Lok CE. Dysfunctional autogenous fistulas: outcomes after angioplasty—are there clinical predictors of patency? *Radiology.* 2004;232:508.
15. Vascular Access Work Group. Clinical practice guidelines for vascular access. *Am J Kidney Dis.* 2006;48:S248.

16. Trumell-Rodrigues L, Vengloan J, Bourquelot P. Interventional radiology in hemodialysis fistulae and grafts: a multidisciplinary approach. *Cardiovasc Interv Radiol*. 2002;25:3.

17. Falk A, Gelbfish GA. Percutaneous treatment of thrombosed arteriovenous fistulae using the Gelbfish-Endovac aspiration thrombectomy device. *J Vasc Access*. 2004;5:139.

18. Ursula CB, Mojibian HR, Aruny JE, Perazella MA. Quiz page. *Am J Kidney Dis*. 2006;47:XLV.

19. Shemesh D, Goldin I, Zaghal I, Berlowitz D, Raveh D, Olsha O. Angioplasty with stent graft versus bare stent for recurrent cephalic arch stenosis in autogenous arteriovenous access for hemodialysis: a prospective randomized clinical trial. *J Vasc Surg*. 2008;48:1524.

20. Vesely TM, Siegel JB. Use of peripheral cutting balloon to treat hemodialysis related stenoses. *J Vasc Interv Radiol*. 2005;16:1593.

21. Miller GA, Friedman A, Khariton A, Preddie DC, Savransky Y. Access flow reduction and recurrent symptomatic cephalic arch stenosis in brachiocephalic hemodialysis arteriovenous fistulas. *J Vasc Access*. 2010;11:281.

22. Chen JC, Kamal DM, Jastrzebski J, Taylor DC. Venovenostomy for outflow venous obstruction in patients with upper extremity autogenous hemodialysis arteriovenous access. *Ann Vasc Surgery*. 2005;19:629.

23. Kian K, Unger SW, Mishler R, Schon D, Lenz O, Asif A. Role of surgical intervention for cephalic arch stenosis in the "fistula first" era. *Semin Dial*. 2008;21:93.

SECTION V
Basic and Translational Science

54

VASCULAR ACCESS SCIENCE— WHAT DOES THE FUTURE HOLD?

ALEXANDER S. YEVZLIN

LEARNING OBJECTIVES

1. Understand the evolving role of neointimal hyperplasia in vascular access science.

2. Describe strategies to improve our understanding of vascular access biology.

3. Understand the genetic targets of vascular access science.

4. Understand the current and future roles of imaging modalities in the treatment of access dysfunction.

5. Describe current and future strategies to inhibit inflammation and delivery systems for these interventions.

INTRODUCTION

Hemodialysis access dysfunction remains a $1 billion per year problem[1] despite recent efforts by CMS, the End-Stage Renal Disease (ESRD) networks, and other national institutions. The United States Renal Data System projects that the US hemodialysis population will increase to 774,000 patients by 2020.[1] Given this growth projection and the limited success of recent clinical investigations to clearly define a solution,[2,3] a comprehensive translational research initiative involving endothelial biologists, nephrologists, surgeons, and interventionalists has been undertaken. The purpose of this chapter is to describe the evolution of our understanding of the key pathologic entities underpinning access dysfunction and their mechanisms of action. Further, this chapter functions to identify key clinical, translational, and basic research pathways to follow in order to improve future vascular access outcomes.

Neointimal hyperplasia (NH) (Figures 54-1 and 54-2) has been described as the primary pathologic lesion in hemodialysis access grafts and fistulas that develop stenosis as well as nonmaturation.[4-6] There is also evidence, though limited, that implicates NH in fistula nonmaturation. NH has been regarded as a purely pathologic entity with substantial research efforts directed at preventing and treating NH in the vascular access.[7,8] Newer research suggests that this understanding of NH may be somewhat myopic.[9,10] This chapter, therefore, also functions to recast our understanding of NH and redefine research goals for an evolving discipline.

NEOINTIMAL HYPERPLASIA: THE TRADITIONAL PERSPECTIVE

Several mechanisms have traditionally been implicated in the genesis of NH in hemodialysis vascular access, including proliferation and migration of smooth muscle cells (SMCs) from the media, aggravation of inflammation, alteration of hemodynamic forces, and activation of the coagulation cascade.[11]

Our seminal understanding of NH pathology derived from studies of coronary and peripheral arterial disease that suggested vascular SMCs in media proliferate and migrate into intima. In addition, adventitial remodeling was also noted in studies that examined coronary arteries. NH in the arterial circulation (as in peripheral arterial grafts) however can be very dissimilar to NH seen in the venous circulation (as in a dialysis fistula).[5]

Nonlaminar blood flow, oscillatory shear stress, and increased turbulence following creation of an arteriovenous (AV) anastomosis result in aggressive NH, and patency of the venous conduits is generally worse than the patency of bypass grafts in the arterial circulation. In case of an arteriovenous graft (AVG), the presence of a foreign body adds further bioincompatibility and augments local

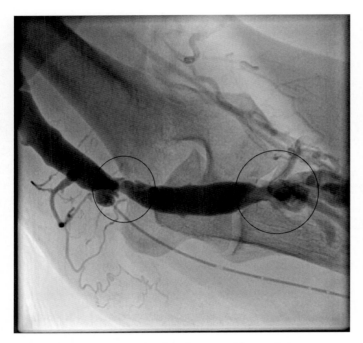

Figure 54-1. Radiograph of dysfunctional hemodialysis access due to neointimal hyperplasia of vascular access.

inflammation that is compounded by repeat injury from dialysis needles and uremia-associated endothelial dysfunction. Changing rheology and increased blood flow actually induce regression of NH in polytetrafluoroethylene (PTFE) grafts.[12] The pathology and pathophysiology of NH have been examined both in humans and in animal models. In one study, human venous tissue obtained from three patents and one thrombosed arteriovenous fistula (AVF) was examined. NH was present together with medial hypertrophy resulting in greater than 80% stenosis. The predominant cell type was myofibroblasts by immunohistochemistry.[6]

In dialysis AVG, histological and immunohistochemical analysis of NH have also revealed SMC and myofibroblast proliferation at the venous anastomosis and downstream vein.[5] Angiogenesis was prominent in the adventitia and neointima at these sites. In addition, there was increased

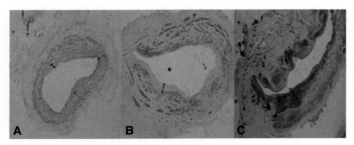

Figure 54-2. Neointimal hyperplastic lesions in a porcine model of AVF (NH represented by black lines). Mild, moderate, and severe NH in (**A**), (**B**), and (**C**), respectively.

growth factor expression by SMCs, myofibroblasts, microvessels, and macrophages in these areas. In other models, cytokines related to oxidative stress have also been shown to be expressed in conjunction with growth factors.[13] A number of other inflammatory cytokines are also likely to play a role in this process of venous NH.[14]

It is anecdotally acknowledged that after primary stenoses have been treated with angioplasty in AVFs, there is a significant increase in subsequent stenosis. Recent findings confirm this clinical observation by noting an increase in the proliferative index in medial and intimal lesions.[4] This suggests that angioplasty-induced vascular injury is likely to enhance growth factor and cytokine expression. Thus, paradoxically, the very procedure performed to treat venous stenoses may in fact be responsible for aggressive dialysis access stenosis. On the basis of the pathogenic mechanisms involved in NH, a mathematic model of venous NH has also been developed.[15] The model anticipates possible access stenosis and may provide an indication for intervention. What is more difficult to track but also significant is that venous endothelium per se may be able to promote NH through one or more paracrine mechanisms.[16]

Genetic factors have also been linked to the development of aggressive NH. Single-nucleotide polymorphisms in the matrix metalloproteinase gene and angiotensin-converting enzyme gene can alter vascular responsiveness and the latter has been investigated with regards to hemodialysis access patency. Polymorphisms of transforming growth factor- (TGF-β), heme oxygenase-1 (HO-1), and the methylene tetrahydrofolate reductase gene also have been linked to AVF patency.[17–20] Among these polymorphisms, HO-1 appears to have the greatest likelihood of having a direct association with access outcomes.

HO-1 is an inducible protein that regulates vascular response to injury, decreasing NH, and inflammation. HO-1 deficiency is linked with NH and inflammation with HO-1 null mice manifesting an increased number of occluded AVF through mechanisms involving matrix metalloproteinases compared with wild-type mice in experimental AVF creation.[21]

Far-infrared therapy also increases blood flow and patency of AVF in HD via HO-1 presumably through activation of thermoreceptors with a concomitant reduction in endothelial inflammation.[22] HO-1 is likely the mechanism too for the salutary effects of rapamycin and paclitaxel in decreasing AVF stenosis. Thus, delivery of HO-1 into the AV anastomosis could have the potential for preventing NH or even inducing regression of NH that is already present.

Inflammation has to be considered an auxiliary if not primary stimulus for NH in dialysis access. The inflammatory activity of surgically harvested thrombosed fistulas has been measured and found to be elevated using a series of inflammatory biomarkers.[23] This finding has been corroborated by other evidence of inflammation around NH lesions, including increased expression of interleukin-6 and vascular cellular adhesion molecule-1.

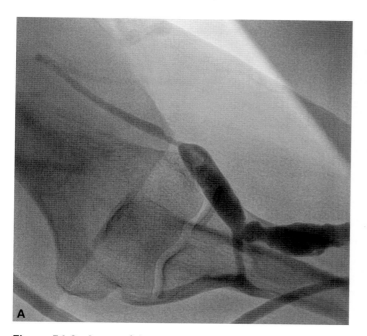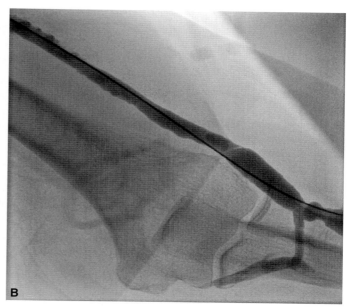

Figure 54-3. Successful percutaneous angioplasty ("mechanical" treatment) of NH lesion leading to total chromic occlusion. (**A**) Preintervention 100% stenosis with collateral, (**B**) postintervention 0% residual stenosis.

Lee et al recently documented significant venous NH prior to AVF or AVG creation in venous segments at the site of AV access creation.[24] These data suggest that uremia, inflammation, and oxidative stress in chronic kidney disease (CKD)/ESRD patients could be responsible for these changes. It is as yet unclear as to whether preexisting NH correlates with patency or a reduction in patency.

CURRENT AND FUTURE TREATMENT MODALITIES

As described above, neointimal hyperplasia has been traditionally regarded as a purely pathological entity. The approach, likewise, to NH in dialysis access so far has been clinically mechanistic (Figures 54-3 and 54-4), consisting of repeat interventions with angioplasties and stent placement. These therapies might be successful in the short term in altering NH. However, long-term patency remains elusive and the ability to *regulate* NH, not just eradicate or prevent it, for any potential benefit is unknown. Inward remodeling (what is currently called "NH") and outward remodeling (what is currently called "vascular maturation"), rather than distinct pathologic processes, can be viewed as two potential pathways for vascular remodeling in response to stress. As our understanding of the true role of NH evolves, broader based investigations will refocus therapeutic efforts from "suppression" of NH to "control" (Figure 54-5).[9]

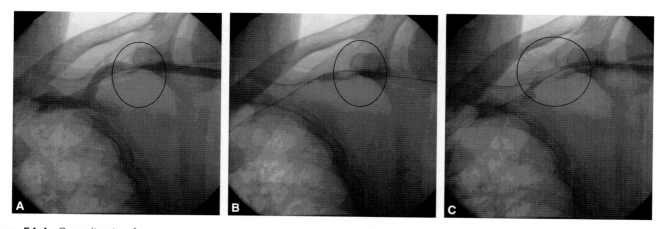

Figure 54-4. Complication from percutaneous angioplasty ("mechanical" treatment) of NH lesion. (**A**) Preintervention stenosis, (**B**) balloon angioplasty, (**C**) postintervention dissection with intimal flap occluding flow and extravasation.

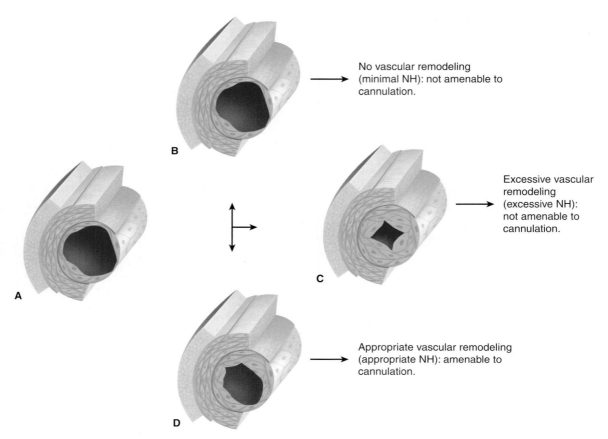

No vascular remodeling (minimal NH): not amenable to cannulation.

Excessive vascular remodeling (excessive NH): not amenable to cannulation.

Appropriate vascular remodeling (appropriate NH): amenable to cannulation.

Figure 54-5. Neointimal hyperplasia of vascular access can develop and progress through several pathways.[9,10] (**A**) Normal vein prior to access creation; (**B**) no vascular remodeling after access creation; (**C**) luminal narrowing (NH) resulting in luminal compromise due to smooth muscle proliferation and inflammation; (**D**) outward dilatation (maturation) resulting in luminal preservation of the AVF.

The effect of short-term local pharmacologic interventions on NH in AV grafts has been evaluated in different animal models (dogs, pigs, and sheep with normal kidney function). A beneficial effect in an animal model, however, does not necessarily translate into a clinical benefit in dialysis patients given differences in vascular properties, responsiveness to drugs among species, effects of uremia, the short-term nature of these studies, and the use of surrogate outcomes. A perivascular paclitaxel wrap inhibited graft stenosis in a pig model;[24,25] however, a clinical trial evaluating a paclitaxel wrap on graft failure was suspended pending a safety review. Similarly, a pilot study demonstrated the safety of a sirolimus-eluting collagen matrix implanted during graft surgery.[26] On the other hand, edifoligide, an E2F transcription factor decoy that modulates muscle proliferation in vitro, did not prevent failure of coronary or peripheral bypass grafts.[27] Other experimental approaches are being evaluated, manifested maybe most significantly by the development of autologous tissue-engineered vascular grafts.[28] It appears that one obvious strategy to consider is the application of these interventions shortly after creation of the AVG to potentially allow processes to initiate NH but to regulate the evolution of NH.

A number of vasoactive drugs have the potential to regulate NH in dialysis vascular access, such as platelet antagonists, calcium channel blockers, angiotensin-converting enzyme inhibitors, and fish oil. Other agents that can alter vascular remodeling include statins, peroxisome proliferator-activated receptor agonists, and immunosuppressive agents. Imatinib mesylate, a phosphotyrosine kinase inhibitor of platelet derived growth factor (PDGF), Bcr-Abl, and C-kit, seems to be a possible therapeutic agent. While delivery of these agents at the time of surgery could be relatively straightforward, repeat delivery, particularly for agents with a short half-life, could be challenging. Initial studies using endovascular balloons with sheathed needles to pierce the vessel wall suggest that repeat perivascular delivery through an endovascular approach is possible.[29]

There has also been interest in exploring nonpharmacologic approaches to affect the course of NH including radiation therapy. Ionizing radiation can induce apoptosis and inhibit the cell cycle. SMCs in their proliferative phase in neointimal tissue are likely to be especially susceptible. In tissue culture, external beam radiation to SMCs inhibited growth in a dose-dependent manner. Venous SMCs were less susceptible than aortic SMCs.[30] Endovascular radiation therapy also inhibited NH in vitro, in porcine models of AVG, in human coronary artery stenosis, and in saphenous vein graft stenosis.[31] Local radiation therapy at the venous anastomotic site delayed site-specific graft stenosis but did not improve cumulative graft survival.[32] A prospective, randomized, controlled study of 1 year of far-infrared therapy improved access flow and patency in patients who received the therapy.[22]

In the Beta Radiation for Treatment of Arterial-Venous Graft Outflow 1 study, 25 patients with dysfunctional AVG were randomly assigned to brachytherapy or sham treatment after angioplasty.[32] Primary patency at 6 months was 42% in the intervention group and 0% in the control group. Interestingly, secondary patency at 6 or 12 months was not affected. Other nonpharmacologic treatments could include local application of physical agents such as photodynamic or ultrasonic therapy via intravascular or external application as well as percutaneous balloon cryoplasty. The last has shown promising results.[33]

It is possible to deliver cells that promote healthy remodeling at the site of NH. This is especially important in considering the aforementioned novel findings from Lee and colleagues that venous endothelium may demonstrate NH even prior to the creation of any surgical shunt. Endothelial cells embedded in absorbable gelatin have been used to wrap around AV anastomoses to augment cytokine production and control NH in porcine AVF models. In vivo seeding with anti-CD34 antibodies accelerates endothelialization of new AVGs in a porcine model.[34] Paradoxically, this therapy resulted in an increase in venous NH at the graft-vein anastomosis, again suggesting that regulating NH is critical and not an all-or-none process in AVG.

Gene transfer of endothelial and inducible nitric oxide synthase, cyclin-dependent kinase inhibitors, retinoblastoma protein, hepatocyte growth factor, and transcription factors such as edifoligide have all been used to inhibit NH in experimental angioplasty models.[30] Gene therapies have focused on other targets as well. In a pig model, adenoviral-mediated delivery of β-adrenergic receptor kinase reduced NH at the venous anastomosis by interfering with Gi signaling.[31] Adenoviral transfer of C-type natriuretic peptide also improved outward remodeling and thickening of venous media in a porcine AVG,[32] while perivascular placement of vascular endothelial growth factor D via an adenoviral vector is currently in phase III clinical trial for the prevention of AVG venous anastomotic stenosis.[33] All these treatments however have (a) the risks of the vector per se; (b) the unpredictability of distribution of vector and target molecule; and (c) a patency-related outcome that, while important, leaves us guessing as to the actual events within the dialysis access that might affect the outcome.

RESEARCH OPPORTUNITIES

Where do we need to go next to understand this unique form of venous biology? Fundamentally, how do we bring together the unique and interesting observations

regarding NH into a synthetic thesis that begets additional and novel ideas regarding therapy and prevention? Traditionally, NH associated with hemodialysis vascular access has been viewed as a vascular SMC lesion. However, with a greater understanding of cellular responses, it is apparent that other events are also occurring. Clearly, a deeper understanding of TGF-β1 signaling is critical to understanding NH. There are studies that have described increased expression of TGF-β1, latent TGF-β1 binding protein-1, and TGF-β1 mRNA in stenotic AVF.[23] Ikegaya et al[35] described elevated erythropoietin receptor and TGF-β1 expression in stenotic AVF in contrast to cutaneous veins and patent AVF in patients who underwent chronic hemodialysis.

TGF-β1 increases plasminogen activator inhibitor-1 (PAI-1) expression. Thus, it is not surprising that PAI-1 expression is increased in stenotic AVF.[36] Interestingly, Lazo-Langner et al[19] were able to demonstrate in a cohort analysis that the risk of dialysis access thrombosis was differentially associated with polymorphisms in the TGF-β1 gene that correlated with TGF-β1 production and that this risk was further modified through an interaction with the PAI-1 genotype present.[19]

Interestingly, mechanisms of TGF-β1 signaling are for the most part unexamined in the context of dialysis access-associated NH or indirectly inferred. Traditional therapies that might antagonize TGF-β1, for example, angiotensin converting enzyme (ACE) inhibition, appear to have little effect in reducing NH or maintaining access patency. However, direct antagonism of type I and II TGF-β1 receptor signaling has yet to be examined as a potential therapeutic alternative for hemodialysis access NH. It should be noted that bone morphogenic protein-7 (BMP-7) might be a therapeutic approach to limit this lesion. Choi and colleagues recently described an AVF model in mice in which BMP-7 administration reduced NH.[37] Additionally, nontraditional sources of TGF-β might also be associated with AVF NH. Jin et al[38] induced AVF in dogs and noted that chymase- and TGF-β (+) mast cells were prominent in proliferating neointima and media. Chymase inhibition reduced neointimal formation.

With a solid body of literature suggesting at least a role for TGF-β1 in hemodialysis access NH, it makes sense to consider the possibility that the venous endothelium is a contributor to the process. Recent data suggest that endothelial cells undergo mesenchymal transition in certain settings.[39–42] The characteristic transformation to myofibroblasts is defined by the loss of cell surface adhesion and the de novo expression of vimentin with a resulting decline in CD31 expression. The presence of myofibroblasts in lesions of NH could well be a manifestation of not just SMCs in transition but also endothelial–mesenchymal transition (End-MT).

This is no doubt exploratory, as the majority of research in End-MT has been focused on embryonic tissues. Yet, it is striking to note that intimal thickening involves transdifferentiation of embryonic endothelial cells.[43] Moreover,

CD40 and CD40 ligand (CD40L) have been implicated, especially the latter, at sites where endothelial cells differentiate into mesenchymal cells. CD40L is manifest in the context of platelet activation and repeated injury to an access via needle sticks could be an obvious stimulus for excess CD40L. It would be fascinating to ascertain the presence of both CD40 and CD40L in a dialysis access at various stages of NH formation, or even immediately following access placement and then after repeated needle placements.

Other markers of potential End-MT could also be assessed in access tissue including NF-kB activated p50/p65 heterodimers, IkB, insulin-like growth factor-II, vitronectin, and certainly an assessment of whether S100A4 is expressed in cells obtained from human AVFs. A constellation of such findings would suggest that End-MT is occurring and possibly contributing to the increased presence of myofibroblasts in the neointimal hyperplastic area.

As noted above, phase II studies are just beginning to examine innovative therapies directed at regulating or preventing NH in dialysis vascular access. A key feature of NH in vascular access is disruption of the internal elastic lamina. Chang and colleagues used gene expression analysis to study the impact of flow velocity and pressure on internal elastic lamina in an aortocaval fistula model.[44] They noted an increase in cathepsin K and S and matrix metalloproteinase 2 (MMP2) mRNA levels, concomitant with increased elastase expression. Immunohistochemical studies localized cathepsin to the venous luminal endothelium lining the internal elastic lamina.

These findings should prompt additional preclinical and clinical studies examining elastase inhibitors including local application of recombinant human elastase to promote vasodilation after fistula creation.[45] Additional elastases and combinations of molecules may be necessary to alter or regulate the vascular transformative process of NH.

Alternatively, different agents that traditionally may not be thought of as anti-NH agents could be tried as therapeutics to affect this process. One example is the novel immunosuppressive agent, FK778. This medication exerts an antiproliferative effect on multiple cell types. Recent work suggests that it has the ability to limit NH in vein graft models.[46,47]

Similarly, discrete signaling cascades that have traditionally not been targeted for intervention merit consideration for their possible role in dialysis access NH. Inhibition of Rho kinase suppresses neointimal formation in models of vascular injury[48-51] and alters endothelial cell migration in certain cell models.[52] However, the identification of specific Rho kinase isoforms present within venous endothelial cells and whether inhibition of Rho kinase affects a true in vivo process are unknown. Furthermore, it remains to be determined if Rho-associated kinase (ROCK) isoforms, ROCK1 and ROCK2, could be present in venous endothelium or dialysis access NH. Indeed ROCK inhibitors are being evaluated as potential therapeutic agents for a number of vascular processes,[53] and there is no reason to exclude them from possible assessment in dialysis vascular access stenosis.

The potential systemic effects of agents that target cathepsin K and S[54,55] have stimulated study of delivery mechanisms to elucidate changes in the vascular access. Novel scaffolds, vectorially directed scaffolds, and nanoparticles with periodic, concentrated delivery of molecules are all areas worthy of more in-depth investigation. Lim and colleagues expanded upon their initial work to improve control of drug release through paclitaxel (Ptx)-loaded poly (lactic-co-glycolic acid) (PLGA) nanoparticles.[56] The Ptx-PLGA-natriuretic peptide (NPs) were prepared and transferred to the luminal surface and inner part of expanded PTFE vascular grafts through a microtube pumping and spin penetration process. This system achieved controlled drug delivery with a reduced initial burst release. The science of molecular packaging and release, targeted and measured levels of drug or molecule in the microenvironment, maintenance of drug or molecule in the microenvironment to reduce systemic side effects, and effect on true clinical outcome are all areas of needed emphasis and inquiry.

Monitoring the effects of an intervention is a difficult puzzle to solve, especially with regards to an outcome that takes time to evolve. With NH, we can measure systemic parameters or treatment parameters, but the event that is of interest is happening in a vessel anastomotic area over a period of time. New imaging methodologies such as surface dissolution imaging and atomic force microscopic topographic imaging could be used for intravital microscopy to assess changes in animal models of venous NH over time. Other nondestructive, nonlinear optical microscopy techniques using harmonic generation and fluorescence[52] are also options for experimental analyses. Intervascular ultrasound (IVUS) has been used in coronary and peripheral intervention to gauge successful therapy. Since IVUS (3D imaging modality) is a fundamentally different source of information than traditional angiography (3D imaging modality), the use of IVUS represents a method of imaging cellular changes that has already entered the clinical arena.

It will be important to move imaging technology into the clinical setting for two reasons. More accurate and precise imaging will provide more knowledge about the evolution of lesions that afflict dialysis vascular access. Second, improvements in imaging that make it less invasive or more feasible to perform in conjunction with cannulation during a dialysis treatment might move imaging into a more precise preemptive or prophylactic technology.

Bioengineering-focused investigations are essential in understanding more about NH. Ex-vivo models of hemodialysis suggest that high blood flow (500 mL/min) can shear off endothelial cells and reduce nitric oxide formation.[57] Such studies represent early investigations in analyzing the impact of shear stress and needle turbulence on not only vascular mediators but also endothelial gene and protein expression in response to these treatment events. It would be interesting to determine if different techniques, for example, buttonhole cannulation, lead to less trauma and changes in activation of various molecular mediators. Alternatively, is there a protective response mediated with some AVF through receptor signaling and desensitization via repeated needle sticks that is not manifested in other individuals who develop NH? Are there different, nontraditional receptor subtypes, for example, cannabinoid receptors,[58,59] activated in the presence of needle jet turbulence or shear stress? These questions are answerable and could lead to better patient predictors of access patency over time.

SUMMARY

The interaction of inflammation, cellular, genetic, and hemodynamic mechanisms at play in NH is complex. Furthermore, our understanding of this complexity thus far has been limited, as reflected in our poor access-related clinical outcomes relative to the rest of the world.[60] In truth, NH may simply be a controllable response to a variety of stimuli, rather than a pathologic entity. NH can be regarded as a mechanism through which the venous endothelium can be manipulated. Programs designed to provide comprehensive access care, from initial placement, to endovascular intervention are working diligently to more rigorously define the fundamental questions that persist about cellular, genetic, inflammatory, and hemodynamic mechanisms of venous endothelial transformation.

REFERENCES

1. U.S. Renal Data System. USRDS 2009 Annual Data Report: Atlas of Chronic Kidney Disease and End-Stage Renal Disease in the United States. Bethesda, MD, National Institutes of Health, National Institute of Diabetes and Digestive and Kidney Diseases; 2009.
2. Dember LM, Beck GJ, Allon M, et al. Effect of clopidogrel on early failure of arteriovenous fistulas for hemodialysis: a randomized controlled trial. *JAMA*. 2008;299:2164–2171.
3. Dixon BS, Beck GJ, Vazquez MA, et al. Effect of dipyridamole plus aspirin on hemodialysis graft patency. *N Engl J Med*. 2009;360:2191–2201.
4. Chang CJ, Ko PJ, Hsu LA, et al. Highly increased cell proliferation activity in the restenotic hemodialysis vascular access after percutaneous transluminal angioplasty: implication in prevention of restenosis. *Am J Kidney Dis*. 2004;43:74–84.
5. Roy-Chaudhury P, Kelly BS, Miller MA, et al. Venous neointimal hyperplasia in polytetrafluoroethylene dialysis grafts. *Kidney Int*. 2001;59:2325–2334.
6. Roy-Chaudhury P, Arend L, Zhang J, et al. Neointimal hyperplasia in early arteriovenous fistula failure. *Am J Kidney Dis*. 2007;50:782–790.
7. Li L, Terry CM, Shiu YT, Cheung AK. Neointimal hyperplasia associated with synthetic hemodialysis grafts. *Kidney Int*. 2008;74:1247–1261.
8. Roy-Chaudhury P, Sukhatme VP, Cheung AK. Hemodialysis vascular access dysfunction: a cellular and molecular viewpoint. *J Am Soc Nephrol*. 2006;17:1112–1127.
9. Yevzlin AS, Chan MR, Becker YT, Roy-Chaudhury P, Lee T, Becker BN. "Venopathy" at work: recasting neointimal hyperplasia in a new light. *Transl Res*. 2010;156(4): 216–225.
10. Lee T, Roy-Chaudhury P. Advances and new frontiers in the pathophysiology of venous neointimal hyperplasia and dialysis access stenosis. *Adv Chronic Kidney Dis*. 2009;16(5):329–338.
11. Roy-Chaudhury P, Spergel LM, Besarab A, Asif A, Ravani P. Biology of arteriovenous fistula failure. *J Nephrol*. 2007;20:150–163.
12. Mattsson EJ, Kohler TR, Vergel SM, Clowes AW. Increased blood flow induces regression of intimal hyperplasia. *Arterioscler Thromb Vasc Biol*. 1997;17:2245–2249.
13. Weiss MF, Scivittaro V, Anderson JM. Oxidative stress and increased expression of growth factors in lesions of failed hemodialysis access. *Am J Kidney Dis*. 2001;37:970–980.
14. Rectenwald JE, Moldawer LL, Huber TS, Seeger JM, Ozaki CK. Direct evidence for cytokine involvement in neointimal hyperplasia. *Circulation*. 2000;102:1697–1702.
15. Budu-Grajdeanu P, Schugart RC, Friedman A, Valentine C, Agarwal AK, Rovin BH. A mathematical model of venous neointimal hyperplasia formation. *Theor Biol Med Model*. 2008;5:2.
16. Allen KE, Varty K, Jones L, Sayers RD, Bell PR, London NJ. Human venous endothelium can promote intimal hyperplasia in a paracrine manner. *J Vasc Surg*. 1994;19:577–584.
17. Fukasawa M, Matsushita K, Kamiyama M, et al. The methylentetrahydrofolate reductase C677T point mutation is a risk factor for vascular access thrombosis in hemodialysis patients. *Am J Kidney Dis*. 2003;41: 637–642.
18. Heine GH, Ulrich C, Sester U, Sester M, Kohler H, Girndt M. Transforming growth factor beta1 genotype polymorphisms determine AV fistula patency in hemodialysis patients. *Kidney Int*. 2003;64:1101–1107.
19. Lazo-Langner A, Knoll GA, Wells PS, Carson N, Rodger MA. The risk of dialysis access thrombosis is related to the transforming growth factor-beta1 production haplotype and is modified by polymorphisms in the plasminogen activator inhibitor-type 1 gene. *Blood*. 2006;108:4052–4058.
20. Lin CC, Yang WC, Lin SJ, et al. Length polymorphism in heme oxygenase-1 is associated with arteriovenous fistula patency in hemodialysis patients. *Kidney Int*. 2006;69: 165–172.
21. Juncos JP, Tracz MJ, Croatt AJ, et al. Genetic deficiency of heme oxygenase-1 impairs functionality and form of an arteriovenous fistula in the mouse. *Kidney Int*. 2008;74: 47–51.
22. Lin CC, Chang CF, Lai MY, Chen TW, Lee PC, Yang WC. Far-infrared therapy: a novel treatment to improve access blood flow and unassisted patency of arteriovenous fistula in hemodialysis patients. *J Am Soc Nephrol*. 2007;18:985–992.
23. Stracke S, Konner K, Kostlin I, et al. Increased expression of TGF-beta1 and IGF-I in inflammatory stenotic lesions of hemodialysis fistulas. *Kidney Int*. 2001;61:1011–1019.
24. Lee T, Chauhan V, Krishnamoorthy M, Wang Y, Arend L, Mistry MJ, El-Khatib M, Banerjee R, Munda R, Roy-Chaudhury P. Severe venous neointimal hyperplasia prior to dialysis access surgery. *Nephrol Dial Transplant*. 2011;26(7):2264–2270. Epub 2011 Jan 10.

25. Kelly B, Melhem M, Zhang J, et al. Perivascular paclitaxel wraps block arteriovenous graft stenosis in a pig model. *Nephrol Dial Transplant.* 2006;21:2425–2431.

26. Paulson WD KN, Kipiani K, Beridze N, DeVita MV, Shenoy S, Iyer SS. Safety and efficacy of locally eluted sirolimus for prolonging AV graft patency (PTFE graft plus Coll-R)-First in man experience. *J Am Soc Nephrol.* 2008;19:252A.

27. Hoel AW, Conte MS. Edifoligide: a transcription factor decoy to modulate smooth muscle cell proliferation in vein bypass. *Cardiovasc Drug Rev.* 2007;25:221–234.

28. McAllister TN, Maruszewski M, Garrido SA, et al. Effectiveness of haemodialysis access with an autologous tissue-engineered vascular graft: a multicentre cohort study. *Lancet.* 2009;373:1440–1446.

29. Ikeno F, Lyons J, Kaneda H, Baluom M, Benet LZ, Rezaee M. Novel percutaneous adventitial drug delivery system for regional vascular treatment. *Catheter Cardiovasc Interv.* 2004;63:222–230.

30. Kim SJ, Masaki T, Rowley R, Leypoldt JK, Mohammad SF, Cheung AK. Different responses by cultured aortic and venous smooth muscle cells to gamma radiation. *Kidney Int.* 2005;68:371–377.

31. Sun S, Beitler JJ, Ohki T, et al. Inhibitory effect of brachytherapy on intimal hyperplasia in arteriovenous fistula. *J Surg Res.* 2003;115: 200–208.

32. Misra S, Bonan R, Pflederer T, Roy-Chaudhury P. BRAVO I: a pilot study of vascular brachytherapy in polytetrafluoroethylene dialysis access grafts. *Kidney Int* 2006;70:2006–2013.

33. Rifkin BS, Brewster UC, Aruny JE, Perazella MA. Percutaneous balloon cryoplasty: a new therapy for rapidly recurrent anastomotic venous stenoses of hemodialysis grafts? *Am J Kidney Dis.* 2005;45:e27–e32.

34. Rotmans JI, Heyligers JM, Verhagen HJ, et al. In vivo cell seeding with anti-CD34 antibodies successfully accelerates endothelialization but stimulates intimal hyperplasia in porcine arteriovenous expanded polytetrafluoroethylene grafts. *Circulation.* 2005;112:12–18.

35. Ikegaya N, Yamamoto T, Takeshita A, et al. Elevated erythropoietin receptor and transforming growth factor-{beta}1 expression in stenotic arteriovenous fistulae used for hemodialysis. *J Am Soc Nephrol.* 2000:928–935.

36. De Marchi S, Falleti E, Giacomello R, et al. Risk factors for vascular disease and arteriovenous fistula dysfunction in hemodialysis patients. *J Am Soc Nephrol.* 1996;7:1169–1177.

37. Kokubo T, Ishikawa N, Uchida H, et al. CKD accelerates development of neointimal hyperplasia in arteriovenous fistulas. *J Am Soc Nephrol.* 2009;20:1236–1245.

38. Jin D, Ueda H, Takai S, et al. Effect of chymase inhibition on the arteriovenous fistula stenosis in dogs. *J Am Soc Nephrol.* 2005;16:1024–1034.

39. Kizu A, Medici D, Kalluri R. Endothelial-mesenchymal transition as a novel mechanism for generating myofibroblasts during diabetic nephropathy. *Am J Pathol.* 2009;175:1371–1373.

40. Potenta S, Zeisberg E, Kalluri R. The role of endothelial-to-mesenchymal transition in cancer progression. *Br J Cancer.* 2008;99:1375–1379.

41. Zeisberg EM, Potenta S, Xie L, Zeisberg M, Kalluri R. Discovery of endothelial to mesenchymal transition as a source for carcinoma-associated fibroblasts. *Cancer Res.* 2007;67:10123–10128.

42. Zeisberg EM, Tarnavski O, Zeisberg M, et al. Endothelial-to-mesenchymal transition contributes to cardiac fibrosis. *Nat Med.* 2007;13:952–961.

43. Arciniegas E, Carrillo LM, De Sanctis JB, Candelle D. Possible role of NFkappaB in the embryonic vascular remodeling and the endothelial mesenchymal transition process. *Cell Adhes Migr.* 2008;2:17–29.

44. Chang CJ, Chen CC, Hsu LA, et al. Degradation of the internal elastic laminae in vein grafts of rats with aortocaval fistulae: potential impact on graft vasculopathy. *Am J Pathol.* 2009;174:1837–1846.

45. Burke SK FF, LaRochelle A, Mendenhall HV. Local application of recombinant human type 1 pancreatic elastase (PRT-201) to an arteriovenous fistula (AVF) increases AVF blood flow in a rabbit model. *J Am Soc Nephrol.* 2008;19:252A.

46. de Graaf R, Kloppenburg G, Tintu A, et al. The new immunosuppressive agent FK778 attenuates neointima formation in an experimental venous bypass graft model. *Vasc Pharmacol.* 2009;50:83–88.

47. Kloppenburg G, de Graaf R, Grauls G, Bruggeman CA, van Hooff JP, Stassen F. FK778 attenuates cytomegalovirus-enhanced vein graft intimal hyperplasia in a rat model. *Intervirology.* 2009;52:189–195.

48. Eto Y, Shimokawa H, Hiroki J, et al. Gene transfer of dominant negative Rho kinase suppresses neointimal formation after balloon injury in pigs. *Am J Physiol Heart.* 2000;278:1744–1750.

49. Matsumoto Y, Uwatoku T, Oi K, et al. Long-term inhibition of rho-kinase suppresses neointimal formation after stent implantation in porcine coronary arteries: involvement of multiple mechanisms. *Arterioscler Thromb Vasc Biol.* 2004;24:181–186.

50. Sawada N, Itoh H, Ueyama K, et al. Inhibition of rho-associated kinase results in suppression of neointimal formation of balloon-injured arteries. *Circulation.* 2000;101:2030–2033.

51. Shibata R, Kai H, Seki Y, et al. Role of rho-associated kinase in neointima formation after vascular injury. *Circulation.* 2001;103:284–289.

52. Lee P-F, Yeh AT, Bayless KJ. Nonlinear optical microscopy reveals invading endothelial cells anisotropically alter three-dimensional collagen matrices. *Exp Cell Res.* 2009;315:396–410.

53. Liao JKMD, Seto MP, Noma KMDP. Rho kinase (ROCK) inhibitors. *J Cardiovasc Pharmacol.* 2007;50: 17–24.

54. Bone HG, McClung MR, Roux C, et al. Odanacatib, a cathepsin-K Inhibitor for osteoporosis: a two-year study in postmenopausal women with low bone density. *J Bone Miner Res.* 2010;25(5)937–947.

55. Saegusa K, Ishimaru N, Yanagi K, et al. Cathepsin S inhibitor prevents autoantigen presentation and autoimmunity. *J Clin Invest.* 2002;110:361–369.

56. Hyun Jung L, Hye Yeong N, Byung Ha L, Dae Joong K, Jai Young K, Jong-sang P. A novel technique for loading of paclitaxel-PLGA nanoparticles onto ePTFE vascular grafts. *Biotechnol Press.* 2007;23:693–697.

57. Huynh TN, Chacko BK, Teng X, et al. Effects of venous needle turbulence during ex vivo hemodialysis on endothelial morphology and nitric oxide formation. *J Biomech.* 2007;40:2158–2166.

58. Begg M, Mo F-M, OffertÃ¡ler Ls, et al. G protein-coupled endothelial receptor for atypical cannabinoid ligands modulates a Ca^{2+}-dependent K^+ current. *J Biol Chem.* 2003;278:46188–46194.

59. Rajesh M, Mukhopadhyay P, Batkai S, et al. CB2-receptor stimulation attenuates TNF-{alpha}-induced human endothelial cell activation, transendothelial migration of monocytes, and monocyte-endothelial adhesion. *Am J Physiol Heart.* 2007;293:H2210–2218.

60. Rayner HC, Pisoni RL, Gillespie BW, et al. Creation, cannulation and survival of arteriovenous fistulae: data from the Dialysis Outcomes and Practice Patterns Study. *Kidney Int.* 2003;63:323–330.

55

FLOW DYNAMICS, MATURITY, AND ACCESS FAILURE

PRABIR ROY-CHAUDHURY & RUPAK K. BANERJEE

LEARNING OBJECTIVES

1. To understand the central role of hemodynamics in arteriovenous fistula (AVF) maturation.
2. To use this information to develop novel therapies to enhance AVF maturation.

INTRODUCTION

The arteriovenous fistula (AVF) is currently the preferred form of permanent dialysis vascular access due to its superior long-term survival and decreased risk of infection.[1] Despite these advantages, AVFs have very significant problems with maturation (defined as adequate increases in blood flow and diameter to allow them to support adequate hemodialysis). Indeed a recent large National Institutes of Health study documented that 60% of AVFs were not suitable for dialysis between 4 and 5 months postsurgery.[2]

At a radiological level, AVF maturation failure presents as a perianastomotic stenosis (Figure 55-1), while at a histological level, we have described the presence of an aggressive neointimal hyperplasia (Figure 55-2).[3] In addition, at a pathogenetic level, it is likely that the pattern of vascular remodeling (outward or inward) plays a critical role in the determination of final luminal stenosis.[4-6] Thus, the presence of significant neointimal hyperplasia or vessel wall thickening when combined with outward or positive remodeling (upper panel; Figure 55-3a) could in fact result in an increase in luminal diameter (clinically this would result in successful AVF maturation). In marked contrast, even a small amount of neointimal hyperplasia when combined with inward or negative remodeling (lower panel; Figure 55-3b) results in a marked decrease in luminal diameter (clinically this would result in AVF maturation failure). At a pathogenetic level, therefore, AVF maturation failure likely depends on the balance between neointimal hyperplasia and the pattern of vascular remodeling.

Identification of the upstream injury events that could influence both these processes is therefore key to (a) understanding the mechanisms responsible for AVF maturation failure and (b) developing novel therapies for the prevention of AVF maturation failure.[5,7,8] In this context, our group and others have described a number of mediators of vascular injury that could impact on AVF maturation failure. These include hemodynamic stressors, surgical injury, the uremic milieu, and direct cannulation injury.[5] Of these, only hemodynamic stress has the potential to influence both vascular remodeling and neointimal hyperplasia. We believe that a better understanding of the linkages between hemodynamic profiles, neointimal hyperplasia, and vascular remodeling is critical to the future development of novel therapies to prevent AVF maturation failure and this will be the focus of the current chapter.

▶ Blood Flow and Shear Stress Patterns Influence Endothelial Function and Luminal Stenosis

We have known for over 25 years that the pattern of flow has a profound effect on endothelial cell morphology. Thus, Figure 55-4 demonstrates that endothelial cells grown under static flow conditions have a polygonal appearance (Figure 55-4a). When grown under laminar flow conditions, these cells have a stellate appearance and orient themselves in the direction of flow (Figure 55-4b). Finally, when these same cells are grown under turbulent flow conditions, they undergo endothelial cell proliferation and activation.[9,10]

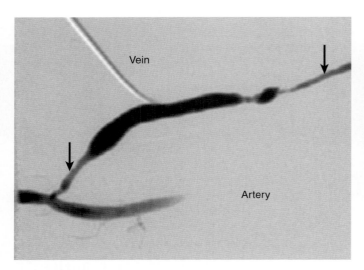

Figure 55-1. Radiology of AVF maturation failure: describes the classical radiological picture of AV fistula maturation failure. Note the tight perianastomotic venous stenoses (arrows) that are responsible for AVF nonmaturation.

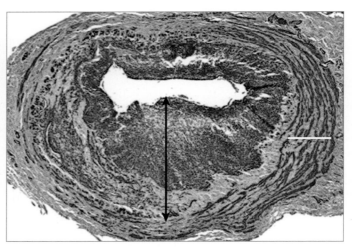

Figure 55-2. Histology of AVF maturation failure: describes the classical histological picture that is seen within the lesions in Figure 55-1 which is an aggressive neointimal hyperplasia (extent of double headed arrow). Note also the presence of some medial hypertrophy. Brown staining for alpha smooth muscle actin. (From Roy-Chaudhury et al. *Am J Kidney Dis.* 2007.)

The most important hemodynamic parameter, however, that likely influences both neointimal hyperplasia and vascular remodeling is hemodynamic shear stress, which in essence is the frictional force per unit area that a fluid exerts as it flows over a surface.[11] At a physical level, shear stress is described by the Poiseuille equation and is directly proportional to flow velocity and inversely proportional to

the third power of the radius. There are two main types of flow and shear stress profiles.

Laminar flow with laminar shear (high values of shear) is described in the right panel of Figure 55-5. In vitro studies suggest that this type of flow and shear profile is associated with endothelial quiescence, the production of prostacyclin and nitric oxide, and a reduction in oxidative

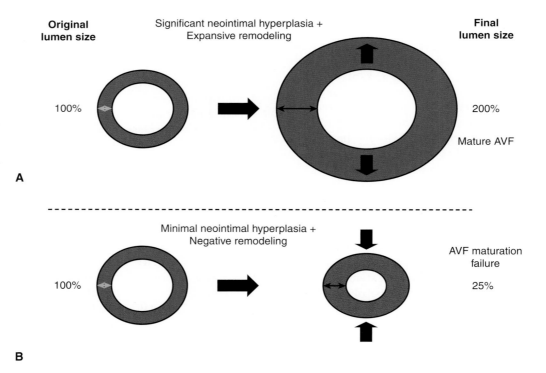

Figure 55-3. Final luminal stenosis is dependent on both neointimal hyperplasia and vascular remodeling: **(A)** documents an increase in lumen size when neointimal hyperplasia is combined with outward vascular remodeling; **(B)** describes a decrease in lumen size when even a small amount of neointimal hyperplasia is combined with inward or negative vascular remodeling. (Adapted from Michael S. Conte MD, UCSF.)

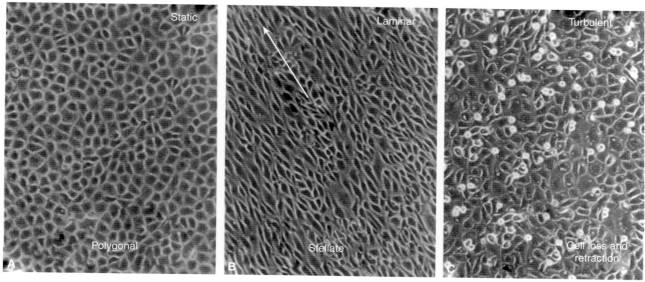

Figure 55-4. Flow patterns and endothelial cell morphology: (**A**) describes the classic polygonal appearance of endothelial cells when grown in culture under static flow conditions; (**B**) documents a stellate morphology when endothelial cells are grown under laminar flow conditions. Note that the cells also orient themselves in the direction of flow (white arrow). Finally, (**C**) shows cell loss and cell retraction under turbulent conditions. (From Davies et al. *PNAS* 1986.)

stress. In marked contrast, disturbed flow (defined as low flow, flow separation, reversed flow, or turbulence) is associated with low or oscillatory shear stress profiles as shown in the left panel of Figure 55-5. In vitro studies suggest that this latter type of flow and shear profile are associated with endothelial activation, reduced production of nitric oxide and prostacyclin, and an increase in oxidative stress.[9-23]

At an in vivo level, laminar flow and shear have been associated with minimal atherosclerosis and neointimal

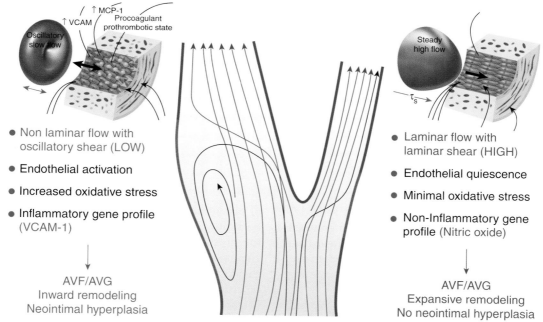

Figure 55-5. Linkages between flow patterns, shear stress, and vascular stenosis: the right panel of the figure describes a laminar flow and shear pattern in the portion of the vessel that is outlined in blue. This flow and shear pattern is in general associated with quiescent endothelial cells, release of nitric oxide, minimal neointimal hyperplasia, and outward remodeling. In contrast the left panel of the figure describes a nonlaminar flow pattern with possible regions of oscillatory shear stress. This flow and shear pattern is in general associated with endothelial cell activation, minimal production of nitric oxide, aggressive neointimal hyperplasia and inward remodeling. (Adapted from Hahn C, Schwartz MA. Mechanotransduction in vascular physiology and atherogenesis. *Nat Rev Mol Cell Biol.* Jan;10(1):53–62.)

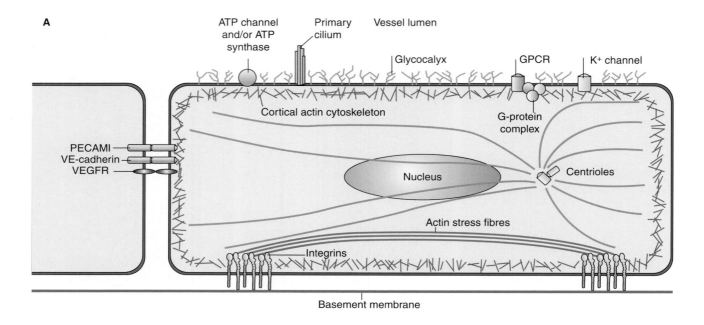

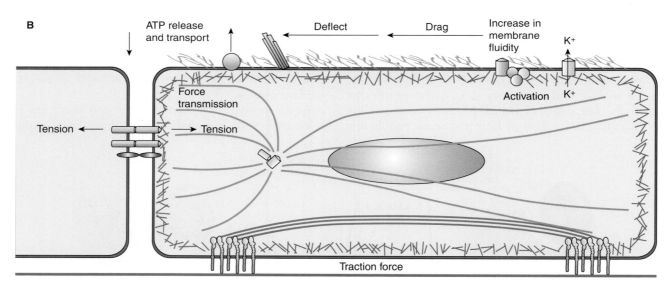

Figure 55-6. Endothelial mechanotransduction pathways: (**A**) describes potential endothelial mechanotransducers that could potentially sense differences in flow and shear stress patterns. These include the glycocalyx, primary cilia, K channels, G proteins, integrins, and ATP complexes; (**B**) documents the changes that occur when these molecules are exposed to fluid shear stress. (From Hahn and Schwartz in *Nat Rev Mol Cell Biol.* 2009.)

hyperplasia and also with outward or positive remodeling, resulting in an absence of luminal stenosis. In contrast, disturbed flow patterns with low or oscillatory shear have been associated in vivo with increased atherosclerosis and neointimal hyperplasia and also with inward remodeling, resulting in luminal stenosis.[18,24–36]

Since the endothelial cell is the cell type, which is exposed to different flow and shear stress profiles, an important question is the mechanism by which the endothelial cell is able to identify differences in flow and shear stress profiles and then convert this into differing signal transduction and cellular activation/quiescence pathways. While the exact mechanisms have not been completely elucidated, we do know that the endothelial cell has an intricate array

of potential surface receptors, which can sense changes in both flow and shear. These include primary cilia, integrins, the glycocalyx, ATP proteins, G proteins, and potassium channels, which when activated by laminar or oscillatory shear can transmit signals to the cytoskeleton and beyond, resulting in either endothelial quiescence or activation (Figure 55-6).[11,37] In addition to direct signal transduction, disturbed flow also results in a greater contact time between cellular elements such as mononuclear cells and potentially activated endothelium, which is already expressing inflammatory adhesion molecules such as E-selectin and vascular cell adhesion molecule (VCAM-1).[38–41] This results in an increased adhesion of inflammatory cells with all the subsequent downstream inflammatory events.

Blood Flow and Shear Stress Profiles in AVFs

The linkages between blood flow, shear stress profiles, and neointimal hyperplasia are not as well defined in the specific setting of AVF. However, we do know that AVF stenoses often occur at swing segments, suggesting that disturbed flow dynamics in these areas could be the initiator of these narrowings.[42] The earliest research in this area was performed by the late Ali Bakran's group in which ex vivo modeling suggested certain sites within an AVF that might be prone to the development of stenoses.[43] More recently, computational fluid dynamic modeling by the Andrea Remuzzi group has identified a number of regions within the anatomical configuration of a standard AVF, which are likely to be exposed to disturbed flow and oscillatory shear stress profiles; even though the overall flow pattern is laminar. Their findings suggest that these regions could be the sites responsible for the initiation of the perianastomotic stenoses that are often responsible for AVF maturation failure.[44] In addition, we have demonstrated that the creation of AVFs in different anatomical configurations (curved versus straight for example) results in very different flow and shear stress profiles.[45,46]

Finally, at a clinical level, a number of studies have established possible linkages between higher intraoperative or immediate postoperative levels of blood flow and maturation success.[47,48] In addition, a meticulous study by Corpataux et al in six patients with a radiocephalic AVF described an immediate increase in shear stress following surgery. This resulted in a compensatory increase in diameter, which returned shear stress levels to normal by 3 months. This study also described an increase in cross-sectional wall area, which was felt to be due to circumferential or tangential strain and not as a result of shear stress changes.[49]

In summary, it is likely that focal regions of disturbed flow and low or oscillatory shear stress are the initiators of endothelial activation, neointimal hyperplasia, and inward remodeling that finally result in the perianastomotic stenoses associated with AVF maturation failure. Initial studies by our group and others suggest that these regions of disturbed flow may be a function of the anatomical configuration of the AVF. In this context, we believe that identification of the "ideal" flow and hemodynamic shear stress profile could perhaps allow us to create future AVFs in an "ideal" anatomical configuration. However, this clearly remains a "work in progress" at the present time.

REFERENCES

1. DOQI. Vascular Access Guidelines. *Am J Kid Dis.* 2006;48:S177–S247.
2. Dember LM, Beck GJ, Allon M, Delmez JA, Dixon BS, Greenberg A, Himmelfarb J, Vazquez MA, Gassman JJ, Greene T, Radeva MK, Braden GL, Ikizler TA, Rocco MV, Davidson IJ, Kaufman JS, Meyers CM, Kusek JW, Feldman HI. Dialysis Access Consortium Study Group. Effect of clopidogrel on early failure of arteriovenous fistulas for hemodialysis: a randomized controlled trial. *JAMA.* 2008;299(18):2164–2171.
3. Roy-Chaudhury P, Arend L, Zhang J, Krishnamoorthy M, Wang Y, Banerjee R, Samaha A, Munda R. Neointimal hyperplasia in early arteriovenous fistula failure. *Am J Kidney Dis.* 2007;50:782–790.
4. Roy-Chaudhury P, Kelly BS, Melhem M, Zhang J, Li J, Desai P, Munda R, Heffelfinger SC. Vascular access in hemodialysis: issues, management, and emerging concepts. *Cardiol Clin.* 2005;23:249–273.
5. Roy-Chaudhury P, Sukhatme VP, Cheung AK. Hemodialysis vascular access dysfunction: a cellular and molecular viewpoint. *J Am Soc Nephrol.* 2006;17:1112–1127.
6. Keren G. Compensatory enlargement, remodeling, and restenosis. *Adv Exp Med Biol.* 1997;430:187–196.
7. Roy-Chaudhury P, Lee TC. Vascular stenosis: biology and interventions. *Curr Opin Nephrol Hypertens.* 2007;16:516–522.
8. Roy-Chaudhury P, Spergel LM, Besarab A, Asif A, Ravani P. Biology of arteriovenous fistula failure. *J Nephrol.* 2007;20:150–163.
9. Dardik A, Chen L, Frattini J, Asada H, Aziz F, Kudo FA, Sumpio BE. Differential effects of orbital and laminar shear stress on endothelial cells. *J Vasc Surg.* 2005;41:869–880.
10. Davies PF, Remuzzi A, Gordon EJ, Dewey CF, Jr., Gimbrone MA, Jr. Turbulent fluid shear stress induces vascular endothelial cell turnover in vitro. *Proc Natl Acad Sci USA.* 1986;83:2114–2117.
11. Hahn C, Schwartz MA. Mechanotransduction in vascular physiology and atherogenesis. *Nat Rev Mol Cell Biol.* 2009;10:53–62.
12. Wasserman SM, Topper JN. Adaptation of the endothelium to fluid flow: in vitro analyses of gene expression and in vivo implications. *Vasc Med.* 2004;9:35–45.
13. Wasserman SM, Mehraban F, Komuves LG, Yang R-B, Tomlinson JE, Zhang Y, Spriggs F, Topper JN. Gene expression profile of human endothelial cells exposed to sustained fluid shear stress. *Physiol Genom.* 2002;12:13–23.
14. Andersson M, Karlsson L, Svensson PA, Ulfhammer E, Ekman M, Jernas M, Carlsson LM, Jern S. Differential global gene expression response patterns of human endothelium exposed to shear stress and intraluminal pressure. *J Vasc Res.* 2005;42:441–452.
15. Ballermann BJ, Dardik A, Eng E, Liu A. Shear stress and the endothelium. *Kidney Int Suppl.* 1998;67:S100–S108.
16. Braddock M, Schwachtgen JL, Houston P, Dickson MC, Lee MJ, Campbell CJ. Fluid shear stress modulation of gene expression in endothelial cells. *News Physiol Sci.* 1998;13:241–246.
17. Chiu JJ, Chen LJ, Chang SF, Lee PL, Lee CI, Tsai MC, Lee DY, Hsieh HP, Usami S, Chien S. Shear stress inhibits smooth muscle cell-induced inflammatory gene expression in endothelial cells: role of NF-kappaB. *Arterioscler Thromb Vasc Biol.* 2005;25:963–969.
18. Hwang J, Saha A, Boo YC, Sorescu GP, McNally JS, Holland SM, Dikalov S, Giddens DP, Griendling KK, Harrison DG, Jo H. Oscillatory shear stress stimulates endothelial production of O_2^- from p47phox-dependent NAD(P)H oxidases, leading to monocyte adhesion. *J Biol Chem.* 2003;278:47291–47298.
19. Wang N, Miao H, Li YS, Zhang P, Haga JH, Hu Y, Young A, Yuan S, Nguyen P, Wu CC, Chien S. Shear stress regulation

of Kruppel-like factor 2 expression is flow pattern-specific. *Biochem Biophys Res Commun.* 2006;341:1244–1251.

20. Berk BC. Atheroprotective signaling mechanisms activated by steady laminar flow in endothelial cells. *Circulation.* 2008;117:1082–1089.

21. Andrews AM, Jaron D, Buerk DG, Kirby PL, Barbee KA. Direct, real-time measurement of shear stress-induced nitric oxide produced from endothelial cells in vitro. *Nitric Oxide.* 2010;23:335–342.

22. Garanich JS, Pahakis M, Tarbell JM. Shear stress inhibits smooth muscle cell migration via nitric oxide-mediated downregulation of matrix metalloproteinase-2 activity. *Am J Physiol Heart Circ Physiol.* 2005;288:H2244–H2252.

23. Dancu MB, Berardi DE, Vanden Heuvel JP, Tarbell JM. Asynchronous shear stress and circumferential strain reduces endothelial NO synthase and cyclooxygenase-2 but induces endothelin-1 gene expression in endothelial cells. *Arterioscler Thromb Vasc Biol.* 2004;24:2088–2094.

24. Berceli SA, Davies MG, Kenagy RD, Clowes AW. Flow-induced neointimal regression in baboon polytetrafluoroethylene grafts is associated with decreased cell proliferation and increased apoptosis. *J Vasc Surg.* 2002;36:1248–1255.

25. Castier Y, Brandes RP, Leseche G, Tedgui A, Lehoux S. p47phox-dependent NADPH oxidase regulates flow-induced vascular remodeling. *Circ Res.* 2005;97:533–540.

26. Glagov S, Zarins C, Giddens DP, Ku DN. Hemodynamics and atherosclerosis. Insights and perspectives gained from studies of human arteries. *Arch Pathol Lab Med.* 1988;112:1018–1031.

27. Guzman RJ, Abe K, Zarins CK. Flow-induced arterial enlargement is inhibited by suppression of nitric oxide synthase activity in vivo. *Surgery.* 1997;122:273–279; discussion 9–80.

28. LaDisa JF Jr, Olson LE, Molthen RC, Hettrick DA, Pratt PF, Hardel MD, Kersten JR, Warltier DC, Pagel PS. Alterations in wall shear stress predict sites of neointimal hyperplasia after stent implantation in rabbit iliac arteries. *Am J Physiol Heart Circ Physiol.* 2005;288:H2465–H2475.

29. Lam CF, Peterson TE, Richardson DM, Croatt AJ, d'Uscio LV, Nath KA, Katusic ZS. Increased blood flow causes coordinated upregulation of arterial eNOS and biosynthesis of tetrahydrobiopterin. *Am J Physiol Heart Circ Physiol.* 2006;290:H786–H793.

30. Lehoux S, Castier Y, Tedgui A. Molecular mechanisms of the vascular responses to haemodynamic forces. *J Intern Med.* 2006;259:381–392.

31. Lehoux S, Tronc F, Tedgui A. Mechanisms of blood flow-induced vascular enlargement. *Biorheology.* 2002;39: 319–324.

32. Mattsson EJ, Kohler TR, Vergel SM, Clowes AW. Increased blood flow induces regression of intimal hyperplasia. *Arterioscler Thromb Vasc Biol.* 1997;17:2245–2249.

33. Meyerson SL, Skelly CL, Curi MA, Shakur UM, Vosicky JE, Glagov S, Schwartz LB, Christen T, Gabbiani G. *J Vasc Surg.* 2001;34(1):90–97. Erratum in: *J Vasc Surg.* 2001;34(4):580.

34. Osterberg K, Mattsson E. Intimal hyperplasia in mouse vein grafts is regulated by flow. *J Vasc Res.* 2005;42:13–20.

35. Tronc F, Wassef M, Esposito B, Henrion D, Glagov S, Tedgui A. Role of NO in flow-induced remodeling of the rabbit common carotid artery. *Arterioscler Thromb Vasc Biol.* 1996;16:1256–1262.

36. Won D, Zhu SN, Chen M, Teichert AM, Fish JE, Matouk CC, Bonert M, Ojha M, Marsden PA, Cybulsky MI. Relative reduction of endothelial nitric-oxide synthase expression and transcription in atherosclerosis-prone regions of the mouse aorta and in an in vitro model of disturbed flow. *Am J Pathol.* 2007;171:1691–1704.

37. Tarbell JM, Pahakis MY. Mechanotransduction and the glycocalyx. *J Intern Med.* 2006;259:339–350.

38. Hinds MT, Park YJ, Jones SA, Giddens DP, Alevriadou BR. Local hemodynamics affect monocytic cell adhesion to a three-dimensional flow model coated with E-selectin. *J Biomech.* 2001;34:95–103.

39. Honda HM, Hsiai T, Wortham CM, Chen M, Lin H, Navab M, Demer LL. A complex flow pattern of low shear stress and flow reversal promotes monocyte binding to endothelial cells. *Atherosclerosis.* 2001;158:385–390.

40. Kim MC, Nam JH, Lee CS. Near-wall deposition probability of blood elements as a new hemodynamic wall parameter. *Ann Biomed Eng.* 2006;34:958–970.

41. Heise M, Kruger U, Ruckert R, Pfitzman R, Neuhaus P, Settmacher U. Correlation of intimal hyperplasia development and shear stress distribution at the distal end-side-anastomosis, in vitro study using particle image velocimetry. *Eur J Vasc Endovasc Surg.* 2003;26: 357–366.

42. Badero OJ, Salifu MO, Wasse H, Work J. Frequency of swing-segment stenosis in referred dialysis patients with angiographically documented lesions. *Am J Kidney Dis.* 2008;51:93–98.

43. Sivanesan S, How TV, Black RA, Bakran A. Flow patterns in the radiocephalic arteriovenous fistula: an in vitro study. *J Biomech.* 1999;32:915–925.

44. Ene-Iordache B, Remuzzi A. Disturbed flow in radial-cephalic arteriovenous fistulae for haemodialysis: low and oscillating shear stress locates the sites of stenosis. *Nephrol Dial Transplant.* 2011;27:358–368.

45. Krishnamoorthy M, Roy-Chaudhury P, Wang Y, Sinha Roy A, Zhang J, Khoury S, Munda R, Banerjee R. Measurement of hemodynamic and anatomic parameters in a swine arteriovenous fistula model. *J Vasc Access.* 2008;9:28–34.

46. Krishnamoorthy MK, Banerjee RK, Wang Y, Zhang J, Roy AS, Khoury SF, Arend LJ, Rudich S, Roy-Chaudhury P. Hemodynamic wall shear stress profiles influence the magnitude and pattern of stenosis in a pig AV fistula. *Kidney Int.* 2008;74:1410–1419.

47. Wong V, Ward R, Taylor J, Selvakumar S, How TV, Bakran A. Factors associated with early failure of arteriovenous fistulae for haemodialysis access. *Eur J Vasc Endovasc Surg.* 1996;12:207–213.

48. Berman SS, Mendoza B, Westerband A, Quick RC. Predicting arteriovenous fistula maturation with intraoperative blood flow measurements. *J Vasc Access.* 2008;9:241–247.

49. Corpataux JM, Haesler E, Silacci P, Ris HB, Hayoz D. Low-pressure environment and remodelling of the forearm vein in Brescia-Cimino haemodialysis access. *Nephrol Dial Transplant.* 2002;17:1057–1062.

56

NEOINTIMAL HYPERPLASIA

TIMMY LEE & DAVINDER WADEHRA

INTRODUCTION

Neointimal hyperplasia is defined as the thickening of the tunica intima secondary to the response to vascular injury. Neointimal hyperplasia is a pathologic lesion seen in a number of disease processes including coronary artery disease (CAD) and lower extremity peripheral vascular disease (PAD), and remains central to the pathology of vein graft restenosis in these disease processes. The vein is the gold standard for vascular graft conduits in CAD and Peripheral Vascular Disease (PVD). Vein grafts adapt to the arterial environment, "arterialization," by limiting formation of neointimal hyperplasia, which characterized histologically by vessel wall thickening with the deposition of smooth muscle cells (SMC) and extracellular matrix (ECM) in all layers of the vein, but particularly within the intima.[1-3] Abnormal vessel wall remodeling in response to high vessel wall sheer stress may lead to excessive neointimal hyperplasia.[4-6] Recent reports have shown that 20% to 50% of saphenous vein grafts in cardiovascular disease (CVD) are complicated by abnormal remodeling, which leads to vein graft thrombosis and eventual failure.[7,8]

Hemodialysis vascular access dysfunction shares similar clinical and pathological characteristics to CAD and PAD. The major cause of hemodialysis vascular access dysfunction in native arteriovenous fistulas (AVF) and polytetrafluoroethylene (PTFE) arteriovenous grafts (AVG) is venous stenosis due to aggressive neointimal hyperplasia (Figure 56-1).[9-13] Unlike CAD and PVD, there has been a lack of basic and translational research focusing on neointimal hyperplasia in the setting of hemodialysis vascular access dysfunction. Consequently, because of the poor understanding of the pathogenesis of neointimal hyperplasia in vascular access dysfunction, there are currently few effective treatments for this important clinical problem. However, AVFs and AVGs, due to their superficial location and frequent use and follow-up, may be the ideal model to test novel therapies for neointimal hyperplasia with future applications to other clinical conditions characterized by neointimal hyperplasia such as CAD, PVD, and postangioplasty restenosis.[9,13]

This remainder of this chapter will primarily focus on hemodialysis vascular access dysfunction and will (1) discuss the pathology of hemodialysis vascular access dysfunction in AVF and AVG, (2) review the pathogenesis and novel mechanisms of neointimal hyperplasia formation in hemodialysis vascular access, (3) discuss current and novel therapies in to treat neointimal hyperplasia in hemodialysis vascular access dysfunction, and (4) explore future areas for clinical and translational research.

PATHOLOGY OF VASCULAR ACCESS DYSFUNCTION

▶ Neointimal Hyperplasia in AVF and AVG Dysfunction

In AVFs, the two main etiologies of failure are an initial failure to mature (early failure) followed by a subsequent venous stenosis (late failure). The pathology of late AVF stenosis, venous neointimal hyperplasia, has been shown

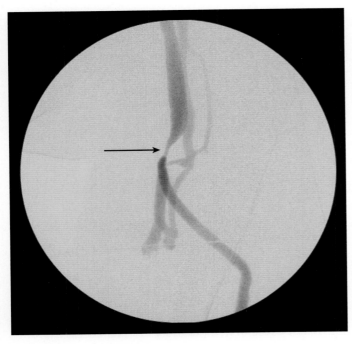

Figure 56-1. Angiogram of PTFE graft with venous stenosis at the vein-graft anastomosis.

significant research interest as a multicenter randomized, controlled, clinical trial reported that 60% of AVFs placed failed to mature for dialysis[16] and other studies have shown a steady increase in recent years (Figure 56-2). The pathology of early AVF failures (nonmaturation) has recently also been demonstrated to be secondary to aggressive venous neointimal hyperplasia with the majority of cells within the neointima staining for myofibroblasts (Figure 56-3).[12] While venous neointimal hyperplasia is the most common lesion in AVF stenosis, arterial inflow stenosis, likely from arterial calcification[17–19] and intimal hyperplasia,[20,21] has been reported to occur at significant rates.[22–28] The location of venous stenoses differs by type of AVFs placed in both early and late AVF failures. Radiocephalic fistulas most commonly fail due to a stenosis within the perianastomotic region (arterial anastomosis and juxta-anastomotic areas combined), while brachiocephalic fistulas often have narrowings at the juxta-anastomosis (portion of the AVF immediately adjacent to the arterial anastomosis).[29] More proximal stenoses can also occur in both cases especially in the case of brachiocephalic fistulas (cephalic arch stenosis).[26,29]

In AVGs, venous stenosis occurs most commonly at the graft-vein and juxta-anastomotic vein segments (Figure 56-1), but recent data suggest that stenosis at the graft–artery anastomosis also occurs frequently.[30] Venous stenosis in AVGs most commonly arises from progressive neointimal hyperplasia, characterized by the presence of alpha smooth muscle cells, myofibroblasts, and an abundance of extracellular matrix components within the neointima.[10,31–33] Angiogenesis (neovascularization) within the adventitia and macrophage layer, lining the perigraft region, are also present

to be similar to AVGs and composed primarily of alpha smooth muscle actin positive cells, together with expression of mediators and cytokines such as transforming growth factor beta (TGF-β), platelet-derived growth factor (PDGF), and endothelin within the media and intima of the vein.[14,15] Early AVF failure has been recent area of

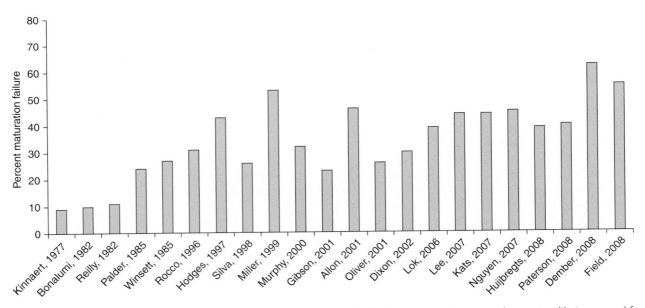

Figure 56-2. Comparison of AVF nonmaturation rates from 1997 to 2008. AVF nonmaturation rates have steadily increased from 1977 to 2008.

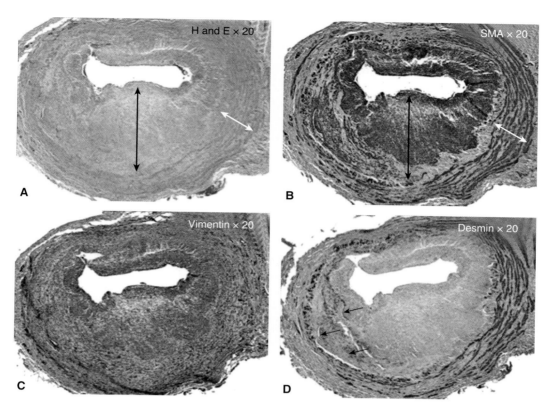

Figure 56-3. A–D, describe H and E (A), SMA (B), vimentin (C), and desmin (D) stains on sequential sections of the venous segment of an AVF with maturation failure. Note the very significant degree of neointimal hyperplasia (black double headed arrows in A and B) with relatively less medial hypertrophy (white double headed arrows in A and B). Note also that while most of the cells within the region of neointimal hyperplasia appear to be SMA +ve, vimentin +ve, desmin −ve myofibroblasts, there are also some SMA +ve, desmin +ve contractile smooth muscle cells present within the neointima (small black arrows in D). +ve, Positive; −ve, negative. (Adapted from Roy-Chaudhury et al. *Am J Kidney Dis* 2008 with permission from Elsevier Inc.)

in AVGs, which is major difference from venous stenosis in AVFs.[10,34] An increased expression of mediators and cytokines such as TGF-β, PDGF, and endothelin within the media, neointima, and adventitia is also present in AVGs.[15,32]

▶ Cellular Phenotypes of Neointimal Cells

While contractile smooth muscle cells, myofibroblasts, fibroblasts, and macrophages all play an important role in the pathogenesis of vascular access dysfunction, the majority of cells that comprise the neointimal lesion (both in AVFs and in AVGs) are myofibroblasts.[31] These cells specifically express vimentin and alpha smooth muscle actin but not markers such as desmin and smoothelin.[14] However, it remains unknown whether these myofibroblasts are fibroblasts that have transformed, migrating from the adventitia, that develop a smooth muscle cell actin expression to become myofibroblasts, or contractile smooth muscle cells migrating from the media which lose desmin expression and acquire vimentin expression. However, targeting of myofibroblasts, rather than fibroblasts or contractile smooth muscle cells, could serve as future novel therapies for hemodialysis access stenosis.

PATHOGENESIS AND NOVEL MECHANISMS OF NEOINTIMAL HYPERPLASIA FORMATION IN HEMODIALYSIS VASCULAR ACCESS DYSFUNCTION

▶ Cascade of Events in the Pathogenesis of Vascular Access Stenosis: Upstream and Down Stream Events

The pathogenesis of venous neointimal hyperplasia in AVG stenosis and late AVF stenosis has been well described and involves a number of events that are best divided and explained as upstream and downstream events.[13,35] Upstream events are the initial events and insults that are responsible for endothelial injury, which lead to a cascade of mediators (downstream events) that regulate endothelial dysfunction, oxidative stress, and inflammation and result ultimately in venous neointimal hyperplasia. Upstream events that are believed to contribute to the pathogenesis of neointimal hyperplasia include:[9,13] (1) surgical trauma at the time of AV surgery, causing vasospasm, ischemia, and hemodynamic changes to the vessel,[36,37] (2) hemodynamic shear stress at the vein–artery or vein–graft anastomosis, resulting low sheer stress, turbulence, and compliance mismatch,[38–40] (3) bioincompatibility of the AVG, causing recruitment of inflammatory cells,[41–44] (4) vessel injury due to dialysis needle punctures,[45] (5) uremia resulting in endothelial dysfunction,[46,47] and (6) repeated balloon angioplasties causing additional endothelial injury.[48,49] Downstream events represent the response to endothelial and vascular injury from upstream events, resulting in the migration of smooth muscle cells from the media to the intima, eventually forming the lesion of venous neointimal hyperplasia.

The pathogenesis of early AVF failure (nonmaturation) still remains poorly understood. Clinically, AVF nonmaturation is seen as early stenosis/thrombosis on physical exam or angiography, poor access flow, or the inability to successfully cannulate with two needles for hemodialysis. At a histological level, there is aggressive neointimal hyperplasia in both animal and human models.[12,50–52] The underlying upstream events, which may contribute to early AVF failure, include: (1) small diameter sizes in the vein and artery,[53–56] (2) surgical injury at the time AVF placement, resulting in adventitial damage and tissue hypoxia,[36,57] (3) previous venipunctures,[45] (4) development of accessory veins after surgery,[58–62] (5) hemodynamic shear stress at the AV anastomosis,[38,39,63,64] (6) genetic predisposition to vascular constriction and neointimal hyperplasia,[65,66] and (7) preexisting venous neointimal hyperplasia.[67–71]

A future paradigm for treatment of vascular access dyfunction could include therapies that simultaneously target "upstream" vascular injury (hemodynamics) and "downstream" events.

▶ Novel Downstream Mechanisms of Neointimal Hyperplasia: Oxidative Stress, Inflammation, Endothelial Dysfunction, and Alternative Origins for Neointimal Cells

The subsequent section will focus on specific downstream events and mechanisms responsible for neointimal hyperplasia organized into three thematic areas with potential targets for therapy: (1) oxidative stress, (2) inflammation, (3) endothelial dysfunction, and (4) alternative origins for neointimal cells.

Oxidative stress

Oxidative stress is defined as a disturbance in the equilibrium between antioxidants and prooxidants, with increased levels of prooxidants resulting in tissue damage.[72] Prooxidants are reactive species (RS) that can be divided into reactive nitrogen species (RNS) and reactive oxygen species (ROS). RS are free radicals that cause oxidative damage due to their unpaired electrons.[73] While RS are necessary for fundamental processes such as cell growth and signaling, an excessive production of RNS and ROS leads to damage of biomolecules.[73] ROS species generated in the vascular wall can directly stimulate vascular smooth muscle cell proliferation and migration, and

enhance the production of proinflammatory cytokines. In conditions of increased oxidative stress, the superoxide anion produced by the nicotinamide adenine dinucleotide phosphate-oxidase (NADPH) oxide can quickly react with the nitric oxide (NO). This decreased availability of nitric oxide, along with endothelial and smooth muscle dysfunction, along with maladaptive remodeling, has been shown to result in increased atherogenicity in cardiovascular diseases[74] and vein graft neointimal hyperplasia in CAD and PVD.

Many of the upstream mechanisms described earlier (specifically hemodynamic shear stress and angioplasty injury) have been documented to result in an increase in the production of free radicals and its downstream products nitrotyrosine and peroxynitrate. Peroxynitrate, generated by the reaction of ROS with NO, is a potent upregulator of the matrix metalloproteinases (MMPs),[75,76] which are key enzymes that cause breakdown of extracellular matrix proteins such as collagen and elastin, facilitate the migration of vascular smooth muscle cells (VSMCs) in neointimal hyperplasia formation.[77] Paradoxically, the same mechanisms have also been shown to facilitate a beneficial dilatation of the feeding artery (through a breakdown of the internal elastic laminae and adaptive vessel remodeling) in both rabbit and mouse AVF models.[78,79] Experimental studies of AVGs in porcine models have demonstrated a differential upregulation of MMP-2 at the graft-vein anastomosis, with early expression (9 days) in the adventitia and a later expression (19 days) within the intima, supporting the concept of cellular migration from the adventitia to the intima (see section on alternative mechanisms below).[80] Furthermore, linkages between hemodynamic shear stress and the expression of oxidative stress markers and cytokines in a porcine model of AVG stenosis have also been reported.[81] In experimental models of AVFs in mouse and rats, MMP-2 and MMP-9 expression was increased at the site of venous stenosis compared to controls.[82,83] Clinical studies of stenotic and thrombotic AVGs and AVFs requiring revision, have described an upregulation of MMPs,[84] and have also documented that the colocalization of oxidative stress markers with inflammatory cytokines such as TGF-β, and PDGF[15] within the neointima of stenotic AVGs and AVFs.

HO-1 is an important enzyme pathway which has been shown to confer protective effects in the vascular endothelium and other organ systems through its antioxidant, antiinflammatory, and antiproliferative actions and properties.[85] A recent study has described an increase in both the magnitude of AVF stenosis and the frequency of thrombosis following the creation of AVFs in HO-1 knockout mice as compared to wild-type animals.[86,87] Furthermore, in the HO-1 knockout mice, there was significant induction of MMP-9 expression in the vein at 1 week compared to wild-type mice, suggesting that MMP expression in vascular tissue and its deleterious effects with regard to promoting cellular migration may be in part be inhibited by HO-1. In a clinical study evaluating gene polymorphisms of HO-1, a higher frequency of AVF failure has been demonstrated in patients with HO-1 gene polymorphisms with long GT repeats (resulting in increased oxidative stress).[65]

Systemic antioxidant therapies have been shown to decrease cardiovascular events in End Stage Renal Disease (ESRD) patients but not in the general population.[88] Treatment with MMP inhibitors has been shown to reduce neointimal hyperplasia in human saphenous veins through reduction in levels of MMP-2 and MMP-9.[89] In regards to vascular access, oral MMP inhibitors have been evaluated in porcine AVG models and shown to reduce neointimal hyperplasia at the graft-vein anastomosis.[77] Finally in animal models, N-acetylcysteine (NAC), an antioxidant has been demonstrated to reduce neointimal hyperplasia in arteries after balloon angioplasty interventions,[90] but there are no clinical studies to date evaluating NAC therapy in vascular access stenosis.

Inflammation

In vein-graft models of CVD and PVD, leukocyte recruitment and the inflammatory response, following placement of the vein-graft, play an important role in vein-graft adaptation.[57] Chronic inflammation within the vein-graft wall is initiated by leukocytes attaching to the endothelial surface and migrating into the graft vessel wall mediated by adherence molecules such as monocyte chemotactic protein (MCP)-1,[91] inflammatory cell adhesion molecule (ICAM),[92,93] Mac-1 (CD11b/CD18),[94] and glycoproteinIbα.[95] The degree of leukocyte migration has been shown to be associated with the level of neointimal thickness the vein graft develops.[96] Leukocyte recruitment is accelerated by cytokines secreted from cells in the graft wall and leukocytes themselves, such as IL-8, IL-1, IL-6, and tumor necrosis factor (TNF-α) in association with ROS and growth factors.[97] Furthermore, recruitment of the surrounding cells and adventitial inflammation also play important roles in neointimal development.[36,98]

There is paucity of data evaluating the role of inflammation in dialysis access in both animal models and clinical studies. In a rat model of AVF, marked upregulation of proinflammatory genes as MCP-1, plasminogen activator inhibitor-1, and endothelin-1, 2 weeks after the creation of AVF was reported, and increased expression of TGF-β1 at 16 weeks.[99] These changes were accompanied by progressive neointimal hyperplasia in variable degrees by 5 weeks after creation of AVF, and by 16 weeks, such neointimal hyperplasia was pronounced.[99] Further support for the role of inflammation in vascular access stenosis comes from a recent study that showed marked upregulation of monocyte chemoattractant protein-1 (MCP-1) in the venous segment of AVF compared to rats deficient in the MCP-1 gene.[100] In clinical studies, the presence of inflammatory cells (macrophages and lymphocytes), cytokines such as TGF-β and insulin-like growth factor-1 (IGF-1), and their association with the magnitude of neointimal hyperplasia within stenotic AVFs has been described.[101]

In AVGs, local bioincompatibility to PTFE graft material likely plays an important role in the inflammatory process. In vitro studies have demonstrated that conditioned media obtained after the interaction of peripheral blood mononuclear cells (PBMCs) with PTFE graft material resulted in a significant upregulation of smooth muscle cell proliferation as compared to control media.[102] This smooth muscle cell proliferation likely occurs as result of accumulation of T-lymphocytes which release cytokines such as TNF-α that stimulate smooth muscle proliferation and fibroblast migration.[103,104] This proliferative response has been shown to attenuated by TNF-α inhibitors.[105] In addition, it has also been reported that macrophages line PTFE graft material in both experimental and clinical AVG stenosis with coexpression of inflammatory cytokines such as basic fibroblast growth factor (bFGF).[14,33] These data suggest that inflammatory cytokines produced by macrophages also likely to play a role in the pathogenesis of neointimal hyperplasia. Recently, calcification within AVGs has been reported which may play a role in vascular access stenosis,[106] but this mechanism needs further evaluation.

There are currently no therapies targeting inflammatory pathways in dialysis access stenosis. Given the known role of inflammation in the development of neointimal hyperplasia, suppression of the immune response is a theoretical target in the treatment of progressive neointimal hyperplasia. In dialysis access, there have been no published experimental or clinical studies evaluating suppression of inflammation to treat neointimal hyperplasia. However, a number of experimental models in vein-grafts for CAD and PVD, evaluating anti-inflammatory therapies such as vaccinia virus protein,[107] flavonoid,[108] FK778,[109] and mTOR inhibitors such as rapamycin,[110-112] have shown attenuation of neointimal hyperplasia.

Endothelial dysfunction

NO is an important player in the prevention of vein-graft failure as it plays a critical role in vasodilatation, antiplatelet activity, and neointimal hyperplasia.[113] An intact and functional endothelium is absolutely necessary for a vessel to properly respond to acute changes in blood flow,[114] such that occurs in vein-graft and dialysis accesses, and NO is an important mediator responsible for these transformations.[115] Transition to an arterial environment with its higher wall shear stress injures the vein-graft endothelium and induces cell apoptosis with subsequent cell proliferation.[116] Physiologic NO is created by healthy endothelial cells via endothelial NOS (eNOS) at the venous levels of shear stress. In the initial stages of vein-graft adaptation, the concentration of NO is physiologically low to preserve the venous identity, and to protect the vascular wall from platelet-derived vasoactive substance and inflammatory responses, as well as to promote smooth muscle cell relaxation.[117,118] Over time, the arterialized condition disrupts venous tissue homeostasis and NO production (lower production) because of endothelial injury.[57] NO limits neointimal hyperplasia by inhibiting proliferation of smooth muscle cells.[119] Increasing levels of NO have been associated with reducing neointimal hyperplasia in vein-grafts.[120–123]

In hemodialysis patients, the presence of uremia has been shown to exacerbate endothelial dysfunction, possibly through the pathways of inflammation and oxidative stress described above.[124,125] In the specific context of dialysis access stenosis, a recent experimental study in mice with AVF, Chronic Kidney Disease (CKD)-created mice (by renal ablation) had accelerated development of neointimal hyperplasia at the Arteriovenous (AV) anastomosis compared to control non-CKD mice with AVF placed.[47] Another study has also demonstrated increased neointimal hyperplasia in the venous limb of AVF in rats with subnephrectomy.[126] This same group also demonstrated that administration of NG-nitro-L-arginine methyl ester (L-NAME), an inhibitor of NOS activity, in experimental models increased neointimal hyperplasia in the venous segment of AVF,[126] likely because asymmetrical dimethylarginine (ADMA), an endogenous inhibitor of NO, accumulates in uremic milieu, leading to an accelerated progression of venous neointimal hyperplasia.[126]

In humans, ADMA has been implicated as an important contributor to endothelial dysfunction.[127,128] ADMA is not excreted in ESRD patients and its levels have been reported to be two to six times higher in this patient population as compared to nonuremic individuals.[128] In a recent study by Wu et al, patients with elevated ADMA levels at the time of percutaneous transluminal angioplasty of an initial AVF stenosis had a significantly increased risk of a recurrent AVF stenosis.[129]

To date, there are no experimental or clinical studies evaluating NO therapies in dialysis access dysfunction. In experimental vein-graft models evaluating saphenous veins, NO-donating aspirin (NO-ASA) has shown promising results in inhibiting neointimal hyperplasia.[122,123]

Alternative origins of neointimal cells

The traditional paradigm for the pathogenesis of neointimal hyperplasia stresses the migration of smooth muscle cells from the media to the intima (through the internal elastic lamina) that undergo a change from a contractile to secretory phenotype (de-differentiation), accompanied by further proliferation and sustained extracellular matrix and fibrous protein and deposition.[1,130] However, a number of groups have reported that following coronary angioplasty or saphenous vein bypass grafting there is also a migration of cells (fibroblasts) from the adventitia, through the media, and into the intima, where these cells transform into "myofibroblasts."[131–133]

In dialysis access, several studies in AVGs, similar to cardiovascular models, have supported the concept of a migration of adventitial cells into the intima where they contribute to final neointimal volume.[32,134] In addition, recent data from experimental AVF stenosis models have shown that smooth muscle cells in the neointima, may in part, originate from bone marrow-derived cells that bind to the site of vascular injury and later differentiate into a smooth muscle cell phenotype in the neointima.[75,135,136]

From a therapeutic standpoint, a more complete understanding about the true source of neointimal cells will help direct novel therapies. The failure of antiproliferative therapies to reduce neointimal hyperplasia in clinical trials is likely due to these therapies inability to target these extrinsic cells.

Hemodynamics and vascular remodeling

In vein grafts, when transplanted into an arterial environment, venous tissue is immediately exposed to intense pulsatile stretch forces and wall sheer stress. These wall stretch forces induce cell apoptosis and results in cellular proliferation.[57,116] In dialysis access, creation of the AV anastomosis may result in hemodynamic stresses at the vein-graft or artery-vein anastomosis with turbulent, low flow, and low and oscillatory-shear stress systems predisposing to neointimal hyperplasia.[39,63,64,137] Substantial vascular remodeling and vasodilatation is required for an AV access to become functional for dialysis.

The pattern (vasoconstriction or vasodilatation) of vessel remodeling may play the most important role in hemodialysis vascular access dysfunction. For example, a small amount of neointimal hyperplasia in the presence of a lack of vasodilatation, or adverse remodeling, could produce a significant venous stenosis. Alternatively, the presence of significant neointimal hyperplasia may not cause venous stenosis in the setting of adequate vasodilatation, positive remodeling (Figure 56-4). While the precise factors associated with adverse remodeling are unknown, adventitial angiogenesis and scar formation have shown to play a role in CAD and PVD models.[138,139] Therefore, the ideal therapy to treat vascular stenosis would block adverse remodeling and proliferation of neointimal hyperplasia and promote vasodilatation.

TRANSLATING SCIENCE TO THERAPIES IN HEMODIALYSIS VASCULAR ACESSS DYSFUNCTION: FROM THE BENCH TO BEDSIDE

Understanding the pathology and pathophysiology of hemodialysis vascular access dysfunction described in the previous sections may allow for targeting of specific mechanistic pathways for further investigation and identify potential therapies to prevent and treat vascular access stenosis. At the current time, there are few therapies that effectively treat hemodialysis vascular access dysfunction.

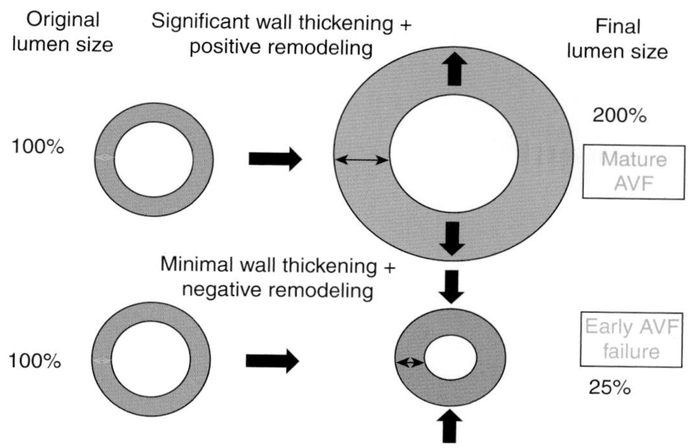

Figure 56-4. Vascular remodeling versus vessel wall thickening: The top panel shows a marked increase in lumen size following creation of an AVF because of vascular dilatation, despite significant vessel wall thickening/neointimal hyperplasia. In marked contrast the bottom panel documents that even a small amount of vessel wall thickening/neointimal hyperplasia can result in a marked reduction of lumen size if this thickening is accompanied by negative vascular remodeling or vasoconstriction. (Adapted from Lee et al. *Adv Chronic Kidney Dis* 2009 with permission from Elsevier Inc.)

▶ Systemic Therapies

There has been significant interest in using systemic agents that have the ability to block smooth muscle cell proliferation and migration. Recently, two randomized controlled trials, as part of the Dialysis Access Consortium (DAC) sponsored by the National Institutes of Health, evaluating antiplatelet agents in AVG and AVF to prevent neointimal hyperplasia were published.[16,140] In the DAC AVG study, dipyridamole and aspirin, modestly reduced the risk of stenosis and improved primary unassisted patency.[140] In the DAC AVF study, clopidogrel reduced frequency of early thrombosis but did not improve AVF suitability defined as successful cannulation with two needles, minimum dialysis blood flow of 300 mL/min, successful AVF use 8/12 dialysis sessions, and use after 120 days from creation.[16] While these two studies have shown some promising results, the clinical significance of these drugs used as standard treatment for hemodialysis access stenosis remains questionable.

Fish oil has shown to prevent AVG stenosis and thrombosis in a randomized, controlled trial.[141] Currently, another study evaluating fish oil and AVG stenosis and thrombosis is ongoing.[142] Other systemic agents, which have shown potential antiproliferative effects targeting neointimal hyperplasia in CVD or PVD models, include peroxisome proliferation-activated receptor γ agonist,[143–145] sirolimus,[146] and imatinib mesylate.[145,147,148]

▶ Radiation Therapy

There has been interest and significant research in recent years on the use of radiation for inhibition of neointimal hyperplasia because of its potent antiproliferative effect on smooth muscle cells, endothelial cells, and macrophages,[149,150] mediated primarily by irradiation-induced vascular cell apoptosis,[37,151] and beneficial effects on vessel wall vasodilatation.[152] Clinical trials in CAD have shown that intracoronary radiation is effective for treatment of coronary restenosis postangioplasty.[153,154] While studies in animals[155–157] and early clinical trials,[158,159] which have shown reduction in neointimal hyperplasia in dialysis access, recent larger clinical trials have not demonstrated significant reduction in neointimal hyperplasia in AVF or AVG.[160,161]

▶ Local Biological Delivery Therapies

Local therapies may be the most beneficial and effective way to successfully modulate the upstream and downstream events involved in the pathology and pathogenesis of dialysis access dysfunction and deliver drugs to the direct site where venous stenosis occurs. The advantages and rationale behind local therapies in dialysis access,[9,13] specifically perivascular therapy, are that (1) local drug delivery targets the adventitia and may block adventitial activation and fibroblast migration, (2) small amounts of potentially toxic drugs can be delivered to the site of stenosis without concerns of systemic toxicity, and (3) this therapy be an ideal model for testing perivascular therapies in other diseases such as CAD and PVD because these therapies can be applied at the time of surgery.

Perivascular therapies in dialysis

Paclitaxel-eluting wraps Paclitaxel inhibits cell division by stabilizing the mitotic spindle.[162] In animal models of dialysis access AVGs, perivascular delivery of paclitaxel at the vein-graft anastomoses has shown to inhibit neointimal hyperplasia.[163–165] A recent multicenter clinical trial evaluating paclitaxel eluting wrap therapy, "Vascular Wrap™" (Angiotech Pharmaceuticals, Inc.; Vancouver, British Columbia, Canada), in AVGs was suspended due to high rates of infection in the paclitaxel-treated group (Figure 56-5). An alternative antiproliferative therapy is the use of sirolimus eluting COLL-R® wraps (Covalon Technologies Ltd: Mississauga, Ontario, Canada). An initial phase II study demonstrated primary unassisted AVG patency of 75% and 38% at 1 and 2 years, respectively, with these wraps.[166]

Endothelial cell-loaded gel foam wraps Endothelial cells produce a number of beneficial mediators such as NO and prostacyclin. In dialysis access, porcine models of AVGs and AVFs, where endothelial cells lined around the vein-graft or vein-artery anastomosis, have shown beneficial effects in vasodilatation.[167,168] In a recent phase I/II clinical trial in hemodialysis patients evaluating allogeneic aortic endothelial cells ("Vascugel") wraps (Pervasis Therapeutics, Cambridge, MA) in AVFs and AVGs at the venous and arterial anastomosis demonstrated safety

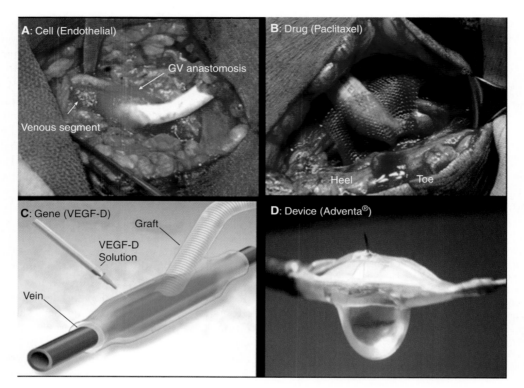

Figure 56-5. Novel local therapies for dialysis access stenosis: (**A**) shows an endothelial cell-loaded gel-foam wrap being placed around the graft-vein anastomosis and proximal venous segment; (**B**) describes the placement of a paclitaxel eluting wrap around the graft-vein anastomosis; (**C**) shows a diagrammatic representation of the biodegradable reservoir that will be used for VEGF-D gene therapy. (**D**) shows a magnified view of the Adventa® catheter that can deliver therapies to the perivascular region through an endovascular approach. (Adapted from Lee et al. *Adv Chronic Kidney Dis* 2009 with permission from Elsevier Inc.)

and feasibility (Figure 56-5).[14] A larger multicenter trial phase III clinical trial is planned in AVGs in the near future.

Gene therapy Vascular endothelial cell growth factor (VEGF) is a subfactor of growth factors that induces endothelial cell proliferation and migration.[169] In experimental models of angioplasty-induced restenosis, the delivery of adenoviral particles encoding for VEGF-C to the site of stenosis has been demonstrated to release NO and prostacyclin and limit neointimal hyperplasia development.[170] In clinical studies in dialysis access, Trinam® (Ark Therapeutics, United Kingdom), a combination of a vascular endothelial growth factor (VEGF-D) gene packaged in an adenoviral vector (Ad 5) and a biodegradable local drug delivery device (Figure 56-5), applied at the vein-graft anastomosis in AVGs in a phase IIb study was initiated in 2009 but terminated in 2010 due to poor patient enrollment.

Recent studies using decoy oligodeoxynucleotide, which binds and inactivates the pivotal cell-cycle transcription factor E2F, which regulates a dozen cell-cycle genes, have shown that intraoperative transfection of human bypass vein grafts with E2F-decoy is safe, feasible, and can achieve sequence-specific inhibition of cell-cycle gene expression and DNA replication.[113,171] Randomized trials in PVD (PREVENT I)[172] and CAD (PREVENT II)[173] vein grafting

testing E2F gene therapy showed good safety, transfection efficiency, and fewer occlusions or revisions in the treatment group. However, subsequent, large, multicenter trials, phase III trials, PREVENT III,[174] and PREVENT IV[175] revealed that E2F decoy (edifoligide) was no more effective than placebo in preventing stenosis in vein-grafts for CAD and PVD. In dialysis access, a randomized, controlled, multicenter phase II clinical trial in AVF grafts using E2F decoy (PREVENT V) was initiated in 2004 but terminated in 2005.

Recombinant elastase therapy Elastases modify the extracellular matrix of blood vessels, leading to immediate and persistent vessel enlargement (in veins and arteries) and increases in blood flow. PRT-201 (Proteon Therapeutics, Inc., Waltham, MA) is a recombinant elastase and has been demonstrated in experimental models to produce increased arterial and venous vasodilatation in AVFs.[176] Currently, a phase II study in humans is ongoing in AVFs and AVGs.

▶ **Endovascular Therapies**

Percutaneous transluminal angioplasty

The current standard treatment for AVF and AVF stenosis is primarily percutaneous transluminal angioplasty (PTA). Initial success rates, when measuring primary patency, to treat stenosis and thrombosis in AVF and AVGs have been very good[26,27,62,177,178] but have poor long-term outcomes. However, vessel injury occurs after the PTA (in CAD models) that leads to further development of neointimal hyperplasia and restenosis.[2,3,48,179,180] In dialysis access, in AVFs that required angioplasty for stenosis, markedly increased cellular proliferation and activity has been seen histologically in postangioplasty restenotic lesions.[49] This suggests, while PTA may be important to treat stenosis in AVF and AVG, drug therapies may need to be applied to site of angioplasty and injury to prolong access patency.

Endovascular stent therapy

The main advantage of stent therapy after PTA is a reduction in adverse remodeling. In dialysis access, placement of bare metal stents after PTA compared to PTA alone has been shown to improve primary patency.[181,182] However, bare-metal stents have yielded poor results due to aggressive development of in-stent restenosis. In both experimental[183,184] and clinical studies in CAD,[185–187] placement of drug-eluting stents (releasing sirolimus or pactlitaxel) have demonstrated reduced in-stent restenosis after angioplasty compared to bare-metal stents. In experimental models of dialysis access in AVGs, drug-eluting stents have shown to reduce neointimal hyperplasia and improve luminal stenosis compared to bare-metal stents.[188] However, unfortunately, there still remain no clinical studies evaluating drug-eluting stents in dialysis access.

Stent grafts (covered stents constructed from the same material of AVGs) have received recent attention in prevention of restenosis due to its ability to prevent elastic recoil and inability of the neointimal cells to penetrate the covered barrier. A recently published multicenter, randomized controlled, clinical trial showed stent grafts, placed after PTA, to treat venous stenosis had better primary unassisted patency compared to PTA alone.[189] Currently, this is the only treatment to date that has shown to be truly effective to treat dialysis access stenosis in a large, randomized, clinical trial. However, this treatment occurs only after a stenosis develops.

▶ Altering Hemodynamics

As mentioned in previous sections hemodynamic sheer stresses play a significant role in development of neointimal hyperplasia. Therefore, altering the sheer stress pattern to prevent turbulent, low-flow, and low-sheer stresses could reduce the development of neointimal hyperplasia. Previous clinical data to date to support such an intervention comes from several studies evaluating cuffed AVG grafts ("Venaflo"; Bard Vascular, Tempe Arizona).[190–192] In a recent randomized trial evaluating cuffed versus noncuffed AVG, cuffed AVGs showed better primary patency and cumulative survival.[193] Finally, results from a newly developed anastomotic implant device, "Optiflow™" (Bioconnect Systems; Ambler, PA), to connect the artery and vein in AVFs and improve hemodynamics by providing a symmetric flow pattern, have shown a primary patency of 83% at 90 days.[194] This primary patency rate higher compared to other similarly published studies.[195]

▶ Other Novel Therapies

Endothelial progenitor cells

Postnatal bone marrow contains a subtype of unique progenitor cells that have the capacity to differentiate into functional endothelial cells. CD34+ hematopoietic progenitor cells have the ability to differentiate into an endothelial phenotype, and have subsequently shown to have the ability to home into sites of vascular damage and play a role in endothelialization of these injured vascular regions.[196–199] Experimental models in CVD have shown re-endothelialization after endothelial progenitor cell (EPC) administration after angioplasty,[200] which may translate into a reduction of neointimal hyperplasia. In dialysis access, only one study to date, in a porcine model, has evaluated anti-CD34-coated AVG grafts implanted between the carotid artery and internal jugular vein.[201] Placement of anti-CD34-coated grafts in an AVG resulted in almost complete endothelialization of the grafts with a difference in reduction neointimal of hyperplasia when compared to noncoated grafts.[201] While there have been limited studies of EPCs in dialysis access, EPCs may have an important therapeutic application in the future.

Bone marrow-derived neointimal cells

Recent data from experimental models have shown that smooth muscle cells in the neointima may originate from bone marrow-derived cells that bind to the site of vascular injury and differentiate into smooth muscle cells.[135,136] Targeting bone marrow-derived cells may provide a novel therapeutic approach for decreasing venous neointimal hyperplasia.

Far-infrared therapy

Far-infrared therapy (FIR) is an electromagnetic wave with wavelengths that range from 5.6 to 1000 μm. The thermal effect of FIR results in vasodilation and increasing blood flow. The nonthermal effects have been shown to induce eNOS expression, inhibit neointimal hyperplasia, and reduce oxidative stress. In the lone clinical study in dialysis access, far-infrared therapy was shown to increase blood flow through AVFs,[202] likely through activation of HO-1 pathways and reduction in endothelial inflammation.[203]

FUTURE PERSEPCTIVES: NEW FRONTIERS IN RESEARCH

▶ Vascular Imaging

A number of imaging modalities are available for evaluation of stenosis in hemodialysis access. Both color Doppler ultrasonography (CDUS) and contrast digital subtraction angiography (DSA) have been the main imaging methods utilized till date. Duplex ultrasound is an attractive method for qualitative and quantitative evaluation of vessels that is noninvasive and safe.[204] It provides for an assessment of blood flow and arterial and vein diameter.[205] Furthermore, duplex ultrasound can detect vascular access stenosis[206,207] at the venous anastomosis, but frequently fails to detect stenoses in the central veins. DSA is currently the gold standard that provides a comprehensive assessment of the vasculature. However, DSA provides images only in a one-dimensional plane and only information about lumen size.

A number of novel imaging techniques are now being utilized to study the pathophysiology of neointimal hyperplasia in AVF and AVG. Computerized tomography (CT)[63,208–210] and magnetic resonance imaging (MRI)[206,211–215] both allow for high resolution imaging in two- and three-dimensional planes and any orientation. Furthermore, CT and MRI allow for collection of information regarding blood flow, anatomical configuration, and calculation of shear stress profiles. Future experimental and clinical studies should evaluate longitudinally the progression of neointimal hyperplasia in AVF and AVG linking with information such as shear stress profiles, anatomical configurations, and other biological data.

Intravascular ultrasound (IVUS) is another novel imaging modality used primarily in CAD to quantify calcification.[216] IVUS also provides multiplanar images, complete assessment of luminal diameters and vessel stenosis, and assessment of the intima, media, and adventitia, and has been evaluated in experimental and clinical studies of AVG[217] and AVF.[218] Utilizing IVUS to gauge successful therapy after angioplasty could provide a new area of research.

Novel Endovascular Drug Delivery Systems

All the technologies of drug delivery for AVF and AVG previously described using perivascular techniques required application of therapy at the time of surgery. However, because stenosis does not only occur in the perioperative period, the ability to deliver drugs, genes, or cells at time point distant to surgical creation but also may play a critical role in treating hemodialysis vascular access stenosis. Currently, there is no technology of this kind available. However, Mercator MedSystems, Inc. (San Leandro, CA) has developed the Adventa endovascular balloon catheter, which has a sheathed microneedle that pierces the vessel after inflation of the balloon (Figure 56-5).[219] This endovascular catheter may allow delivery of these drugs, cells, and genes after PTA therapy in AVF and AVG. Furthermore, this may be a technology that has broader applications to other cardiovascular diseases such as CAD, but first tested in dialysis patients who are a captive audience and have their vessels cannulated thrice-weekly.

Genomics

Recent sequencing of the human genome has opened up fertile areas of investigation for many human diseases. To date, there have been very few studies that have investigated the genetic underpinnings of vascular stenosis in hemodialysis access dysfunction. Experimental and clinical studies evaluating arterial and venous samples utilizing gene expression microarrays may provide new molecular patterns of neointimal hyperplasia development in vascular access as they have in CAD and PVD. Fundamental advancements in our knowledge of the molecular pathophysiology of neointimal hyperplasia development and vascular access stenosis utilizing genomic technology represents an unprecedented opportunity to develop new diagnostic, prognostic, and therapeutic interventions for this important clinical problem of AVF maturation.

Animal Models

In the last decade, small and large animal models of AVF and AVG have provided tremendous insight into the pathology and pathogenesis of hemodialysis vascular access dysfunction.[33,50,80,87,99,126,134,164,215,220] Animal models of AVF and AVG have been used to evaluate hemodynamic sheer stress,[63,64,215] vascular remodeling,[80] and delivery of novel local pharmacologic therapies.[221,222] Recently, AVF animal models with CKD have been developed in rats[47,126] and pigs[223] and have allowed for simulation of uremia seen in ESRD patients. These uremic animal models of AVF have demonstrated that CKD accelerates neointimal hyperplasia after AVF creation.[47] Animal models will play an important future role in (1) elucidation of new pathways using genetically altered "knockout animals," (2) longitudinal assessment of the pathophysiology of neointimal hyperplasia development using imaging techniques and genomic and proteomic studies, and (3) in testing novel therapies and drug delivery systems.

Preexisting Arterial and Venous Vascular Changes

Preexisting arterial changes have been reported to be present in large arteries of CKD patients such as the coronary arteries with progressive worsening of this neointimal hyperplasia and vascular stenosis with more advanced CKD stage.[224] Preexisting arterial changes in small arteries have recently been described in radial arteries used to create AVFs.[20,21,225] These preexisting arterial changes (thicker intima and intima-media ratios) have been associated with worse AVF survival.[20,21] While preexisting venous neointimal hyperplasia has been previously reported,[67–70] a recent study has demonstrated that (1) the lesion of preexisting neointimal hyperplasia can be very severe measured by morphometric analysis, (2) the predominant cellular phenotype within the neointima are myofibroblast (similar to stenotic AVFs),

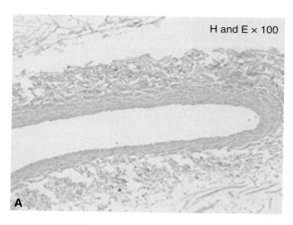

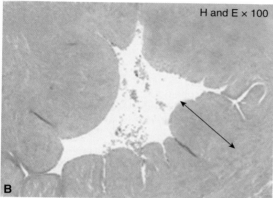

Figure 56-6. Histopathology of (**A**) normal vein without CKD and (**B**) vein of advanced CKD patient. Normal vein shows the absence of neointimal hyperplasia. Note that considerable neointimal hyperplasia is present in this vein sample of advanced CKD patient.

(3) preexisting neointimal hyperplasia is associated with worse AVF maturation outcomes (Figure 56-6).[71] Furthermore, a recent clinical study of vein tissue collected at the time of AVF construction showed elevated levels of MMP-2 expression in veins of patients with eventual AVF nonmaturation.[226] Therefore, understanding the mechanisms that lead to development of venous neointimal hyperplasia and developing targeted therapies to be used prior to vascular access placement may play a important role in the overall paradigm of treating vascular access dysfunction in the future.

▶ Tissue-Engineered Vascular Grafts

In hemodialysis patients who must dialyze with an AVG, PTFE is the most common type of graft material used. PTFE grafts are prone to infection, thrombus, and development of neointimal hyperplasia at the distal anastomosis or outflow vein.[227–233] Thus, in recent years there has been interest in developing tissue-engineered vascular grafts (TEVGs) which are less immunogenic and can tolerate the high hemodynamic loads from increased postoperative flow and repeated venipunctures from large bore needles. To date, TEVGs formed by seeding autologous bone marrow cells onto a copolymer of L-lactide and ε-caprolactone[234] or culturing autologous fibroblasts and endothelial cells[235] without a scaffold, have shown promising results in clinical trials. Furthermore, advances in nanotechnology may bring additional functionality to vascular scaffolds, help optimize internal vascular graft surface and direct the differentiation of stem cells into a specific vascular cell phenotype, and dramatically accelerate vascular tissue assembly.[236] Thus, the potential of developing AVGs which are less thrombogenic and prone to infection, using novel technologies, may significantly improve the morbidity and clinical outcomes of dialysis with an AVG.

CONCLUSION

This is an unprecedented time for research in hemodialysis vascular access dysfunction. The magnitude of vascular access dysfunction will be magnified in the coming years as both the incident and prevalent is projected to increase in the next 10 years[237] and likely the costs of treating vascular access dysfunction as well. Our improvement in the understanding of the pathology and pathophysiology of venous neointimal hyperplasia and alternative mechanisms responsible for venous neointimal hyperplasia is in large part due to the previous large body of work generated from the CVD and PVD community studying veingrafts. This has translated into advances in cellular and molecular pathobiology, biomaterials, and drug delivery techniques for neointimal hyperplasia. Unfortunately, there are still very few effective therapies to treat neointimal hyperplasia in dialysis access. Further advancements in the understanding of neointimal hyperplasia in dialysis access will require a translational research effort, utilizing the advancements of uremic animal models of AVF and AVG[47,83,126,223] and targeted observational studies and clinical trials derived from the knowledge from these animal models. Finally, AVFs and AVGs may be the ideal clinical model to test future novel therapies for neointimal hyperplasia because of the superficial location of the vessels, the frequency of accessing the vessels, the aggressiveness of neointimal hyperplasia development, and the fact that dialysis patients are a captive audience. Knowledge from therapies in dialysis access could be applied to other important clinical settings such as CAD, PVD, and postangioplasty restenosis; these are fields that have provided critical knowledge to advance the science and treatment of hemodialysis access dysfunction to date.

REFERENCES

1. Owens CD, Ho KJ, Conte MS. Lower extremity vein graft failure: a translational approach. *Vasc Med*. Feb 2008; 13(1):63–74.
2. Libby P, Tanaka H. The molecular bases of restenosis. *Prog Cardiovasc Dis*. Sep–Oct 1997;40(2):97–106.

3. Nakatani M, Takeyama Y, Shibata M, et al. Mechanisms of restenosis after coronary intervention: difference between plain old balloon angioplasty and stenting. *Cardiovasc Pathol*. Jan–Feb 2003;12(1):40–48.

4. Cin VG, Pekdemir H, Camsar A, et al. Diffuse intimal thickening of coronary arteries in slow coronary flow. *Jpn Heart J*. Nov 2003;44(6):907–919.

5. Greenwald SE, Berry CL. Improving vascular grafts: the importance of mechanical and haemodynamic properties. *J Pathol*. Feb 2000;190(3):292–299.

6. Sho E, Sho M, Singh TM, et al. Arterial enlargement in response to high flow requires early expression of matrix metalloproteinases to degrade extracellular matrix. *Exp Mol Pathol*. Oct 2002;73(2):142–153.

7. Veith FJ, Gupta SK, Ascer E, et al. Six-year prospective multicenter randomized comparison of autologous saphenous vein and expanded polytetrafluoroethylene grafts in infrainguinal arterial reconstructions. *J Vasc Surg*. Jan 1986;3(1):104–114.

8. Fitzgibbon GM, Kafka HP, Leach AJ, Keon WJ, Hooper GD, Burton JR. Coronary bypass graft fate and patient outcome: angiographic follow-up of 5,065 grafts related to survival and reoperation in 1,388 patients during 25 years. *J Am Coll Cardiol*. Sep 1996;28(3):616–626.

9. Roy-Chaudhury P, Sukhatme VP, Cheung AK. Hemodialysis vascular access dysfunction: a cellular and molecular viewpoint. *J Am Soc Nephrol*. Apr 2006;17(4):1112–1127.

10. Roy-Chaudhury P, Kelly BS, Miller MA, et al. Venous neointimal hyperplasia in polytetrafluoroethylene dialysis grafts. *Kidney Int*. Jun 2001;59(6):2325–2334.

11. Roy-Chaudhury P, Lee TC. Vascular stenosis: biology and interventions. *Curr Opin Nephrol Hypertens*. Nov 2007;16(6):516–522.

12. Roy-Chaudhury P, Arend L, Zhang J, et al. Neointimal hyperplasia in early arteriovenous fistula failure. *Am J Kidney Dis*. Nov 2007;50(5):782–790.

13. Lee T, Roy-Chaudhury P. Advances and new frontiers in the pathophysiology of venous neointimal hyperplasia and dialysis access stenosis. *Adv Chronic Kidney Dis*. Sep 2009;16(5):329–338.

14. Conte MS, Nugent HM, Gaccione P, Guleria I, Roy-Chaudhury P, Lawson JH. Multicenter phase I/II trial of the safety of allogeneic endothelial cell implants after the creation of arteriovenous access for hemodialysis use: the V-HEALTH study. *J Vasc Surg*. Dec 2009;50(6):1359–1368 e1351.

15. Weiss MF, Scivittaro V, Anderson JM. Oxidative stress and increased expression of growth factors in lesions of failed hemodialysis access. *Am J Kidney Dis*. May 2001;37(5):970–980.

16. Dember LM, Beck GJ, Allon M, et al. Effect of clopidogrel on early failure of arteriovenous fistulas for hemodialysis: a randomized controlled trial. *J Am Med Assoc*. May 2008;299(18):2164–2171.

17. Leon C, Asif A. Arteriovenous access and hand pain: the distal hypoperfusion ischemic syndrome. *Clin J Am Soc Nephrol*. Jan 2007;2(1):175–183.

18. Wang N, Yang J, Yu X, et al. Radial artery calcification in end-stage renal disease patients is associated with deposition of osteopontin and diminished expression of alpha-smooth muscle actin. *Nephrology (Carlton)*. Oct 2008;13(5):367–375.

19. Goldsmith DJ, Covic A, Sambrook PA, Ackrill P. Vascular calcification in long-term haemodialysis patients in a single unit: a retrospective analysis. *Nephron*. 1997;77(1):37–43.

20. Kim YO, Choi YJ, Kim JI, et al. The impact of intima–media thickness of radial artery on early failure of radiocephalic arteriovenous fistula in hemodialysis patients. *J Korean Med Sci*. Apr 2006;21(2):284–289.

21. Kim YO, Song HC, Yoon SA, et al. Preexisting intimal hyperplasia of radial artery is associated with early failure of radiocephalic arteriovenous fistula in hemodialysis patients. *Am J Kidney Dis*. Feb 2003;41(2):422–428.

22. Asif A, Gadalean FN, Merrill D, et al. Inflow stenosis in arteriovenous fistulas and grafts: a multicenter, prospective study. *Kidney Int*. May 2005;67(5):1986–1992.

23. Duijm LE, van der Rijt RH, Cuypers PW, et al. Outpatient treatment of arterial inflow stenoses of dysfunctional hemodialysis access fistulas by retrograde venous access puncture and catheterization. *J Vasc Surg*. Mar 2008;47(3):591–598.

24. Duijm LE, Liem YS, van der Rijt RH, et al. Inflow stenoses in dysfunctional hemodialysis access fistulae and grafts. *Am J Kidney Dis*. Jul 2006;48(1):98–105.

25. Duijm LE, Overbosch EH, Liem YS, et al. Retrograde catheterization of haemodialysis fistulae and grafts: angiographic depiction of the entire vascular access tree and stenosis treatment. *Nephrol Dial Transplant*. Feb 2009;24(2):539–547.

26. Beathard GA, Arnold P, Jackson J, Litchfield T. Aggressive treatment of early fistula failure. *Kidney Int*. Oct 2003;64(4):1487–1494.

27. Beathard GA. Fistula salvage by endovascular therapy. *Adv Chronic Kidney Dis*. Sep 2009;16(5):339–351.

28. Maya ID, Oser R, Saddekni S, Barker J, Allon M. Vascular access stenosis: comparison of arteriovenous grafts and fistulas. *Am J Kidney Dis*. Nov 2004;44(5):859–865.

29. Turmel-Rodrigues L, Pengloan J, Baudin S, et al. Treatment of stenosis and thrombosis in haemodialysis fistulas and grafts by interventional radiology. *Nephrol Dial Transplant*. Dec 2000;15(12):2029–2036.

30. Asif A. Effectiveness and safety of dialysis vascular access procedures performed by interventional nephrologists. *Kidney Int*. Apr 2005;67(4):1634; author reply 1634.

31. Roy-Chaudhury P, Wang Y, Krishnamoorthy M, et al. Cellular phenotypes in human stenotic lesions from haemodialysis vascular access. *Nephrol Dial Transplant*. Sep 2009;24(9):2786–2791.

32. Roy-Chaudhury P, McKee L, Miller M, Reaves A, Armstrong J, Duncan H, Munda R, Kelly B, Heffelfinger S. Adventitial fibroblasts contribute to venous neointimal hyperplasia in PTFE grafts [Abstract]. *J Am Soc Nephrol*. 2001;12:301A.

33. Kelly BS, Heffelfinger SC, Whiting JF, et al. Aggressive venous neointimal hyperplasia in a pig model of arteriovenous graft stenosis. *Kidney Int*. Dec 2002;62(6):2272–2280.

34. Swedberg SH, Brown BG, Sigley R, Wight TN, Gordon D, Nicholls SC. Intimal fibromuscular hyperplasia at the venous anastomosis of PTFE grafts in hemodialysis patients. Clinical, immunocytochemical, light and electron microscopic assessment. *Circulation*. Dec 1989;80(6):1726–1736.

35. Alexander JW, Goodman HR, Cardi M, et al. Simultaneous corticosteroid avoidance and calcineurin inhibitor minimization in renal transplantation. *Transplant Int.* Apr 2006;19(4):295–302.

36. Mitra AK, Gangahar DM, Agrawal DK. Cellular, molecular and immunological mechanisms in the pathophysiology of vein graft intimal hyperplasia. *Immunol Cell Biol.* Apr 2006;84(2):115–124.

37. Li L, Terry CM, Shiu Y-TE, Cheung AK. Neointimal hyperplasia associated with synthetic hemodialysis grafts. *Kidney Int.* 2008;74(10):1247–1261.

38. Remuzzi A, Ene-Iordache B, Mosconi L, et al. Radial artery wall shear stress evaluation in patients with arteriovenous fistula for hemodialysis access. *Biorheology.* 2003;40(1–3):423–430.

39. Paszkowiak JJ, Dardik A. Arterial wall shear stress: observations from the bench to the bedside. *Vasc Endovascular Surg.* Jan–Feb 2003;37(1):47–57.

40. Unnikrishnan S, Huynh TN, Brott BC, et al. Turbulent flow evaluation of the venous needle during hemodialysis. *J Biomech Eng.* Dec 2005;127(7):1141–1146.

41. Haruguchi H, Teraoka S. Intimal hyperplasia and hemodynamic factors in arterial bypass and arteriovenous grafts: a review. *J Artif Organs.* 2003;6(4):227–235.

42. Sivanesan S, How TV, Black RA, Bakran A. Flow patterns in the radiocephalic arteriovenous fistula: an in vitro study. *J Biomech.* Sep 1999;32(9):915–925.

43. Ballyk PD, Walsh C, Butany J, Ojha M. Compliance mismatch may promote graft-artery intimal hyperplasia by altering suture-line stresses. *J Biomech.* Mar 1998;31(3):229–237.

44. Hofer M, Rappitsch G, Perktold K, Trubel W, Schima H. Numerical study of wall mechanics and fluid dynamics in end-to-side anastomoses and correlation to intimal hyperplasia. *J Biomech.* Oct 1996;29(10):1297–1308.

45. Ross EA, Verlander JW, Koo LC, Hawkins IF. Minimizing hemodialysis vascular access trauma with an improved needle design. *J Am Soc Nephrol.* Jul 2000;11(7):1325–1330.

46. Croatt AJ, Juncos JP, Hernandez MC, et al. Upregulation of inflammation-related genes and neointima formation in arteriovenous fistula (AVF) model in the rat (Abstract). *J Am Soc Nephrol.* 2008;19:252A.

47. Kokubo T, Ishikawa N, Uchida H, et al. CKD accelerates development of neointimal hyperplasia in arteriovenous fistulas. *J Am Soc Nephrol.* Jun 2009;20(6):1236–1245.

48. Jacobson GM, Dourron HM, Liu J, et al. Novel NAD(P)H oxidase inhibitor suppresses angioplasty-induced superoxide and neointimal hyperplasia of rat carotid artery. *Circ Res.* Apr 2003;92(6):637–643.

49. Chang CJ, Ko PJ, Hsu LA, et al. Highly increased cell proliferation activity in the restenotic hemodialysis vascular access after percutaneous transluminal angioplasty: implication in prevention of restenosis. *Am J Kidney Dis.* Jan 2004;43(1):74–84.

50. Lin T, Horsfield C, Robson MG. Arteriovenous fistula in the rat tail: a new model of hemodialysis access dysfunction. *Kidney Int.* Aug 2008;74(4):528–531.

51. Chi-Jen C, Po-Jen K, Lung-An H, et al. Highly increased cell proliferation activity in the restenotic hemodialysis vascular access after percutaneous transluminal angioplasty: implication in prevention of restenosis. *Am J Kidney Dis.* 2004;43(1):74–84.

52. Wang Y, Krishnamoorthy M, Banerjee R, et al. Venous stenosis in a pig arteriovenous fistula model—anatomy, mechanisms and cellular phenotypes. *Nephrol Dial Transplant.* Feb 2008;23(2):525–533.

53. Leblanc M, Saint-Sauveur E, Pichette V. Native arteriovenous fistula for hemodialysis: What to expect early after creation? *J Vasc Access.* Apr–Jun 2003;4(2):39–44.

54. Allon M, Lockhart ME, Lilly RZ, et al. Effect of preoperative sonographic mapping on vascular access outcomes in hemodialysis patients. *Kidney Int.* Nov 2001;60(5):2013–2020.

55. Robbin ML, Chamberlain NE, Lockhart ME, et al. Hemodialysis arteriovenous fistula maturity: US evaluation. *Radiology.* Oct 2002;225(1):59–64.

56. Robbin ML, Gallichio MH, Deierhoi MH, Young CJ, Weber TM, Allon M. US vascular mapping before hemodialysis access placement. *Radiology.* Oct 2000;217(1):83–88.

57. Muto A, Model L, Ziegler K, Eghbalieh SD, Dardik A. Mechanisms of vein graft adaptation to the arterial circulation. *Circ J.* Aug 2010;74(8):1501–1512.

58. Singh P, Robbin ML, Lockhart ME, Allon M. Clinically immature arteriovenous hemodialysis fistulas: effect of US on salvage. *Radiology.* Jan 2008;246(1):299–305.

59. Asif A, Roy-Chaudhury P, Beathard GA. Early arteriovenous fistula failure: a logical proposal for when and how to intervene. *Clin J Am Soc Nephrol.* Mar 2006;1(2):332–339.

60. Nassar GM, Nguyen B, Rhee E, Achkar K. Endovascular Treatment of the "failing to mature" arteriovenous fistula. *Clin J Am Soc Nephrol.* Mar 2006;1(2):275–280.

61. Faiyaz R, Abreo K, Zaman F, Pervez A, Zibari G, Work J. Salvage of poorly developed arteriovenous fistulae with percutaneous ligation of accessory veins. *Am J Kidney Dis.* Apr 2002;39(4):824–827.

62. Beathard GA, Settle SM, Shields MW. Salvage of the nonfunctioning arteriovenous fistula. *Am J Kidney Dis.* May 1999;33(5):910–916.

63. Krishnamoorthy M, Roy-Chaudhury P, Wang Y, et al. Measurement of hemodynamic and anatomic parameters in a swine arteriovenous fistula model. *J Vasc Access.* Jan–Mar 2008;9(1):28–34.

64. Krishnamoorthy MK, Banerjee RK, Wang Y, et al. Hemodynamic wall shear stress profiles influence the magnitude and pattern of stenosis in a pig AV fistula. *Kidney Int.* Sep 2008;74(11):1410–1419.

65. Lin CC, Yang WC, Lin SJ, et al. Length polymorphism in heme oxygenase-1 is associated with arteriovenous fistula patency in hemodialysis patients. *Kidney Int.* Jan 2006;69(1):165–172.

66. Girndt M, Heine GH, Ulrich C, Kohler H. Gene polymorphism association studies in dialysis: vascular access. *Semin Dial.* Jan–Feb 2007;20(1):63–67.

67. Wali MA, Eid RA, Al-Homrany MA. Smooth muscle changes in the cephalic vein of renal failure patients before use as an arteriovenous fistula (AVF). *J Smooth Muscle Res.* Jun 2002;38(3):75–85.

68. Wali MA, Eid RA, Dewan M, Al-Homrany MA. Intimal changes in the cephalic vein of renal failure patients before arterio-venous fistula (AVF) construction. *J Smooth Muscle Res.* Aug 2003;39(4):95–105.

69. Wali MA, Eid RA, Dewan M, Al-Homrany MA. Pre-existing histopathological changes in the cephalic vein of renal failure patients before arterio-venous fistula (AVF) construction. *Ann Thorac Cardiovasc Surg.* Oct 2006;12(5):341–348.

70. Feinfeld DA, Batista R, Mir R, Babich D. Changes in venous histology in chronic hemodialysis patients. *Am J Kidney Dis.* Oct 1999;34(4):702–705.

71. Lee T, Chauhan V, Krishnamoorthy M, et al. Severe venous neointimal hyperplasia prior to dialysis access surgery. *Nephrol Dial Transplant.* Jul 2011;26(7):2264–2274.

72. Sies H. Oxidative stress: oxidants and antioxidants. *Exp Physiol.* Mar 1997;82(2):291–295.

73. Annuk M, Zilmer M, Fellstrom B. Endothelium-dependent vasodilation and oxidative stress in chronic renal failure: impact on cardiovascular disease. *Kidney Int Suppl.* May 2003(84):S50–S53.

74. Himmelfarb J, Hakim RM. Oxidative stress in uremia. *Curr Opin Nephrol Hypertens.* Nov 2003;12(6):593–598.

75. Castier Y, Lehoux S, Hu Y, Foteinos G, Tedgui A, Xu Q. Characterization of neointima lesions associated with arteriovenous fistulas in a mouse model. *Kidney Int.* Jul 2006;70(2):315–320.

76. Dixon BS. Why don't fistulas mature? *Kidney Int.* 2006;70(8):1413–1422.

77. Rotmans JI, Velema E, Verhagen HJ, et al. Matrix metalloproteinase inhibition reduces intimal hyperplasia in a porcine arteriovenous-graft model. *J Vasc Surg.* Feb 2004;39(2):432–439.

78. Castier Y, Brandes RP, Leseche G, Tedgui A, Lehoux S. p47phox-dependent NADPH oxidase regulates flow-induced vascular remodeling. *Circ Res.* Sep 2005;97(6):533–540.

79. Tronc F, Mallat Z, Lehoux S, Wassef M, Esposito B, Tedgui A. Role of matrix metalloproteinases in blood flow-induced arterial enlargement: interaction with NO. *Arterioscler Thromb Vasc Biol.* Dec 2000;20(12):E120–E126.

80. Misra S, Doherty MG, Woodrum D, et al. Adventitial remodeling with increased matrix metalloproteinase-2 activity in a porcine arteriovenous polytetrafluoroethylene grafts. *Kidney Int.* Dec 2005;68(6):2890–2900.

81. Misra S, Fu AA, Puggioni A, et al. Increased shear stress with upregulation of VEGF-A and its receptors and MMP-2, MMP-9, and TIMP-1 in venous stenosis of hemodialysis grafts. *Am J Physiol Heart Circ Physiol.* May 2008;294(5):H2219–H2230.

82. Chan CY, Chen YS, Ma MC, Chen CF. Remodeling of experimental arteriovenous fistula with increased matrix metalloproteinase expression in rats. *J Vasc Surg.* Apr 2007;45(4):804–811.

83. Yang B, Shergill U, Fu AA, Knudsen B, Misra S. The mouse arteriovenous fistula model. *J Vasc Interv Radiol.* Jul 2009;20(7):946–950.

84. Misra S, Fu AA, Rajan DK, et al. Expression of hypoxia inducible factor-1 alpha, macrophage migration inhibition factor, matrix metalloproteinase-2 and -9, and their inhibitors in hemodialysis grafts and arteriovenous fistulas. *J Vasc Interv Radiol.* Feb 2008;19(2 Pt 1):252–259.

85. Nath KA. Heme oxygenase-1: a provenance for cytoprotective pathways in the kidney and other tissues. *Kidney Int.* Aug 2006;70(3):432–443.

86. Maines MD. Heme oxygenase: function, multiplicity, regulatory mechanisms, and clinical applications. *FASEB J.* Jul 1988;2(10):2557–2568.

87. Juncos JP, Tracz MJ, Croatt AJ, et al. Genetic deficiency of heme oxygenase-1 impairs functionality and form of an arteriovenous fistula in the mouse. *Kidney Int.* Jul 2008;74(1):47–51.

88. Tepel M. Acetylcysteine for the prevention of radiocontrast -induced nephropathy. *Minerva Cardioangiol.* Oct 2003;51(5):525–530.

89. Porter KE, Loftus IM, Peterson M, Bell PR, London NJ, Thompson MM. Marimastat inhibits neointimal thickening in a model of human vein graft stenosis. *Br J Surg.* Oct 1998;85(10):1373–1377.

90. Ghigliotti G, Mereto E, Eisenberg PR, et al. N-acetyl-cysteine reduces neointimal thickening and procoagulant activity after balloon-induced injury in abdominal aortae of New Zealand white rabbits. *Thromb Haemost.* Apr 2001;85(4):724–729.

91. Schepers A, Eefting D, Bonta PI, et al. Anti-MCP-1 gene therapy inhibits vascular smooth muscle cells proliferation and attenuates vein graft thickening both in vitro and in vivo. *Arterioscler Thromb Vasc Biol.* Sep 2006;26(9):2063–2069.

92. Diacovo TG, deFougerolles AR, Bainton DF, Springer TA. A functional integrin ligand on the surface of platelets: intercellular adhesion molecule-2. *J Clin Invest.* Sep 1994;94(3):1243–1251.

93. Zou Y, Hu Y, Mayr M, Dietrich H, Wick G, Xu Q. Reduced neointima hyperplasia of vein bypass grafts in intercellular adhesion molecule-1-deficient mice. *Circ Res.* Mar 2000;86(4):434–440.

94. Diacovo TG, Roth SJ, Buccola JM, Bainton DF, Springer TA. Neutrophil rolling, arrest, and transmigration across activated, surface-adherent platelets via sequential action of P-selectin and the beta 2-integrin CD11b/CD18. *Blood.* Jul 1996;88(1):146–157.

95. Simon DI, Chen Z, Xu H, et al. Platelet glycoprotein ibalpha is a counterreceptor for the leukocyte integrin Mac-1 (CD11b/CD18). *J Exp Med.* Jul 2000;192(2):193–204.

96. Zhang L, Freedman NJ, Brian L, Peppel K. Graft-extrinsic cells predominate in vein graft arterialization. *Arterioscler Thromb Vasc Biol.* Mar 2004;24(3):470–476.

97. Wainwright CL, Miller AM, Wadsworth RM. Inflammation as a key event in the development of neointima following vascular balloon injury. *Clin Exp Pharmacol Physiol.* Nov 2001;28(11):891–895.

98. Fogelstrand P, Osterberg K, Mattsson E. Reduced neointima in vein grafts following a blockage of cell recruitment from the vein and the surrounding tissue. *Cardiovasc Res.* Aug 2005;67(2):326–332.

99. Nath KA, Kanakiriya SK, Grande JP, Croatt AJ, Katusic ZS. Increased venous proinflammatory gene expression and intimal hyperplasia in an aorto-caval fistula model in the rat. *Am J Pathol.* Jun 2003;162(6):2079–2090.

100. Juncos JP, Grande JP, Kang L, et al. MCP-1 contributes to arteriovenous fistula failure. *J Am Soc Nephrol.* Jan 2011;22(1):43–48.

101. Stracke S, Konner K, Kostlin I, et al. Increased expression of TGF-beta1 and IGF-I in inflammatory stenotic lesions of hemodialysis fistulas. *Kidney Int.* Mar 2002;61(3):1011–1019.

102. Miller KM, Anderson JM. Human monocyte/macrophage activation and interleukin 1 generation by biomedical polymers. *J Biomed Mater Res.* Aug 1988;22(8): 713–731.

103. Postlethwaite AE, Seyer JM. Stimulation of fibroblast chemotaxis by human recombinant tumor necrosis factor alpha (TNF-alpha) and a synthetic TNF-alpha 31–68 peptide. *J Exp Med.* Dec 1990;172(6): 1749–1756.

104. Jovinge S, Hultgardh-Nilsson A, Regnstrom J, Nilsson J. Tumor necrosis factor-alpha activates smooth muscle cell migration in culture and is expressed in the balloon-injured rat aorta. *Arterioscler Thromb Vasc Biol.* Mar 1997; 17(3):490–497.

105. Mattana J, Effiong C, Kapasi A, Singhal PC. Leukocyte-polytetrafluoroethylene interaction enhances proliferation of vascular smooth muscle cells via tumor necrosis factor-alpha secretion. *Kidney Int.* Dec 1997;52(6):1478–1485.

106. Mehta RI, Mukherjee AK, Patterson TD, Fishbein MC. *Cardiovasc Pathol.* Jul–Aug 2011;20(4):213–221.

107. Puhakka HL, Turunen P, Gruchala M, et al. Effects of vaccinia virus anti-inflammatory protein 35K and TIMP-1 gene transfers on vein graft stenosis in rabbits. *In Vivo.* May–Jun 2005;19(3):515–521.

108. Cayci C, Wahlquist TC, Seckin SI, et al. Naringenin inhibits neointimal hyperplasia following arterial reconstruction with interpositional vein graft. *Ann Plast Surg.* Jan 2010;64(1):105–113.

109. de Graaf R, Kloppenburg G, Tintu A, et al. The new immunosuppressive agent FK778 attenuates neointima formation in an experimental venous bypass graft model. *Vascul Pharmacol.* Mar–Apr 2009;50(3–4): 83–88.

110. Adkins JR, Castresana MR, Wang Z, Newman WH. Rapamycin inhibits release of tumor necrosis factor-alpha from human vascular smooth muscle cells. *Am Surg.* May 2004;70(5):384–387; discussion 387–388.

111. Schachner T, Oberhuber A, Zou Y, et al. Rapamycin treatment is associated with an increased apoptosis rate in experimental vein grafts. *Eur J Cardiothorac Surg.* Feb 2005;27(2):302–306.

112. Schachner T, Zou Y, Oberhuber A, et al. Local application of rapamycin inhibits neointimal hyperplasia in experimental vein grafts. *Ann Thorac Surg.* May 2004;77(5):1580–1585.

113. Shuhaiber JH, Evans AN, Massad MG, Geha AS. Mechanisms and future directions for prevention of vein graft failure in coronary bypass surgery. *Eur J Cardiothorac Surg.* Sep 2002;22(3):387–396.

114. Langille BL, O'Donnell F. Reductions in arterial diameter produced by chronic decreases in blood flow are endothelium-dependent. *Science.* Jan 1986;231(4736): 405–407.

115. Ignarro LJ, Buga GM, Wood KS, Byrns RE, Chaudhuri G. Endothelium-derived relaxing factor produced and released from artery and vein is nitric oxide. *Proc Natl Acad Sci U S A.* Dec 1987;84(24):9265–9269.

116. Liu SQ, Ruan YY, Tang D, Li YC, Goldman J, Zhong L. A possible role of initial cell death due to mechanical stretch in the regulation of subsequent cell proliferation in experimental vein grafts. *Biomech Model Mechanobiol.* Jun 2002;1(1):17–27.

117. Furchgott RF. Endothelium-derived relaxing factor: discovery, early studies, and identification as nitric oxide. *Biosci Rep.* Aug 1999;19(4):235–251.

118. Joannides R, Haefeli WE, Linder L, et al. Nitric oxide is responsible for flow-dependent dilatation of human peripheral conduit arteries in vivo. *Circulation.* Mar 1995;91(5):1314–1319.

119. Sarkar R, Meinberg EG, Stanley JC, Gordon D, Webb RC. Nitric oxide reversibly inhibits the migration of cultured vascular smooth muscle cells. *Circ Res.* Feb 1996;78(2): 225–230.

120. Kown MH, Yamaguchi A, Jahncke CL, et al. L-arginine polymers inhibit the development of vein graft neointimal hyperplasia. *J Thorac Cardiovasc Surg.* May 2001;121(5):971–980.

121. Ohta S, Komori K, Yonemitsu Y, Onohara T, Matsumoto T, Sugimachi K. Intraluminal gene transfer of endothelial cell-nitric oxide synthase suppresses intimal hyperplasia of vein grafts in cholesterol-fed rabbit: a limited biological effect as a result of the loss of medial smooth muscle cells. *Surgery.* Jun 2002;131(6):644–653.

122. Wan S, Shukla N, Angelini GD, Yim AP, Johnson JL, Jeremy JY. Nitric oxide-donating aspirin (NCX 4016) inhibits neointimal thickening in a pig model of saphenous vein-carotid artery interposition grafting: a comparison with aspirin and morpholinosydnonimine (SIN-1). *J Thorac Cardiovasc Surg.* Oct 2007;134(4): 1033–1039.

123. Shukla N, Angelini GD, Ascione R, Talpahewa S, Capoun R, Jeremy JY. Nitric oxide donating aspirins: novel drugs for the treatment of saphenous vein graft failure. *Ann Thorac Surg.* May 2003;75(5):1437–1442.

124. Bolton CH, Downs LG, Victory JG, et al. Endothelial dysfunction in chronic renal failure: roles of lipoprotein oxidation and pro-inflammatory cytokines. *Nephrol Dial Transplant.* Jun 2001;16(6):1189–1197.

125. Ghiadoni L, Cupisti A, Huang Y, et al. Endothelial dysfunction and oxidative stress in chronic renal failure. *J Nephrol.* Jul–Aug 2004;17(4):512–519.

126. Croatt AJ, Grande JP, Hernandez MC, Ackerman AW, Katusic ZS, Nath KA. Characterization of a model of an arteriovenous fistula in the rat: the effect of L-NAME. *Am J Pathol.* May 2010;176(5):2530–2541.

127. Kielstein JT, Boger RH, Bode-Boger SM, et al. Asymmetric dimethylarginine plasma concentrations differ in patients with end-stage renal disease: relationship to treatment method and atherosclerotic disease. *J Am Soc Nephrol.* Mar 1999;10(3):594–600.

128. Cooke JP. Does ADMA cause endothelial dysfunction? *Arterioscler Thromb Vasc Biol.* Sep 2000;20(9): 2032–2037.

129. Wu CC, Wen SC, Yang CW, Pu SY, Tsai KC, Chen JW. Plasma ADMA predicts restenosis of arteriovenous fistula. *J Am Soc Nephrol.* Jan 2009;20(1):213–222.

130. Davies MG, Hagen PO. Pathophysiology of vein graft failure: a review. *Eur J Vasc Endovasc Surg.* Jan 1995; 9(1):7–18.

131. Scott NA, Cipolla GD, Ross CE, et al. Identification of a potential role for the adventitia in vascular lesion formation after balloon overstretch injury of porcine coronary arteries. *Circulation.* Jun 1996;93(12):2178–2187.

132. Shi Y, O'Brien JE, Fard A, Mannion JD, Wang D, Zalewski A. Adventitial myofibroblasts contribute to neointimal

formation in injured porcine coronary arteries. *Circulation*. Oct 1996;94(7):1655–1664.

133. Shi Y, O'Brien JE, Jr., Mannion JD, et al. Remodeling of autologous saphenous vein grafts. The role of perivascular myofibroblasts. *Circulation*. Jun 1997; 95(12):2684–2693.

134. Li L, Terry CM, Blumenthal DK, et al. Cellular and morphological changes during neointimal hyperplasia development in a porcine arteriovenous graft model. *Nephrol Dial Transplant*. Nov 2007;22(11):3139–3146.

135. Caplice NM, Wang S, Tracz M, et al. Neoangiogenesis and the presence of progenitor cells in the venous limb of an arteriovenous fistula in the rat. *Am J Physiol Renal Physiol*. Aug 2007;293(2):F470–F475.

136. Diao Y, Guthrie S, Xia SL, et al. Long-term engraftment of bone marrow-derived cells in the intimal hyperplasia lesion of autologous vein grafts. *Am J Pathol*. Mar 2008;172(3):839–848.

137. Corpataux JM, Haesler E, Silacci P, Ris HB, Hayoz D. Low-pressure environment and remodelling of the forearm vein in Brescia-Cimino haemodialysis access. *Nephrol Dial Transplant*. Jun 2002;17(6):1057–1062.

138. Kwon HM, Sangiorgi G, Ritman EL, et al. Enhanced coronary vasa vasorum neovascularization in experimental hypercholesterolemia. *J Clin Invest*. Apr 1998;101(8): 1551–1556.

139. O'Brien JE, Jr., Shi Y, Fard A, Bauer T, Zalewski A, Mannion JD. Wound healing around and within saphenous vein bypass grafts. *J Thorac Cardiovasc Surg*. Jul 1997;114(1):38–45.

140. Dixon BS, Beck GJ, Vazquez MA, et al. Effect of dipyridamole plus aspirin on hemodialysis graft patency. *N Engl J Med*. May 2009;360(21):2191–2201.

141. Schmitz PG, McCloud LK, Reikes ST, Leonard CL, Gellens ME. Prophylaxis of hemodialysis graft thrombosis with fish oil: double-blind, randomized, prospective trial. *J Am Soc Nephrol*. Jan 2002;13(1):184–190.

142. Lok CE, Allon M, Donnelly S, et al. Design of the fish oil inhibition of stenosis in hemodialysis grafts (FISH) study. *Clin Trials*. 2007;4(4):357–367.

143. Murthy SN, Obregon DF, Chattergoon NN, et al. Rosiglitazone reduces serum homocysteine levels, smooth muscle proliferation, and intimal hyperplasia in Sprague-Dawley rats fed a high methionine diet. *Metabolism*. May 2005;54(5):645–652.

144. Takagi T, Yamamuro A, Tamita K, Katayama M, Morioka S. Thiazolidinedione treatment attenuates diffuse neointimal hyperplasia in restenotic lesions after coronary stent implantation in type 2 diabetic patients: an intravascular ultrasound study. *J Cardiol*. Apr 2005;45(4):139–147.

145. Davies MG, Owens EL, Mason DP, et al. Effect of platelet-derived growth factor receptor-alpha and -beta blockade on flow-induced neointimal formation in endothelialized baboon vascular grafts. *Circ Res*. Apr 2000; 86(7):779–786.

146. Hausleiter J, Kastrati A, Mehilli J, et al. Randomized, double-blind, placebo-controlled trial of oral sirolimus for restenosis prevention in patients with in-stent restenosis: the Oral Sirolimus to Inhibit Recurrent In-stent Stenosis (OSIRIS) trial. *Circulation*. Aug 2004;110(7):790–795.

147. Rutherford C, Martin W, Salame M, Carrier M, Anggard E, Ferns G. Substantial inhibition of neo-intimal response to balloon injury in the rat carotid artery using a combination of antibodies to platelet-derived growth factor-BB and basic fibroblast growth factor. *Atherosclerosis*. Apr 1997; 130(1–2):45–51.

148. Leppanen O, Rutanen J, Hiltunen MO, et al. Oral imatinib mesylate (STI571/gleevec) improves the efficacy of local intravascular vascular endothelial growth factor-C gene transfer in reducing neointimal growth in hypercholesterolemic rabbits. *Circulation*. Mar 2004;109(9):1140–1146.

149. Fareh J, Martel R, Kermani P, Leclerc G. Cellular effects of beta-particle delivery on vascular smooth muscle cells and endothelial cells: a dose-response study. *Circulation*. Mar 1999;99(11):1477–1484.

150. Rubin P, Williams JP, Riggs PN, et al. Cellular and molecular mechanisms of radiation inhibition of restenosis. Part I: role of the macrophage and platelet-derived growth factor. *Int J Radiat Oncol Biol Phys*. Mar 1998;40(4):929–941.

151. Scott S, O'Sullivan M, Hafizi S, Shapiro LM, Bennett MR. Human vascular smooth muscle cells from restenosis or in-stent stenosis sites demonstrate enhanced responses to p53: implications for brachytherapy and drug treatment for restenosis. *Circ Res*. Mar 2002;90(4): 398–404.

152. Sabate M, Serruys PW, van der Giessen WJ, et al. Geometric vascular remodeling after balloon angioplasty and beta-radiation therapy: A three-dimensional intravascular ultrasound study. *Circulation*. Sep 1999; 100(11):1182–1188.

153. Grise MA, Massullo V, Jani S, et al. Five-year clinical follow-up after intracoronary radiation: results of a randomized clinical trial. *Circulation*. Jun 2002;105(23): 2737–2740.

154. Leon MB, Teirstein PS, Moses JW, et al. Localized intracoronary gamma-radiation therapy to inhibit the recurrence of restenosis after stenting. *N Engl J Med*. Jan 2001;344(4):250–256.

155. Sun S, Beitler JJ, Ohki T, et al. Inhibitory effect of brachytherapy on intimal hyperplasia in arteriovenous fistula. *J Surg Res*. Dec 2003;115(2):200–208.

156. Rodriguez VM, Grove J, Yelich S, Pearson D, Stein M, Pevec WC. Effects of brachytherapy on intimal hyperplasia in arteriovenous fistulas in a porcine model. *J Vasc Interv Radiol*. Dec 2002;13(12):1239–1246.

157. Kelly BS, Narayana A, Heffelfinger SC, et al. External beam radiation attenuates venous neointimal hyperplasia in a pig model of arteriovenous polytetrafluoroethylene (PTFE) graft stenosis. *Int J Radiat Oncol Biol Phys*. Sep 2002;54(1):263–269.

158. Roy-Chaudhury P, Duncan H, Barrett W, et al. Vascular brachytherapy for hemodialysis vascular access dysfunction: exploring an unmet clinical need. *J Invasive Cardiol*. Jan 2003;15 Suppl A:25A–30A.

159. Misra S, Bonan R, Pflederer T, Roy-Chaudhury P. BRAVO I: A pilot study of vascular brachytherapy in polytetrafluoroethylene dialysis access grafts. *Kidney Int*. Dec 2006;70(11):2006–2013.

160. van Tongeren RB, Levendag PC, Coen VL, et al. External beam radiation therapy to prevent anastomotic intimal hyperplasia in prosthetic arteriovenous fistulas: results of a randomized trial. *Radiother Oncol*. Oct 2003; 69(1):73–77.

161. Krueger K, Bendel M, Zaehringer M, Reinicke G, Lackner K. Centered endovascular irradiation to prevent postangioplasty restenosis of arteriovenous fistula in hemodialysis patients; Results of a feasibility study. *Cardiovasc Radiat Med.* Jan–Mar 2004;5(1):1–8.

162. Jordan MA, Toso RJ, Thrower D, Wilson L. Mechanism of mitotic block and inhibition of cell proliferation by taxol at low concentrations. *Proc Natl Acad Sci U S A.* Oct 1993;90(20):9552–9556.

163. Masaki T, Rathi R, Zentner G, et al. Inhibition of neointimal hyperplasia in vascular grafts by sustained perivascular delivery of paclitaxel. *Kidney Int.* Nov 2004; 66(5):2061–2069.

164. Kelly B, Melhem M, Zhang J, et al. Perivascular paclitaxel wraps block arteriovenous graft stenosis in a pig model. *Nephrol Dial Transplant.* Sep 2006;21(9):2425–2431.

165. Kohler TR, Toleikis PM, Gravett DM, Avelar RL. Inhibition of neointimal hyperplasia in a sheep model of dialysis access failure with the bioabsorbable Vascular Wrap paclitaxel-eluting mesh. *J Vasc Surg.* May 2007;45(5):1029–1037; discussion 1037–1028.

166. Paulson WD, Kipshidze N, Kipiani K, et al. Safety and efficacy of locally eluted sirolimus for prolonging AV graft patency (PTFE graft plus Coll-R) first in man experience. *J Am Soc Nephrol.* 2008(19):252A.

167. Nugent HM, Groothuis A, Seifert P, et al. Perivascular endothelial implants inhibit intimal hyperplasia in a model of arteriovenous fistulae: a safety and efficacy study in the pig. *J Vasc Res.* Nov–Dec 2002;39(6):524–533.

168. Nugent HM, Sjin RT, White D, et al. Adventitial endothelial implants reduce matrix metalloproteinase-2 expression and increase luminal diameter in porcine arteriovenous grafts. *J Vasc Surg.* Sep 2007;46(3): 548–556.

169. Ferrara N. Molecular and biological properties of vascular endothelial growth factor. *J Mol Med.* Jul 1999;77(7): 527–543.

170. Hiltunen MO, Laitinen M, Turunen MP, et al. Intravascular adenovirus-mediated VEGF-C gene transfer reduces neointima formation in balloon-denuded rabbit aorta. *Circulation.* Oct 2000;102(18):2262–2268.

171. Mann MJ, Gibbons GH, Kernoff RS, et al. Genetic engineering of vein grafts resistant to atherosclerosis. *Proc Natl Acad Sci U S A.* May 1995;92(10):4502–4506.

172. Mann MJ, Whittemore AD, Donaldson MC, et al. Ex-vivo gene therapy of human vascular bypass grafts with E2F decoy: the PREVENT single-centre, randomised, controlled trial. *Lancet.* Oct 1999;354(9189): 1493–1498.

173. Mann MJ, Dzau VJ. Therapeutic applications of transcription factor decoy oligonucleotides. *J Clin Invest.* Nov 2000;106(9):1071–1075.

174. Conte MS, Bandyk DF, Clowes AW, et al. Results of PREVENT III: a multicenter, randomized trial of edifoligide for the prevention of vein graft failure in lower extremity bypass surgery. *J Vasc Surg.* Apr 2006;43(4):742–751; discussion 751.

175. Alexander JH, Hafley G, Harrington RA, et al. Efficacy and safety of edifoligide, an E2F transcription factor decoy, for prevention of vein graft failure following coronary artery bypass graft surgery: PREVENT IV: a randomized controlled trial. *JAMA.* Nov 2005;294(19):2446–2454.

176. Burke SK, LaRochelle A, Mendenhall HV. Local application of recombinant human type I pancreatic elastase (PRT-201) to an arteriovenous fistula (AVF) increase AVF blood flow in a rabbit model. *J Am Soc Nephrol.* 2008(19):252A.

177. Beathard GA. Percutaneous transvenous angioplasty in the treatment of vascular access stenosis. *Kidney Int.* Dec 1992;42(6):1390–1397.

178. Beathard GA. Angioplasty for arteriovenous grafts and fistulae. *Semin Nephrol.* May 2002;22(3):202–210.

179. Inoue T, Node K. Molecular basis of restenosis and novel issues of drug-eluting stents. *Circ J.* Apr 2009;73(4): 615–621.

180. Okamoto E, Couse T, De Leon H, et al. Perivascular inflammation after balloon angioplasty of porcine coronary arteries. *Circulation.* Oct 2001;104(18):2228–2235.

181. Maya ID, Allon M. Outcomes of thrombosed arteriovenous grafts: comparison of stents vs angioplasty. *Kidney Int.* Mar 2006;69(5):934–937.

182. Chan MR, Bedi S, Sanchez RJ, et al. Stent placement versus angioplasty improves patency of arteriovenous grafts and blood flow of arteriovenous fistulae. *Clin J Am Soc Nephrol.* May 2008;3(3):699–705.

183. Suzuki T, Kopia G, Hayashi S, et al. Stent-based delivery of sirolimus reduces neointimal formation in a porcine coronary model. *Circulation.* Sep 2001;104(10):1188–1193.

184. Heldman AW, Cheng L, Jenkins GM, et al. Paclitaxel stent coating inhibits neointimal hyperplasia at 4 weeks in a porcine model of coronary restenosis. *Circulation.* May 2001;103(18):2289–2295.

185. Morice MC, Serruys PW, Sousa JE, et al. A randomized comparison of a sirolimus-eluting stent with a standard stent for coronary revascularization. *N Engl J Med.* Jun 2002;346(23):1773–1780.

186. Stone GW, Ellis SG, Cox DA, et al. A polymer-based, paclitaxel-eluting stent in patients with coronary artery disease. *N Engl J Med.* Jan 2004;350(3):221–231.

187. Moses JW, Leon MB, Popma JJ, et al. Sirolimus-eluting stents versus standard stents in patients with stenosis in a native coronary artery. *N Engl J Med.* Oct 2003;349(14):1315–1323.

188. Rotmans JI, Pattynama PM, Verhagen HJ, et al. Sirolimus-eluting stents to abolish intimal hyperplasia and improve flow in porcine arteriovenous grafts: a 4-week follow-up study. *Circulation.* Mar 2005;111(12):1537–1542.

189. Haskal ZJ, Trerotola S, Dolmatch B, et al. Stent graft versus balloon angioplasty for failing dialysis-access grafts. *N Engl J Med.* Feb 2010;362(6):494–503.

190. Nyberg SL, Hughes CB, Valenzuela YM, et al. Preliminary experience with a cuffed ePTFE graft for hemodialysis vascular access. *Asaio J.* Jul–Aug 2001;47(4):333–337.

191. Tsoulfas G, Hertl M, Ko DS, et al. Long-term outcome of a cuffed expanded PTFE graft for hemodialysis vascular access. *World J Surg.* Aug 2008;32(8):1827–1831.

192. Sorom AJ, Hughes CB, McCarthy JT, et al. Prospective, randomized evaluation of a cuffed expanded polytetrafluoroethylene graft for hemodialysis vascular access. *Surgery.* Aug 2002;132(2):135–140.

193. Ko PJ, Liu YH, Hung YN, Hsieh HC. Patency rates of cuffed and noncuffed extended polytetrafluoroethylene grafts in dialysis access: a prospective, randomized study. *World J Surg.* Apr 2009;33(4):846–851.

194. Roy-Chaudhury P, Wang Y, Krishnamoorthy M, Dakin A. Optiflow: a novel anastomotic conduit for reducing AV fistula dysfunction. *J Am Soc Nephrol.* 2008;19:253A.

195. Falk A. Maintenance and salvage of arteriovenous fistulas. *J Vasc Interv Radiol.* May 2006;17(5):807–813.

196. Hristov M, Weber C. Endothelial progenitor cells in vascular repair and remodeling. *Pharmacol Res.* Aug 2008; 58(2):148–151.

197. Wallitt EJ, Jevon M, Hornick PI. Therapeutics of vein graft intimal hyperplasia: 100 years on. *Ann Thorac Surg.* Jul 2007;84(1):317–323.

198. Urbich C, Dimmeler S. Endothelial progenitor cells: characterization and role in vascular biology. *Circ Res.* Aug 2004;95(4):343–353.

199. Asahara T, Murohara T, Sullivan A, et al. Isolation of putative progenitor endothelial cells for angiogenesis. *Science.* Feb 1997;275(5302):964–967.

200. Werner N, Junk S, Laufs U, et al. Intravenous transfusion of endothelial progenitor cells reduces neointima formation after vascular injury. *Circ Res.* Jul 2003;93(2):e17–e24.

201. Rotmans JI, Heyligers JM, Verhagen HJ, et al. In vivo cell seeding with anti-CD34 antibodies successfully accelerates endothelialization but stimulates intimal hyperplasia in porcine arteriovenous expanded polytetrafluoroethylene grafts. *Circulation.* Jul 2005; 112(1):12–18.

202. Lin CC, Chang CF, Lai MY, Chen TW, Lee PC, Yang WC. Far-infrared therapy: a novel treatment to improve access blood flow and unassisted patency of arteriovenous fistula in hemodialysis patients. *J Am Soc Nephrol.* Mar 2007; 18(3):985–992.

203. Lin CC, Liu XM, Peyton K, et al. Far infrared therapy inhibits vascular endothelial inflammation via the induction of heme oxygenase-1. *Arterioscler Thromb Vasc Biol.* Apr 2008;28(4):739–745.

204. Wong V, Ward R, Taylor J, Selvakumar S, How TV, Bakran A. Factors associated with early failure of arteriovenous fistulae for haemodialysis access. *Eur J Vasc Endovasc Surg.* Aug 1996;12(2):207–213.

205. Malovrh M. Non-invasive evaluation of vessels by duplex sonography prior to construction of arteriovenous fistulas for haemodialysis. *Nephrol Dial Transplant.* Jan 1998; 13(1):125–129.

206. Bacchini G, Cappello A, La Milia V, Andrulli S, Locatelli F. Color Doppler ultrasonography imaging to guide transluminal angioplasty of venous stenosis. *Kidney Int.* Oct 2000;58(4):1810–1813.

207. Bacchini G, La Milia V, Andrulli S, Locatelli F. Color Doppler ultrasonography percutaneous transluminal angioplasty of vascular access grafts. *J Vasc Access.* Apr–Jun 2007;8(2):81–85.

208. Krishnamoorthy MK, Banerjee RK, Wang Y, et al. Hemodynamic wall shear stress profiles influence the magnitude and pattern of stenosis in a pig AV fistula. *Kidney Int.* Dec 2008;74(11):1410–1419.

209. Ye C, Mao Z, Rong S, et al. Multislice computed tomographic angiography in evaluating dysfunction of the vascular access in hemodialysis patients. *Nephron Clin Pract.* 2006;104(2):c94–c100.

210. Ko SF, Huang CC, Ng SH, et al. MDCT angiography for evaluation of the complete vascular tree of hemodialysis fistulas. *Am J Roentgenol.* Nov 2005;185(5): 1268–1274.

211. Bakker CJ, Peeters JM, Bartels LW, et al. Magnetic resonance techniques in hemodialysis access management. *J Vasc Access.* Oct–Dec 2003;4(4):125–139.

212. Zhang J, Hecht EM, Maldonado T, Lee VS. Time-resolved 3D MR angiography with parallel imaging for evaluation of hemodialysis fistulas and grafts: initial experience. *Am J Roentgenol.* May 2006;186(5):1436–1442.

213. Planken RN, Tordoir JH, Dammers R, et al. Stenosis detection in forearm hemodialysis arteriovenous fistulae by multiphase contrast-enhanced magnetic resonance angiography: preliminary experience. *J Magn Reson Imaging.* Jan 2003;17(1):54–64.

214. Terry CM, Kim SE, Li L, et al. Longitudinal assessment of hyperplasia using magnetic resonance imaging without contrast in a porcine arteriovenous graft model. *Acad Radiol.* Jan 2009;16(1):96–107.

215. Misra S, Woodrum DA, Homburger J, et al. Assessment of wall shear stress changes in arteries and veins of arteriovenous polytetrafluoroethylene grafts using magnetic resonance imaging. *Cardiovasc Intervent Radiol.* Jul–Aug 2006;29(4):624–649.

216. Kostamaa H, Donovan J, Kasaoka S, Tobis J, Fitzpatrick L. Calcified plaque cross-sectional area in human arteries: correlation between intravascular ultrasound and undecalcified histology. *Am Heart J.* Mar 1999;137(3): 482–488.

217. Arbab-Zadeh A, Mehta RL, Ziegler TW, et al. Hemodialysis access assessment with intravascular ultrasound. *Am J Kidney Dis.* Apr 2002;39(4):813–823.

218. Higuchi T, Okuda N, Aoki K, et al. Intravascular ultrasound imaging before and after angioplasty for stenosis of arteriovenous fistulae in haemodialysis patients. *Nephrol Dial Transplant.* Jan 2001;16(1):151–155.

219. Roy-Chaudhury P. The mercator study investigators perivascular dexamethasone for PTFE graft stenosis: The HAPPI (hemodialysis access patency extension with percutaneous transluminal infusion of dexamethasone). *J Am Soc Nephrol.* 2007(18):468A.

220. Misra S, Fu AA, Anderson JL, et al. The rat femoral arteriovenous fistula model: increased expression of matrix metalloproteinase-2 and -9 at the venous stenosis. *J Vasc Interv Radiol.* Apr 2008;19(4):587–594.

221. Kuji T, Masaki T, Goteti K, et al. Efficacy of local dipyridamole therapy in a porcine model of arteriovenous graft stenosis. *Kidney Int.* Jun 2006;69(12):2179–2185.

222. Masaki T, Rathi R, Zentner G, et al. Inhibition of neointimal hyperplasia in vascular grafts by sustained perivascular delivery of paclitaxel. *Kidney Int.* Nov 2004;66(5):2061–2069.

223. Misra S, Fu AA, Puggioni A, et al. Proteomic profiling in early venous stenosis formation in a porcine model of hemodialysis graft. *J Vasc Interv Radiol.* Feb 2009;20(2): 241–251.

224. Nakano T, Ninomiya T, Sumiyoshi S, et al. Association of kidney function with coronary atherosclerosis and calcification in autopsy samples from Japanese elders: the Hisayama study. *Am J Kidney Dis.* Jan 2010;55(1):21–30.

225. Liu BC, Li L, Gao M, Wang YL, Yu JR. Microinflammation is involved in the dysfunction of arteriovenous fistula in patients with maintenance hemodialysis. *Chin Med J (Engl).* Nov 2008;121(21):2157–2161.

226. Lee ES, Shen Q, Pitts RL, Guo M, Wu MH, Yuan SY. Vein tissue expression of matrix metalloproteinase as biomarker

for hemodialysis arteriovenous fistula maturation. *Vasc Endovasc Surg.* Nov 2010;44(8):674–679.

227. Schwab SJ, Raymond JR, Saeed M, Newman GE, Dennis PA, Bollinger RR. Prevention of hemodialysis fistula thrombosis. Early detection of venous stenoses. *Kidney Int.* Oct 1989;36(4):707–711.

228. Schwab SJ. Hemodialysis vascular access: entering a new ara. *Am J Kidney Dis.* Sep 1999;34(3):xxxviii–xxxvxi.

229. Schwab SJ. Reducing the risk of hemodialysis access. *Am J Kidney Dis.* Aug 1999;34(2):362–363.

230. Akoh JA, Patel N. Infection of hemodialysis arteriovenous grafts. *The journal of vascular access.* Apr–Jun 2010;11(2):155–158.

231. Schild AF. Maintaining vascular access: the management of hemodialysis arteriovenous grafts. *J Vasc Access.* Apr–Jun 2010;11(2):92–99.

232. Maya ID, Weatherspoon J, Young CJ, Barker J, Allon M. Increased risk of infection associated with polyurethane dialysis grafts. *Semin Dial.* Nov–Dec 2007;20(6):616–620.

233. Allon M. Current management of vascular access. *Clin J Am Soc Nephrol.* Jul 2007;2(4):786–800.

234. Shin'oka T, Matsumura G, Hibino N, et al. Midterm clinical result of tissue-engineered vascular autografts seeded with autologous bone marrow cells. *J Thorac Cardiovasc Surg.* Jun 2005;129(6):1330–1338.

235. McAllister TN, Maruszewski M, Garrido SA, et al. Effectiveness of haemodialysis access with an autologous tissue-engineered vascular graft: a multicentre cohort study. *Lancet.* Apr 25 2009;373(9673):1440–1446.

236. Mironov V, Kasyanov V, Markwald RR. Nanotechnology in vascular tissue engineering: from nanoscaffolding towards rapid vessel biofabrication. *Trends Biotechnol.* Jun 2008;26(6):338–344.

237. *U.S. Renal Data System, USRDS 2009 Annual Data Report: Atlas of CKD and ESRD in the United States, National Institutes of Health*, National Institute of Diabetes and Digestive and Kidney Diseases, Bethesda, MD, 2009.

57

PHARMACOLOGICAL APPROACHES TO VASCULAR ACCESS DYSFUNCTION

PRABIR ROY-CHAUDHURY, TIMMY LEE, KARTHIK RAMANI & DAVINDER WADEHRA

LEARNING OBJECTIVES

1. To describe novel pharmacological approaches for dialysis vascular access dysfunction.

2. To emphasize the importance of local therapies.

Dialysis vascular access dysfunction remains a huge clinical problem for which there are currently no effective therapies. The last decade, however, has witnessed significant advances in our understanding of the pathobiology of both neointimal hyperplasia and vascular remodeling (outward or inward) and we believe that this knowledge is currently in the process of being converted into novel pharmacologic therapies.[1-11]

The current chapter will divide pharmacological therapies for dialysis access dysfunction into systemic and local approaches. Particular attention will be paid to large randomized studies on arteriovenous fistulae (AVF) and PTFE grafts in this area. Catheters will not be a focus of this chapter.

SYSTEMIC THERAPIES (LARGE RANDOMIZED STUDIES ONLY)

There have been three key randomized studies published in this area over the last few years and each will be discussed in turn.

1. *NIH Dialysis Access Consortium Fistula Study*: In this large well conducted study, over 800 subjects receiving a new AVF were randomized to receive either Clopidogrel 75 mg or placebo for 6 weeks.[12] The primary end point was AVF thrombosis at 6 weeks, while the secondary end point was suitability for hemodialysis between 4 and 5 months postsurgery. Of note, the study was stopped prematurely due to a reduction in the 6-week thrombosis rate from 19% in the placebo group to 12% in the clopidogrel-treated group. Unfortunately, this reduction in thrombosis did not translate into any improvement in the percentage of subjects whose AVF was suitable for hemodialysis. In fact, over 60% of subjects in both the clopidogrel and placebo groups had AVFs that were not suitable for dialysis at between 4 and 5 months postsurgery. This study clearly emphasized that we needed to know more about the natural history and biology of AVF maturation and has resulted in the setting up of a large NIH-funded consortium (Hemodialysis Fistula Maturation Consortium) whose goal is to identify both biological and clinical predictors of AVF success or failure.[13]

2. *NIH Dialysis Access Consortium Graft Study*: Similar to the AVF study, this was also a large well conducted study involving almost 700 subjects who were randomized to receive either placebo or Aggrenox (a combination of aspirin and extended release dipyridamole) starting as soon as possible following surgery and continuing until the first episode of thrombosis or intervention required to maintain patency.[14] The efficacy end point of the study was primary patency at 1 year, which was 23% in the placebo arm and 28% in the treatment (Aggrenox) arm. Or stated another way, the use of Aggrenox delayed the time to first intervention or thrombosis by 6 and 8 weeks. While this result was statistically significant, its clinical significance is unclear and this intervention has not been broadly embraced at present, by the dialysis vascular access community. Of note, enrolled subjects were allowed to be on aspirin and a subset multivariate analysis which looked at 1 year primary patency in subjects on baseline aspirin as compared to those who were not taking baseline aspirin suggested that baseline

aspirin users had a 17% improvement in primary patency (HR = 0.83, CI = 0.68–1.01; $P = 0.06$); a result which appeared to have more clinical significance as compared to the Aggrenox data but which did not reach statistical significance.[15]

3. *Fish Oil Inhibition of Stenosis in Hemodialysis Grafts (FISH)*: This was a randomized study of 201 subjects who were randomized to receive either 4 g of fish oil or placebo for 1 year.[16] The primary end point of the study was primary patency defined as for the NIH graft study above, with secondary end points that included time to loss of patency, rate of loss of patency, time to thrombosis, rate of thrombosis, rate of corrective interventions, and rate of cardiovascular events. The loss of primary patency in the fish oil group was 48% at 1 year as compared to 61% in the placebo group; a result that just missed statistical significance ($P = 0.06$). Intriguingly, this study did achieve statistical significance in all the secondary end points listed above including a reduction in cardiovascular events. Of note, the results from the FISH study were only recently described in preliminary form at the American Society of Nephrology meeting in Philadelphia in November 2011. A full and detailed description of the results is therefore awaited, but compared to the NIH studies the results appear to be far more clinically relevant and may have a greater chance of being translated into clinical practice.

In addition to the above studies, there have been a number of smaller randomized, nonrandomized, and retrospective analyses which have examined the role of a number of agents such as ACE inhibitors,[17] calcium channel blockers,[18] and fish oil[19] that may be effective for the prevention of stenosis and thrombosis in AVFs and PTFE grafts. There are also a number of excellent reviews that address this issue.[18,20–22] None of these therapies, however, are currently considered to be the standard of care for reducing dialysis vascular access dysfunction.

LOCAL THERAPIES

The somewhat equivocal results from these large multicenter studies suggest that conventional systemic therapies may not always be successful for the treatment of the aggressive stenosis that characterizes dialysis vascular access dysfunction. An alternative approach could be the use of local pharmacologic therapies (drugs, cells, genes, and chemicals) that are applied to the arteriovenous (AVF) or graft-vein (PTFE grafts) anastomosis, through either the perivascular (outside-in) or endovascular (inside-out) approach.[2,7,23]

▶ Perivascular Therapies

We believe that perivascular therapies in particular are extremely well suited to this clinical setting in that (a) dialysis access grafts and fistulas could be the ideal clinical model for the use of perivascular therapies since these can be easily applied at the time of surgery; (b) perivascular therapies preferentially target the adventitia which could be an important site for the inward migration of adventitial fibroblasts which could contribute to final neointimal volume; (c) multiple studies have demonstrated that lipophilic molecules in particular when placed over the adventitia rapidly diffuse through all the layers of the vessel wall; and (d) small amounts of otherwise toxic drugs can be safely delivered to the site of stenosis resulting in high local concentrations that have a therapeutic effect at the graft-vein or arteriovenous anastomoses but with minimal systemic toxicity. The following paragraphs describe a number of perivascular interventions for the delivery of pharmacologic therapies (drugs, cells, genes, and chemicals) to the site of venous stenosis that have at the very minimum been used in a "First in Man" study.

a. *Drug eluting perivascular wraps*: Experimental studies in our laboratory and others have previously demonstrated the efficacy of paclitaxel eluting wraps in animal models of AV graft stenosis.[24,25] The rationale behind this approach was the local antiproliferative effect of paclitaxel at the site of venous stenosis. A large multicenter clinical study on the use of paclitaxel wraps, however, was suspended following a DSMB review at the 25% enrollment level due to an imbalance in the incidence of infections between the control (graft only) and treatment arms (graft plus paclitaxel wrap). An alternative approach is the use of sirolimus eluting COLL-R wraps. An initial phase II study demonstrated primary unassisted AV graft patencies of 75% and 38% at 1 and 2 years, in patients treated with the COLL-R wrap albeit in the absence of a control arm.[26] More recently, 30 patients were treated with this wrap following AVF placement. A total of 87% of the fistulae underwent successful maturation with a mean maturation time of 27 days. There were no complications related specifically to the wrap and the peak sirolimus level in this study was 4.13 ng/mL at 6 hours following surgery.[27]

b. *Endothelial cell loaded gel foam wraps*: The rationale behind the use of these wraps is that the endothelial cell (in addition to lining blood vessels) is also a "bioreactor" which produces a large number of beneficial mediators that could reduce neointimal hyperplasia and enhance positive vascular remodeling.[28,29] Initial experimental studies have documented a beneficial effect of these endothelial cell loaded gel-foam wraps in porcine models of AVF and graft stenosis.[28,30] In addition, a recent phase II study was able to demonstrate technical feasibility and safety, with a possible efficacy signal in 65 hemodialysis patients who received a "Vascugel®" wrap loaded with treated human aortic endothelial cells at the time of AVF or graft placement.[31] A subset analysis of this data documented a significant improvement in primary patency in diabetic patients treated with the Vascugel® wraps as opposed to the control wraps.[32]

c. *Vascular endothelial growth factor D gene therapy*: In animal models of angioplasty-induced restenosis, the delivery of adenoviral particles encoding for vascular-endothelial growth factor C to the site of vascular injury has been shown to trigger the release nitric oxide and prostacyclin and reduce neointimal hyperplasia.[33] Preliminary data on the use of VEGF-D gene therapy in patients receiving PTFE grafts (using a packaged an adenoviral vector and a bio-degradable local drug delivery device made from collagen [Trinam®] which is placed at the vein-graft anastomosis at the time of surgery) have been able to document technical feasibility and safety. A large multicenter study using this technology, however, was discontinued due to poor enrollment. Despite this setback, we believe that arteriovenous fistulae and grafts remain perhaps the best clinical setting for the use of gene therapy in view of the ease of local delivery and the relatively low impact of adverse events due to the intervention (compare the downsides of a thrombosed graft with a myocardial infarction as a result of a thrombosed coronary artery).

d. *Recombinant Elastase PRT-201*: PRT 201 is a recombinant elastase that has been shown to result in both arterial and venous dilation and also to increase AV fistula blood flow in a rabbit model when applied to AV fistulas at the time of surgery. The potential clinical benefit of this approach is that, it could enhance AV fistula maturation (through rapid vascular dilation) and so reduce dependency on tunneled dialysis catheters. Recent data from a human phase II study in AVFs using three different doses document technical feasibility and safety together with a possible improvement in patency in the low dose group.[34] A larger phase IIb study in AVFs has just been completed with the results expected soon.

e. *Adventa® catheter*: All of the above technologies require that the identified intervention is applied at the time of AV fistula or AV graft placement. In order to deliver these therapies at a time point distant to surgery (since stenosis does not only occur in the perioperative period), Mercator Med has developed an endovascular balloon with a sheathed microneedle that can be placed over the site of vascular injury at the time of angioplasty. Inflating the balloon to 2 atm. allows the sheathed needle to pierce through the venous wall at the site of vascular injury. This "perivascular" needle can then be used to deliver the drug, cell, gene, or chemical of interest to the site of vascular injury at a time point that is distant from surgical placement of the AV fistula or graft. Our group has used the Adventa® catheter in a small study of hemodialysis patients undergoing PTFE graft angioplasty and has documented the technical feasibility of such an approach.[35]

▶ Endovascular Therapies

Although not suited for application at the time of surgery, endovascular interventions for the pharmacologic treatment of dialysis vascular access dysfunction have the advantages that they can be (a) used at time points that are far removed from the initial surgery and (b) used in a prophylactic mode to ameliorate vascular injury at the time of angioplasty or stent placement. The following paragraphs describe some examples of endovascular pharmacologic therapies that have been used in the clinical setting of either dialysis vascular access stenosis or peripheral vascular disease.

a. *Paclitaxel-coated balloons*: The biological rationale for this approach is that combining angioplasty injury with local delivery of an antiproliferative agent could potentially reduce neointimal hyperplasia. Although these have not been used in the setting of dialysis vascular access stenosis there are good data for the use of these drug-coated balloons in the setting of peripheral vascular disease.[36] More recently a small pilot study describes the use of a paclitaxel-coated balloon in dialysis vascular access grafts postangioplasty with a 6-month primary patency of 70% as compared to 25% for conventional balloon angioplasty.[37]

b. *Drug eluting stents*: The biological rationale for the use of drug eluting stents is that while the scaffold of the stent prevents inward remodeling following angioplasty; the coated drug will prevent the aggressive neointimal hyperplasia that is associated with the presence of the "foreign" stent within the vascular tree. Although there is a lot of data on the use of drug eluting stents in the coronary and peripheral circulations,[38–40] there is only animal data in the setting of dialysis vascular access.[41]

In summary, we believe that all of the above are important studies; in that they open the door for the development of novel local delivery systems (drugs, cells, genes, and chemicals) that target the key downstream pathways for venous stenosis such as oxidative stress, endothelial dysfunction, and neointimal hyperplasia. We hope that these preliminary therapeutic advances will allow us to address the huge "unmet clinical need" for pharmacologic therapies for dialysis vascular access dysfunction.

REFERENCES

1. Lee T, Roy-Chaudhury P. Advances and new frontiers in the pathophysiology of venous neointimal hyperplasia and dialysis access stenosis. *Adv Chronic Kidney Dis.* 2009;16:329–338.
2. Roy-Chaudhury P, Lee, T. Vascular stenosis: biology and interventions. *Curr Opinion Nephrol Hypertens.* 2007;16:516–522.
3. Roy-Chaudhury P, Kelly BS, Narayana A, et al. Hemodialysis vascular access dysfunction from basic biology to clinical intervention. *Adv Ren Replace Ther.* 2002;9:74–84.
4. Roy-Chaudhury P, Kelly BS, Zhang J, et al. Hemodialysis vascular access dysfunction: from pathophysiology to novel therapies. *Blood Purif.* 2003;21:99–110.
5. Roy-Chaudhury P, Melhem M, Husted T, Kelly BS. Solutions for hemodialysis vascular access dysfunction: Thinking out of the box!! *J Vasc Access.* 2005;6:3–8.

6. Roy-Chaudhury P, Spergel LM, Besarab A, Asif A, Ravani P. Biology of arteriovenous fistula failure. *J Nephrol.* 2007;20:150–163.

7. Roy-Chaudhury P, Sukhatme VP, Cheung AK. Hemodialysis vascular access dysfunction: a cellular and molecular viewpoint. *J Am Soc Nephrol.* 2006;17:1112–1127.

8. Dember LM, Dixon BS. Early fistula failure: back to basics. *Am J Kidney Dis.* 2007;50:696–699.

9. Dixon BS. Why don't fistulas mature? *Kidney Int.* 2006;70:1413–1422.

10. Allon M. Current management of vascular access. *Clin J Am Soc Nephrol.* 2007;2:786–800.

11. Allon M, Lok CE. Dialysis fistula or graft: the role for randomized clinical trials. *Clin J Am Soc Nephrol* 2010;5:2348–2354.

12. Dember LM, Beck GJ, Allon M, et al. Effect of clopidogrel on early failure of arteriovenous fistulas for hemodialysis: a randomized controlled trial. *J Am Med Assoc.* 2008;299:2164–2171.

13. Gerald J. Beck AKC, Laura M. Dember, Harold I. Feldman, Jonathan Himmelfarb, Thomas S. Huber, John W. Kusek, Prabir Roy-Chaudhury, Miguel A. Vazquez, Charles E. Alpers, Michelle L. Robbin, Joseph Vita. Progress of the hemodialysis fistula maturation (HFM) study. *J Am Soc Nephrol.* 2011;SA-OR452.

14. Dixon BS, Beck GJ, Vazquez MA, et al. Effect of dipyridamole plus aspirin on hemodialysis graft patency. *N Engl J Med.* 2009;360:2191–2201.

15. Dixon BS, Beck GJ, Dember LM, et al. Use of aspirin associates with longer primary patency of hemodialysis grafts. *J Am Soc Nephrol.* 2011;22:773–781.

16. Lok C, Louise M. Moist, Brenda Hemmelgarn, Marcello Tonelli, Michael Allon, Kenneth Stanley. The fish oil inhibition of stenosis in hemodialysis grafts (FISH) study. *J Am Soc Nephrol.* 2011;OR01.

17. Heine GH, Ulrich C, Kohler H, Girndt M. Is AV fistula patency associated with angiotensin-converting enzyme (ACE) polymorphism and ACE inhibitor intake? *Am J Nephrol.* 2004;24:461–468.

18. Saran R, Dykstra DM, Wolfe RA, Gillespie B, Held PJ, Young EW. Association between vascular access failure and the use of specific drugs: the Dialysis Outcomes and Practice Patterns Study (DOPPS). *Am J Kidney Dis.* 2002;40:1255–1263.

19. Schmitz PG, McCloud LK, Reikes ST, Leonard CL, Gellens ME. Prophylaxis of hemodialysis graft thrombosis with fish oil: double-blind, randomized, prospective trial. *J Am Soc Nephrol.* 2002;13:184–190.

20. Diskin CJ, Stokes TJ, Thomas SG, et al. An analysis of the effect of routine medications on hemodialysis vascular access survival. *Nephron.* 1998;78:365–368.

21. Diskin CJ, Stokes TJ, Jr., Pennell AT. Pharmacologic intervention to prevent hemodialysis vascular access thrombosis. *Nephron.* 1993;64:1–26.

22. Himmelfarb J. Pharmacologic prevention of vascular access stenosis. *Curr Opin Nephrol Hypertens.* 1999;8:569–572.

23. Roy-Chaudhury P, Kelly BS, Melhem M, et al. Vascular access in hemodialysis: issues, management, and emerging concepts. *Cardiol Clin.* 2005;23:249–273.

24. Kelly B MM, Jianhua Zhang, Gerald Kasting, Jinsong Li, Krisnamoorthy M, Sue Heffelfinger, Steven Rudich, Pankaj Desai, Prabir Roy-Chaudhury. Perivascular paclitaxel wraps block arteriovenous stenosis in a pig model. *Nephrol Dial Transplant.* 2006;21:2425–2431.

25. Kohler TR, Toleikis P, Gravett DM, Avelar RL. Inhibition of neointimal hyperplasia in a sheep model of dialysis access failure with the bioabsorbable vascular wrap paclitaexel eluting mesh. *J Vasc Surg.* 2007;45:1029–1038.

26. Paulson WD NK, Kipiani K, Beridze N, DeVita MV, Shenoy S, Iyer SS. Safety and efficacy of locally eluted sirolimus for prolonging AV graft patency (PTFE graft plus Coll-R) first in man experience. In: *American Society of Nephrology.* Philadelphia, 2008;TH-PO643.

27. DeVita M, Eric S. Chemla, Kipshidze Nickolas, Surendra Shenoy, Sriram Iyer. Improved arteriovenous fistula maturation with intra-operative implant of a perianastomotic sirolimus eluting collagen membrane (Coll-R). *J Am Soc Nephrol.* 2011;SA-OR459.

28. Nugent HM, Groothuis A, Seifert P, et al. Perivascular endothelial implants inhibit intimal hyperplasia in a model of arteriovenous fistulae: a safety and efficacy study in the pig. *J Vasc Res.* 2002;39:524–533.

29. Nugent HM, Rogers C, Edelman ER. Endothelial implants inhibit intimal hyperplasia after porcine angioplasty. *Circ Res.* 1999;84:384–391.

30. Nugent HM, Sjin RT, White D, et al. Adventitial endothelial implants reduce matrix metalloproteinase-2 expression and increase luminal diameter in porcine arteriovenous grafts. *J Vasc Surg.* 2007;46:548–556.

31. Conte MS, Nugent HM, Gaccione P, Guleria I, Roy-Chaudhury P, Lawson JH. Multicenter phase I/II trial of the safety of allogeneic endothelial cell implants after the creation of arteriovenous access for hemodialysis use: the V-HEALTH study. *J Vasc Surg.* 2009;50:1359–1368e1.

32. Conte MS, Nugent HM, Gaccione P, Roy-Chaudhury P, Lawson JH. Influence of diabetes and perivascular allogeneic endothelial cell implants on arteriovenous fistula remodeling. *J Vasc Surg.* 2011;54:1383–1389.

33. Hiltunen MO, Laitinen M, Turunen MP, et al. Intravascular adenovirus-mediated VEGF-C gene transfer reduces neointima formation in balloon-denuded rabbit aorta. *Circulation* 2000;102:2262–2268.

34. Dixon B, Eric K. Peden, David B. Leeser, Mahmoud T. El-Khatib, MD, Prabir Roy-Chaudhury, Jeffrey Lawson, Matthew Menard, Marc H. Glickman, Laura M. Dember, Steven K. Burke. Effect of recombinant human type 1 pancreatic elastase (PRT-201) treatment on fistula patency. *J Am Soc Nephrol.* 2011;SA-OR457.

35. Roy-Chaudhury P, Ted Kohler, Rui Avelar. Rationale, design, methods and statistical aspects of a randomized, multicenter, clinical study to assess the effectiveness of maintaining patency and the safety of the vascular wrap™ paclitaxel-eluting mesh implanted with a lifespan® ePTFE vascular graft for hemodialysis vascular access. *J Am Soc Nephrol.* 2007;18:469A.

36. Tepe G, Zeller T, Albrecht T, et al. Local delivery of paclitaxel to inhibit restenosis during angioplasty of the leg. *N Engl J Med.* 2008;358:689–699.

37. Katsanos K, Dimitris Karnabatidis, Panagiotis Kitrou, Stavros Spiliopoulos, Nikolaos Christeas, Dimitris Siablis. Drug-coated balloon angioplasty. In: *Hemodialysis Access.* 38th Annual Vascular and Endovascular Issues, Techniques and Horizons (VEITHsymposium), November 16–20, 2011.

38. Morice MC, Serruys PW, Sousa JE, et al. A randomized comparison of a sirolimus-eluting stent with a standard stent for coronary revascularization. *N Engl J Med.* 2002;346:1773–1780.

39. Stone GW, Ellis SG, Cox DA, et al. A polymer-based, paclitaxel-eluting stent in patients with coronary artery disease. *N Engl J Med.* 2004;350:221–231.

40. Stone GW, Moses JW, Ellis SG, et al. Safety and efficacy of sirolimus- and paclitaxel-eluting coronary stents. *N Engl J Med.* 2007;356:998–1008.

41. Rotmans JI, Pattynama PM, Verhagen HJ, et al. Sirolimus-eluting stents to abolish intimal hyperplasia and improve flow in porcine arteriovenous grafts: a 4-week follow-up study. *Circulation.* 2005;111:1537–1542.

DEVICE INNOVATION

MICHAEL J. KALLOK

1. Understand the processes required to convert ideas into new devices and products.
2. Understand the value of patents and other intellectual property.
3. Describe invention disclosures, patent applications, and the differences between provisional and nonprovisional patent applications.
4. Understand the product development process.
5. Describe the bench and animal testing and the clinical data required to obtain Food and Drug Administration (FDA) approval of new medical devices.
6. Understand the difference between various US FDA regulatory paths.
7. Describe the commercialization of new medical devices.

INTRODUCTION

The field of interventional nephrology (IN) is a procedural-based discipline that is relatively new. Although many of the interventions performed by interventional nephrologists are not new, the technical approach often is novel. Furthermore, many of the devices currently being used to perform IN procedures are inherited from other interventional disciplines and, in many cases, are not ideally designed to meet requirements specific to IN. As a result, there exists a unique opportunity within the field to design novel techniques and devices. The purpose of this chapter is to familiarize practitioners of IN with the steps involved in the conversion of new ideas, which we all have, to new devices, which we would all like to have.

Many people have ideas about new and better ways of doing things, regardless of their occupation or the field in which they work. These ideas might suggest a means to improve efficiency, reduce costs, make procedures safer and easier to perform, or provide a brand new and improved approach to an existing method. Although all professions provide opportunities for new ideas and innovation, the field of medicine is a particularly fertile ground for new medical and surgical treatments, more sensitive and specific diagnoses, and novel devices and drugs that enhance the practice of medicine and patient care. This fact is reflected in the thriving Medical Device and Pharmaceutical Industries in the United States, and the plethora of new devices and drugs that allow physicians to provide better diagnoses and treatments, or allow nurses and other health care workers to deliver better care for their patients.

Ideas originate from our own thoughts, various types of inspiration from others, situations we observe, problems we encounter, and from sources we may not even notice or be aware of. A recent Mayo Clinic Alumni Association publication stated "At least once a day, a Mayo Clinic physician, scientist, or employee submits an idea for a new invention to Mayo's Office of Intellectual Property."[1] Although the Mayo Clinic is a large organization with many employees, university hospitals, and academic institutions likely have a similar number of new ideas. How does one turn the ideas into inventions, and ultimately, into products? If you are fortunate enough to be affiliated with an institution or organization that supports innovators and inventors, then it may be a simple matter to submit your idea and have the office responsible for that activity obtain a patent and make arrangements to develop it and commercialize your idea.

Often inventors have ideas that belong to them personally and not necessarily to their employer. Others do not have access to an intellectual property service at their institution and consequently must navigate this process on their own. In this chapter, we will attempt to outline the steps by which one can protect their intellectual property, develop a product and even launch a business, gain FDA approval, and sell their product. Because the medical device industry is so unique, this chapter will focus on devices rather than drugs or nonmedical products. However, many of the topics apply to any new invention.

Identifying and Protecting Intellectual Property

The most important thing an inventor can do when a novel idea is identified is to document the idea. Write it down in a notebook, sign it, date it, and have someone read it and sign it as a witness. This simple act establishes the date when the idea was first conceived and provides tangible evidence in the form of a written document. This recording of the date first conceived may become important later if a similar product is invented and a dispute over the earliest description of the device arises.

New inventions always belong to the inventor, although rights to manufacture, use, or sell the product which result from the idea can be assigned to an employer, to another person, or to a company. The ability to assign rights to an invention often becomes a valuable consideration for the inventor. Employers may require ideas developed using their resources to be assigned to them, so it is a good idea to understand the intellectual property policies of your employer or institution. Even if you are required to assign intellectual property rights to your employer for ideas developed using their resources or while you are at your job, ideas conceived by you while you are away from your workplace and using your own resources legally belong to you and you may not be required to assign the idea to your employer. If in doubt, you should ask for a copy of your employer's intellectual property policy and ask an attorney for help in understanding your rights and obligations.

After the initial idea is documented, you must continue to think about your invention, how it might work, how you could build it, and what purposes it might have. As your idea description grows and the details of your device become better defined, you have begun a process known as *reduction to practice*. Your chances for a broader patent will increase as you are able to provide more details about how your product works, what purposes it has, how it can be manufactured, and any materials that can be used in its construction, and so on. This process often identifies new embodiments of the invention that broaden the description you are able to protect with a patent.

Maintain good records of your efforts to better describe and refine your idea. Sketches, rough prototypes, photographs, testing for the purpose of demonstrating that it actually works, chemical formulations, and any other details that could be used to more completely define your idea should be written in a notebook with the entries dated and signed. All this documentation will help when you and your patent attorney prepare a patent application.

Filing a Patent Application

Your idea has been developed, described, and documented. Now the question is, should you file a patent application? Patents are property rights granted by the US Constitution. A patent permits the inventor (or assignee) to "exclude others from making, using, offering for sale, or selling the invention throughout the United States or importing the invention into the United States" for a period of 20 years after filing the application in exchange for teaching the public your invention.[2] What this means is that you must describe your invention in enough detail that someone "skilled in the art" can make it based on your description. A person skilled in the art is one who would generally be familiar with the field of the invention and the purpose of the invention.

There are three types of patents:

- **Utility patents** may be granted to anyone who invents or discovers any new and useful process, machine, article of manufacture, or composition of matter, or any new and useful improvement to these;
- **Design** patents may be granted to anyone who invents a new, original, and ornamental design for an article of manufacture; and
- **Plant** patents may be granted to anyone who invents or discovers and asexually reproduces any distinct and new variety of plant.

Most inventors do not realize that obtaining a patent does not give them the right to make and use their invention, but only the right to exclude others from making and using their device. Once a patent is issued, the patentee must enforce the patent usually through legal means without the aid of the US Patent and Trademark Office. Even though you have a patent covering your invention, you must conduct what is known as a freedom to operate analysis, which is an examination of relevant patents in the field that might incorporate features of your invention. Freedom to operate analysis is usually performed by patent attorneys with the inventor's assistance to both identify and analyze patents that may potentially be infringed by your invention.

The patent process can take several years to complete. It begins with the filing of a patent application that is drafted by a patent attorney or patent agent with the help of the inventor. The patent application may be a provisional or nonprovisional application. The difference between these two applications is that a provisional application only generally describes the invention and does not include all the details necessary for the examiner to reach a decision about patentability. A provisional patent application establishes a priority date for the invention that might become important if a dispute about the earliest to invent ever arises. A provisional patent application must be followed by a nonprovisional application within 1 year or abandoned, which forfeits the priority date.

When the nonprovisional patent application is filed, the application is logged into the Patent and Trademark Office, assigned a number, and after approximately 18 months is published and made available in the public domain for everyone to see. Twelve to 18 months after the patent application is published, the patent examiner issues what is known as an office action. The office action is a formal response to the application, citing any reasons why a particular claim of the patent cannot be allowed. Often all claims in a patent are rejected after the first review. Following the first office action, the patent attorney or agent responds to the examiner's critique of the claims, modifying the claims or explaining why a particular claim should be allowed. This negotiating process between the patent attorney and examiner continues until agreement is reached on the language and scope of the claims that are a series of statements that are the essence of what is patented.

The patent law specifies the general field of subject matter that can be patented and the conditions under which a patent may be obtained. Quoting the language of the statute, any person who "invents or discovers any new and useful process, machine, manufacture, or composition of matter, or any new and useful improvement thereof, may obtain a patent," subject to the conditions and requirements of the law.[2] The word "process" is defined by the law as a process, act or method, and primarily includes industrial or technical processes. The term "machine" used in the statute needs no explanation. The term "manufacture" refers to articles that are made, and includes all manufactured articles. The term "composition of matter" relates to chemical compositions and may include mixtures of ingredients as well as new chemical compounds. These classes of subject matter taken together include practically everything that is made by man and the processes for making the products. The courts have interpreted the statute and come to the conclusion that laws of nature, physical phenomena, and abstract ideas are not eligible material to patent. Also, the importance of adding sufficient detail to the patent application is necessary because pure speculative ideas are not patentable.

In order for an invention to be patentable, it must be new as defined in the patent law. Again quoting from the statute,[2] if: (a) "the invention was known or used by others in this country, or patented or described in a printed publication in this or a foreign country, before the invention thereof by the applicant for patent," or (b) "the invention was patented or described in a printed publication in this or a foreign country or in public use or on sale in this country more than 1 year prior to the application for patent in the United States . . ." then it cannot be patented.

An important consideration is that if the invention has been described in a printed publication anywhere in the world, or if it was known or used by others in the United States before the date that the applicant made his/her invention, a patent cannot be obtained. This is particularly relevant to academic inventors who publish the results of their research. In this situation, it is immaterial when the invention was made, or whether the printed publication or public use was by the inventor or by someone else. If the inventor describes the invention in a printed publication or uses the invention publicly, or attempts to sell it, the inventor must apply for a patent within 1 year of publication or use, otherwise any right to a patent will be lost. The inventor must file on the date of public use or disclosure, however, in order to preserve patent rights in many foreign countries.

Even if the subject matter described in the patent application is not exactly illustrated by the prior art, and involves one or more differences over the most nearly similar thing already known, a patent may still be refused if the differences would be obvious. The subject matter which is being patented must be sufficiently different from what has been used or described before that it may be said to be nonobvious to a person having ordinary skill in the area of technology related to the invention. For example, the substitution of one color for another, or changes in size, is ordinarily not patentable.

The preparation of an application for a patent and conducting the proceedings in the United States Patent and Trademark Office (USPTO) to obtain the patent is a task that generally requires the knowledge of patent law and rules and USPTO practice and procedures, as well as knowledge of the scientific or technical matters involved in the particular invention. Inventors may prepare their own applications and file them in the USPTO and conduct the proceedings themselves, but unless they are familiar with the process as well as the laws, they may get into considerable difficulty and jeopardize the issuance of a patent. While a patent may be obtained in many cases by persons not skilled as a patent attorney or agent, there would be no assurance that the patent obtained would adequately protect the particular invention.

Most inventors employ the services of registered patent attorneys or patent agents. The law gives the USPTO the power to make rules and regulations governing acceptance and recognition of patent attorneys and agents to practice before the USPTO. Persons who are not recognized for this practice are not permitted by law to represent inventors before the USPTO. The USPTO maintains a register of attorneys and agents, and to be admitted to this register, patent attorneys usually have an undergraduate degree in engineering, science, or some technical field. Patent attorneys must also pass a special examination.

The USPTO registers both attorneys and persons who are not attorneys. The former persons are now referred to as "patent attorneys" and the latter persons are referred to as "patent agents." Both patent attorneys and patent agents are permitted to prepare an application for a patent and conduct the prosecution in the USPTO. Patent agents, however, cannot conduct patent litigation in the courts or perform various services that the local jurisdiction (state or federal courts) considers as practicing law. For example, a patent agent could not draw up a contract relating to a patent, such as an assignment or a license, if the state in which he/she resides considers drafting contracts as practicing law. Patent agents are often employed at law firms to help patent attorneys with drafting applications. The USPTO maintains a directory of registered patent attorneys and agents at **http://www.uspto. gov/web/offices/dcom/olia/oed/roster/index.html**.

In employing a patent attorney or agent, the inventor executes a power of attorney that is filed in the USPTO. When a registered attorney or agent has been appointed, the USPTO does not communicate with the inventor directly but conducts the correspondence with the attorney or agent since he/she is acting for the inventor thereafter although the inventor is free to contact the USPTO concerning the status of his/her application. The inventor may remove the attorney or agent by revoking the power of attorney.

Since the rights granted by a US patent are valid only within the United States and its territories and have no equivalent rights in a foreign country, an inventor who wishes patent protection in other countries must apply for a patent in each of the other countries or in regional patent offices. Almost every country has its own patent law, and a person desiring a patent in a particular country must make an application for patent in that country, in compliance with the requirements of that country.

The laws of many countries differ in various respects from the patent law of the United States. In most foreign countries, publication of the invention before the date of the application will disqualify the invention from being patented. In most foreign countries, maintenance fees are required to be paid to keep a patent valid. Most foreign countries require that the patented invention be manufactured in that country after a certain period, usually 3 years. If there is no manufacture within this period, the patent may be void in some countries, although in most countries the patent may be valid following the grant of licenses to any authorized person who may apply for a license.

The timely filing of an international application establishes an international filing date in each country which is designated in the international application and provides (1) a search of the field of the invention and (2) a later time period within which the national applications for patent must be filed. A number of patent attorneys specialize in obtaining patents in foreign countries.

Under US law, it is necessary, in the case of inventions made in the United States, to obtain a license from the Director of the USPTO before applying for a patent in a foreign country. Such a license is required if the foreign application is to be filed before an application is filed in the United States or before the expiration of 6 months from the filing of the US application. The filing of an application for a patent constitutes the request for a license and the granting or denial of such request is indicated in the filing receipt mailed to each applicant. After 6 months from the US filing, a license is not required unless the invention has been ordered to be kept secret. If the invention has been ordered to be kept secret, the consent to filing abroad must be obtained from the Director of the USPTO during the period the order of secrecy is in effect.

▶ Developing a Prototype

Because medical devices are regulated by various agencies like the FDA in the United States, Competent Authorities in European countries, and various other regulatory bodies in other parts of the world, there are special considerations that must be followed when developing any new medical device (and new drug). After an initial idea for a new product is formulated, the inventor will likely want to make a first prototype to demonstrate what the actual device will look like. Developing an actual working prototype of your invention is an important first step in developing a new product. Often this is done in a casual, noncontrolled

environment. The best approach, however, is to develop the prototype within the constraints of a formal product development protocol that incorporates design controls. This ensures that when you do reach a final design you have proper documentation for all the steps completed from the first concept through manufacturing. This documentation becomes important in securing regulatory approvals to market your device in the United States and abroad. There are many types of product development protocols, but most are developed to conform to the requirements in the following regulations:

a. FDA Quality System Regulation (QSR), Title 21 Code of Federal Regulations (CFR) Part 820;

b. FDA Medical Device Reporting (MDR) regulation, 21 CFR Part 803;

c. FDA Reports of Corrections and Removals regulation, 21 CFR Part 806; and

d. ISO 13485:2003, Quality Management Systems—Medical Devices—System Requirements for Regulatory Purposes

The basic phases normally used in the design control process are illustrated in the chart below. Each phase is distinct and has various inputs and outputs that drive the process from one phase to another, that is, the output of one phase often becomes part of the input for the next phase. At each phase proper documentation must be maintained because at the end of the process the manufacturer must be able to show the process steps to an independent auditor for the purpose of obtaining regulatory approval.

▶ Design Control Flowchart

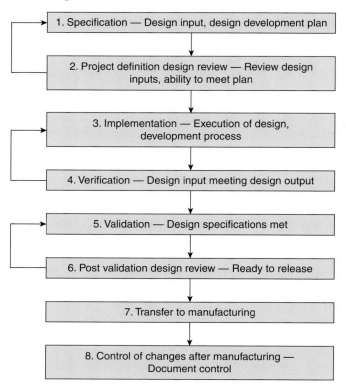

1. Specification — Design input, design development plan

2. Project definition design review — Review design inputs, ability to meet plan

3. Implementation — Execution of design, development process

4. Verification — Design input meeting design output

5. Validation — Design specifications met

6. Post validation design review — Ready to release

7. Transfer to manufacturing

8. Control of changes after manufacturing — Document control

Although the design control process takes a company through a finished design and manufacturing, there are considerations at each stage of the process that need to be followed so that the final design meets all the requirements. The initial prototype phase begins with a concept or problem. The needs of the user and market place are defined by available sources of customer input. These needs are reflected in the Product Requirement Specification, which becomes the document that drives additional development. Sample prototypes are constructed to determine if they meet the initial specification, design iterations are made to refine the design, and the prototype is compared to the specification to see if it meets all the requirements or if not, which requirements need to be modified.

▶ Manufacturing Your Product

After the concept phase is completed as documented by the development of a Product Requirements Specification and construction of an early prototype, a full project plan is developed and formal design controls now apply. The Specification is a living document allowing the conceptual design to be refined. As the design process continues, there are additional design iterations, establishment of detailed engineering specifications, and tolerances. A hazard analysis on the design is conducted and mitigation of hazards defined, and test methods are developed to determine if the design meets all the requirements.

All medical devices and drugs are regulated by the FDA. The FDA has established classes of products for both devices and drugs. The particular classification determines the level of testing required to establish that the product is safe and effective. The testing requirements range from certifying compliance to published standards to extensive bench and animal testing and large randomized clinical trials. For medical devices, FDA has published a document that describes how devices are classified and therefore the level of proof required to obtain FDA approval to market. The Medical Device Amendments of 1976 to the Federal Food, Drug, and Cosmetic Act established three regulatory classes for medical devices. The three classes are based on the degree of control necessary to assure that the various types of devices are safe and effective. The most regulated devices are in Class III. The amendments define a Class III device as one that supports or sustains human life or is of substantial importance in preventing impairment of human health or presents a potential, unreasonable risk of illness or injury. According to the FDA, insufficient information exists on a Class III device so that performance standards (Class II) or general controls (Class I) cannot provide reasonable assurance that the device is safe and effective for its intended use.

Effective June 1, 1997, manufacturers of Class II, Class III, and certain Class I devices are required to follow design control procedures when originally developing devices and for subsequent modifications to those devices, even during the development process. Product modifications that could significantly affect safety and effectiveness are subject to

510(k) submission requirements under 21 CFR 807 as well as design control requirements under 21 CFR 820.30. In accordance with the Quality System Regulation, manufacturers must have a systematic set of requirements and activities for the management of design and development, including documentation of design inputs, risk analysis, design output, test procedures, verification and validation procedures, and documentation of formal design reviews. In this process, the manufacturer must ensure that design input requirements are appropriate so the device will meet its intended use and the needs of the user population. The manufacturer must also establish and maintain procedures for defining and documenting design output in terms that allow an adequate evaluation of conformance to design input requirements. Thus, manufacturers may need to refine their device design requirements as verification and validation results are obtained. The design specifications that result from this process are the design outputs, which form the basis for the device master record (DMR) (see 21 CRF 820.3 [i]). The DMR is subject to inspection by FDA personnel.

Since design control requirements are now in effect and require the manufacturer to conduct verification and validation studies of a type that have traditionally been included in 510(k) submissions, FDA believes that it may be appropriate to forgo a detailed review of the underlying data normally required in 510(k)s. For this reason, FDA is allowing an alternative to the traditional method of demonstrating substantial equivalence for certain device modifications. For these well-defined modifications, the FDA believes that the rigorous design control procedure requirements produce highly reliable results that can form, in addition to the other 510(k) content requirements, a basis for the substantial equivalence determination. Under the Quality Systems Regulation, data that is generated as a result of the design control procedures must be maintained by the manufacturer and be available for FDA inspection.

Under the New 510(k) Paradigm, a manufacturer should refer to 21 CFR 807.81(a)(3) and the FDA guidance document entitled, "Deciding When to Submit a 510(k) for a Change to an Existing Device" to decide if a device modification may be implemented without submission of a new 510(k). If a new 510(k) is needed for the modification and if the modification does not affect the intended use of the device or alter the fundamental scientific technology of the device, then summary information that results from the design control process can serve as the basis for clearing the application.

▶ Gaining FDA Approval for Medical Products

There are two primary processes for medical devices: the first is Premarket Approval, or PMA, and the second is 510(k) clearance. The PMA process is the most rigorous process for FDA approval. The manufacturer is required to demonstrate that the new medical device is safe and effective for the labeling claims made. Under

Section 515 of the act, all devices placed into Class III are subject to PMA requirements. Premarket approval by FDA is the required process of scientific review to ensure the safety and effectiveness of Class III devices. An approved Premarket Approval Application (PMAA)—like an approved New Drug Application (NDA)—is, in effect, a private license granted to the applicant for marketing a particular medical device. A Class III device that fails to meet PMAA requirements is considered to be adulterated under Section 501(f) of the act and cannot be marketed. Premarket approval requirements apply differently to pre-amendments devices, postamendments devices, and transitional Class III devices.

A preamendments device is one that was in commercial distribution before May 28, 1976, the enactment date of the Medical Device Amendments. Manufacturers of Class III preamendments devices are not required to submit a PMAA until 30 months after the promulgation of a final classification regulation or until 90 days after the publication of a final regulation requiring the submission of a PMAA, whichever period is later. FDA may allow more than 90 days after promulgation of a final rule for submission of a PMA.

A postamendments device is one that was first distributed commercially on or after May 28, 1976. Postamendments devices that FDA determines are substantially equivalent to preamendments Class III devices are subject to the same requirements as the preamendments devices. FDA determines substantial equivalence after reviewing an applicant's premarket notification submitted in accordance with Section 510(k) of the act. Postamendments devices determined by FDA to not be substantially equivalent to either preamendments devices or postamendments devices classified into Class I or II are "new" devices and fall automatically into Class III. Before such devices can be marketed, they must have an approved premarket approval application or be reclassified into Class I (general controls) or Class II (standards).

Class III transitional devices and "new" devices (described in the paragraph above) are automatically classified into Class III by statute and require premarket approval by FDA before they may be commercially distributed. Applicants may either submit a PMAA or Product Development Protocol (PDP), or they may petition FDA to reclassify the devices into Class I or Class II. Clinical studies in support of a PMAA, PDP, or a reclassification petition are subject to the investigational device exemption (IDE) regulations (for further details on these regulations, refer to 21 CFR 812 for general devices).

New section 515 (d)(6) of the act added by the FDA Modernization Act of 1997, provides that PMA supplements are required for all changes that affect safety and effectiveness unless such change involves modifications to manufacturing procedures or method of manufacture. These types of manufacturing changes require a 30-day notice or, where FDA finds such notice inadequate, a 135-day PMA supplement.

Under section 510(k) of the Act, a person who intends to introduce a device into commercial distribution is required to submit a premarket notification, or 510(k), to FDA at least 90 days before commercial distribution is to begin. Section 513(i) of the Act states that FDA may issue an order of substantial equivalence only upon making a determination that the device to be introduced into commercial distribution is as safe and effective as a legally marketed device. Under 21 CFR 807.87, FDA established the content requirements for premarket notifications to be submitted by device manufacturers in support of the substantial equivalence decision. FDA has, however, discretion in the type of information it deems necessary to meet those content requirements. For example, to allocate review resources more effectively to the highest risk devices, FDA developed a tiering system based on the complexity and the level of risk posed by medical devices. Under this system, the substantial equivalence determination for low risk devices is based primarily on descriptive information and a labeling review, while the decision for higher risk devices relies on performance data.

In a further effort to manage FDA's workload and allocate resources most appropriately, the Agency exempted Class I devices for which it determined that premarket notification requirements were not necessary to provide reasonable assurance of safety and effectiveness.

Between the passage of the Medical Device Amendments of 1976 and the Food and Drug Administration Modernization Act (FDAMA) of 1997, FDA exempted 574 generic types of Class I devices from the requirement of premarket notification. As a result of the FDAMA, all Class I devices are exempt from the requirement of premarket notification, unless the device is intended for a use that is of substantial importance in preventing impairment to human health or presents a potential unreasonable risk of illness or injury ("reserved" criteria). Therefore, only those Class I devices that meet the reserved criteria remain subject to the premarket notification requirement (see 63 FR 5387, February 2, 1998, for a listing of Class I "reserved" devices).

The FDAMA also gave FDA the authority to directly exempt certain Class II devices rather than first downclassifying them to Class I before they become eligible for exemption. On January 21, 1998, FDA published a listing of Class II devices that no longer require premarket notification (see 63 FR 3142). In the future, additional Class II devices may become exempt from the premarket notification requirement as FDA considers additional devices for exemption.

The last phase of the Agency's effort to evaluate which devices should be subject to 510(k) review involves the preamendments Class III devices. Preamendments Class III devices for which general controls or special controls are sufficient to ensure safety and effectiveness will eventually be down-classified to either Class I [510(k) exempt or reserved] or to Class II, respectively. Those preamendments Class III devices that are not appropriate for reclassification will remain in that class and be subject to either PMA or PDP requirements. It is anticipated that, as a result of this reclassification effort, the premarket notification process will be primarily reserved for Class II devices and a few "reserved" Class I devices. Until a preamendments Class III device type becomes subject to a regulation requiring premarket approval, however, the device type will remain subject to the premarket notification requirement.

▶ Marketing and Selling Your Product

Marketing and selling medical devices are very specialized activities. There are regulations governing advertising, promoting, providing incentives, off label promotion and use, to name a few. Most of these regulations stem from regulatory concerns, Medicare and Medicaid fraud and abuse practices, billing fraud, and other activities that relate to the somewhat unique situation that exists in medicine. The "customer" is normally the patient but they often do not participate in the buying decision; sometimes the health care provider makes the buying decision and at times the hospital makes the decision; reimbursement is normally provided by a third party payor, and they can be either a private insurance company or a government entity. This somewhat complicated business model demands expertise in numerous areas including medical procedures, hospital economics, insurance regulations, operating room, and catheterization laboratory protocols. Most sales representatives undergo extensive training and enter their profession with backgrounds including engineering, medicine, nursing, medical technicians, to name a few. They receive product-specific training upon joining a new company, in addition to training in FDA regulations, dealing with customer complaints and product issues, recalls, billing, and so on. All this required training makes sales of medical devices a very complex process and one that can make or break a medical device Company. An alternative to hiring and training a sales force is to use an established medical products distributor that is a company that employees sales representatives and sells many medical devices for multiple manufacturers. The distributor provides training and support to the sales representatives and makes certain all the relevant regulations are followed. This type of relationship is more costly than establishing a direct sales force, but the overhead associated with hiring and training employees may well offset the costs.

Regarding marketing, manufacturers need to be familiar with the FDA's regulations describing what are known as labeling claims, or the specific conditions for which the device has been approved. Making claims that are not included in the original FDA 510(k) clearance or PMAA approval can result in serious consequences including seizure of product and criminal charges against the company. Use of a device for purposes other than those specifically listed in the labeling constitutes "off label" use. The interesting fact about off label is that the FDA does not have jurisdiction over the practice of medicine and thus does not regulate how a physician uses a device. This does not mean that there are no issues to consider when using a device off label, but simply that the FDA does not regulate this practice. What the FDA does regulate, however, is the promotion of medical devices by manufacturers. Regardless of how a device is used, the manufacturer is only allowed to promote the device for the uses described in the approved labeling.

SUMMARY

The creative process is present in employees working in all occupations, but the field of medicine in particular provides many opportunities for new device innovation because of the nature of the profession. Physicians, nurses, and other health care workers are always looking for ways to help their patients and most people recognize the limitations of existing therapeutic and diagnostic devices. Inventors of new medical devices who want to see their ideas developed into products can expect a long tedious process to that goal, but there are resources available to help. If the employer does not provide formal assistance with intellectual property protection and commercialization of new devices, there are many sources that can provide the necessary expertise. If the inventor does not want to be a business entrepreneur, one can still receive appropriate credit and monetary compensation for their idea.

The first step in the process is to carefully document your idea in writing and having your document witnessed to establish the date when first conceived. After sufficient details are identified, contact a patent attorney to draft a patent application that can either be a provisional application to establish a filing date or a nonprovisional application to secure an actual patent. In addition to patenting your concept, your patent attorney will want to conduct a freedom to operate analysis to determine if there are other patents that your invention would potentially infringe.

Following application for the intellectual property rights, you will need to arrange for the product design and development to be carried out. If you intend to do this yourself, you will need to establish a company, hire appropriate employees, establish a quality system, to name a few. This is a huge undertaking and normally requires finding a company CEO who has done this activity previously. As the inventor you maintain inventorship of the intellectual property, but you normally would assign the invention to the company, usually in exchange for equity. This in effect makes the company the owner of the intellectual property. An alternative approach is to find a contract organization that has experience in medical device design and development, quality systems, regulatory affairs, manufacturing, to name a few. Using contract services minimizes the overhead associated with establishing a company and given the right people, will result in a finished device ready to sell.

REFERENCES

1. Mayo Clinic's Office of Intellectual Property. Bringing Inventive Ideas to Life. *Mayo Alumni.* 2011, Spring.
2. Public Law 106-1 13, 11 3 Stat. 1501 (1999).

SECTION VI
Political and Policy Affairs

The opportunities for training in IN remain rather limited at this time, although these are improving. Many private practices provide interventional training to practicing nephrologists. ASDIN, through its role in providing accreditation to the training centers, creating curriculum and providing guidance for certification, has been instrumental in providing such information to those desirous of training. Vascular access centers, besides providing much needed access care to the patients, have the potential to become major training sites for these practitioners.

▶ Accreditation of Vascular Access Center

During recent times, there has been intense focus on training of interventional nephrology practitioners. The ASDIN has developed standards for certification of trainees and for accreditation of training centers. ASDIN accreditation is available for centers meeting these rigorous standards and is discussed in this text elsewhere in detail (see Chapter 9).[16] The criteria for training center are based upon the availability of proper facilities and equipment, didactic curriculum, expert trainers, and an adequate number of supervised procedures that must be performed as primary operator. For training physicians, there are minimum criteria for certification in each technique, with availability of partial certifications in specific procedures.

▶ Operational Structure of Vascular Access Centers

Common structures for VACs are as follows:

1. *Hospital owned or managed VAC with inpatient and/ or outpatient management of vascular access*

   VAC may be set up by the institution either as within the hospital itself or as a free standing ambulatory surgical center (ASC). The hospital provides the capital for construction and equipment, manages the employees, and supplies and bears the burden of operations. Physician reimbursement remains separate unless he/she is an employee of the hospital. Disadvantages for the operator include lack of autonomy, potential interference by hospital and complexities of local politics. Disadvantages for the patient are largely related to the inconvenience and delay of interacting with a system largely set up to service an inpatient population.[10]

2. *Free standing VAC as an extension of practice*

   As discussed in Chapter 60 on reimbursement, the majority of interventional facilities are currently set up and operated as an extension of a physician's office practice. This results in enhanced autonomy for the physician practice and revenue accrual if run expertly and efficiently. Compliance issues and capital investment are significantly reduced in comparison to the other option for an outpatient facility, an ASC. Since the physician practice now assumes the risk for management and operation of the facility, the potential return to the practice is greater. Disadvantages include the risks inherent in capital investment and the assumption of management responsibilities for the facility and employees. Partnering with a management company can mitigate these burdens, although that may substantially reduce the financial return. Multiple models of varying complexity, involvement and cost are currently available through a variety of vendors. In addition, a VAC operating as an extension of an office practice is a freestanding facility. Should serious complications occur, management involves stabilization of the patient and transport to an inpatient facility all of which needs to be assured in advance.

3. *Ambulatory Surgical Center*

   The ASC is geared toward providing specialty surgery in an outpatient setting. The ASC, is different from a hospital in that it does not provide emergency services, nor does it have the facilities for an overnight stay. While there is significant overlap, it provides facilities for procedures that are considered too intense for doctors' office. There are very strict requirements that must be followed when constructing an ASC. Regulations vary by state law and ASCs are regulated by state agencies. The regulatory oversight applied to an ASC is stricter compared to that for a physician's office practice and reimbursement for performing procedures (physician fees) are strictly segregated from the facility reimbursement. ASCs need to be accredited and are subject to audit by an accreditation agency. The reimbursement structure and differences between ASCs and the physician office are discussed in Chapter 60.

▶ Requirements for Setting up a VAC

The primary purpose of a VAC is to provide expedient, efficient, and expert care to the dialysis patient. The first and foremost requirement for any center that plans to take care of the dialysis patients' vascular access is availability of a dedicated, well-trained interventionalist who combines knowledge in vascular access procedures with knowledge of dialysis, and dialysis patients.

Due to the patient centered nature, the design of the center should provide adequate amenities for patients and visitors. The access procedure suite must be of user-friendly design to allow smooth workflow for both physician and staff. The equipment should include a portable C arm with capability for digital subtraction and road mapping. Ultrasound equipment should be available for central vein access. Supplies to meet the demands of procedures must be ensured, and should be tailored to operator preference, within the consideration of economics. The staff should be knowledgeable and dedicated to the care of dialysis patients and with special knowledge in observation and problem solving relating to dialysis vascular access procedures.

Computerized database should also be available for operations and quality assurance of VAC. Procedures, outcomes, and supplies should be able to be tracked. Additionally, computerized database can help in researching the most efficient, effective, and innovative methods to improve patient care at the VAC. The complications must be tracked to provide a healthy feedback for future improvement. There should be performance measures for the center, as well as for the operator for quality improvement as well as for reporting. There is a possibility for collaboration with academic centers to perform basic research in pathology and pathophysiology of VA failure. The interventionalist can also focus on bringing "bench to bedside" and vice versa. High-quality research is needed in this upcoming subspecialty to disseminate the knowledge about the best processes that could improve outcomes and VAC can contribute to this goal.

The multidisciplinary approach to VA care has been described as "integrated vascular access management."[10] Employing a vascular access coordinator can markedly improve vascular access quality. The interventional nephrologist must interact with the VA surgeon, practicing nephrologist, and dialysis staff to develop a plan of care starting with vascular mapping. Surgeon selection must be based on training in the full spectrum of surgical techniques[17] and a dedication to access care. With this multidisciplinary approach and development of dedicated VAC, it is possible to significantly improve VA-related outcomes.

Economic viability for an access center depends upon performance of a minimum number of procedures to satisfy overhead needs and to maintain a trained and expert staff. Often, the number of patients in an individual practice is not sufficient to sustain a VAC. It is possible, although tedious, to legally joint venture with one or more groups with each group operating out of the same facility while sharing overhead costs. The setup of such centers can be legally complex, but is feasible. Centers must meet local, state, and federal regulations. Policies and procedures must be in place.

▶ Viability of Vascular Access Center: Overview

When making the decision to open an interventional nephrology facility, multiple considerations must be taken into account. The questions to ask include: should the facility be hospital-based or freestanding? Should the facility be owned by a proprietary company or should the facility be owned by the university or a private group of physicians? How one answers these questions is essential to the long-term viability of the center and is dependent upon the patient population served and who will be providing the services. The political environment of the institution or practice must also be considered.

The first and foremost issue of importance is credentialing. In most hospital centers and university centers, interventional procedures can only be performed within a radiology suite. In addition, not only is the access to these suites controlled by the interventional radiology community but credentialing is also likely to be contested. If the

services are to be provided by interventional radiologists wishing to specialize in this area, it may be in the institution's best interests to stay in hospital. However, given the commitment by Centers for Medicare and Medicaid Services to move procedures to the less expensive outpatient environment, this may be a very unstable long-term solution. If the procedures are to be performed by interventional nephrologists credentialing considerations and access to the radiology equipment may mandate the development of a freestanding facility. While most free standing facilities currently function as an extension of a physician's office practice for financial reasons, unless a strong quality assurance program is mandated from the start and immediately implemented, quality control may become a significant issue in the future. External regulatory oversight for this arena is currently weak in most states. However, indications suggest that this may not stay this way in the future.

Several other factors need to be taken into consideration. Certificate of Need (CON) is a state issue and in states that require CON a careful study of surrounding facilities will be necessary to determine whether a CON can be obtained. In addition, an interesting change in the reimbursement climate is underway. The Medicare Modernization Act passed by Congress several years ago mandated that CMS eliminate the difference in reimbursement between hospital-based ASC facilities (POS 22) and freestanding facilities functioning as ASCs (POS 24). This has been progressing over the last several years as CMS has been progressively reducing the reimbursement to hospital owned ASC facilities while increasing the reimbursement to freestanding ASCs. Currently, the CPT codes for radiologic supervision and interpretation cannot be billed within the confines of an ASC. In addition, although an arterial angioplasty can now be performed within the confines of an ASC and billed to the Medicare system the radiology component of the procedure cannot. Also, placement of vascular stents is a growing part of interventional procedures in the access (venous) system. These devices, however, are expensive and often cost more than $2000 per device. Currently they are not reimbursable when placed in an ASC. Should CMS decide that radiology supervision and interpretation components of angioplasty procedures have become a common surgical practice, should they allow the billing for the radiology supervision and interpretation codes within the confines of an ASC and reimburse for the supplies needed to place a stent the reimbursement curve will shift in favor of POS 24 (ASC) rather than POS 11 (access center) However, the question for an institution or investor of whether to spend the excess money to build an access center (POS 11) to the specifications of an ASC (POS 24) for future conversion must be considered by each individual planning to build a center.

The question of how many patients need to be regularly referred for the financial viability of the center is extremely important. If the center is not to be subsidized from the general revenue of the institution or the nephrology or interventional radiology sections, it must at least break even. In the current reimbursement environment, this requires between 400 and 800 patients. In addition, the business plan will be predicated upon how likely it is that patients will actually be referred for procedures to the given center.

The least complex plan is to simply open a center and depend upon the reputation of the institution to promote referral of patients from a surrounding regional area. In the authors' estimation, this is a potentially unstable situation. If access centers remain profitable, it will be in the best interests of nephrology groups to develop their own centers rather than refer patients to someone else's facility. Thus, the institution could find itself with an expensive facility that is markedly underutilized.

If one accepts, the estimation of between 400 and 800 patients required for the viability of the center then the question of how this patient population is accumulated must be asked. Many academic centers do not care for 400 ESRD patients. However, many institutions are surrounded by small individual nephrology practices that could not afford to open their own center. Developing a mutually beneficial plan in which all practices benefit is not mechanically difficult. Politically, however, it is well known and obvious that this may require a great deal of tact and diplomacy.

If the institution is able to maintain a population of 400–800 patients in the aggregate who are routinely referred to the access center, multiple other considerations still remain. First such consideration is whether the institution can utilize existing coding and billing resources or acquire them to maximize interventional reimbursement. This is important because interventional reimbursement is component in nature and individual component CPT procedure codes, separately reimbursed, are put into multiple combinations for each procedure. In the rest of nephrology billing, the coding is much simpler and more straightforward. Whether the skills to perform interventional coding exist or can be developed within the institution is also of primary importance.

Second, one needs to reflect on the management ability of the institution. Many institutions do not own and operate dialysis facilities because of the lack of the expertise required to run these facilities profitably. Many institutions decline to develop these skills. This situation is replicated and magnified in the operation of an access center. Should the institution be able to muster the knowledge and skills mentioned, then the commitment to utilizing them in this alien arena has to be discussed. Alternatively, the institution can choose to hire a consultant to set up the administrative and billing departments necessary for the administration of a successful center. As a further alternative, the institution may wish to partner with a proprietary company to build and manage a facility. At this time, approximately a half dozen alternative partnership options exist within the commercial sector. While choosing this latter option may cost between 15% and 50% of the net profits of the facility, the institution may consider this well worthwhile.

The prevalence of AVF versus AVG in the dialysis population is a foremost consideration as well. Grafts clot at a markedly higher frequency than fistulas. Because of the component nature of billing, the thrombectomy procedure is significantly more remunerative than that of a simple angioplasty. Therefore, a facility servicing a population with a high prevalence of AVG is potentially much more remunerative.

Many dialysis facilities now provide access flow surveillance on a monthly basis. If this is present, it markedly diminishes the necessity of thrombectomy for both grafts and fistulas. To the extent surveillance is utilized, the potential reimbursement per procedure will be much lower because of the lower occurrence of thrombectomy procedures. However, the existence of access surveillance offers the potential to anticipate procedural needs and therefore to electively schedule most of the procedures performed at the center. This allows for much more efficient utilization of the facility. This may well become a positive that outweighs the financial negative of fewer thrombectomies.

In addition, as mentioned above, procedures on fistulas tend to be much more difficult than procedures on grafts. This may well be because fistulas develop dilated areas and dilated collaterals which enable them to stay patent and function even in the face of disease which would make a graft totally dysfunctional and likely to thrombose. Therefore, by the time the fistula presents to the access facility it may be severely diseased. Since these procedures in the author's experience utilize more supplies and more time, the cost per procedure is higher. In the author's experience, this can be largely obviated by an aggressive program of ultrasound surveillance of dialysis fistulas. Accurate performance of this procedure requires a detailed knowledge of the physiology and physical exam of the fistula. The examination of the fistula is essential for the proper interpretation of the ultrasound procedure. The procedure should not be referred to a general ultrasound department with technicians not specifically trained in dialysis vascular access and is probably best performed by an interventionalist. This allows correlation of the functional history and physical anatomy together with ultrasound anatomical data. If an individual skilled in ultrasound evaluation is able to perform the procedure with a periodicity individualized to the patient, the problems in fistulas can be discovered before they become inordinately severe. The institution, quite obviously, may find this an important skill to be added to the fellowship program. As these procedures are separately billable from the dialysis procedure when performed in an office or ASC facility setting, the procedure may also directly add to the financial viability of the center.

► Viability of Access Center Creation: Financial Analysis

Once all of the above considerations are recognized then a spreadsheet must be developed describing the potential financial viability of a center. Because the author (DS) has been asked on multiple occasions over the last dozen years how best to perform this analysis, a toolkit was developed with the Renal Physicians Association (RPA) which can be utilized for this analysis and is available on the RPA website. It can be accessed through the members-only section by doing a search for vascular access practice assessment tool.

Before further discussion, it is best to first take a short digression through the nature of physician reimbursement. In an ASC, the physician fee for performing the procedure and interpretation of the X-rays is coded and billed separately from the reimbursement for the facility overhead and supplies. This mandates a clear-cut division between the procedural reimbursement and the professional component of performing the procedure. In a physician's office practice or its extension this division is obliterated. The physician receives one fee to perform the procedure, read and interpret the X-rays and pay the overhead including all procedural costs such as the building and staff for the facility. This fee is listed in the Medicare physician fee schedule.

Utilizing RPA toolkit

Prior to utilizing the tables in the RPA toolkit, it is important to ensure that the most recent update for the Medicare physician fee schedule is utilized. This can be found by search of the Federal Register and local fiscal intermediary's (also known as medicare administrative contractors or MACs) website. The latter is preferable as there are adjustors for cost-of-living and practice expense in various regions of the country. If necessary, the RVU reimbursement for each procedural code should be updated and the new values inserted into the table. The appropriate table for the characteristics of the individual patient population in consideration should be extracted from the toolkit, filled out and utilized. This will allow an estimation of the profitability of the Center for each 1000 procedures performed. For patients with grafts it can be assumed that there will be approximately 1.5 procedures per patient per year. For patients with fistulas, a calculation of 1.3 procedures per patient per year would be more appropriate. These are very conservative estimates.

We hereby provide an example by using the first table on the RPA toolkit (Table 59-1). First, however, we must caution that these numbers may not be reflective of the practice patterns of your interventionalist and need to be analyzed carefully prior to use.

In the RPA toolkit, the first example is for a population with 50% catheters, 10% graphs, 40% AVF, and with surveillance. On the top, there are 700 patients and using conservative numbers one could expect 910 procedures. With this distribution of patients and without surveillance and only 10% grafts one would expect that only 8% of the procedures would be thrombectomies as listed under procedure type. Down below under reimbursement are the details of reimbursement for the CPT codes for each type of procedure. However, if we just look at the summary data to the right of procedure type we see the total number of procedures by type of procedure, the total reimbursement for each type of procedure, we subtract the supply costs and the costs for the center and its employees and what we end up with is a net profit of $778,037.78. This easily converts to $854,986.57 per 1000 procedures in net revenue. Therefore, this toolkit can be used to estimate the financial viability of a proposed center. We need to further caution that this spreadsheet assumes tight control of staffing costs and equipment costs that are essential for profitability. It is important to factor expenses for anticipated practice patterns, supply costs and staff costs and expected overhead expenses in terms of rent and facility cost.

Coding issues

Interventional nephrology is in a state of evolution and is constantly changing; so is its billing and reimbursement. The current paradigm in billing and reimbursement has evolved from interventional radiology and vascular surgery. The ASDIN has been active in developing this aspect of vascular access care and the current status can be assessed at its website (www.asdin.org). The only certainty is that it is certain to change over time. The viability of a VAC is dependent upon reimbursement and the importance of this issue cannot be underestimated. There is a paucity of experienced billing organizations in this area that represents a significant obstacle to success.

Quality assurance

With increasing availability of expertise and involvement of interventionalists in day-to-day management of VAC, the responsibility to ensure quality care is a major consideration. Quality assurance may be thought of as two components. First, the center must ensure adequate training of its staff and especially its interventional physicians. Second, a program of ongoing quality assurance measurements must be implemented to ensure quality maintenance through monitoring. The computerized database should be used for documentation and billing purposes, timely patient-related communication as well as for quality assurance and improvement.

ASDIN maintains criteria on its website including a process for ASDIN certification of interventional physicians. Minimum numbers of supervised cases are listed and revised on an ongoing basis. To ensure an ongoing level of quality outcomes, it is important to follow performance measures. Existing Society for Interventional Radiology

TABLE 59–1

Example of Financial Analysis Based on RPA Toolkit

Profitability Analysis for a Vascular Access Center: 50% cath, 10% grafts, 40% AVF, With or Without Surveillance

Number of Patients	Estimated Procedures/Year
700	910

Procedure Type	%	Total Number of Procedures	Reimbursement Total	Fixed Supply cost	Total Supply Cost
Thrombectomies	8.00%	73	215,924.80	$696	$50,669
Fistulograms and PTA	39.00%	355	649,943.99	$400	$141,818
Fistulograms	3.00%	27	16,751.28	$119	$3,243
LTTC placements	25.00%	228	147,602.00	$384	$87,360
Exchange	20.00%	182	13,249.60	$480	$87,360
Removals	5.00%	46	6,006.00	$2	$109
	100.00%				

Cost	Total Revenue
	$2,375,959
Labor	$332,634
Rent	$160,000
Overhead	$546,471
Equipment note	$188,257
	$370,559

Annual Net Cashflow
$778,037.78   33%

Reimbursement

Thrombectomy	Number	Medicare Reimbursment	Total with Multiple Procedure Discount*
36147	73	$767	$22,335
36148	73	$242	$7,047
35476	73	$1,636	$47,640
75978	73	$226	$13,162
36870	73	$1,767	$102,910
75710	73	$243	$14,152
75820	4	$118	$412
36215	73	$277	$8,066
75827	4	$57	$199
36010	4	bundled	$0
35475	7	$2,177	$6,339
75962	7	$228	$1,328

Fistulogram and PTA	Number	Medicare Reimbursable	Total with Multiple Procedure Discount*
36147	355	$767	$108,883
36148	43	$242	$4,123
35476	355	$1,636	$464,493
75978	355	$226	$64,166
75710	43	$243	$8,279
36215	43	$277	$4,719
35475	35	$2,177	$30,905
75962	35	$228	$6,473

Fistulogram	Number	Medicare Reimbursment	Total with Multiple Procedure Discount*
36147	27	$767	$16,751

Cath Placement	Number	Medicare Reimbursable	Total with Multiple Procedure Discount*
36558	228	$777	$141,414
76937	228	$34	$6,188
77001	228	$104	$18,928

Exchange	Number	Medicare Reimbursable	Total with Multiple Procedure Discount*
36581	182	$182	$13,250
77001	182	$104	$15,142
35476	140	$1,636	$183,415
75978	140	$87	$9,754

Removal	Number	Medicare Reimbursable	Total with Multiple Procedure Discount*
36589	46	$165	$6,006

Total Revenue $2,375,959

*The financial figures are factored for the multiple procedural discount and are for illustrative purposes only.

TABLE 59–2

Types of Vascular Access Procedure Complications[18]

Type I	Access site hematoma
Type II	Vascular rupture
Type III	Arterial complications
Type IV	Stent related complications
Type V	Catheter insertion complications
Type VI	Adverse reactions to medications
Type VII	Oxygen saturation and apnea
Type VIII	Hypotension/hypertension
Type IX	Cardiac arrhythmia
Type X	Clinical status

(SIR) guidelines for analysis of complication rates have not been found to be reproducible. Therefore, ASDIN has recently issued a position statement paper concerning the categorization and grading of complications of hemodialysis vascular access procedures (Tables 59-2 and 59-3).[18] While acceptable levels of complications have not yet been quantified, safety can only be assured by an ongoing process of complication monitoring.

Challenges in setting up VAC

The primary goal of VAC must be to provide better care to the patients with vascular access dysfunction. VAC has the capability to streamline this care. To operate a VAC, the mission and vision of the center have to be established at the outset and shared by all parties involved. Proper goal development is essential to develop a healthy culture in any organization. Once the goals are set, it is imperative that an analysis of the needs of the community, patient availability for referrals, expected revenues,

and essential expenses is done to ensure smooth functioning of the center. The feasibility of the VAC depends upon unique payment structure in different geographic locations and must be specific to the VAC being contemplated. Infrastructure to provide support for management and operations has to be planned before the VAC can be established. As mentioned above, such support can be developed locally, or is available from established corporations.

Limited availability of trained operators is one of the major hurdles preventing many practices from augmenting their vascular access care. Multiple strategies have been employed to overcome this difficulty. Some experienced management companies have the capability of providing on-site or off-site training as part of the negotiated contract. There are a limited but growing number of academic nephrology programs producing fellows with 3–12 months training in interventional procedures. Recruiting an already trained individual from an existing practice is another strategy. Continued on-site training may be necessary for the operator to become ASDIN certified as independent operator. If this is necessary, it can be quite expensive.

TABLE 59–3

General Severity Grading Scheme of Vascular Access Procedure Complication[18]

Grade 1	Nominal therapy required Unplanned increase in level of care to a nominal degree No clinical consequence or adverse sequelae
Grade 2	Minor therapy required Successful management using percutaneous therapy No significant long-term sequelae
Grade 3	Major therapy required Persistent or unstable complication Surgical repair is required Hospitalization for observation or management of a complication
Grade 4	Significant long-term (>30 days) sequelae Loss of limb or significant loss of limb function

REFERENCES

1. O'neill WC. The new nephrologists. *Am J Kidney Dis.* 2000;35:978–979.
2. NKF-DOQI clinical practice guidelines for vascular access. National Kidney Foundation—Dialysis Outcomes Quality Initiative. *Am J Kidney Dis.* 1997;30:S150–S191.
3. National Kidney Foundation—K DOQI Clinical Practice Guidelines for vascular access: Update 2000. *Am J Kidney Dis.* 2001;37:S137–S181.
4. Asif A, Byers P, Vieira CF, Roth D. Developing a comprehensive diagnostic and interventional nephrology program at an academic center. *Am J Kidney Dis.* 2003;42:229–233.
5. Beathard GA, Litchfield T. Effectiveness and safety of dialysis vascular access procedures performed by interventional nephrologists. *Kidney Int.* 2004;66:1622–1632.
6. Gupta RK, Balogun RA. Native renal biopsies: complications and glomerular yield between radiologists and nephrologists. *J Nephrol.* 2005;18:553–558.
7. Mishler R, Sands JJ, Ofsthun NJ, Teng M, Schon D. Lazarus JM. Dedicated outpatient vascular access center decreases hospitalization and missed outpatient dialysis treatments. *Kidney Int.* 2006;69:393–398.
8. Jackson JW, Lewis JL, Brouillette, JR, Brantley RR. Initial experience of a nephrologist-operated vascular access center. *Semin Dial.* 2008;13:354–368.
9. Arnold WP. Improvement in hemodialysis vascular access outcomes in a dedicated access center. *Semin Dial.* 2008;13:359–363.
10. Beathard GA. Integrated vascular access management. *Blood Purif.* 2003;21:89–98.
11. O'Neill WC. Sonography of the kidney and urinary tract. *Semin Nephrol.* 2002;22:242–253.

12. Asif A, Pflederer TA, Vieira CF, Diego J, Roth D, Agarwal A. Does catheter insertion by nephrologists improve peritoneal dialysis utilization? A multicenter analysis. *Semin Dial.* 2005;18:157–160.

13. Asif A, Besarab A, Roy-Chaudhury P, Spergel LM, Ravani P. Interventional nephrology: from episodic to coordinated vascular access care. *J Nephrol.* 2007;20:399–405.

14. Pervez A, Zaman F, Aslam A, Petty S, Murphy S, Vachharajani T, Abreo K. Port catheter placement by nephrologists in an interventional nephrology training program. *Semin Dial.* 2004;17:61–64.

15. Berns J, O'Neill W. Performance of procedures by nephrologists and nephrology fellows at US Nephrology training programs. *Clin J Am Soc Nephrol.* 2008;19:941–947.

16. Available at: http://asdin.org/displaycommon. cfm?an=1&subarticlenbr=3. Accessed May, 2011.

17. O'Hare AM, Dudley RA, Hynes DM, McCulloch CE, Navarro D, Colin P, Stroupe K, Rapp J, Johansen KL. Impact of surgeon and surgical center characteristics on choice of permanent vascular access. *Kidney Int.* 2003;64:681–689.

18. Vesely TM, Beathard G, Ash S, Hoggard J, Schon D. Classification of complications associated with hemodialysis vascular access procedures. A position statement from the American Society of Diagnostic and Interventional Nephrology. J *Vasc Access.* 2008; 9:12–19.

60

CODING AND REIMBURSEMENT FOR VASCULAR ACCESS PROCEDURES: PAST, PRESENT, AND FUTURE

DONALD SCHON

LEARNING OBJECTIVES

1. Describe history of evolution of coding for interventional nephrology procedures.
2. Discuss current interventional nephrology coding practices and standards.
3. Discuss future of reimbursement in interventional nephrology.

BACKGROUND

Following the evolution of reimbursement for vascular access procedures provides an interesting insight into medicine as a business and highlights the interactions of the stakeholders with the Centers for Medicare and Medicaid Services (CMS). This chapter begins with a short review of this history in the hope of making this difficult and somewhat arcane subject more understandable.

By the mid-1990s, it became apparent that there was a crisis in the arena of vascular access within the United States. The United States had the highest dialysis-related mortality among developed countries and concurrently the lowest rate of arteriovenous fistula (AVF) prevalence. Indeed, 90% of prevalent dialysis patients had arteriovenous grafts (AVG). To overcome this problem and improve morbidity and mortality, the Kidney Disease Outcomes Quality Initiative (KDOQI) guidelines and the Fistula First Breakthrough Initiative (FFBI) evolved with the blessing and support of CMS.[1-3] CMS made a commitment to decreasing costs and improving outcomes. After analysis it became apparent that vascular access maintenance was

poorly done and was unnecessarily expensive. The evolution of the field of interventional nephrology appeared an obvious and important step in the solution of this vexing problem.

The policy makers within CMS pushed to move procedures from the hospital to the ambulatory surgical center (ASC) environment. The ASC setting was particularly attractive because of significant state and federal regulations mandated in order to ensure quality control. However, a significant roadblock unsurmountable at that time was a statutory prohibition against reimbursement for radiology procedures within the confines of an ASC.

▶ Initial Controversies

In the meantime, a separate conflict was developing between the surgical and interventional radiology communities over the growing and numerically much more significant field of peripheral vascular arterial and venous disease. Interventional nephrology procedures are coded with the same current procedural terminology (CPT) codes as those used for vascular procedures within the limbs and therefore interventional nephrology was enmeshed in this controversy from the start.

The surgeons preferred that the procedures remain within the hospital where apparently they felt secure. The radiologists felt that if they could move these procedures to the ASC setting (POS 22 and 24) it would be better long term.

▶ CMS Structure and Reimbursement Guidelines

What was not appreciated within the infant interventional nephrology community was that CMS functionally is split into two arms: policy and reimbursement. Neither was it known by those of us involved that these two arms were independent and did not necessarily communicate effectively. The CMS reimbursement division wanted peripheral vascular procedures moved to the less expensive outpatient venue. They, therefore, began to authorize payment of certain interventional vascular procedures within the ASC setting by alterations of the Medicare Physicians Fee Schedule. However, this was an unsatisfactory solution. The prohibition against using radiology codes in the ASC setting remained. Established CMS policy also permitted use of these CPT codes in the setting of an extension of the physician's office practice, provided there was evidence that it was safe. This place of service (POS 11) as opposed to the ASC setting or place of service (POS 24) had been utilized by ear nose and throat specialists (ENT), plastic surgeons, and gynecologists for years. A standardized procedure already existed for evaluating the safety of procedures performed in an office setting. By utilizing POS 11, CMS was able to promote the movement of vascular procedures to the outpatient setting. This created the very odd situation that arterial angioplasty as deemed safe and reimbursed in the setting the physician's office but until very recently disallowed in the ASC settings.[4] Physicians took advantage of this option and were able to avoid the heavy layers of state and federal regulations applied to ASCs and considerably decrease overhead.

All of a sudden, POS 11 became a highly attractive alternative to an ASC setting and offered a much more profitable opportunity than ever before conceptualized. Entrepreneurs, including entrepreneurial physicians, immediately moved into this market creating centers throughout the United States. With this movement and the dearth of trained interventional nephrologists, the pressure for academic centers to develop interventional nephrology teaching programs became progressively intense.

▶ CMS and Development of Coding

To understand coding and billing practice and requirements, a fundamental knowledge of the reimbursement structure is necessary. CMS administers the Medicare program. It issues National Coverage Decisions (NCD)[4] which are strict, cannot be interpreted nor modified, and are relatively few by intent. This allows flexibility for the expression of variation in regional standards of care and practice. The system is administered contractually through local intermediaries or carriers. These privately owned companies receive contracts through a bidding process and have defined areas of administrative responsibility. Interpretation of what is allowable within the description of any CPT code is mandated by carrier-specific local coverage decisions (LCD). These interpretative mandates are issued with a comment period and modified with provider comments in mind. Regional interpretations may vary significantly. This is discussed in detail in the ASDIN coding manual.[5]

CPT codes are created by a committee of the AMA called the CPT Committee. They are published by and owned by the AMA.[6,7] The committee is composed of representatives of all specialties. Codes are created by a committee of physician representatives of all specialty societies who utilize the codes, are submitted to the CPT Committee of physician representatives, and must be crafted very carefully to avoid confusion. They specify what components of procedures are allowable and what are disallowable for that specific CPT code. Once created, they are very difficult to modify and the process of creation is specific and difficult.

Once created, CPT codes must have a relative value applied. This is applied by another committee of the AMA called the Relative Value Scale Update Committee (RUC). The RUC process is involved and often contentious. The committee is composed of representatives of many but not all specialties and subspecialties. Deliberations are done in closed-door panels. It must be remembered that Medicare reimbursement is done by dividing a fixed amount of money that is designated by statute. It is therefore a zero sum process. Money allocated to a new code decreases reimbursement for all other codes. Therefore, often vested interests come in conflict.

Most procedural coding is composed of set packages or bundles. However, radiology coding of procedures is still done largely by combinations of components of codes. This is discussed in more detail in the ASDIN manual. CMS also owns an agency called the National Correct Coding Initiative (NCCI). The role of NCCI is to promote correct coding and it does so by issuing "coding edits" which define what codes may be billed separately in the same procedure.[8] This again is discussed in detail in the ASDIN coding manual as referenced below.

EVOLUTION OF INTERVENTIONAL NEPHROLOGY CODING PRACTICES

Initially, billing practices were variable and chaotic within the field of interventional nephrology. This was irrespective of whether the procedures were performed by nephrologists, surgeons, or radiologists. Variability in coding practices was surveyed by the infant American Society of Diagnostic and Interventional Nephrology (ASDIN) and found to be unsustainable. In 2005, ASDIN decided to modify and standardize reimbursement in an attempt to promote credibility in the field of interventional nephrology. At that time, Interventional Nephrologists were often held in low esteem by other subspecialties. A committee and manual was created under the direction of Dr. Gerald Beathard and Dr. Don Schon with the sanctioning and guidance of the Renal Physicians Association (RPA). The initial manual reflected the prevailing coding trends at the time within the interventional nephrology community, and was published in 2005 as a combined product of ASDIN and the RPA.[5]

Parallel with this and with the growth of interventional nephrology procedures within the radiology community, radiologists continued to standardize their own approach toward interventional billing. They were instrumental in creating many of the CPT codes necessary to the field and guiding them to and through the CPT and RUC committees. Their societies had a heavy academic influence that contributed a very different philosophy towards reimbursement. Their approach to coding was (and is) published in the Coding Users' Guide of the Society of Interventional Radiology (SIR).[9]

Slowly, the approaches of the two societies began to coalesce. The 2006 to 2007 revision of the ASDIN coding manual began to make significant changes bringing the ASDIN approach closer to that of the radiologists.[10] Soon thereafter, both societies decided to form a combined committee to resolve major coding differences. This committee over an 18-month period discussed, compromised on perspective, and resolved most of the differences between the two societies. The 2009 to 2010 version of the manual reflected this and basically major differences between the two societies no longer exist.[11,12]

CURRENT CODING STANDARDS

The growth of spending for interventional nephrology procedures in POS 11 began to place interventional nephrology procedures on the CMS radar screen. In addition, confusion in the usage of CPT codes generated many questions by professional coding specialists. This necessitated a review by CMS at the request of ASDIN and SIR. Several issues were at stake. They revolved around the definition of an access and attempts by CMS to control a perceived over utilization of certain radiology procedures in general.

In the meantime, the nationwide growth of fistula prevalence had been encouraging and rewarding. This trend, as can be anticipated, resulted in a much higher prevalence of problematic AVF problems sent to access centers than problematic AVG. In some areas of the country, in excess of 60% of procedures performed in access centers were performed on AVF rather than AVG.[13] Prevalent experience and opinion are that procedures on AVF are much more difficult and consuming of time and equipment than procedures performed on AVG. However, the CPT codes used to define and reimburse interventional nephrology procedures were first developed in an era of over 90% grafts. They therefore do not reflect the increased cost in time, effort, and equipment required in AVF procedures. In response to this, ASDIN promoted several important concepts. First, the traditional SIR definition of an access that began at the arterial anastomosis and ended at the origin of the subclavian vein was considered appropriate for AV grafts since procedures performed on AVG were usually straightforward. However, we felt that the definition of an AVF should include the vessel of the main body and end at the elbow in a forearm fistula (ie, the next named vessel) Second procedures performed in the central vessels

should be separately reimbursed. Third, angioplasty procedures performed in the drainage veins of a forearm fistula should be separately reimbursed from angioplasties performed within the defined conduit of the fistula. Fourth, the site of the arterial anastomosis in an AVF was very difficult to define. Therefore coding for an arterial angioplasty (a higher-level code than an angioplasty within the fistula body) should be considered appropriate whenever the balloon must be at least partially inflated within the inflow or feeding artery in order to appropriately perform the angioplasty.

ASDIN in direct meetings with CMS did prevail in two areas.[14] Angioplasty of central vessels is coded separately when performed during the same procedure as an angioplasty on the access. Also, the definition of an arterial angioplasty was not limited. However, the definition of an access was described as starting from the arterial anastomosis up to but not including the central vessels for both AVF as well as an AVG. By defining the access in such a manner, not only did CMS failed to differentiate between AVG and the more difficult AVF procedures but also prohibited the coding of separate angioplasties within the draining vessels of an AVF. In addition, no longer was it considered acceptable to code for an arterial angioplasty at the anastomosis and an angioplasty within the body of the fistula. These principles significantly decreased reimbursement for interventional nephrology procedures performed in access centers. These changed principles were incorporated in the most recent revision of the ASDIN/RPA coding manual for 2010.

However, ASDIN was able to prevail in a separate and potentially more important issue. CMS, in an attempt to control the proliferation of CT, MRI, and PET scanners proposed that all facilities with procedure rooms whose aggregate worth was greater than $1 million would be mandated to run at 90% capacity or have their reimbursement for supplies, personnel, and facility overhead reduced. Depending on the definition of 90% of capacity, this was a potentially devastating threat to the viability of access centers throughout the country. In a face-to-face meeting with CMS, ASDIN made it very clear what the implications of this proposal were for the FFBI and KDOQI guidelines. CMS accepted the concept that procedure rooms with composite equipment rather than a single piece of equipment worth more than $1 million would be excluded from this regulation.[15]

One may ask why is CMS so interested in this area. First of all, the policy side of CMS has invested heavily on the success of Fistula First and KDOQI. Promoting and regulating centers involved in the management of the AVF and AVG are essential tools in their perspective. In addition, if the FFBI and KDOQI goals of 66% AVF prevalence were achieved, significant savings to the Medicare Trust Fund were predicted by CMS itself and the private/academic sector. As example, Schon et al in a paper in the *Clinical Journal of the American Society of Nephrology* in 2006 suggested that if the KDOQI objectives were accomplished, the savings to CMS would be between $400 million and $800 million for each dialysis cohort entering the system.[16,17]

All individuals interested in Interventional Nephrology should keep in mind that this scrutiny by CMS of the private provider sector is not likely to go away.

Currently, the radiology CPT codes still cannot be billed within the confines of an ASC. In addition, although an arterial angioplasty can now be performed within the confines of an ASC and billed to the Medicare system, the radiology component of the procedure cannot. In addition, reimbursement for placement of stents is allowed in the office setting but not in the ASC setting. As stents often cost in excess of $2000 and usage is growing, this is a major impediment to performing procedures in an outpatient ASC. Should CMS decide that stent placement is safe and allowable in an outpatient ASC setting, this would promote performing interventional nephrology procedures in an ASC. In addition, if radiology components of angioplasty procedures have become a common and safe surgical practice and therefore allow the billing for the radiology supervision and interpretation codes within the confines of an ASC, the reimbursement curve may shift in favor of POS 24 rather than POS 11. At this time, this remains a moot point. However, the question for an institution or investor of whether to spend the excess money to build an access center (POS 11) to the specifications of an ASC (POS 24) for future conversion must be considered by each individual planning to build a center.

If an institution is able to maintain a population of 400–800 patients either solely or in the aggregate who are routinely referred to the access center, multiple other questions still need to be asked. The first series include: can the institution utilize existing coding and billing resources (or acquire them) to maximize interventional reimbursement. This is important because interventional reimbursement is component in nature. What is meant by this is that individual component CPT procedure codes, separately reimbursed, are put into multiple combinations for each procedure. In the rest of nephrology billing and coding is much simpler and more straightforward. Whether the skills to perform interventional coding exist or can be developed within the institution is of primary importance. Second, one needs to reflect on the management ability of the institution. Many institutions do not own and operate dialysis facilities because of the lack of the expertise required to run these facilities profitably. Many institutions decline to develop these skills. This situation is replicated and magnified in the operation of an access center. Should the institution be able to muster the knowledge and skills mentioned, then the commitment to utilizing them in this alien arena has to be discussed. Alternatively, the institution can choose to hire a consultant to set up the administrative and billing departments necessary for the administration of a successful center. As a further alternative, the institution may wish to partner with a proprietary company to build and manage a facility. At this time, approximately a half dozen alternative partnership options exist within the commercial sector. While choosing this latter option may cost between 15% and 50% of the net profits of the facility, the individual institution may consider this well worthwhile.

Before discussing this topic it is best to first take a short digression through some of the nuances of physician reimbursement. In an ASC, physician fee for performance of the procedure and interpretation of the X-rays is coded and billed separately from the fees reimbursed for the facility overhead and supplies. This mandates a clear-cut division between the facility and professional reimbursement related to performing the procedure. In a physician's office practice or its extension this division is obliterated. The physician receives one fee to perform the procedure, read and interpret the X-rays, and pay the overhead including all procedural costs including the building and staff for the facility. This fee is listed in the Medicare physician fee schedule.

Because of many requests, the RPA has published a series of tables as a toolkit to guide institutions in evaluating the potential profitability of a proposed access center. These tables are available to members on the RPA website and are discussed in more detail in Chapter 59. Prior to utilizing the tables in the RPA toolkit please make sure that you have the most recent update for the Medicare physician fee schedule. This can be found by search of the Federal Register and your intermediary's (or MAC's) website. The latter is preferable as there are adjustors for cost-of-living and practice expense in various regions of the country. If necessary, the relative value units (RVU) reimbursement for each procedural code should be updated and the new values inserted into the table. The appropriate table for the characteristics of the individual patient population in consideration should be extracted from the tool kit, filled out and utilized.

FUTURE CHANGES IN REIMBURSEMENT

What we have discussed so far is applicable to the present. We are frequently asked to predict what will happen to reimbursement in the future. There are many things we cannot say with confidence or certainty. Radiology procedural coding, upon which our coding is predicated, is one of the only component coding practices left in medicine. CMS and the other specialties strongly wish to bundle these procedures. The first bundled code directly applicable to our procedures was created by the CPT committee and valued by the RUC in 2010. This bundle (CPT code 36147) involved the most frequently performed procedures in interventional nephrology. On average, reimbursement was not diminished for this procedure. However, future outcomes may not be as positive.

The CPT and RUC committees are committees formed by the AMA and whose recommendations are largely but not invariably followed by CMS. During the sequence of creation and valuation of codes the CPT committee recognizes what CPT codes (reflecting procedures performed) are highly associated. It then mandates that the society or societies doing the vast majority of these procedures create a new single code that encompasses (bundles) all of the associated component codes and their most likely variants. This process restricts the billing to the most frequently performed variant. The assumption is that the subsequent reimbursement will be generous to the procedures that are easy to perform and which will compensate the physician for the added costs of procedures that are very difficult to perform. However, the assumption only holds if the easy procedures balance in frequency the difficult ones. Once the CPT code with its description is accepted by the CPT committee, it is then referred to the RUC. This committee as previously mentioned, also a committee of the AMA, is composed of the major specialties and some of the subspecialties. Nephrology does not necessarily have representation and therefore is not always involved in the deliberations. Reimbursement from Medicare is a zero sum process. In other words, the reimbursement pie (or pool of dollars) is divided amongst the represented physician groups. The RUC has no ability to increase the size of the pie. Therefore, all specialties and subspecialties are contending for the same dollars. Therefore, every time a CPT code goes to the RUC it may well come out of committee with less reimbursement than expected and wished for by the specialties performing the procedure(s). The process by which the RUC assigns the relative value units that determine reimbursement is only partially objective with a large subjective component. The meetings of the RUC are closed and attendance is by invitation only. ASDIN has access only through the RPA.

In addition to the discussion above, every 5 years the RUC has the authority to review the value of codes selected on a rotating basis. Thus the theory goes, as technological advancements make procedures easier and quicker the work necessary to their performance decreases and so their relative value should be decreased commensurate to this. The problem is again that the revaluation process is partially objective and partially subjective. It is in the best interest of the competing societies to limit the value of any procedure they do not perform.

Whenever a bundle is created or any codes revalued the societies representing physicians who perform these procedures are asked to discuss the issue together and come up with combined recommendations. In practice, this means that all codes used in interventional nephrology must be negotiated with the Society for Vascular Surgery (SVR) and the American College of Radiology (ACR) and the Society of Interventional Radiology (SIR). It is, therefore, of importance for ASDIN to continue to forge a positive working relationship with both these societies. However, competing agendas often make this difficult. Therefore, it is impossible for us to estimate what will happen to reimbursement in the future. In addition, with the changes anticipated for outcome-based reimbursement and the development of Accountable Care Organizations (ACOs) and the Medical Home further uncertainty exists.

REFERENCES

1. Besarab A, Work J, Brouwer D, et al. KDOQI Clinical Practice Guidelines for Vascular Access. *Am J Kidney Dis.* 2006;48(suppl 1):S184–S186.
2. Arteriovenous Fistula First, Available at: http://www.fistulafirst.org/. Accessed September, 2010.
3. Casey Mary, Armistead N, Lynch J, Vinson B. Fistula First Breakthrough Initiative Annual Report, Mid-Atlantic Renal Coalition, February 26, 2010. Available at: http://fistula.memberpath.com/LinkClick.aspx?fileticket=Q7ZDEJHrhOk%3D&tabid=39. Accessed September, 2010.
4. Ambulatory Surgery Center Association Website. "Medicare's 2011 ASC Payments: Rates and Policies." Ambulatory Surgery Center Association. ASC Association and Ambulatory Surgery Foundation, 2010. Web. September 2010. Available at: http://ascassociation.org/medicare2011/.
5. Procedures: Answers to your Toughest CPT Coding Questions. 2009, Ingenix.
6. Abraham M, Ahlman J, Boudreau A, et al. *CPT: Current Procedural Terminology*, Professional Edition., Chicago, IL: American Medical Society; 2010.
7. Medicare National Coverage Determinations Manual, Coverage Determinations. Available through CMS with annual updates. Available at: https://www.cms.gov/manuals/downloads/ncd103c1_Part4.pdf. Accessed September, 2010.
8. National Correct Coding Initiative Policy Manual for Medicare Services. Updated at least annually and available through the NCCI. Available at: http://www.cms.gov/NationalCorrectCodInitEd/. Accessed September, 2010.
9. *Coding of Procedures in Interventional Nephrology*, 6-22-05. Clinton, MS: Published by the American Society of Diagnostic and Interventional Nephrology; 2005.
10. Interventional Radiology: Coding Users' Guide, sixteenth edition, 2010. Available through the Society of Interventional Radiology and the American College of Radiology.
11. *Coding of Procedures in Interventional Nephrology*, 7/1/06. Clinton, MS: American Society of Diagnostic and Interventional Nephrology; 2006.
12. *Coding of Procedures in Interventional Nephrology*, 3/30/09, with 6/22/2009 clarifications. Clinton, MS: American Society of Diagnostic and Interventional Nephrology; 2009.
13. *Coding of Procedures in Interventional Nephrology*, 6/17/10. Clinton, MS: American Society of Diagnostic and Interventional Nephrology; 2010.
14. *Coding of Procedures in Interventional Nephrology*, 12/23/2009. Clinton, MS: American Society of Diagnostic and Interventional Nephrology; 2009.
15. *Coding of Procedures in Interventional Nephrology*, 2/15/12. Clinton, MS: American Society of Diagnostic and Interventional Nephrology; 2012.

16. Department of Health and Human Services, Centers for Medicare & Medicaid Services, 42 CFR Parts 410, 416, 419, 421, 485, and 48, [CMS-1506-FC; CMS-4125-F], RIN 0938-AO15 applicable January 1, 2007.

17. Schon, D, Blume, SW, Niebaurer, K, Hollenbeak, CS, de Lissovoy, G. Increasing the use of arteriovenous fistula in hemodialysis: economic benefits and economic barriers. *Clin J Am Soc Nephrol.* 2007;2:268–276.

61

QUALITY ASSURANCE AND OUTCOMES MONITORING

TIMOTHY A. PFLEDERER

1. Understand the history of quality improvement efforts in dialysis access and the major organizations involved in those efforts.
2. Define terminology used to describe quality outcomes in hemodialysis and peritoneal dialysis access procedures.
3. Understand key quality parameters related to hemodialysis and peritoneal dialysis procedures.
4. Understand important quality parameters related to processes of care.
5. Understand important quality and patient safety parameters related to facilities providing dialysis access procedural services.
6. Discuss the impact of future healthcare reforms on quality assurance efforts.

INTRODUCTION

There are a number of organizations and societies actively working to ensure that patients have access to high quality dialysis access care in the United States. These groups work to establish quality standards, monitor performance, and provide education. Unfortunately, while quality outcomes information is available in the published literature, current benchmarking data is not readily available.

▶ Centers for Medicare and Medicaid Services (CMS)

The provision of care to end-stage renal disease patients in the United States has been managed through the federal government Medicare program since 1972. The CMS infrastructure to monitor and improve the quality of care is through a number of contracted regional Networks established in 1978.[1] These 18 Networks oversee all aspects of the provision of dialysis care. However, there was no dedicated focus on dialysis access until 2000 when the National Vascular Access Initiative (NVAII) had begun. This initiative was started because of the rising costs of vascular access care and recognition of use of autogenous arteriovenous grafts (AVG) as the predominant permanent hemodialysis access. The goal of NVAII was to increase the use of autologous arteriovenous fistulae (AVF) from the prevalent rate of approximately 25% to the previously published Kidney Disease Outcomes Quality Initiative guideline of 40% nationwide. The effort met this goal in 2005, and CMS intervened with a greater "stretch goal" of increasing prevalent AVF rate to 66% by 2010. This new effort was called the Fistula First Breakthrough Initiative (FFBI)[2] and under this program prevalence of AVF has continued to rise to 57% by the end of 2010. CMS has continued to focus on increasing prevalent AVF but has now also focused more attention on decreasing prevalent catheter use. Additionally, due to concern over the rapidly increasing cost of healthcare in the United States, CMS has endorsed the "triple aim" approach to healthcare reform first developed by the Institute for Healthcare Improvement (IHI): (1) improving the individual experience of care, (2) improving the health of populations, and (3) reducing the per capita costs of care for populations.[3] While CMS' efforts are having positive effect on the quality of dialysis access care, they have not been the only efforts.

▶ National Kidney Foundation (NKF)

The National Kidney Foundation published its Kidney Disease Outcomes Quality Improvement (KDOQI) guidelines in 1997. The NKF brought together experts in anemia, dialysis adequacy, vascular access, and other areas to review available literature and create evidence-based guidelines intended to establish best practices for the care of hemodialysis and peritoneal dialysis patients. The first vascular access guidelines were published in 1997[4] and these have been updated in 2006.[5] These guidelines rapidly became the standard of care in the United States and continue to provide outcomes targets for quality improvement efforts today.

National Quality Forum (NQF)

The National Quality Forum (NQF) is an organization that works to improve the quality of American healthcare by building consensus on national priorities and goals for performance improvement and endorsing national consensus standards for measuring and publicly reporting on performance. NQF advocates a three step process to improving American healthcare: "The first step toward achieving quality is convening expert members across the healthcare industry, including patients to define quality with uniform standards and measures that apply to the many facets of care patients receive. Second, information gleaned from measuring performance is reported and analyzed to pinpoint where patient care falls short. Third, caregivers examine information about the care they are providing and use it to improve."[6] NQF consensus standards are utilized by CMS and others in developing public reporting requirements and pay for performance contracts. There are NQF-endorsed reporting standards related to dialysis and dialysis access.

Other Organizations

The Centers for Disease Control (CDC) has published quality improvement guidelines related to dialysis catheter care and catheter infection. These evidence-based guidelines were updated in 2011.[7] The Infectious Disease Society of America (IDSA) has also published guidelines concerning the diagnosis and management of catheter related infections.[8] A number of United States medical societies have published quality improvement and clinical practice guidelines related to dialysis access. These include the Society of Interventional Radiology (SIR),[9–15] Society of Vascular Surgery (SVS),[16–18] American Society of Diagnostic and Interventional Nephrology (ASDIN),[19] as well as societies outside the United States including those in Australia,[20] Canada,[21] United Kingdom,[22] and Europe.[23]

Coordinated Efforts

Despite this large number of quality improvement guidelines and efforts from numerous agencies and organizations, relatively few practitioners regularly track quality data specific to dialysis access. There is a great need for a coordinated effort toward implementing comprehensive quality standards and continuous quality improvement for patients with kidney disease undergoing procedures related to their dialysis access. Additionally, there is need

for greater transparency in reporting of these outcomes measures.

Every provider who performs dialysis access procedures should monitor their procedure outcomes in a continuous quality improvement (CQI) program. Additionally, metrics related to the process of care should be monitored to allow improvement in how care is delivered. A dialysis access CQI program consists of the following elements: (1) comprehensive data collection on all procedures performed, (2) regular review of key quality indicators related to those procedures, and (3) establishment of quality thresholds for each indicator based upon national standards, published literature, or available benchmarking data.

Data should be monitored in aggregate as well as by individual practitioner and location of service so that improvement opportunities are identified. When performance of an indicator is below the established threshold, focused quality improvement efforts should be applied. Depending on the indicator, quality improvement tools such as peer review, rapid cycle plan-do-study-act (PDSA), six-sigma, or lean methodologies may be useful and appropriate.

The rest of this chapter will discuss the quality indicators that are specific to dialysis access procedures, processes of care, and the facilities where procedures are performed.

QUALITY IMPROVEMENT IN HEMODIALYSIS ACCESS PROCEDURES

Defining quality terms has been a significant barrier to establishing nationally recognized outcomes standards. Definitions vary in the peer-reviewed literature, making it difficult to compare study outcomes directly. Several organizations have attempted to provide standardized reporting guidelines or quality definitions. The Society of Vascular Surgery (SVS), The Society of Interventional Radiology (SIR), NKF_KDOQI, and The North American Vascular Access Consortium have each published guidelines that include definitions of quality outcomes parameters.[24] There are differences in these definitions in part depending on whether the outcome of interest is related to the initial placement of an access or to a procedure performed on an existing access. The use of similar terms for such different outcomes can be confusing. There remains a need to develop consistent, standardized reporting guidelines for use of terms in dialysis access research. However, a definition of those outcomes measures that are most useful for quality improvement efforts can be found by combining these society's current guidelines.

Definitions Related to Access Placement

- *Primary access patency*—the interval from placement of an access to the first procedure required on that access. Primary patency ends with the first subsequent procedure of any type performed on that specific access.

TABLE 61–1

Hemodialysis Access Procedure Quality Metrics

Quality Metric	Suggested Threshold	Comments
Access placement procedures		
Primary access patency		No recommendation available
Secondary (cumulative) access patency	AVG 50% 3[5] AVF	No recommendation available for AVF, but may be similar to AVG
Primary access failure rate	AVG <10%[5] AVF <30%[5]	
Fistula maturation rate	80%	
Primary fistula maturation rate		No recommendation available
Secondary fistula maturation rate		No recommendation available
Existing access procedures		
Procedural success rate		No recommendation available
Clinical success rate	AVG thrombectomy >85%[5]	
Postintervention primary patency	PTA thrombectomy 40% 6 months[5] PTA nonthrombosed 50% 6 months[5]	
Postintervention cumulative patency		No recommendation available

- *Secondary (cumulative) access patency*—the interval from placement of an access to access abandonment, irrespective of the number of procedures done on that access.

- *Primary access failure rate*—the percentage of accesses placed that fail to develop or function and are abandoned before becoming consistently useable for dialysis.

- *Fistula maturation rate*—the percentage of fistulae placed that mature to support adequate dialysis with two needles.

  – *Primary fistula maturation rate*—the percentage of fistula that mature after placement without any additional procedure.

  – *Secondary fistula maturation rate*—the percentage of fistula that mature after placement but required one or more additional procedures to aid maturation.

▶ **Definitions Related to Procedures on Existing Accesses**

- *Procedural (Immediate) success*—anatomic success (restoration of flow and/or <30% residual stenosis) and return of at least one abnormal hemodynamic or clinical indicator (venous pressures, arterial pressures, access flow, physical exam, etc.) to normal or baseline value.

- *Clinical success*—procedural success and the ability to accomplish at least one dialysis session subsequent to the procedure. Applies only to accesses that are in current use.

- *Post intervention primary patency*—interval following intervention until the next intervention on that access. Includes any type of intervention required for any problem with that access.

- *Post intervention cumulative access patency*—interval following intervention until the access is abandoned.

▶ **Definitions Related to Procedural Complications**

There is no standardized method for reporting dialysis vascular access procedure complications. SIR and ASDIN have published endovascular procedure complication reporting guidelines. While the terminology in these two scales differs, they are similar in structure requiring both a name and severity grade to the complications that occur. Tables 61-1 and 61-2 provide these complication scales. Until an agreed upon standard is available, practitioners should utilize one or both scales to track every procedure complication that occurs.

TABLE 61–2

Peritoneal Dialysis Catheter Procedure Quality Metrics

Quality Metric	Suggested Threshold	Comments
Primary outflow failure	<5%	Incidence 5–20%[28]
Secondary outflow failure	<5%	No recommendation available
Pericatheter leak	<5%	Incidence 1–40%[28]
Catheter cuff extrusion	0%	Incidence 3.5–17%[28]
Peritonitis	0%	
Exit site infection	0%	
Tunnel infection	0%	
Bowel perforation	<1%[28]	
Bladder perforation	0%	
Bleeding	<2%[29]	

TABLE 61–3

Process of Care Quality Metrics

Quality Metric	Suggested Threshold	Comments
Prevalent AVF rate	66%[2]	
Prevalent AVG rate		No recommendation available
Prevalent catheter rate		No recommendation available
Prevalent catheter >90 days	<10%[5]	
Incident AVF rate		No recommendation available
Incident graft rate		No recommendation available
Incident catheter rate		No recommendation available
Incident patients seen by nephrologist for <6 months		No recommendation available
Incident patients seen by nephrologist for 6–12 months		No recommendation available
Incident patients seen by nephrologist for >12 months		No recommendation available
Thrombosis rate AVF	<0.25[5]	
Thrombosis rate AVG	<0.50[5]	
Infection rate AVF	<1%[5]	
Infection rate AVG	<10%[5]	
Infection rate catheter	<10% at 3 months and <50% at 1 year[5]	
Total number of procedures performed per patient per year	<1.5	
Time from contact to surgical referral		No recommendation available
Time from surgical referral to consultation		No recommendation available
Time from surgical consult to surgery		No recommendation available
Time from surgery to access maturation or use		No recommendation available
Unplanned hospitalization rate		No recommendation available

► Key Quality Outcome Goals

Every provider involved in hemodialysis access procedures should monitor the outcomes of those procedures in a quality assessment and performance improvement (QAPI) program. While some of the outcome terms defined above relate more to research purposes, all providers should follow some quality outcome metrics. Threshold levels should be set for each outcome parameter so that when performance falls below the threshold specific CQI efforts can be employed. Quality metrics should be monitored by individual provider, recognizing the limitations imposed by lower procedure volumes. Since an important goal is to minimize the number of procedures patients require, procedure number per patient per year should be reported along with applicable quality metrics. Suggested minimal quality metrics and threshold levels are provided in Table 61-3.

QUALITY IMPROVEMENT IN PERITONEAL DIALYSIS ACCESS PROCEDURES

Peritoneal dialysis requires the placement and maintenance of access to the peritoneal space within the abdominal cavity. A peritoneal catheter is placed by surgical, laparoscopic, or fluoroscopic technique. There are many catheter designs but all have an intraperitoneal perforated portion and one or more cuffs implanted in the rectus muscle and/or subcutaneous tunnel. The catheters may exit on the abdomen or chest wall. Most protocols attempt to place the catheters approximately 1–2 weeks before they are needed to be used for dialysis, although catheters can be immediately used if necessary. Placement technique, catheter type, timing of use, and other factors may influence the immediate and long-term outcomes of the catheter. A number of complications may occur during placement and use of the peritoneal catheter. These complications are typically classified as either early (occurring within 30 days of catheter placement) or late (occurring beyond 30 days postcatheter placement). It is the early complications that may relate to the placement procedure and should be followed in a dialysis access CQI program.

► Definition of Terms Related to Procedure Outcomes

- *Primary outflow failure*—failure of adequate catheter inflow or outflow occurring within 7 days of placement. The catheter does not ever function to allow flow that would be adequate for dialysis. This may occur due to catheter malposition, catheter kinking, intraluminal occlusion (ie, thrombus), or extraluminal occlusion (ie, omental wrap).

- *Secondary outflow failure*—failure of adequate catheter inflow or outflow occurring after the catheter is initially used but within the first 30 days postplacement. This is typically due to intraluminal occlusion, extraluminal occlusion, catheter migration, or patient factors (ie, constipation).

- *Pericatheter leak*—leaking of peritoneal dialysate from the peritoneal cavity around the catheter entrance site. The fluid may leak externally from the exit site or be localized within the tunnel, abdominal wall, or inguinal canal.
- *Catheter cuff extrusion*—erosion of the catheter cuff through the skin to the outer abdominal wall.
- *Peritonitis*—infection occurring in the peritoneal space and fluid.
- *Exit site infection*—infection at the site of catheter exit from the skin which does not include the catheter tunnel tract. Exit site infection may occur alone or in association with peritonitis.
- *Tunnel infection*—infection within the catheter subcutaneous tunnel tract with or without evidence of infection at the catheter exit site. Tunnel infection may occur alone or in association with peritonitis.

▶ **Definition of Terms Related to Direct Procedure Complications**

- *Surgical wound infection*—infection at the incision or site of peritoneal dialysis catheter placement with or without involvement of the catheter exit site and tunnel.
- *Bleeding*—any bleeding complication occurring during or within 3 days after catheter placement that requires increased monitoring, transfusion, or other therapeutic intervention.
- *Bowel perforation*—inadvertent puncture of the small or large intestine during the catheter placement procedure.
- *Bladder perforation*—inadvertent puncture of the bladder during the catheter placement procedure.

▶ **Key Quality Outcome Goals**

Providers who place and remove peritoneal dialysis catheters should monitor the outcomes and complications of those procedures. Table 61-3 lists important quality metrics that should be followed and suggested threshold levels that should trigger CQI efforts.

QUALITY IMPROVEMENT RELATED TO PROCESS OF CARE

Patient outcomes depend both on high quality procedures and well-functioning processes to support the placement, development, initial use, and ongoing maintenance of dialysis access. The rates of use of fistula, grafts, and catheters in both incident and prevalent patients should be continually monitored. Catheters in place >90 days (irrespective of presence of permanent access) should also be followed. The involvement of nephrologists in CKD care prior to dialysis initiation should also be monitored with the goal of early involvement of nephrology in this patient population. Infection and thrombosis rates should be monitored

for appropriate access types. The overall number of procedures performed per patient per year can be utilized to assess the efficiency and quality of procedures being done. Because delays in placement of permanent access or procedures to aid maturation can lead to prolonged catheter use, monitoring the time between referral events can be very useful. Some times to monitor include: time to referral for surgery, time to surgical consultation, time to surgery, time to first maturation assistance procedure, time to maturation, and so on. Finally, the rate of unplanned hospitalization related to dialysis access procedure complications should be monitored. Table 61-3 lists suggested quality metrics and threshold levels where data exist for these metrics.

QUALITY IMPROVEMENT IN VASCULAR ACCESS CENTERS

▶ **Introduction**

There has been a dramatic shift in the facility location where dialysis access procedures are performed over the past 10 years. Many procedures that were once done in the hospital are now being done in free-standing access centers. These centers operate either as a physician office or as an ambulatory surgery center. Historically, this setting has less regulation and reporting requirements than the hospital setting. Small studies have shown excellent patient outcomes in these centers.[25-27] Despite reduced regulatory burden, free-standing centers have an obligation to ensure that their operations lead to high quality, safe patient care. In truth, every facility where dialysis access procedures are performed has this same obligation.

▶ **Quality Infrastructure**

Vascular access centers often serve a population of patients from more than one dialysis facility and as such serve as the center of coordination for those patient's procedural care. Two key components to providing high quality access care include an access coordinator and an electronic database.

There are many models for access coordination but an excellent system often involves both an individual at the dialysis facility designated to monitor access issues and an external access coordinator. This access coordinator is often a nurse or other clinical person who has significant experience with dialysis and dialysis vascular access. The access coordinator is sometimes associated with the nephrology practice, hospital, or surgeon's practice. When an access center is providing procedural care, staff from the center may serve as the access coordinator. An access coordinator receives information from dialysis or physician's offices, schedules procedures, and provides postprocedural follow-up as needed. Specific duties include: receiving new patient referrals, taking phone calls about access problems, reviewing surveillance data, monitoring access maturity, tracking catheter use and timely removal, following established protocols to schedule procedures, communicating with the surgeon or interventionalist about problems and protocol outliers, providing postprocedure communication about procedures and plans to dialysis staff and referring physicians, and following procedure data for quality assurance monitoring. Since some procedures will necessarily be done at the hospital or other locations, the best programs coordinate care across all places of service.

An electronic database is essential in order to organize and manage the complex information about patient's access and access procedures. The database may contain information about patient's dialysis, surgical and endovascular procedures, current and previous accesses, co-morbid conditions, and future plans. Critical procedural data includes complications and outcomes—both immediate and delayed. The database will need to monitor greater details about the procedures and patient safety issues for those procedures done at the center. The access center at a minimum must be able to report quality and safety data for procedures done at that facility. If moderate sedation or other types of anesthesia are utilized these need to be monitored for quality outcomes. Patients should be surveyed regularly for their satisfaction with the services provided by the facility.

▶ Radiologic Imaging

When imaging or procedures are offered using ionizing radiation, the patient and staff radiation exposure should be continually monitored. Protocols should be in place to reduce radiation exposure to "As Low As Possible" (ALARA) levels. Radiologic images obtained during the performance of dialysis procedures should be available to all caregivers and archived according to recognized standards.

▶ Patient Safety

There are several patient safety issues that are important in an access center's quality improvement program. The Joint Commission National Patient Safety Goals that have been developed for hospitals and ambulatory care sites are a good guide to topics worth monitoring. Surgical site infections at 7 and 30 days are important indicators of the center's sterile technique, processing, and environment. Adherence to universal protocol and wrong site surgery events should be monitored. Medication errors, adverse medication reactions, patient falls, device or equipment malfunction, and other adverse events should be recorded. Patient hospitalization rate should also be monitored as an indicator of both the appropriateness of patient selection and the quality of the procedures being done. The goal for these safety events is a zero occurrence rate and any event should prompt appropriate CQI efforts. Some safety events are classified as "never events" and any occurrence

should lead to a thorough root cause analysis and formal improvement plan.

▶ Accreditation

More centers are choosing to become accredited as a way of demonstrating and maintaining their quality care. External accreditation is required for ambulatory surgery centers to participate in Medicare patient care. However, even office-based centers can benefit from the rigor of accreditation. The accrediting body provides significant information that is helpful in ensuring your center is operating according to the safest and highest quality standards. Accreditation is currently available through The Joint Commission (TJC), American Association of Ambulatory Healthcare Centers (AAAHC), and the American Association for Accreditation of Ambulatory Surgery Facilities (AAAASF).

▶ Key Quality Parameters

Every hospital, ambulatory surgery center, or access center facility irrespective of accreditation status should have a robust QAPI program specific to dialysis access procedures. The metrics followed should include procedure outcomes, procedure complications, and patient safety parameters. Data should be regularly evaluated and continually subjected to CQI efforts.

CONCLUSION

The provision of dialysis access care has undergone dramatic transformation in the past 10 years. Procedures are being done by physicians of more diverse specialties. Procedures are being done in more diverse locations and increasingly outside of the hospital setting. This increased focus by physicians specializing in dialysis access and move to a lower cost setting should both improve the quality and lower the cost of access care.

Unfortunately, at present, there is no clear data whether this has occurred. What information is available does not reflect well. Prevalent fistula rates have risen significantly but catheter use remains very high. Overall procedural volume, especially angioplasty and stent placement, has increased dramatically. Reported catheter-related infection rates are high. In most studies, nearly 50% of AVF failed to mature. Procedural complications are not monitored or reported. Indeed, there is no uniform quality reporting standard for dialysis access which makes benchmarking and quality improvement challenging. Greater attention and transparency is certainly needed.

The current system is likely to change. Payment for dialysis access care is fragmented with no incentive for coordination that could reduce costs. The physician, dialysis facility, access center, and hospital are each paid independently to provide care. The greatest cost of access care is related to the procedures themselves, hospitalizations, and treatment of complications. Fee for service payments provide perverse incentive to increase procedure volume. Efforts to reduce hospitalization certainly help patients but only reduce a hospital's Medicare Part A revenue. The dialysis facility's efforts in this regard bring only minimal benefit of not missing patient treatments. That is certainly not enough incentive to increase staff or utilize new technology that could impact infections and other problems. And while hospitals are beginning to be penalized for preventable complications occurring during inpatient care, there is no consistent reporting standard to understand the incidence and importance of dialysis access procedure complications.

High costs combined with less than optimal outcomes make clear the need for change in the United States healthcare system. It is very likely that over the next 10 years the payment system will change to pay providers for provision of service across the continuum of patient care. Payment bundles, capitation, and Accountable Care Organizations (ACO) are some of the ways described to accomplish this change. All follow the same basic concepts. First, make a prospective payment from which the provider must then be responsible to provide all included care. So each procedure now instead of adding revenue, removes revenue from the initial prospective payment. It is a cost to the provider. Second, pay for performance. Pay additional incentives for meeting quality outcome targets or institute penalties for missing those targets.

The coming changes in healthcare have the potential to increase the quality and transparency of care, while at the same time reducing costs significantly. Practitioners will be well served by developing the quality processes and infrastructure now to be able to assess their work. Patients will benefit as we continuously improve.

REFERENCES

1. Forum of ESRD Networks' website. Available at: www.esrdnetworks.org. Accessed May 5, 2011.
2. Fistula First website. Available at: http://www.fistulafirst.org. Accessed May 5, 2011.
3. Berwick DM, Nolan TW, Wittington J. The triple aim: care, health, and cost health affairs. *Health Affairs.* 2008;27(3):759–769.
4. Owens JR, Roberts J, Alexander S, et al. NKF-DOQI clinical practice guidelines for hemodialysis adequacy. *Am J Kidney Dis* .1997;30(suppl 2):S15–S64.
5. KDOQI Clinical Practice Guidelines and Clinical Practice Recommendations for 2006 Updates: Hemodialysis adequacy, peritoneal dialysis adequacy and vascular access. *Am J Kidney Dis.* 2006;48(suppl 1):S1–S322.
6. National Quality Forum website. Available at: http://www.qualityforum.org/About_NQF/About_NQF.aspx. Accessed May 5, 2011.
7. O'Grady NP, Alexander M, Burns LA, Dellinger EP, Garland J, Heard SO, Lipsett PA, Masur H, Mermel LA, Pearson ML, Raad II, Randolph A, Rupp ME, Saint S. The Healthcare Infection Control Practices Advisory Committee (HICPAC)14. *Guidelines for the Prevention of Intravascular*

Catheter-Related Infections, 2011. Available at: http://www.cdc.gov/hicpac/BSI/BSI-guidelines-2011.html. Accessed November 1, 2011.
8. Mermel LA, Allon M, Bouza E, Craven DE, Flynn P, O'Grady NP, Raad II, Rijnders BJA, Sherertz RJ, Warren DK. Clinical Practice Guidelines for the diagnosis and management of intravascular catheter-related infection: 2009 Update by the Infectious Diseases Society of America. *Clin Infect Dis.* 2009;49:1–45.
9. Omary RA, Bettmann MA, Cardella JF, et al. Quality improvement guidelines for the reporting and archiving of interventional radiology procedures. *J Vasc Interv Radiol.* 2002;13:879–881.
10. Gray RJ, Sack D, Martin LG, Trerotola SO. Members of the Technology Assessment Committee. Reporting standards for percutaneous interventions in dialysis access. *J Vasc Interv Radiol.* 1999;10:1405–1415.
11. Gray RJ, Subcommittee Chair, Sacks D, Committee Chair, Martin LG, Trerotola SO. Members of the Society of Interventional Radiology Technology Assessment Committee. Reporting standards for percutaneous interventions in dialysis *Access J Vasc Interv Radiol.* 2003;14:S433–S442.
12. Omary RA, Bettmann MA, Cardella JF, Bakal CW, Schwartzberg MS, Sacks D, Rholl KS, Meranze SG, Lewis CA. The Society of Interventional Radiology Standards of Practice Committee. Quality improvement guidelines for the reporting and archiving of interventional radiology procedures. *J Vasc Interv Radiol.* 2003;14:S293–S295.
13. Rutherford RB, Becker GJ. Standards for evaluating and reporting the results of surgical and percutaneous therapy for peripheral arterial disease. *J Vasc Interv Radiol.* 1991;2:169–174.
14. Miller DL, Balter S, Wagner LK, Cardella J, Clark TW, Neithamer CD, Schwartzberg MS, Swan TL, Towbin RB, Rholl KS, Sacks D. SIR Standards of Practice Committee. Quality improvement guidelines for recording patient radiation dose in the medical record. *J Vasc Interv Radiol.* 2004;15:423–429.
15. Dariushnia SR, Michael J. Wallace MJ, Nasir H. Siddiqi NH, Towbin RB, Wojak JC, Kundu S, Cardella JF. Quality improvement guidelines for central venous access. *J Vasc Interv Radiol.* 2010;21:976–981.
16. Sidawy AN, Spergel LM, Besarab A, Allon M, Jennings WC, Padberg FT, Murad MH, Montori VM, O'Hare AM, Calligaro KD, Macsata RA, Lumsden AB, Ascher E. The society for vascular surgery: clinical practice guidelines for the surgical placement and maintenance of arteriovenous hemodialysis access. *J Vasc Surg.* 2008;48:2S–25S.
17. Sidawy AN, Gray R, Besarab A, Henry M, Ascher E, Silva M Jr, Miller A, Scher L, Trerotola S, Gregory RT, Rutherford RB, Kent KC. Recommended standards for reports dealing with arteriovenous hemodialysis accesses. *J Vasc Surg.* 2002;35:603–6110.
18. Murad MH, Sidawy AN, Elamin MB, Rizvi AZ, Flynn DN, McCausland FR, et al. Timing of referral for chronic hemodialysis vascular access placement: a systematic review. *J Vasc Surg.* 2008;48(suppl S):31S–33S.
19. Vesely TM, Beathard G, Ash S, Hoggard J, Schon D. The ASDIN Clinical Practice Committee. Classification of

complications associated with hemodialysis vascular access procedures a position statement from the American Society of Diagnostic and Interventional Nephrology. *Semin Dial.* 2007;20(4):359–364.

20. CARI: Caring for Australians with Renal Impairment. Available at: http://www.cari.org.au/dialysis_va_005_pub. php. Accessed March 23, 2008.

21. Jindal K, Chan CT, Deziel C, Hirsch D, Soroka SD, Tonelli M, et al. Hemodialysis clinical practice guidelines for the Canadian Society of Nephrology. *J Am Soc Nephrol.* 2006; 17(3 suppl 1):S1–S27.

22. The Renal Association Clinical Practice Guidelines. Available at: http://www.renal.org/Clinical/GuidelinesSection/Vascular Access.aspx. Accessed May 5, 2011.

23. Tordoir J, Canaud B, Haage P, Konner K, Basci A, Fouque D, Kooman J, Martin-Malo A, Pedrini L, Pizzarelli F, Tattersall J, Vennegoor M, Wanner C, Wee P, Vanholder R. EBPG on vascular access. *Nephrol Dial Transplant.* 2007;22(suppl 2): ii88–ii117.

24. Lee T, Mokrzycki M, Moist L, Maya I, Vazquez M, Lock CE, North Amercian Vascular Access Consortium. Standardized

definitions for hemodialysis vascular access. *Semin Dial.* 2011;24(5):515–524.

25. Arnold WP. Improvement in hemodialysis access outcomes in a dedicated access center. *Semin Dial.* Nov–Dec 2000; 13(6):359–363.

26. Mishler R, Sands J, Ofsthun N, Teng M, Schon D, Lazarus M. Dedicated outpatient vascular access center decreases hospitalization and missed outpatient dialysis treatments. *Kidney Int.* Jan 2006;69(2):393–398.

27. Kian K, Takesian K, Wyatt C, Vassalotti J, Mishler R, Schon D. Efficiency and outcomes of emergent vascular access procedures performed at a dedicated outpatient vascular access center. Seminars in Dialysis. 2007;20(4): 346–350.

28. Peppelenbosch A, van Kuijk W, Bouvy, N, van der Sande F, Tordoir J. Peritoneal dialysis catheter placement technique and complications. *Nephrol Dial Transplant.* 2008:1(suppl 4); iv23–iv28.

29. Mital S, Fried L, Priaino B. Bleeding complications associated with peritoneal dialysis catheter insertion. *Perit Dial Int.* 2004; 24:478–480.

62

RESEARCH OPPORTUNITIES IN INTERVENTIONAL NEPHROLOGY: WHY, WHAT, AND HOW!

PRABIR ROY-CHAUDHURY, DIRK HENTSCHEL, & ANIL AGARWAL

LEARNING OBJECTIVES

1. To identify research opportunities in interventional nephrology.
2. To develop paradigms for the fostering of high quality research programs in this area.

INTRODUCTION

As repeatedly emphasized in previous chapters, interventional nephrology is in the midst of an exponential growth phase with United States Renal Data System (USRDS) data suggesting that at least 25% of total vascular access procedure costs are billed by nephrologists.[1] An important reason for the growth of interventional nephrology has been the premise that dialysis vascular access care was both fragmented and inadequate prior to the active involvement of nephrologists, at both the procedural and process of care level. Indeed, it is likely that the growth of interventional nephrology as a specialty has played an important role in the success of process of care initiatives such as "Fistula First" which has raised the arteriovenous fistula (AVF) prevalence rate from 34% in December 2003 at the start of this initiative to 59.5% as of August 2011.[2] Despite these positive indicators, however, there remain significant reasons for concern, which highlight

the need for high quality research in this field **(the Why)**. These include:

▶ **Why We Need Research in Dialysis Vascular Access?**

(a) Dismal primary and cumulative patency rates for AVF and arteriovenous grafts (AVG) as compared to other forms of vascular surgery. The 1 year unassisted primary patency for polytetrafluoroethylene (PTFE) dialysis access grafts for example is 23%[3] as compared to 90% for aortobifemoral vascular grafts (Table 62-1), with only 40% of AVFs being suitable for dialysis at between 4 and 5 months postsurgery.[4]

(b) Poor post-intervention primary patency following angioplasty with a 6-month postintervention primary patency of only 50% for nonthrombosed grafts (Table 62-2).[5]

(c) A tunneled dialysis catheter rate of over 80% in patients initiating long-term hemodialysis[6] and an AVF incident rate of only 40% even in the population of patients who had seen a nephrologist for over 12 months prior to initiation of hemodialysis.

While there are clearly multiple biological and process of care reasons for these problems,[7-11] we believe that an important underlying cause for the clinical problems described above is a relative lack of focused basic science, translational, clinical, and process of care (outcome) research in the field of dialysis vascular access. A second key

TABLE 62–1

Postsurgery Primary Patency Results

- CABG (LIMA)   90% @ 10 years
- CABG (SV)   50% @ 10 years
- Aortobifemoral bypass   90% @ 5 years
- BK Femoropopliteal bypass 33% @ 5 years
- AVG Surgery   23% @ 1 year!!!
- AVF Surgery   40% suitable for HD @ 4–5 m

reason could be the fact that dialysis vascular access is in many ways an *orphan disease state*, in that other than nephrologists and a small group of surgeons and interventional radiologists who are dedicated to vascular access, there are very few in the medical profession for whom this is a real problem. Perhaps this is the reason why our gold standard (AV fistula) is a procedure that has remained unchanged for 46 years (since 1966)[12] and why the last major innovation in this field (the PTFE graft circa 1976) continues to have significant problems.

We therefore suggest that it is imperative for this group of physicians to come together to develop research programs in this area. The impact of such an effort would likely be felt far beyond the vascular access arena since dialysis vascular access is in many ways, the ideal clinical model for novel therapies (especially local therapies) for vascular stenosis in all parts of the vascular tree (coronaries, carotids, and peripherals); in view of the fact that (a) AVFs and AVGs are easily accessible for the application of local therapies at the time of surgical placement and (b) the current high event rate could allow for the conduct of more rapid clinical trials, with a smaller number of patients being followed over a shorter time of period.

Finally, the induction of formal, high quality research initiatives into interventional nephrology programs in particular, could potentially transform the standing of this specialty within both nephrology and internal medicine. Thus research programs in this area could go a long way toward enhancing the standing of interventional nephrology in the eyes of nephrology program and division directors, and could be an important step toward making interventional nephrology a true sub-specialty of nephrology akin to transplant nephrology. Such research programs could also help to bring interventional nephrology into academic institutions. This is absolutely essential for the future of interventional nephrology, since sustained long-term growth of this specialty will likely occur only if it has a solid base within academia; while at the same maintaining its close links with the community physician base that has allowed this specialty to grow so rapidly.

Having addressed the *"Why"* the next section of this chapter will attempt to identify core areas of research that are desperately needed to reduce the huge clinical morbidity and economic cost associated with dialysis vascular access dysfunction *(the What)*:

▶ **What Are the Core Areas of Research in Dialysis Vascular Access?**

The first publication that attempted to identify core areas of research in vascular access was the 2006 Kidney Disease Outcomes Quality Initiative (KDOQI) on vascular access, which identified a large number of areas for possible research investigation (summarized in Table 62-3).

In 2010, Kian et al[13] addressed the issue of research within interventional nephrology in an interesting manner. Rather than identifying specific areas in need of research investigation, these authors performed an exhaustive survey of the available literature on vascular access for dialysis between 1997 and 2009. Using relatively broad criteria, they were able to identify 2135 articles, which they then analyzed. Their key findings included (a) over 50% of these articles were observational (case reports or reviews) (b) less than 3% of the articles focused on basic science research or described randomized controlled trials (c) there was a strong multidisciplinary aspect to these publications with nephrologists contributing individually or in a collaborative fashion to over 50% of these papers (d) the greatest annual increase in publications within a specific subject area between 1997 and 2009 was on arteriovenous fistulae and (e) there was a significant increase in the surgical contribution in particular between 1997 and 2009. On a positive note, these data indicate an increasing multidisciplinary interest in dialysis vascular access. On the negative side, the descriptive nature of the majority of the publications, the lack of publications on basic biology, and the paucity of randomized controlled studies all suggest that much work remains to be done.

TABLE 62–2

Postangioplasty Primary Patency Results

- Coronary angioplasty   90% @ 9 months
- Carotid angioplasty   90% @ 1 year
- Iliac angioplasty   70% @ 5 years
- Femoral angioplasty   50% @ 2 years
- PTFE graft angioplasty 50% @ 6 months (p)
                          40% @ 3 months (t)
- AVF angioplasty   50% @ 1 year

TABLE 62–3

KDOQI Research Recommendations

- Patient preparation
- Selection and placement of hemodialysis access
- Cannulation of fistulae and grafts and accession of hemodialysis catheters and port catheter systems
- Detection of access dysfunction; monitoring, surveillance, and diagnostic testing
- Treatment of fistula complications
- Treatment of AVG complications
- Prevention and treatment of catheter and port complications

More recently, a survey sent out to the membership of the American Society of Diagnostic and Interventional Nephrology identified (a) arteriovenous fistula maturation (b) process of care guidelines for the creation and maintenance of dialysis vascular access, and (c) PTFE graft stenosis as the three most pressing areas for research into dialysis vascular access (in the order described).

In addition, the Interventional Nephrology Advisory Group of the American Society of Nephrology in combination with the council of the American Society of Diagnostic and Interventional Nephrology recently submitted a number of areas for research investigation to the Kidney Research National Dialogue sponsored through the National Institute of Diabetes, Digestive and Kidney Diseases.

The above paragraphs clearly document that there are a large number of potential areas for research in this field and also at least some consensus on a priority ranking of subjects for investigation. What is needed, however, is a mechanism to be able to do this successfully *(the How)* and this will be addressed in the next section.

▶ *How* Can We Develop Research Programs in Dialysis Vascular Access?

While there are many approaches to investigative research in dialysis vascular access, the key issue in many ways is the establishment of a system or a process that encourages long-term active research in this field. One approach that has been espoused by the Interventional Nephrology Advisory Group of the American Society of Nephrology as a way to lay a firm foundation for a long-term commitment to research activity in this field is to support the establishment of a number of academic dialysis access centers (ADAC).[14] These centers will (a) establish basic or translational research programs focused on dialysis vascular access, (b) develop clinical research programs (both investigator initiated and industry sponsored), and (c) establish dedicated (1 year) interventional nephrology training programs where nephrology fellows will be trained not just to do procedures but also in the biology, epidemiology, and process of care of dialysis vascular access. We believe that establishment of such ADACs will not only increase the opportunities for well-funded high quality research in this area but will also play a key role in allowing interventional nephrology to grow; by establishing a place for this subspecialty of nephrology within academic institutions. In addition, while these ADACs are likely to have a home within divisions of nephrology, it is critical that they retain a multidisciplinary nature.

In summary, we believe that this is the time to aggressively develop a formal structure for focused research into dialysis vascular access. We know the problems and we are asking the questions that need to be asked. In addition, we are lucky that the last decade has seen phenomenal advances in bioengineering, drug delivery, nanotechnology, and cellular therapies, all of which can impact on dialysis vascular access. We therefore need to apply these biological and technological advances (combined with outcomes and process of care research) to the clinical problem of dialysis vascular access, so that we can improve upon the care that we provide to our patients. Developing high quality research programs focused on dialysis vascular access are essential to be able to achieve this.

REFERENCES

1. USRDS 2009 Annual Data Report: Atlas of End-Stage Renal Disease in the United States. National Institutes of Health, National Institute of Diabetes and Digestive and Kidney Diseases, Bethesda, MD, 2009.
2. Fistula First. 2011. Available at: http://www.fistulafirst.org. Accessed Feb. 21, 2012.
3. Dixon BS, Beck GJ, Vazquez MA, et al. Effect of dipyridamole plus aspirin on hemodialysis graft patency. *N Engl J Med.* 2009;360:2191–2201.
4. Dember LM, Beck GJ, Allon M, et al. Effect of clopidogrel on early failure of arteriovenous fistulas for hemodialysis: a randomized controlled trial. *JAMA.* 2008;299:2164–2171.
5. DOQI. Vascular Access Guidelines. *Am J Kid Dis.* 2006;48:S177–S247.
6. USRDS. USRDS 2008 Annual Data Report: Atlas of End-Stage Renal Disease in the United States. National Institutes of Health, National Institute of Diabetes and Digestive and Kidney Diseases, Bethesda, MD, 2008.
7. Lee T, Roy-Chaudhury P. Advances and new frontiers in the pathophysiology of venous neointimal hyperplasia and dialysis access stenosis. *Adv Chronic Kidney Dis.* 2009;16:329–338.
8. Roy-Chaudhury P, Lee TC. Vascular stenosis: biology and interventions. *Curr Opin Nephrol Hypertens.* 2007;16:516–522.
9. Asif A, Ravani P, Roy-Chaudhury P, Spergel LM, Besarab A. Vascular mapping techniques: advantages and disadvantages. *J Nephrol.* 2007;20:299–303.
10. Roy-Chaudhury P, Kelly BS, Melhem M, et al. Vascular access in hemodialysis: issues, management, and emerging concepts. *Cardiol Clin.* 2005;23:249–273.
11. Lopez-Vargas PA, Craig JC, Gallagher MP, et al. Barriers to timely arteriovenous fistula creation: a study of providers and patients. *Am J Kidney Dis.* 2011;57:873–882.
12. Brescia MJ, Cimino J, Appel K, et al. Chronic hemodialysis using venipuncture and a surgically created arteriovenous fistula. *New Eng J Med.* 1966;275:1089–1092.
13. Kian K, Asif A. Status of research in vascular access for dialysis. *Nephrol Dial Transplant.* 2010;25:3682–3686.
14. Roy-Chaudhury P, Yevzlin A, Bonventre JV, Agarwal A, Almehmi A, Besarab A, Dwyer A, Hentschel DM, Kraus M, Maya I, Pflederer T, Schon D, Wu S, Work J. Academic interventional nephrology: a model for training, research, and patient care. *CJASN* e pub Feb 2012.

Note: Page numbers followed by *f* indicate figures; and page numbers followed by *t* indicate tables.